BOWES & CHURCH'S

Food Values

of Portions Commonly Used

BOWES & CHURCH'S

Food Values

of Portions
Commonly Used

SEVENTEENTH EDITION

REVISED BY

Jean A. T. Pennington, Ph.D., R.D.

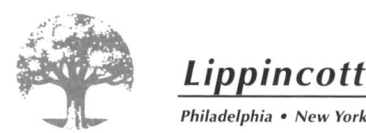

Lippincott
Philadelphia • New York

Executive Editor: Margaret Biblis
Assistant Editor: Patricia Moore
Project Editor: Barbara Ryalls
Senior Production Manager: Helen Ewan
Production Coordinator: Nannette Winski
Design Coordinator: Doug Smock
Indexer: Ann Cassar

Edition 17

9   8   7   6   5   4   3   2

Library of Congress Cataloging-in-Publication Data

Bowes, Anna de Planter.
    Bowes & Church's food values of portions commonly used. — 17th ed. / revised
by Jean A.T. Pennington.
        p.   cm.
    Includes bibliographical references and index.
    1. Nutrition—Tables.   2. Food—Composition—Tables.   I. Pennington, Jean A. Thompson.
II. Church, Helen Nichols.   III. Title.
    TX551.B64   1998   97-24666
    613.2'8—dc21   CIP

The information provided in this book should be used by the healthcare practitioner under appropriate supervision in accordance with professional standards of care used with regard to the unique circumstances that apply in each practice situation. Care has been taken to confirm the accuracy of information presented. The author, editors, and publisher cannot accept any responsibility for errors or omissions or for any consequences from application of the information in this book and make no warranty express or implied, with respect to the contents of the book.

   The author has attempted to provide readers with the most accurate food composition data available as of the date of manuscript submission. However, the field of food composition is a dynamic one. The nutrient composition of foods varies because of genetic, environmental, and processing variables; changes in product formulation and package size; sampling techniques; and advances in analytical methodologies. The information in these tables should be used as reasonable approximations of the nutrient composition of foods. Individuals who are on restricted or specialized diets for medical purposes may need to contact food manufacturers for more specific information.

The Seventeenth Edition of *Bowes and Church's Food Values of Portions Commonly Used* is dedicated to the authors of previous editions:

Anna dePlanter Bowes, M.A. (editions one through eight, 1937–1956)

Charles F. Church, M.D. (editions one, and nine through twelve, 1937–1975)

Helen Nichols Church, B.A., R.D. (editions nine through fourteen, 1963–1985)

and to:

Carmella Genene Pennington (1971–1994) for her love, patience, and support.

Preface to the First Edition

The purpose of this book is to supply authoritative data on the nutritional values of foods in a form for quick and easy reference.

In teaching nutrition to students of medicine, dentistry, dental hygiene and public health nursing, food values based on common measures of portions frequently served have been found most useful. This basis of calculation is particularly well suited to the practical study of comparative food values, as well as to the approximate analysis of diets from records of daily food intake. For calculations of diets from weighed portions the actual weight of each food is given in grams or ounces.

Anna dePlanter Bowes
Charles F. Church
November 1937
Philadelphia, PA

Preface to the Seventeenth Edition

This Seventeenth Edition of *Bowes and Church's Food Values of Portions Commonly Used* is a reference food composition database "to supply authoritative data on the nutritional values of foods in a form for quick and easy reference." This was the goal established for the first edition by Ms. Anna dePlanter Bowes and Dr. Charles F. Church in 1937 and has remained the goal for all subsequent editions. The database and accompanying information provided herein are intended to assist dietitians and nutritionists in providing dietary information to their patients and clients. The information in this book may also be of use to research nutritionists, students of nutrition and dietetics, and individuals who are on special diets or who want to know more about the composition of foods.

The various features of this publication and changes from the Sixteenth Edition are identified in the *Explanatory Notes*. I have attempted to provide current information for a wide range of commonly consumed foods as well as various foods of interest and curiosity and to remove all commercially discontinued foods and questionable values. I apologize for any errors that may have occurred. Your comments, suggestions, and corrections are always welcomed.

I gratefully acknowledge: the expert review of this edition provided by Sally Schakel, R.D. of the Nutrition Coordinating Center, University of Minnesota in Minneapolis; the industry nutritionists, home economists, and consumer affairs representatives who responded to my request for food composition data for this and previous editions; and the editorial assistance and computer support provided by Andrew Allen, Patricia Moore, Robert Fleishmann, Barbara Ryalls, and others at Lippincott-Raven Publishers.

Jean A.T. Pennington, Ph.D., R.D.
February 1997
Chevy Chase, Maryland

Contents

SUPPLEMENTARY TABLES

Features of the Seventeenth Edition

Front Material

The front material provides information on standards for nutrient intake in the United States (US) established by the Food and Nutrition Board of the National Academy of Sciences (NAS) in 1989; the standards for the nutrition labeling of food developed by the Food and Drug Administration (FDA); the Dietary Guidelines for Americans developed by the US Department of Agriculture (USDA) and the Department of Health and Human Services (DHHS); and the USDA Food Guide Pyramid. The table on *US Daily Values,* developed by FDA, replaces the information on *US Recommended Dietary Allowances,* also developed by FDA, that was presented in the Sixteenth Edition of this book. The *US Daily Values* are the current standards used by food companies to provide nutrient information on food labels.

Main Table

The main food composition table in this database, entitled *Nutrient Content of Foods,* provides values for 30 nutrients in about 8,100 foods. This edition has about the same number of foods as the Sixteenth Edition to maintain the size of the database and hence not increase the cost of the book. Nutrient values for different flavors of some foods (e.g., gelatin desserts, icings, puddings, granola bars, ice cream, juice drinks) were averaged (as indicated in the footnotes) so that the food would be listed only once. The nutrient values for the different flavored items were similar, and the averaging saved space as it allows for one food entry to represent three or more similar foods. In addition, each food is listed only once, although some foods may be applicable to several food group sections. The index may be used to locate foods for which classification may not be apparent, and the section *Food Name Synonyms and Cross-References* provides a means to locate foods known by several different names.

The foods are grouped into 34 sections on the basis of food type with concerns for common usage. The foods within each of the 34 groupings are arranged in a hierarchical structure and are listed alphabetically. Upper case is used for brand names and trademark names; lower case is otherwise used for food names and for proper nouns and adjectives (eg, french fries, danish, brussels sprouts, and chinese cabbage). Each food is identified by name, description (eg, color, maturity, preservation method, and cooking method), brand name (if applicable), serving portion, and gram weight of the serving portion. Abbreviations are used to save space and provide as complete a description as is possible for each food. The abbreviated words and symbols used with the food names and descriptions are listed in the *Abbreviations and Symbols* section. Foods are presented primarily in their table-ready form, although ingredient items (eg, flour, baking soda, herbs) are also listed in the database. Where available, brand names are used to help identify products such as ready-to-eat breakfast cereals, desserts, candy bars, soups, and entrees. The serving portions are those provided by food companies or the USDA food composition database.

The sections on *Special Dietary Foods* and *Special Dietary Formulas, Commercial and Hospital* in the Sixteenth Edition were merged to form the section called *Special Dietary Products* in the Seventeenth Edition. Thus, the Seventeenth Edition contains 34 food group sections, whereas the Sixteenth Edition contained 35 sections. The original *Special Dietary Foods* section included retail meal replacement products for reducing diets, and some products formulated to be *low in* or *free of* specific nutrients. The current section on *Special Dietary Products* includes formulated products used for medical purposes and meal replacement foods used for weight reduction. There are also some changes in the food subgroupings (ie, the alphabetical hierarchies) between the Sixteenth and Seventeenth editions within the 34 sections of the database to reflect changes in the availability of commercial products within the past 4 to 5 years (ie, new products and product deletions).

The heading at the top of each page of the main table indicates the nutrients and units of measurement for the numerical values listed in the two lines. For two sections, *Infant Formulas* and *Special Dietary Products,* there are four lines of nutrient data per food to include the complete nutrient profiles that were available for these formulated products.

Supplementary Tables

The supplementary tables, following the main table, provide information on the levels of amino acids, alcohol, caffeine, gluten, iodine, pectin, phytosterol, purines, salicylates, selenium, sugars, theobromine, vitamin D, vitamin E, alpha-tocopherol, and vitamin K in foods. The tables on the iodine and selenium content of foods are new for this edition. There is also a table for the levels of calories and carbohydrates in chewing gum, mints, candies, and medications. The supplementary tables present information on food components for which there was not enough data to warrant a listing in the main table. The foods in the supplementary tables are listed by the major food groupings used for the main table. All of the foods in the amino acid supplementary table are listed in the main table. Many of the foods in the other supplementary tables are also listed in the main table and the serving portions, if used, are usually consistent. Some of the nutrients in the supplementary tables are listed per 100 grams of food, rather than by serving portions.

Data Sources

The nutrient values included in this reference database have been obtained directly from the USDA Database for Standard Reference, Release 11 (1996); food companies; trade associations; and the scientific literature. All the data obtained from the USDA-revised Agriculture Handbook No. 8 sections (ie, sections 8-1 through 8-21 and the yearly supplements) that were included in the Sixteenth Edition were updated by deriving them from the USDA Database for Standard Reference, Release (1996). To do this, all USDA-derived foods in the Sixteenth Edition and all USDA-derived foods that became available since the Sixteenth Edition were identified by USDA code numbers and derived electronically from Release 11. The use of Release 11 ensures that the data obtained from USDA are as accurate as possible.

No values have been calculated from food ingredients or imputed with the following exceptions: the cholesterol content of some plant products was assigned a value of zero, and the dietary fiber content of some animal products was assigned a value of zero if the original source did not provide a value; if the vitamin A value in IUs (international units) was zero, the vitamin A value in REs (retinol equivalents) was assigned a zero value; if the value for total fat was zero, the values for saturated fatty acids, monounsaturated fatty acids, and polyunsaturated fatty acids were also assigned zero values; and if the value for total carbohydrate was zero, the value for sugars was assigned a zero value.

The *Ref* (reference) codes in the right-hand column of

the main table and the amino acid table indicate the data sources for the nutrient values. For data obtained from USDA Release 11, the reference codes are 801 through 821, indicating the sections of the hardcopy version of the USDA database (*Agriculture Handbook No 8*, revised, 1976 to 1992, and the 1989 to 1991 yearly supplements published from 1990 to 1992, respectively). Other reference codes are *I* (industry) for data from food companies and trade associations and *L* for data from the scientific literature. In some cases, two or more sources were used to provide data for a food in the main table. This was done if the food was clearly identified (usually by brand name) and if the two sources showed similar or identical values for nutrients in common. In these cases, MUL (more than one source) is listed in the *Ref* column. The sources of information for the supplementary tables are indicated in the footnotes for each table.

As has been done for previous editions, food companies were contacted and asked to provide updated nutrient values for the foods they produce. For this Seventeenth Edition, 87 food companies were contacted via phone and letter. Updated information was provided from 52 companies. For companies that provided data for the Sixteenth Edition, but were unable to respond to the request for updated information (40 companies), the data that they provided for the Sixteenth Edition were reviewed and selectively reused in this edition.

Since the Sixteenth Edition, there have been changes in nutrition labeling regulations developed by USDA and FDA. The changes in regulations identifying which nutrients are mandatory and which are voluntary for food labels have affected the type of data provided by food companies for this Seventeenth Edition. For this edition, the companies provided more information than in previous years for dietary fiber, saturated fat, sugars, and cholesterol, but far less information on thiamin, riboflavin, or niacin. Some companies had previously provided full nutritional profiles for the vitamins and minerals in their foods, but for this edition, most companies were only able to provide vitamins A and C, calcium, and iron. This is certainly understandable because food companies must now bear the expense of providing nutrition labeling for all their products, and of necessity, focus on the nutrients that must be present on labels (as opposed to those that may be listed voluntarily).

The food companies were asked to provide mean (ie, average) values for the nutrients in their food products; however, many of the companies were only able to provide nutrition labeling values. Nutrition labeling information was used for some foods in this edition, rather than exclude the foods from the database. In contrast to mean values, labeling values are rounded and adjusted to be in compliance with government labeling regulations. The values for vitamins and minerals (ie, vitamins A and C, calcium, and iron) are provided as percent Daily Values for nutrition labeling. For this edition, these Daily Values were back-calculated to obtain weight values for the vitamins and minerals. Therefore, the data derived from labeling values are not as precise as mean values, but they do adequately represent the nutrient content of foods.

The data on total sugars, which appeared in a supplementary table in the Sixteenth Edition, is now in the main table because of the increased availability of information on this food component from food companies. The format for the main table nutrients was altered from that of the Sixteenth Edition to provide for the inclusion of sugars. Unfortunately, the USDA Release 11 does not include information on total sugars; however, USDA had provided information on the total sugars content of 249 foods in a provisional table published in 1986. Where possible, these foods were matched to the USDA foods in the main table, and the values for total sugars were included for 175 of these foods. The sugar values for all 249 foods (in mg per 100 g) are also provided in a supplementary table.

Back Material

The back material of the book includes the sources consulted for this edition, Latin names for plants and animals, a bibliography of publications on the composition of foods, a list of food name synonyms and cross-references, and an index. The list of food name synonyms and cross-references is new for this edition. The purpose of this list is to assist users in locating foods with various names (including regional names) or various arrangements of the same name (eg, lima beans vs. beans, lima vs. butterbeans).

The bibliography includes 167 papers and books on food composition published between January 1992 (when the Sixteenth Edition was submitted to the publisher) and February 1997 (when the Seventeenth Edition was submitted to the publisher). The references are listed alphabetically by the authors' last names. Key words are listed in bold to identify food components (analytes) and the foods analyzed.

Cautionary Notes

The information and level of detail in this database are limited to that provided by the sources. The collection and aggregation of data from various sources invariably results in some unevenness in food descriptions and some apparent inconsistencies of nutrient values and serving sizes. The attempt to include both generic and brand-specific products in a database causes some confusion, because descriptions for generic foods are somewhat vague, and the foods may not be recognized by data users. Likewise, data for commercial products identified only by trademark names are only useful if the database user is familiar with the products.

Those unfamiliar with the use of food composition tables are requested to note the following:

- These tables should be used as approximate guides to the nutrient content of foods. Persons on special diets for various disease conditions may require more specific nutrient composition data from food manufacturers.
- Blank spaces indicate a lack of data from the original source. Blank spaces should not be assumed to be zeros, as this could underestimate the dietary intake of various food components.
- The nutrient values presented here are mean values or values used for nutrition labeling. Some of the values have large standard deviations and wide ranges. Causes of nutrient variations in foods include soil type, season, geography, genetics, animal diets, processing, method of preparation, changes in product formulations, sampling schemes, and methods of analysis.
- Because of nutrient variation and the fact that the data are collected from various sources (ie, food companies, trade associations, USDA, and the scientific literature), apparent inconsistencies may occur. For example, portion sizes and gram weights of similar foods may vary among sources, and nutrient values may vary according to season, sampling area, or analytical methodology.
- The values presented here may not be representative of the entire US food supply. Representativeness depends upon the sampling schemes and the number of samples collected and analyzed.
- The mineral content of water varies from one geographic location to another. The mineral content of beverages made by addition of water to powders or frozen concentrates and of foods cooked in water (eg, rice, oatmeal, pasta, and vegetables) may vary depending on the mineral content of the water used. Likewise, the mineral content of commercial beverages (eg, beer, carbonated sodas, and juice drinks) depends on the mineral content of the water in the area where the beverages are bottled. Individuals on medically restricted diets may need to obtain information on the mineral content of their home tap water and on the mineral content of the specific beverages they consume.
- Information presented in these tables may not be the same as that provided on food labels because of industry changes in serving sizes or industry product reformulation with different ingredients or different proportions of ingredients.

Recommended Dietary Allowances,[1] Revised 1989

Food and Nutrition Board, National Academy of Sciences
National Research Council

Designed for the maintenance of good nutrition of practically
all healthy people in the United States

Age (years) or Condition	Weight[2] (kg)	Weight[2] (lb)	Height[2] (cm)	Height[2] (in)	Protein (g)	Vitamin A (µg RE)[3]	Vitamin D (µg)[4]	Vitamin E (mg α-TE)[5]	Vitamin K (µg)	Vitamin C (mg)	Thiamin (mg)	Riboflavin (mg)	Niacin (mg NE)[6]	Vitamin B$_6$ (mg)	Folate (µg)	Vitamin B$_{12}$ (µg)	Calcium (mg)	Phosphorus (mg)	Magnesium (mg)	Iron (mg)	Zinc (mg)	Iodine (µg)	Selenium (µg)
INFANTS																							
0.0-0.5	6	13	60	24	13	375	7.5	3	5	30	0.3	0.4	5	0.3	25	0.3	400	300	40	6	5	40	10
0.5-1.0	9	20	71	28	14	375	10	4	10	35	0.4	0.5	6	0.6	35	0.5	600	500	60	10	5	50	15
CHILDREN																							
1-3	13	29	90	35	16	400	10	6	15	40	0.7	0.8	9	1.0	50	0.7	800	800	80	10	10	70	20
4-6	20	44	112	44	24	500	10	7	20	45	0.9	1.1	12	1.1	75	1.0	800	800	120	10	10	90	20
7-10	28	62	132	52	28	700	10	7	30	45	1.0	1.2	13	1.4	100	1.4	800	800	170	10	10	120	30
MALES																							
11-14	45	99	157	62	45	1,000	10	10	45	50	1.3	1.5	17	1.7	150	2.0	1,200	1,200	270	12	15	150	40
15-18	66	145	176	69	59	1,000	10	10	65	60	1.5	1.8	20	2.0	200	2.0	1,200	1,200	400	12	15	150	50
19-24	72	160	177	70	58	1,000	10	10	70	60	1.5	1.7	19	2.0	200	2.0	1,200	1,200	350	10	15	150	70
25-50	79	174	176	70	63	1,000	5	10	80	60	1.5	1.7	19	2.0	200	2.0	800	800	350	10	15	150	70
51+	77	170	173	68	63	1,000	5	10	80	60	1.2	1.4	15	2.0	200	2.0	800	800	350	10	15	150	70
FEMALES																							
11-14	46	101	157	62	46	800	10	8	45	50	1.1	1.3	15	1.4	150	2.0	1,200	1,200	280	15	12	150	45
15-18	55	120	163	64	44	800	10	8	55	60	1.1	1.3	15	1.5	180	2.0	1,200	1,200	300	15	12	150	50
19-24	58	128	164	65	46	800	10	8	60	60	1.1	1.3	15	1.6	180	2.0	1,200	1,200	280	15	12	150	55
25-50	63	138	163	64	50	800	5	8	65	60	1.1	1.3	15	1.6	180	2.0	800	800	280	15	12	150	55
51+	65	143	160	63	50	800	5	8	65	60	1.0	1.2	13	1.6	180	2.0	800	800	280	10	12	150	55
Pregnant					60	800	10	10	65	70	1.5	1.6	17	2.2	400	2.2	1,200	1,200	320	30	15	175	65
Lactating																							
1st 6 months					65	1,300	10	12	65	95	1.6	1.8	20	2.1	280	2.6	1,200	1,200	355	15	19	200	75
2nd 6 months					62	1,200	10	11	65	90	1.6	1.7	20	2.1	260	2.6	1,200	1,200	340	15	16	200	75

[1] The allowances, expressed as average daily intakes over time, are intended to provide for individual variations among most normal persons as they live in the United States under usual environmental stresses. Diets should be based on a variety of common foods in order to provide other nutrients for which human requirements have been less well defined.

[2] Weights and heights of Reference Adults are actual medians for the U.S. population of the designated age, as reported by NHANES II. The median weights and heights of those under 19 years of age were taken from Hamill PVV, TA Drizd, CL Johnson, RB Reed, AF Roche, WM Moore. Physical growth: National Center for Health Statistics percentiles. Am J Clin Nutr 32:607–629, 1979.

[3] Retinol equivalents. 1 retinol equivalent = 1 µg retinol or 6 µg β-carotene.

[4] As cholecalciferol. 10 µg cholecalciferol = 400 IU of vitamin D.

[5] α-Tocopherol equivalents. 1 mg d-α tocopherol = 1 α-TE.

[6] 1 NE (niacin equivalent) = 1 mg of niacin or 60 mg of dietary tryptophan.

From: Recommended Dietary Allowances, 10th ed. National Academy Press. Washington DC. 1989, p. 285.

Estimated Safe and Adequate Daily Dietary Intakes of Selected Vitamins and Minerals[1]

Category	Age (years)	Vitamins		Trace Elements[2]				
		Biotin (μg)	Pantothenic Acid (mg)	Copper (mg)	Manganese (mg)	Fluoride (mg)	Chromium (μg)	Molybdenum (μg)
Infants	0–0.5	10	2	0.4–0.6	0.3–0.6	0.1–0.5	10–40	15–30
	0.5–1	15	3	0.6–0.7	0.6–1.0	0.2–1.0	20–60	20–40
Children and adolescents	1–3	20	3	0.7–1.0	1.0–1.5	0.5–1.5	20–80	25–50
	4–6	25	3–4	1.0–1.5	1.5–2.0	1.0–2.5	30–120	30–75
	7–10	30	4–5	1.0–2.0	2.0–3.0	1.5–2.5	50–200	50–150
	11+	30–100	4–7	1.5–2.5	2.0–5.0	1.5–2.5	50–200	75–250
Adults		30–100	4–7	1.5–3.0	2.0–5.0	1.5–4.0	50–200	75–250

[1] Because there is less information on which to base allowances, these figures are not given in the main table of RDA and are provided here in the form of ranges of recommended intakes.

[2] Since the toxic levels for many trace elements may be only several times usual intakes, the upper levels for the trace elements given in this table should not be habitually exceeded.

From: Recommended Dietary Allowances, 10th ed. National Academy Press. Washington DC. 1989, p. 284.

Estimated Sodium, Chloride, and Potassium Minimum Requirements of Healthy Persons

Age	Weight (kg)	Sodium (mg)[1,2]	Chloride (mg)[1,2]	Potassium (mg)[3]
MONTHS				
0-5	4.5	120	180	500
6-11	8.9	200	300	700
YEARS				
1	11.0	225	350	1,000
2-5	16.0	300	500	1,400
6-9	25.0	400	600	1,600
10-18	50.0	500	750	2,000
>18[4]	70.0	500	750	2,000

[1] No allowance has been included for large, prolonged losses from the skin through sweat.

[2] There is no evidence that higher intakes confer any health benefit.

[3] Desirable intakes of potassium may considerably exceed these values (~3,500 mg for adults).

[4] No allowance included for growth. Values for those below 18 years assume a growth rate at the 50th percentile reported by the National Center for Health Statistics and averaged for males and females.

From: Recommended Dietary Allowances, 10th ed. National Academy Press. Washington DC. 1989, p. 253.

Amino Acid Requirement Estimates[1]

Amino Acid	Requirements, mg/kg/day, by age group			
	Infants, 3-4 mo[2]	Children, ~2 yr[3]	Children, 10-12 yr[4]	Adults[5]
Histidine	28			8-12
Isoleucine	70	31	28	10
Leucine	161	73	42	14
Lysine	103	64	44	12
Methionine plus cystine	58	27	22	13
Phenylalanine plus tyrosine	125	69	22	14
Threonine	87	37	28	7
Tryptophan	17	12.5	3.3	3.5
Valine	93	38	25	10
Total without histidine	714	352	214	84

[1] From Energy and Protein Requirements. Report of a Joint FAO/WHO/UNU Expert Consultation. Technical Report Series 724. World Health Organization. Geneva. 1985.

[2] Based on amounts of amino acids in human milk or cow's milk formulas fed at levels that supported good growth.

[3] Based on achievement of nitrogen balance sufficient to support adequate lean tissue gain (16 N/kg per day).

[4] Based on upper range of requirement for positive nitrogen balance.

[5] Based on highest estimate of requirement to achieve nitrogen balance.

From: Recommended Dietary Allowances, 10th ed. National Academy Press. Washington DC. 1989, p. 57.

Median Heights and Weights and Recommended Energy Intakes

Age (years) or Condition	Weight		Height		REE[1] (kcal/day)	Average Energy Allowance (kcal)[2]		
	(kg)	(lb)	(cm)	(in)		Multiples of REE	Per kg	Per day[3]
INFANTS								
0.0-0.5	6	13	60	24	320		108	650
0.5-1.0	9	20	71	28	500		98	850
CHILDREN								
1-3	13	29	90	35	740		102	1,300
4-6	20	44	112	44	950		90	1,800
7-10	28	62	132	52	1,130		70	2,000
MALES								
11-14	45	99	157	62	1,440	1.70	55	2,500
15-18	66	145	176	69	1,760	1.67	45	3,000
19-24	72	160	177	70	1,780	1.67	40	2,900
25-50	79	174	176	70	1,800	1.60	37	2,900
51+	77	170	173	68	1,530	1.50	30	2,300
FEMALES								
11-14	46	101	157	62	1,310	1.67	47	2,200
15-18	55	120	163	64	1,370	1.60	40	2,200
19-24	58	128	164	65	1,350	1.60	38	2,200
25-50	63	138	163	64	1,380	1.55	36	2,200
51+	65	143	160	63	1,280	1.50	30	1,900
Pregnant								
1st trimester								+0
2nd trimester								+300
3rd trimester								+300
Lactating								
1st 6 months								+500
2nd 6 months								+500

[1] Resting energy expenditure.
[2] In the range of light to moderate activity, the coefficient of variation is ±20%.
[3] Figure is rounded.

From: Recommended Dietary Allowances, 10th ed. National Academy Press. Washington DC. 1989, p. 33.

Weight for Height of Adults in the United States[1]

Height		Weight, kg (lb)					
		Males, by percentile			Females, by percentile		
(cm)	(in)	15th	50th	85th	15th	50th	85th
147	58				45 (99)	55 (122)	72 (159)
152	60				49 (107)	60 (132)	75 (164)
157	62	57 (125)	64 (142)	76 (168)	51 (112)	60 (132)	77 (170)
163	64	58 (129)	67 (148)	79 (174)	54 (118)	63 (139)	79 (175)
168	66	61 (134)	71 (158)	83 (183)	55 (122)	64 (141)	81 (179)
173	68	65 (143)	76 (167)	88 (195)	59 (130)	67 (148)	83 (184)
178	70	67 (149)	79 (173)	93 (206)	61 (133)	69 (152)	78 (171)
183	72	73 (161)	83 (183)	99 (218)			
188	74	77 (171)	88 (194)	99 (217)			
193	76	85 (187)	103 (227)	106 (234)			

[1] Unpublished data from NHANES II (1976–1980) provided by the National Center for Health Statistics. Values rounded to nearest whole number. Subjects were ages 18 to 74 years. Height determined without shoes. Weight includes clothing weight, ranging from an estimated 0.09 to 0.28 kg (0.20 to 0.62 lb).

From: Recommended Dietary Allowances, 10th ed. National Academy Press. Washington DC, 1989, p. 15.

Daily Values (DV) for Nutrition Labeling[1]

Food Component	Daily Value (DV)
MANDATORY COMPONENTS OF THE NUTRITION LABEL:	
Total Fat	65 g
Saturated Fat	20 g
Cholesterol	300 mg
Sodium	2,400 mg
Total Carbohydrate	300 mg
Dietary Fiber	25 g
Vitamin A	5,000 IU
Vitamin C	60 mg
Calcium	1,000 mg
Iron	18 mg
VOLUNTARY COMPONENTS OF THE NUTRITION LABEL:	
Vitamin D	400 IU
Vitamin E	30 IU
Vitamin K	80 mcg
Thiamin	1.5 mg
Riboflavin	1.7 mg
Niacin	20 mg
Vitamin B-6	2.0 mg
Folic Acid	400 mcg
Vitamin B-12	6.0 mcg
Biotin	300 mcg
Pantothenic Acid	10 mg
Phosphorus	1,000 mg
Iodine	150 mcg
Magnesium	400 mg
Zinc	15 mg
Selenium	70 mcg
Copper	2.0 mg
Manganese	2.0 mg
Chromium	120 mcg
Molybdenum	75 mcg
Chloride	3,400 mg
Potassium	3,500 mg

[1] Daily Values are based on a caloric intake of 2,000 kcal per day. This listing is for foods for adults and children four or more years of age.

From: *Code of Federal Regulations, Food and Drugs,* Title 21, Part 101.9, Nutrition labeling of food. The Office of the Federal Register, National Archives and Records Administration. Washington DC. US Government Printing Office. 1996.

USDA/DHHS Dietary Guidelines for Americans, 1995[1]

- Eat a variety of foods.

- Balance the food you eat with physical activity—maintain or improve your weight.

- Choose a diet with plenty of grain products, vegetables, and fruits.

- Choose a diet low in fat, saturated fat, and cholesterol.

- Choose a diet moderate in sugars.

- Choose a diet moderate in salt and sodium.

- If you drink alcoholic beverages, do so in moderation.

---

[1] From: US Department of Agriculture, US Department of Health and Human Services. *Nutrition and Your Health: Dietary Guidelines for Americans,* fourth edition. Home and Garden Bulletin No. 232. 1995, inside cover.

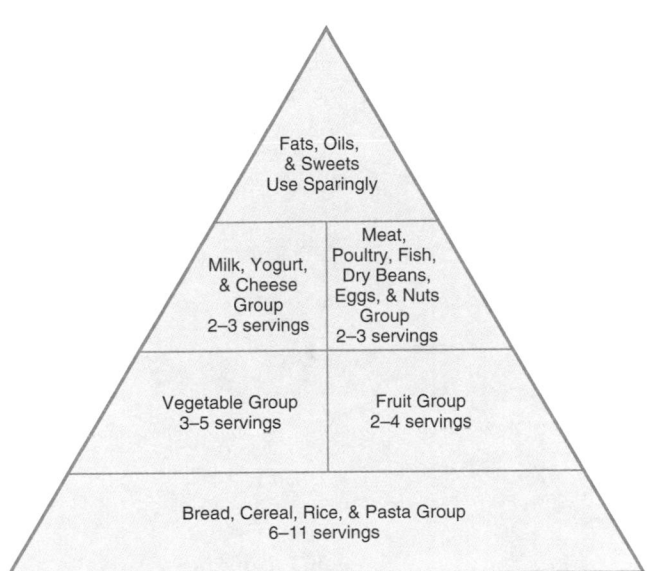

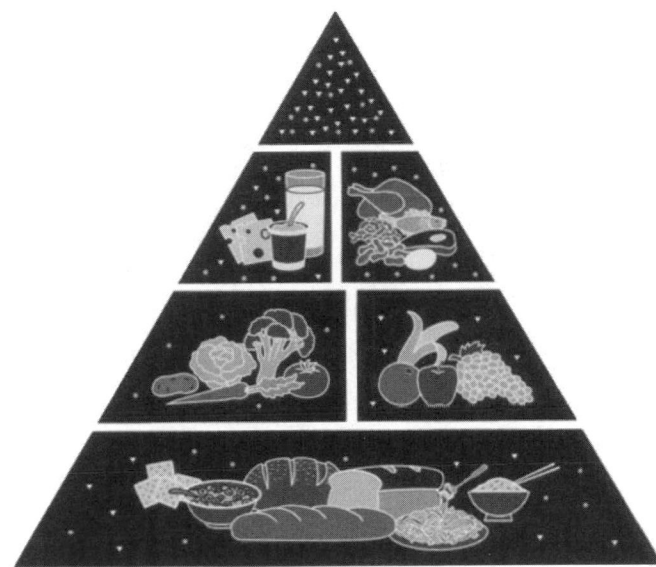

WHAT COUNTS AS A SERVING?

Grain Product Group

- 1 slice of bread
- 1 ounce of ready-to-eat cereal
- ½ cup of cooked cereal, rice, or pasta

Vegetable Group

- 1 cup of raw leafy vegetables
- ½ cup of other vegetables, cooked or chopped raw
- ¾ cup of vegetable juice

Fruit Group

- 1 medium apple, banana, orange
- ½ cup of chopped, cooked, or canned fruit
- ¾ cup of fruit juice

Milk Group

- 1 cup of milk or yogurt
- 1½ ounces of cheese
- 2 ounces of processed cheese

Meats & Beans Group

- 2-3 ounces of cooked lean meat, poultry, or fish
- ½ cup of cooked dry beans or 1 egg counts as 1 ounce of lean meat
- 2 tablespoons of peanut butter or ⅓ cup of nuts counts as 1 ounce of meat

Abbreviations, Symbols, and Reference Codes

am	American	IU	international units
amt	amount	jce	juice
ap	as purchased	jr	junior food
arg	arginine	K	potassium
avg	average	kcal	calories/calorie
bbq	barbecue	L	liter
bio	biotin	lb	pound
blank space	lack of information	leu	leucine
Ca	calcium	lys	lysine
cal	calories/calorie	marb	marbled
calif	California	marg	margarine
chln	choline	mcg	micrograms
cho	carbohydrate	mct	medium-chain triglycerides
choc	chocolate	med	medium
chol	cholesterol	met	methionine
cinn	cinnamon	mg	milligrams
ckd	cooked	Mg	magnesium
Cl	chloride	Mn	manganese
cmprt	compartment	micro ckd	microwave cooked
cnd[1]	canned	mL	milliliter
combo	combination	Mo	molybdenum
conc	concentrate	mod	modified
cond	condensed	mufa	monounsaturated fatty acids
Cr	chromium	Na	sodium
crm	cream	nfdm	nonfat dry milk solids
Cu	copper	nia	niacin
cys	cystine	orig	original
dfibr	dietary fiber (generally total dietary fiber)	oz	ounce
dia	diameter	P	phosphorus
enr	enriched	pant	pantothenic acid
F	fluoride	phe	phenylalanine
Fe	iron	pkg	package
flav	flavor	pkt	packet
fl oz	fluid ounce	prep	prepared
fol	folic acid	pro	protein
frzn[1]	frozen	pufa	polyunsaturated fatty acids
g	grams/gram	rd	round
his	histidine	RE	retinol equivalents
H_2O	water	recon	reconstituted
hp	heaping	red cal	reduced cal
hydg	hydrogenated	ref	reference
I	iodine	refrig	refrigerated
imit	imitation	reg	regular
inos	myo-inositol	rtd	ready-to-drink
inst	instant	rte	ready-to-eat
iso	isoleucine	rth	ready-to-heat

[1] Canned (cnd) *and* frozen (frzn) *refer to commercially canned and frozen foods.*

rts	ready-to-serve/ready-to-spread		veg	vegetable/vegetables
sce	sauce		vit A	vitamin A
Se	selenium		vit B-1	vitamin B-1 (thiamin)
sec	second		vit B-2	vitamin B-2 (riboflavin)
sep	separable		vit B-6	vitamin B-6 (pyridoxine)
sfa	saturated fatty acids		vit B-12	vitamin B-12 (cobalamin)
sq	square		vit C	vitamin C (ascorbic acid)
std	standard		vit D	vitamin D
str	strained baby food		vit E	vitamin E (tocopherol)
sub	substitute		vit E (AT)	vitamin E as alpha-tocopherol
suc	sucrose		vit K	vitamin K
sugr	sugars/sugar		vol	volume
t	teaspoon		whpd	whipped
T	tablespoon		wt	weight
thr	threonine		w/	with
tr	trace		w/o	without
try	tryptophan		Zn	zinc
tyr	tyrosine		&	and
unenr	unenriched		0	zero/none
val	valine		/	per/or
van	vanilla			

Reference Codes for the Nutrient Data

456—USDA Agriculture Handbook No. 456, 1975 (see source #1)
      USDA Nutrient Data Base for Standard Reference, Release 11, 1996 (see source #18)
801—Dairy and Egg Products, Agriculture Handbook Number (Agr Hnd No) 8-1
802—Spices and Herbs, Agr Hnd No 8-2
803—Baby Foods, Agr Hnd No 8-3
804—Fats and Oils, Agr Hnd No 8-4
805—Poultry Products, Agr Hnd No 8-5
806—Soups, Sauces, and Gravies, Agr Hnd No 8-6
807—Sausages and Luncheon Meats, Agr Hnd No 8-7
808—Breakfast Cereals, Agr Hnd No 8-8
809—Fruit and Fruit Juices, Agr Hnd No 8-9
810—Pork Products, Agr Hnd No 8-10
811—Vegetables and Vegetable Products, Agr Hnd No 8-11
812—Nut and Seed Products, Agr Hnd No 8-12
813—Beef Products, Agr Hnd No 8-13
814—Beverages, Agr Hnd No 8-14
815—Finfish and Shellfish Products, Agr Hnd No 8-15
816—Legumes and Legume Products, Agr Hnd No 8-16
817—Lamb, Veal, and Game, Agr Hnd No 8-17
818—Baked Products, Agr Hnd No 8-18
819—Snacks and Sweets, Agr Hnd No 8-19
820—Cereal Grains and Pastas, Agr Hnd No 8-20
821—Fast Foods, Agr Hnd No 8-21

B&C—16th edition of *Bowes & Church's Food Values of Portions Commonly Used*

I—Food companies and trade associations

L—Scientific literature

MUL—More than one source

Conversion Tables

Volume Measures

1 t = ⅓ T	– ⅙ fl oz	= 4.9 ml
3 t = 1 T	= ½ fl oz	= 14.8 ml
2 T = ⅛ cup	= 1 fl oz	= 29.6 ml
4 T = ¼ cup	= 2 fl oz	= 59.1 ml
5⅓ T = ⅓ cup	= 2⅔ fl oz	= 78.9 ml
8 T = ½ cup	= 4 fl oz	= 118.3 ml
10⅔ T = ⅔ cup	= 5⅓ fl oz	= 157.7 ml
12 T = ¾ cup	= 6 fl oz	= 177.4 ml
14 T = ⅞ cup	= 7 fl oz	= 207.0 ml
16 T = 1 cup	= 8 fl oz	= 236.6 ml

1 ml = .034 fl oz	= 1 cc	= .001 liter
1 liter = 34 fl oz	= 1000 ml	

1 pint = 2 cups	= .473 liter	= 473 ml
1 quart = 2 pt	= .946 liter	= 946 ml
1 gallon = 4 quarts	= 3.785 liter	= 3785 ml
1 liter = 1.057 quarts	= 0.264 gallon	= 1000 ml

Weight Measures

1 g = .035 oz = .001 kg = 1000 mg = 1,000,000 mcg
1 mg = .001 g = 1000 mcg
1 oz = 28.35 g (often rounded to 28 g)
1 lb = 16 oz = 453.59 g = .454 kg
1 kg = 2.21 lb = 1000 g
1 kg = 100 g = 3.52 oz

Heat Measures

1 kilojoule = 0.239 kilocalories
1 kilocalorie = 4.184 kilojoules

The relationship between volume measures and weight measures is variable depending on the food. For example, note the weights of 1 cup of the following foods:

Food	Weight of 1 level cup
almonds, chopped	127 g
cottage cheese	233 g
orange juice	244 g
peas, green, canned	172 g
pickle relish	243 g
chicken noodle soup	230 g
milk, whole	244 g
mayonnaise	221 g
shredded wheat	35 g
puffed wheat	12 g
peanut butter	251 g

The volume weight of water is a commonly used reference point for other food measures.

1 T water	= 15 g	= 15 cc
1 cup water	= 237 g	
1 fl oz water	= 29.54 g (often rounded to 30 g)	
1 cc water	= 1 g	= 1 ml
1 liter water	= 1 kg	= 1000 g
1 quart water	= 946 g	= .946 kg

Nutrient Content of Foods

1. BEVERAGES
1.1 ALCOHOLIC & MALT BEVERAGES

	KCAL / WT (g)	H₂O (g) / FAT (g)	PRO (g) / SFA (g)	CHO (g) / MUFA (g)	SUGR (g) / PUFA (g)	DFIB (g) / CHOL (mg)	A (RE) / A (IU)	C (mg) / B-1 (mg)	B-2 (mg) / NIA (mg)	B-6 (mg) / B-12 (mcg)	FOL (mcg) / PANT (mg)	Na (mg) / K (mg)	Ca (mg) / P (mg)	Mg (mg) / Fe (mg)	Zn (mg) / Cu (mg)	Mn (mg) / REF
ale, Elk Mountain Amber Ale	190		2.7	17.4								9				
12 fl oz	355	0.0	0.0	0.0	0.0	0										I
ale, Northstone Amber	149		2.0	11.6								16				
12 fl oz	360	0.0	0.0	0.0	0.0	0										I
beer	146	328.6	1.1	13.2		0.7	0	0	.09	.18	21	18	18	21	.07	.043
12 fl oz	356	0.0	0.0	0.0	0.0	0	0	.02	1.6	.07	.21	89	43	.11	.032	814
Big Sky	148		1.0	12.6								7				
12 fl oz	360	0.0	0.0	0.0	0.0	0										I
Black & Tan	192		2.5	22.6								9				
12 fl oz	355	0.0	0.0	0.0	0.0	0										I
Bud Dry	130	331.0	1.1	8.2	0.0	0.0			.07	.17		12	11	17	.01	.030
12 fl oz	356	0.0	0.0	0.0	0.0	0		.00	2.1	.00	.14	102	151	.01	.010	I
Bud Ice	148		1.3	9.2								9				
12 fl oz	355	0.0	0.0	0.0	0.0	0										I
Budweiser	147	331.0	1.2	11.4	0.0	0.0			.11	.16		12	12	19	.01	.030
12 fl oz	357	0.0	0.0	0.0	0.0	0		.00	2.2	.00	.21	111	147	.01	.010	I
Busch	143		1.1	10.9								9				
12 fl oz	355	0.0	0.0	0.0	0.0	0										I
Busch Ice	169		1.3	12.8								9				
12 fl oz	355	0.0	0.0	0.0	0.0	0										I
Elk Mountain Red	160		2.2	14.2								9				
12 fl oz	355	0.0	0.0	0.0	0.0	0										I
Faust	168		2.4	15.4								9				
12 fl oz	355	0.0	0.0	0.0	0.0	0										I
Genuine Draft	143		1.0	13.1								7				
12 fl oz	360	0.0	0.0	0.0	0.0	0										I
High Life	143		1.0	13.1								7				
12 fl oz	360	0.0	0.0	0.0	0.0	0										I
High Life Ice	156		1.1	11.0								9				
12 fl oz	360	0.0	0.0	0.0	0.0	0										I
Hurricane	158		1.6	9.2								9				
12 fl oz	355	0.0	0.0	0.0	0.0	0										I
Icehouse	132		1.2	8.7								8				
12 fl oz	360	0.0	0.0	0.0	0.0	0										I
Icehouse 5.5	149		1.3	9.8								9				
12 fl oz	360	0.0	0.0	0.0	0.0	0										I
King Cobra	177		1.7	14.1								9				
12 fl oz	355	0.0	0.0	0.0	0.0	0										I
Lowenbrau Special/Dark	158		1.4	14.3								7				
12 fl oz	360	0.0	0.0	0.0	0.0	0										I
Magnum	155		1.1	9.0								8				
12 fl oz	360	0.0	0.0	0.0	0.0	0										I
Meister Brau	128		1.0	11.4								6				
12 fl oz	360	0.0	0.0	0.0	0.0	0										I
Michelob	157		1.3	13.5								9				
12 fl oz	355	0.0	0.0	0.0	0.0	0										I
Michelob Amber Block	159		1.4	14.3								9				
12 fl oz	355	0.0	0.0	0.0	0.0	0										I
Michelob Classic Dark	163		1.5	14.8								9				
12 fl oz	355	0.0	0.0	0.0	0.0	0										I
Michelob Dry	130		1.2	7.9								9				
12 fl oz	355	0.0	0.0	0.0	0.0	0										I
Michelob Golden Draft	151		1.6	13.1								9				
12 fl oz	355	0.0	0.0	0.0	0.0	0										I
Michelob Malt	160		1.4	9.8								9				
12 fl oz	355	0.0	0.0	0.0	0.0	0										I
Miller	150		1.1	13.2								4				
12 fl oz	360	0.0	0.0	0.0	0.0	0										I

	KCAL	H₂O (g)	PRO (g)	CHO (g)	SUGR (g)	DFIB (g)	A (RE)	C (mg)	B-2 (mg)	B-6 (mg)	FOL (mcg)	Na (mg)	Ca (mg)	Mg (mg)	Zn (mg)	Mn (mg)
	WT (g)	FAT (g)	SFA (g)	MUFA (g)	PUFA (g)	CHOL (mg)	A (IU)	B-1 (mg)	NIA (mg)	B-12 (mcg)	PANT (mg)	K (mg)	P (mg)	Fe (mg)	Cu (mg)	REF
Milwaukee's Best	128		0.9	11.4								6				
12 fl oz	360	0.0	0.0	0.0	0.0	0										I
Milwaukee's Best Ice	135		0.9	6.9								5				
12 fl oz	360	0.0	0.0	0.0	0.0	0										I
Muenchener	178		2.5	11.9								9				
12 fl oz	355	0.0	0.0	0.0	0.0	0										I
Natural Ice	158		1.3	9.4								9				
12 fl oz	355	0.0	0.0	0.0	0.0	0										I
Natural Pilsner	145		1.1	11.1								9				
12 fl oz	355	0.0	0.0	0.0	0.0	0										I
Red Dog	147		0.7	14.1								4				
12 fl oz	360	0.0	0.0	0.0	0.0	0										I
Red Wolf	160		1.5	11.6								9				
12 fl oz	355	0.0	0.0	0.0	0.0	0										I
Ziegenbock	154		1.3	11.1								9				
12 fl oz	355	0.0	0.0	0.0	0.0	0										I
beer light	99	337.0	0.7	4.6		0.0	0	0	.11	.12	15	11	18	18	.11	.057
12 fl oz	354	0.0	0.0	0.0	0.0	0	0	.03	1.4	.04	.13	64	42	.14	.085	814
Big Sky Light	104		1.0	11.0								6				
12 fl oz	360	0.0	0.0	0.0	0.0	0										I
Bud Ice Light	96		0.8	3.5								9				
12 fl oz	355	0.0	0.0	0.0	0.0	0										I
Bud Light	110	336.0	0.9	6.6		0.0			.07	.16		12	11	17	.01	.030
12 fl oz	356	0.0	0.0	0.0	0.0	0		.00	1.6	.00	.18	90	139	.01	.010	I
Busch Light	110		0.8	6.7								9				
12 fl oz	355	0.0	0.0	0.0	0.0	0										I
Genuine Draft Light	110		0.8	7.0								6				
12 fl oz	360	0.0	0.0	0.0	0.0	0										I
High Life Light	110		1.0	7.0								6				
12 fl oz	360	0.0	0.0	0.0	0.0	0										I
Meister Brau Light	103		0.9	4.8								6				
12 fl oz	360	0.0	0.0	0.0	0.0	0										I
Michelob Golden Draft Light	110		1.0	6.7								9				
12 fl oz	355	0.0	0.0	0.0	0.0	0										I
Michelob Light	134		1.0	11.5								9				
12 fl oz	355	0.0	0.0	0.0	0.0	0										I
Miller Lite	96		0.9	3.2								6				
12 fl oz	360	0.0	0.0	0.0	0.0	0										I
Miller Lite Ice 5.0	113		0.9	4.0								7				
12 fl oz	360	0.0	0.0	0.0	0.0	0										I
Miller Lite Ice 5.5	125		1.0	4.2								7				
12 fl oz	360	0.0	0.0	0.0	0.0	0										I
Milwaukee's Best Light	98		0.8	3.5								6				
12 fl oz	360	0.0	0.0	0.0	0.0	0										I
Natural Light	110		0.9	6.7								9				
12 fl oz	355	0.0	0.0	0.0	0.0	0										I
Southpaw Light	123		0.8	6.3								6				
12 fl oz	360	0.0	0.0	0.0	0.0	0										I
bloody mary (tomato jce, vodka, &	115	127.3	0.7	4.9		0.4	50	20	.03	.11	20	332	10	12	.13	.073
lemon jce)—*5 fl oz cocktail*	148	0.1	0.0	0.0	0.0	0	508	.05	0.6	.00	.24	216	21	.55	.102	814
bourbon & soda	104	100.8	0.0	0.0	0.0	0.0	0	0	.00	.00	0	16	3	1	.09	.007
4 fl oz cocktail	116	0.0	0.0	0.0	0.0	0	0	.00	0.0	.00	.00	2	2	.02	.014	814
daiquiri, cnd	259	154.4	0.0	32.5		0.0	0	3	.00	.01	2	83	0	2	.06	.010
6.8 fl oz can	207	0.0	0.0	0.0	0.0	0	4	.00	0.0	.00	.01	23	4	.02	.033	814
daiquiri (rum, lime jce, & sugar)	112	41.9	0.1	4.1		0.0	0	1	.00	.00	1	3	2	1	.04	.008
2 fl oz cocktail	60	0.1	0.0	0.0	0.0	0	2	.01	0.0	.00	.01	13	4	.09	.026	814
distilled spirits, all types, 80 proof	97	28.0	0.0	0.0	0.0	0.0	0	0	.00	.00	0	0	0	0	.02	.008
1.5 fl oz jigger	42	0.0	0.0	0.0	0.0	0	0	.00	0.0	.00	.00	1	2	.02	.009	814
gin, 90 proof	110	26.1	0.0	0.0	0.0	0.0	0	0	.00	.00	0	1	0	0	.00	.000
1.5 fl oz jigger	42	0.0	0.0	0.0	0.0	0	0	.00	0.0	.00	.00	0	0	.00	.002	814
gin & tonic (tonic water, gin, & lime jce)	171	193.0	0.0	15.8		0.0	0	1	.00	.00	1	9	5	2	.18	.002
7.5 fl oz	225	0.0	0.0	0.0	0.0	0	2	.00	0.0	.00	.01	11	2	.04	.018	814

	KCAL / WT (g)	H₂O (g) / FAT (g)	PRO (g) / SFA (g)	CHO (g) / MUFA (g)	SUGR (g) / PUFA (g)	DFIB (g) / CHOL (mg)	A (RE) / A (IU)	C (mg) / B-1 (mg)	B-2 (mg) / NIA (mg)	B-6 (mg) / B-12 (mcg)	FOL (mcg) / PANT (mg)	Na (mg) / K (mg)	Ca (mg) / P (mg)	Mg (mg) / Fe (mg)	Zn (mg) / Cu (mg)	Mn (mg) / REF
liqueur																
coffee, 53 proof	175	16.1	0.1	24.3		0.0	0	0	.01	.00	0	4	1	2	.02	.009
1.5 fl oz	52	0.2	0.1	0.0	0.1	0	0	.00	0.1	.00	.00	16	3	.03	.021	814
coffee w/ cream, 34 proof	154	21.9	1.3	9.8		0.0	20	0	.03	.01	0	43	8	1	.08	.016
1.5 fl oz	47	7.4	4.5	2.1	0.3	7	82	.00	0.0	.06	.04	15	24	.06	.019	814
creme de menthe	186	14.2	0.0	20.8		0.0	0	0	.00	.00	0	3	0	0	.02	.020
1.5 fl oz	50	0.1	0.0	0.0	0.1	0	0	.00	0.0	.00	.00	0	0	.04	.040	814
malt beverage, nonalcoholic	32	353.2	1.1	5.1									25	31	.03	.047
12 fl oz	360	0.0	0.0	0.0	0.0	0							110	.05	.040	814
Bush NA	60		0.6	13.0									9			
12 fl oz	355	0.0	0.0	0.0	0.0	0										I
O'Doul's	70	343.0	0.7	14.0	0.0	0.0			.11	.24		12	17	25	.01	.030
12 fl oz	361	0.0	0.0	0.0	0.0	0		.00	2.6	.00	.29	139	165	.01	.010	I
Sharp's	58		0.4	12.1									3			
12 fl oz	360	0.0	0.0	0.0	0.0	0										I
manhattan (whiskey & vermouth)	128	37.7	0.1	1.8		0.0	0	0	.00	.00	0	2	1	1	.03	.024
2 fl oz cocktail	57	0.0	0.0	0.0	0.0	0	0	.01	0.1	.00	.00	15	4	.05	.016	814
martini (gin & vermouth)	156	47.3	0.0	0.2		0.0	0	0	.00	.00	0	2	1	1	.01	.017
2.5 fl oz	70	0.0	0.0	0.0	0.0	0	0	.00	0.0	.00	.00	13	2	.06	.004	814
pina colada, cnd	526	121.9	1.3	61.3		0.2	4	3	.01	.04	13	158	2	13	.44	.708
6.8 fl oz can	222	16.9	14.6	1.0	0.3	0	53	.04	0.2	.00	.12	184	80	.07	.193	814
pina colada (pineapple jce, rum, sugar,	262	91.8	0.6	39.9		0.8	0	7	.02	.06	14	8	11	11	.18	.744
& coconut cream)—4.5 fl oz cocktail	141	2.7	1.2	0.2	0.5	0	3	.04	0.2	.00	.06	100	10	.31	.116	814
rum, 80 proof	97	28.0	0.0	0.0	0.0	0.0	0	0	.00	.00	0	0	0	0	.03	.008
1.5 fl oz jigger	42	0.0	0.0	0.0	0.0	0	0	.00	0.0	.00	.00	1	2	.05	.021	814
screwdriver (orange jce & vodka)	175	178.5	1.1	18.3		0.4	13	66	.03	.07	75	2	15	17	.09	.023
7 fl oz cocktail	213	0.0	0.0	0.0	0.0	0	134	.14	0.3	.00	.27	326	30	.17	.079	814
tequila sunrise, cnd	232	166.3	0.6	23.8		0.0	21	41	.03	.11	22	120	0	15	1.27	.030
6.8 fl oz can	211	0.2	0.0			0	205	.08	0.4	.00	.19	21	21	.04	.089	814
tequila sunrise (orange jce, tequila, lime	189	137.3	0.5	14.8		0.3	17	33	.03	.09	18	7	10	12	.10	.024
jce, & grenadine)—5.5 fl oz cocktail	172	0.2	0.0	0.0	0.0	0	167	.07	0.3	.00	.15	179	17	.48	.072	814
tom collins (club soda, gin, lemon jce, &	122	202.9	0.0	2.9		0.0	0	4	.00	.01	2	38	9	2	.18	.004
sugar)—7.5 fl oz cocktail	222	0.0	0.0	0.0	0.0	0	2	.01	0.0	.00	.01	18	2	.02	.018	814
vodka, 80 proof	97	28.0	0.0	0.0	0.0	0.0	0	0	.00	.00	0	0	0	0	.00	.000
1.5 fl oz jigger	42	0.0	0.0	0.0	0.0	0	0	.00	0.0	.00	.00	0	2	.00	.004	814
whiskey, 86 proof	105	26.8	0.0	0.0		0.0	0	0	.00	.00	0	0	0	0	.02	.006
1.5 fl oz	42	0.0	0.0	0.0	0.0	0	0	.00	0.0	.00	.00	1	2	.01	.009	814
whiskey sour																
cnd	249	160.7	0.0	28.0		0.2	2	3	.01	.00	0	92	0	2	.13	.013
6.8 fl oz can	209	0.0	0.0	0.0	0.0	0	27	.02	0.0	.00	.02	23	13	.02	.019	814
lemon jce, whiskey, & sugar	122	69.4	0.2	5.0		0.2	1	11	.00	.02	5	10	5	4	.05	.015
3 fl oz cocktail	90	0.1	0.0	0.0	0.0	0	7	.19	0.1	.00	.04	48	6	.07	.027	814
prep from bottled mix	158	77.0	0.0	13.9		0.0	1	2	.01	.00	0	66	1	1	.06	.006
2 fl oz mix & 1.5 fl oz whiskey	106	0.0	0.0	0.0	0.0	0	14	.01	0.0	.00	.01	19	6	.08	.010	814
prep from powdered mix—17 g pkt w/	169	71.2	0.1	16.4		0.0	0	0	.00	.00	0	47	46	4	.05	.006
1.5 fl oz water & 1.5 fl oz whiskey	103	0.0	0.0	0.0	0.0	0	5	.00	0.0	.00	.01	4	4	.08	.034	814
whiskey sour mix, bottled	55	50.8	0.1	13.9		0.0	1	2	.01	.00	0	66	1	1	.05	.000
2 fl oz cocktail	65	0.1	0.0	0.0	0.0	0	14	.01	0.0	.00	.01	18	4	.07	.000	814
whiskey sour mix, powder	65	0.1	0.1	16.5		0.0	1	0	.00	.00	0	47	46	3	.02	.000
1 pkt	17	0.0	0.0	0.0	0.0	0	5	.00	0.0	.00	.01	3	2	.07	.022	814
wine, cooking																
red, Regina	25		0.0	3.0	0.0						190					
2 T	30 ml	0.0	0.0	0.0	0.0	0										I
sauterne, Regina	20		0.0	3.0								190				
2 T	30 ml	0.0	0.0	0.0	0.0	0										I
sherry, Regina	35		0.0	5.0	1.0							190				
2 T	30 ml	0.0	0.0	0.0	0.0	0										I
wine, dessert, dry	44	25.2	0.1	1.4				0	.01	.00	0	3	3	3	.02	.041
2 fl oz	59	0.0	0.0	0.0	0.0	0		.01	0.1	.00	.01	32	4	.08	.016	814

	KCAL / WT (g)	H₂O (g) / FAT (g)	PRO (g) / SFA (g)	CHO (g) / MUFA (g)	SUGR (g) / PUFA (g)	DFIB (g) / CHOL (mg)	A (RE) / A (IU)	C (mg) / B-1 (mg)	B-2 (mg) / NIA (mg)	B-6 (mg) / B-12 (mcg)	FOL (mcg) / PANT (mg)	Na (mg) / K (mg)	Ca (mg) / P (mg)	Mg (mg) / Fe (mg)	Zn (mg) / Cu (mg)	Mn (mg) / REF
wine, dessert, sweet	90	42.8	0.1	7.0		0.0	0	0	.01	.00	0	5	5	5	.04	.070
2 fl oz	59	0.0	0.0	0.0	0.0	0	0	.01	0.1	.00	.02	54	5	.14	.027	814
wine, table all types	72	91.6	0.2	1.4		0.0	0	0	.02	.02	1	8	8	10	.07	.149
3.5 fl oz	103	0.0	0.0	0.0	0.0	0	0	.00	0.1	.01	.03	92	14	.42	.014	814
red	74	91.2	0.2	1.8		0.0	0	0	.03	.04	2	5	8	13	.09	.615
3.5 fl oz	103	0.0	0.0	0.0	0.0	0	0	.01	0.1	.01	.04	115	14	.44	.021	814
rose	73	91.6	0.2	1.4	2.6	0.0	0	0	.02	.02	1	5	8	10	.06	.108
3.5 fl oz	103	0.0	0.0	0.0	0.0	0	0	.00	0.1	.01	.03	102	15	.39	.054	814
white	70	92.3	0.1	0.8	0.6	0.0	0	0	.01	.01	0	5	9	10	.07	.473
3.5 fl oz	103	0.0	0.0	0.0	0.0	0	0	.00	0.1	.00	.02	82	14	.33	.022	809

1.2 CARBONATED BEVERAGES

	KCAL / WT (g)	H₂O (g) / FAT (g)	PRO (g) / SFA (g)	CHO (g) / MUFA (g)	SUGR (g) / PUFA (g)	DFIB (g) / CHOL (mg)	A (RE) / A (IU)	C (mg) / B-1 (mg)	B-2 (mg) / NIA (mg)	B-6 (mg) / B-12 (mcg)	FOL (mcg) / PANT (mg)	Na (mg) / K (mg)	Ca (mg) / P (mg)	Mg (mg) / Fe (mg)	Zn (mg) / Cu (mg)	Mn (mg) / REF
All Sport	70		0.0	20.0	19.2	0.0				.20	40	55				
8 fl oz[1]	240	0.0	0.0	0.0	0.0	0		.15	2.0	.60		50	61			I
Birch Beer, Canada Dry	150		0.0	40.0	40.0							40				
12 fl oz	360															I
Bitter Lemon, Canada Dry	150		0.0	38.0	38.0							15				
12 fl oz	360	0.0	0.0	0.0	0.0											I
Blue Cream Soda, Nehi	178			48.3	48.3							50				
12 fl oz.	360	0.0	0.0	0.0	0.0							28	0			I
Cactus Cooler, Canada Dry	150		0.0	40.0	40.0							40				
12 fl oz	360	0.0	0.0	0.0	0.0											I
Cherry Coca-Cola	104			28.0				0				4				
8 fl oz	240	0.0	0.0	0.0	0.0								37			I
Cherry RC	160		0.0	43.0	43.0							50				
12 fl oz	360	0.0	0.0	0.0	0.0	0						15	46			I
Coca-Cola Classic	97		0.0	27.0				0				9				
8 fl oz	240	0.0	0.0	0.0	0.0								41			I
Coke II	105			29.0								4				
8 fl oz	240											0	38			I
cola	152	330.8	0.0	38.5		0.0	0	0	.00	.00	0	15	11	4	.04	.130
12 fl oz	370	0.0	0.0	0.0	0.0	0	0	.00	0.0	.00	.00	4	44	.11	.041	814
Cola Champagne, Nehi	192			52.0	52.0							50				
12 fl oz	360	0.0	0.0	0.0	0.0							23	0			I
cream soda	189	321.7	0.0	49.3		0.0	0	0	.00	.00	0	45	19	4	.26	.048
12 fl oz	371	0.0	0.0	0.0	0.0	0	0	.00	0.0	.00	.00	4	0	.19	.030	814
creme soda, Mug	170		0.0	48.0	48.0	0.0						65				
12 fl oz	360	0.0	0.0	0.0	0.0	0							0			I
Dr. Nehi	143		0.0	38.8	38.8							50				
12 fl oz	360	0.0	0.0	0.0	0.0								0			I
Dr. Pepper	150		0.0	40.0	40.0							55				
12 fl oz	360	0.0	0.0	0.0	0.0							43	52			I
Draft Cola, Royal Crown	180			49.1	49.1							50				
12 fl oz	360	0.0	0.0	0.0	0.0							31	61			I
fruit flavored soda, Nehi	182		0.0	48.9	48.9							50				
12 fl oz[2]	360	0.0	0.0	0.0	0.0							26	0			I
fruit flavors, Minute Maid	113			30.4								8				
8 fl oz[3]	240											13	0			I
fruit punch, Nehi	180		0.0	51.0	51.0							50				
12 fl oz	360	0.0	0.0	0.0	0.0							48	0			I
ginger ale	124	333.8	0.0	31.8		0.0	0	0	.00	.00	0	26	11	4	.18	.048
12 fl oz	366	0.0	0.0	0.0	0.0	0	0	.00	0.0	.00	.00	4	0	.66	.066	814
Fanta	86		0.0	23.0				0				4				
8 fl oz	240	0.0	0.0	0.0	0.0							11				I
Nehi	140		0.0	36.6	36.6							50				
12 fl oz	360	0.0	0.0	0.0	0.0							0	0			I
Par-T-Pak	130			32.1	32.1							50				
12 fl oz	360	0.0	0.0	0.0	0.0							1	0			I

	KCAL	H₂O (g)	PRO (g)	CHO (g)	SUGR (g)	DFIB (g)	A (RE)	C (mg)	B-2 (mg)	B-6 (mg)	FOL (mcg)	Na (mg)	Ca (mg)	Mg (mg)	Zn (mg)	Mn (mg)
	WT (g)	FAT (g)	STA (g)	MUFA (g)	PUFA (g)	CHOL (mg)	A (IU)	B-1 (mg)	NIA (mg)	B-12 (mcg)	PANT (mg)	K (mg)	P (mg)	Fe (mg)	Cu (mg)	REF
grape	160	330.3	0.0	41.7		0.0	0	0	.00	.00	0	56	11	4	.26	.048
12 fl oz	372	0.0	0.0	0.0	0.0	0	0	.00	0.0	.00	.00	4	0	.30	.082	814
Fanta	117		0.0	31.0								9				
8 fl oz	240	0.0	0.0	0.0	0.0							0	0			I
Nehi	180		0.0	48.3	48.3							50				
12 fl oz	360	0.0	0.0	0.0	0.0	0						24	72			I
Hi-Spot, Canada Dry	150			41.0	41.0							60				
12 fl oz	360	0.0	0.0	0.0	0.0											I
Jamaica Cola, Canada Dry	150		0.0	40.0	40.0							15				
12 fl oz	360	0.0	0.0	0.0	0.0											I
Kick	180		0.0	48.7	48.7							50				
12 fl oz	360	0.0	0.0	0.0	0.0							69	0			I
lemon-lime	147	329.4	0.0	38.3		0.0	0	0	.00	.00	0	40	7	4	.18	.048
12 fl oz	368	0.0	0.0	0.0	0.0	0	0	.00	0.1	.00	.00	4	0	.26	.044	814
Lockjaw Fruit, Nehi	180			44.0	44.0							50				
12 fl oz[4]	360	0.0	0.0	0.0	0.0							59	0			I
Maxxvm Cola, Nehi	184			49.7	49.7							50				
12 fl oz	360	0.0	0.0	0.0	0.0							15	72			I
Mello Yello	119		0.0	32.0				0				9				
8 fl oz	240	0.0		0.0	0.0							22	0			I
Mountain Dew	170		0.0	46.0	46.0	0.0						70				
12 fl oz	360	0.0	0.0	0.0	0.0	0						0	0			I
Mr. Pibb	97		0.0	26.0				0				7				
8 fl oz	240	0.0		0.0	0.0							14	29			I
orange	179	325.9	0.0	45.8		0.0	0	0	.00	.00	0	45	19	4	.37	.048
12 fl oz	372	0.0	0.0	0.0	0.0	0	0	.00	0.0	.00	.00	7	4	.22	.056	814
Crush	180		0.0	50.0	50.0							45				
12 fl oz	360	0.0	0.0	0.0	0.0											I
Fanta	118		0.0	32.0				0				9				
8 fl oz	240	0.0		0.0	0.0							0	0			I
Minute Maid	118		0.0	32.0				0				0				
8 fl oz	240	0.0		0.0	0.0							14	0			I
Nehi	190		0.0	51.6	51.6							50				
12 fl oz	360	0.0	0.0	0.0	0.0	0						29	60			I
Sunkist	190		0.0	52.0	52.0							45	0			
12 fl oz	360	0.0	0.0	0.0	0.0							0		.00		I
pepper type	151	329.0	0.0	38.3		0.0	0	0	.00	.00	0	37	11	0	.15	.129
12 fl oz	368	0.4	0.3			0	0	.00	0.0	.00	.00	4	40	.15	.022	814
Pepsi	150		0.0	41.0	41.0	0.0						35				
12 fl oz	360	0.0	0.0	0.0	0.0	0						10	53	.00		I
Pepsi, wild cherry	160		0.0	43.0	43.0	0.0						35				
12 fl oz	360	0.0	0.0	0.0	0.0	0						10	53	.00		I
quinine water, Nehi	130		0.0	34.1	34.1							50				
12 fl oz	360	0.0	0.0	0.0	0.0							0	0			I
RC Cola	160		0.0	43.2	43.2							50				
12 fl oz	360	0.0	0.0	0.0	0.0	0						15	68			I
root beer	152	330.4	0.0	39.2		0.0	0	0	.00	.00	0	48	19	4	.26	.048
12 fl oz	370	0.0	0.0	0.0	0.0	0	0	.00	0.0	.00	.00	4	0	.19	.026	814
Barq's	111		0.0	30.0								24				
8 fl oz	240	0.0		0.0	0.0							0	0			I
Barrelhead, Canada Dry	150		0.0	40.0	40.0							40				
12 fl oz	360	0.0	0.0	0.0	0.0									.		I
Hires	170		0.0	45.0	45.0							70				
12 fl oz	360	0.0	0.0	0.0	0.0											I
Mug	160		0.0	43.0	43.0	0.0						65				
12 fl oz	360	0.0	0.0	0.0	0.0	0							0			I
Nehi	180		0.0	48.6	48.6							50				
12 fl oz	360	0.0	0.0	0.0	0.0	0						41	0			I
Seven-Up	144		0.0	36.2	36.2	0.0						32				
12 fl oz	360	0.0	0.0	0.0	0.0	0										I

	KCAL / WT (g)	H₂O (g) / FAT (g)	PRO (g) / SFA (g)	CHO (g) / MUFA (g)	SUGR (g) / PUFA (g)	DFIB (g) / CHOL (mg)	A (RE) / A (IU)	C (mg) / B-1 (mg)	B-2 (mg) / NIA (mg)	B-6 (mg) / B-12 (mcg)	FOL (mcg) / PANT (mg)	Na (mg) / K (mg)	Ca (mg) / P (mg)	Mg (mg) / Fe (mg)	Zn (mg) / Cu (mg)	Mn (mg) / REF
Slice																
cherry spice	145		0.0	39.5	39.0	0.0						35				
12 fl oz	360	0.0	0.0	0.0	0.0	0							34			I
cola	160		0.0	43.0	43.0	0.0						35				
12 fl oz	360	0.0	0.0	0.0	0.0	0							51	.00		I
fruit flavors	177		0.0	47.6	47.6	0.0						59				
12 fl oz[5]	360	0.0	0.0	0.0	0.0	0										I
red	190		0.0	51.0	50.0	0.0						55				
12 fl oz	360	0.0	0.0	0.0	0.0	0										I
Sprite	96		0.0	26.0				0				23				
8 fl oz	240	0.0	0.0	0.0	0.0							0	0			I
Tahitian Treat, Canada Dry	170		0.0	45.0	45.0							40				
12 fl oz	360	0.0	0.0	0.0	0.0											I
tonic water, Par-T-Pak	130			35.1	35.1							50				
12 fl oz	360	0.0	0.0	0.0	0.0							13	0			I
tonic water/quinine water	124	333.4	0.0	32.2		0.0	0	0	.00	.00	0	15	4	0	.37	.004
12 fl oz	366	0.0	0.0	0.0	0.0	0	0	.00	0.0	.00	.00	0	0	.04	.022	814
Upper 10	160		0.0	41.6	41.6							50				
12 fl oz[6]	360	0.0	0.0	0.0	0.0							59				I
Vanilla Cream, Canada Dry	160		0.0	44.0	44.0							40				
12 fl oz	360	0.0	0.0	0.0	0.0											I
Wink, Canada Dry	160		0.0	43.0	43.0							35				
12 fl oz	360	0.0	0.0	0.0	0.0											I

1.3 CARBONATED BEVERAGES, LOW CALORIE

	KCAL / WT (g)	H₂O (g) / FAT (g)	PRO (g) / SFA (g)	CHO (g) / MUFA (g)	SUGR (g) / PUFA (g)	DFIB (g) / CHOL (mg)	A (RE) / A (IU)	C (mg) / B-1 (mg)	B-2 (mg) / NIA (mg)	B-6 (mg) / B-12 (mcg)	FOL (mcg) / PANT (mg)	Na (mg) / K (mg)	Ca (mg) / P (mg)	Mg (mg) / Fe (mg)	Zn (mg) / Cu (mg)	Mn (mg) / REF
club soda	0	354.6	0.0	0.0	0.0	0.0	0	0	.00	.00	0	75	18	4	.35	.004
12 fl oz	355	0.0	0.0	0.0	0.0	0	0	.00	0.0	.00	.00	7	0	.04	.021	814
club soda, Par-T-Pak	0			0.0	0.0							55				
12 fl oz	360	0.0	0.0	0.0	0.0							73	0			I
diet cherry Coca-Cola	1		0.1	0.1				0				4				
8 fl oz[7]	240	0.0	0.0	0.0	0.0							12	18			I
diet cherry ginger ale, Canada Dry	5		0.0	0.0	0.0							90				
12 fl oz	360	0.0	0.0	0.0	0.0											I
Diet Coke	1		0.1	0.1				0				4				
8 fl oz[7]	248	0.0	0.0	0.0	0.0							12	18			I
diet cola, aspartame sweetened	4	354.3	0.4	0.4	0.0	0.0	0	0	.08	.00	0	21	14	4	.28	.124
12 fl oz	355	0.0	0.0	0.0	0.0	0	0	.02	0.0	.00	.00	0	32	.11	.039	814
diet cola, sodium saccharin sweetened	0	354.3	0.0	0.4	0.0	0.0	0	0	.00	.00	0	57	14	4	.18	.060
12 fl oz	355	0.0	0.0	0.0	0.0	0	0	.00	0.0	.00	.00	7	39	.14	.089	814
diet creme soda, Mug	5		0.0	0.0	0.0	0.0						80				
12 fl oz[8]	360	0.0	0.0	0.0	0.0								0			I
Diet Dr. Pepper	0		0.0	0.0	0.0							55				
12 fl oz	360	0.0	0.0	0.0	0.0											I
Diet Kick Citrus	15		0.0	3.1	3.1							50				
12 fl oz	360	0.0	0.0	0.0	0.0							83	21			I
Diet Mello Yello	3			0.2								0				
8 fl oz[9]	240											35	0			I
Diet Mountain Dew	0		0.0	0.0	0.0	0.0						35				
12 fl oz	360	0.0	0.0	0.0	0.0	0						70	0			I
Diet Mr. Pibb	1			0.3								2				
8 fl oz[7]	240											20	29			I
diet orange																
Crush	20		0.0	5.0	5.0							45				
12 fl oz	360	0.0	0.0	0.0	0.0											I
Minute Maid	2		0.2	0.0	0.0			0				0				
8 fl oz[10]	240											43	0			I
Sunkist	0		0.0	0.0	0.0							100				
12 fl oz	360	0.0	0.0	0.0	0.0											I

							Vitamins					Minerals				
	KCAL	H_2O (g)	PRO (g)	CHO (g)	SUGR (g)	DFIB (g)	A (RE)	C (mg)	B-2 (mg)	B-6 (mg)	FOL (mcg)	Na (mg)	Ca (mg)	Mg (mg)	Zn (mg)	Mn (mg)
	WT (g)	FAT (g)	SFA (g)	MUFA (g)	PUFA (g)	CHOL (mg)	A (IU)	B-1 (mg)	NIA (mg)	B-12 (mcg)	PANT (mg)	K (mg)	P (mg)	Fe (mg)	Cu (mg)	REF
Diet Pepsi	0		0.0	0.0	0.0	0.0						35				
12 fl oz[11]	360	0.0	0.0	0.0	0.0	0						30	41			I
Diet RC	2		0.0	0.0	0.0							0				
12 fl oz	360	0.0	0.0	0.0	0.0							65	41			I
Diet Rite black cherry	4		0.0	0.0	0.0							2				
12 fl oz	360	0.0	0.0	0.0	0.0							92				I
Diet Rite Cola	2			0.0	0.0							0				
12 fl oz[12]	360	0.0	0.0	0.0	0.0	0						65	40			I
Diet Rite fruit-flavored soda	4		0.0	0.0	0.0							1				
12 fl oz[13]	360	0.0	0.0	0.0	0.0	0						92	0			I
diet root beer, Hires	5		0.0	0.0	0.0							100				
12 fl oz	360	0.0	0.0	0.0	0.0											I
diet root beer, Mug	0		0.0	0.0	0.0	0.0						65				
12 fl oz[14]	360	0.0	0.0	0.0	0.0	0							0			I
Diet Slice, lemon lime	0		0.0	1.0	0.0	0.0						35				
12 fl oz[15]	360	0.0	0.0	0.0	0.0	0							0			I
Diet Slice, mandarin orange	0		0.0	1.0	0.0	0.0						50				
12 fl oz[16]	360	0.0	0.0	0.0	0.0	0						85	0			I
Diet Sprite	3		0.1	0.0	0.0			0				0				
8 fl oz[17]	240	0.0	0.0	0.0	0.0							67	0			I
Diet Upper 10	4		0.0	0.0	0.0							0				
12 fl oz	360	0.0	0.0	0.0	0.0	0						57	0			I
Fresca	3		0.1	0.2				0				1				
8 fl oz[17]	240	0.0	0.0	0.0	0.0							55	0			I
seltzer, flavored, Schweppes	0		0.0	0.0	0.0							15	0			
12 fl oz	360	0.0	0.0	0.0	0.0							0		.00		I
Tab	1		0.0	0.3								4				
8 fl oz[18]	240	0.0	0.0	0.0	0.0							12	30			I
vichy water, Schweppes	0		0.0	0.0	0.0							0				
12 fl oz	360	0.0	0.0	0.0	0.0							0		.00		I

1.4 CEREAL GRAIN BEVERAGES

	KCAL	H_2O (g)	PRO (g)	CHO (g)	SUGR (g)	DFIB (g)	A (RE)	C (mg)	B-2 (mg)	B-6 (mg)	FOL (mcg)	Na (mg)	Ca (mg)	Mg (mg)	Zn (mg)	Mn (mg)
	WT (g)	FAT (g)	SFA (g)	MUFA (g)	PUFA (g)	CHOL (mg)	A (IU)	B-1 (mg)	NIA (mg)	B-12 (mcg)	PANT (mg)	K (mg)	P (mg)	Fe (mg)	Cu (mg)	REF
powder	9	0.1	0.1	1.9		0.2	0	0	.00	.02	1	2	1	6	.01	.025
1 t	2.3	0.1	0.0	0.0	0.0	0	0	.01	0.4	.00	.02	42	13	.11	.005	814
powder, reg/coffee flavor, Postum	10		0.0	1.0	0.0	0.0	0	0				0	0			
1 t (amt for 8 fl oz)	3	0.0	0.0	0.0	0.0	0	0					110		.00		I
powder, Roma Kaffree	8	0.0	0.1	1.8	0.1		0					3	1		.01	
1 t	2.0	0.0	0.0	0.0	0.0	0	0					20	8	.08		I
prep from powder w/ water	9	177.7	0.2	1.8		0.0	0	0	.00	.02	1	7	5	7	.05	.027
6 fl oz water & 1 t powder	180	0.0	0.0	0.0	0.0	0	0	.01	0.4	.00	.02	43	13	.11	.016	814
prep from powder w/ whole milk	120	161.0	6.1	10.4		0.2	57	2	.30	.08	9	91	220	30	.70	.030
6 fl oz milk & 1 t powder	185	6.1	3.8	1.8	0.3	24	229	.07	0.5	.65	.57	318	183	.20	.022	814

1.5 COFFEE

	KCAL	H_2O (g)	PRO (g)	CHO (g)	SUGR (g)	DFIB (g)	A (RE)	C (mg)	B-2 (mg)	B-6 (mg)	FOL (mcg)	Na (mg)	Ca (mg)	Mg (mg)	Zn (mg)	Mn (mg)
	WT (g)	FAT (g)	SFA (g)	MUFA (g)	PUFA (g)	CHOL (mg)	A (IU)	B-1 (mg)	NIA (mg)	B-12 (mcg)	PANT (mg)	K (mg)	P (mg)	Fe (mg)	Cu (mg)	REF
brewed	4	175.8	0.2	0.7		0.0	0	0	.00	.00	0	4	4	9	.04	.048
6 fl oz	177	0.0	0.0	0.0	0.0	0	0	.00	0.4	.00	.00	96	2	.09	.012	814
ground, Folgers			0.5	0.8							0					
1 T[19]	4	0.0	0.0	0.0	0.0	0						71	7			I
iced, cappuccino, Maxwell House Cappio	130		2.0	24.0	21.0	0.0	0	0				120	0			
8 fl oz	240 ml	2.5	1.5			5	0					280		.00		I
iced, cappuccino, mocha/van, Maxwell	140		2.0	27.0	24.5	0.0	0	0				113	90			
House Cappio—8 fl oz[20]	240 ml	2.5	1.5			5	0					275		.00		I
inst powder	4	0.1	0.2	0.7		0.0	0	0	.00	.00	0	1	3	6	.01	.031
1 rd t	1.8	0.0	0.0	0.0	0.0	0	0	.00	0.5	.00	.00	64	5	.08	.003	814
Cafe Amaretto, General Foods Intl	60		8.0	5.0	0.0		0				105	0				
1 1/3 T (amt for 8 fl oz)	13	3.0	0.5			0	0					150		.00		I
Cafe Francais, General Foods Intl	60		7.0	5.0	0.0		0				25	0				
1 1/3 T (amt for 8 fl oz)	13	3.5	0.5			0	0					270		.00		I
Cafe Vienna, General Foods	70		11.0	10.0	0.0		0				110	0				
Intl—1 1/3 T (amt for 8 fl oz)	16	2.5	0.5			0	0					130		.00		I
Cafe Vienna, sugar-free, General Foods	30		3.0	0.0	0.0		0				75	0				
Intl—1 1/3 T (amt for 8 fl oz)	7	1.5	0.5			0	0					110		.00		I

	KCAL	H₂O (g)	PRO (g)	CHO (g)	SUGR (g)	DFIB (g)	A (RE)	C (mg)	B-2 (mg)	B-6 (mg)	FOL (mcg)	Na (mg)	Ca (mg)	Mg (mg)	Zn (mg)	Mn (mg)
	WT (g)	FAT (g)	SFA (g)	MUFA (g)	PUFA (g)	CHOL (mg)	A (IU)	B-1 (mg)	NIA (mg)	B-12 (mcg)	PANT (mg)	K (mg)	P (mg)	Fe (mg)	Cu (mg)	REF
cappuccino flavor, sugar sweetened	61	0.2	0.4	10.6		0.0	0	0	.01	.00	0	97	4	7	.04	.028
2 rd t	14	2.1	1.8	0.1	0.0	0	0	.02	0.3	.00	.01	116	26	.14	.015	814
decaffeinated	4	0.1	0.2	0.8		0.0	0	0	.02	.00	0	0	3	6	.00	.022
1 rd t	1.8	0.0	0.0	0.0	0.0	0	0	.00	0.5	.00	.00	63	5	.07	.001	814
Folgers	8		0.5	1.4					.05			1				
1 t	2.2	0.0	0.0	0.0	0.0	0			0.7			86	8			I
french flavor, sugar sweetened	57	0.3	0.5	6.6			0	0		.00	0	24	4	5	.01	.028
2 rd t	12	3.4	2.9	0.2	0.1	0	0	.00	0.7	.00	.00	136	41	.08	.003	814
French Van Cafe, General Foods Intl	60		10.0	8.0	0.0		0				55	0				
1 ⅓ T (amt for 8 fl oz)	14	2.5	0.5			0	0					75		.00		I
French Van Cafe, sugar-free, General	35		4.0		0.0		0				55	0				
Foods Intl—1 ⅓ T (amt for 8 fl oz)	7	2.0	0.5			0	0					70		.00		I
Hazelnut Belgian Cafe, General Foods	70		12.0	9.0	0.0		0				65	0				
Intl—1 ⅓ T (amt for 8 fl oz)	16	2.0	0.5			0	0					130		.00		I
Italian Cappuccino, General Foods Intl	50		10.0	8.0	0.0		0				50	0				
1 ⅓ T (amt for 8 fl oz)	16	1.5	0.5			0	0					85		.00		I
Kahlua Cafe, General Foods Intl	60		10.0	7.0	0.0		0				55	0				
1 ⅓ T (amt for 8 fl oz)[21]	13	2.0	0.5			0	0					80		.00		I
mocha flavor, sugar sweetened	51	0.2	0.5	8.4		0.1	0	0	.00	.00	0	31	4	8	.11	.051
2 rd t	12	1.9	1.6	0.1	0.0	0	0	.00	0.3	.00	.01	119	29	.23	.050	814
Orange Cappuccino, General Foods Intl	70		11.0	9.0	0.0		0				100	0				
1 ⅓ T (amt for 8 fl oz)	16	2.0	0.5			0	0					140		.00		I
Orange Cappuccino, sugar-free, General	30		3.0	0.0	0.0		0				75	0				
Foods Intl—1 ⅓ T (amt for 8 fl oz)	7	1.5	0.5			0	0					110		.00		I
Swiss Mocha, General Foods Intl	60		8.0	6.0	0.0		0				50	0				
1 ⅓ T (amt for 8 fl oz)	13	2.5	0.5			0	0					140		.00		I
Swiss Mocha, sugar-free, General Foods	30		4.0	0.0	0.0		0				30	0				
Intl—1 ⅓ T (amt for 8 fl oz)	7	2.0	0.5			0	0					105		.00		I
Viennese Choc Cafe, General Foods Intl	60		10.0	9.0	0.0		0				30	0				
1 ⅓ T (amt for 8 fl oz)	13	2.0	1.0			0	0					75		.00		I
w/ chicory	6	0.1	0.2	1.3		0.0	0	0	.01	.00	0	5	2	4	.01	.022
1 rd t	1.8	0.0	0.0	0.0	0.0	0	0	.00	0.4	.00	.00	61	5	.09	.001	814
prep from inst powder	4	177.2	0.2	0.7		0.0	0	0	.00	.00	0	5	5	7	.05	.032
6 fl oz water & 1 rd t powder	179	0.0	0.0	0.0	0.0	0	0	.00	0.5	.00	.00	64	5	.09	.013	814
cappuccino flavor, sugar sweetened	61	177.8	0.4	10.8		0.0	0	0	.01	.00	0	104	8	10	.08	.029
6 fl oz water & 2 rd t powder	192	2.1	1.8	0.1	0.0	0	0	.02	0.3	.00	.01	119	27	.15	.027	814
Cappuccino, plain/flavored, Maxwell	93		1.5	17.5	16.8	0.0	0	0				68	60			
House Cappio—1 pkt in 8 fl oz water[22]	229	1.5	0.3			0	0					149		.00		I
decaffeinated	4	177.2	0.2	0.7		0.0	0	0	.03	.00	0	5	5	7	.05	.023
6 fl oz water & 1 rd t powder	179	0.0	0.0	0.0	0.0	0	0	.00	0.5	.00	.00	63	5	.07	.013	814
french flavor, sugar sweetened	57	177.7	0.6	6.6		0.0	0	0	.00	.00	0	30	8	2	.04	.000
6 fl oz water & 2 rd t powder	189	3.4	2.9	0.2	0.1	0	0	.00	0.7	.00	.00	136	42	.02	.011	814
mocha flavor, sugar sweetened	51	176.7	0.6	8.5	4.9	0.2	0	0	.00	.00	0	36	8	9	.15	.053
6 fl oz water & 2 rd t powder	188	1.9	1.6	0.1	0.0	0	0	.00	0.3	.00	.01	118	28	.24	.060	814
w/ chicory	7	177.2	0.2	1.3		0.0	0	0	.01	.00	0	11	5	5	.05	.023
6 fl oz water & 1 rd t powder	179	0.0	0.0	0.0	0.0	0	0	.00	0.4	.00	.00	61	5	.09	.013	814

1.6 JUICE DRINKS & FRUIT FLAVORED BEVERAGES

	KCAL	H₂O (g)	PRO (g)	CHO (g)	SUGR (g)	DFIB (g)	A (RE)	C (mg)	B-2 (mg)	B-6 (mg)	FOL (mcg)	Na (mg)	Ca (mg)	Mg (mg)	Zn (mg)	Mn (mg)
apple cider mix, sugar-free, Swiss Miss	14		0.0	3.4	0.4	0.0		81				78	5			
amt for 8 fl oz	4	0.0	0.0	0.0	0.0	0								.05		I
apple cider mix, Swiss Miss	84		0.0	20.3	18.5	0.9		65				58	3			
amt for 8 fl oz	22	0.3	0.0			0								.05		I
apple cranberry drink, cnd, Motts	170		0.0	40.0	37.0							0				
2 fl oz	60	0.0	0.0	0.0								65				I
apple raspberry drink, cnd, Mott's	130		0.0	31.0	29.0							0				
2 fl oz	60	0.0	0.0	0.0								75				I
Capri Sun jce drink	103		0.0	27.2	27.2	0.0	0	0				20	0			
6.75 fl oz[23]	200 ml	0.0	0.0	0.0	0.0	0	0					30				I
citrus fruit jce drink, from frzn conc	114	217.7	0.7	28.5		0.0	10	67	.03	.06	5	7	22	15	.12	.181
8 fl oz	248	0.0	0.0	0.0	0.0	0	104	.03	0.4	.00	.33	278	25	2.78	.079	814
cranapple drink, Ocean Spray	130		0.0	32.0				60				4	13	4	.07	
6 fl oz	190	0.0	0.0	0.0	0.0							51	5	.10	.014	I

	KCAL / WT (g)	H₂O (g) / FAT (g)	PRO (g) / SFA (g)	CHO (g) / MUFA (g)	SUGR (g) / PUFA (g)	DFIB (g) / CHOL (mg)	A (RE) / A (IU)	C (mg) / B-1 (mg)	B-2 (mg) / NIA (mg)	B-6 (mg) / B-12 (mcg)	FOL (mcg) / PANT (mg)	Na (mg) / K (mg)	Ca (mg) / P (mg)	Mg (mg) / Fe (mg)	Zn (mg) / Cu (mg)	Mn (mg) / REF
cranberry-apple jce drink, bottled	123	152.4	0.2	31.5		0.2	0	59	.04	.04	0	4	13	4	.07	.331
6 fl oz	184	0.0	0.0	0.0	0.0	0	6	.01	0.1	.00	.10	50	6	.11	.013	814
cranberry-apricot jce drink, bottled	118	153.6	0.4	29.8		0.2	85	0	.02	.04	1	4	17	6	.07	.230
6 fl oz	184	0.0	0.0	0.0	0.0	0	852	.01	0.2	.00	.07	112	9	.28	.028	814
cranberry-grape jce drink, bottled	103	157.5	0.4	25.8		0.2	0	59	.03	.05	1	6	15	6	.07	.291
6 fl oz	184	0.2	0.1	0.0	0.0	0	9	.02	0.2	.00	.10	44	7	.02	.013	814
cranberry jce cocktail																
bottled	108	162.4	0.0	27.4		0.2	0	67	.02	.04	0	4	6	4	.13	.367
6 fl oz	190	0.2	0.0	0.0	0.1	0	8	.02	0.1	.00	.11	34	4	.28	.034	814
from frzn conc	103	160.6	0.0	26.2		0.2	2	19	.02	.03	0	6	9	4	.07	.077
6 fl oz	187	0.0	0.0	0.0	0.0	0	19	.01	0.0	.00	.26	26	2	.17	.019	814
low cal, bottled	34	169.5	0.0	8.4		0.0	0	57	.02	.03	0	5	16	4	.04	.304
6 fl oz[24]	178	0.0	0.0	0.0	0.0	0	7	.02	0.1	.00	.10	39	2	.07	.025	814
crangrape drink, Ocean Spray	110		0.0	26.0				60	.03			7	7	4		
6 fl oz	190	0.0	0.0	0.0	0.0			.02	0.2			37	7	.25	.022	I
cranraspberry drink, Ocean Spray	110		0.0	27.0				60				6				
6 fl oz	190	0.0	0.0	0.0								35				I
Crystal Light, low cal mix	5		0.0	0.0	0.0		0	6				0	0			
⅛ tub (amt for 8 fl oz)[25]	1.4	0.0	0.0	0.0	0.0	0	0					28		.00		I
fruit punch, cnd, Mott's In-A-Minute	140		0.0	34.0	32.0							0				
2 fl oz	60	0.0	0.0	0.0	0.0							90				I
fruit punch, cnd, Sunkist	180		0.0	49.0	49.0							35	0			
12 fl oz	360	0.0	0.0	0.0	0.0									.00		I
fruit punch drink																
cnd	87	163.7	0.0	22.1	21.0	0.2	2	55	.04	.00	2	41	15	4	.22	.372
6 fl oz	186	0.0	0.0	0.0	0.0	0	26	.04	0.0	.00	.03	47	2	.39	.095	814
from frzn conc	114	217.9	0.0	28.9		0.2	2	108	.03	.01	2	10	10	5	.10	.252
8 fl oz	247	0.0	0.0	0.0	0.0	0	27	.02	0.1	.00	.02	32	2	.22	.074	814
from powder	97	236.8	0.0	24.9	30.4	0.0	0	31	.01	.00	0	37	42	3	.08	.008
2 rd t in 8 fl oz water	262	0.0	0.0	0.0	0.0	0	0	.00	0.0	.00	.00	3	52	.13	.047	814
fruit punch jce drink, from frzn conc	124	216.5	0.2	30.3		0.2	2	14	.16	.03	0	12	17	10	.55	.149
8 fl oz	248	0.5	0.1	0.1	0.1	0	15	.00	0.1	.00	.07	191	0	.57	.060	814
grape apple drink, cnd, Mott's	140		0.0	34.0	33.0							0				
2 fl oz	60	0.0	0.0	0.0	0.0							105				I
grape drink, cnd	85	166.2	0.0	21.6		0.0	0	64	.01	.01	1	11	6	4	.21	.068
6 fl oz	188	0.0	0.0	0.0	0.0	0	2	.01	0.0	.00	.01	9	2	.32	.023	814
grape jce drink, cnd	94	163.6	0.2	24.3		0.2	0	30	.02	.04	2	2	6	8	.06	.203
6 fl oz	188	0.0	0.0	0.0	0.0	0	4	.02	0.2	.00	.02	66	8	.19	.026	814
Hawaiian Punch																
Fruit Juicy Red	120		0.0	30.0	30.0	0.0	0	60	.00			160	0			
8 fl oz	240	0.0	0.0	0.0	0.0	0	0	.00	0.0			50	110	.00		I
Fruit Juicy Red, no sugar added	15		0.0	4.0	4.0	0.0	0	60	.00			170				
8 fl oz	240	0.0	0.0	0.0	0.0	0	0	.00	0.0			50		.00		I
Typhoon Blastus	123		0.0	30.8	29.5	0.0	0	60				100	0			
8 fl oz[26]	240	0.0	0.0	0.0	0.0	0	0					44	110	.00		I
Kool-Aid																
Bursts	100		0.2	24.3	24.3	0.0	0	0				31	0			
6.75 fl oz[27]	200 ml	0.0	0.0	0.0	0.0	0						15		.00		I
mix prep w/ sugar & water	100		0.0	25.0	25.0	0.0	0	6				18	0			
8 fl oz[28]	240	0.0	0.0	0.0	0.0	0						0		.00		I
mix, sugar-free	5		0.0	0.0	0.0	0.0	0	6				2	0			
⅛ pkg (amt for 8 fl oz)[29]	1.2	0.0	0.0	0.0	0.0	0	0					0		.00		I
mix, sweetened	60		0.0	16.2	16.2	0.0	0	6				0	0			
⅛ pkg (amt for 8 fl oz)[30]	17	0.0	0.0	0.0	0.0	0	0					0		.00		I
lemonade																
flavored drink, from powder	112	237.0	0.0	28.7		0.0	0	34	.00	.00	0	19	29	3	.08	.000
2 T mix in 8 fl oz water	266	0.0	0.0	0.0	0.0	0	0	.00	0.0	.00	.00	3	3	.05	.027	814

Columns are paired per item: the first line gives the top label, the second line (serving row) gives the lower label. Vitamins group = A, C, B-2, B-6, FOL. Minerals group = Na, Ca, Mg, Zn, Mn.

Item	KCAL / WT (g)	H_2O (g) / FAT (g)	PRO (g) / SFA (g)	CHO (g) / MUFA (g)	SUGR (g) / PUFA (g)	DFIB (g) / CHOL (mg)	A (RE) / A (IU)	C (mg) / B-1 (mg)	B-2 (mg) / NIA (mg)	B-6 (mg) / B-12 (mcg)	FOL (mcg) / PANT (mg)	Na (mg) / K (mg)	Ca (mg) / P (mg)	Mg (mg) / Fe (mg)	Zn (mg) / Cu (mg)	Mn (mg) / REF
from frzn conc	96	214.3	0.2	25.2	22.1	0.2	5	9	.05	.01	5	7	7	5	.10	.012
8 fl oz	240	0.0	0.0	0.0	0.0	0	50	.01	0.0	.00	.03	36	5	.38	.043	814
from mix	103	236.8	0.0	26.9	14.5	0.0	0	8	.00	.01	3	13	71	3	.11	.000
8 fl oz	264	0.0	0.0	0.0	0.0	0	0	.01	0.0	.00	.02	34	34	.16	.021	814
from mix, aspartame sweetened	5	236.3	0.0	1.2		0.0	0	6	.00	.00	0	7	50	2	.07	.002
8 fl oz	238	0.0	0.0	0.0	0.0	0	0	.00	0.0	.00	.00	0	24	.10	.017	814
from mix, sugar-free, Country Time	5		0.0	0.0	0.0		0	6				0	0			
8 fl oz[31]	239	0.0	0.0	0.0	0.0		0					40		.00		I
from mix, Wyler's	78		0.0	19.4				19	.00			39	0		.00	
8 fl oz	240	0.0	0.0	0.0	0.0		0	.00	0.0				0	.00	.000	I
mix, sweetened, Country Time	70		0.0	16.7	16.7	0.0	0	6				13	0			
amt for 8 fl oz[32]	18	0.0	0.0	0.0	0.0	0	0					3		.00		I
limeade, from frzn conc, prep w/ water	101	219.6	0.0	27.2		0.2	0	7	.00	.00	2	5	7	2	.05	.000
8 fl oz	247	0.0	0.0	0.0	0.0	0	0	.00	0.1	.00	.05	32	2	.07	.012	814
orange & apricot jce drink, cnd	128	216.8	0.8	31.8		0.3	145	50	.03	.07	15	5	13	10	.13	.010
8 fl oz	250	0.3	0.0	0.1	0.1	0	1450	.05	0.5	.00	.19	200	20	.25	.088	814
orange breakfast drink, from frzn conc	85	165.6	0.2	21.2		0.0	2	104	1.96	.13	61	19	220	21	.09	.026
6 fl oz	188	0.0	0.0	0.0	0.0	0	11	.20	0.5	.00	.36	254	62	.15	.182	814
orange breakfast drink, from powder	86	163.9	0.0	21.9		0.0	413	91	.03	.00	107	9	47	2	.07	.011
3 rd t in 6 fl oz water	186	0.0	0.0	0.0	0.0	0	1376	.00	0.0	.00	.00	37	28	.15	.028	814
orange drink, cnd	95	161.6	0.0	24.0	13.4	0.2	4	63	.01	.02	4	30	11	4	.17	.028
6 fl oz	186	0.0	0.0	0.0	0.0	0	33	.01	0.1	.00	.03	33	2	.52	.006	814
orange gelatin drink, from powder	67	119.0	6.1	10.5		0.0	0	50	.00	.00	0	33	3	1	.03	.000
1 pkt in 4 fl oz water	136	0.3	0.0	0.1	0.1	0	0	.00	0.0	.00	.00	3	0	.00	.007	814
orange gelatin drink powder w/ nutra-sweet, Knox—0.37 oz pkt	39		5.7	4.0				113	.00			17	0			
	10	0.1				0	0	.00	0.0			0	0	.00	.000	I
orange juice beverage, Citrus Hill Lite Premium—6 fl oz	60		0.0	14.0				72	.07	.12	40	10	40	24		
	180	0.0	0.0	0.0	0.0			.12	0.8		.40	210	45		.080	I
pineapple & grapefruit jce drink, cnd	118	219.8	0.5	29.0		0.3	10	115	.04	.11	26	35	18	15	.15	1.032
8 fl oz	250	0.3	0.0	0.0	0.1	0	88	.07	0.7	.00	.13	153	15	.78	.112	814
pineapple & orange jce drink, cnd	125	217.3	3.3	29.5		0.3	133	56	.05	.12	27	8	13	15	.15	.902
8 fl oz	250	0.0	0.0	0.0		0	1328	.07	0.5	.00	.14	115	10	.68	.103	814
pink grapefruit jce cocktail, Ocean Spray	80		0.0	20.0				100				15	14	8	.11	
6 fl oz	180	0.0	0.0	0.0	0.0							125	16	.24	.060	I
Sun Sip Punch	90		0.0	23.0		0.0		60				35				
6 fl oz[33]	180	0.0	0.0	0.0	0.0	0	1000	.30					0			I
Sunny Delight Citrus Punch	125		0.0	31.5	29.0	0.0		60				160				
8 fl oz[34]	240	0.0	0.0	0.0	0.0	0	1000	.23				42	70			I
Tang mix, orange/mango	100		0.0	24.5	24.5			60	.17	.20	80	0	60			
2 T (amt for 8 fl oz)[35]	26	0.0	0.0	0.0	0.0	0	500		2.0			25		.00		I
Tang mix, orange, sugar-free	5		0.0	0.0	0.0			60	.17	.20	80	65	0			
amt for 8 fl oz	2.5	0.0	0.0	0.0	0.0	0	500		2.0			1		.00		I
Thirst Quencher, bottled	60	225.3	0.0	15.2	14.2	0.0	0	0	.00	.00	0	96	0	2	.05	.000
8 fl oz	241	0.0	0.0	0.0	0.0	0	0	.01	0.0	.00	.00	27	22	.12	.048	814
tropical punch, from powder, Wyler's	85		0.0	21.1				17	.00			18	0			
8 fl oz	240	0.1					0	.00	0.0						.00	I
wild strawberry, from powder, Wyler's	85		0.0	20.7				0	.00			43	0	0	.00	.000
8 fl oz	240	0.3					0	.00	0.0			0	0	.00	.000	I

1.7 TEA, HOT/ICED

brewed

Item	KCAL / WT (g)	H_2O (g) / FAT (g)	PRO (g) / SFA (g)	CHO (g) / MUFA (g)	SUGR (g) / PUFA (g)	DFIB (g) / CHOL (mg)	A (RE) / A (IU)	C (mg) / B-1 (mg)	B-2 (mg) / NIA (mg)	B-6 (mg) / B-12 (mcg)	FOL (mcg) / PANT (mg)	Na (mg) / K (mg)	Ca (mg) / P (mg)	Mg (mg) / Fe (mg)	Zn (mg) / Cu (mg)	Mn (mg) / REF
black, 3 min	2	177.5	0.0	0.5		0.0	0	0	.02	.00	9	5	0	5	.04	.390
6 fl oz	178	0.0	0.0	0.0	0.0	0	0	.00	0.0	.00	.02	66	2	.04	.018	814
black, Lipton	0		0.0	0.0	0.0	0.0	0	0				0				
1 tea bag[36]	2.0	0.0	0.0	0.0	0.0	0	0							.00		I
green w/ passion fruit, Lipton	80		0.0	19.0	19.0	0.0						5				
8 fl oz	240 ml	0.0	0.0	0.0	0.0											I
herb	2	177.5	0.0	0.4	0.0	0.0	0	0	.01	.00	1	2	4	2	.07	.078
6 fl oz	178	0.0	0.0	0.0	0.0	0	0	.02	0.0	.00	.02	16	0	.14	.027	814

	KCAL / WT (g)	H₂O (g) / FAT (g)	PRO (g) / SFA (g)	CHO (g) / MUFA (g)	SUGR (g) / PUFA (g)	DFIB (g) / CHOL (mg)	A (RE) / A (IU)	C (mg) / B-1 (mg)	B-2 (mg) / NIA (mg)	B-6 (mg) / B-12 (mcg)	FOL (mcg) / PANT (mg)	Na (mg) / K (mg)	Ca (mg) / P (mg)	Mg (mg) / Fe (mg)	Zn (mg) / Cu (mg)	Mn (mg) / REF
iced																
diet lemon/diet peach, Lipton	0		0.0	0.0	0.0	0.0						5				
8 fl oz	250	0.0	0.0	0.0	0.0	0										I
lemonade/peach/raspberry flavors,	110		0.0	26.0	26.0	0.0						5				
Lipton—8 fl oz	250	0.0	0.0	0.0	0.0	0										I
w/ sugar & lemon, Lipton	100		0.0	25.0	25.0	0.0		60	.00			10	0	0	.00	.000
8.45 fl oz	250						0	.00	0.0			0	0	.00	.000	I
iced, inst powder	2	0.0	0.1	0.4		0.0	0	0	.00	.01	1	1	0	3	.02	.518
1 t	0.7	0.0	0.0	0.0	0.0	0	0	.00	0.1	.00	.03	46	3	.03	.006	814
Lipton	0		0.0				0	.00				0	0		.00	
1 t (amt for 8 fl oz)	0.7	0.0	0.0	0.0	0.0		0	.00	0.0					.00		I
sweetened, Crystal Light	70		0.0	17.0	17.0	0.0	0	6				0	0			
amt for 8 fl oz	18	0.0	0.0	0.0	0.0	0	0					10		.00		I
w/ lemon flavor	4	0.1	0.1	1.1		0.0	0	0	.02	.01	1	7	0	2	.02	.429
1 rd t	1.4	0.0	0.0	0.0	0.0	0	0	.00	0.1	.00	.03	48	1	.01	.005	814
w/ lemon flavor, Lipton	0		0.0				0	.00							.00	
amt for 8 fl oz	1.3	0.0	0.0	0.0	0.0	0	0	.00						.00		I
w/ nutrasweet, Lipton	5		0.0	1.0			0	.00							.00	
1 T (amt for 8 fl oz)	2.0	0.0	0.0	0.0	0.0	0	0	.00	0.0					.00		I
w/ sodium saccharin & lemon flavor	5	0.1	0.1	1.3		0.0	0	0	.01	.00	5	17	0	2	.01	.486
2 t	1.6	0.0	0.0	0.0	0.0	0	0	.00	0.1	.00	.02	41	2	.14	.002	814
w/ sugar & lemon flavor	89	0.1	0.1	22.4		0.0	0	0	.05	.01	10	1	1	3	.02	.682
3 rd t	23	0.1	0.0	0.0	0.0	0	0	.00	0.1	.00	.03	50	3	.04	.006	814
w/ sugar & lemon, Lipton	90		0.0	22.0	22.0	0.0	0	.00				0			.00	
amt for 8 fl oz	23	0.0	0.0	0.0	0.0	0	0	.00	0.0					.00		I
prep from inst powder	2	236.3	0.0	0.5		0.0	0	0	.00	.00	1	7	5	5	.07	.519
1 t powder in 8 fl oz water	237	0.0	0.0	0.0	0.0	0	0	.00	0.1	.00	.03	47	2	.05	.019	814
w/ lemon flavor	5	236.6	0.0	1.0		0.0	0	0	.02	.00	1	14	5	5	.07	.431
1 rd t powder in 8 fl oz water	238	0.0	0.0	0.0	0.0	0	0	.00	0.1	.00	.03	50	2	.02	.019	814
w/ sodium saccharin & lemon flavor	5	236.3	0.0	1.2		0.0	0	0	.01	.00	5	24	5	5	.07	.488
2 t powder in 8 fl oz water	238	0.0	0.0	0.0	0.0	0	0	.00	0.1	.00	.02	40	2	.14	.017	814
w/ sugar & lemon flavor	88	236.2	0.3	22.0		0.0	0	0	.05	.01	10	8	5	5	.08	.673
3 rd t powder in 8 fl oz water	259	0.0	0.0	0.0	0.0	0	0	.00	0.1	.00	.03	49	3	.05	.021	814

1.8 WATER

	KCAL / WT (g)	H₂O (g) / FAT (g)	PRO (g) / SFA (g)	CHO (g) / MUFA (g)	SUGR (g) / PUFA (g)	DFIB (g) / CHOL (mg)	A (RE) / A (IU)	C (mg) / B-1 (mg)	B-2 (mg) / NIA (mg)	B-6 (mg) / B-12 (mcg)	FOL (mcg) / PANT (mg)	Na (mg) / K (mg)	Ca (mg) / P (mg)	Mg (mg) / Fe (mg)	Zn (mg) / Cu (mg)	Mn (mg) / REF
bottled, Perrier	0	191.8	0.0	0.0	0.0	0.0	0	0	.00	.00	0	2	27	0	.00	.000
6.5 fl oz	192	0.0	0.0	0.0	0.0	0	0	.00	0.0	.00	.00	0	0	.00	.000	814
bottled, Poland Spring	0	237.0	0.0	0.0	0.0	0.0	0	0	.00	.00	0	2	2	2	.00	.000
8 fl oz	237	0.0	0.0	0.0	0.0	0	0	.00	0.0	.00	.00	0	0	.02	.000	814
municipal tap	0	236.8	0.0	0.0	0.0	0.0	0	0	.00	.00	0	7	5	2	.07	.002
8 fl oz	237	0.0	0.0	0.0	0.0	0	0	.00	0.0	.00	.00	0	0	.02	.014	814

1. Values are averages for blue ice, cherry slam, fruit punch, grape, lemon lime, and orange.
2. Values are averages for kiwi-strawberry, lemon, lemon-lime, lime-lemon, mango melon, passion plum, peach, pina colada, pineapple, strawberry, and watermelon.
3. Values are averages for berry, black cherry, fruit punch, grape, grapefruit, lemonade, peach, pineapple, raspberry, and strawberry.
4. Values are averages for blue raspberry, green apple, red cherry, and yellow lemon.
5. Values are averages for cherry lime, fruit punch, grape, lemon lime, mandarin orange, pineapple, and strawberry.
6. The sodium free product contains 0 mg sodium and 25 mg potassium.
7. Contains 125 mg aspartame.
8. Contains 178 mg aspartame.
9. Contains 126 mg aspartame.
10. Contains 150 mg aspartame.
11. Contains 177 mg aspartame.
12. This product is available with caffeine (48 mg caffeine/12 fl oz) and caffeine-free (0 mg caffeine/12 fl oz).
13. Values are averages for cranberry, cranberry apple, golden peach, fruit punch, key lime, kiwi strawberry, lemonade, lemon-lime, mango melon, passion plum, pink grapefruit, red raspberry, tangerine, and white grape.
14. Contains 189 mg aspartame.
15. Contains 186 mg aspartame.
16. Contains 240 mg aspartame.
17. Contains 118 mg aspartame.
18. Contains 19 mg aspartame.
19. Values for decaffeinated product are approximately the same, except that the caffeine is 1 mg instead of 59 mg.
20. Values are averages for mocha and vanilla flavored products.
21. Contains Kahlua coffee liqueur without alcohol.
22. Values are averages for cinnamon, mocha, plain, and vanilla.
23. Values are averages for all 12 flavors of product.
24. Sweetened with calcium saccharin and corn sweeteners.

25. Values are averages for citrus blend, cranberry breeze, decaffeinated iced tea, fruit punch, iced tea, lemon lime, lemonade, pink grapefruit, and raspberry ice.
26. Values are averages for megamonsoon grape, stormin tropical strawberry, tidal wave tropical fruit, and surquake orange,
27. Values are averages for all 8 flavors of product.
28. Values are averages for all 16 flavors. Made with ⅛ pkg (0.5g) of unsweetened mix.
29. Values are averages for all 9 flavors of product.
30. Values are averages for all 13 flavors of product.

31. Includes lemonade and pink lemonade sugar-free mixes.
32. Values are averages for lemonade, lemonade punch, and pink lemonade.
33. Values are averages for cranberry citrus, concord grape, pineapple orange, and red berry fruit.
34. Values are averages for California and Florida styles.
35. Values are averages for orange and mango.
36. Values apply to regular tea, decaffeinated tea, English tea, green tea, herbal teas, flavored teas, and jasmine tea.

	KCAL	H₂O (g)	PRO (g)	CHO (g)	SUGR (g)	DFIB (g)	A (RE)	C (mg)	B-2 (mg)	B-6 (mg)	FOL (mcg)	Na (mg)	Ca (mg)	Mg (mg)	Zn (mg)	Mn (mg)
	WT (g)	FAT (g)	SFA (g)	MUFA (g)	PUFA (g)	CHOL (mg)	A (IU)	B-1 (mg)	NIA (mg)	B-12 (mcg)	PANT (mg)	K (mg)	P (mg)	Fe (mg)	Cu (mg)	REF

2. CANDY & GUM

After Eight Mints	29	0.5	0.2	6.1		0.2	0	0	.00	.00	0	1	2	4	.05	.017
2 mints	8	1.1	0.7	0.4	0.0	0	2	.00	0.0	.00	.00	13	5	.12	.020	819
Almond Joy	241	3.8	2.1	28.6	22.3	2.3	0	0	.07	.03	4	72	30	32	.39	.279
1.7 oz bar	49	13.1	8.5	2.6	1.2	2	0	.02	0.2	.06	.12	120	69	.66	.137	MUL
Alpine White w/ Almonds	349	0.7	6.2	31.2		3.3	16	0	.26			45	143			
2.2 oz bar	62	22.9	11.8	8.5	1.6	8	52	.05	0.1			259		.35		819
Baby Ruth	289	2.9	4.5	39.1		1.7	0	0	.06	.04	19	136	25	48	.78	.451
2.1 oz bar	60	12.7	7.4	3.9	2.0	2	0	.06	1.7	.03	.20	238	91	.13	.297	819
Bar None	224	1.7	3.5	22.4		1.4	10	0	.12	.03	12	45	62	31	.53	.215
1.5 oz bar	43	14.6	9.4	3.4	0.9	7	57	.03	0.7	.18	.24	168	86	.52	.112	I
Bit-O-Honey	186	3.4	1.4	38.9	23.1		0	0	.12			124	27			
1.7 oz bar	48	3.8					0	.00	0.0			60		.14		819
Bounty, dark choc	139		0.9	17.3				0	.01			22	5			
1 oz	28	7.4					7	.01	0.1					.49		I
Bounty, milk choc	139		1.1	17.2				0	.03			29	20			
1 oz bar	28	7.3					22	.01	0.1					.30		I
Breathsavers sugar free mints	10		0.0	2.0	0.0							0				
1 mint[1]	2.0	0.0	0.0	0.0	0.0	0										I
butter mints, Kraft	60		0.0	14.0	14.0	0.0	0	0				25	0			
7 pieces	15	0.0	0.0	0.0	0.0	0	0					0		.00		I
Butterfinger	293	1.3	7.6	40.0		1.5	0	0	.04	.04	16	121	16	48	.70	.438
2.16 oz bar	61	11.4	6.3	3.3	1.7	1	0	.05	1.5	.01	.16	230	79	.45	.291	819
butterscotch	112	0.2	0.0	27.0		0.0	10	0	.01	.00	0	12	1	0	.01	.010
1 oz (5 pieces)	28	1.0	0.3	0.1	0.0	3	39	.00	0.0	.00	.00	1	1	.02	.010	819
butterscotch chips, Hershey	82		0.6	9.7	9.2	0.1	0	0				12	20			
1 T	15	4.5	4.0			1	0							.00		I
butterscotch morsels, Nestle	80		0.0	9.0	9.0	0.0	0	0				15	0			
1 T	14	4.0	3.5			0	0							.00		I
candied fruit																
cherries	96	3.4	0.1	24.6												
1 oz (8 cherries)	28	0.1														456
citron	89	5.0	0.1	22.7								82	24			
1 oz	28	0.1										34	7	.20		456
figs	84	5.9	1.0	20.6												
1 oz	28	0.1														456
grapefruit peel	90	4.9	0.1	22.9												
1 oz	28	0.1														456
lemon peel	90	4.9	0.1	22.9												
1 oz	28	0.1														456
orange peel	90	4.9	0.1	22.9												
1 oz	28	0.1														456
pear	85	5.9	0.4	21.3												
1 oz	28	0.2														456
pineapple	90	5.0	0.2	22.7												
1 oz	28	0.1														456

| | KCAL | H₂O (g) | PRO (g) | CHO (g) | SUGR (g) | DFIB (g) | Vitamins A (RE) | C (mg) | B-2 (mg) | B-6 (mg) | FOL (mcg) | Minerals Na (mg) | Ca (mg) | Mg (mg) | Zn (mg) | Mn (mg) |
	WT (g)	FAT (g)	SFA (g)	MUFA (g)	PUFA (g)	CHOL (mg)	A (IU)	B-1 (mg)	NIA (mg)	B-12 (mcg)	PANT (mg)	K (mg)	P (mg)	Fe (mg)	Cu (mg)	REF
candy corn	182	3.8	0.1	44.8				0	.00			106	7			
¼ cup	50	1.0	0.3	0.5			0	.00	0.0			2	3	.55		456
caramel, choc flavored roll	230	4.7	1.2	55.9		0.5	1	0	.04	.01	1	17	15	20	.34	.068
2.25 oz bar	64	1.6	0.4	0.7	0.5	0	5	.01	0.0	.04	.09	65	25	.26	.186	819
Caramello, Cadburry's	214	0.4	2.8	28.6	21.6	0.7	0	0	.18	.02	3	62	83	19	.43	.068
1.6 oz bar	45	9.8	6.3			12	0	.02	0.5	.28	.22	147	72	.32	.080	MUL
caramels	271	6.0	3.3	54.7		0.9	6	0	.13	.02	4	174	98	12	.31	.008
2.5 oz (6 pieces)	71	5.8	4.7	0.6	0.1	5	23	.01	0.2	.00	.42	152	81	.10	.013	819
caramels, Kraft	170		2.0	32.0	27.0	0.0	0	0				110	80			
5 pieces	41	3.0	1.0			5	0					120		.00		I
carob	470	1.3	7.1	49.0		3.3	7	0	.15	.11	24	93	264	31	3.07	.122
3 oz bar	87	27.3	25.2	0.4	0.3	3	21	.09	0.9	.87	.65	551	110	1.12	.159	819
Cherry Nibs, Y&S	106	0.3	0.8	26.2		0.0	1	0	.01	.00	0	67	18	2	.05	.043
1 oz	28	0.7				0	6	.01	0.0	.00	.00	18	88	.17	.258	I
Chews, all flavors, Lance	117	1.4	0.0	28.0												
1.1 oz	30	0.6	0.6	0.0	0.0	0										I
choc baking chips, red fat, Hershey's	63		0.6	10.7	9.4	0.7	0	0				0	4			
Bake Shoppe—1 T²	15	3.5	3.4			0	0					47		.33		I
choc, Bittersweet, Hershey	77		0.9	8.2		1.0	0	0				1	6			
½ bar (.5 oz)	14	4.5	2.8			1	0					61		.50		I
choc chips, semi-sweet	1351	1.8	11.9	178.1	90.7	16.6	3	0	.25	.00	7	32	91	324	4.57	2.258
1 cup (6 oz pkg)	168	84.7	50.1	28.1	2.7	0	59	.15	1.2	.10	.30	1032	371	8.84	1.976	819
Bakers	60		1.0	9.0	8.0	0	0				0	0				
½ oz (27 chips)	14	3.5	2.0			0	0					60		.36		I
Hershey	80		0.7	9.6	7.8	0.8	0	0				2	5			
1 T	15	4.3	2.7			1	0							.38		I
mint, Nestle	70		0.0	9.0	7.0	2.0	0	0				0	0			
1 T	14	4.0	2.0			0	0							.00		I
Nestle	70		0.4	9.0	7.7	1.2	0	0				0	0			
1 T³	14	4.0	2.3			0	0							.00		I
choc chunks, semi-sweet, Hershey	76		0.7	8.9	8.4	0.2	0	0				2	4			
6 pieces	14	4.2	2.6			1	0							.30		I
choc coated																
almonds	161	0.6	3.5	11.2				0	.15			17	58			
1 oz (6-8 almonds)	28	12.4	2.1	8.2			0	.03	0.5			155	97	.80		456
choc fudge	122	1.7	1.1	20.7				0	.04			65	29			
1 oz	28	4.5	1.5	2.5			0	.01	0.1			55	31	.40		456
choc fudge w/ nuts	128	1.7	1.4	19.1				0	.04			58	29			
1 oz	28	5.9	1.5	2.6			0	.02	0.1			62	39	.40		456
coconut	124	1.8	0.8	20.4				0	.02			56	14			
1 oz	28	5.0	2.9	1.9	0.0		0	.01	0.1			47	22	.30		456
fondant	128	2.7	0.8	28.1		0.4	1	0	.02	.00	0	9	6	22	.16	.140
1 large patty (1.23 oz)	35	3.3	1.9	1.1	0.1	0	7	.01	0.2	.00	.02	59	33	.55	.150	819
mint	45	0.6	0.2	8.9				0	.01			20	6			
1 small	11	1.2	0.4	0.7			0	.00	0.0			10	6	.10		456
peanuts	208	0.8	5.2	19.8		1.7	0	0	.07	.08	3	16	42	36	.75	.332
10 pieces	40	13.4	5.8	5.2	1.7	4	0	.05	1.7	.18	.23	201	85	.52	.234	819
peanuts, Goobers	200	0.7	5.3	19.0		2.4	0	0	.08	.08	3	16	50	46	.85	.324
1.38 oz pkg	39	13.1	4.8	5.7	2.0	4	0	.05	2.0	.11	.22	196	115	.52	.316	819
raisins	39	1.1	0.4	6.8		0.4	1	0	.02	.01	1	4	9	5	.08	.029
10 pieces	10	1.5	0.9	0.5	0.1	0	4	.01	0.0	.02	.03	51	14	.17	.034	819
raisins, Raisinets	185	2.9	2.1	32.0		2.3	4	0	.10	.05	2	16	49	20	.36	.132
1.58 oz pkg	45	7.2	3.3	2.7	0.9	2	17	.04	0.2	.09	.13	231	65	.54	.154	819
van creams	123	2.1	1.1	19.9				0	.02			52	36			
1 oz	28	4.8	1.4	2.8			0	.01	0.0			50	31	.20		456
Choc Crisps, Planters	140		2.0	21.0	13.0						30					
13 pieces	30	7.0	2.0	2.5	0.5	0										I
choc disks, sugar-coated	132	0.3	1.5	20.6				0	.06			20	38			
1 oz	28	5.6	3.1	2.0			30	.02	0.1			71	40	.40		456
choc flavored chips, semi-sweet, Bakers	70		0.0	10.0	9.0	0	0				10	0				
½ oz (27 chips)	14	3.0	3.0			0	0					70		.36		I

	KCAL	H₂O (g)	PRO (g)	CHO (g)	SUGR (g)	DFIB (g)	A (RE)	C (mg)	B-2 (mg)	B-6 (mg)	FOL (mcg)	Na (mg)	Ca (mg)	Mg (mg)	Zn (mg)	Mn (mg)
	WT (g)	FAT (g)	SFA (g)	MUFA (g)	PUFA (g)	CHOL (mg)	A (IU)	B-1 (mg)	NIA (mg)	B-12 (mcg)	PANT (mg)	K (mg)	P (mg)	Fe (mg)	Cu (mg)	REF
choc, semi-sweet	228	0.3	2.0	30.1	15.3	2.8	1	0	.04	.00	1	5	15	55	.77	.381
1 oz	28	14.3	8.5	4.7	0.5	0	10	.03	0.2	.02	.05	174	63	1.49	.333	819
Bakers	130		2.0	17.0	13.0	2.0	0	0				0	0			
1 oz square	28	9.0	5.0			0	0					140		1.44		I
coated raisins, Nestle	70		0.6	11.0	9.0	0.7	0	0				0	0			
1.3 T	15	3.0	1.5			0	0							.00		I
Hershey	75		0.7	9.0	7.3	0.7	0					2	4			
½ bar (.5 oz)	14	4.0	2.5			1	0					47		.33		I
Nestle	70		0.8	9.0		2.0	0	0				0	0			
.5 oz baking bar	14	4.0	2.5			0	0							.40		I
choc, sweet																
dark	207	0.2	1.6	24.4	20.0	2.3	1	0	.10	.02	1	7	10	46	.61	.203
1.45 oz bar	41	14.0	8.2	4.6	0.4	0	8	.01	0.3	.00	.03	119	60	1.13	.235	819
German's, Bakers	60		1.0	8.0	8.0	0	0				0	0				
2 squares (.46 oz)	13	3.5	2.0			0	0					50		.36		I
Special Dark, Hershey	227	0.5	2.0	24.8	19.2	2.1	0	0	.10	.02	2	3	11	47	.62	.328
1.5 oz bar	41	13.3	8.3	4.1	0.4	1	0	.01	0.3	.00	.03	136	66	.96	.328	MUL
choc, white, Bakers	160		2.0	17.0	17.0	0.0	0	0				25	40			
1 oz square	28	9.0	6.0			5	0					80		.00		I
Chunky	198	1.2	3.6	22.8		1.9	4	0	.16	.05	9	21	57	29	.74	.198
1.4 oz bar	40	11.7	9.3	0.1	1.8	4	25	.03	0.8	.15	.20	214	83	.50	.248	819
confectioner's coating																
butterscotch	147	0.3	0.6	18.9		0.0	0	0	.00	.00	1	27	10	1	.03	.002
1 oz	28	8.2	6.8	1.0	0.1	0	0	.02	0.0	.03	.03	53	7	.02	.004	819
peanut butter	141	1.6	5.2	12.7		0.3	1	0	.06	.06	27	71	31	31	.57	.397
1 oz	28	8.4	3.7	2.7	1.5	0	6	.01	2.3	.02	.32	143	88	.48	.113	819
white	458	1.1	5.0	50.4		0.0	1	0	.24	.05	14	77	169	10	.63	.011
3 oz bar	85	27.3	16.5	7.7	0.9	18	30	.05	0.6	.64	.52	243	150	.20	.051	819
Cookies 'n Creme, Hershey	227		3.9	24.5	20.7	0.1	0	0				87	125			
1.6 oz bar	43	12.6	7.3			6	0							.47		I
Cookies 'n Mint, Hershey	226		3.5	27.0	20.6	1.4	0	0				79	73			
1.5 oz bar	43	11.5	5.6			8	0							.78		I
Crunch baking pieces, Nestle	70		0.8	10.0	8.0	0.0	0	0				25	0			
1.5 T	15	3.0	2.0			0	0									I
Crunch, Nestle	209	0.5	2.4	26.1		1.0	8	0	.22	.16	32	53	68	23	.57	.182
1.4 oz bar	40	10.5	6.1	3.4	0.3	5	28	.14	1.6	.15	.17	138	81	.20	.145	819
divinity	38	1.0	0.1	9.8		0.0	0	0	.01	.00	0	5	0	0	.00	.003
.4 oz piece	11	0.0	0.0	0.0	0.0	0	0	.00	0.0	.00	.00	2	0	.01	.004	819
Fifth Avenue, Hershey	197	1.0	3.6	26.4	18.0	0.9	0	0	.13	.05	31	66	30	36	.62	.211
2 oz bar	57	8.5	3.2	4.9	2.9	2	0	.01	1.9	.10	.43	187	86	.52	.125	MUL
fondant	57	1.1	0.0	14.8		0.0	0	0	.00	.00	0	6	0	0	.01	.002
.56 oz piece	16	0.0	0.0	0.0	0.0	0	0	.00	0.0	.00	.00	3	0	.01	.006	819
fudge																
brown sugar w/ nuts	55	1.1	0.4	10.9		0.1	2	0	.01	.01	2	14	16	7	.09	.090
.49 oz piece	14	1.4	0.2	0.3	0.8	1	11	.01	0.0	.00	.04	52	12	.25	.059	819
choc	65	1.6	0.3	13.5		0.1	8	0	.01	.00	0	11	7	4	.07	.023
.6 oz piece	17	1.4	0.9	0.4	0.1	2	32	.00	0.0	.01	.02	18	10	.08	.030	819
choc marshmallow	84	1.6	0.5	14.3		0.0	16	0	.02	.00	0	21	7	7	.11	.045
.7 oz piece	20	3.4	2.0	1.0	0.1	5	66	.00	0.0	.01	.02	28	13	.19	.045	819
choc marshmallow w/ nuts	96	1.6	0.7	15.1		0.4	16	0	.02	.01	2	21	11	10	.16	.090
.78 oz piece	22	4.3	2.1	1.3	0.7	5	67	.01	0.0	.01	.03	37	18	.23	.068	819
choc w/ nuts	81	1.3	0.6	13.8		0.2	9	0	.02	.02	2	11	10	9	.14	.096
.67 oz piece	19	3.1	1.1	0.8	1.0	3	38	.01	0.0	.01	.03	30	18	.14	.065	819
peanut butter	59	1.7	0.6	12.5		0.1	2	0	.01	.01	2	12	7	4	.07	.035
.56 oz piece	16	1.0	0.2	0.5	0.3	1	7	.00	0.2	.01	.03	21	10	.04	.014	819
van	59	1.7	0.2	13.2		0.0	8	0	.01	.00	0	11	6	1	.02	.002
.56 oz piece	16	0.9	0.5	0.2	0.0	3	33	.00	0.0	.01	.02	8	5	.01	.006	819
van w/ nuts	62	1.2	0.4	11.3		0.1	7	0	.01	.01	2	9	7	4	.07	.061
.53 oz piece	15	2.0	0.6	0.5	0.8	2	30	.01	0.0	.01	.03	17	11	.06	.033	819

	KCAL / WT (g)	H₂O (g) / FAT (g)	PRO (g) / SFA (g)	CHO (g) / MUFA (g)	SUGR (g) / PUFA (g)	DFIB (g) / CHOL (mg)	A (RE) / A (IU)	C (mg) / B-1 (mg)	B-2 (mg) / NIA (mg)	B-6 (mg) / B-12 (mcg)	FOL (mcg) / PANT (mg)	Na (mg) / K (mg)	Ca (mg) / P (mg)	Mg (mg) / Fe (mg)	Zn (mg) / Cu (mg)	Mn (mg) / REF
Fudgies, Kraft	180		1.0	32.0	27.0	0.0	0	0				90	20			
5 pieces	41	5.0	2.5			0	0					140		.36		I
Golden Almond																
Hershey	499	1.3	9.6	44.2		4.4	34	0	.48	.05	22	57	298	101	1.55	.764
3.2 oz bar	91	34.4				11	134	.05	1.0	.39	.34	429	246	1.36	.355	I
III, Hershey	471	2.5	5.9	50.8		5.2	20	1	.25	.10	11	79	275	61	1.00	.355
3.2 oz bar	91	30.0				17	82	.06	0.1	.41	.53	413	200	.55	.255	I
Solitaires w/ almonds, Hershey	455	1.2	9.9	40.0		4.2	8	0	.42	.04	18	46	305	100	1.56	.705
3 oz pkg	85	31.4	13.4	13.8	2.9	10	43	.05	0.9	.40	.33	428	255	1.19	.323	819
gum	10	0.0	0.0	2.9	2.1			0		.00		0				
1 stick	3	0.0	0.0	0.0	0.0			.00				0				819
Breathsavers Ice Breaker, sugarless, peppermint—1 stick	10		0.0	2.0	0.0							0				
peppermint—1 stick	3	0.0	0.0	0.0	0.0	0										I
Bubble Yum	25		0.0	6.0	6.0							0				
1 piece[4]	8	0.0														I
Bubble Yum, sugarless	15		0.0	3.0	0.0							0				
1 piece[5]	5	0.0	0.0	0.0	0.0	0										I
Care Free, sugarless	5		0.0	2.0	0.0							0				
1 stick[6]	2.5	0.0	0.0	0.0	0.0	0										I
Care Free, sugarless, bubble	10		0.0	2.0	0.0							0				
1 stick[7]	3	0.0	0.0	0.0	0.0	0										I
Fruit Stripe	10		0.0	2.0	2.0							0				
1 stick[8]	3	0.0	0.0	0.0	0.0											I
Stick Free, sugarless	10		0.0	2.0	0.0							0				
1 stick[6]	3	0.0	0.0	0.0	0.0	0										I
gum drops	135	0.3	0.0	34.6		0.0	0	0	.00	.00	0	15	1	0	.00	.003
10 small	35	0.0	0.0	0.0	0.0	0	0	.00	0.0	.00	.00	2	0	.14	.004	819
Gummi Savers	130		2.0	30.0	20.0							0				
11 pieces[9]	39	0.0	0.0	0.0	0.0	0										I
Gummy Bears, Amazin' Fruit	129		2.2	30.0	18.6	0.2	0	0				45	3			
1.39 oz	39	0.0	0.0	0.0	0.0	0	0									I
hard candy	106	0.4	0.0	27.8		0.0	0	0	.00	.00	0	11	1	1	.00	.003
1 oz	28	0.0	0.0	0.0	0.0	0	0	.00	0.0	.00	.00	1	1	.09	.008	819
Hundred Grand	200	2.2	2.1	30.4		0.6	10	0	.19	.14	28	89	49	16	.42	.141
1.5 oz bar	43	7.8	4.8	2.5	0.3	8	35	.12	1.4	.11	.12	97	58	.13	.105	819
jelly beans	103	1.8	0.0	26.1	16.5	0.0	0	0	.00	.00	0	7	1	1	.01	.010
10 large (1 oz)	28	0.1	0.0	0.1	0.0	0	0	.00	0.0	.00	.00	10	1	.31	.008	819
Kit Kat Wafer, Hershey	219	0.6	2.9	26.7	22.4	0.8	0	0	.11	.02	0	32	72	18	.42	.126
1.5 oz bar	42	11.2	7.2	3.2	0.3	8	0	.02	0.2	.26	.24	126	73	.36	.099	MUL
Krackel choc bar, Hershey	218	0.9	2.7	25.3	20.7	0.9	0	0	.12	.01	3	57	72	23	.50	.127
1.5 oz bar	41	11.8	7.4	2.9	2.3	8	0	.02	0.2	.24	.23	140	91	.37	.160	MUL
Life Savers																
all fruit flavors	20		0.0	5.0	0.0						0					
2 pieces	5	0.0	0.0	0.0	0.0	0										I
mint flavors	20		0.0	5.0	0.0						0					
3 pieces	5	0.0	0.0	0.0	0.0											I
super size	60		0.0	16.0	15.0							0				
4 candies[10]	16	0.0	0.0	0.0	0.0											I
super size, Butter Rum	60		0.0	15.0	13.0							65				
4 candies	16	0.0	0.0	0.0	0.0	0										I
Life Savers Delites, sugar-free	38		0.0	14.0	0.0							35				
5 candies[11]	15	0.0	0.0	0.0	0.0											I
lollipop	22	0.1	0.0	5.9		0.0	0	0	.00	.00	0	2	0	0	.00	.001
1 lollipop	6	0.0	0.0	0.0	0.0	0	0	.00	0.0	.00	.00	0	0	.02	.002	819
lollipop, swirled flavors, Life Savers	45		0.0	11.0	11.0							0				
1 pop	11	0.0	0.0	0.0	0.0											I
M&M's	236	0.8	2.1	34.2		1.2	25	0	.10	.01	2	29	50	20	.46	.102
1.69 oz pkg (69 pieces)	48	10.1	6.3	3.3	0.3	7	97	.03	0.1	.13	.14	128	72	.53	.134	819
M&M's Peanut	253	0.9	4.6	29.6		1.7	12	0	.10	.04	20	24	49	30	.66	.091
1.74 oz pkg (25 pieces)	49	12.9	5.1	5.4	2.1	4	46	.07	1.0	.12	.13	169	93	.56	.206	819

	KCAL / WT (g)	H₂O (g) / FAT (g)	PRO (g) / SFA (g)	CHO (g) / MUFA (g)	SUGR (g) / PUFA (g)	DFIB (g) / CHOL (mg)	A (RE) / A (IU)	C (mg) / B-1 (mg)	B-2 (mg) / NIA (mg)	B-6 (mg) / B-12 (mcg)	FOL (mcg) / PANT (mg)	Na (mg) / K (mg)	Ca (mg) / P (mg)	Mg (mg) / Fe (mg)	Zn (mg) / Cu (mg)	Mn (mg) / REF
maple sugar candy	99	2.2	0.0	25.5		0.0	1	0	.00	.00	0	3	25	5	1.70	1.238
1 oz piece	28	0.1	0.0	0.0	0.0	0	7	.00	0.0	.00	.01	77	1	.45	.028	819
Mars Almond	234	2.3	4.0	31.4		1.1	23	1	.16	.03	7	85	84	36	.56	.211
1.76 oz bar	50	11.5	2.7	5.6	2.8	5	81	.02	0.5	.15	.19	163	114	.55	.125	819
marshmallows	23	1.2	0.1	5.9		0.0	0	0	.00	.00	0	3	0	0	.00	.001
1 regular	7	0.0	0.0	0.0	0.0	0	0	.00	0.0	.00	.00	0	1	.02	.007	819
cocoa flavored teddy bears, Kraft	100		1.0	23.0	16.0	0.0	0	0				25	0			
½ cup	30	0.0	0.0	0.0	0.0	0	0					50		.00		I
miniature	146	7.5	0.8	37.4		0.0	0	0	.00	.00	0	22	1	1	.02	.004
1 cup, not packed	46	0.1	0.0	0.0	0.0	0	0	.00	0.0	.00	.00	2	4	.11	.045	819
miniature, Kraft	100		25.0	17.0	0.0	0	0				30	0				
½ cup¹²	30	0.0	0.0	0.0	0.0	0	0					0		.00		I
milk choc	226	0.6	3.0	26.0	24.0	1.5	24	0	.13	.02	4	36	84	26	.61	.132
1.55 oz bar	44	13.5	8.1	4.4	0.5	10	81	.03	0.1	.17	.19	169	95	.61	.169	819
Hershey	233		3.2	24.9	21.7	1.1	0	0				38	86			
1.5 oz bar	43	13.4	8.5			9	0							.41		I
Hugs, Hershey	208		2.8	22.1	20.2	0.5	0	0				37	85			
8 pieces (1.4 oz)	38	12.0	6.1			9	0					147		.17		I
Kisses, Hershey	211		2.9	22.6	19.7	1.0	0	0				34	78			
8 pieces (1.4 oz)	41	7.7				8	0					152		.37		I
Mini Kisses, Hershey	82		1.1	8.7	7.6	0.4	0	0				13	30			
11 pieces	15	4.7	3.0			3	0							.14		I
w/ almonds	231	0.7	4.0	23.4	21.5	2.7	6	0	.19	.02	5	33	99	40	.59	.275
1.55 oz bar	44	15.1	7.5	5.9	1.0	8	33	.03	0.3	.23	.19	195	116	.72	.186	819
w/ almonds, Hershey	228		4.5	20.5	17.7	1.2	0	0				36	87			
1.5 oz bar	41	14.2	7.0			7	0							.64		I
w/ peanuts	154	0.3	4.0	12.6				0	.07			19	49			
1 oz	28	10.8	4.5	4.2			50	.07	1.4			138	83	.40		456
w/ rice cereal	203	0.8	2.6	26.0	19.0	1.1	4	0	.12	.02	4	59	70	20	.46	.131
1.45 oz bar	41	10.9	6.5	3.5	0.3	8	23	.02	0.2	.16	.25	141	79	.31	.128	819
milk choc chips	862	2.2	11.6	99.5	91.7	5.7	92	1	.51	.07	13	138	321	101	2.32	.502
1 cup	168	51.6	31.0	16.7	1.8	37	311	.13	0.5	.66	.71	647	363	2.34	.647	819
Baker's	70		1.0	9.0	8.0	0.0	0	0				10	20			
½ oz (27 chips)	14	4.0	2.0			0	0					50		.00		I
Hershey	78		0.9	9.2	8.7	0.0	0	0				10	25			
1 T	15	4.6	2.7			2	0					49		.13		I
Nestle Toll House	70		0.6	9.0	8.0	0.0	0	0				0	0			
1 T	14	4.0	2.5			3	0							.00		I
Milky Way	258	3.8	2.7	43.7		0.8	35	1	.14	.03	5	146	79	21	.43	.122
2.15 oz bar	61	9.8	4.8	3.7	0.4	9	127	.02	0.2	.27	.23	147	98	.46	.091	819
Milky Way Snack Bar	76	1.1	0.8	12.9		0.2	10		.04	.01	1	43	23	6	.13	.036
.6 oz	18	2.9	1.4	1.1	0.1	3	37	.01	0.1	.08	.07	43	29	.14	.027	819
mint choc chips, Hershey	78		0.8	9.7	8.0	0.9	0	0				1	4			
1 T	15	4.2	2.6			1	0					44		.40		I
mints	100	2.1	0.0	24.7				0	.00			58	4			
¼ cup	28	0.6					0	.00	0.0			1	2	.30		456
Mounds	253	8.1	2.0	31.2	20.9	3.1	0	0	.03	.02	2	79	8	36	.55	.398
1.9 oz bar	53	13.3	10.8	3.5	0.4	1	0	.01	0.0	.00	.07	111	64	1.13	.297	MUL
Mr. Goodbar, Hershey	252	0.9	6.2	25.1		2.1	5	0	.13	.06	35	17	54	47	.88	.392
1.75 oz bar	49	15.8	8.8	5.5	0.7	10	20	.02	2.3	.22	.39	221	137	.59	.245	819
Oh Henry	244	3.3	6.2	36.7		2.0	5	0	.09	.04	19	134	62	35	.70	.310
2 oz bar	57	9.6	3.8	3.8	1.5	5	27	.01	1.6	.19	.29	184	103	.32	.000	819
party mints, Kraft	60		0.0	14.0	14.0	0.0	0	0				35	0			
7 pieces	15	0.0	0.0	0.0	0.0	0	0					0		.00		I
peanut bar	235	0.7	7.0	21.3		1.5	23	0	.06	.05	27	108	35	33	.62	.394
1.6 oz bar	45	15.2	1.9	7.5	4.8	3	229	.05	3.6	.01	.28	183	69	.44	.132	819
Lance	259	0.9	9.0	24.6					.04			94	25			
1.7 oz bar	50	13.8	2.4	6.8	4.5	0		.01	0.9			500		.06		I
Planters	230		6.0	22.0	13.0	2.0						70				
1.6 oz bar	45	14.0	1.5			0						210				I

	KCAL / WT (g)	H₂O (g) / FAT (g)	PRO (g) / SFA (g)	CHO (g) / MUFA (g)	SUGR (g) / PUFA (g)	DFIB (g) / CHOL (mg)	A (RE) / A (IU)	C (mg) / B-1 (mg)	B-2 (mg) / NIA (mg)	B-6 (mg) / B-12 (mcg)	FOL (mcg) / PANT (mg)	Na (mg) / K (mg)	Ca (mg) / P (mg)	Mg (mg) / Fe (mg)	Zn (mg) / Cu (mg)	Mn (mg) / REF
peanut brittle	128	0.5	2.1	19.6		0.6	13	0	.01	.03	20	128	9	14	.27	.168
1 oz	28	5.4	1.4	2.4	1.3	4	54	.05	1.0	.00	.15	59	31	.39	.100	819
peanut brittle, Kraft	170		3.0	29.0	21.0	1.0	0	0				310	0			
5 pieces	38	5.0	1.0			0	0					75		.00		I
Peanut Butter & Jelly Crisps, Planters	140		3.0	20.0	9.0	1.0						80				
12 pieces	31	6.0	1.0	2.5	1.5	0										I
Peanut Butter Chips, Reese's	79		3.1	7.0	5.7	0.6	0	0				35	18			
1 T	15	4.3	3.6			0	0							.17		I
Peanut Butter Crisps, Planters	150		4.0	18.0	9.0	2.0						100				
12 pieces	31	8.0	1.5	4.0	1.5	0										I
Peanut Butter Cups, Reese's	270	3.2	5.2	27.3	23.6	1.6	0	0	.11	.04	14	158	39	43	.70	.400
2 pieces (1. 8 oz)	50	15.6	5.5	4.9	1.9	3	0	.02	1.9	.23	.32	176	120	.58	.200	MUL
Peanut Clusters, Little Debbie	193	1.8	2.9	22.6	15.9	0.9		0	.04			119	24			
1.4 oz pkg	39	11.1	2.2			1	5	.07	1.2					.55		I
Peppermint Pattie, York	165	3.8	0.9	33.6	26.6	0.8	0	0	.04	.01	2	10	6	26	.32	.168
1.5 oz patty	42	3.0	1.8			0	0	.01	0.4	.01	.02	49	40	.41	.181	MUL
praline	177	3.9	1.1	24.2		1.1	2	0	.02	.03	5	24	12	20	.79	.657
1.38 oz piece	39	9.5	0.7	5.9	2.4	0	18	.12	0.1	.00	.25	82	43	.46	.196	819
Rainbow Morsels, Nestle	130		1.0	21.0	16.0	1.0	0	0				0	0			
1 oz	28	5.0	3.5			0	0							.40		I
raspberry chips, Hershey	80		0.7	9.6	7.8	0.8	0	0				2	5			
1 T	15	4.3	2.7			1	0							.38		I
Reese's Pieces, Hershey	226	1.2	6.4	28.2	24.3	1.3	0	0	.11	.06	26	74	36	37	.51	.202
1.6 oz pkg	46	9.7	8.3	1.1	1.1	1	0	.02	2.6	.15	.40	202	106	.33	.060	MUL
Rolo caramels w/ milk choc, Hershey	219	1.1	2.6	28.4	25.5	0.4	0	0	.14	.04	4	93	81	16	.37	.106
9 pieces (1.9 oz)	53	10.6	6.5	2.5	2.2	9	0	.03	0.1	.37	.27	132	85	.25	.053	MUL
sesame crunch	181	0.8	4.1	17.6		2.7	0	0	.07	.20	24	8	247	88	1.32	.654
20 pieces	35	11.7	1.6	4.4	5.1	0	2	.19	1.3	.00	.04	154	155	1.49	.332	819
Skittles Fruit Chews, M&M Mars	263	2.5	0.1	58.9	0.0		0	43	.01	.00	0	10	0	1	.02	.025
2.3 oz (59 pieces)	65	2.8	0.6	1.9	0.1	0	0	.00	0.0	.00	.00	3	1	.01	.029	I
Skor toffee bar, Hershey	219	1.7	1.8	22.7	21.0	0.6	0	0	.13	.01	2	108	51	13	.30	.059
1.4 oz bar	39	13.4	8.6			20	0	.01	0.0	.11	.12	93	58	.20	.051	MUL
Skor toffee bits, Hershey	67		0.2	7.3	6.9	0.1	0					73	5			
1 T	13	4.1	2.4			10	0							.03		I
Snickers	292	3.3	4.9	36.1		1.5	24	0	.10	.07	45	162	57	41	.87	.080
2.16 oz bar	61	15.0	5.5	6.4	3.0	8	93	.13	2.2	.08	.10	206	113	.46	.288	819
Solitaires, Hershey	445		9.3	36.6	29.0	3.1	0	0				44	147			
2.8 oz pkg	78	29.0	11.9			10	0							1.79		I
Star Crunch, Little Debbie	139	1.9	1.0	21.7	12.5	0.4		0	.04			84	11			
1.1 oz pkg	31	5.9	1.3			0	1	.06	0.4					.43		I
Starburst Fruit Chews	234	4.0	0.2	49.9	0.0		0	31	.00	.00	0	33	2	1	.00	.009
2.07 oz pk (6 pieces)	59	4.9	0.7	2.1	1.8	0	0	.00	0.0	.00	.02	1	4	.08	.007	819
sugar-coated almonds	129	0.6	2.2	19.9				0	.08			6	28			
1 oz	28	5.3	0.4				0	.01	0.3			72	47	.50		456
Sweet Escapes																
caramel peanut butter crisp	151		2.3	24.3	17.7	0.8	0	0				144	47			
1.4 oz bar	39	5.0	2.2			2	0					77		.22		I
choc toffee crisp	192		2.5	27.0	21.2	0.7	0	0				86	66			
1.4 oz bar	39	8.2	4.2			5	0							1.00		I
triple choc wafer	122		1.6	27.2	23.6	0.7	0	0				55	30			
1.4 oz bar	39	4.9	2.6			2	0					110		.59		I
Symphony	209	0.5	3.1	22.7		0.8	5	0	.15	.02	3	34	94	22	.45	.072
1.4 oz bar	40	13.0				11	28	.04	0.1	.16	.17	154	100	.40	.124	819
taffy	56	0.7	0.0	13.7	0.0		5	0	.00	.00	0	13	0	0	.00	.007
.5 oz piece	15	0.5	0.3	0.1	0.0	1	20	.00	0.0	.00	.00	1	0	.01	.004	819
Three Musketeers	250	3.5	1.9	46.1		1.0	16	0	.08	.01	0	116	50	17	.33	.096
2.13 oz bar	60	7.7	3.9	2.6	0.3	7	63	.02	0.1	.13	.14	80	55	.44	.093	819
toffee	65	0.1	0.1	7.7	6.6	0.0	38	0	.01	.00	0	22	4	0	.02	.001
.42 oz piece	12	3.9	2.5	1.1	0.1	13	152	.00	0.0	.01	.02	6	4	.01	.004	819

| | KCAL | H₂O (g) | PRO (g) | CHO (g) | SUGR (g) | DFIB (g) | A (RE) | C (mg) | B-2 (mg) | B-6 (mg) | FOL (mcg) | Na (mg) | Ca (mg) | Mg (mg) | Zn (mg) | Mn (mg) |
	WT (g)	FAT (g)	SFA (g)	MUFA (g)	PUFA (g)	CHOL (mg)	A (IU)	B-1 (mg)	NIA (mg)	B-12 (mcg)	PANT (mg)	K (mg)	P (mg)	Fe (mg)	Cu (mg)	REF
truffles	59	1.7	0.7	5.4		0.3	17	0	.03	.00	0	9	19	6	.13	.027
.42 oz piece	12	4.1	2.6	1.2	0.1	6	62	.01	0.0	.04	.05	37	21	.12	.035	819
Turtles, Demet's	82	1.0	1.1	9.9		0.4	6	0	.04	.01	2	16	27	9	.24	.111
.6 oz piece	17	4.7	1.8	1.9	0.8	4	28	.03	0.1	.07	.09	52	33	.23	.059	819
Twix, caramel	283	2.4	2.6	37.2		0.6	14	0	.13	.02	4	109	51	18	.44	.160
2 oz pkg (2 pieces)	57	13.8	5.0	7.6	0.5	3	54	.09	0.7	.10	.16	115	68	.46	.123	819
Twix, peanut butter	265	0.9	5.1	26.3		1.7	9	0	.07	.07	13	136	39	37	.70	.434
1.77 oz pkg (2 pieces)	50	16.1	5.7	7.4	2.1	3	36	.05	2.0	.07	.24	178	95	.46	.158	819
Twizzlers																
Cherry Bites	136		1.3	31.0	16.5	0.4	0	0				118	3			
1.43 oz	40	0.8	0.1			0	0							.08		I
Cherry Nibs	136		1.1	30.6	16.9	0.5	0	0				83	2			
1.39 oz	39	1.0	0.2			0	0							.08		I
Cherry Pull-n-Peel	116		1.2	26.5	14.3	0.3	0	0				97	2			
1.21 oz	34	0.6	0.3			0	0							.11		I
Cherry Twists	136		1.3	31.0	16.5	0.4	0	0				118	3			
1.43 oz	40	0.8	0.1			0	0							.08		I
Strawberry	263		2.3	65.8		0.1	0	0	.03	.01	0	197	25	4	.11	.106
2.5 oz pkg	71	1.1				0	0	.01	0.1	.00	.00	45	220	.35	.646	819
vanilla milk chips, Hershey	80		1.2	9.5	8.8	0.0	0	0				31	39			
1 T	15	4.1	3.4			1	0							.03		I
Whatchamacallit, Hershey	216	1.0	4.3	29.0	21.2	1.0	0	0	.13	.03	5	99	55	27	.33	.206
1.7 oz bar	48	9.2	4.5	4.9	1.9	5	0	.29	1.0	.19	.22	148	96	.43	.062	MUL
white baking bar, Nestle	80		1.0	8.0	8.0	0.0	0	0				15	40			
.5 oz	14	5.0	3.0			3	0							.00		I
White Morsels, Nestle	80		0.6	9.0	9.0	0.0	0	0				20	20			
1 oz	28	4.0	3.5			0	0							.00		I

1. Includes peppermint, spearmint, vanilla mint, and wintergreen.
2. Contains 3 g of Salatrim per serving, only 55% of which is used by the body, thereby providing 2 g of available total fat and saturated fat. The regular semi-sweet chocolate chips contain 4 g of available total fat and 2.5 g saturated fat.
3. Values are averages for regular size, mini, and mega chocolate chips.
4. Includes original flavor, cotton candy, cyclone fruits, and grape.
5. Includes original flavor, peppermint, and wild cherry.
6. Includes peppermint and spearmint.
7. Includes original flavor and wild cherry.
8. Includes regular gum and bubble gum.
9. Includes assorted 5 flavors, mixed berry, tangy fruits, and wacky frootz.
10. Includes five flavors, pep-o-mint, tangy fruits, wild cherry, and wint-o-green.
11. Values are averages for butter toffee, European collection, orchard fruit, and summer blends; contains 13.3 grams sugar alcohol.
12. One half cup is equivalent to about four large marshmallows.

3. CEREALS, COOKED

| | KCAL | H₂O | PRO | CHO | SUGR | DFIB | A | C | B-2 | B-6 | FOL | Na | Ca | Mg | Zn | Mn |
	WT	FAT	SFA	MUFA	PUFA	CHOL	A	B-1	NIA	B-12	PANT	K	P	Fe	Cu	REF
banana nut multigrain, inst, Nabisco	150		3.0	31.0	14.0	3.0						200				
1 pkt dry	40	2.0	0.0	1.0	0.5	0						160				I
barley, pearled, ckd	193	108.0	3.5	44.3		6.0	2	0	.10	.18	25	5	17	35	1.29	.407
1 cup	157	0.7	0.1	0.1	0.3	0	11	.13	3.2	.00	.21	146	85	2.09	.165	820
buckwheat groats, roasted, ckd	182	149.7	6.7	39.5		5.3	0	0	.08	.15	28	8	14	101	1.21	.798
1 cup	198	1.2	0.3	0.4	0.4	0	0	.08	1.9	.00	.71	174	139	1.58	.289	820
bulgur, ckd	151	141.5	5.6	33.8		8.2	0	0	.05	.15	33	9	18	58	1.04	1.108
1 cup	182	0.4	0.1	0.1	0.2	0	0	.10	1.8	.00	.63	124	73	1.75	.137	820
corn grits, inst																
white, enr	508	13.7	12.1	109.1		2.2	0	0	.52	.20	7	1	3	37	.56	.145
1 pkt prep	137	1.6	0.2	0.4	0.7	0	0	.88	6.8	.00	.66	188	100	5.36	.103	808
white, enr, Quaker	96	2.4	2.4	22.1	0.1	1.5	0	0	.09	.06	2	305	6	10	.19	
1 oz pkt dry	28	0.3	0.0	0.0	0.1	0	0	.16	1.5	.00	.53	41	31	8.75	.030	I

	KCAL / WT (g)	H₂O (g) / FAT (g)	PRO (g) / SFA (g)	CHO (g) / MUFA (g)	SUGR (g) / PUFA (g)	DFIB (g) / CHOL (mg)	A (RE) / A (IU)	C (mg) / B-1 (mg)	B-2 (mg) / NIA (mg)	B-6 (mg) / B-12 (mcg)	FOL (mcg) / PANT (mg)	Na (mg) / K (mg)	Ca (mg) / P (mg)	Mg (mg) / Fe (mg)	Zn (mg) / Cu (mg)	Mn (mg) / REF
white w/ butter flavor, enr, Quaker	101	2.5	2.3	20.9	0.2	1.3		0	.09	.04	1	323	2	8	.11	
1 oz pkt dry	28	1.4	0.4	0.4	0.4	0	54	.15	1.4	.00	.12	54	25	8.23	.020	I
white w/ cheddar cheese flavor, enr, Quaker—1 oz pkt dry	102	2.1	2.4	20.5	0.6	1.2		0	.08	.05	4	522	13	10	.21	.000
	28	1.6	0.5	0.4	0.2	1	4	.14	1.3	.06	.11	47	39	8.10	.030	I
white w/ imit bacon bits, enr, Quaker	98	2.0	2.8	21.7	0.1	1.5	0	0	.09	.06	2	341	11	9	.26	.000
1 oz pkt dry	28	0.5	0.1	0.1	0.2	0	0	.16	1.4	.00	.11	71	39	8.32	.020	I
white w/ imit ham bits, enr, Quaker	95	2.2	2.8	20.9	0.1	1.4	0	0	.09	.06	8	527	14	14	.24	.000
1 oz pkt dry	28	0.5	0.1	0.1	0.1	0	0	.15	1.4	.06	.11	60	37	8.20	.050	I
corn grits, quick, dry																
white, enr, Albers	140		3.0	31.0	0.0	1.0	0	0	.10			0	0			
¼ cup (1.4 oz)	40	0.5	0.0				0	.15	1.2					1.08		I
white, enr, Quaker	128	3.9	3.2	29.3	0.4	1.8	0	0	.13	.10	4	1	2	18	.34	
½ cup	37	0.5	0.1	0.1	0.3	0	0	.21	1.8	.00	.12	54	61	1.30	.040	I
yellow, enr, Quaker	125	4.3	3.1	28.8	0.4	2.1	0	0	.14	.10	18	1	1	15	.27	
¼ cup (1.3 oz)	37	0.6	0.2	0.2	0.3	0	211	.19	1.6	.00	.12	62	46	1.52	.030	I
corn grits, reg/quick, enr, ckd	145	206.4	3.4	31.5		0.5	0	0	.15	.06	2	0	0	10	.17	.041
1 cup	242	0.5	0.1	0.1	0.2	0	0	.24	2.0	.00	.15	53	29	1.55	.029	808
corn grits, reg/quick, unenr, ckd	145	206.4	3.4	31.5		0.5	0	0	.02	.06	2	0	0	10	.17	.041
1 cup	242	0.5	0.1	0.1	0.2	0	0	.05	0.5	.00	.15	53	29	.48	.029	808
corn grits, reg, white, enr, Quaker	142	4.3	3.5	32.5	0.4	2.0	0	0	.14	.11	4	1	2	20	.38	
¼ cup dry	41	0.6	0.1	0.1	0.3	0	0	.24	2.0	.00	.13	60	68	1.44	.050	I
couscous, ckd	200	129.9	6.8	41.6		2.5	0	0	.05	.09	27	9	14	14	.47	.150
1 cup	179	0.3	0.1	0.0	0.1	0	0	.11	1.8	.00	.66	104	39	.68	.073	820
Cream of Rice, ckd	95	160.1	1.6	20.9		0.2	0	0	.00	.05	5	2	5	5	.29	.264
¾ cup	183	0.2	0.0	0.1	0.0	0	0	.00	0.7	.00	.14	37	31	.37	.062	808
Cream of Rice, Nabisco	170		3.0	38.0	0.0						0					
¼ cup dry	46	0.0	0.0	0.0	0.0	0										I
Cream of Rye, Roman Meal	116		3.8	26.8	5.3							0	13			
⅓ cup dry	36	0.9				0								1.10		I
Cream of Wheat																
apple 'n cinn, inst, Nabisco	130		2.0	29.0	13.0	1.0						300				
1 pkt dry	35	0.0	0.0	0.0	0.0	0						45				I
brown sugar cinn, inst, Nabisco	130		2.0	29.0	12.0	1.0						220				
1 pkt dry	35	0.0	0.0	0.0								60				I
cinn toast, inst, Nabisco	130		2.0	29.0	12.0	1.0						170				
1 pkt dry	35	0.0	0.0	0.0	0.0	0						40				I
inst, ckd	116	152.8	3.3	23.7		2.2	0	0	.00	.02	7	5	45	11	.31	
¾ cup	181	0.4	0.1	0.0	0.2	0	0	.18	1.3	.00	.13	36	33	9.05	.069	808
inst, mix & eat	102	116.6	2.7	21.4		0.4	376	0	.28	.57	101	241	20	7	.24	
1 pkt prep	142	0.3	0.0	0.0	0.2	0	1252	.43	5.0	.00	.13	38	20	8.09	.041	808
inst, mix & eat, flavored	132	117.4	2.4	29.0		0.4	377	0	.30	.45	101	242	41	9	.22	
1 pkt prep	150	0.4	0.1		0.2	0	1251	.45	4.9	.00	.12	56	20	8.10	.057	808
inst, Nabisco	100		3.0	21.0	0.0	1.0						170				
1 pkt dry	28	0.0	0.0	0.0	0.0							25				I
maple brown sugar, inst, Nabisco	130		2.0	29.0	13.0						180					
1 pkt dry	35	0.0	0.0	0.0	0.0							40				I
quick, ckd	97	155.0	2.7	20.0		0.9	0	0	.00	.02	7	104	38	9	.25	
¾ cup	179	0.4	0.1	0.0	0.2	0	0	.18	1.1	.00	.13	34	75	7.70	.050	808
reg, ckd	100	163.7	2.8	20.7		1.3	0	0	.00	.03	8	2	38	8	.24	
¾ cup	188	0.4	0.1	0.1	0.2	0	0	.19	1.1	.00	.14	32	32	7.71	.056	808
req/quick, Nabisco	120		3.0	25.0	0.0	1.0						0				
3 T dry	33	0.0	0.0	0.0	0.0	0										I
farina																
ckd, enr	88	153.8	2.4	18.6	0.2	2.4	0	0	.09	.02	4	0	4	4	.12	.165
¾ cup	175	0.2	0.0	0.0	0.1	0	0	.14	1.0	.00	.10	23	21	.88	.019	808
ckd, unenr	88	153.8	2.4	18.6		2.4	0	0	.02	.02	4	0	4	4	.12	.165
¾ cup	175	0.2	0.0	0.0	0.1	0	0	.02	0.2	.00	.10	23	21	.04	.019	808
quick, enr, Quaker	155	4.6	4.7	34.3	0.1	1.2	0	0	.15	.02	9	1	6	6	.23	
¼ cup (1.6 oz) dry	44	0.2	0.0	0.2	0.1	0	0	.21	2.4	.00	.16	43	39	14.39	.030	I

	KCAL	H₂O (g)	PRO (g)	CHO (g)	SUGR (g)	DFIB (g)	A (RE)	C (mg)	B-2 (mg)	B-6 (mg)	FOL (mcg)	Na (mg)	Ca (mg)	Mg (mg)	Zn (mg)	Mn (mg)
	WT (g)	FAT (g)	SFA (g)	MUFA (g)	PUFA (g)	CHOL (mg)	A (IU)	B-1 (mg)	NIA (mg)	B-12 (mcg)	PANT (mg)	K (mg)	P (mg)	Fe (mg)	Cu (mg)	REF
Malt-O-Meal (wheat cereal w/ malt)																
choc flavored, ckd	99		2.8	21.9		0.8			.26			0	4	10	.21	
1 cup (from 1 oz dry)	240	0.3	0.1	0.1	0.1	0		.38	5.0			65	35	8.10	.070	I
ckd	100		3.6	21.1		0.8			.25	.02	6	1	4	8	.21	
1 cup (from 1 oz dry)	240	0.4	0.1	0.1	0.2	0		.37	5.0		.14	34	36	8.10	.010	I
w/ 40% oat bran, ckd	128		5.7	25.0		2.9			.26			1				
1 cup (from 1 oz dry)	240	1.7						.38	5.0			110	119	8.10		I
Maltex, ckd	135	151.5	4.3	29.7		2.2	0	0	.07	.06	17	7	13	43	1.40	
¾ cup	187	0.7	0.1	0.1	0.3	0	0	.19	1.8	.00	.17	200	135	1.35	.252	808
Maypo, ckd	128	148.9	4.3	23.9		4.3	527	22	.54	.72	7	7	94	38	1.12	
¾ cup	180	1.8	0.3	0.5	0.7	0	1753	.54	7.0	2.16	.25	158	185	6.30	.119	808
millet, ckd	286	171.4	8.4	56.8		3.1	0	0	.20	.26	46	5	7	106	2.18	.653
1 cup	240	2.4	0.4	0.4	1.2	0	0	.25	3.2	.00	.41	149	240	1.51	.386	820
multigrain, Quaker	133	4.4	4.5	29.4	0.2	4.8		0	.06	.10	11	1	14	46	1.28	
½ cup dry	40	1.0	0.2	0.2	0.5	0	3	.12	1.4	.00	.20	165	138	1.19	.180	I
oat bran cereal, Quaker/Mother's	212	2.3	8.6	41.3	9.2	6.5		6	.44	.52	104	205	31	101	3.89	
1 ¼ cup (2 oz) dry	57	3.0	0.6	1.0	1.2	0	519	.39	5.2	.00	.49	258	302	16.20	.180	I
oatmeal, inst	104	151.3	4.4	18.1		3.0	453	0	.28	.74	150	285	163	42	.87	1.035
1 pkt prep	177	1.8	0.3	0.6	0.7	0	1510	.53	5.5	.00	.35	99	133	6.30	.097	808
apple & cinn	125	117.1	3.2	26.1		2.5	305	0	.35	.41	94	121	104	30	.70	.915
1 pkt prep	149	1.4	0.3	0.5	0.6	0	1019	.30	4.1	.00	.15	106	113	3.89	.085	808
apples & cinn, Quaker	128	2.2	3.3	26.9	10.3	2.6		0	.36	.42	84	122	106		.69	
1.2 oz pkt dry	35	1.5	0.4	0.5	0.6	0	1050	.31	4.2	.00	.15	108	116	4.00	.080	I
bran & raisins	158	156.0	4.9	30.4		5.5	480	0	.64	.76	156	248	174	57	1.35	1.589
1 pkt prep	195	1.9	0.4			0	1599	.57	8.1	.00	.45	236	207	7.62	.285	808
choc chip cookie, Quaker Kid's Choice	158	2.8	3.9	31.6	11.8	2.6		0	.36	.42	84	198	107		.82	
1.5 oz pkt dry	42	2.5	0.5	0.8	0.6	0	1050	.31	4.2	.00	.19	114	122	4.01	.090	I
cinn & spice	177	117.9	4.8	35.1		2.6	473	0	.34	.77	153	280	172	52	.97	1.473
1 pkt prep	161	1.9	0.4	0.6	0.7	0	1578	.56	5.7	.00	.38	105	145	6.63	.119	808
cinn & spice, Quaker	172	2.6	4.1	35.7	15.5	2.8		0	.36	.42	84	242	108	40	.92	
1.6 oz pkt dry	46	2.1	0.4	0.7	0.8	0	1050	.31	4.2	.00	.19	115	138	4.01	.100	I
cookies 'n cream, Quaker	162	2.7	3.7	31.2	11.7	2.4		0	.36	.42	84	198	107		.76	
1.5 oz pkt dry	42	3.1	0.7	1.2	0.8	0	1050	.31	4.2	.01	.18	114	123	4.01	.080	I
fruit & cream banana, Quaker	135	2.2	3.2	26.1	10.1	2.3		0	.36	.42	84	170	106		.67	
1.2 oz pkt dry	35	2.5	0.5	0.8	0.6	0	1050	.31	4.2	.01	.14	102	113	4.00	.070	I
fruit & cream blueberry, Quaker	135	2.2	2.9	26.2	9.9	2.0		0	.36	.42	84	157	106		.64	
1.2 oz pkt dry	35	2.5	0.6	0.8	0.6	0	1050	.31	4.2	.02	.13	89	106	4.00	.070	I
fruity marshmallow, Quaker	148	2.7	3.6	30.5	12.6	2.6		0	.36	.42	84	185	106		.08	
1.4 oz pkt dry	40	1.9	0.4	0.7	0.6	0	1050	.31	4.2	.00	.17	113	122	4.00	.090	I
low sodium, Quaker	103	2.6	4.0	18.5	0.3	2.5		0	.36	.42	84	78	107		.84	
1 oz pkt dry	28	2.0	0.4	0.7	0.8	0	1050	.31	4.2	.00	.17	105	126	8.23	.080	I
maple & brown sugar	153	116.1	4.2	31.4		2.6	302	0	.34	.40	81	234	105	39	.90	1.203
1 pkt prep	155	1.8	0.4	0.6	0.7	0	1008	.30	4.0	.00	.34	112	132	3.86	.098	808
maple & brown sugar, Quaker	160	2.6	4.4	32.7	13.1	2.7		0	.36	.42	84	240	108		.90	
1.5 oz pkt dry	43	1.9	0.4	0.7	0.8	0	1050	.31	4.2	.00	.36	116	138	4.01	.100	I
oatmeal raisin cookie, Quaker Kid's	156	3.1	3.4	32.1	14.5	2.5		0	.36	.42	84	225	107		.71	
Choice—*1.5 oz pkt dry*	42	2.1	0.4	0.6	0.5	0	1050	.31	4.2	.00	.16	122	109	4.01	.090	I
peaches & cream, Quaker	135	2.2	2.7	26.4	11.5	2.4		0	.36	.42	84	176	106		.57	
1.25 oz pkt dry	35	2.6	0.5	0.8	0.5	0	1050	.31	4.2	.02	.12	99	100	4.00	.070	I
radical raspberry, Quaker Kid's Choice	154	2.8	3.6	29.1	10.7	2.7		1	.36	.42	84	179	106		.78	
1.4 oz pkt dry	40	3.2	0.7	1.7	0.6	0	1050	.31	4.2	.02	.17	116	129	4.00	.080	I
raisins & spice	161	118.5	4.3	31.9		2.2	441	0	.36	.75	150	226	166	36	.71	
1 pkt prep	158	1.7	0.3	0.6	0.6	0	1468	.51	5.5	.00	.37	150	133	6.59	.100	808
raisins & spice, Quaker	158	3.3	3.6	32.8	14.7	2.6		0	.36	.42	84	250	107		.78	
1.5 oz pkt dry	43	1.9	0.4	0.7	0.7	0	1050	.31	4.2	.00	.16	148	121	4.00	.100	I
raisins, dates, & walnuts, Quaker	135	3.0	3.3	27.3	11.7	2.5		0	.36	.42	84	237	107		.72	
1.3 oz pkt dry	37	2.0	0.4	0.6	0.8	0	1050	.31	4.2	.00	.16	130	109	4.00	.100	I
s'mores, Quaker Kid's Choice	159	2.7	3.7	32.0	13.1	2.4		0	.36	.42	84	217	107		.75	
1.5 oz pkt dry	42	2.4	0.5	0.8	0.5	0	1050	.31	4.2	.00	.17	106	113	4.01	.080	I
strawberries & cream, Quaker	135	2.2	2.7	26.5	11.4	2.0		0	.36	.42	84	173	106		.56	
1.25 oz pkt dry	35	2.5	0.6	0.8	0.6	0	1050	.31	4.2	.02	.12	98	99	4.00	.070	I

	KCAL / WT (g)	H₂O (g) / FAT (g)	PRO (g) / SFA (g)	CHO (g) / MUFA (g)	SUGR (g) / PUFA (g)	DFIB (g) / CHOL (mg)	A (RF) / A (IU)	C (mg) / B-1 (mg)	B-2 (mg) / NIA (mg)	B-6 (mg) / B-12 (mcg)	FOL (mcg) / PANT (mg)	Na (mg) / K (mg)	Ca (mg) / P (mg)	Mg (mg) / Fe (mg)	Zn (mg) / Cu (mg)	Mn (mg) / REF
twisted strawberry & banana, Quaker	148	2.7	3.6	30.6	12.6	2.6		0	.36	.42	84	175	106		.80	
1.4 oz pkt dry	40	1.9	0.4	0.7	0.6	0	1050	.31	4.2	.00	.17	115	121	4.00	.090	I
oatmeal, microwave																
apple spice, Quaker Quick 'n Hearty	166	2.9	3.7	34.8	15.2	3.0		0	.36	.42	84	306	108	36	.84	
1.6 oz pkt dry	45	2.0	0.4	0.7	0.6	0	1050	.31	4.2	.00	.21	136	132	3.97	.100	I
brown sugar cinn, Quaker Quick 'n Hearty—1.5 oz pkt dry	155	3.0	2.9	31.4	11.6	2.6		0	.36	.42	84	255	108	40	.90	
	42	2.2	0.4	0.8	0.7	0	1050	.31	4.2	.00	.21	125	140	3.97	.090	I
cinn double raisin, Quaker Quick 'n Hearty—1.66 oz pkt dry	169	4.2	4.0	35.0	15.5	2.9		0	.36	.42	84	275	108	40	.84	
	47	2.2	0.4	0.8	0.7	0	1050	.31	4.2	.00	.19	188	139	3.97	.120	I
honey bran, Quaker Quick 'n Hearty	151	2.9	3.9	30.6	11.4	2.7		0	.36	.42	84	253	108	41	.90	
1.4 oz pkt dry	41	2.1	0.4	0.7	0.7	0	1050	.31	4.2	.00	.22	118	142	3.97	.100	I
Quaker Quick 'n Hearty	106	2.8	3.8	19.1	0.3	2.4		0	.36	.42	84	153	108	38	.86	
1 oz pkt dry	29	2.2	0.4	0.7	0.7	0	1050	.31	4.2	.00	.20	110	136	8.53	.090	I
oatmeal, old fashioned, Quaker	148	3.8	5.5	27.3	0.6	3.7	0	0	.05	.04	20	1	19	108	1.28	
½ cup dry	40	3.0	0.4	0.8	0.9	0	0	.22	0.3	.00	.28	143	183	1.86	.150	I
oatmeal, quick/reg/inst, ckd	145	199.6	6.1	25.3	0.9	4.0	5	0	.05	.05	9	2	19	56	1.15	1.369
1 cup	234	2.3	0.4	0.7	0.9	0	37	.26	0.3	.00	.47	131	178	1.59	.129	808
Ralston, ckd	101	163.6	4.2	21.3		4.6	0	0	.13	.09	13	4	10	44	1.06	
¾ cup	190	0.6	0.1	0.1	0.3	0	0	.15	1.5	.08	.25	116	110	1.23	.150	808
Wheat Hearts, General Mills	130		5.0	26.0	1.0	2.0	0	0	.34	.00	0	0	0	32	1.20	
¼ cup dry	36	1.0	0.0	0.0	0.0	0	0	.45	6.0	.00	.00	130	100	10.80	.040	I
Wheatena, ckd	102	155.4	3.6	21.5		4.9	0	0	.04	.03	13	4	7	36	1.26	1.496
¾ cup	182	0.9	0.1	0.1	0.5	0	0	.02	1.0	.00	.08	140	109	1.02	.095	808
Whole Wheat Natural, Quaker	134	3.7	4.6	30.3	0.4	4.0		0	.05	.05	19	2	14	50	1.10	
½ cup (1.4 oz) dry	40	0.8	0.1	0.1	0.4	0	36	.14	1.9	.00	.28	168	142	1.15	.170	I

4. CEREALS, READY-TO-EAT

	KCAL / WT (g)	H₂O (g) / FAT (g)	PRO (g) / SFA (g)	CHO (g) / MUFA (g)	SUGR (g) / PUFA (g)	DFIB (g) / CHOL (mg)	A (RF) / A (IU)	C (mg) / B-1 (mg)	B-2 (mg) / NIA (mg)	B-6 (mg) / B-12 (mcg)	FOL (mcg) / PANT (mg)	Na (mg) / K (mg)	Ca (mg) / P (mg)	Mg (mg) / Fe (mg)	Zn (mg) / Cu (mg)	Mn (mg) / REF
All-Bran, Kellogg's	81	1.1	3.9	23.0	6.0	10.0		15	.43	.50	100	284	100	140	3.75	
½ cup (1.09 oz)	31	1.1	0.2	0.2	0.7	0	750	.38	5.0	1.50	.49	310	300	4.50	.400	I
All-Bran w/ extra fiber, Kellogg's	50	1.0	3.2	19.7	0.0	13.3		15	.43	.50	100	110	100	100	3.75	
½ cup (.9 oz)	26	0.5	0.1			0	750	.38	5.0	1.50		260	250	4.50	.300	I
almond crunch w/ raisins, Healthy Choice—1 cup (2.05 oz)	209	1.8	4.6	49.5	12.0	4.9		0	.60	.70	100	300	28	60	.16	
	58	2.0	0.0	0.0		0	500	.53	7.0	2.10	3.50	180	150	6.30		I
Alpha-Bits, Post	130		3.0	27.0	13.0	1.0		0	.43	.50	100	210	0	24	1.50	
1 cup (1.1 oz)	32	1.0	0.0			0	1250	.38	5.0	1.50		60	60	2.70	.080	I
Apple Cinnamon Cherrios, General Mills	120		2.0	25.0	13.0	1.0		15	.43	.50	100	160	20	16	14.75	
¾ cup (1.06 oz)	30	2.0	0.0	1.0	0.0	0	750	.38	5.0	.00	.00	65	60	4.50	.000	I
Apple Jacks, Kellogg's	120	0.9	1.6	29.6	16.4	0.6		15	.43	.50	100	148	3	8	3.75	
1 cup (1.16 oz)	33	0.1	0.0			0	750	.38	5.0			34	40	4.50	.080	I
Apple Raisin Crisp, Kellogg's	178	2.8	3.3	45.0	15.0	4.2		0	.43	.50	100	360	14	8	1.50	
1 cup (1.87 oz)	53	0.0	0.0	0.0	0.0	0	750	.38	5.0	1.50		135	80	1.80	.040	I
Apple Zaps, Quaker	118	0.8	1.2	26.5	14.1	0.7		12	.43	.50	100	132	3	15	3.76	
1 cup (1.06 oz)	30	1.0	0.5	0.5	0.2	0	1002	.38	5.0	.00	.10	53	45	4.51	.040	I
Banana Nut Crunch, Post	250		5.0	43.0	11.0	4.0		0	.43	.50	100	200	20	40	1.50	
1 cup (2.08 oz)	59	6.0	1.0			0	1250	.38	5.0	1.50		190	150	1.80	.030	I
Basic 4, General Mills	210		4.0	42.0		3.0		15	.43	.50	100	330	250	32	3.75	
1 cup (1.94 oz)	55	3.0	0.0	1.0	1.0	0	1250	.38	5.0	.00	.00	170	250	4.50	.120	I
Berry Basic, Sunbelt	235	1.7	5.2	41.3	12.7	4.2		2	1.80			171	20			
1.94 oz	55	5.4	1.4			1	54	.63	1.9					4.35		I
Berry Berry Kix, General Mills	120		1.0	26.0	9.0	0.0		15	.43	.50	100	180	40	0	3.75	
¾ cup (1.06 oz)	30	1.5	0.0	1.0	0.0	0	750	.38	5.0	.00	.00	25	40	4.50	.000	I
Blueberry Morning, Post	230		4.0	45.0	14.0	2.0		0	.43	.50	100	250	0	24	.90	
1 ¼ cups (2 oz)	57	3.5	0.5			0	1250	.38	5.0	1.50		105	80	1.80	.080	I
Body Buddies, Natural Fruit, General Mills—1 cup (1.06 oz)	120		2.0	26.0	6.0	0.0		15	.43	.50	100	290	400	0	1.50	
	30	1.0	0.0	0.5	0.0	0	750	.38	5.0	1.50	1.00	30	40	8.10	.200	I

	KCAL	H₂O (g)	PRO (g)	CHO (g)	SUGR (g)	DFIB (g)	A (RE)	C (mg)	B-2 (mg)	B-6 (mg)	FOL (mcg)	Na (mg)	Ca (mg)	Mg (mg)	Zn (mg)	Mn (mg)
	WT (g)	FAT (g)	SFA (g)	MUFA (g)	PUFA (g)	CHOL (mg)	A (IU)	B-1 (mg)	NIA (mg)	B-12 (mcg)	PANT (mg)	K (mg)	P (mg)	Fe (mg)	Cu (mg)	REF
Boo Berry, General Mills	120		1.0	27.0	14.0	0.0		15	.43	.50	100	210	20	0	3.75	
1 cup (1.06 oz)	30	0.5	0.0	0.0	0.0	0	0	.38	5.0	.00	.00	15	20	4.50	.000	I
bran 100%	75	0.8	3.5	20.4		8.3	0	27	.76	.90	20	194	20	132	2.43	2.528
½ cup (1 oz)	28	1.4	0.2	0.2	0.8	0	0	.67	8.9	2.66	.54	277	340	3.44	.442	808
Bran 100%, Nabisco	80		4.0	23.0	7.0	8.0		0	.43	.50	100	120	20	80	3.75	
⅓ cup (1.02 oz)	29	0.5	0.0			0	1250	.38	5.0	.00		270	250	8.10	.300	I
Bran Buds, Kellogg's	83	0.9	2.8	24.0	8.0	12.0		15	.43	.50	100	200	20	80	3.75	
⅓ cup (1.06 oz)	30	0.7	0.1	0.2	0.4	0	750	.38	5.0	1.50	.00	269	150	4.50	.200	I
bran flakes (40 % bran)																
Malt-O-Meal	93	0.7	3.2	22.5				15	.43	.50	100	205	13	49	2.71	
⅔ cup (1 oz)	28	0.9	0.1	0.2	0.5	0	1250	.38	5.0			170	150	4.50	.170	I
Post	90		3.0	22.0	5.0	6.0		0	.43	.50	100	210	0	60	1.50	
⅔ cup (1 oz)	28	0.5	0.0			0	1250	.38	5.0	1.50		180	150	8.10	.200	I
Ralston Purina	91	0.7	3.2	22.3		3.9	371	15	.42	.50	99	261	13	67	1.16	1.286
¾ cup (1 oz)	28	0.4				0	1235	.36	4.9	1.48	.39	164	156	4.45	.204	808
Bran'ola, Post	200		4.0	43.0	15.0	5.0		0	.43	.50	100	240	0	60	1.50	
½ cup (1.87 oz)	53	3.0	0.5			0	1250	.37	5.0	1.50		200	150	4.50	.040	I
Bran'ola Raisin, Post	200		4.0	44.0	18.0	5.0		0	.43	.50	100	220	0	40	1.50	
½ cup (1.9 oz)	55	3.0	0.5			0	1250	.38	5.0	1.50		220	100	4.50	.160	I
Cap'n Crunch																
crunchberries/wildberry colors, Quaker	105	0.6	1.2	22.3	12.0	0.6		0	.43	.50	100	180	5	14	3.76	
¾ cup (1 oz)	26	1.4	0.4	0.8	0.3	0	33	.38	5.0	.00	.09	49	43	4.51	.040	I
peanut butter, Quaker	112	0.5	2.0	21.5	9.2	0.8		0	.43	.50	100	204	3	19	3.75	
¾ cup (1 oz)	27	2.3	0.6	1.2	0.6	0	37	.38	5.0	.00	.12	62	52	4.50	.070	I
Quaker	107	0.6	1.4	23.1	11.6	0.9		0	.43	.50	100	208	5	9	3.75	
¾ cup (1 oz)	27	1.4	0.5	0.3	0.2	0	36	.38	5.0	.00	.10	35	28	4.51	.040	I
Cheerios, General Mills	110		3.0	23.0	1.0	3.0		15	.43	.50	100	280	40	32	3.75	
1 cup (1.06 oz)	30	2.0	0.0	0.5	0.5	0	1250	.38	5.0	.00	.00	90	100	8.10	.040	I
Cinnamon Mini-Buns, Kellogg's	120	0.7	1.0	26.6	12.0	0.7		15	.43	.50	100	208	4	8	3.80	
¾ cup (1.06 oz)	30	0.6	0.2	0.1	0.3	0	750	.38	5.0	1.50		36	20	4.50		I
Cinnamon Toast Crunch, General Mills	130		1.0	24.0	10.0	1.0		15	.43	.50	100	210	40	8	3.75	
¾ cup (1.06 oz)	30	3.5	0.5	1.0	0.0	0	750	.38	5.0	.00	.00	45	60	4.50	.040	I
Cocoa Blasts, Quaker	129	0.8	1.3	29.1	16.1	0.8		13	.47	.55	110	133	9	19	4.13	
1 cup (1.2 oz)	33	1.2	0.5	0.6	0.2	0	1100	.41	5.5	.00	.09	71	55	4.95	.080	I
Cocoa Krispies, Kellogg's	120	0.7	1.6	27.2	13.0	0.4		15	.43	.50	100	210	4	8	1.50	
¾ cup (1.09 oz)	31	0.8	0.6	0.1	0.1	0	750	.38	5.0			60	20	1.80	.040	I
Cocoa Pebbles, Post	120		1.0	25.0	13.0	1.0		0	.43	.50	100					
¾ cup (1.02 oz)	29	1.0	1.0			0	1250	.38	5.0	1.50						I
Cocoa Puffs, General Mills	120		1.0	27.0	14.0	0.0		15	.43	.50	100	190	20	0	3.75	
1 cup (1.06 oz)	30	1.0	0.0	0.5	0.0	0	0	.38	5.0	1.50	.00	40	40	4.50	.040	I
Complete Bran Flakes, Kellogg's	93	1.0	2.9	23.8	5.0	4.9		15	.43	.50	100	226	13	60	3.75	
¾ cup (1.02 oz)	29	0.6	0.1	0.1	0.4	0	750	.38	5.0	1.50		170	150	8.10	.120	I
corn flakes																
Country, General Mills	120		2.0	26.0	2.0	0.0		15	.43	.50	100	290	40	0	3.75	
1 cup (1.06 oz)	30	0.5	0.0	0.0	0.0	0	750	.38	5.0	.00	.00	35	40	8.10	.000	I
Kellogg's	102	0.8	2.3	24.0	1.9	1.1		15	.43	.50	100	304	1	3	.19	
1 cup (1 oz)	28	0.2	0.1	0.0	0.1	0	750	.38	5.0		.05	25	11	8.10	.020	I
Malt-O-Meal	106	0.6	2.0	24.8				15	.43	.50	100	268			1.56	
1 cup (1 oz)	28	0.2	0.0	0.1	0.1	0	1250	.38	5.0			28		2.70	.020	I
Post Toasties	100		2.0	24.0	2.0	1.0		0	.43	.50	100	270	0	0	.00	
1 cup (1 oz)	28	0.0	0.0	0.0	0.0	0	1250	.38	5.0	1.50		30	0	.36	.000	I
Corn Pops, Kellogg's	117	0.9	1.4	27.9	14.0	0.4		15	.43	.50	100	119	4	2	1.50	
1 cup (1.09 oz)	31	0.2	0.0	0.1	0.1	0	750	.38	5.0			27	8	1.80	.020	I
Corn Quakes, Quaker	121	0.8	1.3	25.5	10.9	0.7		12	.43	.50	100	218	10	16	3.75	
¾ cup (1.06 oz)	30	1.7	0.5	1.0	0.3	0	1000	.38	5.0	.00	.10	58	54	4.50	.040	I
Count Chocula, General Mills	120		1.0	26.0	14.0	0.0		15	.43	.50	100	190	20	0	3.75	
1 cup (1.06 oz)	30	1.0	0.0			0	0	.38	5.0	1.50	.00	65	20	4.50	.040	I

	KCAL / WT (g)	H₂O (g) / FAT (g)	PRO (g) / SFA (g)	CHO (g) / MUFA (g)	SUGR (g) / PUFA (g)	DFIB (g) / CHOL (mg)	A (RE) / A (IU)	C (mg) / B-1 (mg)	B-2 (mg) / NIA (mg)	B-6 (mg) / B-12 (mcg)	FOL (mcg) / PANT (mg)	Na (mg) / K (mg)	Ca (mg) / P (mg)	Mg (mg) / Fe (mg)	Zn (mg) / Cu (mg)	Mn (mg) / REF
Cracklin' Oat Bran, Kellogg's	190	1.3	3.8	35.6	15.0	5.6		15	.43	.50	100	168	22	60	1.50	1.476
¾ cup (1.7 oz)	49	6.3	1.5	3.4	1.4	0	750	.38	5.0	.00	.37	230	166	1.80	.120	MUL
Crisp 'n Crackling Rice, Malt-O-Meal	108	0.6	1.9	24.8		0.4		15	.43	.50	100	252		9	1.65	
1 cup (1 oz)	28	0.3	0.1	0.1	0.1	0	1250	.38	5.0			43	34	2.18	.080	I
crisp rice, low Na	113	0.8	1.5	25.5		0.4	0	0	.05	.04	3	3	19	11	.42	.320
1 cup (1 oz)	28	0.1	0.0	0.0	0.0	0	0	.00	0.4	.00	.15	22	29	.86	.068	808
Crispix, Kellogg's	109	0.9	2.0	25.0	2.9	0.6		15	.43	.50	100	240	3	7	1.50	
1 cup (1.02 oz)	29	0.3	0.1	0.1	0.1	0	750	.38	5.0			35	20	1.80	.040	I
crispy rice	111	0.7	1.8	24.8	2.5	0.3	371	15	.59	.69	138	206	5	12	.46	.363
1 cup (1 oz)	28	0.1	0.0	0.0	0.0	0	1235	.52	6.9	.08	.11	27	31	.70	.061	808
Crispy Wheaties 'n Raisins, General Mills—1 cup (1.9 oz)	190		4.0	44.0	20.0	4.0		0	.43	.50	100	270	40	40	.60	
	55	1.0	0.0	0.0	0.0	0	1250	.38	5.0	.00	.00	220	100	4.50	.160	I
Crunchy Bran, Quaker	90	0.7	1.9	22.7	5.5	5.0		0	.43	.50	100	253	21	14	3.75	
¾ cup (.95 oz)	27	0.9	0.2	0.2	0.4	0	38	.08	5.0	.00	.10	56	36	8.51	.070	I
CW Post	122	0.6	2.3	21.0		2.1	371	0	.42	.50	99	48	13	19	.47	
¼ cup (1 oz)	28	3.7	0.5	1.7	1.3	0	1235	.36	4.9	1.48	.23	57	65	4.45	.109	808
CW Post w/ raisins	121	1.1	2.4	20.1		3.7	371	0	.42	.50	99	44	14	20	.45	
¼ cup (1 oz)	28	4.0	3.0	0.5	0.4	0	1235	.36	4.9	1.48	.21	71	63	4.45	.108	808
Double Dip Crunch, Kellogg's	111	0.9	1.0	26.4	10.9	0.4		15	.43	.50	100	170	2		1.50	
¾ cup (1.02 oz)	29	0.1	0.0	0.0	0.1	0	750	.38	5.0			21		1.80		I
Dutch Apple, Betty Crocker	220		4.0	46.0	17.0	1.0		15	.43	.50	100	310	40	24	3.75	
1 cup (1.09 oz)	55	2.0	0.0	0.0	0.0	0	750	.38	5.0	.00	.00	100	100	4.10	.040	I
Fiber One, General Mills	60		2.0	24.0	0.0	13.0		9	.43	.50	100	125	40	60	1.20	
½ cup (1.06 oz)	30	1.0	0.0			0	0	.38	5.0	.00	.00	230	150	4.50	.200	I
Frankenberry, General Mills	120		1.0	27.0	14.0	0.0		15	.43	.50	100	210	20	0	3.75	
1 cup (1.06 oz)	30	1.0	0.0	0.5	0.0	0	0	.38	5.0	1.50	.00	15	20	4.50	.000	I
French Toast Crunch, General Mills	120		1.0	26.0	12.0	0.0		15	.43	.50	100	170	60	0	3.75	
¾ cup (1.06 oz)	30	1.5	0.0	0.0	0.0	0	750	.38	5.0	.00	.00	20	40	4.50	.000	I
Froot Loops, Kellogg's	120	0.8	1.6	28.2	15.0	0.6		60	.43	.50	100	150	3	8	3.75	
1 cup (1.1 oz)	32	0.9	0.4	0.2	0.3	0	750	.38	5.0		.10	34	20	4.50	.020	I
Frosted Bran, Kellogg's	110	0.9	2.4	27.0	9.8	3.0		15	.43	.50	100	213	10	40	3.80	
¾ cup (1.09 oz)	31	1.0	0.1	0.3	0.7	0	750	.38	5.0	1.50		126	10	4.50	.080	I
Frosted Cheerios, General Mills	120		2.0	25.0	13.0	1.0		15	.43	.50	100	210	20	16	3.75	
1 cup (1.06 oz)	30	1.0	0.0	0.0	0.0	0	750	.38	5.0	.00	.00	60	60	4.50	.000	I
Frosted Flakes, Kellogg's	119	0.8	1.0	28.4	13.0	0.5		15	.43	.50	100	200	1	2	.16	
¾ cup (1.09 oz)	31	0.2	0.1	0.0	0.1	0	750	.38	5.0			20	9	4.50	.010	I
Frosted Flakes, Quaker	116	0.6	1.5	27.6	12.1	1.0		16	.44	.52	103	281	1	8	.15	
¾ cup (1.09 oz)	31	0.4	0.1	0.1	0.2	0	1292	.39	5.2	.00	.06	30	17	4.65	.020	I
Frosted Krispies, Kellogg's	98	0.6	1.2	23.5	9.6	0.3		15	.43	.50	100	190	2	7	.30	
¾ cup (.9 oz)	26	0.2	0.1	0.1	0.1	0	750	.38	5.0			20	20	1.80	.030	I
Frosted Mini-Wheats, bite size, Kellogg's	201	3.1	5.5	48.0	12.0	6.3	0	0	.43	.50	100	2	9	60	1.50	
1 cup (2.08 oz)	59	1.0	0.2	0.2	0.6	0	0	.38	5.0	1.50		200	150	16.20	.200	I
Frosted Mini-Wheats, Kellogg's	180	2.7	4.8	41.0	10.0	5.0	0	0	.43	.50	100	1	18	60	1.50	
5 biscuits (1.8 oz)	51	0.8	0.2	0.1	0.6	0	0	.38	5.0	1.50		170	150	14.40	.160	I
Frosted Rice Krinkles	108	0.5	1.3	25.5		0.2	371	0	.42	.50	99	176	4	8	1.48	.304
⅞ cup (1 oz)	28	0.1	0.0	0.0	0.0	0	1235	.36	4.9	1.48	.13	14	20	1.76	.047	808
Frosted Wheat Bites, Nabisco	102		4.0	44.0	12.0	5.0	0	0	.43	.50	100	10	20	40	1.50	
1 cup (1.8 oz)	52	1.0	0.0			0	0	.38	5.0	1.50		170	150	1.80	.160	I
Fruit & Fibre w/ dates, raisins & walnuts, Post—1 cup (2.1 oz)	210		4.0	46.0	15.0	6.0		0	.51	.60	120					
	60	3.0	0.5			0	1500	.45	6.0	1.80						I
Fruit & Fibre w/ peaches, raisins & almonds, Post—1 cup (2.1 oz)	210		4.0	46.0	15.0	6.0		0	.51	.60	120	270	20	80	1.50	
	60	3.0	0.5			0	1500	.45	6.0	1.80		280	20	5.40	.300	I
Fruit Wheats																
Blueberry, Nabisco	170		4.0	41.0	10.0	4.0	0	0	.43	.50	100	15	20	40	1.50	
¾ cup (1.8 oz)	51	0.5	0.0			0	750	.38	5.0	1.50		170	100	1.80	.160	I
Raspberry, Nabisco	160		4.0	40.0	10.0	4.0	0	0	.43	.50	100	15	20	40	1.50	
¾ cup (1.7 oz)	49	0.5	0.0			0	750	.38	5.0	1.50		160	100	1.80		I
Strawberry, Nabisco	170		4.0	41.0	12.0	4.0	0	0	.43	.50	100	15	20	40	1.50	
¾ cup (1.8 oz)	51	0.5	0.0			0	200	.38	5.0	1.50		160	100	1.80	.160	I
Fruitany Ohs, Quaker	121	0.8	1.5	27.0	13.4	0.8		12	.44	.52	103	160	3	18	3.88	
1 cup (1.1 oz)	31	1.1	0.3	0.5	0.5	0	1034	.39	5.2	.00	.11	55	55	4.65	.050	I

						Vitamins					Minerals				
KCAL	H₂O (g)	PRO (g)	CHO (g)	SUGR (g)	DFIB (g)	A (RE)	C (mg)	B-2 (mg)	B-6 (mg)	FOL (mcg)	Na (mg)	Ca (mg)	Mg (mg)	Zn (mg)	Mn (mg)
WT (g)	FAT (g)	SFA (g)	MUFA (g)	PUFA (g)	CHOL (mg)	A (IU)	B-1 (mg)	NIA (mg)	B-12 (mcg)	PANT (mg)	K (mg)	P (mg)	Fe (mg)	Cu (mg)	REF
Fruity Marshmallow Krispies, Kellogg's															
106	0.8	1.3	25.3	13.0	0.3		15	.43	.50	100	167	2	7	.32	
¾ cup (1 oz)															
28	0.1	0.0	0.0	0.1	0	750	.38	5.0			16	24	1.80	.040	I
Fruity Pebbles, Post															
110		1.0	24.0	12.0	0.0		0	.43	.50	100	150	0	0	1.50	
¾ cup (.95 oz)															
27	1.0	0.5			0	1250	.38	5.0	1.50		20	0	1.81	.040	I
Golden Crisp, Post															
110		1.0	25.0	15.0	0.0		0	.43	.50	100	40	0	16	1.50	
¾ cup (.95 oz)															
27	0.0	0.0	0.0	0.0	0	1250	.38	5.0	1.50		35	40	1.80	.040	I
Golden Grahams, General Mills															
120		1.0	25.0	11.0	0.0		15	.43	.50	100	280	0	8	3.75	
¾ cup (1.06 oz)															
30	1.0	0.0	0.0	0.0	0	750	.38	5.0	.00	.00	55	40	4.50	.000	I
Golden Multi-Grain Flakes, Healthy															
Choice—*¾ cup (1.09 oz)* 107	0.9	2.6	26.1	6.0	2.9		0	.60	.70	100	180	9	32	1.50	
31	0.4	0.0	0.2	0.2	0	500	.53	7.0	2.10	3.50	100	80	6.30	.080	I
granola															
banana nut, Sunbelt															
254	1.7	5.2	38.1	11.8	3.2			.20			49	36			
1.9 oz															
55	9.2	4.0			1		.12	1.2					1.05		I
fruit & nut, Sunbelt															
246	2.6	4.9	38.7	16.4	3.4		0	.29			61	42			
1.9 oz															
55	8.0	2.5			1		.12	0.1					1.16		I
fruit, low-fat, General Mills															
210		4.0	44.0	19.0	3.0	0	0	.03	.00	0	210	20	24	.60	
⅔ cup (1.9 oz)															
55	2.5	0.0	1.0	0.5	0	0	.12	0.0	.00	.00	150	150	1.44	.040	I
Hearty, Post															
280		5.0	45.0	15.0	4.0		0	.43	.50	100	150	20	40	.90	
⅔ cup (2.15 oz)															
61	9.0	1.0			0	1250	.37	5.0	1.50		115	150	4.50	.200	I
homemade															
131	1.5	4.1	14.8		2.9	1	0	.08	.09	24	7	23	50	1.14	
¼ cup (1 oz)															
28	6.9	1.3	2.2	3.0	0	10	.21	0.6	.00	.17	151	129	1.18	.171	808
low-fat, Kellogg's															
190	1.7	4.1	39.3	12.0	2.9		2	.43	.50	100	120	19	40	3.80	
½ cup (1.7 oz)															
49	2.9	0.5	0.6	1.9	0	750	.38	5.0	1.50		122	100	1.80	.080	I
low-fat, Sunbelt															
220	3.2	4.4	43.3	19.9	3.0	0	0	.13			83	27			
1.9 oz															
55	3.2	0.9			0	0	.09	1.1					1.05		I
Nature Valley															
126	1.2	3.0	18.4		1.8	0	0	.03	.04	4	45	21	27	.56	.665
⅓ cup (1 oz)															
28	4.9	0.6	3.3	1.0	0	0	.09	0.3	.00	.23	93	81	.87	.081	808
oats & honey, Quaker 100% Natural															
219	1.2	5.3	31.4	13.1	3.3		0	.12	.07	15	20	61	51	1.05	
½ cup (1.7 oz)															
48	9.2	3.8	4.1	1.2	1	3	.13	0.8	.10	.32	225	158	1.21	.300	I
oats, honey, & raisins, Quaker 100%															
Natural—*½ cup (1.8 oz)* 225	2.0	5.1	34.4	16.1	3.3		0	.12	.08	14	19	59	49	.99	
51	8.6	3.6	3.8	1.1	1	4	.13	0.8	.10	.29	250	152	1.24	.300	I
w/ almonds, Sun Country															
266	0.8	6.7	38.3	11.6	3.0		0	.10	.07	19	19	49	52	1.14	
½ cup (2 oz)															
57	9.5	1.3	3.3	1.8	0	0	.18	0.5	.04	.32	221	168	2.48	.170	I
w/ raisins & dates, Sun Country															
262	1.7	5.9	43.3	17.5	3.6		0	.13	.08	19	15	46	50	.96	
½ cup (2.1 oz)															
60	8.2	1.2	2.8	1.6	0	0	.17	0.5	.12	.32	257	178	2.50	.160	I
w/ raisins, low-fat, Kellogg's															
220	3.2	4.9	47.2	16.0	3.0		4	.43	.50	100	150	20	40	3.80	
⅔ cup (2.1 oz)															
60	3.0	1.0	0.7	1.3	0	750	.38	5.0	1.50		170	150	1.80	.120	I
w/ raisins, low-fat, Quaker 100% Natural	213	2.1	4.6	44.3	18.3	3.0		0	.06	.08	13	145	33	44	1.02
⅔ cup (1.9 oz)															
55	3.0	0.8	1.3	0.7	0	10	.16	1.0	.00	.25	189	130	1.43	.170	I
Grape-Nut Flakes, Post															
100		3.0	24.0	5.0	3.0		0	.43	.50	100	140	0	32	1.20	
¾ cup (1.02 oz)															
29	1.0	0.0			0	1250	.38	5.0	1.50		80	80	8.10	.160	I
Grape-Nuts, Post															
200		6.0	47.0	7.0	5.0		0	.43	.50	100	350	20	60	1.20	
½ cup (2 oz)															
58	1.0	0.0			0	1250	.38	5.0	1.50		160	150	8.10	.200	I
Great Grains Crunchy Pecan, Post															
220		5.0	38.0	8.0	4.0		0	.43	.50	100	150	20	40	1.20	
⅔ cup (1.87 oz)															
53	6.0	1.0			0	1250	.38	5.0	1.50		120	150	2.70	.200	I
Great Grains Raisins, Dates & Pecans,															
Post—*⅔ cup (1.9 oz)* 210		4.0	39.0	13.0	4.0		0	.51	.60	120	150	20	40	1.20	
54	5.0	0.5			0	1500	.45	6.0	1.80		150	150	3.60	.200	I
Heartland Natural															
122	1.1	2.8	19.1		1.7	2	0	.04	.05	16	71	18	36	.74	
¼ cup (1 oz)															
28	4.3	1.1	1.2	1.7	0	16	.09	0.4	.00	.23	94	101	1.06	.072	808
w/ coconut															
123	0.9	2.9	19.0		2.0	2	0	.04	.04	15	57	18	37	.73	
¼ cup (1 oz)															
28	4.6	1.7	1.1	1.5	0	15	.09	0.5	.00	.22	102	101	1.44	.142	808
w/ raisins															
119	1.4	2.7	19.3		1.5	2	0	.04	.05	11	57	17	36	.72	
¼ cup (1 oz)															
28	4.0	1.0	1.1	1.6	0	16	.08	0.4	.00	.23	106	96	1.02	.118	808
Honey & Nut Toasty O's, Malt-O-Meal															
107	0.7	3.1	22.6		1.5		15	.43	.50	0	172	28	31	1.08	
¾ cup (1 oz)															
28	1.2	0.3			0	1250	.38	5.0	1.50		93	105	4.50	.110	I
Honey Bran															
95	0.7	2.5	22.9		3.1	371	15	.42	.50	19	162	13	37	.72	1.072
⅞ cup (1 oz)															
28	0.6	0.2	0.1	0.2	0	1235	.36	4.9	1.48	.16	120	106	4.45	.133	808
Honey Bunches of Oats, Post															
120		2.0	25.0	6.0	1.0		0	.43	.50	100	190	0	16	.30	
¾ cup (1.06 oz)															
30	1.5	0.5			0	1250	.38	5.0	1.50		50	40	2.70	.080	I
Honey Bunches of Oats w/ almonds, Post															
130		3.0	24.0	6.0	1.0		0	.43	.50	100	180	0	24	.30	
¾ cup (1.09 oz)															
31	3.0	0.5			0	1250	.38	5.0	1.50		65	60	2.70	.080	I

	KCAL	H₂O (g)	PRO (g)	CHO (g)	SUGR (g)	DFIB (g)	A (RE)	C (mg)	B-2 (mg)	B-6 (mg)	FOL (mcg)	Na (mg)	Ca (mg)	Mg (mg)	Zn (mg)	Mn (mg)
	WT (g)	FAT (g)	SFA (g)	MUFA (g)	PUFA (g)	CHOL (mg)	A (IU)	B-1 (mg)	NIA (mg)	B-12 (mcg)	PANT (mg)	K (mg)	P (mg)	Fe (mg)	Cu (mg)	REF
Honey Crunch Corn Flakes, Kellogg's	110		2.0	26.0	10.0	1.0		15	.43	.50	100	270	0			
¾ cup (1.06 oz)	30	1.0	0.0			0	750	.38	5.0			35		1.80		I
Honey Frosted Wheaties, General Mills	110		1.0	27.0	12.0	0.0		15	.43	.50	100	200	20	0	3.75	
¾ cup (1.06 oz)	30	0.0	0.0	0.0	0.0	0	750	.38	5.0	.00	.00	35	20	4.50	.000	I
Honey Graham Oh!s, Quaker	112	0.5	1.4	22.8	11.1	0.7		12	.43	.50	100	178	12	13	3.76	
¾ cup (1 oz)	27	1.9	0.6	1.1	0.3	0	1004	.38	5.0	.00	.08	45	42	4.52	.040	I
Honey Nut Cheerios, General Mills	120		3.0	24.0	11.0	2.0		15	.43	.50	100	270	0	24	3.75	
1 cup (1.06 oz)	30	1.5	0.0	0.5	0.0	0	750	.38	5.0	.00	.00	95	100	4.50	.040	I
Honey Nut Clusters, General Mills	210		4.0	46.0	16.0	3.0	0	9	.43	.50	100	270	40	32	.60	
1 cup (1.9 oz)	55	2.5	0.0			0		.38	5.0	.00	.00	130	100	4.50	.080	I
Honeycomb, Post	110		2.0	26.0	11.0	1.0	0		.43	.50	100	190	0	8	1.50	
1 ⅓ cups (1.02 oz)	29	0.0	0.0	0.0	0.0	0	1250	.38	5.0	1.50		35	20	2.70	.040	I
Just Right w/ fiber nuggets, Kellogg's	209	1.8	4.3	47.2	11.9	2.8			.43	.50	100	320	9	32	.90	
1 cup (1.98 oz)	56	1.5	0.0	0.9	0.3	0		.38	5.0	1.50		120	6	16.20	.080	I
Just Right w/ fruit & nuts, Kellogg's	210	4.1	4.0	48.3	15.0	3.0			.43	.20	100	290	0	40	1.20	
1 cup (2.1 oz)	60	1.5	0.0			0		.38	5.0	1.50		170	100	16.20	.080	I
Kaboom, General Mills	120		3.0	24.0	6.0	1.0		15	.43	.50	100	280	40	16	3.75	
1 ¼ cups (1.06 oz)	30	1.5	0.0	0.0	0.0	0	750	.38	5.0	.00	.00	65	80	8.10	.000	I
King Vitaman, Quaker	120	0.6	2.3	26.1	6.3	1.2		13	.44	.52	104	260	4	26	3.91	
1.5 cups (1.1 oz)	31	1.1	0.3	0.4	0.3	0	1044	.39	5.2	1.57	.16	86	79	8.74	.080	I
Kix, General Mills	120		2.0	26.0	3.0	1.0		15	.43	.50	100	270	40	8	3.75	
1 ⅓ cups (1.06 oz)	30	0.5	0.0	0.0	0.0	0	1250	.38	5.0	.00	.00	45	40	8.10	.000	I
Life, oat cinn, Quaker	120	1.3	2.9	25.6	9.5	1.9		0	.46	.54	107	145	85	27	4.02	
¾ cup (1.1 oz)	32	1.2	0.2	0.4	0.4	0	10	.40	5.4	.00	.14	72	117	4.82	.070	I
Life, Quaker	121	1.3	3.2	25.2	6.4	2.0		0	.45	.53	107	175	98	31	4.00	
¾ cup (1.1 oz)	32	1.3	0.2	0.4	0.6	0	11	.40	5.3	.00	.21	79	136	8.96	.090	I
Lucky Charms, General Mills	120		2.0	25.0	13.0	1.0		15	.43	.50	100	210	20	16	3.75	
1 cup (1.06 oz)	30	1.0	0.0	0.0	0.0	0	750	.38	5.0	.00	.00	60	60	4.10	.000	I
Marshmallow Alpha-Bits, Post	120		2.0	25.0	14.0	1.0	0		.43	.50	100	160	0	16	1.50	
1 cup (1.02 oz)	29	1.0	0.0			0	1250	.37	5.0	1.50		45	60	2.70	.040	I
Marshmallow Safari, Quaker	119	0.6	1.7	25.3	14.2	1.3		12	.43	.50	100	192	26	17	3.75	
¾ cup (1.06 oz)	30	1.5	0.4	0.8	0.4	0	1000	.38	5.0	.00	.12	42	59	4.50	.070	I
muesli, 5 whole grains, Sunbelt	206	5.0	5.3	41.9	15.3	3.8		2	.18			105	26			
1.9 oz	55	1.9	0.3			0	194	.14	2.8					2.04		I
Multi-Grain Cheerios, General Mills	110		3.0	24.0	6.0	3.0		15	.43	.50	100	240	40	24	3.75	
1 cup (1.06 oz)	30	1.0	0.0	0.0	0.0	0	750	.38	5.0	.00	.00	100	100	8.10	.040	I
muselix, apple & almond crunch, Kellogg's—¾ cup (1.87 oz)	203	2.2	5.2	39.4	8.9	4.5						260	33	60	3.00	
	53	4.8				0				1.50	2.00	201	150	4.50	.080	I
muselix, raisin & almond crunch w/ dates, Kellogg's—⅔ cup (1.9 oz)	200	5.7	4.0	40.0	17.0	3.8		0	.43	.50	100	160	20	40	3.75	
	55	3.2	0.0	2.0	1.0	0	200	.38	5.0	1.50	2.50	230	150	4.50	.080	I
Nutri-Grain, almond raisin, Kellogg's	180	3.0	3.9	38.0	7.0	3.9	0	0	.43	.50	100	174	149	16	3.75	
1 ¼ cup (1.7 oz)	49	2.8	0.1	1.3	1.4	0	0	.38	5.0	1.50		180	200	1.40	.080	I
Nutri-Grain, wheat, Kellogg's	100	1.1	3.0	24.0	0.4	3.8	0	15	.43	.50	100	221	9	24	3.75	
¾ cup (1.06 oz)	30	1.0	0.1	0.2	0.7	0	0	.38	5.0	1.50		109	100	1.08	.040	I
oat bran, Common Sense	109	1.0	3.9	23.2	6.3	4.0	0		.43	.50	100	270	14	40	3.75	
¾ cup (1.06 oz)	30	1.2	0.3	0.6	0.3	0	750	.38	5.0	1.50		120	150	8.10	.080	I
Oatmeal Crisp																
almond, General Mills	220		6.0	42.0	15.0	4.0	0	9	.43	.50	100	250	20	60	3.75	
1 cup (1.9 oz)	55	5.0	0.5	2.5	1.0	0	0	.38	5.0	.00	.00	190	150	4.50	.160	I
apple, General Mills	210		4.0	46.0	19.0	4.0	0	9	.43	.50	100	280	20	40	3.75	
1 cup (1.9 oz)	55	2.0	0.0	0.5	0.0	0	0	.38	5.0	.00	.00	160	100	4.50	.120	I
raisin, General Mills	210		4.0	44.0	19.0	3.0	0		.43	.50	100	210	20	40	3.75	
1 cup (1.9 oz)	55	2.5	0.0	1.0	0.0	0	750	.38	5.0	.00	.00	220	100	4.50	.160	I
Oatmeal Squares, Quaker	216	1.3	7.3	43.3	9.3	4.3		7	.48	.56	113	263	36	70	4.22	
1 cup (2 oz)	56	2.6	0.5	0.8	1.1	0	563	.42	5.6	.00	.44	228	186	16.20	.240	I
100% Natural, cinn & raisin, Nature Valley—¾ cup (1.9 oz)	240		5.0	38.0	14.0	3.0	0		.03	.00	0	90	40	40	.90	
	55	8.0	1.0			0	0	.15	0.4	.00	.00	80	150	1.08	.120	I
100% Natural, oat, fruit & nut, Nature Valley—⅔ cup (1.9 oz)	250		6.0	34.0	13.0	3.0	0	0	.07	.00	0	75	40	40	.90	
	55	11.0	2.0			0	0	.15	0.4	.00	.00	190	150	1.44	.160	I
Product 19, Kellogg's	100	0.9	2.3	25.1	3.5	1.0		60	1.70	2.00	400	280	3	16	15.00	
1 cup (1.06 oz)	30	0.2	0.0			0	750	1.50	20.0	6.00	10.00	50	40	18.00	.030	I

	KCAL / WT (g)	H₂O (g) / FAT (g)	PRO (g) / SFA (g)	CHO (g) / MUFA (g)	SUGR (g) / PUFA (g)	DFIB (g) / CHOL (mg)	A (RE) / A (IU)	C (mg) / B-1 (mg)	B-2 (mg) / NIA (mg)	B-6 (mg) / B-12 (mcg)	FOL (mcg) / PANT (mg)	Na (mg) / K (mg)	Ca (mg) / P (mg)	Mg (mg) / Fe (mg)	Zn (mg) / Cu (mg)	Mn (mg) / REF
puffed rice	56	0.4	0.9	12.6	0.0	0.2	0	0	.25	.01	3	0	1	4	.14	.210
	14	0.1	0.0			0	0	.36	4.9	.00	.04	16	14	4.44	.024	808
Malt-O-Meal	54	0.7	1.0	12.2		0.1			.26			0				
1 cup (.5 oz)	14	0.2	0.0	0.1	0.1	0		.38	5.0			18	20	4.51		I
Quaker	54	0.6	1.0	12.3	0.0	0.2	0	0	.01	.00	1	1	1	4	.15	
1 cup (.5 oz)	14	0.1	0.1	0.0	0.1	0	0	.06	0.9	.00	.05	16	17	.41	.130	I
puffed wheat	51	0.4	2.1	11.1	0.2	0.6	0	0	.25	.02	4	1	4	20	.33	.246
1 cup (.5 oz)	14	0.2	0.0			0	0	.36	4.9	.00	.07	49	50	4.44	.057	808
Malt-O-Meal	53	0.7	2.5	10.4		1.2			.26			0		21	.51	
1 cup (.5 oz)	14	0.4	0.1	0.1	0.2	0		.38	5.0			57		4.50	.040	I
Quaker	55	0.6	2.4	11.5	0.2	1.4	0	0	.04	.02	5	1	4	20	.46	
1.25 cup (.5 oz)	15	0.3	0.1	0.1	0.2	0	2	.06	1.8	.06	.07	55	50	.70	.090	I
Quisp/Sweet Crunch, Quaker	109	0.7	1.4	23.0	11.8	0.7		0	.43	.51	102	194	5	14	3.82	
1 cup (1 oz)	27	1.5	0.4	0.5	0.5	0	33	.38	5.1	.00	.09	36	42	4.58	.060	I
raisin bran																
General Mills	200		4.0	41.0	19.0	3.0	0	0	.43	.50	100	250	60	40	.90	
¾ cup (1.9 oz)	55	4.0	0.5	2.5	0.5	0	0	.38	5.0	.00	.00	220	150	4.50	.160	I
Kellogg's	197	5.5	6.0	47.1	18.0	8.2		0	.43	.50	100	390	35	80	3.75	
1 cup (2.15 oz)	61	1.5	0.0	0.5	1.0	0	750	.38	5.0	1.50		350	200	4.50	.300	I
Malt-O-Meal	129	3.0	3.3	29.7		4.6		6	.43	.50	100	199	16	49	2.57	
¾ cup (1.4 oz)	40	1.7				0	1250	.38	5.0			226	143	4.50	.160	I
Post	190		4.0	46.0	20.0	8.0		0	.60	.70	140	300	20	100	2.25	
1 cup (2.08 oz)	59	1.0	0.0			0	1750	.53	7.0	2.10		380	250	6.30	.300	I
Ralston Purina	121	2.8	3.0	31.5		5.1	377	1	.42	.49	101	330	18	57	1.14	1.440
¾ cup (1.3 oz)	38	0.2	0.0	0.0	0.1	0	1257	.38	5.0	1.52	.28	195	168	18.54	.207	808
Reese's Peanut Butter Puffs, General Mills—¾ cup (1.06 oz)	130		2.0	23.0	12.0	0.0		15	.43	.50	100	210	20	0	3.75	
	30	3.0	0.5	1.5	1.0	0	750	.38	5.0	1.50	.00	45	40	4.10	.000	I
Rice Krispies																
apple cinn, Kellogg's	108	0.9	1.5	25.8	11.0	0.0		15	.43	.50	100	216	2	8	.30	
¾ cup (1.02 oz)	29	0.1	0.0			0	750	.38	5.0			30	20	1.80		I
frosted, Kellogg's	106	0.6	1.3	25.3		0.3	242	16	.45	.53	112	205	2	7	.34	.210
1 cup (1 oz)	28	0.2	0.1	0.1	0.1	0	808	.39	5.4	.00	.19	22	22	1.93	.028	808
Kellogg's	120	0.8	2.3	28.5	3.0	0.5		15	.43	.50	100	350	3	16	.60	
1 ¼ cup (1.16 oz)	33	0.2	0.0			0	750	.38	5.0			39	40	1.80	.040	I
Treats, Kellogg's	120	1.1	1.1	25.7	8.6	0.3		15	.43	.50	100	190	2	6		
¾ cup (1.06 oz)	30	1.5	0.3	1.0	0.2	0	750	.38	5.0	1.50		19	20	1.80		I
S'mores Grahams, General Mills	120		1.0	26.0	13.0	0.0		15	.43	.50	100	220	0	8	3.75	
¾ cup (1.06 oz)	30	1.0		0.5		0	750	.38	5.0	.00	.00	45	20	4.10	.040	I
shredded wheat	102	1.1	3.1	23.0		2.8	0	0	.08	.07	14	1	12	48	.71	.870
1 oz	28	0.5	0.1	0.1	0.2	0	0	.08	1.3	.00	.23	93	103	.89	.142	808
1 biscuit	86	1.3	2.6	19.3	0.1	2.4	0	0	.07	.06	12	2	9	32	.79	.737
(.8 oz)	24	0.4	0.1	0.1	0.2	0	0	.06	1.3	.00	.20	87	85	1.01	.159	808
Nabisco	160		5.0	38.0	0.0	5.0	0	0	.00	.16	16	0	20	60	1.20	
2 biscuits (1.06 oz)	46	0.5	0.0			0	0	.12	0.2	.00		200	150	1.44	.160	I
Quaker	216	3.4	7.0	50.4	0.5	7.3	0	0	.07	.16	32	3	28	107	1.58	
3 biscuits (2.2 oz)	63	1.3	0.4	0.2	0.8	0		.14	3.3	.00	.51	223	225	2.07	.320	I
spoon size, Nabisco	170		5.0	41.0	0.0	5.0	0	0	.03	.16	16	0	20	60	1.20	
1 cup (1.73 oz)	49	0.5	0.0			0	0	.12	3.0	.00		200	200	1.44	.160	I
Shredded Wheat 'n Bran, Nabisco	200		7.0	47.0	1.0	8.0	0	0	.03	.16	24	0	20	80	2.25	
1 ¼ cups (2.08 oz)	59	1.0	0.0			0	0	.15	4.0	.00		250	250	2.70	.200	I
Shredded Wheat Squares																
apple cinn, Kellogg's	182	5.2	4.0	44.1	11.7	4.7		0	.43	.50	100	20	20	40	1.50	
¾ cup (1.9 oz)	55	1.0	0.2	0.3	0.5	0	0	.38	5.0	1.50		166	150	16.20	.120	I
blueberry, Kellogg's	181	2.9	4.0	43.0	11.0	5.0		0	.43	.50	100	20	15	60	1.50	
¾ cup (1.9 oz)	54	1.0	0.2	0.2	0.5	0	0	.38	5.0	2.00		180	150	16.20	.120	I
raisin, Kellogg's	180	5.0	4.2	41.3	11.0	5.0		0	.43	.50	100	3	10	40	1.50	
¾ cup (1.87 oz)	53	1.5	0.2	0.1	0.5	0	0	.38	5.0	1.50		250	150	16.20	.120	I
strawberry, Kellogg's	170	4.3	4.0	39.5	8.7	4.6		0	.43	.50	100	15	20	60	1.50	
¾ cup (1.76 oz)	50	1.5	0.0			0	0	.38	5.0	1.50		170	150	16.20	.120	I

	KCAL	H₂O (g)	PRO (g)	CHO (g)	SUGR (g)	DFIB (g)	A (RE)	C (mg)	B-2 (mg)	B-6 (mg)	FOL (mcg)	Na (mg)	Ca (mg)	Mg (mg)	Zn (mg)	Mn (mg)
	WT (g)	FAT (g)	SFA (g)	MUFA (g)	PUFA (g)	CHOL (mg)	A (IU)	B-1 (mg)	NIA (mg)	B-12 (mcg)	PANT (mg)	K (mg)	P (mg)	Fe (mg)	Cu (mg)	REF
Smacks, Kellogg's	103	0.8	1.7	23.7	14.7	1.0		15	.43	.50	100	51	3	14	.31	
¾ cup (.95 oz)	27	0.5	0.3	0.1	0.2	0	750	.38	5.0			40	35	1.80	.040	I
Special K, Kellogg's	110	0.9	6.4	22.4	3.0	1.0		15	.60	.70	100	250	5	18	3.75	
1 cup (1.09 oz)	31	0.3	0.0	0.0	0.2	0	750	.53	7.0	1.50	.15	54	60	8.10	.030	I
Streusel, Betty Crocker	120		2.0	25.0	8.0	1.0		15	.43	.50	100	180	20	16	3.75	
¾ cup (1.06 oz)	30	1.5	0.0	0.0	0.0	0	750	.38	5.0	.00	.00	60	60	4.10	.040	I
Sugar Corn Pops, Kellogg's	107	0.8	1.0	25.7		0.4	210	14	.39	.48	99	111	2	2	1.40	.068
1 cup (1 oz)	28	0.2	0.1	0.1	0.0	0	700	.36	4.7	.00	.08	20	6	1.68	.028	808
Sugar Frosted Corn Flakes, Malt-O-Meal	109	0.3	1.4	26.0		0.6		15	.43	.50	100	186			1.10	
¾ cup (1 oz)	28	0.2	0.0	0.1	0.1	0	1250	.38	5.0			24		1.94	.010	I
Sugar Frosted Flakes, Ralston Purina	109	0.4	1.5	25.2		0.6	371	15	.42	.50	2	182	3	2	.60	.017
¾ cup (1 oz)	28	0.4	0.2	0.1	0.1	0	1235	.36	4.9	1.48	.01	18	7	.70	.019	808
Sugar Puffs, Malt-O-Meal	109	0.6	2.5	24.7		1.0			.43	.50	100	23		18	.45	
1 cup (1 oz)	28	0.4	0.1	0.1	0.2	0	1248	.37	5.0	1.50		51	54	4.48	.070	I
Sun Crunchers, General Mills	220		5.0	45.0	16.0	2.0		15	.43	.50	100	370	80	40	.60	
1 cup (1.94 oz)	55	3.0	0.0	0.0	0.0	0	750	.38	5.0	.00	.00	130	150	4.10	.160	I
Sweet Puffs, Quaker	133	0.8	2.3	29.9	16.4	1.2		0	.04	.02	6	80	3	19	.42	
1 cup (1.2 oz)	34	0.7	0.1	0.2	0.3	0		.05	1.5	.05	.11	50	48	.66	.080	I
Tasteeos, Ralston Purina	110	0.6	3.6	22.1		3.0	371	15	.42	.50	99	213	13	31	.80	
1¼ cups (1 oz)	28	0.8	0.3	0.2	0.2	0	1235	.36	4.9	1.48	.14	83	112	8.01	.165	808
Team Flakes, Nabisco	220	2.2	4.0	49.0	10.0	1.0		15	.43	.50	0	360	0	24	.90	.731
1¼ cups (2 oz)	57		0.0	0.3	0.4	0	1250	.38	5.0	1.50		80	80	8.10	.120	MUL
Temptations, french van almond, Kellogg's—3/4 cup (.9 oz)	103	0.7	1.8	21.4	7.6	1.0		15	.43	.50		179	9			
	26	1.4	0.9	0.0	0.5	0	750	.38	5.0			35		4.50		I
Temptations, honey roasted pecan, Kellogg's—⅔ cup (1.02 oz)	118	0.8	1.7	23.6	9.0	7.0		15	.43	.50	100	240	0			
	29	2.2	0.5	1.1	0.6	0	750	.38	5.0			28		4.50		I
Toasted Brown Sugar Squares, Healthy Choice—1 cup (1.9 oz)	186	2.7	5.1	44.2	9.0	5.0	0		.60	.70	100	2	18	60	1.50	
	54	1.0	0.2	0.6	0.3	0	500	.53	7.0	2.10	3.50	210	200	6.30	.120	I
Toasty O's, Malt-O-Meal	107	1.3	3.8	20.3		1.8		15	.43	.50		236	41	32	.80	
1¼ cups (1 oz)	28	2.0	0.3	0.8	0.7	0	1250	.38	5.0	1.50		92	108	8.10	.130	I
Tootie Fruities, Malt-O-Meal	113	0.6	1.5	24.7		0.6		15	.43	.50	100	121		8	3.74	
1 cup (1 oz)	28	1.1	0.2	0.6	0.2	0	1248	.37	5.0			30	29	4.48	.030	I
Total Corn Flakes, General Mills	110		2.0	25.0	3.0	0.0		60	1.70	2.00	400	210	200	0	15.00	
1.3 cups (1.06 oz)	30	0.5	0.0	0.0	0.0	0	1250	1.50	20.0	6.00	10.00	30	100	18.00	.000	I
Total, General Mills	110		3.0	24.0	5.0	3.0		60	1.70	2.00	400	200	250	24	15.00	
¾ cup (1.06 oz)	30	1.0	0.0	0.0	0.0	0	1250	1.50	20.0	6.00	10.00	100	200	18.00	.080	I
Total Raisin Bran, General Mills	180		4.0	43.0	19.0	5.0		0	1.70	2.00	400	240	200	40	15.00	
1 cup (1.9 oz)	55	1.0	0.0	0.0	0.0	0	1250	1.50	20.0	6.00	10.00	290	250	18.00	.160	I
Triples, General Mills	120		2.0	25.0	6.0	0.0		15	.43	.50	100	190	40	0	3.75	
1 cup (1.06 oz)	30	1.0	0.0	0.0	0.0	0	1250	.38	5.0	.00	.00	30	20	8.10	.040	I
Trix, General Mills	120		1.0	26.0	13.0	0.0		15	.43	.50	100	200	20	0	3.75	
1 cup (1.06 oz)	30	1.5	0.0	1.0	0.0	0	750	.38	5.0	.00	.00	20	20	4.10	.000	I
Wheaties, General Mills	110		3.0	24.0	4.0	3.0		15	.43	.50	100	220	0	32	.60	
1 cup (1.06 oz)	30	1.0	0.0	0.0	0.0	0	1250	.38	5.0	.00	.00	110	100	8.10	.080	I

5. CHEESE & CHEESE PRODUCTS
5.1 CHEESE

Food / Serving	KCAL / WT (g)	H2O (g) / FAT (g)	PRO (g) / SFA (g)	CHO (g) / MUFA (g)	SUGR (g) / PUFA (g)	DFIB (g) / CHOL (mg)	A (RE) / A (IU)	C (mg) / B-1 (mg)	B-2 (mg) / NIA (mg)	B-6 (mg) / B-12 (mcg)	FOL (mcg) / PANT (mg)	Na (mg) / K (mg)	Ca (mg) / P (mg)	Mg (mg) / Fe (mg)	Zn (mg) / Cu (mg)	Mn (mg) / REF
american & swiss, processed,	101		5.8	0.7				0	.10			443	172			
Land O'Lakes—1 oz	28	8.3	5.2	2.2	0.3	26	269	.01	0.0			36	179	.13		I
american processed	106	11.1	6.3	0.5		0.0	82	0	.10	.02	2	406	174	6	.85	.004
1 oz	28	8.9	5.6	2.5	0.3	27	343	.01	0.0	.20	.14	46	211	.11	.009	801
extra melt, Land O'Lakes	104		5.6	0.7				0	.10			428	160			
1 oz	28	8.8	5.5	2.3	0.3	27	291	.01	0.0			38	173	.15		I
Harvest Moon	70		4.0	0.0	0.0			0	.07			320	100	0	60	
⅔ oz slice	19	6.0	4.0			20	200			.12		15	150	.00		I
Kraft	110		5.0	1.0	0.0	0.0		0	.10			460	150	0	.60	
1 oz slice	28	9.0	6.0			25	300			.12		25	200	.00		I
Old English	110		6.0	1.0	0.0	0.0		0	.10			460	150	0	.60	
1 oz slice	28	9.0	6.0			30	300			.12		20	200	.00		I
sharp, Land O'Lakes	102		5.9	0.5				0	.09			440	171		.00	
1 oz	28	8.6	5.4	2.2	0.3	27	279	.01	0.0			29	269	.16		I
blue	100	12.0	6.1	0.7		0.0	65	0	.11	.05	10	396	150	7	.75	.003
1 oz	28	8.1	5.3	2.2	0.2	21	204	.01	0.3	.35	.49	73	110	.09	.011	801
brick	105	11.7	6.6	0.8		0.0	86	0	.10	.02	6	159	191	7	.74	.003
1 oz	28	8.4	5.3	2.4	0.2	27	307	.00	0.0	.36	.08	38	128	.12	.007	801
brie	95	13.7	5.9	0.1		0.0	52	0	.15	.07	18	178	52	6	.67	.010
1 oz	28	7.8	4.9	2.3	0.2	28	189	.02	0.1	.47	.20	43	53	.14	.005	801
camembert	85	14.7	5.6	0.1		0.0	71	0	.14	.06	18	239	110	6	.67	.011
1 oz	28	6.9	4.3	2.0	0.2	20	262	.01	0.2	.37	.39	53	98	.09	.006	801
caraway	107	11.1	7.1	0.9		0.0	82	0	.13	.02	5	196	191	6	.83	.006
1 oz	28	8.3	5.3	2.3	0.2	26	299	.01	0.1	.08	.05	26	139	.18	.007	801
cheddar	114	10.4	7.1	0.4	0.5	0.0	86	0	.11	.02	5	176	204	8	.88	.003
1 oz	28	9.4	6.0	2.7	0.3	30	300	.01	0.0	.23	.12	28	145	.19	.009	801
	403	36.8	24.9	1.3	1.8	0.0	303	0	.38	.07	18	621	721	28	3.11	.010
3.5 oz	100	33.1	21.1	9.4	0.9	105	1059	.03	0.1	.83	.41	98	512	.68	.031	801
	455	41.5	28.1	1.4	2.0	0.0	342	0	.42	.08	21	701	815	31	3.51	.011
1 cup, not packed	113	37.4	23.8	10.6	1.1	119	1197	.03	0.1	.93	.47	111	579	.77	.035	801
extra sharp, processed, Land O'Lakes	100		6.0	1.0								370				
1 oz	28	9.0	6.0	2.0	0.0	30						30				I
fat-free, shredded, Kraft Healthy	45		10.0	1.0	0.0	0.0		0	.14			220	250	8	1.20	
Favorites—¼ cup	29	0.0	0.0	0.0	0.0	5	400			.24		20	150	.00		I
low-fat	49	17.9	6.9	0.5		0.0	18	0	.06	.01	3	174	118	5	.52	.002
1 oz	28	2.0	1.2	0.6	0.1	6	66	.00	0.0	.14	.05	19	137	.12	.006	801
low sodium	113	11.1	6.9	0.5		0.0	82	0	.11	.02	5	6	199	8	.88	.003
1 oz	28	9.2	5.9	2.6	0.3	28	297	.01	0.0	.24	.09	32	137	.20	.010	801
nacho blend w/ peppers, Kraft	110		7.0	0.0	0.0	0.0		0	.10			250	200	0	1.20	
1 oz	28	9.0	6.0			30	300			.24		15	150	.00		I
sharp, red fat, Kraft	80		9.0	1.0	0.0	0.0		0	.14			220	250	8	1.20	
1 oz	28	5.0	3.0			20	300			.24		20	150	.00		I
cheddar & bacon, processed,	110		6.0	1.0								350				
Land O'Lakes—1 oz	28	9.0	5.0	3.0	0.0	25						30				I
cheddar/colby/monterey, red fat, Kraft	80		9.0	0.0	0.0	0.0		0	.14			220	250	8	1.20	
1 oz	28	5.0	3.5			20	300			.24		15	150	.00		I
cheshire	110	10.7	6.6	1.4		0.0	69	0	.08	.02	5	198	182	6	.79	.003
1 oz	28	8.7	5.5	2.5	0.2	29	279	.01	0.0	.23	.12	27	131	.06	.012	801
colby	112	10.8	6.7	0.7		0.0	78	0	.11	.02	5	171	194	7	.87	.003
1 oz	28	9.1	5.7	2.6	0.3	27	293	.00	0.0	.23	.06	36	129	.22	.012	801
cottage cheese																
1% fat	164	186.4	28.0	6.1		0.0	25	0	.37	.15	28	918	138	12	.86	.007
1 cup	226	2.3	1.5	0.7	0.1	10	84	.05	0.3	1.43	.49	193	302	.32	.063	801
2% fat	203	179.2	31.1	8.2		0.0	45	0	.42	.17	30	918	155	14	.95	.007
1 cup	226	4.4	2.8	1.2	0.1	19	158	.05	0.3	1.61	.55	217	340	.36	.063	801
creamed	29	22.1	3.5	0.8	0.2	0.0	13	0	.05	.02	3	113	17	1	.10	.001
1 rd T	28	1.3	0.8	0.4	0.0	4	46	.01	0.0	.17	.06	24	37	.04	.008	801

	KCAL / WT (g)	H₂O (g) / FAT (g)	PRO (g) / SFA (g)	CHO (g) / MUFA (g)	SUGR (g) / PUFA (g)	DFIB (g) / CHOL (mg)	A (RE) / A (IU)	C (mg) / B-1 (mg)	B-2 (mg) / NIA (mg)	B-6 (mg) / B-12 (mcg)	FOL (mcg) / PANT (mg)	Na (mg) / K (mg)	Ca (mg) / P (mg)	Mg (mg) / Fe (mg)	Zn (mg) / Cu (mg)	Mn (mg) / REF
creamed	117	89.2	14.1	3.0	0.7	0.0	54	0	.18	.08	14	457	68	6	.42	.003
4 oz	113	5.1	3.2	1.5	0.2	17	184	.02	0.1	.70	.24	95	149	.16	.032	801
creamed	217	165.8	26.2	5.6	1.3	0.0	101	0	.34	.14	26	850	126	11	.78	.006
1 cup, not packed	210	9.5	6.0	2.7	0.3	31	342	.04	0.3	1.31	.45	177	277	.29	.059	801
creamed w/ fruit	279	162.9	22.4	30.1		0.0	81	0	.29	.12	22	915	108	9	.66	.007
1 cup	226	7.7	4.9	2.2	0.2	25	278	.04	0.2	1.12	.38	151	236	.25	.063	801
dry curd	123	115.7	25.0	2.7		0.0	12	0	.21	.12	21	19	46	6	.68	.004
1 cup, not packed	145	0.6	0.4	0.2	0.0	10	44	.04	0.2	1.20	.24	47	151	.33	.041	801
nonfat, Knudsen	80		15.0	4.0	2.0	0.0		0	.17			370	60			
½ cup	122	0.0	0.0	0.0	0.0	10	200	.00		.60		75	150	.00		I
cream cheese	99	15.2	2.1	0.8	0.5	0.0	124	0	.06	.01	4	84	23	2	.15	.001
1 oz (2 T)	28	9.9	6.2	2.8	0.4	31	405	.00	0.0	.12	.08	34	30	.34	.005	801
soft, fat-free, Philadelphia Brand	30		5.0	2.0	1.0	0.0		0	.03			160	100	0	.30	
2 T	33	0.0	0.0	0.0	0.0	5	500			.12		65	150	.00		I
soft, flavored, Philadelphia Brand	103		1.7	2.7	1.0	0.0		0	.50			138	23	0	.00	
2 T[1]	31	9.3	6.3		0.3	30	333			.00		53	23	.00		I
soft, light, Philadelphia Brand	70		3.0	2.0	2.0	0.0		0				150	40	0	.00	
2 T	32	5.0	3.5			15	400			.00		55	40	.00		I
soft, Philadelphia Brand	100		2.0	1.0	1.0	0.0		0	.03			100	20	0	.00	
2 T	30	10.0	7.0			30	300			.00		40	20	.00		I
whipped, Philadelphia Brand	110		2.0	1.0	1.0	0.0		0	.03			95	20	0	.00	
3 T	31	11.0	7.0			35	400			.00		35	20	.00		I
edam	101	11.8	7.1	0.4		0.0	72	0	.11	.02	5	274	207	8	1.06	.003
1 oz	28	7.9	5.0	2.3	0.2	25	260	.01	0.0	.44	.08	53	152	.12	.010	801
farmers, Kraft	100		6.0	1.0	0.0	0.0		0	.03			190	200	8	1.20	
1 oz	28	8.0	6.0			25	300			.48		25	150	.00		I
feta	75	15.7	4.0	1.2		0.0	36	0	.24	.12	9	316	140	5	.82	.008
1 oz	28	6.0	4.2	1.3	0.2	25	127	.04	0.3	.48	.27	18	96	.18	.009	801
fontina	110	10.8	7.3	0.4		0.0	82	0	.06	.02	2	227	156	4	.99	.004
1 oz	28	8.8	5.4	2.5	0.5	33	333	.01	0.0	.48	.12	18	98	.07	.007	801
gjetost	132	3.8	2.7	12.1		0.0	78	0	.39	.08	1	170	113	20	.32	.011
1 oz	28	8.4	5.4	2.2	0.3	27	316	.09	0.2	.69	.95	399	126	.15	.023	801
goat																
hard	128	8.2	8.7	0.6		0.0	135	0	.34	.02	1	98	254	15	.45	.071
1 oz	28	10.1	7.0	2.3	0.2	30	451	.04	0.7	.03	.12	14	207	.53	.178	801
semi-soft	103	12.9	6.1	0.7		0.0	113	0	.19	.02	1	146	84	8	.19	.026
1 oz	28	8.5	5.9	1.9	0.2	22	378	.02	0.3	.06	.05	45	106	.46	.160	801
soft	76	17.2	5.3	0.3		0.0	80	0	.11	.07	3	104	40	5	.26	.028
1 oz	28	6.0	4.1	1.4	0.1	13	267	.02	0.1	.05	.19	7	73	.54	.208	801
gouda	101	11.8	7.1	0.6		0.0	49	0	.09	.02	6	232	198	8	1.11	.003
1 oz	28	7.8	5.0	2.2	0.2	32	183	.01	0.0	.44	.10	34	155	.07	.010	801
gruyere	117	9.4	8.5	0.1		0.0	85	0	.08	.02	3	95	287	10	1.11	.005
1 oz	28	9.2	5.4	2.8	0.5	31	346	.02	0.0	.45	.16	23	172	.05	.009	801
havarti, Kraft	120		6.0	0.0	0.0	0.0		0	.10			240	150	0	.90	
1 oz	28	11.0	7.0			35	300			.12		10	100	.00		I
italian blend, grated, Kraft	25		3.0	0.0	0.0	0.0	0	0	.00			95	80	0	.30	
2 t	6	1.5	1.0			5	0			.24		0	60	.00		I
jalapeno jack, processed, Land O'Lakes	90		5.0	1.0								430				
1 oz	28	8.0	5.0	2.0	0.0	20						25				I
limburger	93	13.7	5.7	0.1		0.0	90	0	.14	.02	16	227	141	6	.60	.011
1 oz	28	7.7	4.7	2.4	0.1	26	363	.02	0.0	.29	.33	36	111	.04	.006	801
monterey	106	11.6	6.9	0.2		0.0	72	0	.11	.02	5	152	212	8	.85	.003
1 oz	28	8.6	5.4	2.5	0.3	25	269	.00	0.0	.23	.06	23	126	.20	.009	801
monterey jack, hot pepper, Land O'Lakes	110		7.0	0.0	0.0							150				
1 oz	28	9.0	5.0	3.0	0.0	20						25				I
mozzarella																
low moisture	90	13.7	6.1	0.7		0.0	78	0	.08	.02	2	118	163	6	.70	.003
1 oz	28	7.0	4.4	2.0	0.2	25	256	.00	0.0	.21	.02	21	117	.06	.006	801
part skim	72	15.2	6.9	0.8		0.0	50	0	.09	.02	2	132	183	7	.78	.003
1 oz	28	4.5	2.9	1.3	0.1	16	166	.01	0.0	.23	.02	24	131	.06	.007	801

	KCAL	H₂O (g)	PRO (g)	CHO (g)	SUGR (g)	DFIB (g)	A (RE)	C (mg)	B-2 (mg)	B-6 (mg)	FOL (mcg)	Na (mg)	Ca (mg)	Mg (mg)	Zn (mg)	Mn (mg)
	WT (g)	FAT (g)	SFA (g)	MUFA (g)	PUFA (g)	CHOL (mg)	A (IU)	B-1 (mg)	NIA (mg)	B-12 (mcg)	PANT (mg)	K (mg)	P (mg)	Fe (mg)	Cu (mg)	REF
part skim, low moisture	79	13.8	7.8	0.9		0.0	54	0	.10	.02	3	150	207	7	.89	.003
1 oz	28	4.9	3.1	1.4	0.1	15	178	.01	0.0	.26	.03	27	149	.07	.008	801
string, Kraft	80		7.0	1.0	0.0	0.0		0	.07			240	150	0	1.20	
1 oz stick	28	6.0	3.5			20	200			.48		20	100	.00		I
whole milk	80	15.3	5.5	0.6		0.0	68	0	.07	.02	2	106	147	5	.63	.002
1 oz	28	6.1	3.7	1.9	0.2	22	225	.00	0.0	.19	.02	19	105	.05	.006	801
muenster	104	11.8	6.6	0.3		0.0	90	0	.09	.02	3	178	203	8	.80	.002
1 oz	28	8.5	5.4	2.5	0.2	27	318	.00	0.0	.42	.05	38	133	.12	.009	801
neufchatel	74	17.6	2.8	0.8		0.0	75	0	.06	.01	3	113	21	2	.15	.001
1 oz	28	6.6	4.2	1.9	0.2	22	321	.00	0.0	.07	.16	32	39	.08	.005	801
parmesan, grated	23	0.9	2.1	0.2		0.0	9	0	.02	.01	0	93	69	3	.16	.001
1 T	5	1.5	1.0	0.4	0.0	4	35	.00	0.0	.07	.03	5	40	.05	.002	801
parmesan, hard	111	8.3	10.1	0.9		0.0	42	0	.09	.03	2	454	336	12	.78	.006
1 oz	28	7.3	4.7	2.1	0.2	19	171	.01	0.1	.34	.13	26	197	.23	.009	801
pimento, processed	106	11.1	6.3	0.5		0.0	91	1	.10	.02	2	405	174	6	.84	.005
1 oz	28	8.8	5.6	2.5	0.3	27	358	.01	0.0	.20	.14	46	211	.12	.009	801
pizza cheese																
four cheese, shredded, Kraft	90		7.0	1.0	0.0	0.0		0	.10			230	200	8	1.20	
¼ cup	27	7.0	4.5			20	200			.48		20	150	.00		I
mozzarella & provolone, shredded, Kraft	90		6.0	1.0	1.0	0.0		0	.07			210	150	0	.90	
¼ cup	27	7.0	4.5			20	200			.48		20	100	.00		I
mozzarella, shredded, Kraft	100		6.0	1.0	0.0	0.0		0	.07			190	150	0	.96	
¼ cup	27	8.0	5.0			25	300			.36		25	100	.00		I
port du salut	100	12.9	6.7	0.2		0.0	105	0	.07	.02	5	151	184	7	.74	.003
1 oz	28	8.0	4.7	2.6	0.2	35	378	.00	0.0	.43	.06	38	102	.12	.006	801
provolone	100	11.6	7.3	0.6		0.0	75	0	.09	.02	3	248	214	8	.92	.003
1 oz	28	7.5	4.8	2.1	0.2	20	231	.01	0.0	.41	.13	39	141	.15	.007	801
queso anejo, mexican	106	10.8	6.1	1.3		0.0	18	0	.06	.01	0	321	193	8	.83	.010
1 oz	28	8.5	5.4	2.4	0.3	30	63	.01	0.0	.39	.07	25	126	.13	.002	801
queso asadero, mexican	101	12.0	6.4	0.8		0.0	18	0	.06	.02	2	186	187	7	.86	.010
1 oz	28	8.0	5.1	2.3	0.2	30	63	.01	0.1	.28	.07	24	126	.14	.007	801
queso chihuahua, mexican	106	11.1	6.1	1.6		0.0	18	0	.06	.02	1	175	185	7	.99	.020
1 oz	28	8.4	5.3	2.4	0.3	30	64	.01	0.0	.29	.08	15	125	.13	.007	801
ricotta, part skim	171	92.3	14.1	6.4	1.7	0.0	140	0	.23	.02	16	155	337	18	1.66	.012
½ cup	124	9.8	6.1	2.9	0.3	38	536	.03	0.1	.36	.30	155	226	.55	.042	801
ricotta, whole milk	216	88.9	14.0	3.8	1.7	0.0	166	0	.24	.05	15	104	257	14	1.44	.007
½ cup	124	16.1	10.3	4.5	0.5	63	608	.02	0.1	.42	.26	130	196	.47	.026	801
romano	110	8.8	9.0	1.0		0.0	40	0	.10	.02	2	340	302	12	.73	.006
1 oz	28	7.6	4.9	2.2	0.2	29	162	.01	0.0	.32	.12	24	215	.22	.009	801
romano, grated, Kraft	25		2.0	0.0	0.0	0.0		0	.00			90	60	0	.00	
2 t	5	1.5	1.0			5	0			.00		0	40	.00		I
roquefort, sheep's milk	105	11.2	6.1	0.6		0.0	85	0	.17	.04	14	513	188	8	.59	.009
1 oz	28	8.7	5.5	2.4	0.4	26	297	.01	0.2	.18	.49	26	111	.16	.010	801
swiss	107	10.5	8.1	1.0	0.2	0.0	72	0	.10	.02	2	74	272	10	1.11	.005
1 oz	28	7.8	5.0	2.1	0.3	26	240	.01	0.0	.48	.12	31	171	.05	.009	801
swiss, processed	95	12.0	7.0	0.6		0.0	65	0	.08	.01	2	388	219	8	1.02	.004
1 oz	28	7.1	4.5	2.0	0.2	24	229	.00	0.0	.35	.07	61	216	.17	.008	801
taco cheese, cheddar & monterey,	100		6.0	1.0	0.0	0.0		0	.10			180	150	0	.90	
shredded, Kraft—*¼ cup*	26	8.0	6.0			25	400			.24		25	100	.00		I
tilsit, whole milk	96	12.2	6.9	0.5		0.0	82	0	.10	.02	6	213	198	4	.99	.004
1 oz	28	7.4	4.8	2.0	0.2	29	296	.02	0.1	.60	.10	18	142	.07	.007	801

5.2 CHEESE PRODUCTS

	KCAL	H₂O (g)	PRO (g)	CHO (g)	SUGR (g)	DFIB (g)	A (RE)	C (mg)	B-2 (mg)	B-6 (mg)	FOL (mcg)	Na (mg)	Ca (mg)	Mg (mg)	Zn (mg)	Mn (mg)
cheese fondue	247	66.5	15.4	4.1		0.0	123	0	.21	.06	4	143	514	25	2.12	.107
½ cup[2]	108	14.5	9.4	3.8	0.5	49	447	.03	0.2	.90	.25	113	330	.42	.028	801
cheese food																
american	93	12.2	5.6	2.1	2.8	0.0	62	0	.13	.04	2	337	163	9	.85	.003
1 oz	28	7.0	4.4	2.0	0.2	18	259	.01	0.0	.32	.16	79	130	.24	.009	801

	KCAL / WT (g)	H₂O (g) / FAT (g)	PRO (g) / SFA (g)	CHO (g) / MUFA (g)	SUGR (g) / PUFA (g)	DFIB (g) / CHOL (mg)	A (RE) / A (IU)	C (mg) / B-1 (mg)	B-2 (mg) / NIA (mg)	B-6 (mg) / B-12 (mcg)	FOL (mcg) / PANT (mg)	Na (mg) / K (mg)	Ca (mg) / P (mg)	Mg (mg) / Fe (mg)	Zn (mg) / Cu (mg)	Mn (mg) / REF
american, cold pack	94	12.2	5.6	2.4		0.0	57	0	.13	.04	2	274	141	8	.85	.003
1 oz	28	6.9	4.4	2.0	0.2	18	200	.01	0.0	.36	.28	103	113	.24	.009	801
american, Kraft	70		4.0	2.0	1.0	0.0		0	.10			290	100	0	.30	
¾ oz slice	21	5.0	3.0			15	300		.12			50	100	.00		I
american, Kraft	100			4.0	3.0	0.0		0	.17			290	150	8	.60	
2 T	31	8.0	5.0			25	300		.36			130	100	.00		I
italian herb, Land O'Lakes	90		6.0	2.0								430				
1 oz	28	7.0	4.0	2.0	0.0	20						70				I
jalapeno, Land O'Lakes	90		6.0	2.0								400				
1 oz	28	7.0	4.0	2.0	0.0	20						70				I
onion, Land O'Lakes	90		6.0	2.0								410				
1 oz	28	7.0	4.0	2.0	0.0	20						70				I
pepperoni, Land O'Lakes	90		6.0	1.0								430				
1 oz	28	7.0	4.0	2.0	0.0	20						65				I
processed, Land O'Lakes	88		5.2	2.4				0	.16			343	168			
1 oz	28	6.4	4.1	1.6	0.2	20	204	.02	0.1			98	133	.16		I
salami, Land O'Lakes	90		6.0	2.0								410				
1 oz	28	7.0	4.0	2.0	0.0	20						70				I
sharp cheddar, cold pack, Land O'Lakes	93		5.5	2.3				0	.12			270	139			
1 oz	28	6.9	4.3	1.8	0.2	18	197	.01	0.0			102	112	.24		I
sharp cheddar w/ wine, cold pack, Land O'Lakes—1 oz	93		5.5	2.3				0	.12			270	139			
	28	6.9	4.3	1.8	0.2	18	197	.01	0.0			102	112	.24		I
swiss	92	12.4	6.2	1.3		0.0	69	0	.11	.01	2	440	205	8	1.01	.003
1 oz	28	6.8	4.4	1.9	0.2	23	243	.00	0.0	.65	.14	81	149	.17	.009	801
swiss, Kraft	70		4.0	1.0	1.0	0.0		0	.07			320	150	0	.30	
¾ oz slice	21	5.0	3.5			15	200		.36			50	100	.00		I
cheese nuggets, mozzarella, frzn, Banquet—6 pieces (3 oz)	210		9.0	20.0	3.0	2.0	0	0				1060	150			
	85	11.0	4.0			10	0							.36		I
cheese product																
american flavor, Harvest Moon	50		4.0	1.0	1.0	0.0		0	.07			280	150	0	.30	
⅔ oz	19	3.0	2.0			10	100		.24			45	100	.00		I
american flavor, Light 'n Lively	50		5.0	2.0	1.0	0.0		0	.10			290	150	0	.60	
¾ oz	21	2.5	1.5			10	200		.24			50	100	.00		I
cheddar, Spreadery	80		5.0	3.0	2.0	0.0		0	.17			290	150	8	.60	
2 T[3]	31	4.5	3.0			15	100		.11			170	150	.00		I
Cheddarella, Land O'Lakes	100		7.0	0.0	0.0							180				
1 oz	28	8.0	5.0	2.0	0.0	25						20				I
Country Crock	66		4.9	2.3								207				
1 oz[4]	28	3.9				16										I
jalapeno pepper, hot/mild, mexican, Velveeta—1 oz	80			2.5	2.0	0.0		0	.14			480	150	8	.60	
	28	6.0	4.0			20	450		.24			95	250	.00		I
mozzarella cheese substitute	70	13.4	3.3	6.7		0.0	124	0	.13	.01	3	194	173	12	.54	.008
1 oz	28	3.5	1.1	1.8	0.5	0	413	.01	0.1	.23	.02	129	165	.11	.031	801
neufchatel, Spreadery	77		3.0	1.3	1.0	0.0		0	.03			207	20	0	.00	
2 T[5]	30	6.7	4.7			20	265		.00			38	20	.00		I
cheese sauce																
aged cheddar, Land O'Lakes	50		1.9	2.0				0	.04			213	57			
1 oz	28	3.8	1.6	1.4	0.2	6	63	.01	0.0			28	84	.04		I
cheddar, conito aged, Land O'Lakes	31		0.6	2.5				0	.03			157	20			
1 oz	28	2.1	0.5	1.0	0.2	1	12	.01	0.0			20	37	.01		I
cheddar, La Chedda	36		1.1	2.5				0	.04			183	37			
1 oz	28	2.3	0.8	1.0	0.2	4	30	.01	0.0			28	59	.02		I
cheddar, mild, Land O'Lakes	39		0.7	2.5				0	.02			211	22			
1 oz	28	2.9	0.7	1.4	0.2	2	15	.01	0.0			20	26	.02		I
cheddar, sharp, Land O'Lakes	38		1.4	2.3				0	.03			180	41			
1 oz	28	2.5	1.1	0.9	0.1	5	45	.01	0.1			20	69	.03		I
cheddar, Stouffers	145	34.8	5.4	3.9				0	.11			285	157			
2 oz	57	12.0				26	137	.02	0.1			63		.17		I
conito jalapeno, Land O'Lakes	39		0.8	2.7				1	.04			192	24			
1 oz	28	2.7	0.6	1.4	0.2	1	37	.01	0.1			36	48	.05		I

	KCAL / WT (g)	H_2O (g) / FAT (g)	PRO (g) / SFA (g)	CHO (g) / MUFA (g)	SUGR (g) / PUFA (g)	DFIB (g) / CHOL (mg)	A (RE) / A (IU)	C (mg) / B-1 (mg)	B-2 (mg) / NIA (mg)	B-6 (mg) / B-12 (mcg)	FOL (mcg) / PANT (mg)	Na (mg) / K (mg)	Ca (mg) / P (mg)	Mg (mg) / Fe (mg)	Zn (mg) / Cu (mg)	Mn (mg) / REF
homemade	59	20.1	3.1	1.6		0.0	48	0	.07	.01	2	148	93	6	.38	.012
2 T[6]	30	4.5	2.4	1.4	0.4	11	182	.01	0.1	.10	.07	43	69	.10	.006	801
nacho jalapeno style, Land O'Lakes	46		0.6	2.1				0	.02			215	15			
1 oz	28	3.9	0.8	2.0	0.3	1	17	.01	0.0			17	51	.02		I
nacho, mild, Land O'Lakes	46		0.6	2.1				0	.02			214	15			
1 oz	28	3.8	0.8	2.0	0.3	1	15	.01	0.0			17	51	.02		I
parmesano, microwave, Knorr	50	36.4	1.5	3.3								680				
1.7 oz	47	3.7														I
Queso Caliente w/ diced peppers, Land O'Lakes—1 oz	37		1.2	2.7				1	.04			204	36			
QuesOle!, Land O'Lakes	28	2.3	1.0	0.8	0 1	4	17	.01	0.1			37	84	.08		I
1 oz	46		0.6	2.1				0	.02			216	15			
squeezable, Cheez Whiz	28	3.9	0.8	2.0	0.3	1	52	.01	0.0			20	51	.03		I
2 T	100		2.0	4.0	1.0	0.0		0	.03			470	40	0	.00	
	33	8.0	4.0			15	100			.00		30	200	.00		I
cheese spread																
american	46	7.6	2.6	1.4		0.0	30	0	.07	.02	1	215	90	5	.41	.003
1 T	16	3.4	2.1	1.0	0.1	9	126	.01	0.0	.06	.11	39	114	.05	.005	801
american	82	13.5	4.7	2.5		0.0	54	0	.12	.03	2	381	159	8	.73	.006
1 oz	28	6.0	3.8	1.8	0.2	16	223	.01	0.0	.11	.19	69	202	.09	.009	801
American Easy Cheese	100		6.0	2.0	2.0	0.0						400				
2 T	34	7.0	4.0	1.5	0.0	25										I
american flavor, Harvest Moon	60		3.0	2.0	2.0	0.0			.07			300	100	0	.30	
¾ oz	21	4.5	3.0			15	200			.12		60	80	.00		I
cheddar, Country Crock	64		4.9	2.4								188				
1 oz	28	3.8				15										I
Cheez Whiz	90		5.0	2.0	2.0	0.0		0	.10			560	150	0	.60	
2 T	33	7.0	5.0			20	300			.24		75	300	.00		I
Easy Cheese, Nabisco	100		5.0	3.0	2.5	0.0						413				
2 T[7]	34	7.0	4.0			25										I
Golden Melt, Land O'Lakes	84		5.2	2.3				0	.13			382	160			
1 oz	28	6.0	3.8	1.5	0.2	19	198	.02	0.1			84	228	.13		I
Golden Velvet, Land O'Lakes	81		5.0	2.4				0	.13			379	156			
1 oz	28	5.7	3.6	1.5	0.2	18	186	.02	0.1			84	226	.13		I
italiana, Velveeta, Kraft	80			2.0	2.0	0.0		0	.14			430	100	0	.30	
1 oz	28	6.0	4.0			20	200			.36		75	200	.00		I
jalapeno peppers, Cheez Whiz	90		5.0	2.0	1.0	0.0		0	.10			530	150	0	.60	
2 T	33	8.0	5.0			25	300			.12		60	300	.00		I
jalapeno peppers, Kraft	80		5.0	2.0	2.0	0.0		0	.14			470	150		.60	
1 oz	28	6.0	4.0		1.0	20	100			.24		90	250	.00		I
limburger, Mohawk Valley	80		4.0	0.0	0.0	0.0		0	.03			500	150	0	.60	
2 T	32	7.0	4.5			20	300			.00		15	250	.00		I
salsa, hot/mild, Cheez Whiz	90		5.0	2.0	1.0	0.0		0	.07			535	150	0	.60	
2 T	33	7.0	5.0			25	300			.12		65	300	.00		I
sharp, Old English	90		5.0	1.0	0.0	0.0		0	.07			520	150	0	.60	
2 T	32	8.0	5.0			25	500			.12		15	300	.00		I
sharp, Squeez-A-Snak	90		5.0	1.0	0.0	0.0		0	.07			440	150	0	.90	
2 T	32	8.0	5.0			25	300			.24		15	250	.00		I
Velveeta	80		5.0	3.0	2.0	0.0		0	.14			420	150		.60	
1 oz	28	6.0	4.0			20	300			.24		80	250	.00		I

1. Values are averages for cream cheese with chives and onion, herb and garlic, olive and pimento, pineapple, smoked salmon, and strawberries.
2. Contains table wine, Swiss cheese, and all-purpose enriched flour.
3. Includes medium cheddar, sharp cheddar, and Vermont sharp white cheddar.
4. Values are averages for cheddar and bacon, cheddar Mexican style, cheddar with port wine, classic ranch, garden vegetable, and herb and garlic.
5. Values are averages for neufchatel classic ranch, garden vegetables, and garlic and herb.
6. Thin white sauce made with cheddar cheese and salt.
7. Values are averages for cheddar, cheddar 'n bacon, nacho, and sharp cheddar.

	KCAL	H₂O (g)	PRO (g)	CHO (g)	SUGR (g)	DFIB (g)	A (RE)	C (mg)	B-2 (mg)	B-6 (mg)	FOL (mcg)	Na (mg)	Ca (mg)	Mg (mg)	Zn (mg)	Mn (mg)
	WT (g)	FAT (g)	SFA (g)	MUFA (g)	PUFA (g)	CHOL (mg)	A (IU)	B-1 (mg)	NIA (mg)	B-12 (mcg)	PANT (mg)	K (mg)	P (mg)	Fe (mg)	Cu (mg)	REF

6. CHIPS, PRETZELS, POPCORN, & OTHER SNACK FOODS

	KCAL	H₂O	PRO	CHO	SUGR	DFIB	A	C	B-2	B-6	FOL	Na	Ca	Mg	Zn	Mn
banana chips	147	1.2	0.7	16.6		2.2	2	2	.00	.07	4	2	5	22	.21	.442
1 oz	28	9.5	8.2	0.6	0.2	0	24	.02	0.2	.00	.18	152	16	.35	.058	819
beef & chicken stick, smoked	110	3.8	4.3	1.1			34	1	.09	.04	0	296	14	4	.48	.017
.7 oz stick	20	9.9	4.2	4.1	0.9	27	302	.03	0.9	.20	.07	51	36	.68	.026	819
beef jerky, chopped & formed	82	4.7	6.6	2.2		0.4	0	0	.03	.04	27	443	4	10	1.62	.022
1 large piece	20	5.1	2.2	2.3	0.2	10	0	.03	0.3	.20	.03	119	81	1.08	.045	819
beef jerky, Lance	27	1.3	3.0	1.1					.06			183	3			
.3 oz	7	1.2						.01	0.7			45		.44		I
beef, sliced, Armour Star	60		8.0	2.0	2.0	0.0	0	0				1370	0			
7 slices	30	1.5	0.5			25	0							.72		I
beef snack, Lance	91	2.6	4.1	0.3					.05			340	7			
.6 oz	16	8.0						.16	1.0			58		.77		I
Bugles																
baked, Betty Crocker	130		2.0	23.0	2.0	0.0	0	0				350	0			
1 ½ cups	30	3.5	0.5			0	0					20		.00		I
Betty Crocker	150		1.0	20.0	1.0	0	0					340	0			
1 ⅓ cups	30	7.0	6.0			0	0					20		.00		I
cheddar cheese, baked, Betty Crocker	130		2.0	23.0	2.0	0.0	0	0				430	0			
1 ½ cups	30	3.5	0.5			0	0					40		.00		I
nacho, Betty Crocker	160		2.0	18.0	2.0	0	0					300	0			
1 ⅓ cups	30	9.0	7.0			0	0					40		.00		I
ranch, Betty Crocker	160		2.0	18.0	2.0	0	0					310	0			
1 ⅓ cups	30	9.0	8.0			0	0					50		.00		I
sour cream & onion, Betty Crocker	160		2.0	18.0	2.0	0.0	0	0				260	0			
1 ⅓ cups	30	9.0	8.0			0	0					35		.00		I
cheese balls, Lance	188	0.7	1.7	16.2					.11			417	42			
1.1 oz	32	13.1	3.3	7.9	1.8	5		.13	0.3			32		.51		I
cheese puffs/twists	157	0.4	2.2	15.3		0.3	10	0	.10	.04	34	298	16	5	.11	.020
1 oz	28	9.8	1.9	5.7	1.3	1	75	.07	0.9	.04	.11	47	31	.67	.018	819
cheese straws	272	13.0	6.7	20.7				0	.10			433	155			
10 pieces	60	17.9	6.4				230	.01	0.2			38	124	.40		456
cheese twist, crunchy, Lance	225	1.0	2.9	24.9					.04			512	35			
1.5 oz	43	16.0	4.8	10.2	1.0	2		.01	0.5			66		.36		I
Cheez Balls, Planters	150		2.0	15.0	1.0	1.0						300				
1 oz	28	10.0	2.0	3.5	0.5											I
Cheez Balls, red fat, Planters	140		3.0	18.0	1.0							380				
1 oz	28	6.0	1.5	2.0	0.5											I
Cheez Curls, Planters	150		2.0	15.0	1.0							310				
1 oz	28	10.0	2.0	3.5	0.0											I
Cheez Curls, red fat, Planters	130		3.0	19.0	1.0							350				
1 oz	28	5.0	1.5	2.0	0.5											I
Chex Mix	119	1.0	3.1	18.2		1.6	4	13	.14	.44	0	285	10	18	.59	.435
⅔ cup (1 oz)	28	4.8	1.5			0	41	.44	4.7	3.47	.13	75	52	6.92	.125	819
Combos Pretzel Cheddar Snacks	131	0.5	2.8	18.9			2	0	.16	.01	2	317	56	6	.21	.127
1 oz	28	4.8				1	19	.09	0.9	.03	.14	37	41	.26	.034	819
corn-based cones	145	0.6	1.6	17.8		0.3	9	0	.07	.01	1	290	1	3	.06	.025
1 oz	28	7.6	6.4	0.5	0.2	0	90	.09	0.4	.00	.06	23	12	.72	.011	819
corn-based cones, nacho	152	0.5	1.8	16.2		0.3	11	0	.03	.03	1	270	10	7	.14	.022
1 oz	28	9.0	7.6	0.6	0.2	1	89	.06	0.4	.00	.11	35	22	.36	.017	819
corn-based snack, onion-flavor	142	0.6	2.2	18.5		1.1	3	1	.09	.04	5	278	8	8	.09	.057
1 oz	28	6.4	1.2	3.8	0.9	0	34	.06	0.9	.00	.07	41	20	1.05	.033	819
corn cakes	70	0.8	1.5	15.0		0.3	4	0	.01	.03	3	88	3	21	.36	.327
2 cakes	18	0.4	0.1	0.1	0.2	0	44	.04	0.9	.00	.15	28	28	.25	.076	819
blueberry crunch, Quaker	49	0.4	0.7	11.5	3.9	0.3		0	.00	.03	3	3	1	9	.13	
1 cake	13	0.2	0.0	0.1	0.1	0	19	.02	0.4	.00	.08	16	20	.08	.020	I
butter flavor, Quaker	34	0.5	0.7	7.5	0.0	0.3		0	.00	.03	3	45	1	9	.13	
1 cake	9	0.2	0.1	0.1	0.1	0	19	.02	0.4	.00	.08	17	20	.08	.020	I

	KCAL / WT (g)	H2O (g) / FAT (g)	PRO (g) / SFA (g)	CHO (g) / MUFA (g)	SUGR (g) / PUFA (g)	DFIB (g) / CHOL (mg)	A (RE) / A (IU)	C (mg) / B-1 (mg)	B-2 (mg) / NIA (mg)	B-6 (mg) / B-12 (mcg)	FOL (mcg) / PANT (mg)	Na (mg) / K (mg)	Ca (mg) / P (mg)	Mg (mg) / Fe (mg)	Zn (mg) / Cu (mg)	Mn (mg) / REF
caramel, Quaker	50	0.4	0.7	11.5	3.8	0.3		0	.00	.03	3	28	1	9	.13	
1 cake	13	0.2	0.0	0.1	0.1	0	19	.02	0.3	.00	.08	15	20	.08	.020	I
monterey jack, Quaker	38	0.3	0.9	8.2	0.4	0.3		0	.02	.04	3	82	9	10	.16	
1 cake	10	0.3	0.1	0.1	0.1	1	23	.02	0.3	.02	.10	27	27	.09	.020	I
strawberry crunch, Quaker	49	0.4	0.7	11.5	3.9	0.3		0	.00	.03	3	3	1	9	.13	
1 cake	13	0.2	0.0	0.1	0.1	0	170	.02	0.4	.00	.08	16	20	.08	.020	I
white cheddar, Quaker	38	0.3	0.9	8.1	0.4	0.3		0	.01	.04	3	89	8	10	.16	
1 cake	10	0.3	0.1	0.1	0.1	0	22	.02	0.3	.02	.10	25	27	.09	.020	I
corn chips	153	0.3	1.9	16.1		1.4	3	0	.04	.07	6	179	36	22	.36	.108
1 oz	28	9.5	1.3	2.7	4.7	0	27	.01	0.3	.00	.11	40	52	.37	.046	819
barbecue	148	0.3	2.0	15.9		1.5	17	0	.06	.07	11	216	37	22	.30	.219
1 oz	28	9.3	1.3	2.7	4.6	0	173	.02	0.5	.00	.04	67	59	.44	.047	819
barbecue, Lance	257	0.8	3.0	25.3					.07			364	41			
1.7 oz	50	16.0	3.7	9.7	2.7	0		.02	0.8			43		.37		I
Lance	262	0.4	3.2	25.9								355	32			
1.7 oz	50	17.2	4.4	10.5	2.3	0		.03	0.7			50		.59		I
Planters	160		2.0	16.0	1.0	2.0						170				
1 oz[1]	28	10.0	1.5	2.5	6.0	0										I
Corn Crisps																
fresh roasted corn, Pringles	140	0.3	2.0	17.0				1	.02			210	2	24	.30	
1 oz	28	7.0	1.0	2.0	4.0	0	260	.01	0.7			71	60	.60	.030	I
smooth ranch, Pringles	140		2.0	17.0								230				
1 oz	28	7.0	1.0	2.0	4.0											I
tangy cheese, Pringles	140	0.3	2.0	17.0				2	.03			210	10	24	.30	
1 oz	28	7.0	1.0	2.0	4.0	1	320	.01	0.6			80	71	.30	.020	I
Doo Dads Snack Mix, Nabisco	260	1.7	5.9	36.7		3.9	25	0	.15	.12	23	724	42	34	1.28	1.006
1 cup (2 oz)	57	10.5	2.0			1	86	.21	3.1	.01	.33	158	169	1.42	.183	819
meat sticks, Armour Big Ones	130		5.5	1.0	1.0	0.0	0	0				580	0			
1 oz stick[2]	28	12.0	4.5			35	0							.36		I
oriental mix, rice-based	156	0.7	4.9	14.6		3.7	0	0	.04	.02	11	117	15	33	.75	.361
1 oz	28	7.3	1.1	2.8	3.0	0	1	.09	0.9	.00	.13	93	74	.69	.038	819
popcorn, butter																
94% fat-free, Pop Secret	20		1.0	4.0	0.0	1.0	0	0				40	0			
1 cup	5	0.0	0.0	0.0	0.0	0	0					10		.00		I
frzn, Pillsbury	212		2.9	20.0		1.1		3	.03			485	10			
3 cups	40	13.6					53	.05	0.7			95	72	.64		I
frzn, Pillsbury Microwave	210		3.0	20.4		1.0		3	.03			415	8			
3 cups	40	13.2					54	.05	0.7			96	73	.68		I
light, movie theater, Redenbacher	113		2.6	18.9	0.0	4.5	0	0				321	2			
Microwave—2 T unpopped	31	5.1	1.0			0	0							.63		I
light, snack size, Redenbacher Microwave	183		4.1	30.0	0.0	7.2	0	0				539	2			
1.76 oz	50	8.4	1.7		0.1	0	0							1.00		I
movie theater, Smartpop Microwave	92		2.8	20.3	0.0	4.9	0	0				307	16			
2 T unpopped	30	2.1	0.4			0	0							.12		I
no salt added, Redenbacher Microwave	176		2.5	18.7	0.0	4.5	0	0				2	2			
2 T unpopped	37	12.1	2.6			0	0							.62		I
Pop Secret	35		4.0	0.0	0	0				50	0					
1 cup	7	2.5				0	0					15		.00		I
Redenbacher Microwave	168		2.1	15.4	0.0	3.7		0				388	1			
2 T unpopped	34	12.5	2.7			0								.51		I
snack size, Redenbacher Microwave	287		3.4	24.8	0.0	5.9	0	0				647	2			
2 oz	57	22.0	4.8			0	0							.83		I
popcorn, butter toffee, Fiddle Faddle	150		2.0	21.0	13.0	1.0						160				
¾ cup	32	7.0	3.5			10										I
popcorn, butter/zesty, Redenbacher	177		2.2	16.3	0.0	3.9	0	0				429	1			
Microwave—2 T unpopped	36	13.2	2.9			0								.55		I
popcorn cakes	77	1.0	1.9	16.0		0.6	1	0	.04	.04	4	58	2	32	.80	.197
2 cakes	20	0.6	0.1	0.2	0.3	0	14	.01	1.2	.00	.09	65	55	.37	.114	819
butter, mini, Quaker	48	0.5	1.6	10.9	0.2	1.6		0	.04	.03	3	142	1	19	.49	
6 mini cakes	14	0.5	0.1	0.1	0.2	0	28	.03	0.3	.00	.05	40	43	.38	.060	I

| | KCAL | H₂O (g) | PRO (g) | CHO (g) | SUGR (g) | DFIB (g) | A (RE) | C (mg) | B-2 (mg) | B-6 (mg) | FOL (mcg) | Na (mg) | Ca (mg) | Mg (mg) | Zn (mg) | Mn (mg) |
	WT (g)	FAT (g)	SFA (g)	MUFA (g)	PUFA (g)	CHOL (mg)	A (IU)	B-1 (mg)	NIA (mg)	B-12 (mcg)	PANT (mg)	K (mg)	P (mg)	Fe (mg)	Cu (mg)	REF
butter, Redenbacher Microwave	134		2.2	13.0	0.6	1.5	0	0				79	6			
2 cakes	17	1.0	0.2			0	0							.16		I
caramel, mini, Quaker	54	0.5	1.3	12.4	4.1	2.3		0	.03	3.00	3	70	2	15	.40	
5 mini cakes	15	0.5	0.1	0.1	0.2	0	25	.02	0.2	.00	.05	34	36	.31	.050	I
caramel, Quaker	47	0.4	1.0	11.2	3.8	1.0		0	.02	.02	3	25	1	10	.26	
1 cake	13	0.3	0.0	0.1	0.1	0	19	.02	0.2	.00	.03	24	23	.22	.030	I
caramel, Redenbacher Microwave	34		1.0	7.9	2.1	0.7	0	0				16	2			
1 cake	10	0.1	0.0			0	0							.07		I
cheddar cheese, mini, Quaker	54	0.5	1.7	11.2	0.8	1.5		0	.05	.04	3	192	9	20	.50	
6 mini cakes	15	0.9	0.2	0.2	0.2	1	31	.03	0.3	.02	.10	57	50	.38	.060	I
mini, Redenbacher Microwave	55		1.5	11.4	1.2	1.2	1	0				68	5			
8 mini cakes[3]	15	0.7	0.1			0								.14		I
white cheddar, Redenbacher Microwave	63			13.0	0.0	1.5	0	6				83				
2 cakes	17	0.9	0.1			0	0							.16		I
popcorn, caramel	151	1.0	1.3	27.7	13.8	1.8	4	0	.02	.01	1	72	15	12	.20	.077
1 cup (1.24 oz)	35	4.5	1.3	1.0	1.6	2	18	.02	0.8	.00	.03	38	29	.61	.042	819
fat-free, Fiddle Faddle	110			28.0	16.0	1.0						210				
1 cup	30	0.0	0.0	0.0	0.0	0										I
Fiddle Faddle	150		2.0	20.0	12.0	1.0						180				
¾ cup	31	7.0	3.0			10										I
Redenbacher Microwave	179		1.0	23.0	12.3	1.8	0	0				47	18			
2 T unpopped	38	10.0	2.3			0	0							.25		I
w/ peanuts	113	0.9	1.8	22.9		1.1	2	0	.04	.05	5	84	19	23	.35	.217
1 oz	28	2.2	0.3	0.8	0.9	0	18	.01	0.6	.00	07	101	36	1.11	.084	819
popcorn, cheese	147	0.7	2.6	14.4		2.8	12	0	.07	.07	3	249	32	25	.56	.200
2.6 cups (1 oz)	28	9.3	1.8	2.7	4.3	3	68	.03	0.4	.15	.13	73	101	.63	.039	819
cheddar, Pop Secret	30			3.0	0.0	0	0					45	0			
1 cup	6	2.0	0.5			0	0					15		.00		I
cheddar, white/golden, Redenbacher	169		1.9	14.5	0.0	3.3	0	0				372	2			
Microwave—2 T unpopped	33	13.0	2.9			0	0							.45		I
Lance	135	0.4	2.1	12.8					.05			242	40			
.9 oz	25	8.0	2.3	4.9	0.7	4	290	.09	0.3			78		.94		I
nacho, Pop Secret	30			3.0	0.0	0	0					50	0			
1 cup	6	2.0	0.5			0	0					15		.00		I
white cheddar, Lance	140	0.9	2.2	11.6				1	.05			169	17			
.9 oz	25	9.7	2.9	5.8	1.2	4	136	.03	0.3			92		.67		I
popcorn, herb & garlic, Redenbacher	176		2.2	16.3	0.0	3.9	0					499	1			
Microwave—*2 T unpopped*	36	13.1	2.8			0	0							.55		I
popcorn, light butter, Pop Secret	25			4.0	0.0	0	0					35	0			
1 cup	5	1.0	0.0			0	0					15		.00		I
popcorn, light butter, Redenbacher	122		2.7	19.8	0.0	4.7	0	0				357	2			
Microwave—*2 T unpopped*	32	5.7	1.2			0	0							.66		I
popcorn, light, Pop Secret	25			4.0	0.0	0	0					45	0			
1 cup	5	1.0	0.0			0	0					15		.00		I
popcorn, lightly salted, mini, Quaker	52	0.5	1.7	11.7	0.2	1.8		0	.04	.04	4	119	1	21	.55	
7 mini cakes	15	0.6	0.1	0.1	0.3	0	31	.03	0.3	.00	.06	44	47	.42	.070	I
popcorn, plain																
94% fat-free, Pop Secret	20		1.0	4.0	0.0	1.0	0	0				40	0			
1 cup	5	0.0	0.0	0.0	0.0	0	0					10		.00		I
air-popped	107	1.1	3.4	21.8		4.2	6	0	.08	.07	6	1	3	37	.96	.264
3.5 cups (1 oz)	28	1.2	0.2	0.3	0.5	0	55	.06	0.5	.00	.12	84	84	.74	.118	819
frzn, Pillsbury	212		3.0	20.0		1.1		3	.03			426	9			
3 cups	40	13.2					54	.05	0.7			96	73	.68		I
frzn, Pillsbury Microwave	210		3.0	20.1		1.0		3	.03			415	8			
3 cups	40	13.2					54	.05	0.7			96	73	.64		I
Lance	66	1.5	0.3	9.6	1.4	0.4			.03			135	3			
.5 oz	14	2.5	0.6	1.5	0.4	0	66	.01	0.6			44		.45		I
light, Redenbacher Microwave	118		2.6	19.2	0.0	4.6	0	0				382	2			
2 T unpopped	30	5.5	1.1			0	0							.64		I
no salt added, Redenbacher Microwave	174		2.6	18.9	0.0	4.5	0	0				2	2			
2 T unpopped	37	11.8	2.5			0								.63		I

	KCAL	H₂O (g)	PRO (g)	CHO (g)	SUGR (g)	DFIB (g)	Vitamins					Minerals				
	WT (g)	FAT (g)	SFA (g)	MUFA (g)	PUFA (g)	CHOL (mg)	A (RE) / A (IU)	C (mg) / B-1 (mg)	B-2 (mg) / NIA (mg)	B-6 (mg) / B-12 (mcg)	FOL (mcg) / PANT (mg)	Na (mg) / K (mg)	Ca (mg) / P (mg)	Mg (mg) / Fe (mg)	Zn (mg) / Cu (mg)	Mn (mg) / REF
oil-popped	140	0.8	2.5	16.0	0.4	2.8	4	0	.04	.06	5	248	3	30	.74	.246
2.6 cups (1 oz)	28	7.9	1.4	2.3	3.8	0	43	.04	0.4	.00	.09	63	70	.78	.062	819
Pop Secret	35			4.0	0.0	0		0				65	0			
1 cup	7	2.5	0.5			0		0				15		.00		I
Redenbacher Microwave	164		2.4	17.5	0.0	4.2	0	0				512	0			
2 T unpopped	36	11.2	2.4			0	0									I
Redenbacker	92		3.0	22.2	0.0	5.3	0	0				2	2			
2 T unpopped	31	1.4	0.2			0								.74		I
salt free, frzn, Pillsbury Microwave	167		3.3	22.7		0.9		3	.03			6	3			–
3 cups	36	7.0					61	.04	0.8			108	79	.72		I
Smartpop Microwave	96		2.7	19.5	0.0	4.7	0	0				445	2			
2 T unpopped	30	2.9	0.5			0	0							.65		I
snack size, Smartpop Microwave	155		4.6	33.9	0.0	8.1	0	0				539	3			
1.76 oz	50	3.7	0.6			0	0							1.13		I
popcorn, sugar-coated	134	1.4	2.1	29.9				0	.02			0	2			
1 cup	35	1.2	0.4						0.4				47	.50		456
pork skins	155	0.5	17.4	0.0	0.0	0.0	11	0	.08	.01	0	521	9	3	.16	.020
1 oz	28	8.9	3.2	4.2	1.0	27	37	.03	0.4	.18	.12	36	24	.25	.027	819
pork skins, barbecue	153	0.6	16.4	0.5			52	0	.12	.04	9	756	12	0	.20	.021
1 oz	28	9.0	3.3	4.3	1.0	33	428	.02	1.0	.04	.12	51	62	.29	.099	819
potato chips, barbecue	139	0.5	2.2	15.0		1.2	6	10	.06	.18	24	213	14	21	.27	.142
1 oz	28	9.2	2.3	1.9	4.6	0	62	.06	1.3	.00	.17	357	53	.55	.102	I
potato chips, barbecue, Lance	190	0.6	3.0	18.0					.06			138	7			
1.1 oz	32	12.0	3.0	7.4	1.6	0		.05	0.8			345		.72		I
potato chips, cheese	141	0.5	2.4	16.4		1.5	2	15	.04	.10	0	225	20	21	.26	.126
1 oz	28	7.7	2.4	2.2	2.7	1	9	.04	1.4	.00	.22	433	85	.52	.071	819
potato chips, cheese, from dried potatoes	156	0.5	2.0	14.3		0.9	0	2	.03	.15	5	214	31	15	.18	.016
1 oz	28	10.5	2.7	2.0	5.3	1	0	.05	0.7	.00	.10	108	46	.45	.016	819
potato chips, light	134	0.3	2.0	19.0		1.7	0	7	.08	.19	8	139	6	25	.02	.125
1 oz	28	5.9	1.2	1.4	3.1	0	0	.06	2.0	.00	.08	494	55	.38	.170	819
potato chips, light, from dried potatoes	142	0.4	1.6	18.4		1.0	0	3	.02	.22	7	121	10	18	.17	.099
1 oz	28	7.3	1.5	1.7	3.8	0	0	.05	1.2	.00	.07	285	44	.43	.040	819
potato chips, plain	152	0.5	2.0	15.0		1.3	0	9	.06	.19	13	168	7	19	.31	.125
1 oz[4]	28	9.8	3.1	2.8	3.5	0	0	.05	1.1	.00	.11	361	47	.46	.087	819
from dried potatoes	158	0.4	1.7	14.5		1.0	0	2	.03	.04	2	186	7	16	.17	.098
1 oz	28	10.9	2.7	2.1	5.7	0	0	.06	0.9	.00	.06	286	45	.43	.045	819
rippled, idaho, Pringles	170	0.5	2.0	13.0				2	.01			150	7	17	.20	
1.1 oz	32	11.0	3.0	2.0	6.0	0		.07	0.9			300	48	.40	.030	I
rippled, Lance	195	0.3	2.3	12.4				7	.03			118	7			
1.1 oz	32	15.0	3.8	9.2	2.0	0		.04	0.8			266		.37		I
potato chips, sour cream 'n onion	151	0.5	2.3	14.6		1.5	6	11	.06	.19	18	177	20	21	.28	.115
1 oz	28	9.6	2.5	1.7	4.9	2	48	.05	1.1	.28	.23	377	50	.45	.085	819
from dried potatoes	155	0.6	1.9	14.5		0.3	28	3	.03	.13	7	204	18	16	.20	.115
1 oz	28	10.5	2.7	2.0	5.3	1	214	.05	0.7	.00	.23	141	48	.40	.018	819
Lance	190	0.6	3.0	18.0					.06			125	20			
1.1 oz	32	12.0	3.1	7.3	1.6	2		.06	0.8			374		.72		I
Potato Crisps																
barbecue, light, Pringles	130		1.0	17.0				2				100	0			
14 pieces (.9 oz)	26	6.0	1.0	1.0	4.0	0	0	.03	0.8			238		.36		I
barbecue, Pringles	150		2.0	15.0	1.0	1.0	0	4				200	0			
14 pieces (1 oz)	28	10.0	3.0			0	0	.03	0.8			275		.00		I
Cheez-Ums, Pringles	150		2.0	15.0	1.0	1.0	0	4	.03			190	0			
14 pieces (1 oz)	28	10.0	3.0			1	0	.03	0.8			275		.00		I
light, Pringle's	130		1.0	17.0			0	2	.00			100	0			
14 pieces (.9 oz)	26	6.0	1.0	4.0	1.0	0	0	.03	0.8			238		.36		I
light ranch, Pringles	130		1.0	17.0			0	2	.03			110	20			
14 pieces (.9 oz)	26	6.0	1.0	1.0	4.0	1	0	.03	0.8			238		.36		I
light sour cream 'n onion, Pringles	130		1.0	17.0			0	2	.03			110	20			
14 pieces (1 oz)	28	6.0	1.0	1.0	4.0	0	0	.03	0.8			238		.36		I
plain, Pringles	160		2.0	15.0		1.0	0	4	.00			170	0			
14 pieces (1 oz)	28	11.0	3.0			0	0	.03	0.8			275		.00		I

	KCAL / WT (g)	H₂O (g) / FAT (g)	PRO (g) / SFA (g)	CHO (g) / MUFA (g)	SUGR (g) / PUFA (g)	DFIB (g) / CHOL (mg)	A (RE) / A (IU)	C (mg) / B-1 (mg)	B-2 (mg) / NIA (mg)	B-6 (mg) / B-12 (mcg)	FOL (mcg) / PANT (mg)	Na (mg) / K (mg)	Ca (mg) / P (mg)	Mg (mg) / Fe (mg)	Zn (mg) / Cu (mg)	Mn (mg) / REF
plain, rippled, Pringles	160		2.0	15.0		1.0	0	4	.00			150	0			
12 pieces (1 oz)	28	11.0				0	0	.03	0.8			301		.00		I
ranch, Pringles	150		2.0	15.0	1.0	1.0	0	4				130	0			
14 pieces (1 oz)	28	10.0	3.0			0	0					275		.00		I
sour cream 'n onion, Pringles	160		2.0	15.0	1.0	1.0	0	4	.00			135	0			
14 pieces (1 oz)	28	10.0	3.0			1	0	.03	0.8			275		.00		I
potato sticks	148	0.6	1.9	15.1		1.0	0	13	.03	.09	11	71	5	18	.28	.120
1 oz	28	9.8	2.5	1.7	5.1	0	0	.03	1.4	.00	.11	351	49	.64	.089	819
pretzel air crisps, Nabisco	110		2.0	23.0	2.0							550				
22 crisps	28	0.0	0.0	0.0	0.0	0										I
pretzel twists, Planters	100		3.0	23.0	1.0	1.0						420				
1 oz.	28	0.5	0.0	0.0	0.0	0										I
pretzels	108	0.9	2.6	22.5		0.9	0	0	.18	.03	24	486	10	10	.24	.507
1 oz	28	1.0	0.2	0.4	0.3	0	0	.13	1.5	.00	.08	41	32	1.22	.075	819
choc coated	128	0.7	2.1	19.9			1	0	.06	.05	3	159	21	11	.26	.157
2.6 minisize (1 oz)	28	4.7	2.2	1.5	0.6	0	3	.03	0.2	.00	.21	63	41	.56	.085	819
Keebler	52		1.4	10.5					.06			336	3			
33 mini (.5 oz)	14	0.4	0.1		0.0	0		.07	0.9			22		.73		I
whole wheat	101	1.1	3.1	22.7		2.2	0	0	.08	.08	15	57	8	8	.17	.745
2 small (1 oz)	28	0.7	0.2	0.3	0.2	0	0	.12	1.8	.00	.23	120	35	.75	.078	819
Red Hot Sausage, Lance	53	11.3	3.6	1.2					.02			366	4			
.7 oz	21	3.7						.02	1.0			7		.67		I
rice cakes																
apple cinn, mini, Quaker	54	0.5	1.0	3.6		0.3	0	0	.01	.05	2	31	2	16	.23	
5 mini cakes	14	0.4	0.1	0.1	0.1	0	0	.05	0.8	.00	.15	12	38	.19	.030	I
banana crunch, mini, Quaker	54	0.5	0.9	12.0	3.6	0.3	0	0	.01	.05	2	39	1	16	.23	
5 mini cakes	14	0.3	0.1	0.1	0.1	0	0	.04	0.7	.00	.15	28	37	.15	.030	I
banana nut, Quaker	50	0.4	0.7	11.4	5.0	0.2	0	0	.01	.04	2	44	1	12	.17	
1 cake	13	0.3	0.1	0.1	0.1	0	0	.03	0.5	.00	.11	21	29	.12	.030	I
caramel corn, mini, Quaker	53	0.5	0.9	12.1	3.2	0.4		0	.01	.05	3	25	1	13	.19	
5 mini cakes	14	0.3	0.1	0.1	0.1	0	13	.03	0.5	.00	.12	23	31	.12	.030	I
Chico San	35		0.4	8.0		0.4	0	0	.01				0			
1 cake	9	0.2					14	.00	0.6			25		.10		I
choc crunch, mini, Quaker	54	0.5	1.0	11.9	3.2	0.4	0	0	.01	.05	2	10	2	18	.26	
5 mini cakes	14	0.4	0.1	0.1	0.1	0	0	.06	0.8	.00	.16	32	41	.29	.050	I
choc crunch, Quaker	50	0.4	0.9	11.2	3.8	0.4	0	0	.01	.05	2	12	2	16	.22	
1 cake	13	0.3	0.1	0.1	0.1	0	0	.05	0.7	.00	.13	27	36	.28	.050	I
cinn crunch, mini, Quaker	54	0.5	0.9	12.0	3.7	0.3	0	0	.01	.05	2	23	1	16	.23	
5 mini cakes	14	0.3	0.1	0.1	0.1	0	0	.04	0.7	.00	.15	25	37	.16	.030	I
cinn, Quaker	50	0.4	0.8	11.3	3.8	0.3	0	0	.01	.05	2	24	1	14	.20	
1 cake	13	0.3	0.1	0.1	0.1	0	0	.04	0.6	.00	.13	25	33	.14	.030	I
honey nut, mini, Quaker	54	0.5	1.0	12.0	3.2	0.3	0	0	.01	.05	2	23	2	16	.23	
5 mini cakes	14	0.4	0.1	0.1	0.1	0	0	.05	0.8	.00	.15	31	38	.17	.030	I
monterey jack, mini, Quaker	53	0.5	1.3	11.4	0.6	0.4	0	0	.02	.06	4	101	11	16	.26	
6 mini cakes	14	0.4	0.2	0.2	0.1	1	20	.04	0.6	.02	.17	40	44	.15	.030	I
Quaker	35	0.3	0.8	7.5	0.1	0.3	0	0	.01	.05	2	14	1	14	.20	
1 cake	9	0.3	0.1	0.1	0.1	0	0	.04	0.6	.00	.13	25	33	.13	.030	I
unsalted, Quaker	34	0.4	0.9	7.3	0.1	0.3	0	0	.01	.01	2	1	1	11	.23	
1 cake	9	0.3	0.1	0.1	0.1	0	0	.00	0.7	.00	.09	25	32	.13	.040	I
white cheddar, mini, Quaker	53	0.5	1.3	11.3		0.4	0	0	.02	.06	4	120	11	16	.25	
6 mini cakes	14	0.4	0.2	0.2	0.1	1	19	.04	0.6	.02	.17	40	44	.15	.030	I
rice cakes, brown	70	1.0	1.5	14.7		0.8	1	0	.03	.03	4	59	2	24	.54	.671
2 cakes	18	0.5	0.1	0.2	0.2	0	8	.01	1.4	.00	.18	52	65	.27	.080	819
& buckwheat	68	1.1	1.6	14.4		0.7	0	0	.02	.02	4	21	2	27	.45	1.112
2 cakes	18	0.6	0.1	0.2	0.2	0	0	.01	1.5	.00	.21	54	68	.21	.068	819
& corn	69	1.1	1.5	14.6		0.5	0	0	.02	.03	3	52	2	21	.40	.914
2 cakes	18	0.6	0.1	0.2	0.2	0	0	.01	1.2	.00	.17	50	58	.21	.076	819
& rye	69	1.2	1.5	14.4		0.7	0	0	.02	.03	1	20	4	26	.54	.536
2 cakes	18	0.7	0.1	0.2	0.3	0	1	.02	1.3	.00	.20	56	68	.32	.070	819
& sesame seed	71	1.1	1.4	14.7		1.0	0	1	.02	.03	3	41	2	24	.54	.774
2 cakes	18	0.7	0.1	0.2	0.2	0	0	.01	1.3	.00	.26	52	68	.28	.070	819

						Vitamins					Minerals				
KCAL	H₂O (g)	PRO (g)	CHO (g)	SUGR (g)	DFIB (g)	A (RE)	C (mg)	B-2 (mg)	B-6 (mg)	FOL (mcg)	Na (mg)	Ca (mg)	Mg (mg)	Zn (mg)	Mn (mg)
WT (g)	FAT (g)	SFA (g)	MUFA (g)	PUFA (g)	CHOL (mg)	A (IU)	B-1 (mg)	NIA (mg)	B-12 (mcg)	PANT (mg)	K (mg)	P (mg)	Fe (mg)	Cu (mg)	REF
multigrain 70	1.1	1.5	14.4		0.5	0	0	.03	.02	4	45	4	25	.46	.940
2 cakes 18	0.6	0.1	0.2	0.3	0	0	.01	1.2	.00	.18	53	67	.35	.077	819
sesame sticks, wheat-based 153	0.6	3.1	13.2		0.8	3	0	.02	.02	6	422	48	13	.33	.256
1 oz 28	10.4	1.8	3.1	4.9	0	25	.03	0.4	.00	.07	50	39	.21	.115	819
taro chips 141	0.6	0.7	19.3		2.0	0	1	.01	.12	6	97	17	24	.11	.000
12 chips (1 oz) 28	7.1	1.8	1.3	3.7	0	0	.05	0.1	.00	.19	214	37	.34	.079	819
tortilla chips 142	0.5	2.0	17.8		1.8	6	0	.05	.08	3	150	44	25	.43	.108
1 oz 28	7.4	1.4	4.4	1.0	0	56	.02	0.4	.00	.22	56	58	.43	.034	819
nacho 141	0.5	2.2	17.7		1.5	12	1	.05	.08	4	201	42	23	.34	.116
1 oz 28	7.3	1.4	4.3	1.0	1	105	.04	0.4	.01	.08	61	69	.41	.050	819
nacho cheese, Mexican Original 143	0.4	2.2	19.2	0.5	1.5	0	0				184	56			
1 oz 29	6.3	1.2			1	0								.28	I
nacho, Lance 156	0.6	2.6	18.8					.09			240	30			
1.1 oz 32	8.0	2.1	4.4	1.5	2		.04	0.8			36			.70	I
nacho, light 126	0.4	2.5	20.3		1.4	12	0	.08	.07	7	284	45	27		.124
1 oz 28	4.3	0.8	2.5	0.6	1	108	.06	0.1	.00		77	90	.46	.041	819
ranch 139	0.5	2.2	18.3		1.1	8	0	.07	.06	5	174	40	25	.35	.111
1 oz 28	6.7	1.3	4.0	0.9	0	73	.03	0.4	.00	.17	69	68	.41	.033	819
round, Lance 148	0.5	2.0	17.8								207	20			
1 oz 28	7.9	2.1	4.6	1.1	0						31				I
taco flavor 136	0.5	2.2	17.9		1.5	26	0	.06	.08	6	223	44	25	.36	.125
1 oz 28	6.9	1.3	4.1	1.0	1	257	.07	0.6	.00	.08	62	68	.57	.053	819
yellow corn, Mexican Original 165	0.5	2.3	22.3	0.2	1.8	0	0				73	49			
1.2 oz 33	7.4	1.2			0	0							2.90		I
trail mix 131	2.6	3.9	12.7			1	0	.06	.08	20	65	22	45	.91	.293
1 oz 28	8.3	1.6	3.6	2.7	0	5	.13	1.3	.00	.25	194	98	.86	.279	819
tropical 115	2.6	1.8	18.6			1	2	.03	.09	12	3	16	27	.33	.274
1 oz 28	4.8	2.4	0.7	1.5	0	14	.13	0.4	.00	.35	201	53	.75	.150	819
w/ choc chips 137	1.9	4.0	12.7			1	0	.06	.07	18	34	31	46	.89	.301
1 oz 28	9.0	1.7	3.8	3.2	1	12	.12	1.2	.00	.27	184	110	.96	.239	819

1. Values are for regular and king size chips.
2. Values are averages for barbeque, hot 'n spicy, original, and teriyaki.
3. Values are averages for barbeque, butter, caramel, nacho cheese, peanut, and white cheddar.
4. Values for product made with cottonseed oil. If partially hydrogenated soybean oil is used, SFA = 1.5 g, MUFA = 5.0 g, and PUFA = 2.6 g.

7. CREAMS & CREAM SUBSTITUTES

cream topping, Kraft 20		0.0	1.0	1.0	0.0	0	0				0	0			
2 T 7	1.5	1.0			5	0					5		.00		I
creamer, liquid															
Coffee-Mate, non-dairy, Carnation 20		0.0	2.0	0.0	0.0		0	.00	.00	0	0	0	0	.01	
1T 15	1.0	0.0	0.1	0.0	0	18	.00	0.0	.00	.00	25	7	.01	.000	I
Coffee Rich, non-dairy 22	10.4	0.0	2.2		0.0						11	0	0	.00	
½ fl oz 14	1.6	0.3	0.7	0.5	0						6	5	.02	.000	I
Farm Rich 18	11.5	0.0	1.1		0.0	0	.00				7	0	0	.00	
½ fl oz 14	1.5	0.3	0.3	0.4	0	0	.00	0.0			14	9	.01	.003	I
Mocha Mix, non-dairy 19	11.3	0.1	1.2		0.0						7	1	0		
½ fl oz 14	1.6	0.3	0.6	0.7	0						19	8	.06		I
Poly Rich, non-dairy 22	10.5	0.0	2.2		0.0						7	0	0	.00	
½ fl oz 14	1.3	0.3	0.6	0.5	0						12	5	.02	.003	I
creamer, liquid/frzn															
w/ hydg veg oils 20	11.6	0.1	1.7		0.0	1	0	.00	.00	0	12	1	0	.00	.000
½ fl oz[1] 15	1.5	0.3	1.1	0.0	0	13	.00	0.0	.00	.00	29	10	.00	.000	801
w/ lauric acid oils 20	11.6	0.1	1.7		0.0	1	0	.00	.00	0	12	1	0	.00	.006
½ fl oz[2] 15	1.5	1.4	0.0	0.0	0	13	.00	0.0	.00	.00	29	10	.00	.004	801
creamer, powdered 11	0.0	0.1	1.1		0.0	0	0	.00	.00	0	4	0	0	.01	.004
1 t[2] 2.0	0.7	0.7	0.0	0.0	0	4	.00	0.0	.00	.00	16	8	.02	.002	801
Coffee-Mate Lite, non-dairy, Carnation 10		0.0	2.0	0.0	0.0		0				0	0			.000
1 t 2.0	0.3	0.1	0.0	0.0	0	0			.00		18	7	.00		I

	KCAL	H_2O (g)	PRO (g)	CHO (g)	SUGR (g)	DFIB (g)	Vitamins A (RE)	C (mg)	B-2 (mg)	B-6 (mg)	FOL (mcg)	Minerals Na (mg)	Ca (mg)	Mg (mg)	Zn (mg)	Mn (mg)
	WT (g)	FAT (g)	SFA (g)	MUFA (g)	PUFA (g)	CHOL (mg)	A (IU)	B-1 (mg)	NIA (mg)	B 12 (mcg)	PANT (mg)	K (mg)	P (mg)	Fe (mg)	Cu (mg)	REF
Coffee-Mate, non-dairy, Carnation	10		0.0	1.0	0.0	0.0		0			0	0	0			
1 t	2.0	0.6	0.5	0.0	0.0	0	0			.00		18	7	.00		I
Swiss Miss 'n Rich	10		0.1	1.2	0.0	0.0	0	0				4	0			
1 t	2.0	0.5	0.1			0	0							.00		I
half & half (milk & cream)	20	12.1	0.4	0.6		0.0	16	0	.02	.01	0	6	16	2	.08	.000
1 T	15	1.7	1.1	0.5	0.1	6	65	.01	0.0	.05	.04	19	14	.01	.002	801
light (coffee/table) cream	29	11.1	0.4	0.5		0.0	27	0	.02	.00	0	6	14	1	.04	.000
1 T	15	2.9	1.8	0.8	0.1	10	108	.00	0.0	.03	.04	18	12	.01	.001	801
medium (25% fat) cream	37	10.3	0.4	0.5		0.0	35	0	.02	.00	0	6	14	1	.04	.000
1 T	15	3.8	2.3	1.1	0.1	13	141	.00	0.0	.03	.04	17	11	.01	.001	801
sour cream																
cultured	26	8.5	0.4	0.5		0.0	23	0	.02	.00	1	6	14	1	.03	.000
1 T	12	2.5	1.6	0.7	0.1	5	95	.00	0.0	.04	.04	17	10	.01	.002	801
fat-free, Breakstone/Sealtest/	35			6.0	2.0	0.0		0				25	40			
Knudsen Free—*2 T*	32	0.0	0.0	0.0	0.0	200	.00				70		.00		I	
half & half, cultured	20	12.0	0.4	0.6		0.0	17	0	.02	.00	2	6	16	2	.07	.000
1 T	15	1.8	1.1	0.5	0.1	6	68	.01	0.0	.04	.05	19	14	.01	.002	801
imitation	59	20.2	0.7	1.9		0.0	0	0	.00	.00	0	29	1	2	.33	.031
1 oz	28	5.5	5.0	0.2	0.0	0	0	.00	0.0	.00	.00	46	13	.11	.016	801
light, Land O'Lakes	18		0.8	1.8				0	.04			17	17			
1 T	15	0.7	0.5	0.2	0.0	3	116	.01	0.0			38	17	.02		I
light, Sealtest/Knudsen Light	40		2.0	2.0	2.0	0.0		0	.07			20	40			
2 T	31	2.5	2.0			10	200	.00		.12		65	30	.00		I
sour cream dairy blend, light,	20		1.0	2.0								15				
Land O'Lakes—*1 T*	16	1.0				5						35				I
sour cream dip																
flavored, Breakstone	54		1.0	2.0	1.0	0.0		0				174	24			
2 T[3]	31	4.2	2.9			21	100					43		.00		I
flavored, Knudsen Premium	57		1.3	2.3	1.3	0.0		0				177	27			
2 T[4]	31	4.3	3.0			18	100					48		.00		I
flavored, Kraft	60		1.0	3.4	0.0	0	0					229	0			
2 T[5]	27	4.1	3.0			0	0					22		.00		I
flavored, Kraft Premium	52		1.0	1.9	0.0		0					194	33			
2 T[6]	31	4.6	2.8			13	120					37		.00		I
flavored, Land O'Lakes	40		1.0	2.0								140				
3 T (1.7 oz)	48	3.0										40				I
french onion, Sealtest	50		1.0	2.0	1.0	0.0		0				160	20			
2 T	31	4.0	3.0			20	100					40		.00		I
whipped topping																
from mix, Dream Whip	20		0.0	2.0	2.0	0.0	0	0				10	0			
2 T[7]	10	1.0	1.0			0	0					15		.00		I
from mix, prep w/ whole milk	8	2.7	0.1	0.7		0.0	2	0	.00	.00	0	3	4	0	.01	.000
1 T	4	0.5	0.4	0.0	0.0	0	14	.00	0.0	.01	.01	6	3	.00	.000	801
frzn	13	2.0	0.1	0.9		0.0	3	0	.00	.00	0	1	0	0	.00	.002
1 T	4	1.0	0.9	0.1	0.0	0	34	.00	0.0	.00	.00	1	0	.00	.001	801
frzn, Cool Whip Extra Creamy	30		0.0	2.0	2.0	0.0	0	0				5	0			
2 T	9	2.0	2.0	0.0	0.0	0	0					5		.00		I
frzn, Cool Whip Lite	20		0.0	2.0	1.0	0.0	0	0				0	0			
2 T	8	1.0	1.0	0.0	0.0	0	0					5		.00		I
frzn, Cool Whip, non-dairy	25		0.0	2.0	1.0	0.0	0	0				0	0			
2 T	9	1.5	1.5	0.0	0.0	0	0					0		.00		I
Kraft	20		0.0	1.0	1.0	0.0	0	0				0	0			
2 T	7	1.5	1.0			0	0					0		.00		I
liquid, Richwhip	20	4.2	0.0	1.2								4	0	0	.00	
¼ oz[8]	7	1.6	1.3									0	0	.00	.000	I
pressurized	11	2.4	0.0	0.6		0.0	2	0	.00	.00	0	2	0	0	.00	.002
1 T	4	0.9	0.8	0.1	0.0	0	19	.00	0.0	.00	.00	1	1	.00	.001	801
pressurized, Richwhip	20	4.2	0.0	1.1								3	0	0	.00	
¼ oz	7	1.7	1.4									1	0	.00	.000	I

	KCAL	H₂O (g)	PRO (g)	CHO (g)	SUGR (g)	DFIB (g)	A (RE)	C (mg)	B-2 (mg)	B-6 (mg)	FOL (mcg)	Na (mg)	Ca (mg)	Mg (mg)	Zn (mg)	Mn (mg)
	WT (g)	FAT (g)	SFA (g)	MUFA (g)	PUFA (g)	CHOL (mg)	A (IU)	B-1 (mg)	NIA (mg)	B-12 (mcg)	PANT (mg)	K (mg)	P (mg)	Fe (mg)	Cu (mg)	REF
prewhipped, Richwhip	12	2.0	0.1	1.0		0.0		0	.00			1	0	0	.00	
1 T	4	0.9	0.9			0	0	.00	0.0			1	2	.01	.003	I
red cal, D-Zerta	10		0.0	1.0	0.0	0.0	0	0				10	0			
amt for 2 T	2.0	1.0	0.5			0	0					10		.00		I
whipping cream																
heavy, fluid	52	8.7	0.3	0.4	0.4	0.0	63	0	.02	.00	1	6	10	1	.03	.000
1 T	15	5.5	3.5	1.6	0.2	21	221	.00	0.0	.03	.04	11	9	.00	.001	801
light, fluid	44	9.5	0.3	0.4		0.0	44	0	.02	.00	1	5	10	1	.04	.000
1 T	15	4.6	2.9	1.4	0.1	17	169	.00	0.0	.03	.04	15	9	.00	.001	801
pressurized	8	1.8	0.1	0.4		0.0	6	0	.00	.00	0	4	3	0	.01	.000
1 T	3	0.7	0.4	0.2	0.0	2	27	.00	0.0	.01	.01	4	3	.00	.000	801

1. Contains hydrogenated vegetable oil and soy protein; vegetable oils are usually soybean, cottonseed, safflower, or blends thereof.
2. Contains lauric acid oils and sodium caseinate; lauric oils include modified coconut oil, hydrogenated coconut oil, and/or palm kernel oil.
3. Values are averages for bacon and onion, chesapeake clam, french onion, jalapeno cheddar, and toasted onion.
4. Values are averages for bacon & onion, french onion, and nacho cheese.
5. Values are averages for avocado, bacon and horseradish, clam, French onion, green onion, jalapeno, and ranch.
6. Values are averages for bacon & horseradish, bacon & onion, blue cheese, clam, creamy cucumber, creamy onion, french onion, jalapeno cheese, and nacho cheese.
7. Prepared with 2% fat milk and vanilla flavoring.
8. 1 fl oz if whipped.

8. DESSERTS
8.1 BROWNIES & BAR COOKIES

	KCAL	H₂O (g)	PRO (g)	CHO (g)	SUGR (g)	DFIB (g)	A (RE)	C (mg)	B-2 (mg)	B-6 (mg)	FOL (mcg)	Na (mg)	Ca (mg)	Mg (mg)	Zn (mg)	Mn (mg)
	WT (g)	FAT (g)	SFA (g)	MUFA (g)	PUFA (g)	CHOL (mg)	A (IU)	B-1 (mg)	NIA (mg)	B-12 (mcg)	PANT (mg)	K (mg)	P (mg)	Fe (mg)	Cu (mg)	REF
brownie	227	7.6	2.7	35.8		1.2	11	0	.12	.02	7	175	16	17	.40	.237
1 large brownie (2 ¾" x ⅞")	56	9.1	2.4	4.7	1.4	10	39	.14	1.0	.08	.31	83	57	1.26	.125	818
from mix	140	4.3	1.4	20.4		0.9	4	0	.05	.01	3	83	6	11	.19	.159
1 brownie (2" sq)	33	6.6	1.3	2.0	2.8	9	15	.04	0.5	.02	.05	61	26	.56	.074	818
fudge, Little Debbie	269	5.6	2.4	39.2	24.0	1.0		0	.09			167	20			
2.2 oz brownie	61	12.7	2.7			13	15	.13	0.9					1.10		I
fudge, Pillsbury	139	5.4	1.3	21.6				0	.05			112	4			
1.2 oz brownie	34	5.3					0	.04	0.8			60	20	.86		I
fudge w/ choc chips, Pillsbury	178	7.6	1.6	25.0				0	.09			112	4			
Microwave—1.6 oz brownie	44	8.7					1	.07	0.7			103	25	.82		I
homemade	112	3.0	1.5	12.0			48	0	.05	.02	4	82	14	13	.23	.141
1 brownie (2 ¼" x 1 ½")	24	7.0	1.8	2.6	2.3	18	184	.03	0.2	.04	.08	42	32	.44	.093	818
Lance	201	5.6	2.0	34.4				3	.05			135	14			
1.7 oz brownie	50	7.1	1.6	3.6	1.9	5	2	.02	0.2			11		.41		I
Brownie Lights, Little Debbie	185	7.6	3.2	38.8	27.0	1.2		0	.09			198	21			
1.9 oz pkg	54	2.9	0.4			1	3	.10	0.8					.92		I
brownie mix																
Betty Crocker	180		2.0	27.0	19.0	0.0	0	0	.07			110	0			
¹⁄₂₀ pkg	40	7.0	1.5	2.0	3.5	20	0	.03	0.4			110		.72		I
double fudge, Duncan Hines Brownies	120	1.0	1.0	22.0					.04			100	6	12	.20	
Plus—¹⁄₂₄ pkg (1 brownie)	28	3.0	1.0	1.0	1.0	0		.04	0.5				22	1.10	.060	I
flavored, Betty Crocker	197		2.1	27.2	19.1	0.6	0	0	.06			124	1			
¹⁄₁₈ pkg[1]	40	9.1	2.1	2.4	3.7	24	0	.03	0.3			118		.80		I
fudge, Duncan Hines	100	0.8	1.0	18.0					.03			85	5	10	.20	
¹⁄₂₄ pkg (1 brownie)	23	2.0	1.0					.03	0.5				18	.90	.070	I
fudge, Robin Hood/Gold Medal Pouch	170		2.0	24.0	17.0	1.0	0	0	.06			105	0			
¹⁄₁₀ pkg (1 brownie)	40	7.0	1.5			20		.03	0.0			115		.72		I
low-fat, Sweet Rewards	130		2.0	27.0	18.0	1.0	0	0	.03			120	0			
¹⁄₁₈ pkg	38	2.5	0.5	0.5	0.5	0		.03	0.4			110		1.08		I
milk choc chunks, Duncan Hines	120	0.7	1.0	20.0					.04			90	10	11	.10	
Brownies Plus—¹⁄₂₄ pkg (1 brownie)	28	4.0	2.0	1.0	1.0	5		.07	0.5				24	1.00	.060	I
peanut butter, Duncan Hines Brownies	120	0.8	3.0	16.0					.03			100	6	15	.20	
Plus—¹⁄₂₄ pkg (1 brownie)	25	5.0	1.0	3.0	1.0	0		.04	1.1			55	30	.90	.080	I

	KCAL	H_2O (g)	PRO (g)	CHO (g)	SUGR (g)	DFIB (g)	Vitamins A (RE)	C (mg)	B-2 (mg)	B-6 (mg)	FOL (mcg)	Minerals Na (mg)	Ca (mg)	Mg (mg)	Zn (mg)	Mn (mg)
	WT (g)	FAT (g)	SFA (g)	MUFA (g)	PUFA (g)	CHOL (mg)	A (IU)	B-1 (mg)	NIA (mg)	B-12 (mcg)	PANT (mg)	K (mg)	P (mg)	Fe (mg)	Cu (mg)	REF
red fat, Sweet Rewards	150		2.0	27.0	19.0	0.0	0	0	.07			110	0			
1/20 pkg (1 brownie)	40	4.0	1.0			20	0	.03	0.4			90		1.08		I
turtle, Duncan Hines	160	1.4	2.0	27.0					.09			120	30	17	.30	
1/16 pkg (1 brownie)	37	5.0	2.0	2.0	1.0	1		.04	0.5			98	48	.90	.100	I
walnut, Duncan Hines	120		1.0	19.0								85				
1/24 pkg (1 brownie)	26	4.0	1.0	1.0	2.0	0										I
brownie snack bar, fat-free, Sweet	100		2.0	24.0	16.0	1.0	0	0				120	0			
Rewards—*1.1 oz bar*	32	0.0	0.0	0.0	0.0	0	0					140		1.08		I
caramel cookie bar, Little Debbie	156	2.0	1.0	22.0	14.8	0.3		0	.05			86	13			
1.2 oz	33	7.7	4.9			0	0	.06	0.5					.50		I
coconut bar	45	0.3	0.6	5.8				0	.01			13	7			
1 bar (3 x 1 1/4 x 1/4")	9	2.2	0.8				14	.00	0.0			21	11	.13		456
date bar mix, Betty Crocker	150		1.0	23.0	14.0	1.0	0	0	.03			90	0			
1/12 pkg	33	6.0	2.0	0.0	0.0	0	0	.06	0.0			95		.71		I
double fudge supreme snack bar,	100		2.0	25.0	15.0	1.0	0	0				90	20			
fat-free, Sweet Rewards—*1.1 oz bar*	32	0.0	0.0	0.0	0.0		0					140		1.08		I
Supreme Dessert Bar mix, Betty Crocker	164		1.8	23.0	13.7	0.0	0	0	.03			122	0			
1/16 pkg[2]	40	7.0	2.0			14	0	.05	0.3			49		.40		I

8.2 CAKES

angel food	73	9.4	1.7	16.4		0.4	0	0	.14	.01	1	212	40	3	.02	.024
1/12 cake (1 oz)	28	0.2	0.0	0.0	0.1	0	0	.03	0.3	.02	.06	26	66	.15	.022	818
choc swirl, from mix, Supermoist	150		3.0	34.0	24.0	0.0	0	0	.07			300	60			
1/12 pkg	40	0.0	0.0	0.0	0.0	0	0	.00	0.0			85		.00		I
confetti, from mix, Supermoist	150		3.0	34.0	24.0	0.0	0	0	.07			300	60			
1/12 pkg	40	0.0	0.0	0.0	0.0	0	0	.00	0.0			85		.00		I
from mix	129	16.4	3.0	29.4		0.1	0	0	.10	.00	3	255	42	4	.07	.032
1/12 cake	50	0.1	0.0	0.0	0.1	0	0	.05	0.1	.01	.06	68	116	.12	.034	818
from mix, Duncan Hines 1-Step	130		3.0	30.0	22.0	0.0	0	0	.10			320	20			
1/12 cake	49	0.0	0.0	0.0	0.0	0	0	.00	0.0			150				I
from mix, Duncan Hines 2-Step	140		4.0	30.0	24.0	1.0	0	0	.10			115	20			
1/12 cake[3]	50	0.0	0.0	0.0	0.0	0	0	.00	0.0			85				I
homemade	142	16.9	4.0	31.5			0	0	.17	.00	2	96	3	5	.07	.058
1/12 of 10" cake	53	0.1	0.0	0.0	0.0	0	0	.05	0.4	.05	.05	116	13	.40	.025	818
lemon custard, from mix, Supermoist	140		3.0	33.0	22.0	0.0	0	0	.07			290	60			
1/12 pkg	38	0.0	0.0	0.0	0.0	0	0	.00	0.0			50		.00		I
angel food cake mix, Supermoist	140		3.0	31.0	23.0	0.0	0	0	.07			270	150			
One-Step—*1/12 pkg*	38	0.0	0.0	0.0	0.0	0	0	.00	0.0			210		.00		I
banana, fat-free, from mix, Sweet	170		3.0	39.0	27.0	0.0	0	0	.10			280	60			
Rewards—*1/8 cake*	44	0.0	0.0	0.0	0.0	0	0	.12	0.8			45		.72		I
boston cream pie																
from mix, Betty Crocker	200		3.0	38.0	28.0	0.0	0	0	.10			300	100			
1/10 cake	80	4.0	1.5			25	0	.06	0.4			80		.72		I
frzn	232	41.8	2.2	39.5		1.3	21	0	.25	.02	7	132	21	6	.15	.046
1/6 of 19.5 oz cake	92	7.8	2.3	4.1	0.9	34	74	.38	0.2	.15	.28	36	45	.35	.078	818
frzn, Mrs. Smith's	170		2.0	29.0	19.0	0.0						140				
1/8 of 8" cake	69	5.0	1.5	2.5	1.0	25						35				I
homemade	293	32.1	4.3	43.0			51	0	.18	.03	8	309	93	16	.44	.169
1/12 of 9" cake	93	12.3	3.9	5.0	2.6	43	180	.13	1.0	.15	.26	95	91	1.23	.085	818
butter choc, from mix, Supermoist	270		4.0	34.0	21.0	1.0		0	.10			380	40			
1/12 cake	80	13.0	7.0	4.0	1.0	75	300	.09	0.8			160		1.44		I
butter pecan, from mix, Supermoist	250		3.0	34.0	20.0	0.0	0	0	.14			300	80			
1/12 cake	80	11.0	2.5	3.0	4.0	55	0	.09	0.8			35		.72		I
butter yellow, from mix, Supermoist	260		3.0	37.0	23.0	0.0		0	.10			330	60			
1/12 cake	80	11.0	6.0	3.5	0.5	75	300	.09	0.8			35		.72		I
caramel w/ caramel icing, homemade	398	21.9	3.9	62.1				0	.07			265	88			
1/12 cake	105	15.5	4.7				210	.02	0.1			67	100	1.60		456
carrot cake																
from mix	239	21.6	3.6	32.7		1.4	173	2	.12	.06	8	249	77	5	.22	.216
1/12 of 9" cake	70	11.0	1.8	3.4	5.0	51	790	.09	0.8	.81	.19	84	122	.92	.024	818

	KCAL	H_2O (g)	PRO (g)	CHO (g)	SUGR (g)	DFIB (g)	Vitamins A (RE)	C (mg)	B-2 (mg)	B-6 (mg)	FOL (mcg)	Minerals Na (mg)	Ca (mg)	Mg (mg)	Zn (mg)	Mn (mg)
	WT (g)	FAT (g)	SFA (g)	MUFA (g)	PUFA (g)	CHOL (mg)	A (IU)	B-1 (mg)	NIA (mg)	B-12 (mcg)	PANT (mg)	K (mg)	P (mg)	Fe (mg)	Cu (mg)	REF
from mix, Supermoist	300		4.0	41.0	25.0	0.0	0	0	.14			360	60			
1/10 cake	80	13.0	3.0	3.5	5.0	65	0	.12	0.8			80		1.08		I
w/ cream cheese icing, homemade	484	22.9	5.1	52.4		1.3	426	1	.17	.08	13	273	28	20	.54	.381
1/12 of 9″ cake	111	29.3	5.4	7.2	15.1	60	3827	.15	1.1	.11	.25	124	79	1.39	.152	818
cheesecake	257	36.5	4.4	20.4		0.3	129	0	.15	.04	12	166	41	9	.41	.112
1/6 of 17 oz cake	80	18.0	9.2	6.2	1.1	44	442	.02	0.2	.14	.46	72	74	.50	.016	818
from mix, Jell-O No Bake Dessert	340		5.8	49.4	34.8	1.0		0				448	170			
1/8 cake[4]	99	13.4	4.2			5	440					284		.72		I
from mix, no-bake type	271	43.8	5.4	35.1		1.9	98	0	.26	.05	18	376	170	19	.46	.119
1/8 of 9″ cake	99	12.6	7.0	3.9	0.6	42	362	.12	0.5	.31	.61	209	232	.47	.029	818
homemade	457	52.4	8.7	32.3			411	1	.27	.06	15	362	74	10	.70	.109
1/12 of 9″ cake	128	33.3	18.4	10.3	2.6	155	1354	.04	0.5	.32	.24	131	123	1.60	.047	818
w/ cherry topping, homemade	408	69.9	7.1	37.6			342	1	.23	.06	14	288	61	10	.57	.116
1/12 of 9″ cake	142	26.3	14.4	8.2	2.2	121	1275	.04	0.5	.24	.22	132	101	1.75	.062	818
cherry chip, from mix, Supermoist	190		3.0	37.0								270				
1/12 cake	80	3.0	1.0	2.0	0.0	0						35				I
cherry fudge w/ choc icing	187	32.7	1.7	27.0		0.9	32	10	.13	.06	6	160	34	13	.43	.137
1/8 of 20 oz cake	71	8.9	3.0	3.3	2.0	39	158	.02	0.5	.21	.46	118	75	.78	.109	818
choc cake																
from mix	198	20.8	3.6	31.9		1.4	16	0	.10	.02	7	370	70	21	.45	.322
1/12 of 9″ cake	65	7.6	1.7	3.1	2.3	35	54	.06	0.6	.07	.14	153	132	2.08	.177	818
homemade	340	23.2	5.0	50.7		1.5	38	0	.20	.04	10	299	57	30	.66	.266
1/12 of 9″ cake	95	14.3	5.2	5.7	2.6	55	133	.13	1.1	.15	.29	133	101	1.53	.197	818
w/ choc icing	235	14.7	2.6	34.9		1.8	18	0	.09	.02	5	214	28	22	.44	.205
1/8 of 18 oz cake	64	10.5	3.0	5.8	1.2	29	61	.02	0.4	.08	.15	128	78	1.41	.155	818
choc chip, from mix, Supermoist	280		3.0	35.0	20.0	0.0	0	0	.14			290	80			
1/12 cake	80	14.0	3.0	4.5	5.0	55	0	.09	0.8			55		.72		I
choc, fat-free, from mix, Sweet Rewards	170		3.0	38.0	24.0	1.0	0	0	.10			390	60			
1/8 cake	44	0.0	0.0	0.0	0.0	0	0	.09	0.8			220		1.44		I
choc fudge, from mix, Supermoist	250		3.0	34.0	20.0	1.0	0	0	.10			430	60			
1/12 cake	80	11.0	3.0	4.0	4.0	55	0	.09	0.4			115		1.08		I
choc, german, from mix, Supermoist	250		3.0	34.0	20.0	1.0	0	0	.14			410	20			
1/12 cake	80	11.0	3.0	4.0	4.0	55	0	.09	0.4			80		1.08		I
choc pudding type, from mix	270	23.3	3.5	34.2		1.5	24	0	.13	.03	8	402	64	19	.49	.259
1/12 of 9″ cake	77	14.3	3.0	4.7	5.9	53	81	.08	0.9	.32	.21	161	146	1.45	.121	818
choc swirl, double, from mix, Supermoist	250		4.0	35.0	22.0	1.0	0	0	.14			390	60			
1/12 cake	80	11.0	3.0	3.0	4.0	55	0	.09	0.8			140		1.80		I
choc swirl, from mix, Supermoist	250		4.0	36.0	20.0	0.0	0	0	.14			290	80			
1/12 cake	80	11.0	2.5	3.5	4.0	55	0	.09	0.8			90		1.08		I
coffee cake																
cheese (cream/neufchatel)	258	24.5	5.3	33.7		0.8	54	0	.10	.04	44	258	45	11	.45	.131
1/6 of 16 oz cake	76	11.6	3.8	5.7	1.2	26	178	.08	0.5	.11	.19	220	75	.49	.040	818
cinn w/ crumb topping	263	13.8	4.3	29.4		1.3	18	0	.14	.02	20	221	34	14	.51	.284
1/9 of 20 oz cake	63	14.7	3.6	8.3	1.8	20	61	.13	1.1	.07	.41	77	68	1.20	.079	818
cinn w/ crumb topping, from mix	178	17.1	3.1	29.6		0.7	22	0	.10	.03	7	236	76	10	.25	.174
1/8 of cake	56	5.4	1.0	2.2	1.8	27	78	.09	0.9	.08	.15	63	120	.80	.083	818
cinn w/ crumb topping, homemade	240	12.6	3.9	30.2			99	0	.12	.05	9	233	67	24	.49	.423
1/12 of 8″ sq cake	60	12.1	2.2	4.6	4.7	36	383	.11	0.7	.09	.24	143	83	1.33	.155	818
creme filled, w/ choc icing	298	26.2	4.5	48.4		1.8	14	0	.07	.04	41	291	34	14	.40	.171
1/6 of 19 oz cake	90	9.7	2.5	5.3	1.3	23	48	.07	0.8	.05	.17	72	68	.46	.063	818
easy mix, dry, Aunt Jemima	168	1.8	1.9	29.5	17.2	0.7	0	0	.12	.01	1	243	59	9	.16	
1/3 cup (1.4 oz)	39	5.0	0.9	1.9	0.2	1	0	.14	1.2	.00	.08	27	88	1.03	.060	I
fruit, from mix, Aunt Jemima	156	15.8	2.6	25.8		1.3	10	0	.10	.02	10	193	23	9	.33	.120
1/8 of 14 oz cake	50	5.1	1.2	2.9	0.7	11	70	.02	1.3	.03	.33	45	59	1.22	.015	818
cottage pudding																
homemade	186	14.4	3.5	29.3				0	.09			161	49			
1/8 cake	54	6.1	1.7				80	.08	0.6			48	62	.80		456
w/ choc sce, homemade	235	20.6	3.9	42.0				0	.10			172	53			
1/8 cake & 1 T sce	74	6.5	2.0				70	.09	0.7			104	81	1.00		456

									Vitamins					Minerals		
	KCAL	H_2O (g)	PRO (g)	CHO (g)	SUGR (g)	DFIB (g)	A (RE)	C (mg)	B-2 (mg)	B-6 (mg)	FOL (mcg)	Na (mg)	Ca (mg)	Mg (mg)	Zn (mg)	Mn (mg)
	WT (g)	FAT (g)	SFA (g)	MUFA (g)	PUFA (g)	CHOL (mg)	A (IU)	B 1 (mg)	NIA (mg)	B-12 (mcg)	PANT (mg)	K (mg)	P (mg)	Fe (mg)	Cu (mg)	REF
w/ strawberry sce, homemade	204	25.6	3.6	33.9				8	.11			163	51			
⅛ cake & 1 T sce	70	6.2	1.7				80	.08	0.8			65	65	.80		456
devil's food																
from mix, Duncan Hines Deluxe	190	0.6	2.0	33.0					.07			360	65	20	.35	
1/12 pkg	43	5.0	2.0	2.0	1.0	0		.07	0.7			140	115	1.98	.176	I
from mix, red fat, Sweet Rewards	220		4.0	35.0	20.0	1.0	0	0	.14			370	40			
1/12 cake	43	7.0	2.0			55	0	.09	0.8			150		1.08		I
from mix, Supermoist	240		3.0	33.0	20.0	1.0	0	0	.10			360	40			
1/12 cake	80	11.0	3.0	3.5	3.5	55	0	.06	0.8			150		1.44		I
w/ choc icing, frzn	323	17.9	3.7	47.3				0	.07			357	46			
⅙ cake	85	15.0	7.7				370	.02	0.2			101	78	.70		456
w/ whipped cream filling & choc icing,	315	25.2	3.0	37.2				0	.07			162	68			
frzn—*⅙ cake*	85	18.6	6.2				230	.02	0.2			96	104	.50		456
fruitcake	139	10.9	1.2	26.5	18.5	1.6	8	0	.04	.02	1	116	14	7	.12	.095
1 piece (1.5 oz)	43	3.9	0.5	1.8	1.4	2	34	.02	0.3	.03	.10	66	22	.89	.022	818
fruitcake, homemade	302	15.6	3.0	54.4			13	4	.10	.09	8	121	55	29	.59	.520
1/36 of 10″ cake	84	9.7	1.2	4.0	3.8	24	60	.14	0.9	.04	.29	260	66	1.56	.223	818
fudge, from mix, Duncan Hines Butter	320	3.0	3.0	40.0	28.0	2.0	0	0	.14			300	20			
Recipe—*1/12 cake*[5]	79	17.0	7.0		2.0	80	0	.03	1.2			190		1.44		I
fudge marble, from mix, Supermoist	250		3.0	35.0	21.0	0.0	0	0	.14			270	80			
1/12 cake	80	11.0	2.5	3.5	4.0	55	0	.09	0.8			40		.72		I
german choc w/ coconut-nut icing,	404	29.9	3.9	55.2		1.5	23	0	.14	.02	4	369	53	19	.49	.003
from mix—*1/12 of 9″ cake*	111	20.6	5.3	8.7	5.5	53	79	.11	1.1	.10	.14	151	173	1.22	.119	818
gingerbread																
classic, from mix, Betty Crocker	230		3.0	38.0	20.0	0.0	0	0	.10			370	60			
⅛ cake	80	7.0	2.0	2.5	0.5	25	0	.12	0.8			150		1.44		I
from mix	207	22.2	2.7	34.0		0.8	11	0	.12	.03	7	307	46	11	.27	.241
1/9 of 9″ sq cake	67	6.8	1.7	3.8	0.9	23	37	.13	1.0	.05	.15	161	113	2.22	.107	818
homemade	263	20.7	2.9	36.4			10	0	.12	.14	6	242	53	52	.29	.505
1/9 of 8″ sq cake	74	12.1	3.1	5.3	3.1	24	36	.14	1.3	.04	.28	325	40	2.13	.144	818
golden, from mix, Duncan Hines Butter	320	1.5	3.0	42.0	29.0	2.0	0	0	.10			190	60			
Recipe—*1/12 cake*[6]	80	16.0	7.0		2.0	80	0	.06	1.2			70		.72		I
honey spice, from mix	363	23.4	4.2	62.7				0	.09			252	73			
1/12 cake	103	11.1	3.3				160	.02	0.2			84	199	.80		456
lemon chiffon, from mix, Betty Crocker	140		3.0	26.0	16.0	0.0		0	.10			140	20		.36	
1/16 cake	55	3.0	0.5	1.0	1.0	25	0	.06	0.4			45				I
lemon, fat-free, from mix, Sweet Rewards	170		2.0	39.0	27.0	0.0	0	0	.10			270	40			
⅛ cake	44	0.0	0.0	0.0	0.0	0	0	.12	0.8			35		.72		I
lemon, from mix, Supermoist	250		3.0	36.0	21.0	0.0	0	0	.14			260	80			
1/12 cake	80	11.0	2.5	4.0	4.0	55	0	.09	0.8			35		1.08		I
lemon pudding cake, from mix, Betty	180		2.0	33.0	24.0	0.0		0	.06			210	20			
Crocker—*⅛ cake*	80	4.0	1.0	2.0	0.0	35	0	.03	0.0			35		.36		I
marble cake, from mix	253	21.8	3.1	34.5		1.3	24	0	.11	.03	7	242	40	9	.30	.227
1/12 of 9″ cake	73	12.4	2.3	4.0	5.4	53	80	.07	0.6	.10	.19	69	142	.88	.062	818
milk choc, from mix, Supermoist	250		3.0	33.0	21.0	1.0	0	0	.14			320	60			
1/12 cake	80	12.0	3.0	4.0	4.0	55	0	.06	0.4			140		1.08		I
party swirl, from mix, Supermoist	250		3.0	35.0	21.0	0.0	0	0	.14			280	80			
1/12 cake	80	11.0	2.5	3.5	4.0	55	0	.09	0.8			40		.72		I
peanut butter choc swirl, from mix,	240		4.0	34.0	19.0	0.0	0	0	.10			320	80			
Supermoist—*1/12 cake*	80	10.0	2.5	3.0	3.5	55	0	.09	1.2			80		1.08		I
pineapple upside-down, from mix,	400		3.0	63.0	43.0		0	.10			350	60				
Betty Crocker—*⅙ cake*	125	15.0	4.0	7.0	2.0	35	200	.12	0.8			90		.72		I
pineapple upside-down, homemade	367	37.1	4.0	58.1		0.9	75	1	.18	.04	8	367	138	15	.36	.402
1/9 of 8″ cake	115	13.9	3.4	6.0	3.8	25	291	.18	1.4	.09	.23	129	94	1.70	.100	818
pound																
butter, frzn, Pepperidge Farms	131		1.5	15.5				0	.03			116	7			
1.1 oz	30	7.0					0	.01	0.2			17		.20		I

	KCAL / WT (g)	H_2O (g) / FAT (g)	PRO (g) / SFA (g)	CHO (g) / MUFA (g)	SUGR (g) / PUFA (g)	DFIB (g) / CHOL (mg)	A (RE) / A (IU)	C (mg) / B-1 (mg)	B-2 (mg) / NIA (mg)	B-6 (mg) / B-12 (mcg)	FOL (mcg) / PANT (mg)	Na (mg) / K (mg)	Ca (mg) / P (mg)	Mg (mg) / Fe (mg)	Zn (mg) / Cu (mg)	Mn (mg) / REF
chol free, frzn, Pepperidge Farm	113		1.4	13.5				0	.03			91	5			
1 oz	28	5.9					62	.00	0.1			19		.10		I
fat-free	80	8.8	1.5	17.3		0.3	8	0	.09	.00	1	97	12	3	.09	.039
1 oz	28	0.3	0.1	0.0	0.1	0	27	.04	0.2	.00	.10	31	41	.58	.016	818
golden, from mix, Betty Crocker	270		4.0	45.0	26.0	0.0		0	.14			220	40			
⅛ cake	80	8.0	3.5	3.0	0.5	55	0	.12	0.8			40		1.08		I
made w/ butter	116	7.4	1.6	14.6		0.1	47	0	.07	.01	3	119	11	3	.14	.027
¹⁄₁₀ of 10.75 oz cake	30	6.0	3.3	1.7	0.3	66	182	.04	0.4	.05	.10	36	41	.41	.011	818
made w/ veg shortening	117	6.9	1.6	15.8		0.3	11	0	.08	.01	3	120	19	4	.12	.026
¹⁄₁₀ of 10.6 oz cake	30	5.4	1.4	3.0	0.7	17	35	.04	0.4	.04	.09	32	40	.49	.016	818
modified, made w/ butter, homemade	206	12.6	3.2	28.4			96	0	.11	.02	7	161	39	6	.26	.112
¹⁄₁₆ of loaf cake[7]	54	9.0	5.2	2.7	0.5	62	372	.11	0.9	.10	.19	47	52	.93	.033	818
modified, made w/ marg, homemade	206	12.6	3.2	28.5			104	0	.14	.02	6	172	39	6	.26	.111
¹⁄₁₆ of loaf cake[7]	54	9.0	1.9	3.8	2.6	41	396	.11	0.9	.10	.19	49	52	.92	.032	818
old-fashioned, made w/ butter, homemade—*¹⁄₁₆ of loaf cake[8]*	229	10.8	3.3	25.2			134	0	.14	.02	8	153	13	5	.27	.102
	53	13.1	7.6	3.9	0.7	92	524	.10	0.8	.13	.22	37	44	.90	.031	818
old fashioned, made w/ marg, homemade—*¹⁄₁₆ of loaf cake[8]*	230	10.8	3.4	25.3			147	0	.14	.03	8	169	13	5	.26	.102
	53	13.0	2.7	5.6	3.9	60	560	.10	0.8	.13	.21	39	44	.88	.029	818
pudding cake, from mix, Betty Crocker	170		2.0	33.0	21.0	1.0	0	0	.03			180	20			
⅛ cake	80	3.5	1.0	2.0	0.0	25	0	.03	0.4			120		.72		I
rainbow chip, from mix, Supermoist	250		3.0	34.0	20.0	0.0	0	0	.10			310	80			
¹⁄₁₂ cake	80	11.0	3.0	3.5	4.0	55	0	.09	0.8			40		.72		I
shortcake, biscuit-type, homemade	225	18.5	4.0	31.5			12	0	.18	.02	7	329	133	10	.31	.215
1 shortcake	65	9.2	2.5	3.9	2.4	2	47	.20	1.7	.05	.16	69	93	1.65	.049	818
sour cream white, from mix, Supermoist	280		4.0	39.0	22.0	0.0	0	0	.10			380	80			
¹⁄₁₀ cake	80	12.0	3.0	3.0	4.5		0	.12	0.8			45		.72		I
spice, from mix, Supermoist	250		3.0	35.0	20.0	0.0	0	0	.14			310	100			
¹⁄₁₂ cake	80	11.0	2.5	3.5	4.0	55	0	.09	0.8			45		1.08		I
sponge	110	11.3	2.1	23.2		0.2	17	0	.10	.02	5	93	27	4	.19	.080
¹⁄₁₂ of 16 oz cake	38	1.0	0.3	0.4	0.2	39	59	.09	0.7	.09	.18	38	52	1.03	.024	818
sponge, homemade	187	18.5	4.6	36.4			49	0	.19	.04	12	144	26	6	.37	.105
¹⁄₁₂ of 10" cake	63	2.7	0.8	1.0	0.4	107	163	.10	0.8	.23	.34	89	63	1.00	.035	818
strawberry swirl, from mix, Supermoist	290		4.0	42.0	25.0	0.0	0	0	.14			330	80			
¹⁄₁₀ cake	80	12.0	3.0	3.0	4.5	65	0	.12	0.8			40		1.08		I
van, french, from mix, Supermoist	250		3.0	35.0	20.0	0.0	0	0	.10			280	80			
¹⁄₁₂ cake	80	10.0	2.5	3.0	3.5	55	0	.09	0.8			40		.72		I
van, golden, from mix, Supermoist	280		3.0	35.0	20.0	0.0	0	0	.10			260	60			
¹⁄₁₂ cake	80	14.0	3.0	4.5	6.0	55	0	.09	0.8			35		1.08		I
white																
from mix	190	19.1	2.5	34.3		0.4	0	0	.10	.01	3	301	86	6	.21	.125
¹⁄₁₂ of 9" cake	62	4.8	0.7	2.0	1.8	0	1	.08	0.4	.06	.08	59	149	.61	.038	818
from mix, Supermoist	230		3.0	35.0	19.0	0.0	0	0	.07			290	60			
¹⁄₁₂ cake	80	9.0	2.5	3.0	3.5	0	0	.09	0.8			30		.72		I
homemade	264	17.2	4.0	42.3		0.6	12	0	.18	.02	5	242	96	9	.24	.146
¹⁄₁₂ of 9" cake	74	9.2	2.4	3.9	2.3	1	41	.14	1.1	.06	.14	70	69	1.12	.044	818
made w/ egg whites, from mix, Duncan Hines—*¹⁄₁₂ cake*	240		2.0	36.0	21.0		0	0	.10			220	60			
	62	10.0	2.0		3.0	0	0	.09	0.8			80				I
made w/ whole eggs, from mix, Duncan Hines—*¹⁄₁₂ cake*	250		3.0	36.0	21.0		0	0	.10			220	60			
	66	12.0	2.5		3.0	45	0	.09	0.8							I
Olympic Party, from mix, Supermoist	240		3.0	33.0	19.0	0.0	0	0	.10			280	60			
¹⁄₁₂ cake	80	11.0	3.0	2.5	3.5	0	0	.09	0.8			25		.72		I
pudding type, from mix	244	19.6	2.5	35.7		0.3	0	0	.10	.01	3	305	35	5	.12	.120
¹⁄₁₂ of 9" cake	69	10.2	1.9	3.8	4.1	0	0	.10	1.0	.05	.08	42	123	.60	.026	818
red fat, from mix, Sweet Rewards	210		3.0	35.0	20.0	0.0	0	0	.10			300	60			
¹⁄₁₂ cake	43	6.0	1.5			0	0	.09	0.8			30		.72		I
w/ coconut icing, homemade	399	23.2	4.9	70.8		1.1	12	0	.21	.03	6	318	101	13	.37	.310
¹⁄₁₂ of 9" cake	112	11.5	4.4	4.1	2.4	1	43	.14	1.2	.07	.19	111	78	1.30	.075	818
yellow																
from mix	202	18.8	3.0	34.3		0.5	16	0	.12	.04	6	299	64	6	.21	.086
¹⁄₁₂ of 9" cake	63	5.9	1.0	2.4	2.0	37	54	.07	0.7	.12	.20	46	151	.78	.034	818

	KCAL	H₂O (g)	PRO (g)	CHO (g)	SUGR (g)	DFIB (g)	A (RE)	C (mg)	B-2 (mg)	B-6 (mg)	FOL (mcg)	Na (mg)	Ca (mg)	Mg (mg)	Zn (mg)	Mn (mg)
	WT (g)	FAT (g)	SFA (g)	MUFA (g)	PUFA (g)	CHOL (mg)	A (IU)	B-1 (mg)	NIA (mg)	B-12 (mcg)	PANT (mg)	K (mg)	P (mg)	Fe (mg)	Cu (mg)	REF
from mix, Duncan	250		3.0	36.0	22.0		0	0	.14			290	80			
¹⁄₁₂ cake[9]	71	11.0	2.0	3.0	5.0	45	0	.09	0.8			80		1.08		I
from mix, Supermoist	240		4.0	34.0	20.0	0.0	0	0	.10			290	80			
¹⁄₁₂ cake	80	10.0	2.5	2.5	4.0	55	0	.09	0.8			30		.72		I
homemade	245	17.1	3.6	36.0		0.5	27	0	.16	.02	7	233	99	8	.31	.129
¹⁄₁₂ of 8" cake	68	9.9	2.7	4.2	2.4	37	95	.12	1.0	.11	.21	62	80	1.12	.038	818
light, 3% fat, from mix	181	25.6	3.0	36.8		0.6	1	0	.12	.01	2	279	69	6	.15	.100
¹⁄₁₂ of 9" cake	69	2.4	1.1	0.9	0.2	0	6	.06	0.6	.06	.10	41	143	.58	.030	456
light, 6% fat, from mix	195	23.7	3.6	36.7		0.6	26	0	.14	.03	6	279	75	6	.29	.102
¹⁄₁₂ of 9" cake	69	3.7	1.5	1.4	0.3	53	84	.07	0.6	.14	.23	43	164	.75	.030	818
light, from mix	115	0.9	1.3	23.8		0.4	1	0	.06	.01	1	171	44	3	.09	.065
1 oz	28	1.6	0.7	0.6	0.1	0	4	.05	0.4	.03	.09	18	92	.37	.018	818
pudding type, from mix	243	20.7	3.1	33.2		0.3	23	0	.13	.02	7	299	54	5	.25	.115
¹⁄₁₂ of 9" cake	69	11.0	2.2	4.1	4.0	50	75	.11	1.0	.12	.13	40	126	.82	.027	818
red fat, from mix, Sweet Rewards	220		3.0	36.0	20.0	0.0	0	0	.14			300	80			
¹⁄₁₂ cake	43	6.0	1.5			55	0	.09	0.8			30		.72		I
w/ choc icing	243	14.0	2.4	35.5		1.2	17	0	.10	.02	5	216	24	19	.40	.166
¹⁄₈ of 18 oz cake	64	11.1	3.0	6.2	1.3	35	58	.08	0.8	.08	.15	114	103	1.33	.120	818
w/ van icing	239	14.1	2.2	37.6		0.2	12	0	.04	.02	6	220	40	4	.16	.061
¹⁄₈ of 18 oz cake	64	9.3	1.5	3.9	3.3	36	40	.06	0.3	.13	.22	34	92	.68	.022	818

8.3 CAKES, SNACK

	KCAL	H₂O (g)	PRO (g)	CHO (g)	SUGR (g)	DFIB (g)	A (RE)	C (mg)	B-2 (mg)	B-6 (mg)	FOL (mcg)	Na (mg)	Ca (mg)	Mg (mg)	Zn (mg)	Mn (mg)
	WT (g)	FAT (g)	SFA (g)	MUFA (g)	PUFA (g)	CHOL (mg)	A (IU)	B-1 (mg)	NIA (mg)	B-12 (mcg)	PANT (mg)	K (mg)	P (mg)	Fe (mg)	Cu (mg)	REF
Apple Delights, Little Debbie	145	4.9	1.4	23.9	12.1	0.5		0	.08			155	9	1		
1.3 oz pkg	36	5.1	1.6	1.9	1.2	4	5	.13	0.0							I
Banana Twins, Little Debbie	246	10.6	1.6	38.9	25.5	0.2		0	.08			172	10			
2.2 oz pkg	62	10.2	2.3	3.5	3.5	8	847	.09	0.8					.93		I
Be My Valentine, choc, Little Debbie	268	7.7	1.8	38.4	27.6	0.7		0	.06			164	16			
2.2 oz pkg	62	13.2	3.0			1	1	.07	0.5					.56		I
Be My Valentine, van, Little Debbie	273	8.2	1.3	37.9	27.2	0.1			.06			166	7			
2.2 oz pkg	62	13.7	3.2	5.0	5.0	0		.09	0.6					.68		I
Cherry Cordials, Little Debbie	161	4.7	0.8	22.9	16.5	0.6			.04			101	6			
1.3 oz pkg	37	8.1	1.8			0	28	.06	0.5					.67		I
Choc Cake Deluxe, Little Debbie	257	9.5	3.0	30.6	21.4	1.2		0	.08			161	14			
2.1 oz pkg	59	14.8	2.8			4	46	.09	0.6					.89		I
choc chip cake, Little Debbie	293	9.0		41.6	32.8	0.6		0	.07			205	8			
2.4 oz pkg	68	14.5	3.3			1	2	.09	0.7					.75		I
choc, creme filled w/ icing	188	9.9	1.7	30.1		0.4	3	0	.15	.01	4	213	37	21	.28	.169
1 snack cake	50	7.3	1.6	2.7	2.1	9	9	.11	1.2	.06	.13	61	47	1.68	.097	818
Choc Twins, Little Debbie	243	12.9	1.9	42.5	27.9	0.5		0	.08			243	18			
2.4 oz pkg	67	8.4	2.1			18	18	.10	0.9					1.00		I
Christmas Tree Cakes, Little Debbie	194	5.0	0.8	26.7	21.6	0.1		0	.04			99	3			
1.5 oz pkg	43	9.8	2.3			0	0	.06	0.4					.47		I
coconut creme cakes, Little Debbie	214	6.4	1.2	30.2	23.8	0.2		0	.05			144	0			
1.7 oz pkg	49	10.3	2.9			2	2	.07	0.5					.64		I
Coconut Rounds, Little Debbie	153	3.8	1.0	22.9	12.7	0.8		0	.05			89	3			
1.2 oz pkg	35	7.0	3.1			0	0	.08	0.6					.77		I
coffee cake, apple streusel, Little Debbie	227	10.4	2.5	39.1	23.3			0	.12			193	15			
2.1 oz pkg	60	7.2	1.5			8	9	.17	1.3					1.50		I
creme-filled choc cupcake, Little Debbie	185	7.1	1.7	25.9	17.6	0.9		0	.05			134	10			
1.6 oz	45	9.4	2.0			4	4	.05	0.4					.45		I
cupcake																
choc w/ icing, low-fat	131	9.8	1.8	28.9		1.8	0	0	.06	.00	2	178	15	11	.24	.096
1 cupcake	43	1.6	0.5	0.8	0.2	0	0	.02	0.3	.00	.10	96	79	.66	.076	818
w/ choc icing, from mix	172	10.7	2.2	28.4				0	.05			161	62			
1 cupcake	48	6.0					80	.02	0.1			56	95	.40		456
w/ choc icing, homemade	173	10.1	2.0	27.9				0	.04			108	30			
1 cupcake	47	6.5					80	.01	0.1			54	49	.30		456
w/ white icing, homemade	172	9.7	1.6	29.8				0	.03			107	24			
1 cupcake	47	5.5					90	.01	0.0			29	35	.10		456

	KCAL	H₂O (g)	PRO (g)	CHO (g)	SUGR (g)	DFIB (g)	Vitamins — A (RE)	C (mg)	B-2 (mg)	B-6 (mg)	FOL (mcg)	Minerals — Na (mg)	Ca (mg)	Mg (mg)	Zn (mg)	Mn (mg)
	WT (g)	FAT (g)	SFA (g)	MUFA (g)	PUFA (g)	CHOL (mg)	A (IU)	B-1 (mg)	NIA (mg)	B-12 (mcg)	PANT (mg)	K (mg)	P (mg)	Fe (mg)	Cu (mg)	REF
Devil Cremes, Little Debbie	190	7.7	1.3	28.9	18.1	0.4		0	.06			165	7			
1.7 oz pkg	47	7.6	1.8			2	2	.09	0.7					.75		I
Devil Squares, Little Debbie	265	7.6	1.9	39.0	30.3	0.8		0	.07			181	16			
2.2 oz pkg	62	12.4	2.9			2	2	.08	0.6					.87		I
Easter Basket Cake, choc, Little Debbie	282	10.2	2.0	41.5	29.4	0.7		0	.07			190	18			
2.4 oz pkg	68	13.3	3.0			2	2	.08	0.6					.68		I
Easter Basket Cake, van, Little Debbie	307	9.4	1.6	44.3	31.3	0.2		0	.07			176	8			
2.5 oz pkg	71	14.7	3.4			0	0	.11	0.8					1.44		I
Fall Party, choc, Little Debbie	292	8.5	1.9	42.5	32.3	0.2		0	.07			182	8			
2.4 oz pkg	68	13.9	3.2			0	0	.10	0.8					1.02		I
Fall Party, van, Little Debbie	312	8.8	1.6	44.4	35.1	0.2		0	.07			177	6			
2.5 oz pkg	71	15.2	3.5			0	0	.11	0.8					.85		I
Fancy Cakes, Little Debbie	298	9.1	1.5	41.7	32.9	0.2		0	.07			189	6			
2.4 oz	68	14.8	3.4			0	0	.10	0.7					.82		I
frosted fudge cake, Little Debbie	186	5.7	1.4	25.2	19.5	0.8		0	.04			130	8			
1.5 oz pkg	43	9.9	2.2			6	6	.05	0.4					.56		I
Holiday Cakes, choc, Little Debbie	290	8.9	1.9	42.4	32.2	0.7		0	.07			184	8			
2.4 oz pkg	68	13.8	4.7			0	0	.10	0.8					1.09		I
Holiday Cakes, van, Little Debbie	294	9.3	1.6	44.4	35.0	0.2		0	.07			169	6			
2.5 oz pkg	71	14.8	3.4			0	0	.11	0.8					.82		I
Holiday Roll, cherry creme, Little Debbie	271	10.3	1.6	40.1	29.2	0.9		0	.05			176	26			
2.3 oz pkg	66	13.1	3.0			14	14	.08	0.6					.73		I
Jelly Creme Pie, Little Debbie	156	3.5	0.8	22.7	14.7	0.3		0	.04			103	4			
1.2 oz pkg	35	7.5	1.5			0	30	.07	0.5					.56		I
Kids Cups, Sports/Soft Rocks/ABCs	367		3.3	49.0	36.0	0.0		0	0			313	60			
2 cupcakes[10]	88	18.0	3.0			70	0							1.08		I
Marshmallow Pie, banana, Little Debbie	162	4.1	1.4	28.4	17.1	0.4		1	.05			70	11			
1.4 oz pkg	39	4.8	1.3			0	20	.05	0.9					.35		I
Marshmallow Pie, choc, Little Debbie	166	3.0	1.6	29.4	16.2	1.7		1	.08			84	11			
1.4 oz pkg	39	4.6	1.3			0	20	.12	0.9					.90		I
Marshmallow Supremes, Little Debbie	128	3.7	1.1	21.7	15.1	0.7		0	.02			66	5			
1.1 oz pkg	32	5.1	1.1			1	1	.04	0.2					.29		I
Raisin Creme Pie, Little Debbie	140	4.1	0.9	23.1	15.5	0.3						118	5			
1.2 oz pkg	34	5.4	1.3			1								.78		I
Raspberry Angel Cake, Little Debbie	124	12.4	2.0	27.2	18.4	0.3		0	.03			116	25			
1.5 oz pkg	43	0.9	0.2			0	20	.03	0.4					.34		I
spice cake, Little Debbie	302	9.3	1.5	43.8	35.7	0.5		0	.06			233	7			
2.5 oz pkg	70	14.3	3.6			8	49	.08	0.6					.84		I
sponge snack cake, creme filled	157	8.7	1.3	27.5		0.2		0	.06	.01	2	157	19	3	.13	.075
1 snack cake	43	4.9	1.2	1.9	1.5	7	7	.07	0.5	.05	.10	39	33	.55	.023	818
Strawberry Shortcake Roll, Little Debbie	232	10.3	1.2	40.3	28.9	0.2		0	.06			161	9			
2.2 oz pkg	61	8.2	2.0			15	306	.09	0.6					.73		I
Swiss Cake Rolls, Little Debbie	254	8.3	1.4	38.8	29.8	0.5		0	.06			178	21			
2.2 oz	61	11.6	2.8			15	16	.09	0.7					.92		I
Tiger Cake, Little Debbie	307	8.8	1.9	44.0	33.7	0.8		0	.08			194	8			
2.5 oz pkg	71	15.1	3.5			0	0	.11	0.8					1.14		I
Zebra Cake, Little Debbie	325	9.3	1.7	46.0	36.2	0.3		0	.07			185	7			
2.6 oz	74	16.0	3.7			0	0	.11	0.8					.96		I

8.4 COOKIES

	KCAL	H₂O (g)	PRO (g)	CHO (g)	SUGR (g)	DFIB (g)	A (RE)	C (mg)	B-2 (mg)	B-6 (mg)	FOL (mcg)	Na (mg)	Ca (mg)	Mg (mg)	Zn (mg)	Mn (mg)
	WT (g)	FAT (g)	SFA (g)	MUFA (g)	PUFA (g)	CHOL (mg)	A (IU)	B-1 (mg)	NIA (mg)	B-12 (mcg)	PANT (mg)	K (mg)	P (mg)	Fe (mg)	Cu (mg)	REF
Almond Toast, Stella D'Oro	110		2.0	21.0	10.0	1.0						85				
2 cookies	29	2.5	0.5	1.0	0.0	30										I
Angel Wings, Stella D'Oro	140		2.0	13.0	3.0	1.0						80				
2 cookies	25	9.0	3.0			5										I
Angelica Goodies, Stella D'Oro	100		2.0	15.0	6.0	0.0						45				
1 cookie	23	4.0	1.0			15										I
Anginette, Stella D'Oro	140		2.0	23.0	17.0	1.0						10				
4 cookies	31	4.0	1.0	1.0	2.0	40										I
animal crackers	126	1.1	2.0	21.0	6.4	0.3	0	0	.09	.01	4	111	12	5	.18	.120
11 pieces (1 oz)	28	3.9	1.0	2.2	0.5	0	0	.10	1.0	.01	.11	28	32	.78	.045	818

							Vitamins					Minerals				
	KCAL	H_2O (g)	PRO (g)	CHO (g)	SUGR (g)	DFIB (g)	A (RE)	C (mg)	B-2 (mg)	B-6 (mg)	FOL (mcg)	Na (mg)	Ca (mg)	Mg (mg)	Zn (mg)	Mn (mg)
	WT (g)	FAT (g)	SFA (g)	MUFA (g)	PUFA (g)	CHOL (mg)	A (IU)	B-1 (mg)	NIA (mg)	B-12 (mcg)	PANT (mg)	K (mg)	P (mg)	Fe (mg)	Cu (mg)	REF
animal crackers, Barnum's	140		2.0	23.0	8.0	1.0						160				
12 pieces	31	4.0				0										I
Animal, Little Debbie	186	1.4	2.7	34.0	9.7	4.1						146	8			
1.5 oz pkg	43	4.4	1.2			0								.78		I
Anisette Sponge, Stella D'Oro	90		2.0	19.0	9.0	1.0						80				
2 cookies	27	1.0	0.0	0.0	0.0	40										I
Anisette Toast, Stella D'Oro	130		2.0	27.0	17.0	1.0						150				
3 cookies	35	1.0	0.0	0.0	0.0	35										I
apple newton, fat-free, Nabisco	100		1.0	24.0	14.0	1.0						60				
2 cookies	29	0.0	0.0	0.0	0.0	0										I
apple oatmeal, Lance	215	4.5	1.8	35.1					.10			213	46			
1.7 oz	47	7.0	1.9	2.8	1.9	5		.12	0.9			28		.59		I
arrowroot biscuit, National	20		0.0	3.0	1.0	1.0						15				
1 cookie	5	0.5														I
blueberry newton, fat-free, Nabisco	100		2.0	23.0	9.0	1.0						90				
2 cookies	29	0.0	0.0	0.0	0.0	0										I
Breakfast Treats, choc, Stella D'Oro	100		2.0	15.0	7.0	1.0						70				
1 cookie	23	3.5	1.0			10										I
Breakfast Treats, Stella D'Oro	100		1.0	16.0	7.0	1.0						80				
1 cookie	23	3.0	1.0			10										I
Brown Edge Wafers, Nabisco	140		1.0	21.0	10.0	1.0						90				
5 cookies	29	6.0	1.5			5										I
butter cookies	23	0.2	0.3	3.4		0.0	8	0	.02	.00	0	18	1	1	.02	.009
1 cookie (2" dia)	5	0.9	0.5	0.3	0.0	4	30	.02	0.2	.01	.02	6	5	.11	.010	818
Buttercup, Keebler	71		1.2	10.8					.05			90	4			
3 cookies	15	2.4	0.6		0.2	0		.05	0.6			22		.38		I
Cameo Creme Sandwich, Nabisco	130		1.0	21.0	10.0	1.0						105				
2 cookies	28	5.0	1.0			0										I
Chinese Dessert, Stella D'Oro	170		2.0	21.0	8.0	1.0						90				
1 cookie	33	9.0	2.0			5										I
choc chip																
(12-17% fat)	45	0.4	0.6	7.3		0.4	0	0	.03	.03	1	38	2	3	.07	.045
1 cookie (2 ¼" dia)	10	1.5	0.4	0.8	0.2	0	0	.03	0.3	.00	.01	12	8	.31	.025	818
(18-28% fat)	48	0.4	0.5	6.7		0.3	0	0	.03	.01	1	32	3	3	.06	.045
1 cookie (2 ¼" dia)	10	2.3	0.8	1.1	0.2	0	0	.02	0.3	.00	.02	14	11	.28	.021	818
bite size, Lance	127	1.5	1.8	20.7	6.2	0.6			.03			105	29			
1 oz	28	4.1	1.9			16	140	.07	1.4			0	45	.88		I
chewy, Chips Ahoy	170		1.0	23.0	14.0	1.0						125				
3 cookies	36	8.0	2.5			5										I
Chips Ahoy	160		2.0	21.0	10.0	1.0						110				
3 cookies	32	8.0	2.5			0										I
chunky, Chips Ahoy	80		1.0	10.0	6.0	0.0						35				
1 cookie	16	4.0	1.5			5										I
Duncan Hines	110		1.0	15.6								90				
2 cookies	25	5.0	2.0	2.5	0.5	0										I
from mix	79	0.6	0.9	10.3		0.2	3	0	.04	.00	1	47	8	6	.11	.050
2" cookie	16	4.1	1.3	2.1	0.4	7	10	.02	0.3	.01	.03	34	15	.34	.047	818
from refrig dough	59	0.4	0.6	8.2		0.2	2	0	.02	.00	1	28	3	3	.07	.057
1 cookie (2 ¼" dia)	12	2.7	0.9	1.4	0.3	3	7	.02	0.2	.01	.02	24	9	.30	.024	818
homemade w/ butter	78	0.9	0.9	9.3			24	0	.03	.01	2	55	6	9	.15	.106
1 cookie (2 ¼" dia)	16	4.5	2.3	1.3	0.7	11	95	.03	0.2	.01	.04	35	16	.40	.062	818
homemade w/ marg	78	0.9	0.9	9.3		0.4	26	0	.03	.01	2	58	6	9	.15	.106
1 cookie (2 ¼" dia)	16	4.5	1.3	1.7	1.3	5	102	.03	0.2	.01	.04	36	16	.39	.061	818
Keebler Old Fashioned	78		0.9	10.9					.03			78	4			
1 cookie	16	3.5	1.0		0.3	0		.02	0.4			22		.37		I
Little Debbie	181	2.8	1.7	23.5	12.2	0.5		0	.08			129	9			
1.3 oz pkg	38	9.4	2.7			5	6	.13	1.0					1.22		I
Pillsbury	68	2.4	0.7	9.3				0	.04			55	2			
1 cookie	16	3.4					4	.03	0.3			17	9	.28		I
red fat, Chips Ahoy	140		2.0	22.0	10.0	1.0						150				
3 cookies	31	5.0	1.5			0										I

	KCAL	H₂O (g)	PRO (g)	CHO (g)	SUGR (g)	DFIB (g)	Vitamins A (RE)	C (mg)	B-2 (mg)	B-6 (mg)	FOL (mcg)	Minerals Na (mg)	Ca (mg)	Mg (mg)	Zn (mg)	Mn (mg)
	WT (g)	FAT (g)	SFA (g)	MUFA (g)	PUFA (g)	CHOL (mg)	A (IU)	B-1 (mg)	NIA (mg)	B-12 (mcg)	PANT (mg)	K (mg)	P (mg)	Fe (mg)	Cu (mg)	REF
red fat, Snackwell's	130		2.0	22.0	10.0	1.0						180				
3 cookies	29	3.5	1.5	1.0	0.0	0										I
soft type	69	1.7	0.5	8.9		0.5	0	0	.03	.02	1	49	2	5	.07	.056
1 cookie	15	3.6	1.1	2.0	0.4	0	0	.02	0.2	.00	.04	14	8	.36	.024	818
choc chip cookie mix, Duncan Hines	130	0.9	1.0	20.1					.06			80	11	10	.17	
⅟₁₈ pkg (2 cookies)	28	5.0	3.0	1.0	1.0	0		.04	0.5			50	21	.50	.084	I
choc chip snaps, Nabisco	150		2.0	24.0	10.0	1.0						115				
7 cookies	32	5.0	1.5	1.5	0.0	0										I
choc choc chip, Pillsbury	66	2.4	0.6	9.6				0	.04			37	2			
1 cookie	16	3.1					1	.03	0.3			38	11	.32		I
choc coated graham crackers	137	0.7	1.6	18.9		0.9	1	0	.06	.02	3	82	16	16	.27	.206
2 crackers (1 oz)	28	6.6	3.1	2.6	0.4	0	3	.04	0.6	.00	.06	59	38	1.01	.122	818
choc fudge, Little Debbie	113	3.8	1.7	23.7	13.4	0.6	0	0	.05			139	9			
1.1 oz pkg	32	1.9	0.4			0	0	.09	0.5					.80		I
choc fudge sandwich, Keebler	83		0.9	11.7					.03			63	3			
1 cookie	17	3.7	1.0		0.2	0		.03	0.5			27		.44		I
choc graham snacks, Teddy Grahams	140		2.0	22.0	9.0	1.0						150				
25 pieces	30	5.0	1.0			0										I
Choc Nilla Wafers, red fat, Nabisco	120		2.0	24.0	12.0	1.0						120				
8 wafers	29	2.0	0.0			0										I
Choc-O-Lunch, Lance	176	0.6	2.7	26.0					.07			148				
1.3 oz	37	7.0	2.1	4.2	0.6			.02	0.5			59		.77		I
choc sandwich																
w/ choc creme, red fat, Snackwell's	110		1.0	20.0	11.0	1.0						220				
2 cookies	26	2.5	0.5	1.0	0.0	0						50				I
w/ creme filling	47	0.2	0.5	7.0		0.3	0	0	.02	.00	1	60	3	5	.08	.053
1 cookie	10	2.1	0.4	1.2	0.3	0	0	.01	0.2	.00	.02	18	10	.39	.035	818
w/ creme filling, choc coated	82	0.3	0.6	11.2		0.9	0	0	.03	.01	1	55	6	7	.10	.063
1 cookie	17	4.5	1.3	2.5	0.5	0	1	.02	0.2	.02	.05	41	15	.53	.054	818
w/ extra creme filling	65	0.2	0.5	8.9		0.3	0	0	.02	.00	1	64	3	4	.08	.050
1 cookie	13	3.3	0.6	1.9	0.4	0	0	.01	0.2	.00	.01	16	12	.37	.045	818
w/ van creme, red fat, Snackwell's	110		1.0	21.0	11.0	1.0						190				
2 cookies	26	2.5	0.5	1.0	0.0	0										I
choc snaps, Nabisco	140		2.0	22.0	8.0	1.0						170				
8 cookies	30	5.0	2.0	2.0	0.5	0										I
Choc Truffle Cakes, fat free, Snackwell's	60		1.0	14.0	8.0	1.0						60				
1 cookie	19	0.0	0.0	0.0	0.0	0										I
choc wafers	123	1.3	1.9	20.5	11.5	1.0	1	0	.08	.01	3	164	9	15	.31	.197
5 wafers (1 oz)[11]	28	4.0	1.0	2.1	0.5	1	2	.06	0.8	.02	.10	60	37	1.14	.131	818
choc wafers, Nabisco Famous	140		2.0	24.0	11.0	1.0						230				
5 wafers	32	4.0	1.5	1.5	0.5	5										I
Commodore, Keebler	60		0.8	9.5					.03			61	7			
1 cookie	13	2.0	0.5		0.1	0		.03	0.5			21		.43		I
Como Delight, Stella D'Oro	140		2.0	18.0	8.0	1.0						60				
1 cookie	32	7.0	2.0			40										I
Cookie Cakes																
devil's food, fat-free, Snackwell's	50		1.0	13.0	9.0	1.0						25				
1 cookie	16	0.0	0.0	0.0	0.0	0										I
double fudge, fat-free, Snackwell's	50		1.0	12.0	6.0	1.0						70				
1 cookie	16	0.0	0.0	0.0	0.0	0										I
golden devil's food, Snackwell's	50		1.0	12.0	8.0	0.0						30				
1 cookie	16	0.5	0.0	0.0	0.0	0										I
Cookie Mates, Keebler	51		0.7	7.8					.03			53	4			
2 cookies	11	1.9	0.3		0.1	0		.04	0.4			18		.37		I
cookie mix, Robin Hood/Gold Medal Pouch—⅟₁₈ pkg (2 cookies)[12]	160		2.3	20.3	12.0	0.3	0	0	.03			124	0			
	32	7.3	2.0			10		.06	0.4			65		.72		I
Cookie Wreaths, Little Debbie	93	0.6	0.6	11.5	6.7	0.1	0	0	.03			57	2			
.6 oz pkg	18	5.0	1.2			0	0	.06	0.4					.49		I
cranberry newtons, fat-free, Nabisco	90		2.0	21.0	8.0	1.0						90				
2 cookies	29	0.0	0.0	0.0	0.0	0										I

	KCAL / WT (g)	H₂O (g) / FAT (g)	PRO (g) / SFA (g)	CHO (g) / MUFA (g)	SUGR (g) / PUFA (g)	DFIB (g) / CHOL (mg)	A (RE) / A (IU)	C (mg) / B-1 (mg)	B-2 (mg) / NIA (mg)	B-6 (mg) / B-12 (mcg)	FOL (mcg) / PANT (mg)	Na (mg) / K (mg)	Ca (mg) / P (mg)	Mg (mg) / Fe (mg)	Zn (mg) / Cu (mg)	Mn (mg) / REF
creme sandwich, red fat, Snackwell's	110		1.0	21.0	10.0	1.0						100				
2 cookies	26	2.5	0.5	0.0	1.0	0										I
creme wafers, fudge covered, Nabisco	150		1.0	19.0	15.0	0.0						20				
3 cookies	28	8.0	2.0			0										I
double fudge, Keebler Old Fashioned	77		1.0	10.9					.02			68	5			
1 cookie	16	3.2	0.8		0.2	0		.02	0.5			21		.56		I
Dunkaroos, Betty Crocker Kid Snacks	127		1.0	20.3	13.6	1.0	0	0				80	0			
1 tray[13]	28	4.5	1.0			0	0							.36		I
Easter Puffs, Little Debbie	144	4.1	0.7	24.3	18.5	0.3		0	.02			65	3			
1.2 oz pkg	35	5.6	1.2			1	1	.03	0.2					.28		I
Egg Jumbo, Stella D'Oro	90		2.0	18.0	9.0	1.0						60				
2 cookies	24	1.0	0.0	0.0	0.0	30										I
fig bar	56	2.6	0.6	11.3		0.7	1	0	.03	.01	2	56	10	4	.06	.055
1 bar	16	1.2	0.2	0.6	0.2	0	7	.03	0.3	.00	.06	33	10	.46	.024	818
fig bar, Lance	188	7.6	2.6	35.3	21.0	2.8			.09			135	38			
1 ¾ oz	50	4.0		2.4	0.6	0	66	.08	0.5			137		2.70		I
fig newton, Nabisco	110		1.0	20.0	13.0	1.0						120				
2 cookies	31	2.5	1.0	1.0	0.0	0										I
Figaroos, Little Debbie	154	6.2	1.2	31.0	20.2	1.2		0	.06			109	17			
1.5 oz pkg	43	3.5	0.8			0	14	.10	0.8					.99		I
fortune	30	0.6	0.3	6.7		0.1	0	0	.01	.00	1	22	1	1	.01	.015
1 cookie	8	0.2	0.1	0.1	0.0	1	1	.01	0.1	.00	.02	3	3	.12	.005	818
fortune, LaChoy	112		1.6	26.3	11.3	0.7	0	0				11	4			
4 cookies	30	0.2	0.1				0		0.0					.17		I
french van creme, Keebler	83		0.8	12.1								69	3			
1 cookie	17	3.6	0.9		0.3	0						10		.37		I
Fruit Chewy Newton, fat-free, Nabisco	100		1.0	23.0	15.0	2.0						115				
2 cookies	29	0.0	0.0	0.0	0.0	0										I
fruit, peach, Little Debbie	134	8.0	0.9	33.0	21.6	0.6		4	.04			113	3			
1.5 oz pkg	43	0.1	0.0			0	46	.09	0.6					.69		I
fruit, strawberry, Little Debbie	134	8.0	0.9	33.0	21.2	0.5		1	.04				3			
1.5 oz pkg	43	0.1	0.0			.0	6	.09	0.6					.86		I
fudge, cake type	73	2.5	1.1	16.4		0.6	0	0	.04	.01	2	40	7	7	.12	.068
1 cookie	21	0.8	0.2	0.4	0.1	0	0	.05	0.3	.02	.04	29	17	.52	.061	818
fudge, caramel & peanut, Heyday	110		2.0	13.0	11.0	1.0						40				
1 cookie	22	5.0	1.0	2.0	0.5	0										I
fudge covered graham, Nabisco	140		1.0	19.0	10.0	1.0						125				
3 cookies	28	7.0	1.5			0										I
Fudge Rounds, Little Debbie	140	3.5	1.1	23.1	14.3	0.7		0	.04			85	6			
1.2 oz pkg	34	5.7	1.1			2	3	.07	0.5					.58		I
Fudge Striped Shortbread, Nabisco	160		2.0	21.0	11.0	1.0						150				
3 cookies	32	8.0	1.5			0										I
German Choc Rings, Little Debbie	135	2.4	1.1	17.7	11.3	1.3		0	.04			63	8			
1 oz pkg	29	7.5	4.0			1	1	.04	0.3					.49		I
ginger, Little Debbie	92	1.3	1.0	15.0	7.4	0.2		0				61	12			
.7 oz pkg	21	3.2	0.5			4	4	.08						.88		I
gingerbread, from mix, Betty Crocker	150		1.0	25.0	16.0	0.0		0	.03			170	20			
2 cookies	30	4.5	1.0	2.0	0.5	0	0	.06	0.4			100		.72		I
gingersnaps	118	1.5	1.6	21.8		0.6	0	0	.08	.05	2	185	22	14	.16	.441
4 cookies (1 oz)	28	2.8	0.5	1.6	0.4	0	0	.06	0.9	.00	.10	98	24	1.81	.086	818
gingersnaps, Nabisco Old Fashioned	120		1.0	22.0	10.0	1.0						210				
4 cookies	28	2.5	0.5	1.0	0.0	0										I
Golden Bars, Stella D'Oro	100		1.0	16.0	7.0	0.0						60				
1 cookie	25	3.5	1.0			20										I
Golden Creme Cake, Little Debbie	161	9.0	1.5	24.6	16.1	0.6		1	.08			144	82			
1.5 oz pkg	42	6.3	1.6			4	55	.03	0.6					.55		I
graham, Bugs Bunny, Nabisco	140		2.0	23.0	7.0	1.0						160				
10 cookies	31	5.0	1.0	1.5		0										I
graham crackers																
cinn, Honey Maid	140		2.0	26.0	11.0	1.0						210				
5 square crackers	32	3.0	0.5			0										I

	KCAL	H₂O (g)	PRO (g)	CHO (g)	SUGR (g)	DFIB (g)	A (RE)	C (mg)	B-2 (mg)	B-6 (mg)	FOL (mcg)	Na (mg)	Ca (mg)	Mg (mg)	Zn (mg)	Mn (mg)
	WT (g)	FAT (g)	SFA (g)	MUFA (g)	PUFA (g)	CHOL (mg)	A (IU)	B-1 (mg)	NIA (mg)	B-12 (mcg)	PANT (mg)	K (mg)	P (mg)	Fe (mg)	Cu (mg)	REF
cinn, low-fat, Honey Maid	110		2.0	24.0	10.0	1.0						160				
4 square crackers	28	1.0	0.0	0.0	0.0	0										I
honey, Keebler	66		1.1	10.7					.05			74	4			
2 crackers	15	1.8	0.5		0.2	0		.02	0.1			22		.53		I
honey, low-fat, Honey Maid	110		2.0	23.0	8.0	1.0						190				
4 square crackers	28	1.5	0.0	0.5		0										I
Honey Maid	120		2.0	22.0	8.0	1.0						180				
4 square crackers	28	3.0	0.5	1.0		0										I
Kitchen Rich	61		0.9	9.1					.03			56	3			
2 crackers	13	2.3	0.4		0.1	0		.01	0.4			23		.39		I
oatmeal crunch, Honey Maid	120		2.0	22.0	7.0	1.0						140				
4 square crackers	28	2.5	0.0	1.0		0										I
plain/honey	120	1.2	2.0	21.8		0.8	0	0	.09	.02	5	172	7	9	.23	.228
4 crackers (1 oz)[14]	28	2.9	0.7	1.4	0.4	0	0	.06	1.2	.00	.15	38	29	1.06	.057	818
graham snacks																
cinn crisps, Honey Maid	130		2.0	27.0	11.0	1.0						190				
18 crisps	31	1.5	0.0	0.0	0.0	0										I
cinn, fat free, Snackwells	110		2.0	26.0	9.0	1.0						90				
20 pieces	30	0.0	0.0	0.0	0.0	0										I
cinn, Teddy Grahams	140		2.0	23.0	8.0	1.0						150				
25 pieces	30	4.0	1.0	1.5	0.0	0										I
honey, crisps, Honey Maid	130		2.0	27.0	11.0	1.0						210				
18 crisps	31	1.5	0.0	0.0	0.0	0										I
honey, Teddy Grahams	140		2.0	22.0	8.0	1.0						150				
25 pieces	30	4.0	1.0	1.5	0.5	0										I
Homeplate, Keebler	60		0.9	9.8					.04			65	4			
1 cookie	13	1.7	0.5		0.1	0		.04	0.4			21		.34		I
ice cream cone																
cake/wafer	17	0.2	0.3	3.2		0.1	0	0	.01	.00	0	6	1	1	.03	.023
1 cone	4	0.3	0.0	0.1	0.1	0	0	.01	0.2	.00	.02	4	4	.14	.008	818
sugar	40	0.3	0.8	8.4		0.2	0	0	.04	.01	1	32	4	3	.08	.073
1 cone	10	0.4	0.1	0.1	0.1	0	0	.05	0.5	.00	.04	15	10	.44	.027	818
sugar, Keebler	47		0.9	10.3					.10			28	3			
1 cone	12	0.2	0.0		0.0	0		.06	0.7			25		.65		I
Van Cups, Keebler	19		0.5	4.1					.02			21	3			
1 cone	5	0.0	0.0	0.0	0.0	0		.01	0.4			7		.28		I
waffle cone, Keebler	97		1.7	20.4					.06			0	4			
1 cone	24	0.7				0		.01	0.1			25		.17		I
Keebies, Keebler	86		1.0	12.6					.04			69	7			
1 cookie	18	3.6	1.1		0.2	0		.00	0.4			27		.58		I
Krisp Kreem Wafers, Keebler	52		0.4	6.8					.04			15	2			
2 cookies	10	2.6	0.5		0.2	0		.00	0.2			9		.17		I
Lady Stella Assortment, Stella D'Oro	130		1.0	19.0	8.0	1.0						65				
3 cookies	28	5.0	1.5	1.5	0.0	5										I
ladyfingers	40	2.1	1.2	6.6		0.1	18	0	.05	.01	4	16	5	1	.13	.026
1 ladyfinger	11	1.0	0.3	0.4	0.1	40	61	.03	0.2	.08	.12	12	19	.39	.010	818
Lemon Creme Wafers, Little Debbie	161	1.0	1.5	22.5	14.1	0.4		1	.07			53	15			
1.2 oz pkg	32	7.7	1.3			0	23	.09	0.7					.53		I
macaroon, homemade	97	2.5	0.9	17.3		0.4	0	0	.03	.02	1	59	2	5	.17	.227
1 cookie (2" x 3/8")	24	3.0	2.7	0.1	0.0	0	0	.00	0.0	.01	.06	37	10	.18	.034	818
Mallomars, Nabisco	120		1.0	17.0	13.0	1.0						35				
2 cookies	26	5.0	3.0	1.5	0.0	0										I
Margherite Combination, Stella D'Oro	140		2.0	22.0	9.0	1.0						75				
2 cookies	32	6.0	1.5	2.0	0.0	10										I
Margherite, Stella D'Oro	140		2.0	22.0	8.0	1.0						90				
2 cookies	32	5.0	1.5			15										I
marshmallow, choc coated	55	1.3	0.5	8.8		0.3	0	0	.03	.00	1	22	6	5	.08	.037
1 sm cookie (1 ¾" x ¾")	13	2.2	0.6	1.2	0.3	0	0	.01	0.1	.02	.04	24	13	.33	.034	818
Marshmallow Puffs Fudge Cakes, Nabisco—1 cookie	90		1.0	14.0	11.0	0.0						45				
	21	4.0	1.0	1.5	0.0	0										I

	KCAL	H₂O (g)	PRO (g)	CHO (g)	SUGR (g)	DFIB (g)	A (RE)	C (mg)	B-2 (mg)	B-6 (mg)	FOL (mcg)	Na (mg)	Ca (mg)	Mg (mg)	Zn (mg)	Mn (mg)
	WT (g)	FAT (g)	SFA (g)	MUFA (g)	PUFA (g)	CHOL (mg)	A (IU)	B-1 (mg)	NIA (mg)	B-12 (mcg)	PANT (mg)	K (mg)	P (mg)	Fe (mg)	Cu (mg)	REF
Marshmallow Twirls Fudge Cakes, Nabisco—*1 cookie*	130		1.0	20.0	15.0	1.0						75				
	30	6.0	1.5			0										I
milk choc chip, Duncan Hines	110		1.0	15.0								95				
2 cookies	25	5.0	2.0	2.5	0.5	0										I
molasses	65	0.9	0.8	11.1		0.1	0	0	.04	.04	1	69	11	8	.07	.189
1 med cookie (3" x ⅜")	15	1.9	0.3	1.1	0.3	0	0	.05	0.5	.00	.06	52	14	.96	.056	818
Mystic Mint Sandwich, Nabisco	90		1.0	11.0	8.0	0.0						65				
1 cookie	17	4.0	1.0	2.0	0.0	0										I
Nekot w/ lemon cream cheese, Lance	258	1.0	2.9	32.7				3	.17			116	19			
1.8 oz	50	12.9	5.0	7.0	0.9	3	2	.04	1.5			51		1.32		I
Nekot w/ peanut butter, Lance	208	1.1	6.2	24.2					.13			99	15			
1.5 oz	43	10.0	4.9	4.1	0.4	2		.09	1.1			78		.76		I
Newton Cobblers, Nabisco	60		1.0	18.0	8.0	1.0						45				
1 cookie[15]	23	0.0	0.0	0.0	0.0	0										I
Nilla Wafers, Nabisco	140		2.0	24.0	12.0	0.0						105				
8 cookies	32	5.0	1.0	1.5		0										I
Nilla Wafers, red fat, Nabisco	120		1.0	24.0	12.0	1.0						105				
8 wafers	29	2.0	0.5	0.5	0.0	0										I
Nutter Butter, peanut butter sandwich, Nabisco—*2 cookies*	130		2.0	19.0	8.0	1.0						110				
	28	6.0	1.0	2.5	1.0	5										I
Nutter Butter, peanut creme patties, Nabisco—*5 patties*	160		4.0	17.0	10.0	1.0						80				
	31	9.0	1.5			0										I
Nutty Bar, Little Debbie	296	1.3	3.8	33.2	21.4	1.3		0	.07			119	9			
2 oz pkg	57	17.8	3.0			0	0	.14	2.0					.80		I
oatmeal	81	1.0	1.1	12.4		0.5	0	0	.04	.01	1	69	7	6	.14	.151
1 cookie	18	3.3	0.6	1.9	0.5	0	3	.05	0.4	.00	.04	26	25	.46	.024	818
bite size, Lance	124	2.0	1.8	20.1	4.8	0.6			.03			94	6			
1 oz	28	4.5	1.1			1		.06	2.2			3	32	.48		I
from mix	74	0.9	1.2	10.4		0.6	3	0	.03	.01	2	75	5	8	.14	.171
2" cookie	16	3.1	0.8	1.7	0.4	7	13	.04	0.2	.01	.06	30	28	.37	.031	818
from refrig dough	57	0.7	0.7	7.9		0.3	2	0	.02	.01	1	39	4	4	.09	.114
1 cookie	12	2.5	0.6	1.4	0.4	3	8	.02	0.2	.00	.03	20	14	.29	.015	818
homemade	67	0.9	1.0	10.0			27	0	.03	.01	2	90	16	6	.14	.159
1 cookie (2 ⅝" dia)	15	2.7	0.5	1.2	0.8	5	107	.04	0.2	.01	.05	27	25	.41	.025	818
Keebler Old Fashioned	52		0.4	6.8					.04			15	2			
1 cookie	18	2.6	0.5		0.2	0		.00	0.2			9		.17		I
soft type	61	1.6	0.9	9.9		0.4	1	0	.03	.01	1	52	14	5	.07	.063
1 cookie	15	2.2	0.4	1.2	0.4	1	5	.03	0.3	.00	.04	20	31	.42	.083	818
Oatmeal Creme, Lance	249	6.4	2.6	37.3				0	.06			162	14			
2 oz	57	10.0	2.9	5.1	2.1	3	335	.34	0.5			6		.92		I
Oatmeal Creme Pies, Little Debbie	166	2.9	1.4	25.8	13.5	0.6		0	.06			193	10			
1.3 oz pkg	38	7.1	1.6			0	0	.12	0.7					.99		I
Oatmeal Lights, Little Debbie	131	5.0	1.5	28.3	15.7	0.6		0	.05			193	10			
1.3 oz pkg	38	2.3	0.5			0	0	.10	0.6					.91		I
oatmeal raisin																
Duncan Hines	110		1.0	15.0								75				
2 cookies	25	5.0	1.0	3.0	1.0	0										I
fat-free	92	3.5	1.7	22.3		2.1	0	0	.07	.02	2	84	11	10	.18	.225
2 cookies (1 oz)	28	0.4	0.1	0.1	0.2	0	0	.04	0.3	.00	.10	60	30	.62	.061	818
homemade	65	1.0	1.0	10.3			25	0	.02	.01	2	81	15	6	.13	.148
1 cookie (2 ⅝" dia)	15	2.4	0.5	1.0	0.8	5	96	.04	0.2	.01	.05	36	24	.40	.027	818
Little Debbie	163	3.7	1.8	25.1	14.3	0.9		0	.06			172	10			
1.3 oz pkg	38	6.6	1.5			0	2	.12	0.0					1.10		I
Pillsbury	65	2.8	1.0	9.0				0	.03			62	3			
1 cookie	16	2.8					2	.03	0.2			26	15	.27		I
red fat, Snackwell's	110		2.0	20.0	10.0	1.0						135				
2 cookies	27	2.5	0.5			0										I
oatmeal raisin cookie mix, Duncan Hines	130	1.3	2.0	18.0					.04			65	20	13	.20	
⅟₁₈ pkg (2 cookies)	28	6.0	1.0	4.0	1.0	0		.07	0.4			70	42	.50	.060	I
oatmeal spice, Little Debbie	115	3.8	1.6	24.3	15.5	0.8		0	.04			122	9			
1.1 oz pkg	32	1.7	0.4			0	0	.09	0.5					.86		I

	KCAL / WT (g)	H₂O (g) / FAT (g)	PRO (g) / SFA (g)	CHO (g) / MUFA (g)	SUGR (g) / PUFA (g)	DFIB (g) / CHOL (mg)	A (RE) / A (IU)	C (mg) / B-1 (mg)	B-2 (mg) / NIA (mg)	B-6 (mg) / B-12 (mcg)	FOL (mcg) / PANT (mg)	Na (mg) / K (mg)	Ca (mg) / P (mg)	Mg (mg) / Fe (mg)	Zn (mg) / Cu (mg)	Mn (mg) / REF
Oreo Double Stuff, Nabisco	140		1.0	19.0	12.0	1.0						150				
2 cookies	28	7.0	1.5	2.5	0.0	0										I
Oreo, fudge covered, Nabisco	110		1.0	14.0	10.0	1.0						85				
1 cookie	21	6.0	1.5	2.5	0.0	0										I
Oreo, Nabisco	160		2.0	23.0	13.0	1.0						220				
2 cookies	33	7.0	1.5	3.0	0.5											I
Oreo, red fat, Nabisco	130		2.0	25.0	13.0	1.0						210				
3 cookies	32	3.5	1.0	1.5	0.5	0										I
peanut butter	72	0.9	1.4	8.8		0.3	1	0	.03	.01	5	62	5	7	.08	.042
1 cookie	15	3.5	0.8	1.3	1.2	0	4	.03	0.6	.01	.07	25	13	.38	.030	818
from refrig dough	60	0.5	1.1	6.9		0.1	2	0	.02	.01	1	52	13	5	.09	.055
1 cookie	12	3.3	0.7	1.7	0.6	4	6	.02	0.5	.01	.04	41	32	.22	.020	818
Keebler Old Fashioned	84		1.6	9.9					.03			102	11			
1 cookie	17	4.4	1.0		0.7	0		.04	1.0			35		.65		I
Pillsbury	68	2.6	1.3	8.4				0	.04			70	3			
1 cookie	16	3.3					5	.03	0.6			29	16	1.55		I
sandwich	67	0.4	1.2	9.2		0.3	0	0	.04	.01	2	52	7	7	.15	.128
1 cookie	14	3.0	0.6	1.5	0.6	0	1	.05	0.5	.01	.06	27	26	.36	.033	818
soft type	69	1.7	0.8	8.7		0.3	0	0	.02	.01	1	50	2	5	.08	.065
1 cookie	15	3.7	0.8	2.0	0.7	0	0	.04	0.3	.00	.05	16	13	.13	.012	818
peanut butter bars, Little Debbie	269	1.9	4.2	31.8	19.3	1.2	0		.07			193	10			
1.9 oz pkg	54	15.1	2.7			0	0	.16	2.5					1.19		I
peanut butter cookie mix, Duncan Hines	140	0.8	2.5	15.1					.04			115	9	11	.16	
¹⁄₁₈ pkg (2 cookies)	26	7.3	1.0	4.0	2.0	0		.03	1.1			60	25	.31	.052	I
peanut butter cookie mix, homemade	95	1.2	1.8	11.8			31	0	.04	.02	4	104	8	8	.16	.114
1 cookie (3" dia)	20	4.8	0.9	2.2	1.4	6	120	.04	0.7	.02	.07	46	23	.45	.037	818
Peanut Butter Creme Wafer, Lance	232	1.0	5.1	30.3					.11				12			
1.7 oz	50	10.0	3.0	4.0	3.0	0		.10	1.4			67		2.52		I
Pecan Passion Shortbread, Nabisco	90		1.0	9.0	3.0	0.0						40				
1 cookie	16	5.0	1.0	2.5	0.0	5										I
Pinwheels, choc & marshmallow cakes	130		1.0	21.0	16.0	1.0						35				
1 cookie	30	5.0	2.5	1.5	0.0	0										I
Pitter Patter, Keebler	88		1.8	11.5					.02			97	6			
1 cookie	18	3.8	0.7		0.5	0		.04	0.6			39		.41		I
Pumpkin Delights, Little Debbie	147	3.8	1.2	23.9	12.8	0.3		0	.07			141	8			
1.2 oz pkg	35	5.2	1.4			3	323	.13	1.0					1.19		I
raisin, soft type	60	2.0	0.6	10.2		0.2	2	0	.03	.01	1	51	7	3	.05	.044
1 cookie	15	2.0	0.5	1.1	0.3	0	6	.03	0.3	.01	.05	21	12	.34	.062	818
raspberry newton, fat-free, Nabisco	100		1.0	23.0	14.0	1.0						115				
2 cookies	29	0.0	0.0	0.0	0.0	0										I
Roman Egg Biscuits, Stella D'Oro	140		2.0	21.0	9.0	1.0						125				
1 cookie	34	5.0	2.0			20										I
sesame, Stella D'Oro	150		2.0	21.0	8.0	1.0						85				
3 cookies	32	6.0	1.5	2.0	0.5	10										I
shortbread	40	0.3	0.5	5.2		0.1	1	0	.03	.00	1	36	3	1	.04	.034
1 cookie (1 ⅝" sq)	8	1.9	0.5	1.1	0.2	2	3	.03	0.3	.01	.02	8	9	.22	.012	818
homemade w/ butter	60	0.3	0.7	6.2			34	0	.03	.00	1	51	2	1	.05	.041
1 cookie (1 ½" dia)	11	3.7	2.3	1.0	0.2	10	136	.04	0.3	.01	.02	8	8	.29	.010	818
homemade w/ marg	60	0.3	0.7	6.2			38	0	.03	.00	1	56	2	1	.04	.041
1 cookie (1 ½" dia)	11	3.7	0.7	1.6	1.2	0	147	.04	0.3	.00	.02	8	8	.28	.009	818
Lorna Doone	140		2.0	19.0	6.0	1.0						130				
4 cookies	29	7.0	1.0	2.5		5										I
pecan	76	0.5	0.7	8.2		0.3	0	0	.03	.00	1	39	4	3	.08	.086
1 cookie (2" dia)	14	4.6	1.0	2.6	0.7	5	2	.04	0.3	.00	.05	10	12	.34	.021	818
Smiley Faces, Little Debbie	135	1.1	1.7	19.1	4.8	0.4	0	0	.03			115	12			
1 oz pkg	28	5.8	1.6			4	0	.09	0.7					.39		I
Social Tea Biscuits, Nabisco	120		2.0	20.0	7.0	1.0						105				
6 cookies	28	4.0	0.5	1.0		5										I
strawberry newton, fat-free, Nabisco	100		1.0	23.0	16.0	1.0						115				
2 cookies	29	0.0	0.0	0.0	0.0	0										I
sugar	72	0.7	0.8	10.2		0.1	4	0	.03	.01	2	54	3	2	.06	.044
1 cookie	15	3.2	0.8	1.8	0.4	8	14	.03	0.4	.02	.05	9	12	.32	.012	818

	KCAL	H₂O (g)	PRO (g)	CHO (g)	SUGR (g)	DFIB (g)	A (RE)	C (mg)	B-2 (mg)	B-6 (mg)	FOL (mcg)	Na (mg)	Ca (mg)	Mg (mg)	Zn (mg)	Mn (mg)
	WT (g)	FAT (g)	SFA (g)	MUFA (g)	PUFA (g)	CHOL (mg)	A (IU)	B-1 (mg)	NIA (mg)	B-12 (mcg)	PANT (mg)	K (mg)	P (mg)	Fe (mg)	Cu (mg)	REF
from refrig dough	58	0.6	0.6	7.9		0.1	1	0	.01	.00	1	56	11	1	.03	.035
1 cookie	12	2.8	0.7	1.6	0.3	4	4	.02	0.3	.01	.02	20	22	.22	.005	818
homemade w/ butter	66	1.2	0.8	8.4			31	0	.04	.00	2	64	10	2	.06	.045
1 cookie (3" dia)	14	3.3	2.0	0.9	0.2	12	125	.04	0.3	.01	.03	10	13	.33	.011	818
homemade w/ marg	66	1.2	0.8	8.4		0.2	35	0	.04	.00	2	69	10	2	.06	.044
1 cookie (3" dia)	14	3.3	0.7	1.4	1.0	4	135	.04	0.3	.01	.03	11	13	.33	.011	818
Keebler Old Fashioned	83		1.0	13.0					.04			71	3			
1 cookie	18	3.1	0.9		0.4	0		.05	0.5			13		.45		I
Pillsbury	66	2.6	0.7	9.6				0	.05			69	1			
1 cookie	16	2.7					2	.04	0.4			8	6	.30		I
sugar cookie mix, Duncan Hines	130	0.8	1.2	16.8					.05			65	4	1	.02	
¹⁄₁₈ pkg (2 cookies)	24	6.0	1.0	4.0	1.0	0		.06	0.6			10	10	.26	.000	I
sugar wafers																
Biscos	140		1.0	21.0	13.0	1.0						40				
8 cookies	28	6.0	1.5	2.5	0.0	0										I
w/ creme filling	145	0.3	1.2	19.9		0.2	0	0	.06	.00	2	42	5	3	.10	.078
8 wafers (1 oz)	28	6.9	1.2	4.1	0.9	0	0	.03	0.7	.00	.05	17	16	.55	.026	818
w/ peanut butter filling	66	0.3	1.4	9.4				0	.01			24	6			
2 cookies	14	2.7					28	.01	0.4			25	16	.12		456
Swiss Fudge, Stella D'Oro	130		1.0	17.0	10.0	1.0						65				
2 cookies	26	6.0	1.5			15										I
Van-O-Lunch, Lance	180		2.0	26.0								150				
1.3 oz	37	7.0	2.0	4.0	1.0	0						20				I
vanilla creme sandwich, Cookie Break	160		1.0	23.0	11.0	1.0						115				
3 cookies	32	6.0	1.5	2.5	0.0	0										I
vanilla sandwich w/ creme filling	48	0.2	0.5	7.2		0.2	0	0	.02	.00	0	35	3	1	.04	.029
1 cookie (1 ¾" dia)	10	2.0	0.4	1.2	0.3	0	0	.03	0.3	.00	.04	9	8	.22	.011	818
vanilla wafers																
(12-17% fat)	125	1.4	1.4	20.9		0.5	5	0	.09	.02	3	88	14	4	.10	.074
7 wafers (1 oz)	28	4.3	1.0	1.7	1.0	16	17	.08	0.9	.03	.12	27	29	.67	.028	818
(18-21% fat)	134	1.2	1.2	20.2		0.6	0	0	.06	.01	2	87	7	3	.09	.109
5 wafers (1 oz)	28	5.5	1.4	3.1	0.7	0	0	.10	0.8	.01	.09	30	18	.63	.035	818
Keebler	74		0.8	10.1					.05			56	7			
4 cookies	15	3.3	0.9		0.3	0		.02	0.4			18		.33		I
Waffle Cremes, Biscos	180		1.0	24.0	17.0	1.0						35				
4 cookies	34	9.0	2.0	4.0	0.0	0										I
Yo-Yo's, Little Debbie	135	5.5	1.1	20.8	12.0	0.5		0				126	6			
1.2 oz pkg	34	6.0	1.4			1	1	.06						.54		I

8.5 DOUGHNUTS

	KCAL	H₂O (g)	PRO (g)	CHO (g)	SUGR (g)	DFIB (g)	A (RE)	C (mg)	B-2 (mg)	B-6 (mg)	FOL (mcg)	Na (mg)	Ca (mg)	Mg (mg)	Zn (mg)	Mn (mg)
	WT (g)	FAT (g)	SFA (g)	MUFA (g)	PUFA (g)	CHOL (mg)	A (IU)	B-1 (mg)	NIA (mg)	B-12 (mcg)	PANT (mg)	K (mg)	P (mg)	Fe (mg)	Cu (mg)	REF
cake	198	9.8	2.3	23.4	7.9	0.7	8	0	.11	.03	4	257	21	9	.26	.160
1 doughnut	47	10.8	1.8	4.5	3.8	17	27	.10	0.9	.11	.13	60	126	.92	.048	818
choc coated/frosted	204	6.2	2.1	20.6		0.9	13	0	.05	.02	7	184	15	17	.26	.170
1 doughnut	43	13.3	3.6	7.4	1.6	25	45	.05	0.6	.16	.17	49	87	1.06	.092	818
choc, sugared/glazed	175	6.8	1.9	24.1		0.9	11	0	.03	.02	7	143	89	14	.24	.155
1 doughnut	42	8.4	2.3	4.6	1.0	24	37	.02	0.2	.07	.14	50	68	.95	.080	818
sugared/glazed	192	8.8	2.3	22.9		0.7	1	0	.09	.01	5	181	27	8	.20	.150
1 doughnut	45	10.3	2.4	5.4	1.2	14	5	.10	0.7	.09	.16	46	53	.48	.045	818
wheat, sugared/glazed	162	13.4	2.8	19.2		1.0	9	0	.11	.03	7	160	22	10	.31	.299
1 doughnut	45	8.7	1.4	3.6	3.1	9	29	.10	0.8	.10	.18	67	47	.50	.050	818
cruller, glazed	169	7.3	1.3	24.4		0.5	1	0	.09	.01	3	141	11	5	.11	.143
1 cruller (3" dia)	41	7.5	1.9	4.3	0.9	5	7	.07	0.6	.03	.12	32	50	.63	.029	818
glazed, Rich's Ever Fresh	141	8.9	2.4	17.2					.08				49			
1.2 oz doughnut	34	7.0						.10	1.0					.69		I
honey oat bran, from dough, Rich's	130	19.9	3.8	22.7		1.9			.11			188	13	24		
1.7 oz doughnut	50	2.6				0	0	.13	1.4			105	78	1.30		I
jelly, Rich's Ever Fresh	213	12.1	3.6	26.0					.14				88			
2.17 oz doughnut	62	9.5						.18	1.7					1.24		I

							Vitamins					Minerals				
	KCAL	H₂O (g)	PRO (g)	CHO (g)	SUGR (g)	DFIB (g)	A (RE)	C (mg)	B-2 (mg)	B-6 (mg)	FOL (mcg)	Na (mg)	Ca (mg)	Mg (mg)	Zn (mg)	Mn (mg)
	WT (g)	FAT (g)	SFA (g)	MUFA (g)	PUFA (g)	CHOL (mg)	A (IU)	B-1 (mg)	NIA (mg)	B-12 (mcg)	PANT (mg)	K (mg)	P (mg)	Fe (mg)	Cu (mg)	REF
sticks, Little Debbie	218	6.6	1.6	26.3		0.8		0	.08			221	33			
1.7 oz pkg	47	11.8	2.7			9	21	.07	0.2					1.03		I
yeast																
glazed	242	15.2	3.8	26.6		0.7	6	0	.13	.03	13	205	26	13	.46	.158
1 doughnut	60	13.7	3.5	7.7	1.7	4	21	.22	1.7	.05	.28	65	56	1.22	.101	818
w/ creme filling	307	32.5	5.4	25.5		0.7	7	0	.13	.02	12	263	21	17	.68	.162
1 doughnut	85	20.8	5.7	11.5	2.5	20	25	.29	1.9	.08	.14	68	65	1.56	.096	818
w/ jelly filling	289	30.3	5.0	33.1		0.7	7	1	.12	.02	14	249	21	17	.64	.160
1 doughnut	85	15.9	4.0	9.0	2.0	22	26	.27	1.8	.05	.11	67	72	1.50	.116	818

8.6 FROZEN DESSERTS

							Vitamins					Minerals				
frozen yogurt																
soft serve	115	45.9	2.9	17.9		1.6	31	0	.15	.05	8	71	106	19	.35	.087
½ cup	72	4.3	2.6	1.3	0.2	4	115	.03	0.2	.21	.49	188	100	.90	.094	819
strawberry, Land O'Lakes	110		3.0	20.0								60				
½ cup	97	3.0	2.0	1.0	0.0	10										I
van, soft serve	114	47.0	2.9	17.4		0.0	41	1	.16	.06	4	63	103	10	.30	.006
½ cup	72	4.0	2.5	1.1	0.2	1	153	.03	0.2	.21	.46	152	93	.22	.029	819
fruit & juice bars	75	72.0	1.1	18.6		0.0	3	9	.02	.02	6	4	5	4	.05	.152
3 fl oz bar	92	0.1	0.0	0.0	0.0	0	27	.01	0.1	.00	.04	49	6	.17	.000	819
ice cream																
butter pecan, Haagen-Dazs	236	44.4	4.2	23.8					.17			78	91			
½ cup	87	13.9					426	.06	0.4			145	98	.35		I
choc	143	36.8	2.5	18.6		0.8	79	0	.13	.04	11	50	72	19	.38	.092
½ cup	66	7.3	4.5	2.1	0.3	22	275	.03	0.1	.19	.37	164	71	.61	.089	819
choc choc chip, Haagen-Dazs	236	44.4	4.3	22.6			1		.17			35	76			
½ cup	89	14.3					424	.01	0.7			204	102	1.48		I
choc, Haagen-Dazs	232	51.0	4.2	20.2					.18	.60		45	84			
½ cup	91	14.9					525	.01				200	96	.46		I
coffee, Haagen-Dazs	271	63.3	4.8	26.9					.28			58	118			
½ cup	112	16.0					713	.03	0.1			203	116	.45		I
french van, soft serve	185	51.4	3.5	19.1		0.0	132	1	.16	.04	8	52	113	10	.45	.004
½ cup	86	11.2	6.4	3.0	0.4	78	464	.04	0.1	.43	.44	152	100	.18	.026	819
Healthy Choice	120		3.0	22.0	19.0	1.0	0					59	100			
½ cup[16]	71	2.0	1.0			5	200							.00		I
honey van, Haagen-Dazs	213	52.1	3.8	18.7					.18			45	92			
½ cup	89	13.7					522	.04	0.5			133	95	.18		I
macadamia nut, Haagen-Dazs	361	59.0	5.4	26.2					.24			87	118			
½ cup	118	26.1					590	.06	1.3			186	130	.41		I
rum raisin, Haagen-Dazs	220	54.3	3.7	18.4					.17			40	80			
½ cup	92	14.7					527	.03	0.6			145	84	.28		I
strawberry	127	39.6	2.1	18.2		0.2	51	5	.17	.03	8	40	79	9	.22	.051
½ cup	66	5.5	3.4			19	211	.03	0.1	.20	.48	124	66	.14	.024	819
strawberry, Haagen-Dazs	270	68.4	4.8	25.5					.22			43	114			
½ cup	116	16.6					557	.03	0.8			173	114	.08		I
van, Haagen-Dazs	220	51.7	4.0	19.4					.19			45	88			
½ cup	90	14.0					444	.03	0.7			122	91	.08		I
van, reg (10% fat)	133	40.3	2.3	15.6		0.0	77	0	.16	.03	3	53	84	9	.46	.005
½ cup	66	7.3	4.5	2.1	0.3	29	270	.03	0.1	.26	.38	131	69	.06	.015	819
van, rich (16% fat)	178	42.3	2.6	16.6		0.0	136	1	.12	.03	4	41	87	8	.30	.006
½ cup	74	12.0	7.4	3.4	0.4	45	476	.03	0.1	.27	.27	118	70	.04	.018	819
van swiss almond, Haagen-Dazs	218	42.4	4.1	17.6					.16			40	78			
½ cup	80	14.4					386	.03	1.0			124	83	.32		I
ice cream bar																
choc w/ dark choc coating, Haagen-Dazs	361	42.6	4.9	29.4				0	.21			54	76			
1 bar	103	24.7					52	.02	0.6			247	128	.93		I
van w/ dark choc coating, Haagen-Dazs	332	39.4	4.5	27.4				0	.13			54	77			
1 bar	95	22.6					56	.03	0.8			192	119			I

	KCAL	H₂O (g)	PRO (g)	CHO (g)	SUGR (g)	DFIB (g)	A (RE)	C (mg)	B-2 (mg)	B-6 (mg)	FOL (mcg)	Na (mg)	Ca (mg)	Mg (mg)	Zn (mg)	Mn (mg)
	WT (g)	FAT (g)	SFA (g)	MUFA (g)	PUFA (g)	CHOL (mg)	A (IU)	B-1 (mg)	NIA (mg)	B-12 (mcg)	PANT (mg)	K (mg)	P (mg)	Fe (mg)	Cu (mg)	REF
van w/ milk choc almond coating,	318	38.6	4.1	23.1				1	.11			47	105			
Haagen-Dazs—*1 bar*	90	23.1					46	.02	0.7			164	120	.63		I
van w/ milk choc coating, Haagen-Dazs	329	38.1	4.0	23.7				0	.12			49	101			
1 bar	91	24.2					55	.02	0.6			165	112	1.00		I
ice milk, van	92	45.0	2.5	15.0		0.0	31	1	.17	.04	4	56	92	10	.29	.005
½ cup	66	2.8	1.7	0.8	0.1	9	109	.04	0.1	.44	.33	139	72	.07	.008	819
ice milk, van, soft serve	111	61.2	4.3	19.2		0.0	26	1	.17	.04	5	62	138	12	.47	.007
½ cup	88	2.3	1.4	0.7	0.1	11	91	.05	0.1	.44	.39	194	106	.05	.024	819
ices, water																
fruit, aspartame-sweetened	12	47.5	0.3	3.2		0.0	0	0	.00	.00	0	3	1	1	.02	.011
1 bar	51	0.1				0	1	.00	0.1	.00	.00	13	0	.07	.009	819
ice pop	42	47.2	0.0	11.2		0.0	0	0	.00	.00	0	7	0	1	.01	.004
2 fl oz bar	59	0.0	0.0	0.0	0.0	0	0	.00	0.0	.00	.00	2	0	.00	.005	819
lime	76	39.5	0.2	19.2		0.0	0	1	.00	.00	0	13	1	1	.01	.012
2 fl oz bar	59	0.0	0.0	0.0	0.0	0	0	.00	0.0	.00	.00	2	1	.09	.008	819
pineapple-coconut	108	70.4	0.0	22.9		0.7	0	13	.00	.02	1	34	0	5	.11	.155
½ cup	96	2.5				0	0	.01	0.0	.00	.04	16	9	3.39	.042	819
Mocha Mix, all flavors	148		0.6	17.9								81				
½ cup[17]	67	7.6	2.1	2.6	1.9	0						105				I
Mr. Freeze bars, assorted/tropical	50		0.0	14.0	14.0	0.0	0	0				20				
3 oz[18]	85	0.0	0.0	0.0	0.0	0	0					0		.00		I
Mr. Freeze bars, sugar-free	20		0.0	5.0	0.0	0.0	0	0				45	0			
3 oz[18]	85	0.0	0.0	0.0	0.0	0	0							.00		I
sherbet, fruit flavors, Land O'Lakes	127		1.2	27.3				1	.06			24	44			
½ cup	97	1.7	1.0	0.4	0.1	4	66					174	34			I
sherbet, orange	132	63.5	1.1	29.2		0.5	13	4	.07	.03	4	44	52	8	.46	.011
½ cup	96	1.9	1.1	0.5	0.1	5	73	.02	0.1	.12	.14	92	38	.13	.027	819
Simple Pleasures																
choc	134	56.0	8.9	22.6		1.3			.26	.05		73	185	23	.82	
½ cup	89	0.9	0.5	0.3	0.0	5	502	.04	0.1	.38	.30	190	143	.60	.070	I
choc chip	144	59.0	6.5	24.4				0	.18	.04		54	172	17	.04	
½ cup	93	2.3	0.9	0.6	0.9	13	518	.03	0.1	.62	.31	140	142	.38	.310	I
coffee	116	60.0	8.7	19.5					.25	.04		69	185	16	.72	
½ cup	89	0.4	0.2	0.2	0.1	13	461	.04	0.2	.73	.36	158	134	.24	.220	I
cookies'n cream	145	56.0	6.1	25.2		1.2		0	.17	.04		85	152	16	.62	
½ cup	90	2.2	0.7	1.3	0.2	11	511	.05	0.4	.41	.24	125	114	.44	.040	I
light, choc caramel sundae	86	52.0	4.8	19.0		0.9		0	.19	.05		82	125	21	.48	
½ cup[19]	78	0.5	0.2	0.1	0.0	9	381	.39	0.2	.44	.50	258	111	.60	.070	I
light, chocolate	74	52.0	5.4	15.8		1.3		0	.21	.06		74	140	23	.54	
½ cup[19]	74	0.5	0.3	0.1	0.0	10	364	.03	0.2	.45	.58	286	126	.62	.080	I
light, vanilla	72	53.0	4.6	15.0				0	.20	.05		68	128	13	.41	
½ cup[19]	74	0.4	0.2	0.1	0.1	9	346	.05	0.1	.88	.56	201	105			I
light, vanilla fudge swirl	90	51.0	4.9	19.8		0.8		0	.19	.06		81	130	16	.42	
½ cup[19]	77	0.3	0.1	0.1	0.0	10	371	.05	0.1	.87	.52	236	111	.24	.030	I
mint choc choc chip	138	59.0	6.5	24.6		2.0		0	.16	.04		51	163	27	.77	
½ cup	92	1.6	1.1	0.6	0.1	4	481	.03	0.2	.29	.23	194	130	.72	.110	I
peach	118	59.0	6.9	21.7				19	.22	.04		59	145	12	.54	
½ cup	89	0.4	0.4	0.2	0.0	5	406	.03	0.1	.56	.21	121	109	.12		I
pecan praline	127	60.0	5.9	22.4				0	.15	.04		63	158	13	.67	
½ cup	91	1.5	0.3	0.8	0.5	4	453	.03	0.1	.59	.24	115	116	.15	.030	I
rum raisin	128	57.0	7.8	23.0					.24	.06		65	168	14	.71	
½ cup	89	0.5	0.2	0.2	0.1	13	422	.04	0.1	.64	.29	145	128	.20	.030	I
strawberry	111	61.0	7.0	20.0				7	.23	.05		57	150	12	.58	
½ cup	89	0.3				5	386	.03	0.2	.64	.24	121	107	.20		I
toffee crunch	131	56.0	8.2	23.2					.25	.06		105	176	13	.06	
½ cup	89	0.6	0.3	0.2	0.0	6	422	.04	0.1	.00	.26	128	124	.13		I
van	116	61.0	5.9	21.1					.17	.05		50	162	12	.67	
½ cup	89	0.7	0.2	0.1	0.0	12	518	.04	0.1	.00	.29	114	122	.14		I

	KCAL / WT (g)	H₂O (g) / FAT (g)	PRO (g) / SFA (g)	CHO (g) / MUFA (g)	SUGR (g) / PUFA (g)	DFIB (g) / CHOL (mg)	A (RE) / A (IU)	C (mg) / B-1 (mg)	B-2 (mg) / NIA (mg)	B-6 (mg) / B-12 (mcg)	FOL (mcg) / PANT (mg)	Na (mg) / K (mg)	Ca (mg) / P (mg)	Mg (mg) / Fe (mg)	Zn (mg) / Cu (mg)	Mn (mg) / REF
sorbet & cream																
key lime & cream, Haagen-Dazs	153	54.9	2.0	28.8					.05			29	54			
½ cup	90	5.2					320	.03	0.5			84	50	.15		I
orange & cream, Haagen-Dazs	169	55.7	2.2	25.2				6	.09			27	52			
½ cup	90	6.7					321	.04	0.7			97	49	.02		I
raspberry & cream, Haagen-Dazs	149	60.1	2.2	22.6					.11			25	57			
½ cup	91	5.6					323	.02	0.6			96	53	.18		I

8.7 FRUIT COBBLERS & TURNOVERS

	KCAL / WT (g)	H₂O (g) / FAT (g)	PRO (g) / SFA (g)	CHO (g) / MUFA (g)	SUGR (g) / PUFA (g)	DFIB (g) / CHOL (mg)	A (RE) / A (IU)	C (mg) / B-1 (mg)	B-2 (mg) / NIA (mg)	B-6 (mg) / B-12 (mcg)	FOL (mcg) / PANT (mg)	Na (mg) / K (mg)	Ca (mg) / P (mg)	Mg (mg) / Fe (mg)	Zn (mg) / Cu (mg)	Mn (mg) / REF
apple brown betty/crisp, homemade	230	86.7	2.5	45.5		2.4	44	3	.10	.06	7	257	39	10	.23	.185
½ cup	141	5.1	1.0	2.2	1.5	0	193	.12	1.1	.00	.13	137	35	1.06	.072	819
apple fritters, frzn, Mrs. Paul's	263		3.3	35.2				5	.09			565	33			
2 fritters	113	12.1					23	.12	1.2			44		1.70		I
cobbler, frzn, Marie Callender's	368		2.8	45.0	24.8	1.0	0	18				166	0			
¼ cobbler[20]	120	18.4	4.2			0	0							1.26		I
strudel, apple	195	30.9	2.3	29.2		1.6	6	1	.02	.03	4	191	11	6	.13	.135
1 strudel	71	8.0	2.1	4.4	1.0	20	21	.03	0.2	.11	.13	69	23	.30	.021	818
Sweets-n-Apples, frzn, Mrs. Paul's	158		1.0	37.1				8	.11			62	28			
4 oz	113	0.6					5434	.06	0.5			120		1.10		I
turnover																
apple, Pillsbury	170	23.0	2.0	22.8				0	.06			320	6			
1 turnover	57	7.9					0	.09	0.9			33	123	.75		I
blueberry, Pillsbury	166	24.1	2.0	21.4				0	.06			316	6			
1 turnover	57	7.9					5	.09	0.9			23	123	.77		I
cherry, Pillsbury	173	22.3	2.1	23.2				5	.07			314	6			
1 turnover	57	7.9					52	.09	0.9			32	124	.91		I

8.8 GELATIN DESSERTS

	KCAL / WT (g)	H₂O (g) / FAT (g)	PRO (g) / SFA (g)	CHO (g) / MUFA (g)	SUGR (g) / PUFA (g)	DFIB (g) / CHOL (mg)	A (RE) / A (IU)	C (mg) / B-1 (mg)	B-2 (mg) / NIA (mg)	B-6 (mg) / B-12 (mcg)	FOL (mcg) / PANT (mg)	Na (mg) / K (mg)	Ca (mg) / P (mg)	Mg (mg) / Fe (mg)	Zn (mg) / Cu (mg)	Mn (mg) / REF
dry mix																
all flavors	324	0.9	6.6	77.0		0.0	0	0	.02	.01	3	216	3	2	.01	.014
3 oz pkg	85	0.0	0.0	0.0	0.0	0	0	.00	0.0	.00	.01	6	121	.13	.100	819
aspartame-sweetened	293	5.7	47.0	28.3		0.0	0	0	.09	.04	12	1840	2	1	.06	.042
.35 oz pkg	85	0.0	0.0	0.0	0.0	0	0	.01	0.0	.00	.05	12	1099	.02	.864	819
Jell-O 1-2-3 dessert, strawberry	130		2.0	26.0	22.0	0.0	0	0				45	0			
amt to make ⅔ cup	31	1.5	1.0			0	0					0		.00		I
Royal	70		2.0	17.0	16.0	0.0						112				
.7 oz (½ cup prep)[21]	19	0.0	0.0	0.0	0.0	0										I
Snackwell's	80		2.0	19.0	18.0	0.0						109				
.7 oz (½ cup prep)[22]	21	0.0	0.0	0.0	0.0	0										I
sugar-free, Royal	10		1.0	1.0		0.0						78				
.09 oz (½ cup prep)[21]	2.5	0.0	0.0	0.0	0.0	0										I
from mix																
all flavors	83	118.4	1.7	19.6		0.0	0	0	.00	.00	0	59	3	1	.04	.004
½ cup	140	0.0	0.0	0.0	0.0	0	0	.00	0.0	.00	.00	1	31	.04	.034	819
all flavors, Jell-O Brand	80		2.0	19.0	19.0	0.0	0	0				54	0			
½ cup[23]	140	0.0	0.0	0.0	0.0	0	0					0		.00		I
all flavors, sugar-free, Jell-O Brand	10		1.0	0.0	0.0	0.0	0	0				56	0			
½ cup[24]	121	0.0	0.0	0.0	0.0	0	0							.00		I
aspartame-sweetened	10	137.2	1.5	1.0		0.0	0	0	.00	.00	0	67	3	1	.04	.003
½ cup	140	0.0	0.0	0.0	0.0	0	0	.00	0.0	.00	.00	0	38	.01	.038	819
strawberry, low calorie, D-Zerta	10		2.0	0.0	0.0	0.0	0	0				5	0			
amt to make ½ cup	2.5	0.0	0.0	0.0	0.0	0	0					45		.00		I
w/ fruit	73	86.4	1.2	17.9		0.6	3	4	.03	.13	4	30	5	7	.05	.041
½ cup	106	0.2	0.1	0.0	0.1	0	30	.03	0.2	.00	.05	110	22	.14	.054	819
Gel Snack Cups, Del Monte	70		0.0	19.0	19.0	1.0	0	0				40	0			
3.5 oz container[25]	99	0.0	0.0	0.0	0.0	0	0							.00		I

	KCAL / WT (g)	H₂O (g) / FAT (g)	PRO (g) / SFA (g)	CHO (g) / MUFA (g)	SUGR (g) / PUFA (g)	DFIB (g) / CHOL (mg)	A (RE) / A (IU)	C (mg) / B-1 (mg)	B-2 (mg) / NIA (mg)	B-6 (mg) / B-12 (mcg)	FOL (mcg) / PANT (mg)	Na (mg) / K (mg)	Ca (mg) / P (mg)	Mg (mg) / Fe (mg)	Zn (mg) / Cu (mg)	Mn (mg) / RFF
Gel Snacks, Kraft Handi-Snacks	80		0.0	20.0	20.0	0.0	0	0				40	0			
3.5 oz container[26]	99	0.0	0.0	0.0	0.0	0	0					39		.00		I
Gelatin Gels, 10% fruit jce, Swiss Miss	79		1.4	18.3	17.8	0.0		0				38	3			
3.5 oz container	99	0.0	0.0	0.0	0.0	0								.08		I
Gelatin Snacks, Jell-O Brand	80		1.0	18.0	18.0	0.0	0	0				45	0			
3.5 oz container[27]	99	0.0	0.0	0.0	0.0	0	0					0		.00		I
Gelatin Snacks, sugar-free, Jell-O Brand	10		1.0	0.0	0.0	0.0	0	0				50	0			
3.2 oz container[28]	92	0.0	0.0	0.0	0.0	0	0					0		.00		I

8.9 GRANOLA, CEREAL, AND SNACK BARS[29]

	KCAL / WT (g)	H₂O (g) / FAT (g)	PRO (g) / SFA (g)	CHO (g) / MUFA (g)	SUGR (g) / PUFA (g)	DFIB (g) / CHOL (mg)	A (RE) / A (IU)	C (mg) / B-1 (mg)	B-2 (mg) / NIA (mg)	B-6 (mg) / B-12 (mcg)	FOL (mcg) / PANT (mg)	Na (mg) / K (mg)	Ca (mg) / P (mg)	Mg (mg) / Fe (mg)	Zn (mg) / Cu (mg)	Mn (mg) / RFF
almond, chewy, Sunbelt	128	2.0	2.2	16.7	7.8	1.3		0	.06			62	25			
1 oz bar[30]	28	6.5	1.6			0	6	.06	0.2					.50		I
almond, hard	119	0.7	1.8	14.9		1.2	1	0	.02	.01	3	61	8	19	.38	.328
.83 oz bar	24	6.1	3.0	1.9	0.9	0	9	.07	0.1	.00	.11	66	55	.60	.030	819
apple berry, Quaker Chewy	109	1.8	1.5	22.5	10.1	1.3		0	.02	.03	4	79	9	16	.38	
1 oz bar	28	1.9	0.6	1.0	0.4	0	1	.06	0.3	.00	.10	61	49	.55	.060	I
apple cereal bar, Fruit Boosters	124	6.7	0.9	27.2	17.5	0.5		0	.04			66	3			
1.3 oz bar	37	1.9	0.4			0	0	.08	0.6					.67		I
apple cinn, chewy, low-fat, Sunbelt	135	2.6	1.9	27.1	14.4	1.2		0	.03			106	19			
1.2 oz bar[31]	35	2.7	0.5			0	10	.07	0.1					.42		I
apple cinn, Kellogg Nutri-Grain	136	5.3	2.0	27.0	11.0	1.0		0	.43	.50	40	110	14	8	1.50	
1.3 oz bar	37	2.8	0.6	1.9	0.3	0	750	.38	5.0			73	40	1.80		I
banana snack bar, Snackwell's	130		2.0	27.0	16.0	0.0						100				
1.3 oz bar	37	2.0	0.0	0.0	1.0	0										I
blueberry cereal bar, Fruit Boosters	125	6.3	0.9	27.5	17.3	0.6		0	.04			67	3			
1.3 oz bar	37	2.0	0.4			0	3	.09	0.6					.67		I
blueberry, Kellogg Nutri-Grain	136	5.4	2.0	27.0	11.0	1.0		0	.43	.50	40	110	18	8	1.50	
1.3 oz bar	37	2.8	0.6	1.9	0.3	0	750	.38	5.0			73	40	1.80		I
Breakfast Bar																
choc chip, chewy, Carnation	150		2.0	24.0	11.0	0.0		15	.43	.50	100	80	500	100	3.75	
1.27 oz bar	36	6.0	2.0			0	1250	.34	5.0	1.50	2.50	40	300	4.50	.500	I
choc chunk granola, Carnation	130		2.0	26.0	12.0	0.5		15	.43	.50	100	40	500	100	3.75	
1.27 oz bar	36	2.5	1.0			0	1250	.38	5.0	1.50	2.50	55	300	4.50	.500	I
honey & oats granola, Carnation	130		2.0	26.0	11.0	0.5		15	.43	.50	100	45	500	100	3.75	
1.3 oz bar	36	2.5	0.5			0	1250	.38	5.0	1.50	2.50	45	300	4.50	.500	I
peanut butter w/ choc chips, Carnation	150		3.0	22.0	10.0	0.5		15	.43	.50	100	85	500	100	3.75	
1.27 oz bar	36	5.0	1.5			0	1250	.38	5.0	.15	2.50	60	300	4.50	.500	I
cereal bar, Snackwell's	120		1.0	29.0	16.2	1.0						106				
1.3 oz bar[32]	37	0.0	0.0	0.0	0.0	0										I
cherry, Kellogg Nutri-Grain	136	5.4	2.0	27.0	12.0	1.0		0	.43	.50	40	110	14	8	1.50	
1.3 oz bar	37	2.8	0.6	1.9	0.3	0	750	.38	5.0			70	40	1.80		I
chewy, low-fat, Nature Valley	110		2.0	21.3	7.5	1.2	0	0				68	0			
1 oz bar[33]	28	2.0	0.1			0	0					65		.36		I
chewy/soft	126	1.8	2.1	19.1		1.3	0	0	.05	.03	7	79	30	21	.43	.434
1 oz bar	28	4.9	2.1	1.1	1.5	0	0	.08	0.1	.11	.15	92	65	.73	.077	819
Chips Ahoy!, Nabisco	120		2.0	20.0	10.0	1.0						45				
1 oz bar	28	4.0	1.0			0										I
Chips Ahoy! snack bar, Nabisco	150		2.0	25.0	17.0	1.0						90				
1.3 oz bar	37	5.0	2.0			10										I
choc chip																
chewy/soft	119	1.5	2.1	19.6		1.4	1	0	.04	.03	6	77	26	22	.43	.369
1 oz bar	28	4.7	2.9	1.0	0.6	0	12	.06	0.3	.05	.15	96	65	.72	.113	819
chewy/soft w/ choc coating	130	1.0	1.6	17.9		1.0	2	0	.07	.03	7	56	29	18	.36	.260
1 oz bar	28	7.0	4.0	2.2	0.5	1	11	.03	0.2	.16	.14	88	56	.65	.098	819
chewy, Sunbelt	155	2.3	2.0	23.1	12.1	1.5		0	.03			67	19			
1.25 oz bar[34]	35	7.0	1.4			0	9	.07	0.2					.63		I
fudge dipped, chewy, Sunbelt	201	2.2	2.2	27.7	16.2	1.7		0	.03			73	20			
1.5 oz bar[35]	43	10.3	3.4			0	9	.07	0.2					.65		I

	KCAL / WT (g)	H₂O (g) / FAT (g)	PRO (g) / SFA (g)	CHO (g) / MUFA (g)	SUGR (g) / PUFA (g)	DFIB (g) / CHOL (mg)	A (RE) / A (IU)	C (mg) / B-1 (mg)	B-2 (mg) / NIA (mg)	B-6 (mg) / B-12 (mcg)	FOL (mcg) / PANT (mg)	Na (mg) / K (mg)	Ca (mg) / P (mg)	Mg (mg) / Fe (mg)	Zn (mg) / Cu (mg)	Mn (mg) / REF
hard	105	0.6	1.8	17.3		1.1	1	0	.02	.01	3	83	18	17	.46	.362
.83 oz bar	24	3.9	2.7	0.6	0.3	0	10	.04	0.1	.00	.12	60	49	.73	.063	819
Quaker Chewy	120	1.6	1.5	20.6	9.3	1.2	0	0	.02	.02	5	68	7	14	.42	
1 oz bar	28	3.9	1.5	1.8	0.5	0	0	.06	0.3	.00	.09	57	52	.56	.080	I
Quaker Dipps	164	1.3	1.8	24.3	14.8	1.1		0	.04	.02	3	91	26	11	.45	
1.2 oz bar	35	7.0	3.7	2.6	0.4	2	24	.05	0.3	.06	.12	81	68	.54	.070	I
choc chunk, low-fat, Quaker Chewy	111	1.7	1.6	22.1	9.6	1.1		0	.02	.02	5	80	9	18	.40	
1 oz bar	28	2.2	0.7	1.0	0.4	0	2	.06	0.4	.00	.09	63	53	.68	.070	I
choc, graham, & marshmallow, chewy/soft—1 oz bar	121	1.7	1.7	20.1		1.1	1	0	.04	.01	6	90	25	20	.37	.363
	28	4.4	2.6	0.8	0.7	0	13	.04	0.3	.00	.11	78	57	.73	.079	819
choc mint, low-fat, Quaker Chewy	112	1.6	1.6	22.0	9.5	1.1		0	.02	.02	5	80	9	18	.41	
1 oz bar	28	2.2	0.7	1.0	0.4	0	2	.06	0.4	.00	.09	63	53	.68	.070	I
cinn, red fat, Nature Valley	200		4.0	35.0	14.0	3.0	0	0				170	0			
2 bars (1.66 oz)	47	6.0	1.0			0	0					110		1.08		I
cookies & cream, low-fat, Quaker Chewy	111	1.6	1.6	22.1	9.1	1.0		0	.02	.02	4	96	8	14	.35	
1 oz bar	28	2.1	0.5	0.9	0.4	0	0	.06	0.3	.00	.09	61	46	.52	.050	I
crisped rice, choc chip	115	2.0	1.4	20.7		0.6	50	0	.17	.20	40	79	6	14	.24	.283
1 oz bar	28	3.8	1.5	1.1	1.0	0	500	.15	2.0	.00	.00	48	38	1.79	.088	819
crunchy almond & brown sugar, low-fat, Kellogg's—.7 oz bar	81	1.1	1.7	16.0	6.0	1.3		0	.17	.20		61	7	16	.60	
	21	1.6	0.2	0.4	0.9	0	500	.15	2.0			52	60	1.80	.120	I
fudge dipped, Snackwell's	110		2.0	22.0	14.0						40					
1 oz bar[36]	28	3.0	2.5			0										I
golden snack bar, Snackwell's	130		2.0	27.0	17.0	0.0						110				
1.3 oz bar	37	2.0	0.5			20										I
hard	134	1.1	2.9	18.3		1.5	4	0	.03	.02	7	83	17	27	.58	.504
1 oz bar	28	5.6	0.7	1.2	3.4	0	43	.07	0.4	.00	.23	95	79	.84	.111	819
macaroon, fudge-dipped, chewy, Sunbelt	278	3.7	2.8	33.6	18.5	2.9		0	.05			100	26			
2 oz bar	57	16.2	7.4			0	9	.08	0.2					.80		I
macaroon, fudge-iced, chewy, Sunbelt	180	3.2	1.9	27.2	17.2	1.5		0	.03			84	18			
1.4 oz bar[37]	41	8.0	3.7			0	6	.05	0.1					.53		I
mixed berry, Kellogg Nutri-Grain	140	5.4	2.0	27.0	12.0	1.0		0	.43	.50	40	110	0	8	1.50	
1.3 oz bar	37	3.0	0.5			0	750	.38	5.0				40	1.80		I
nut & raisin, chewy/soft	129	1.7	2.3	18.0		1.6	1	0	.05	.03	9	72	24	26	.45	.340
1 oz bar	28	5.8	2.7	1.2	1.6	0	12	.05	0.7	.07	.12	111	68	.62	.108	819
Nutter Butter, Nabisco	120			21.0	10.0	1.0						45				
1 oz bar	28	4.0	1.0			0										I
oatmeal cookie, low-fat, Quaker Chewy	111	1.9	1.5	22.1	9.6	1.0	0	0	.02	.02	4	105	9	14	.32	
1 oz bar	28	2.1	0.5	0.9	0.4	0	0	.06	0.3	.00	.08	62	43	.55	.050	I
oatmeal raisin, chewy, low-fat, Sunbelt	130	3.2	2.0	26.9	15.1	1.3		0	.03			99	20			
1.2 oz bar[38]	35	2.3	0.4			1	11	.08	0.2					.53		I
oats 'n honey, red fat, Nature Valley	200		4.0	35.0	14.0	3.0	0	0				170	0			
2 bars (1.66 oz)	47	6.0	1.0			0	0					110		1.08		I
oats & honey, chewy, Sunbelt	123	2.0	1.8	18.7	8.6	1.2		0	.03			62	16			
1 oz bar[39]	28	5.2	1.7			0	8	.06	0.1					.45		I
Oreo, Nabisco	120		2.0	21.0	10.0	1.0						70				
1 oz bar	28	4.0	1.0			0										I
peach, Kellogg Nutri-Grain	136	5.4	2.0	27.0	11.0	1.0		0	.43	.50	40	110	18	8	1.50	
1.3 oz bar	37	2.8	0.6	1.9	0.3	0	750	.38	5.0			73	40	1.80		I
peanut																
fudge-dipped, chewy, Sunbelt	273	3.4	4.3	33.2	18.0	2.2		0	.05			96	29			
2 oz bar	57	15.1	3.6			0	9	.11	1.2					.74		I
fudge-iced, Sunbelt	197	2.5	3.2	28.3	16.7	1.8		0	.03			88	20			
1.6 oz bar[40]	44	9.0	2.2			0	7	.08	0.9					.53		I
hard	115	0.6	2.6	15.3		1.0	1	0	.02	.02	6	67	9	26	.50	.338
.83 oz bar	24	5.1	0.6	1.4	2.9	0	8	.05	0.4	.00	.14	73	72	.60	.067	819
peanut butter																
& choc chip, chewy/soft	122	1.7	2.8	17.6		1.2	1	0	.03	.03	9	93	23	25	.48	.383
1 oz bar	28	5.7	1.6	2.4	1.3	0	3	.03	0.9	.13	.15	107	74	.55	.113	819
& choc chip, Quaker Chewy	122	1.7	2.5	18.6	8.3	1.2	0	0	.02	.02	5	104	10	17	.41	
1 oz bar	28	4.6	1.3	2.3	0.8	0	0	.06	0.9	.00	.08	70	59	.54	.070	I

	KCAL	H₂O (g)	PRO (g)	CHO (g)	SUGR (g)	DFIB (g)	Vitamins					Minerals				
							A (RE)	C (mg)	B-2 (mg)	B-6 (mg)	FOL (mcg)	Na (mg)	Ca (mg)	Mg (mg)	Zn (mg)	Mn (mg)
	WT (g)	FAT (g)	SFA (g)	MUFA (g)	PUFA (g)	CHOL (mg)	A (IU)	B-1 (mg)	NIA (mg)	B-12 (mcg)	PANT (mg)	K (mg)	P (mg)	Fe (mg)	Cu (mg)	REF
chewy/soft	121	2.1	3.0	18.3		1.2	1	0	.04	.03	9	116	26	24	.53	.397
1 oz bar	28	4.5	1.0	1.9	1.2	0	4	.06	0.9	.06	.15	82	71	.60	.187	819
hard	116	0.6	2.4	15.0		0.7	0	0	.02	.02	4	68	10	13	.30	.221
.83 oz bar	24	5.7	0.8	1.7	2.9	.0	4	.05	0.5	.00	.09	70	33	.58	.052	819
red fat, Nature Valley	200		5.0	33.0	13.0	2.0	0	0				170	0			
2 bars (1.66 oz)	47	6.0	1.0			0	0					130		.36		I
soft w/ choc coating	188	1.2	3.8	19.8		1.0	13	0	.08	.04	9	71	40	25	.54	.500
1.3 oz bar	37	11.5	6.3	2.4	0.7	4	48	.04	1.2	.00	.20	125	84	.54	.120	819
raisin, chewy/soft	127	1.8	2.2	18.8		1.2	0	0	.05	.03	6	80	29	20	.37	.357
1 oz bar	28	5.0	2.7	0.8	0.9	0	0	.07	0.3	.05	.14	103	62	.69	.079	819
raspberry cereal bar, Fruit Boosters	127	6.0	0.9	27.8	17.8	0.6	0	0	.04			75	3			
1.3 oz bar	37	1.9	0.4			0	0	.09	0.6					.67		I
raspberry, Kellogg Nutri-Grain	136	5.4	2.0	27.0	11.0	1.0	0	0	.43	.50	40	110	14	8	1.50	
1.3 oz bar	37	2.8	0.6	1.0	0.3	0	750	.38	5.0			72	40	1.80		I
Rice Krispies Treat Squares, Kelloggs	91	1.3	1.0	17.0	8.0	0.0	0	0	.17	.20	24	105	0			
.8 oz square	22	2.0	0.5	0.4	1.1	0	200	.15	2.0	.20				.36		MUL
S'mores, low-fat, Quaker Chewy	111	1.6	1.5	22.3	10.5	1.0	0	0	.02	.02	4	82	9	14	.38	
1 oz bar	28	2.1	0.7	1.0	0.4	0	0	.06	0.3	.00	.09	57	51	.58	.050	I
strawberry cereal bar, Fruit Boosters	126	6.1	0.9	27.6	17.5	0.5		1	.04			68	3			
1.3 oz bar	37	1.9	0.4			0	5	.09	0.6					.78		I
strawberry, Kellogg Nutri-Grain	140	5.4	2.0	26.0	13.0	1.0	0	0	.43	.50	40	110	17		1.50	
1.3 oz bar	37	2.8	0.6	1.9	0.3	0	750	.38	5.0			56	40	1.80		I
Sweet Rewards snack bar, fat-free	120		1.0	29.0	19.0	1.0	0	0				80	0			
1.3 oz bar[41]	37	0.0	0.0	0.0	0.0	0	0					43		.72		I

8.10 PASTRIES

	KCAL	H₂O (g)	PRO (g)	CHO (g)	SUGR (g)	DFIB (g)	A (RE)	C (mg)	B-2 (mg)	B-6 (mg)	FOL (mcg)	Na (mg)	Ca (mg)	Mg (mg)	Zn (mg)	Mn (mg)
	WT (g)	FAT (g)	SFA (g)	MUFA (g)	PUFA (g)	CHOL (mg)	A (IU)	B-1 (mg)	NIA (mg)	B-12 (mcg)	PANT (mg)	K (mg)	P (mg)	Fe (mg)	Cu (mg)	REF
charlotte russe w/ whipped cream filling,	326	51.9	6.7	38.2				0	.11			49	52			
homemade—*1 serving[42]*	114	16.6	8.3				840	.03	0.1			73	104	.80		456
cream puff																
bavarian, Rich's	130	12.7	1.7	17.0				0	.07			43	7	5	.15	
1 cream puff	38	6.1				17	19	.01	0.3			23	27	.50	.060	I
custard, Rich's	163	40.5	4.2	17.2		0.1		0	.11			170	0	12		
1 cream puff	71	8.6				58	109	.04	0.4			106	65	.50		I
w/ custard filling, homemade	335	69.5	8.7	29.8		0.5	259	0	.36	.08	20	443	86	16	.78	.146
1 cream puff	130	20.2	4.8	8.5	5.4	174	969	.16	1.1	.47	.67	150	142	1.52	.046	818
croissant	231	13.2	4.7	26.1		1.5	78	0	.14	.03	16	424	21	9	.43	.188
1 med croissant	57	12.0	6.7	3.3	0.7	43	307	.22	1.2	.17	.49	67	60	1.16	.046	818
apple	145	26.0	4.2	21.1		1.4	42	0	.09	.02	7	156	17	7	.59	.120
1 med croissant	57	5.0	2.5	1.4	0.4	28	154	.13	0.9	.13	.34	51	33	.63	.023	818
cheese	236	12.0	5.2	26.8		1.5	89	0	.19	.04	19	316	30	14	.54	.194
1 med croissant	57	11.9	5.5	3.7	1.5	36	346	.30	1.2	.18	.48	75	74	1.23	.057	818
danish pastry																
apple, Pillsbury's Best	185	19.4	2.1	24.6				0	.07			201	12			
1 danish	57	8.7					5	.12	0.9			37	34	.76		I
caramel w/ nuts, Pillsbury	156	9.0	2.0	19.3				0	.06			244	9			
1 danish	39	8.0					0	.09	0.8			29	106	.59		I
cheese (cream/neufchatel)	266	22.3	5.7	26.4		0.7	44	0	.18	.03	18	320	25	11	.56	.198
1 pastry (4 ¼" dia)	71	15.5	4.9	7.8	1.7	32	144	.13	1.4	.17	.19	70	77	1.14	.055	818
cinn	262	15.8	4.5	29.0		0.8	7	0	.17	.03	21	241	46	12	.47	.235
1 pastry (4 ¼" dia)	65	14.6	3.7	8.1	1.9	20	24	.20	1.9	.11	.21	81	70	1.27	.065	818
cinn raisin w/ icing, Pillsbury	147	10.0	1.6	19.7				0	.06			224	8			
1 danish	39	7.0					3	.09	0.7			27	96	.48		I
fruit	263	19.2	3.8	33.9		1.3	11	3	.16	.02	11	251	33	11	.38	.180
1 pastry (4 ¼" dia)[43]	71	13.1	3.3	7.3	1.7	15	37	.19	1.4	.06	.45	59	63	1.26	.046	818
nut	280	13.3	4.6	29.7		1.3	9	1	.16	.06	18	236	61	21	.57	.549
1 pastry (4 ¼" dia)[44]	65	16.4	3.5	8.2	3.7	30	34	.14	1.5	.11	.21	62	72	1.17	.127	818
orange w/ icing, Pillsbury	146	10.4	1.6	19.3				1	.06			241	5			
1 danish	39	7.1					4	.09	0.7			17	100	.50		I

	KCAL / WT (g)	H₂O (g) / FAT (g)	PRO (g) / SFA (g)	CHO (g) / MUFA (g)	SUGR (g) / PUFA (g)	DFIB (g) / CHOL (mg)	A (RE) / A (IU)	C (mg) / B-1 (mg)	B-2 (mg) / NIA (mg)	B-6 (mg) / B-12 (mcg)	FOL (mcg) / PANT (mg)	Na (mg) / K (mg)	Ca (mg) / P (mg)	Mg (mg) / Fe (mg)	Zn (mg) / Cu (mg)	Mn (mg) / REF
eclair																
choc, Rich's	196	19.0	2.6	25.5				0	.10			65	11	8	.23	
1 eclair	57	9.2				25	29	.02	0.4			35	41	.74	.100	I
custard, Rich's	163	40.5	4.2	17.2		0.1		0	.11			170	0	12		
1 eclair	71	8.6				65	102	.04	0.4			106	65	.50		I
w/ custard filling & choc glaze, homemade—1 eclair	262	52.4	6.4	24.2		0.6	191	0	.27	.06	14	337	63	15	.61	.128
	100	15.7	4.1	6.5	3.9	127	718	.12	0.8	.34	.49	117	107	1.18	.058	819
honey bun																
frzn, Morton	250		3.0	35.0	16.0	2.0	0	0				160	0			
2.28 oz	65	10.0	2.5			0	0							1.44		I
Little Debbie	223	10.4	2.6	23.1	11.7	0.6	0	0	.08			150	75			
1.8 oz pkg	50	13.4	3.5			2	0	.15	2.0					.65		I
mini, frzn, Morton	160		2.0	19.0	6.0	1.0	0	0				100	0			
1.3 oz	38	8.0	2.0			0	0							.72		I
Pecan Spinwheel, sweet roll, Little Debbie—*1 oz pkg*	109	5.7	1.6	16.4	9.0	0.6			.11			78	11			
	28	4.2	0.7			0	14	.12	0.8					.67		I
sweet roll/buns																
cheese (cream/neufchatel)	238	19.4	4.7	28.8		0.8	41	0	.09	.04	20	236	78	13	.42	.139
1 roll	66	12.1	3.8	6.1	1.4	37	135	.10	0.5	.11	.20	87	65	.50	.063	818
cinn raisin	223	14.9	3.7	30.5		1.4	38	1	.16	.06	14	230	43	10	.35	.180
1 roll (2 ¾" sq)	60	9.8	2.5	5.5	1.3	40	129	.19	1.4	.07	.20	67	46	.96	.053	818
cinn, Rich's	293	18.6	4.0	38.0					.20				122			
2.5 oz roll	71	14.6						.25	2.4					1.72		I
cinn w/ icing, Hungry Jack	144	11.0	1.6	18.6				0	.07			660	6			
1 roll	39	7.0					2	.09	0.7			16	115	.47		I
cinn w/ icing, Pillsbury	117	9.8	1.5	17.1				0	.07			262	7			
1 roll	34	4.8					2	.09	0.8			20	109	.64		I
cinn w/ icing, from refrig dough	109	6.8	1.6	16.8			0	0	.07	.01	2	250	10	4	.10	.125
1 roll	30	4.0	1.0	2.2	0.5	0	1	.12	1.1	.01	.08	19	104	.79	.021	818
mini honey, Rich's	133	8.4	1.8	17.5					.09				56			
1.36 oz roll	39	6.6						.11	1.1					.78		I
raisin & nut	196	15.4	3.8	29.6			60	0	.16	.05	18	185	36	16	.38	.319
1 roll	57	7.3	1.4	2.7	2.8	13	233	.16	1.3	.06	.19	123	63	1.46	.118	818
cinn, Pillsbury's Best Quick	211	13.8	2.4	29.4				0	.11			266	13			
1 roll	57	9.3					12	.16	1.1			29	82	1.11		I
toaster pastry																
apple cinn, frosted, Kellogg's Pop Tarts	200	6.5	2.3	37.0	15.0	1.0		0	.17	.20	40	190	12	8	.30	
1.8 oz pastry	52	5.0	0.9	3.0	1.0	0	500	.15	2.0			47	20	1.80		I
apple cinn, frosted, low fat, Kellogg's Pop Tarts—*1.8 oz pastry*	191	6.5	2.2	40.0	20.0	1.0		0	.17	.20	40	206	6			
	52	2.9	0.6	1.5	0.8	0	500	.15	2.0			28	20	1.80		I
apple spice, Pillsbury	199	14.8	2.8	28.1				0	.11			190	8			
1.9 oz pastry	54	8.6					11	.16	1.4			38	69	.97		I
blueberry, frosted, Kellogg's Pop Tarts	203	6.5	2.0	38.0	17.0	1.0		0	.17	.20	40	180	12	8	.60	
1.8 oz pastry	52	5.0	1.0	3.6	0.4	0	500	.15	2.0			50	44	1.80		I
blueberry, Kellogg's Pop Tarts	200	6.6	2.0	36.0	14.0	1.0		0	.17	.20	40	200	13	8	.60	
1.8 oz pastry	52	5.0	1.1	3.4	0.5	0	500	.15	2.0			50	46	1.80	.080	I
blueberry, low fat, Kellogg's Pop Tarts	192	6.5	2.3	39.0	17.0	1.0		0	.17	.20	40	240	6			
1.8 oz pastry	52	2.9	0.6	1.5	0.8	0	500	.15	3.0			29	20	1.80		I
blueberry, Pillsbury	194	12.3	2.2	27.9				0	.11			201	6			
1.9 oz pastry	54	7.6					1	.11	1.1			39	45	.70		I
brown sugar cinn	206	5.4	2.5	34.0		0.5	112	0	.29	.21	40	212	17	12	.32	.161
1 pastry	50	7.1	1.8	4.0	0.9	0	493	.19	2.3	.06	.13	57	67	2.02	.066	818
brown sugar cinn, frosted, Kellogg's Pop Tarts—*1.8 oz pastry*	210	5.3	3.0	34.0	15.0	1.0		0	.17	.20	40	190	14		.57	
	50	7.0	1.1	3.9	2.0	0	500	.15	2.0			55	46	1.80		I
brown sugar cinn, Kellogg's Pop Tarts	210	5.2	3.0	32.0	13.0	1.0		0	.17	.20	40	200	16	8	.60	
1.8 oz pastry	50	7.0	1.0	1.4	4.6	0	500	.15	2.0			70	40	1.80	.040	I

	KCAL / WT (g)	H₂O (g) / FAT (g)	PRO (g) / SFA (g)	CHO (g) / MUFA (g)	SUGR (g) / PUFA (g)	DFIB (g) / CHOL (mg)	A (RE) / A (IU)	C (mg) / B-1 (mg)	B-2 (mg) / NIA (mg)	B-6 (mg) / B-12 (mcg)	FOL (mcg) / PANT (mg)	Na (mg) / K (mg)	Ca (mg) / P (mg)	Mg (mg) / Fe (mg)	Zn (mg) / Cu (mg)	Mn (mg) / REF
brown sugar cinn, low fat, Kellogg's Pop	190	5.5	2.0	38.0	18.0	1.0		0	.17	.20	40	240	7			
Tarts—*1.8 oz pastry*	50	2.8	0.6	1.5	0.7	0	500	.15	2.0			31	20	1.80		I
cherry, frosted, Kellogg's Pop Tarts	204	6.5	2.0	38.0	17.0	1.0		0	.17	.20	40	170	13		.90	
1.8 oz pastry	52	5.0	1.0	3.5	0.5	0	500	.15	2.0			50	42	1.80	.080	I
cherry, Kellogg's Pop Tarts	204	6.5	2.0	37.0	15.0	1.0		0	.17	.20	40	190	14	8	.60	
1.8 oz pastry	52	5.0	0.9	3.0	1.0	0	500	.15	2.0			60	44	1.80	.080	I
cherry, low fat, Kellog's Pop Tarts	192	6.5	2.0	39.0	17.0	1.0		0	.17	.20	40	230	6			
1.8 oz pastry	52	2.9	0.6	1.5	0.8	0	500	.15	2.0			29	20	1.80		I
cherry, Pillsbury	194	15.4	2.8	26.2				0	.11			201	8			
1.9 oz pastry	54	8.6					12	.16	1.4			41	71	1.03		I
choc, frosted, Kellogg's Pop Tarts	201	6.5	3.0	38.0	17.0	1.0		0	.17	.20	40	220	20	15		
1.8 oz pastry	52	5.0	1.0	2.7	1.3	0	500	.15	2.0			80	43	1.80	.080	I
choc fudge, frosted, low fat, Kellogg's Pop	190	6.5	2.7	39.0	18.0	2.0		0	.17	.20	40	249	13	16		
Tarts—*1.8 oz pastry*	52	3.0	0.5	1.2	0.9	0	500	.15	2.0			62	40	1.80	.080	I
choc van creme, frosted, Kellogg's Pop	200	6.5	3.0	37.0	18.0	1.0		0	.17	.20	40	220	16	11	.60	
Tarts—*1.8 oz pastry*	52	5.0	1.0	3.2	0.8	0	500	.15	2.0			60	36	1.80	.040	I
cinn, Pillsbury	193	17.3	2.2	25.9				0	.11			198	5			
1.9 oz pastry	54	8.4					0	.13	0.5			36	45	.70		I
fruit	204	6.4	2.4	37.0		1.1	149	0	.19	.20	42	218	14	9	.34	.154
1 pastry[45]	52	5.3	0.8	2.1	2.0	0	501	.15	2.0	.03	.29	58	58	1.81	.098	818
grape, frosted, Kellogg's Pop Tarts	200	6.5	2.0	37.0	18.0	1.0		0	.17	.20	40	180	12	11	.60	
1.8 oz pastry	52	5.0	0.9	3.1	1.0	0	500	.15	2.0			60	46	1.80	.050	I
milk choc graham, Kellogg's Pop Tarts	210	6.4	3.0	35.0	16.0	1.0		0	.17	.20	40	227	19	16		
1.8 oz pastry	52	5.8	1.5	3.2	1.1	0	500	.15	2.0			82	40	1.80	.040	I
raspberry, frosted, Kellogg's Pop Tarts	210	6.5	2.0	37.0	18.0	1.0		0	.17	.20	40	180	11	8	.60	
1.8 oz pastry	52	4.5	1.0	2.2	1.3	0	500	.15	2.0			44	46	1.80	.040	I
raspberry, Pillsbury	187	17.8	2.2	26.5				0	.11			201	6			
1.9 oz pastry	54	7.5					2	.13	1.1			41	46	.70		I
S'mores, Kellogg's Pop Tarts	200	6.5	3.0	36.0	17.0	1.0		0	.17	.20	40	210	0	8		
1.8 oz pastry	52	5.0	1.0	3.0	1.0	0	500	.15	2.0			65	40	1.80	.040	I
Snackwell's	168		2.0	36.8	20.5	1.0						193				
1.7 oz pastry[46]	48	1.0	0.0	0.0	0.0	0										I
strawberry, frosted, Kellogg's Pop Tarts	200	6.5	2.0	37.0	17.0	1.0		0	.17	.20	40	180	11			
1.8 oz pastry	52	5.0	1.0	3.0	1.0	0	500	.15	2.0			44	20	1.80		I
strawberry, frosted, low fat, Kellogg's	190	6.5	2.1	39.0	19.0	1.0		0	.17	.20	40	220	5			
Pop Tarts—*1.8 oz pastry*	52	3.0	0.6	1.4	1.0	0	500	.15	2.0			26	20	1.80		I
strawberry, Kellogg's Pop Tarts	200	6.5	2.0	37.0	14.0	1.0		0	.17	.20	40	190	12			
1.8 oz pastry	52	5.0	1.0	3.2	0.8	0	500	.15	2.0			60	20	1.80		I
strawberry, low fat, Kellogg's Pop Tarts	192	6.5	2.0	39.0	18.0	1.0		0	.17	.20	40	240	6			
1.8 oz pastry	52	2.9	0.6	1.5	0.8	0	500	.15	2.0			28	20	1.80		I
strawberry, Pillsbury	187	12.2	2.2	27.1				1	.11			202	6			
1.9 oz pastry	54	7.5					1	.13	1.1			41	46	.70		I
Toastettes Tarts, Nabisco	190		2.0	34.8	17.3	1.0						205				
1.7 oz tart[47]	48	5.0	1.5	1.5	0.0	0										I

8.11 PIES

	KCAL / WT (g)	H₂O (g) / FAT (g)	PRO (g) / SFA (g)	CHO (g) / MUFA (g)	SUGR (g) / PUFA (g)	DFIB (g) / CHOL (mg)	A (RE) / A (IU)	C (mg) / B-1 (mg)	B-2 (mg) / NIA (mg)	B-6 (mg) / B-12 (mcg)	FOL (mcg) / PANT (mg)	Na (mg) / K (mg)	Ca (mg) / P (mg)	Mg (mg) / Fe (mg)	Zn (mg) / Cu (mg)	Mn (mg) / REF
apple																
frzn	296	65.3	2.4	42.5		2.0	38	4	.03	.05	5	333	14	9	.20	.227
⅛ of 9" pie	125	13.8	2.6	7.4	2.6	0	155	.04	0.3	.00	.15	81	30	.56	.057	818
frzn, Banquet	300		3.0	41.0	22.0	2.0	0	0				370	0			
⅕ pie (4 oz)	113	13.0	6.0			5	0							.72		I
frzn, Mrs. Smith's	310		2.0	44.0	18.0	1.0						380				
⅛ of 9" pie	131	14.0	2.5	8.0	2.5	0						70				I
homemade	411	73.3	3.7	57.5			19	3	.17	.05	6	327	11	11	.29	.287
⅛ of 9" pie	155	19.4	4.7	8.4	5.2	0	90	.23	1.9	.00	.14	122	43	1.74	.082	818
red fat/no sugar added, frzn, Mrs.	210		2.0	32.0	10.0	2.0						290				
Smith's—*⅙ of 8" pie*	123	8.0	1.5	5.0	1.5	0						85				I
apple cranberry, frzn, Mrs. Smith's	280		2.0	43.0	19.0	1.0						300				
⅙ of 8" pie	123	11.0	2.0	6.0	2.0	0						60				I

							Vitamins					Minerals				
	KCAL	H_2O (g)	PRO (g)	CHO (g)	SUGR (g)	DFIB (g)	A (RE)	C (mg)	B-2 (mg)	B-6 (mg)	FOL (mcg)	Na (mg)	Ca (mg)	Mg (mg)	Zn (mg)	Mn (mg)
	WT (g)	FAT (g)	SFA (g)	MUFA (g)	PUFA (g)	CHOL (mg)	A (IU)	B-1 (mg)	NIA (mg)	B-12 (mcg)	PANT (mg)	K (mg)	P (mg)	Fe (mg)	Cu (mg)	REF
apple pie filling, cnd	75	54.3	0.1	19.4		0.7	1	1	.01	.01	0	33	3	1	.03	.020
⅛ can	74	0.1	0.0	0.0	0.0	0	10	.01	0.0	.00	.03	33	5	.21	.041	819
banana cream																
from mix	231	46.8	3.1	29.1		0.6	92	0	.13	.03	6	267	67	11	.30	.067
⅛ of 9″ pie	92	11.9	6.4	3.8	0.6	25	375	.09	0.7	.19	.24	104	154	.42	.040	818
frzn, Banquet	350		3.0	39.0		1.0	0	0				290	40			
⅓ pie (4.7 oz)	132	21.0	5.0			5	0							.36		I
frzn, Mrs. Smith's	280		2.0	37.0	25.0	1.0						170				
¼ of 8″ pie	108	14.0	4.0	9.0	1.5	0						95				I
homemade	398	70.9	6.5	48.7		1.0	104	2	.31	.20	16	355	111	24	.71	.225
⅛ of 9″ pie	148	20.1	5.6	8.5	4.9	75	386	.21	1.6	.37	.57	244	136	1.54	.077	818
blackberry, frzn, Mrs. Smith's	280		2.0	43.0	21.0	0.0						320				
⅙ of 8″ pie	123	11.0	2.0		2.0	0						65				I
blackberry, homemade	287	60.2	3.1	40.6				5	.02			316	22			
⅛ pie	118	13.0	3.2				110	.02	0.4			118	31	.60		456
blueberry																
frzn	290	65.6	2.3	43.6		1.3	43	3	.04	.05	5	406	10	6	.20	.259
⅛ of 9″ pie	125	12.5	2.3	6.7	2.4	0	175	.01	0.4	.00	.11	63	26	.38	.061	818
frzn, Mrs. Smith's	260		2.0	39.0	17.0	1.0						320				
⅙ of 8″ pie	123	11.0	2.0	6.0	2.0	0						50				I
homemade	360	75.3	4.0	49.2			6	1	.19	.05	7	272	10	12	.29	.441
⅛ of 9″ pie	147	17.5	4.3	7.5	4.5	0	62	.22	1.8	.00	.18	74	44	1.81	.098	818
butterscotch, homemade	354	58.8	6.0	42.3			107	1	.27	.07	14	335	128	22	.69	.220
⅛ of 9″ pie	127	18.2	5.1	7.6	4.3	77	382	.18	1.3	.38	.54	221	135	1.64	.098	818
cherry																
frzn	325	57.8	2.5	49.8		1.0	63	1	.04	.05	10	308	15	10	.22	.175
⅛ of 9″ pie	125	13.8	2.6	7.5	2.5	0	296	.03	0.3	.00	.40	101	36	.60	.050	818
frzn, Banquet	290		3.0	39.0	14.0	2.0		0				310	0			
⅕ pie (4 oz)	113	14.0	6.0			5	200							.36		I
frzn, Mrs. Smith's	310		3.0	45.0	19.0	1.0						400				
⅛ of 9″ pie	131	14.0	2.5	8.0	2.5	0						110				I
homemade	486	82.4	5.0	69.3			86	2	.23	.06	13	344	18	16	.36	.360
⅛ of 9″ pie	180	22.0	5.4	9.6	5.8	0	736	.27	2.3	.00	.22	139	54	3.33	.139	818
red fat/no sugar added, frzn, Mrs.	220		3.0	35.0	10.0	1.0						310				
Smith's—*⅙ of 8″ pie*	123	8.0	1.5	4.0	1.5	0						125				I
special recipe deep dish, frzn, Mrs.	340		3.0	51.0	25.0	1.0						370				
Smith's—*1/10 of 10″ pie*	139	14.0	2.5	8.0	2.5	0						150				I
cherry berry, special recipe deep dish, frzn,	360		3.0	53.0	27.0	1.0						400				
Mrs. Smith's—*1/10 of 10″ pie*	139	15.0	3.0	9.0	3.0	0						120				I
cherry pie filling, cnd	85	51.6	0.4	21.7		0.4	16	3	.01	.03	3	7	8	5	.04	.022
⅛ can	74	0.1	0.0	0.0	0.0	0	152	.02	0.1	.00	.05	78	11	.18	.059	819
choc cream																
frzn	344	49.2	2.9	38.0		2.3	0	0	.12	.02	8	154	41	24	.26	.226
⅙ of 8″ pie	113	21.9	6.0	12.3	2.6	6	2	.04	0.8	.05	.44	144	77	1.21	.056	818
frzn, Banquet	360		3.0	43.0	33.0	3.0		0				240	40			
⅓ pie (4.7 oz)	132	20.0	5.0			5	0							1.08		I
frzn, Mrs. Smith's	330		3.0	42.0	30.0	1.0						200				
¼ of 8″ pie	108	17.0	4.0	10.0	1.5	0						180				I
homemade	400	66.2	6.8	44.3			104	1	.29	.07	14	348	115	37	.91	.298
⅛ of 9″ pie	142	22.9	7.4	9.4	4.8	75	375	.20	1.5	.37	.53	209	156	1.80	.186	818
choc mousse, from mix	247	47.2	3.3	28.1			96	0	.14	.03	3	437	73	30	.57	.199
⅛ of 9″ pie	95	14.6	7.8	4.8	0.8	21	392	.05	0.6	.20	.19	271	219	1.03	.193	818
choc silk, from mix, Jell-O Brand No	310		5.0	38.0	20.0	1.0		0				490	150			
Bake—*⅙ pie*[48]	120	16.0	6.0			5	500					260		1.08		I
coconut cream																
from mix	259	46.7	2.6	26.8		0.5	94	1	.10	.04	4	309	68	16	.36	.179
⅛ of 9″ pie	94	16.5	9.6	4.8	0.8	24	381	.03	0.1	.20	.24	133	159	.38	.075	818

	KCAL / WT (g)	H₂O (g) / FAT (g)	PRO (g) / SFA (g)	CHO (g) / MUFA (g)	SUGR (g) / PUFA (g)	DFIB (g) / CHOL (mg)	A (RE) / A (IU)	C (mg) / B-1 (mg)	B-2 (mg) / NIA (mg)	B-6 (mg) / B-12 (mcg)	FOL (mcg) / PANT (mg)	Na (mg) / K (mg)	Ca (mg) / P (mg)	Mg (mg) / Fe (mg)	Zn (mg) / Cu (mg)	Mn (mg) / REF
from mix, Jell-O Brand No Bake	330		4.0	37.0	26.0	1.0		0				410	80			
⅙ pie[48]	94	19.0	9.0			5	500					180		.36		I
frzn	191	27.6	1.3	23.8		0.8	13	0	.05	.04	3	163	19	13	.41	.355
⅙ of 7″ pie	64	10.6	4.8	4.3	0.9	0	58	.03	0.1	.12	.20	42	54	.51	.052	818
frzn, Banquet	350		3.0	39.0	30.0	2.0		0				250	40			
⅓ pie (4.7 oz)	132	20.0	6.0			5	0							.36		I
frzn, Mrs. Smith's	340		2.0	40.0	23.0	0.0						260				
¼ of 8″ pie	114	19.0	5.0	11.0	2.0	0						55				I
homemade	396	58.1	6.4	45.5			105	1	.28	.08	15	356	113	21	.81	.366
⅛ of 9″ pie	133	21.3	7.6	8.0	4.5	77	379	.18	1.3	.37	.57	184	140	1.49	.076	818
coconut custard	270	51.2	6.1	31.4		1.9	28	0	.15	.01	4	348	84	19	.71	.218
⅙ of 8″ pie	104	13.7	6.0	5.8	1.2	36	114	.09	0.4	.09	.25	182	127	.83	.066	818
coconut custard, frzn, Mrs. Smith's	280		7.0	35.0	18.0	0.0						350				
⅕ of 8″ pie	142	12.0	5.0	5.0	1.5	75						230				I
custard, egg	221	63.9	5.8	21.8		1.7	53	0	.22	.05	21	252	84	12	.55	.063
⅙ of 8″ pie	105	12.2	2.9	6.1	2.0	35	187	.04	0.3	.45	.70	111	118	.61	.025	818
custard, egg, homemade	262	73.9	6.5	34.0			81	1	.29	.06	13	257	107	17	.62	.109
⅛ of 9″ pie	127	11.3	3.5	4.6	2.4	88	281	.12	0.8	.30	.51	159	124	.99	.039	818
fruit, fried	404	48.1	3.8	54.5		3.3	4	2	.14	.04	4	479	28	13	.29	.287
1 snack pie (5″ x 3 ¾″)[49]	128	20.6	3.1	9.5	6.9	0	35	.18	1.8	.10	.14	83	55	1.56	.060	818
key lime, frzn, Mrs. Smith's	380		5.0	58.0	45.0	0.0						240				
⅕ of 8″ pie	125	14.0	5.0	7.0	1.5	15						200				I
lemon cream, frzn, Banquet	360		3.0	43.0	31.0	2.0		0				240	40			
⅓ pie (4.7 oz)	132	20.0	5.0			5	0							.36		I
lemon cream, frzn, Mrs. Smith's	300		2.0	40.0	28.0	0.0						160				
¼ of 8″ pie	108	15.0	4.0	9.0	1.5	0						80				I
lemon meringue																
frzn	303	47.1	1.7	53.3		1.4	59	4	.24	.03	9	165	63	17	.55	.068
⅙ of 8″ pie	113	9.8	1.8	4.1	3.3	51	198	.07	0.7	.17	.90	101	119	.69	.001	818
frzn, Mrs. Smith's	300		2.0	56.0	38.0	0.0						220				
⅕ of 8″ pie	136	8.0	2.0	4.0	2.0	65						20				I
homemade	362	55.0	4.8	49.7			56	4	.20	.03	11	307	15	8	.36	.163
⅛ of 9″ pie	127	16.4	4.0	7.1	4.2	67	203	.15	1.2	.15	.27	83	53	1.27	.053	818
mince, frzn, Mrs. Smith's	300		2.0	48.0	24.0	2.0						400				
⅙ of 8″ pie	123	11.0	2.0	6.0	2.0	0						140				I
mince, homemade	477	61.7	4.3	79.2		4.3	3	10	.17	.11	8	419	36	23	.36	.434
⅛ of 9″ pie	165	17.8	4.4	7.7	4.7	0	36	.25	2.0	.00	.17	335	69	2.46	.186	818
peach																
frzn	261	63.6	2.2	38.5		1.0	26	1	.04	.03	5	316	9	7	.11	.204
⅙ of 8″ pie	117	11.7	2.2	6.3	2.2	0	123	.07	0.2	.00	.11	146	29	.58	.067	818
frzn, Banquet	260		3.0	36.0	17.0	2.0		6				340	0			
⅕ pie (4 oz)	113	12.0	5.0			5	0							.36		I
frzn, Mrs. Smith's	260		2.0	38.0	17.0	1.0						310				
⅙ of 8″ pie	123	11.0	2.0	6.0	2.0	0						115				I
homemade	301	56.1	3.0	45.1				4	.05			316	12			
⅛ pie	118	12.6	3.1				860	.02	0.8			176	34	.60		456
special recipe deep dish, frzn, Mrs.	330		3.0	48.0	27.0	1.0						370				
Smith's—1/10 of 10″ pie	139	14.0	2.5	8.0	2.5	0						160				I
peanut butter cream, frzn, Mrs. Smith's	350		4.0	38.0	26.0	0.0						230				
¼ of 8″ pie	108	20.0	5.0	10.0	1.5	0						105				I
pecan	452	21.8	4.5	64.6		4.0	53	1	.14	.02	7	479	19	20	.64	.892
⅙ of 8″ pie	113	20.9	4.2	12.1	3.4	36	198	.10	0.3	.09	.48	84	87	1.18	.220	818
frzn, Mrs. Smith's	520		5.0	73.0	45.0	1.0						450				
⅙ of 8″ pie	136	23.0	4.0	13.0	6.0	70						90				I
homemade	503	23.8	6.0	63.7			109	0	.22	.07	17	320	39	32	1.24	.869
⅛ of 9″ pie	122	27.1	4.9	13.6	7.0	106	410	.23	1.0	.21	.58	162	115	1.81	.257	818
Lance	352	13.6	4.2	44.5					.09			204				
3 oz pie	85	17.5				38		.03	0.3			48		2.38		I
pineapple chiffon, homemade	233	33.3	5.3	31.7				1	.07			207	19			
⅛ pie	81	9.8	2.6				280	.03	0.3			79	62	.70		456

	KCAL	H₂O (g)	PRO (g)	CHO (g)	SUGR (g)	DFIB (g)	A (RE)	C (mg)	B-2 (mg)	B-6 (mg)	FOL (mcg)	Na (mg)	Ca (mg)	Mg (mg)	Zn (mg)	Mn (mg)
	WT (g)	FAT (g)	SFA (g)	MUFA (g)	PUFA (g)	CHOL (mg)	A (IU)	B-1 (mg)	NIA (mg)	B-12 (mcg)	PANT (mg)	K (mg)	P (mg)	Fe (mg)	Cu (mg)	REF
pineapple custard	251	61.9	4.6	36.6				1	.10			212	57			
⅛ *pie*	114	9.9	3.0				210	.05	0.5			111	74	.50		456
pineapple, homemade	299	56.6	2.6	45.0				1	.02			320	15			
⅛ *pie*	118	12.6	3.1				20	.05	0.5			85	25	.60		456
pumpkin																
frzn	229	63.3	4.3	29.8		2.9	523	2	.17	.06	16	307	65	16	.49	.262
⅙ *of 8" pie*	109	10.4	2.2	5.5	1.7	22	4921	.06	0.2	.43	.55	168	77	.86	.052	818
frzn, Mrs. Smith's	230		5.0	36.0	18.0	1.0						320				
⅛ *of 9" pie*	131	8.0	2.0	4.0	1.5	45						210				I
hearty, frzn, Mrs. Smith's	230		5.0	37.0	17.0	2.0						320				
⅛ *of 9" pie*	131	7.0	1.5	4.0	1.5	45						180				I
homemade	316	90.7	7.0	40.9			1212	3	.31	.07	17	349	146	29	.71	.307
⅛ *of 9" pie*	155	14.4	4.9	5.7	2.8	65	11833	.14	1.2	.14	.69	288	152	1.97	.102	818
raisin, homemade	319	50.2	3.1	50.7				1	.04			336	21			
⅛ *pie*	118	12.6	3.1				10	.04	0.4			227	47	1.10		456
raspberry, red fat, frzn, Mrs. Smith's	280		2.0	43.0	20.0	0.0						320				
⅙ *of 8" pie*	123	11.0	2.0	6.0	2.0	0						70				I
rhubarb, homemade	299	55.9	3.0	45.1				4	.05			319	76			
⅛ *pie*	118	12.6	3.1				60	.02	0.4			188	31	.80		456
strawberry, frzn, Mrs. Smith's	290		2.0	46.0	28.0	1.0						190				
⅕ *of 8" pie*	136	11.0	2.5	7.0	1.5	0						90				I
strawberry, homemade	184	54.3	1.8	28.7				23	.04			180	15			
⅛ *pie*	93	7.3	1.8				40	.02	0.4			112	23	.70		456
strawberry rhubarb, frzn, Mrs. Smith's	280		2.0	44.0	21.0	0.0						380				
⅙ *of 8" pie*	123	11.0	2.0	6.0	2.0							135				I
sweet potato, frzn, Mrs. Smith's	280		4.0	43.0	22.0	1.0						220				
⅙ *of 8" pie*	123	11.0	2.5	5.0	2.5	40						210				I
sweet potato, homemade	243	67.6	5.1	27.0				5	.14			249	79			
⅛ *pie*	114	12.9	4.6				2730	.06	0.3			186	96	.60		456
van cream, homemade	350	59.2	6.0	41.1		0.8	107	1	.27	.06	14	328	113	16	.67	.161
⅛ *of 9" pie*	126	18.1	5.1	7.6	4.3	78	386	.18	1.2	.38	.52	159	131	1.29	.049	818

8.12 PUDDINGS, CUSTARDS, & PIE FILLINGS

	KCAL	H₂O (g)	PRO (g)	CHO (g)	SUGR (g)	DFIB (g)	A (RE)	C (mg)	B-2 (mg)	B-6 (mg)	FOL (mcg)	Na (mg)	Ca (mg)	Mg (mg)	Zn (mg)	Mn (mg)
	WT (g)	FAT (g)	SFA (g)	MUFA (g)	PUFA (g)	CHOL (mg)	A (IU)	B-1 (mg)	NIA (mg)	B-12 (mcg)	PANT (mg)	K (mg)	P (mg)	Fe (mg)	Cu (mg)	REF
all flavors																
from cook & serve mix, Jell-O Brand	148		4.3	27.0	21.9	0.0		0				177	150			
½ *cup*[50]	113	2.8	1.8			10	200					239		.27		I
from cook & serve mix, sugar-free, Jell-O Brand—½ *cup*[51]	85		4.5	11.5	6.0	0.0		0				170	150			
	133	2.5	1.5			10	250					260		.54		I
from inst mix, fat-free, sugar-free, Jell-O Brand—½ *cup*[52]	73		4.3	12.7	6.0	0.0		0				395	150			
	113	0.0	0.0	0.0	0.0	0	200					247		.24		I
from inst mix, Jell-O Brand	155		4.0	29.4	24.0	0.0		0				414	150			
½ *cup*[53]	147	2.9	1.7			10	20					223		.16		I
apple tapioca, homemade	293	175.0	0.5	73.5				0	.00			128	8			
1 cup	250	0.3					30	.00	0.0			65	10	.50		456
banana																
from inst mix w/ lowfat milk	153	109.5	4.1	29.1		0.0	66	1	.20	.05	6	435	150	18	.49	.004
½ *cup*	147	2.5	1.5	0.7	0.2	9	250	.05	0.1	.44	.39	193	318	.09	.015	819
from inst mix w/ whole milk	166	108.0	4.0	28.8		0.0	37	1	.20	.05	6	434	147	18	.47	.004
½ *cup*	147	4.3	2.6	1.2	0.2	16	154	.05	0.1	.44	.39	188	315	.09	.018	819
from reg mix w/ lowfat milk	143	106.0	4.1	25.5		0.0	70	1	.20	.05	6	232	154	18	.50	.006
½ *cup*	140	2.4	1.5	0.7	0.1	10	252	.04	0.1	.36	.39	193	118	.07	.014	819
from reg mix w/ whole milk	157	104.4	4.1	25.3		0.0	38	1	.20	.05	6	231	151	18	.49	.006
½ *cup*	140	4.2	2.6	1.2	0.2	17	154	.04	0.1	.35	.39	189	116	.07	.017	819
rte	180	102.2	3.4	30.1		0.1	43	1	.21	.03	3	278	121	11	.40	.011
5 oz can	142	5.1	0.8	2.2	1.9	0	141	.03	0.2	.26	.23	156	98	.18	.040	819
rte, Snack Pack	119		1.5	18.3	13.8	0.0		0				155	47			
3.5 oz	99	4.5	1.9			2								.25		I

	KCAL / WT (g)	H₂O (g) / FAT (g)	PRO (g) / SFA (g)	CHO (g) / MUFA (g)	SUGR (g) / PUFA (g)	DFIB (g) / CHOL (mg)	A (RE) / A (IU)	C (mg) / B-1 (mg)	B-2 (mg) / NIA (mg)	B-6 (mg) / B-12 (mcg)	FOL (mcg) / PANT (mg)	Na (mg) / K (mg)	Ca (mg) / P (mg)	Mg (mg) / Fe (mg)	Zn (mg) / Cu (mg)	Mn (mg) / REF
bread, homemade	212	79.3	6.6	31.0		1.3	82	1	.28	.09	16	291	144	24	.66	.215
½ cup	126	7.4	2.9	2.7	1.2	83	304	.11	0.8	.33	.53	282	137	1.39	.096	819
butterscotch																
rte, Rich's	133	58.6	1.7	18.3					.09			128	26	5	.14	
3 oz	85	5.9						.02				85	47	.20	.020	I
rte, Snack Pack	130		1.5	21.2	13.7	0.0			.08			164	45			
3.5 oz	99	4.4	1.2			2	33	.02	0.1					.17		I
rte, Swiss Miss	156		2.5	24.1	19.3	0.0		0				182	62			
4 oz	113	5.6	1.4			1								.00		I
choc																
fat-free, rte, Swiss Miss	98		2.3	21.7	16.4	0.0		0				141	54			
4 oz	113	0.2	0.0			0								.42		I
from inst mix w/ lowfat milk	150	109.7	4.6	27.8		0.6	56	1	.21	.06	6	417	153	26	.62	.062
½ cup	147	2.8	1.6	0.9	0.2	9	253	.05	0.1	.46	.40	247	353	.43	.093	819
from inst mix w/ whole milk	158	104.5	4.4	26.7		1.4	30	1	.20	.05	6	403	145	26	.60	.060
½ cup	142	4.4	2.6	1.3	0.3	16	152	.05	0.1	.43	.38	236	339	.41	.091	819
from mix, red cal, D-Zerta	60		5.0	11.0	5.0	1.0		1				65	150			
½ cup[54]	130	0.0	0.0	0.0	0.0	0	200					290		.36		I
from reg mix w/ lowfat milk	151	104.9	4.7	28.0		0.4	68	1	.21	.05	6	149	160	30	.65	.061
½ cup	142	2.8	1.8	0.8	0.1	10	253	.05	0.2	.35	.40	240	138	.51	.105	819
from reg mix w/ whole milk	158	105.6	4.5	25.6		1.4	37	1	.25	.05	6	146	158	21	.64	.061
½ cup	142	4.8	3.0	1.4	0.2	17	156	.04	0.1	.35	.39	231	132	.51	.106	819
homemade w/ lowfat milk	206	106.1	4.9	40.5		1.4	79	1	.22	.05	6	138	155	39	.79	.174
½ cup	157	3.9	2.0	1.3	0.4	9	290	.05	0.2	.36	.41	256	149	.71	.187	819
homemade w/ whole milk	221	104.7	4.9	40.3		1.3	49	1	.22	.05	6	137	152	38	.77	.174
½ cup	157	5.7	3.1	1.8	0.5	17	193	.05	0.2	.35	.40	253	148	.71	.190	819
rte	189	98.4	3.8	32.4		1.4	16	3	.22	.04	4	183	128	30	.60	.098
5 oz can	142	5.7	1.0	2.4	2.0	4	51	.04	0.5	.00	.20	256	114	.72	.165	819
rte, Rich's	141	57.4	1.7	18.2					.08			136	22	13	.25	
3 oz	85	7.1						.02	0.2			111	53	.64	.030	I
rte, Snack Pack	143		2.0	21.7	17.4	0.0		0				139	58			
3.5 oz	99	5.4	1.4			1								.72		I
rte, Swiss Miss	166		3.1	25.8	23.0	0.0		0				177	83			
4 oz	113	5.7	1.5		0.0	1								.73		I
choc caramel swirl, Snack Pack	143		1.8	22.7	16.3	0.0		0				143	53			
3.5 oz	99	5.1	1.5			1								.59		I
choc caramel swirl, Swiss Miss	169		1.9	26.1	19.7	0.0		0				178	66			
4 oz	113	6.3	1.5			1								.40		I
choc fudge																
fat-free, rte, Swiss Miss	101		2.2	22.5	16.6	0.0	20	0				147	54			
4 oz	113	0.2	0.0			0								.42		I
rte, Snack Pack	147		2.1	22.9	17.4	0.0		0				153	50			
3.5 oz	99	5.2	1.6			1								.39		I
rte, Swiss Miss	175		3.3	27.9	21.5	0.0		0				207	79			
4 oz	113	5.6	1.6			1								.22		I
choc marshmallow, rte, Snack Pack	134		2.0	20.5	15.9	0.0		0				121	36			
3.5 oz	99	4.9	1.4			1								.36		I
choc mousse, homemade	446	125.4	8.7	33.1		1.2	323	1	.41	.13	32	87	202	44	1.43	.123
½ cup	202	32.9	18.5	10.3	1.7	299	1133	.08	0.3	.93	1.17	297	259	1.29	.149	819
choc peanut butter swirl, Snack Pack	146		2.5	21.4	14.6	0.0		0				143	53			
3.5 oz	99	5.6	1.3			2								.59		I
choc-van parfait, fat-free, rte, Swiss Miss	96		1.9	21.4	16.1	0.0		0				143	53			
4 oz	113	0.3	0.0			0								.19		I
choc-van swirls, rte, Swiss Miss	169		2.3	26.4	21.1	0.0		0				159	61			
4 oz	113	6.0	1.5			1								.51		I
coconut cream																
from inst mix w/ lowfat milk	157	109.4	4.3	28.2		0.1	69	1	.20	.06	6	362	150	21	.49	.028
½ cup	147	3.4	2.0	0.9	0.3	9	250	.05	0.1	.44	.40	194	295	.22	.037	819

	KCAL / WT (g)	H₂O (g) / FAT (g)	PRO (g) / SFA (g)	CHO (g) / MUFA (g)	SUGR (g) / PUFA (g)	DFIB (g) / CHOL (mg)	A (RE) / A (IU)	C (mg) / B-1 (mg)	B-2 (mg) / NIA (mg)	B-6 (mg) / B-12 (mcg)	FOL (mcg) / PANT (mg)	Na (mg) / K (mg)	Ca (mg) / P (mg)	Mg (mg) / Fe (mg)	Zn (mg) / Cu (mg)	Mn (mg) / REF
from inst mix w/ whole milk	172	107.9	4.3	28.1		0.1	37	1	.20	.05	6	362	147	21	.49	.028
½ cup	147	5.1	3.1	1.4	0.4	16	154	.05	0.1	.44	.39	190	294	.22	.038	819
from reg mix w/ lowfat milk	146	105.8	4.3	24.9		0.3	70	1	.20	.20	6	228	158	22	.52	.052
½ cup	140	3.5	2.5	0.7	0.1	10	252	.04	0.1	.36	.41	223	125	.28	.035	819
from reg mix w/ whole milk	160	104.4	4.2	24.8		0.3	31	1	.20	.20	6	227	155	22	.50	.052
½ cup	140	5.3	3.6	1.2	0.2	17	154	.04	0.1	.35	.40	220	123	.28	.038	819
creamy chilled dessert mixes, Betty Crocker—4.4 oz⁵⁵ [55]	298		4.2	43.2	28.4	0.4		0	.10			352	76			
	125	12.6	4.2			29	340	.03	0.2			178		.58		I
custard																
baked, homemade	209	111.0	7.2	15.1		0.0	85	1	.32	.07	14	109	158	20	.75	.010
½ cup	141	6.6	3.3	2.1	0.5	123	313	.05	0.1	.44	.67	216	159	.42	.020	819
fat-free, rte, Snack Pack	83		1.7	18.6	13.5	0.0	0	0				140	43			
3.5 oz⁵⁶ [56]	99	0.2	0.0			0	0							.24		I
from mix, Jell-O Americana	140		5.0	25.0	23.0	0.0	0					190	200			
½ cup⁵⁷ [57]	113	2.5	1.5			10	200					300		.00		I
from mix, made w/ lowfat milk	149	98.8	5.6	23.5		0.0	74	1	.29	.09	11	200	197	27	.70	.007
½ cup	133	3.7	1.9	1.2	0.3	74	295	.07	0.2	.61	.81	287	176	.35	.025	819
from mix, made w/ whole milk	162	97.4	5.5	23.4		0.0	44	1	.29	.08	11	198	194	25	.69	.007
½ cup	133	5.5	3.0	1.7	0.3	81	200	.07	0.2	.60	.80	283	174	.35	.028	819
rte, Swiss Miss	153		4.5	21.7	20.5	0.0	0					138	120			
4 oz	113	5.3	1.2			4								.00		I
flan/creme caramel																
from mix, Knorr	160		5.0	23.0				1	.31	.09	11	198	199	26	1.00	
½ cup	110	6.0				81	230	.08	0.2	.70	.80	284	174	.30	.030	I
from mix, made w/ lowfat milk	136	100.1	4.0	25.5		0.1	63	1	.20	.05	5	67	153	17	.48	.003
½ cup	133	2.4	1.5	0.7	0.1	9	249	.04	0.1	.36	.39	194	116	.08	.013	819
from mix, made w/ whole milk	150	98.7	4.0	25.4		0.1	35	1	.20	.05	5	65	150	16	.47	.003
½ cup	133	4.1	2.5	1.2	0.2	16	153	.04	0.1	.35	.38	192	114	.08	.016	819
homemade	220	103.9	6.9	34.9		0.0	87	1	.31	.07	14	86	132	17	.72	.012
½ cup	153	6.3	3.0	2.1	0.5	141	314	.04	0.1	.43	.65	185	145	.50	.028	819
w/ sce, from mix, Knorr	190		4.0	34.0								70				
½ cup & 1 T sce	115	4.0				20										I
lemon																
from cook & serve mix, Jell-O Brand	140		1.0	29.0	23.0	0.0	0					75	0			
½ cup⁵⁸ [58]	113	2.0	0.5			75	100					5		.00		I
from inst mix w/ lowfat milk	154	109.1	4.1	29.7		0.0	69	1	.20	.05	6	394	148	16	.49	.004
½ cup	147	2.5	1.5	0.7	0.1	9	250	.05	0.1	.44	.39	190	304	.09	.013	819
from inst mix w/ whole milk	169	107.6	4.0	29.5		0.0	38	1	.20	.05	6	392	146	16	.47	.004
½ cup	147	4.3	2.6	1.2	0.2	16	154	.05	0.1	.44	.39	187	301	.09	.016	819
from reg mix w/ sugar, egg yolk, and water—½ cup	164	106.1	1.0	36.4		0.0	35	0	.05	.02	9	93	12	3	.23	.012
	146	1.9	0.6	0.7	0.2	77	117	.01	0.0	.19	.24	7	31	.26	.020	819
rte	178	101.7	0.1	35.5		0.1	0	0	.01	.00	0	199	3	1	.04	.011
5 oz can	142	4.3	0.6	1.8	1.6	0	0	.00	0.0	.00	.01	1	7	.10	.021	819
rte, Snack Pack	124		0.4	23.7	20.6	0.0	2					47	6			
3.5 oz	99	3.1	0.9			0								.20		I
milk choc, Snack Pack	143		2.0	22.3	17.5	0.0	0					136	53			
3.5 oz	99	5.1	1.5			2								.63		I
mousse, choc, from reg mix, Knorr	80		1.0	8.0								45				
½ cup⁵⁹ [59]	113	5.0				5										I
prune whip, homemade	203	74.4	5.7	48.0				3	.18			213	29			
1 cup	130	0.3					600	.03	0.7			377	43	1.70		456
pudding cup, Del Monte	123		1.5	22.3	17.2	0.0	0	0				119	60			
3.5 oz container⁶⁰ [60]	99	3.3	0.3			0								.00		I
pudding snacks, fat-free, rte, Jell-O Brand Free—4 oz container⁶¹ [61]	100		2.8	23.0	17.5	0.0	0					215	80			
	113	0.0	0.0	0.0	0.0	0	100					166		.27		I
pudding snacks, rte, Jell-O Brand	159		2.6	26.3	21.6	0.0	0					176	94			
4 oz container⁶² [62]	113	5.1	1.9			0	100					171		.41		I

	KCAL	H₂O (g)	PRO (g)	CHO (g)	SUGR (g)	DFIB (g)	Vitamins A (RE)	C (mg)	B-2 (mg)	B-6 (mg)	FOL (mcg)	Minerals Na (mg)	Ca (mg)	Mg (mg)	Zn (mg)	Mn (mg)
	WT (g)	FAT (g)	SFA (g)	MUFA (g)	PUFA (g)	CHOL (mg)	A (IU)	B-1 (mg)	NIA (mg)	B-12 (mcg)	PANT (mg)	K (mg)	P (mg)	Fe (mg)	Cu (mg)	REF
rennin dessert																
choc, from mix w/ lowfat milk	110	109.3	4.4	18.4		0.7	60	1	.21	.06	7	71	171	27	.69	.090
½ cup	136	2.9	1.7	0.8	0.1	10	252	.05	0.1	.45	.40	248	133	.41	.110	819
choc, from mix w/ whole milk	125	107.8	4.4	18.1		0.7	33	1	.21	.06	7	69	169	27	.68	.090
½ cup	136	4.5	2.8	1.3	0.2	16	155	.05	0.1	.44	.39	243	132	.41	.113	819
van, from mix w/ lowfat milk	101	109.2	4.1	16.4		0.0	69	1	.20	.05	7	61	161	17	.48	.004
½ cup	133	2.4	1.5	0.7	0.1	9	251	.05	0.1	.44	.39	189	126	.07	.016	819
van, from mix w/ whole milk	116	107.7	4.0	16.2		0.0	33	1	.20	.05	7	61	158	16	.47	.004
½ cup	133	4.1	2.5	1.2	0.2	17	154	.05	0.1	.44	.38	186	124	.07	.019	819
van, homemade	112	112.6	4.0	15.3		0.0	37	1	.20	.05	5	96	151	16	.48	.004
½ cup	137	4.1	2.5	1.2	0.2	16	153	.05	0.1	.44	.38	185	115	.08	.016	819
rice																
from reg mix w/ 2% milk, Jell-O	160		5.0	30.0	19.0	0.0		0				160	150			
Americana—½ cup	149	2.5	1.5			10	200					190		.36		I
from reg mix w/ lowfat milk	161	105.4	4.8	30.2		0.1	52	1	.20	.05	6	158	151	19	.56	.082
½ cup	144	2.3	1.5	0.6	0.1	9	249	.11	0.6	.36	.42	190	127	.55	.026	819
from reg mix w/ whole milk	176	104.0	4.8	30.1		0.1	29	1	.20	.05	6	157	148	19	.55	.082
½ cup	144	4.0	2.5	1.2	0.2	16	154	.11	0.6	.35	.41	186	124	.55	.029	819
homemade	217	100.9	5.5	40.1		0.8	38	1	.21	.09	6	85	155	24	.68	.219
½ cup	152	4.3	2.6	1.2	0.2	17	154	.12	0.8	.24	.50	269	143	1.00	.084	819
rte	231	96.4	2.8	31.2		0.1	50	1	.10	.04	4	121	74	11	.70	.179
5 oz can	142	10.6	1.7	4.6	4.0	1	162	.03	0.2	.30	.33	85	97	.43	.031	819
S'mores, Snack Pack	136		1.8	21.3	18.1	0.0		0				94	36			
3.5 oz	99	4.9	1.4			1								.36		I
tapioca																
from mix w/ 2% milk, Jell-O Americana	140		4.0	26.0	20.0	0.0		0				170	150			
½ cup	147	2.5	1.5			10	200					190		.00		I
from reg mix w/ lowfat milk	147	105.5	4.1	27.8		0.0	69	1	.20	.05	6	172	149	17	.49	.010
½ cup	141	2.4	1.5	0.7	0.1	8	251	.04	0.1	.35	.39	189	117	.08	.017	819
from reg mix w/ whole milk	161	104.1	4.1	27.6		0.0	38	1	.20	.05	6	171	147	17	.48	.010
½ cup	141	4.1	2.5	1.2	0.2	17	154	.04	0.1	.35	.39	186	116	.08	.018	819
homemade	190	110.8	7.1	25.8		0.0	87	1	.32	.08	14	289	158	20	.74	.015
½ cup	152	6.5	3.3	2.1	0.5	125	315	.05	0.1	.56	.67	216	160	.49	.024	819
rte	169	105.4	2.8	27.5		0.1	0	1	.14	.14	6	168	119	11	.38	.027
5 oz can	142	5.3	0.9	2.2	1.9	1	0	.03	0.4	.16	.30	148	112	.33	.038	819
rte, Snack Pack	125		1.4	20.9	14.5	0.0		0				144	61			
3.5 oz	99	3.9	1.6			1								.24		I
rte, Swiss Miss	138		2.1	24.3	19.6	0.0		0				180	84			
4 oz	113	3.6	0.9			1								.10		I
van																
fat-free, rte, Swiss Miss	93		1.7	21.0	14.4	0.0		0				168	52			
4 oz	113	0.2	0.0			0								.02		I
from inst mix w/ lowfat milk	148	105.8	4.0	28.1		0.0	64	1	.20	.05	6	406	146	17	.47	.010
½ cup	142	2.4	1.4	0.7	0.1	9	241	.05	0.1	.43	.38	185	283	.10	.033	819
from inst mix w/ whole milk	162	104.4	3.8	28.0		0.0	36	1	.19	.05	6	406	143	17	.47	.010
½ cup	142	4.1	2.5	1.2	0.2	16	149	.05	0.1	.43	.37	182	280	.10	.034	819
from reg mix w/ lowfat milk	141	106.0	4.2	26.2		0.0	70	1	.20	.05	6	224	153	18	.50	.006
½ cup	140	2.4	1.5	0.7	0.1	10	252	.04	0.1	.36	.39	193	118	.07	.014	819
from reg mix w/ whole milk	155	104.4	4.1	25.9		0.0	38	1	.20	.05	6	224	150	18	.49	.006
½ cup	140	4.2	2.6	1.2	0.2	17	154	.04	0.1	.35	.39	190	115	.07	.017	819
homemade	130	94.3	4.1	19.6		0.0	37	1	.20	.04	5	113	145	16	.47	.006
½ cup	123	4.1	2.5	1.2	0.2	16	154	.03	0.1	.23	.38	185	114	.09	.018	819
rte	147	80.5	2.6	24.7		0.1	7	0	.16	.01	0	153	99	9	.28	.009
½ cup	113	4.1	0.6	1.7	1.5	8	24	.02	0.3	.11	.20	128	77	.15	.034	819
rte, Rich's	129	58.5	1.6	18.4					.08			162	26	5	.17	
3 oz	85	5.9						.02	0.0			85	48	.17	.030	I
rte, Snack Pack	135		1.7	21.0	17.0	0.0		0				147	47			
3.5 oz	99	4.9	1.3		1.0	1								.01		I

						Vitamins					Minerals				
KCAL	H₂O (g)	PRO (g)	CHO (g)	SUGR (g)	DFIB (g)	A (RE)	C (mg)	B-2 (mg)	B-6 (mg)	FOL (mcg)	Na (mg)	Ca (mg)	Mg (mg)	Zn (mg)	Mn (mg)
WT (g)	FAT (g)	SFA (g)	MUFA (g)	PUFA (g)	CHOL (mg)	A (IU)	B-1 (mg)	NIA (mg)	B-12 (mcg)	PANT (mg)	K (mg)	P (mg)	Fe (mg)	Cu (mg)	REF
rte, Swiss Miss															
156		2.5	24.1	19.3	0.0		0				181	83			
4 oz	113	5.6	1.4			1							.07		I
van-choc parfait, Swiss Miss															
164		2.9	24.5	22.4	0.0		0				196	88			
4 oz	113	6.0	1.6			1							.41		I
van sundae, Swiss Miss															
175		2.0	26.5	22.1	0.0		0				174	64			
4 oz	113	6.8	1.7			1							.44		I

8.13 SAUCES, SYRUPS, & TOPPINGS FOR DESSERTS

KCAL / WT	H₂O / FAT	PRO / SFA	CHO / MUFA	SUGR / PUFA	DFIB / CHOL	A(RE) / A(IU)	C / B-1	B-2 / NIA	B-6 / B-12	FOL / PANT	Na / K	Ca / P	Mg / Fe	Zn / Cu	Mn / REF
apple pie syrup, fat-free, Hershey															
100		0.3	25.4	17.0	0.0	0	0				88	11			
2 T 38	0.0	0.0	0.0	0.0		0					11		.08		I
butterscotch topping, Kraft															
130			28.0	18.0	0.0		0				150	0			
2 T 41	1.5	1.0			5	200					40		.00		I
cake & cookie decorator, all flavors															
except choc, Pillsbury—*1 T* 72	2.5	0.0	13.7				0	.00			0	0			
18	2.0					0	.00	0.0			5	0	.00		I
cake & cookie decorator, choc, Pillsbury															
1 T 64	2.9	0.2	12.2				0	.00			0	0			
16	1.8					0	.00	0.0			5	11	.13		I
caramel sce, Knorr															
1 T 60	5.4	0.0	14.7								5				
21	0.0	0.0	0.0	0.0	0										I
caramel syrup, fat-free, Hershey															
2 T 100		0.8	25.0	16.9	0.0	0	0				93	14			
38	0.0	0.0	0.0	0.0		0							.08		I
caramel topping, Kraft															
2 T 120			28.0	19.0	0.0	0	0				90	60			
41	0.0	0.0	0.0	0.0	0	0					90		.00		I
choc fudge topping															
1 T 73	4.5	0.9	12.4		0.3	5	0	.05	.01	1	27	21	10	.17	.063
21	2.8	1.2	0.8	0.7	3	19	.01	0.0	.06	.06	45	36	.25	.063	819
choc fudge topping, Hershey															
2 T 141		1.7	20.6	16.4	0.7	0	0				50	38			
38	5.8	3.7			7	0							.31		I
choc mint syrup, fat-free, Hershey															
2 T 109		0.7	25.7	16.3	0.9	0	0				26	6			
38	0.4	0.0				0							.04		I
choc syrup															
2 T (1 fl oz) 83	14.1	0.7	22.4	25.4	0.7	1	0	.02	.00	2	36	5	25	.28	.145
38	0.3	0.2	0.1	0.0	0	11	.00	0.1	.00	.00	85	49	.80	.195	819
Hershey 102		0.9	23.8	20.9	1.0	0	0				27	5			
2 T 39	0.4	0.3			0	0							.45		I
lite, Hershey 49		0.6	11.5	9.6	0.7	0	0				48	0			
2 T 35	0.1	0.0			0	0							.35		I
choc topping, Kraft															
110		2.0	26.0	20.0	1.0	0	0				30	20			
2 T 39	0.0	0.0	0.0	0.0	0	0					190		.36		I
double choc fudge topping, Hershey															
125		1.8	24.4	19.6	0.8	0	0				73	34			
2 T 39	2.2	1.1			3	0							.35		I
double choc syrup, fat-free, Hershey															
113		0.7	25.4	16.0	0.9	0	0				26	6			
2 T 38	0.4	0.0			0	0							.04		I
hot fudge topping															
fat-free, Hershey 100		1.4	22.8	17.7	1.0	0	0				135	31			
2 T 39	0.3	0.0			0	0							.10		I
Hershey 126		1.7	19.7	15.4	0.5	0	0				181	43			
2 T 37	4.5	2.0			4	0							.27		I
Kraft 140		1.0	24.0	17.0	1.0	0	0				100	40			
2 T 41	4.0	2.0			0	0					85		.36		I
icing/frosting, from mix															
Betty Crocker 134		1.0	23.4	20.8	0.0		0	.00			48	0			
2 T[63] 34	4.3	1.2			0	100	.00	0.0			43		.07		I
choc creamy, made w/ butter 160	5.6	0.5	30.1		0.8	25	0	.01	.03	0	63	5	13	.27	.109
¹⁄₁₂ pkg prep 42	5.5	2.4	1.1	0.1	10	143	.00	0.0	.00	.01	60	21	.39	.097	819
choc creamy, made w/ marg 161	5.6	0.5	30.1		0.8	29	0	.01	.03	0	69	5	13	.27	.109
¹⁄₁₂ pkg prep 42	5.5	0.7	1.7	1.2	0	154	.00	0.0	.00	.01	61	21	.39	.096	819
Duncan Hines 160	6.9	0.4	24.1					.02			91	6			
¹⁄₁₂ pkg prep[64] 38	7.3	2.0	4.6	0.4	0		.01	0.1					.61		I
van creamy, made w/ butter 182	5.0	0.1	30.4		0.0	41	0	.01	.00	0	90	4	1	.05	.017
¹⁄₁₂ pkg prep 43	7.2	3.1	2.3	1.4	10	199	.01	0.2	.00	.02	9	12	.11	.022	819
van creamy, made w/ marg 182	5.0	0.1	30.4		0.0	46	0	.01	.00	0	95	4	1	.05	.017
¹⁄₁₂ pkg prep 43	7.1	1.4	2.9	2.5	0	211	.01	0.1	.00	.02	9	12	.10	.021	819

	KCAL	H₂O (g)	PRO (g)	CHO (g)	SUGR (g)	DFIB (g)	A (RE)	C (mg)	B-2 (mg)	B-6 (mg)	FOL (mcg)	Na (mg)	Ca (mg)	Mg (mg)	Zn (mg)	Mn (mg)
	WT (g)	FAT (g)	SFA (g)	MUFA (g)	PUFA (g)	CHOL (mg)	A (IU)	B-1 (mg)	NIA (mg)	B-12 (mcg)	PANT (mg)	K (mg)	P (mg)	Fe (mg)	Cu (mg)	REF
white, fluffy, made w/ water	63	9.2	0.4	16.3		0.0	0	0	.01	.00	1	41	1	1	.01	.001
¹⁄₁₂ pkg prep	26	0.0	0.0	0.0	0.0	0	0	.00	0.2	.00	.01	20	1	.02	.007	819
icing/frosting, homemade																
choc creamy, made w/ butter	200	4.3	0.7	38.8		0.8	50	0	.01	.00	1	95	9	13	.20	.100
¹⁄₁₂ recipe	50	5.8	3.5	1.7	0.2	15	203	.00	0.1	.02	.02	45	24	.38	.113	819
choc creamy, made w/ marg	201	4.3	0.7	38.9		0.8	56	0	.01	.01	1	103	9	13	.20	.099
¹⁄₁₂ recipe	50	5.7	1.3	2.5	1.7	1	219	.00	0.1	.01	.02	46	24	.38	.111	819
glaze	97	4.8	0.2	19.8		0.0	22	0	.01	.00	0	25	6	1	.02	.002
¹⁄₁₂ recipe	27	2.1	0.5	0.9	0.6	1	86	.00	0.0	.02	.02	8	5	.02	.009	819
van creamy, made w/ butter	165	8.1	0.3	37.5		0.0	18	0	.01	.00	0	31	11	1	.04	.003
¹⁄₁₂ recipe	48	2.0	1.2	0.6	0.1	6	73	.00	0.0	.03	.03	14	9	.03	.017	819
van creamy, made w/ marg	194	4.4	0.2	38.0		0.0	54	0	.01	.00	0	98	6	1	.02	.003
¹⁄₁₂ recipe	48	5.2	1.1	2.3	1.6	0	211	.00	0.0	.02	.02	9	5	.03	.017	819
white, boiled (7 min)	102	5.5	0.5	25.8		0.0	0	0	.03	.00	0	54	1	1	.01	.004
¹⁄₁₂ recipe	32	0.0	0.0	0.0	0.0	0	0	.00	0.0	.01	.01	20	1	.02	.012	819
icing/frosting, rts																
Betty Crocker Whipped Delux	107		0.1	15.4	14.4	0.0	0	0	.00			34	0			
2 T[65]	24	5.0	1.6			0	0	.00	0.0			26		.15		I
caramel pecan, Pillsbury Supreme	155	9.5	0.2	20.8				0	.00			68	2			
amt for ¹⁄₁₂ cake	37	8.4					3	.01	0.0			34	6	.05		I
choc chip, Pillsbury Supreme	155	5.1	0.2	27.0				0	.00			69	1			
amt for ¹⁄₁₂ cake	38	5.4					1	.00	0.0			20	5	.08		I
choc creamy	151	6.5	0.4	24.0		0.2	75	0	.01	.00	0	70	3	8	.11	.091
¹⁄₁₂ tub	38	6.7	2.1	3.4	0.8	0	249	.00	0.0	.00	.01	74	30	.54	.076	819
choc fudge funfetti, Pillsbury	141	6.6	0.5	21.7				0	.00			79	1			
¹⁄₁₂ can	36	6.0					0	.00	0.1			98	15	.86		I
choc fudge, Pillsbury	109	5.3	0.4	16.6				0	.00			63	1			
amt for ¹⁄₈ cake	28	4.7					0	.00	0.1			78	12	.69		I
choc fudge, Pillsbury Supreme	150	7.0	0.5	23.7				0	.00			82	1			
amt for ¹⁄₁₂ cake	38	6.4					0	.00	0.1			93	39	.47		I
choc mint, Pillsbury Supreme	148	7.5	0.5	22.8				0	.00			83	1			
amt for ¹⁄₁₂ cake	38	6.4					0	.00	0.1			107	16	.92		I
coconut almond, Pillsbury Supreme	151	7.4	0.6	17.1				0	.02			59	7			
amt for ¹⁄₁₂ cake	35	9.3					0	.01	0.1			59	17	.23		I
coconut nut	157	8.0	0.6	20.1		0.5	0	0	.01	.02	2	74	5	7	.16	.320
¹⁄₁₂ tub	38	9.1	2.7	4.6	1.3	0	0	.01	0.1	.00	.10	71	24	.21	.048	819
coconut pecan, Pillsbury Supreme	152	7.4	0.5	16.8				0	.00			59	4			
amt for ¹⁄₁₂ cake	35	9.6					3	.02	0.0			54	14	.18		I
cream cheese	157	5.7	0.0	25.3		0.0	44	0	.00	.00	0	90	1	1	.00	.004
¹⁄₁₂ tub	38	6.6	1.9	3.4	0.9	0	146	.00	0.0	.00	.00	13	1	.06	.008	819
cream cheese, Pillsbury Supreme	160	5.2	0.0	26.3				0	.00			117	1			
amt for ¹⁄₁₂ cake	38	6.2					0	.00	0.0			10	1	.02		I
Creamy Deluxe	147		0.0	23.8	22.3	0.0	0	0	.00			54	0			
2 T[66]	35	5.7	1.6			0	0	.00	0.0			39		.00		I
double dutch, Pillsbury Supreme	145	8.0	0.7	22.0				0	.00			46	1			
amt for ¹⁄₁₂ cake	38	6.5					0	.00	0.1			138	22	1.22		I
lemon, Pillsbury Supreme	160	5.2	0.0	26.3				0	.00			79	0			
amt for ¹⁄₁₂ cake	38	6.2					0	.00	0.0			10	1	.02		I
low fat, choc, Creamy Deluxe	120		1.0	27.0	25.0	0.0	0	0	.00			50	0			
2 T	36	1.0	0.5			0	0	.00	0.0			70		.36		I
low fat, milk choc, Creamy Deluxe	120		1.0	27.0	25.0	0.0	0	0	.00			55	0			
2 T	36	0.5	0.5			0	0	.00	0.0			80		.00		I
low fat, van, Creamy Deluxe	120			28.0	24.0	0.0						25				
2 T	34	0.5	0.5			0						10				I
milk choc, Pillsbury Supreme	153	7.0	0.4	23.7				0	.00			61	1			
amt for ¹⁄₁₂ cake	38	6.4					0	.00	0.1			79	15	.40		I
mocha, Pillsbury Supreme	153	6.4	0.2	24.5				0	.00			60	1			
amt for ¹⁄₁₂ cake	38	6.2					0	.00	0.1			64	9	.46		I
red fat, Sweet Rewards	130		0.0	26.0	23.0	0.0	0	0	.00			47	0			
1 T[67]	36	2.5	1.0			0	0	.00	0.0			55		.12		I

	KCAL	H₂O (g)	PRO (g)	CHO (g)	SUGR (g)	DFIB (g)	A (RE)	C (mg)	B-2 (mg)	B-6 (mg)	FOL (mcg)	Na (mg)	Ca (mg)	Mg (mg)	Zn (mg)	Mn (mg)
	WT (g)	FAT (g)	SFA (g)	MUFA (g)	PUFA (g)	CHOL (mg)	A (IU)	B-1 (mg)	NIA (mg)	B-12 (mcg)	PANT (mg)	K (mg)	P (mg)	Fe (mg)	Cu (mg)	REF
sour cream	157	5.4	0.0	25.7		0.0	46	0	.01	.00	0	78	1	1	.00	.020
¹⁄₁₂ tub	38	6.5	1.9	3.4	0.9	0	152	.00	0.3	.00	.02	74	2	.03	.004	819
sour cream van, Pillsbury Supreme	163	4.4	0.2	26.9				1	.00			78	3			
amt for ¹⁄₁₂ cake	38	6.2					32	.01	0.0			18	5	.05		I
strawberry, Pillsbury Supreme	161	5.2	0.0	26.4			0		.00			78	0			
amt for ¹⁄₁₂ cake	38	6.2					0	.00	0.0			10	1	.02		I
van creamy	159	5.0	0.0	26.4		0.0	86	0	.00	.00	0	34	1	0	.00	.015
¹⁄₁₂ tub	38	6.4	1.9	3.3	0.9	0	283	.00	0.0	.00	.00	14	15	.04	.003	819
van funfetti, Pillsbury	150	5.1	0.0	24.5			0		.00			72	1			
¹⁄₁₂ can	36	5.7					0	.00	0.0			9	0	.02		I
van, Pillsbury	116	4.2	0.0	18.8			0		.00			57	0			
amt for ¹⁄₁₂ cake	28	4.5					0	.00	0.0			7	0	.02		I
van, Pillsbury Supreme	160	5.2	0.0	26.3			0		.00			74	0			
amt for ¹⁄₁₂ cake	38	6.2					0	.00	0.0			10	0	.02		I
marshmallow cream	88	5.2	0.5	22.5		0.0	0	0	.00	.00	0	13	1	1	.01	.002
1 oz	28	0.1	0.0	0.0	0.0	0	0	.00	0.0	.00	.00	1	2	.06	.027	819
marshmallow creme, Kraft	40		0.0	10.0	8.0	0.0	0	0				10	0			
2 T	12	0.0	0.0	0.0	0.0	0	0					0		.00		I
pineapple/strawberry topping, Kraft	110		0.0	28.5	20.5	0.0	0	4				15	0			
2 T	41	0.0	0.0	0.0	0.0	0	0					20		.00		I
pineapple topping	106	13.9	0.0	27.9		0.4	1	25	.00	.01	1	26	9	1	.20	.299
2 T	42	0.0	0.0	0.0	0.0	0	9	.01	0.0	.00	.01	133	3	.20	.014	819
strawberry topping	107	13.9	0.1	27.8		0.4	1	10	.01	.01	1	9	10	2	.21	.017
2 T	42	0.0	0.0	0.0	0.0	0	8	.00	0.1	.00	.05	31	5	.41	.012	819
walnut syrup topping	167	7.6	1.8	21.9		0.7	2	0	.05	.08	9	17	16	26	.43	.426
2 T	41	9.0	0.8	2.0	5.6	0	17	.07	0.2	.00	.09	86	46	.43	.195	819

1. Values are averages for caramel, chocolate chip, chocolate chunk, cookies & cream, dark chocolate fudge, dark chocolate with Hershey's syrup, frosted supreme, fudge, German chocolate, hot fudge, peanut butter candies with Reese's Pieces, walnut, and white chocolate swirl.
2. Values are averages for caramel oatmeal, chocolate chunk, chocolate peanut butter, Easy Layer, Hershey cookie, raspberry, S'mores, strawberry, swirl cheesecake, and Sunkist lemon dessert.
3. Values apply to chocolate, confetti, lemon custard, strawberry, and white angel food cake mixes.
4. Values are averages for blueberry, cherry, homestyle, real, and strawberry; prepared with 2% fat milk, margarine, and sugar.
5. Values are for fudge cake made with margarine; if butter is used, polyunsaturated fat is 1.5 g and cholesterol is 100 mg.
6. Values are for cake made with margarine; if butter is used, polyunsaturated fat is 1.5 g and cholesterol is 100 mg.
7. Made with unequal weights of flour, sugar, fat, and eggs.
8. Made with equal weights of flour, sugar, fat, and eggs.
9. Values also apply to banana, butterscotch, caramel, french vanilla, fudge marble, key lime, lemon, orange, peach, pineapple, raspberry, spice, strawberry, tropical fruit, and wild cherry vanilla.
10. Values are averages for the three flavors.
11. 28 wafers (168g) = 1 ½ cups wafer crumbs.
12. Values are averages for chocolate chip, double chocolate chunk, oatmeal chocolate chip, and peanut butter.
13. Values are averages for chocolate chip cookies with chocolate frosting, cookies & creme, chocolate cookies with vanilla frosting, and cinnamon graham cookies with vanilla frosting.
14. Nine crackers (126 g) are equivalent to 1 ½ cups of cracker crumbs.
15. Values are averages for apple cinnamon and peach apricot.
16. Values are averages for 17 flavors.
17. Values are averages for chocolate chip, Dutch chocolate, mocha almond fudge, Neopolitan, strawberry swirl, toasted almond, vanilla, and vanilla chocolate almond.
18. Two 1.5 oz bars or three 1 oz bars.
19. Contains polydextrose as part of the carbohydrate; polydextrose yields 1 calorie per gram.
20. Values are averages for apple, berry, blueberry, cherry, and peach.
21. Values are averages for cherry, lemon, lime, orange, raspberry, strawberry, and strawberry banana.
22. Values are averages for cherry, lime, orange, raspberry, and strawberry.
23. Values are averages for all 22 flavors.
24. Values are averages for 13 flavors.
25. Values are averages for blueberry, cherry, grape, and strawberry.
26. Includes blue raspberry, cherry, orange, and strawberry.
27. Includes berry blue, cherry, grape, orange, raspberry, strawberry, and strawberry banana.
28. Includes cherry, orange, raspberry, and strawberry.
29. Foods in this section are granola bars unless otherwise specified as breakfast bars, cereal bars, or snack bars.
30. Contains 0.64 g sorbitol.
31. Contains 0.95 g sorbitol.
32. Values are averages for apple cinnamon, blueberry, raspberry, strawberry, and strawberry banana.
33. Values are averages for apple brown sugar, chocolate chip, honey nut, oatmeal raisin, orchard blend, and triple berry.
34. Contains 0.74 g sorbitol.
35. Contains 0.77 g sorbitol.
36. Includes caramel, oatmeal raisin, and original flavors.
37. Contains 0.78 g sorbitol.
38. Contains 0.84 g sorbitol.
39. Contains 0.67 g sorbitol.
40. Contains 0.70 g sorbitol.
41. Values are average for blueberry with drizzle, raspberry, and strawberry with drizzle.
42. Four ladyfingers with ⅓ cup whipped cream filling.
43. Includes apple, cinnamon, raisin, lemon, raspberry, and strawberry.
44. Includes almond, raisin nut, and cinnamon nut.
45. Includes apple, blueberry, cherry, and strawberry.

46. Values are averages for iced apple cinnamon, iced blueberry, iced fudge, and iced strawberry.
47. Values are averages for frosted tarts (blueberry, brown sugar cinnamon, cherry, fudge, and strawberry) and unfrosted strawberry.
48. Prepared with 2% fat milk and margarine.
49. Includes apple, blueberry, cherry, lemon, peach, and strawberry.
50. Values are averages for banana cream, butterscotch, chocolate, chocolate fudge, coconut cream, flan, milk chocolate, and vanilla; prepared with 2% fat milk.
51. Values are for chocolate and vanilla; prepared with 2% fat milk.
52. Values are averages for banana, butterscotch, chocolate, chocolate fudge, pistachio, and vanilla; prepared with nonfat milk.
53. Values are averages for banana cream, butter pecan, butterscotch, chocolate, chocolate fudge, coconut cream, french vanilla, lemon, milk chocolate, pistachio, and vanilla; prepared with 2% fat milk.
54. Prepared with nonfat milk.
55. Values are averages for banana cream, chocolate french silk, coconut cream, cookies & creme, and Sunkist lemon supreme.
56. Values are averages for chocolate, tapioca, and vanilla.
57. Prepared with 2% fat milk.
58. Prepared with sugar, egg yolks, and water.
59. Values are averages for chocolate, dark chocolate, milk chocolate, and white chocolate.

60. Values are averages for banana, butterscotch, chocolate, chocolate fudge, tapioca, and vanilla.
61. Values are averages for chocolate, chocolate vanilla swirl, vanilla, and vanilla chocolate swirl.
62. Values are averages for banana, chocolate, chocolate caramel swirl, chocolate vanilla swirl, tapioca, vanilla, and vanilla chocolate swirl.
63. Values are averages for chocolate, coconut pecan, creamy chocolate fudge, creamy vanilla, and white.
64. Values are averages for chocolate, cream cheese, dark dutch fudge, milk chocolate, milk chocolate polka dot, vanilla, and vanilla pink polka dot.
65. Values are averages for chocolate, cream cheese, fluffy white, lemon, milk chocolate, strawberry, and vanilla.
66. Values are averages for butter pecan, butter cream, caramel chocolate chip, cherry, chocolate, chocolate chip, chocolate chip cookie dough, chocolate chocolate chip, chocolate with dinosaurs, coconut pecan, cream cheese, dark chocolate, french vanilla, lemon, milk chocolate, rainbow chip, sour cream chocolate, sour cream white, strawberry cream cheese, vanilla, vanilla with bears, vanilla with stars, and white chocolate.
67. Values are averages for chocolate, milk chocolate, and vanilla.

						Vitamins					Minerals				
KCAL	H₂O (g)	PRO (g)	CHO (g)	SUGR (g)	DFIB (g)	A (RE)	C (mg)	B-2 (mg)	B-6 (mg)	FOL (mcg)	Na (mg)	Ca (mg)	Mg (mg)	Zn (mg)	Mn (mg)
WT (g)	FAT (g)	SFA (g)	MUFA (g)	PUFA (g)	CHOL (mg)	A (IU)	B-1 (mg)	NIA (mg)	B-12 (mcg)	PANT (mg)	K (mg)	P (mg)	Fe (mg)	Cu (mg)	REF

9. EGGS, EGG DISHES, & EGG SUBSTITUTES

egg, chicken

	KCAL/WT	H₂O/FAT	PRO/SFA	CHO/MUFA	SUGR/PUFA	DFIB/CHOL	A/A	C/B-1	B-2/NIA	B-6/B-12	FOL/PANT	Na/K	Ca/P	Mg/Fe	Zn/Cu	Mn/REF
boiled, hard/soft	78	37.3	6.3	0.6		0.0	84	0	.26	.06	22	62	25	5	.53	.013
1 large	50	5.3	1.6	2.0	0.7	212	280	.03	0.0	.56	.70	63	86	.59	.006	801
fried	92	31.5	6.2	0.6		0.0	114	0	.24	.07	17	162	25	5	.55	.013
1 large	46	6.9	1.9	2.7	1.3	211	394	.03	0.0	.42	.56	61	89	.72	.007	801
omelet, plain	93	46.3	6.3	0.6		0.0	114	0	.24	.07	18	165	26	5	.56	.013
1 large egg	61	7.0	1.9	2.8	1.3	214	399	.03	0.0	.43	.57	62	90	.73	.008	801
poached	75	37.5	6.2	0.6		0.0	95	0	.21	.06	18	140	25	5	.55	.013
1 large	50	5.0	1.5	1.9	0.7	212	316	.02	0.0	.40	.56	60	89	.72	.007	801
scrambled w/ milk	101	44.6	6.8	1.3		0.0	119	0	.27	.07	18	171	43	7	.61	.013
1 large egg	61	7.4	2.2	2.9	1.3	215	416	.03	0.0	.47	.61	84	104	.73	.009	801
white, fresh/frzn	17	29.0	3.5	0.3		0.0	0	0	.15	.00	1	54	2	4	.00	.001
white of 1 large egg	33	0.0	0.0	0.0	0.0	0	0	.00	0.0	.07	.04	47	4	.01	.002	I
whole, dried, stabilized (glucose reduced)	31	0.1	2.4	0.1		0.0	31	0	.06	.02	10	27	11	2	.29	.007
1 T	5	2.2	0.7	0.9	0.3	101	103	.02	0.0	.53	.34	26	36	.41	.014	801
whole, fresh/frzn	75	37.7	6.2	0.6		0.0	96	0	.25	.07	24	63	25	5	.55	.012
1 large	50	5.0	1.6	1.9	0.7	213	318	.03	0.0	.50	.63	61	89	.72	.007	I
yolk, fresh	61	8.3	2.8	0.3		0.0	99	0	.11	.07	25	7	23	2	.53	.012
yolk of 1 large egg	17	5.2	1.6	2.0	0.7	218	331	.03	0.0	.53	.65	16	83	.60	.004	I

egg, chicken dishes

	KCAL/WT	H₂O/FAT	PRO/SFA	CHO/MUFA	SUGR/PUFA	DFIB/CHOL	A/A	C/B-1	B-2/NIA	B-6/B-12	FOL/PANT	Na/K	Ca/P	Mg/Fe	Zn/Cu	Mn/REF
corn pudding, frzn, Stouffers	153	82.5	4.7	18.1				3	.19			463	45			
4 oz	113	6.8				47	102	.10	1.0			203		.57	.	I
quiche, bacon & onion, Pour-a-Quiche	230		13.0	6.0								385				
4.3 oz	123	18.0				240						170				I
quiche, ham, Pour-a-Quiche	230		13.0	4.0								360				
4.3 oz	123	17.0				235						165				I
quiche, spinach & onion, Pour-a-Quiche	220		12.0	6.0								365				
4.3 oz	123	16.0				230						210				I
quiche, three cheeses, Pour-a-Quiche	236		12.9	4.2				1	.30			326	289			
4.3 oz	123	18.7				250	696	.06	0.1			154	253	.96		I
souffle, broccoli & cheese, frzn, Stouffers	151	84.8	8.4	7.7				9	.31			509	130			
4 oz[1]	113	9.6				141	328	.08	0.5			158		.90		I

	KCAL	H₂O (g)	PRO (g)	CHO (g)	SUGR (g)	DFIB (g)	A (RE)	C (mg)	B-2 (mg)	B-6 (mg)	FOL (mcg)	Na (mg)	Ca (mg)	Mg (mg)	Zn (mg)	Mn (mg)
	WT (g)	FAT (g)	SFA (g)	MUFA (g)	PUFA (g)	CHOL (mg)	A (IU)	B-1 (mg)	NIA (mg)	B-12 (mcg)	PANT (mg)	K (mg)	P (mg)	Fe (mg)	Cu (mg)	REF
souffle, cheese	207	61.8	9.4	5.9				0	.23			346	191			
1 cup	95	16.2	8.2				760	.05	0.2			115	185	1.00		456
souffle, spinach	219	100.6	11.0	2.8				3	.30	.12	62	763	230	38	1.29	1.098
1 cup[2]	136	18.4	7.1	6.8	3.1	184	3461	.09	0.5	1.36	.88	201	231	1.35	.120	811
souffle, spinach, frzn, Stouffers	151	84.8	8.4	7.7				9	.31			509	130			
4 oz	113	9.6				141	328	.08	0.5			158		.90		I
egg, other poultry																
duck, whole	130	49.6	9.0	1.0		0.0	279	0	.28	.17	56	102	45	12	.99	.027
1 egg	70	9.6	2.6	4.6	0.9	619	930	.11	0.1	3.78	1.30	156	154	2.69	.043	801
goose, whole	267	101.4	20.0	1.9		0.0	553	0	.55	.34	109	199	87	22	1.92	.055
1 egg	144	19.1	5.2	8.3	2.4	1227	1843	.21	0.3	7.34	2.53	302	299	5.24	.089	801
quail, whole	14	6.7	1.2	0.0		0.0	8	0	.07	.01	6	13	6	1	.13	.003
1 egg	9	1.0	0.3	0.4	0.1	76	27	.01	0.0	.14	.16	12	20	.33	.006	801
turkey, whole	135	57.3	10.8	0.9		0.0	131	0	.37	.10	56	120	78	11	1.25	.030
1 egg	79	9.4	2.9	3.6	1.3	737	438	.09	0.0	1.34	1.49	112	134	3.24	.049	801
egg substitutes																
Better 'n Egg, frzn, Morningstar Farms	23	50.3	5.0	0.2	0.2	0.0	640	0	.26	.11	30	90	7		.51	
¼ cup	57	0.3	0.1	0.1	0.1	2		.01	0.0	.60	.80	68	29	.63		I
Country Morning, Land O'Lakes	173		14.6	1.3				0	.52			180	52			
½ cup	121	12.1				594	1138	.06				133	197	2.07		I
Egg Beaters, frzn/refrig, Fleischmann's	30		6.0	1.0	0.0							100				
¼ cup	60	0.0	0.0	0.0	0.0	0										I
Eggstrodnaire	30		5.0					.23	.02	7	75	15	6	.17		
1.5	43	1.0				40	45	.01	0.1	.22	.21	75	31	.23	.005	I
Eggstrodnaire	74		9.6	3.1					.44			128	27	9		
3 oz	85	2.5				98	94		0.4	.23	.16	138	46	.55		I
Eggstrodnaire	102		12.9	4.2				0	.50	.02		360	37	12	.16	
3.5 oz	99	3.5				105	144	.01	0.1	.29	.20	172	133	7.33	.180	I
frzn	96	43.9	6.8	1.9		0.0	81	0	.23	.08	10	120	44	9	.59	.004
¼ cup[3]	60	6.7	1.2	1.5	3.7	1	810	.07	0.1	.20	1.00	128	43	1.19	.013	801
liquid	40	38.9	5.6	0.3		0.0	102	0	.14	.00	7	83	25	4	.61	.003
1.5 fl oz[4]	47	1.6	0.3	0.4	0.8	0	1015	.05	0.1	.14	1.27	155	57	.99	.011	801
powdered	44	0.4	5.6	2.2		0.0	37	0	.18	.01	13	80	33	6	.18	.008
0.35 oz[5]	10	1.3	0.4	0.5	0.2	57	123	.02	0.1	.35	.34	74	48	.32	.021	801
Scramblend, Land O'Lakes	143		12.1	3.0				0	.38			173	77			
½ cup	121	9.1				466	1071	.06				150	190	1.67		I
Scramblers, Morningstar	37	47.5	6.2	2.2	1.3	0.3		0	.39	.13		97	31		.80	
¼ cup	57	0.4				2	311	.29	0.0	1.77	1.85	50	60	1.07		I

1. Contains whole eggs, broccoli, cream sauce, Swiss cheese, onions, and lemon juice topped with parmesan bread crumbs.
2. Contains whole milk, spinach, egg white, cheddar cheese, egg yolk, butter, flour, salt, and pepper.
3. Contains egg whites, corn oil, and nonfat dry milk.
4. Contains egg white, hydrogenated soybean oil, and soy protein.
5. Contains egg white solids, whole egg solids, sweet whey solids, nonfat dry milk, and soy protein.

10. ENTREES & MEALS
10.1 BOX MIX ENTREES

	KCAL	H₂O (g)	PRO (g)	CHO (g)	SUGR (g)	DFIB (g)	A (RE)	C (mg)	B-2 (mg)	B-6 (mg)	FOL (mcg)	Na (mg)	Ca (mg)	Mg (mg)	Zn (mg)	Mn (mg)
angel hair pasta																
w/ herb sce, dry mix, Pasta Roni	203	5.5	6.8	38.8	3.5	1.7		1	.20	.07	9	707	47	26	.73	
2 oz	56	2.7	0.7	1.5	0.4	0	562	.39	2.6	.19	.29	134	117	1.48	.170	I
w/ lemon & butter, dry mix, Pasta Roni	253	6.9	8.7	48.3	4.7	2.2		1	.25	.09	12	842	65	33	.93	
2.5 oz	70	3.3	0.9	1.8	0.6	1	551	.50	3.3	.29	.38	196	162	1.87	.210	I
w/ parmesan cheese, dry mix, Pasta Roni	212	5.3	7.0	36.7	4.1	1.6		1	.21	.07	9	756	59	26	.72	
2 oz	56	4.5	1.1	2.8	0.4	1	172	.39	2.5	.07	.33	147	121	1.40	.160	I
beans, cajun & sce, Lipton	260		10.0	53.0	1.0	6.0		1	.07		100	460	20			
½ cup	72	1.5	0.0			0	400	.52	3.0					3.60		I

	KCAL / WT (g)	H₂O (g) / FAT (g)	PRO (g) / SFA (g)	CHO (g) / MUFA (g)	SUGR (g) / PUFA (g)	DFIB (g) / CHOL (mg)	A (RE) / A (IU)	C (mg) / B-1 (mg)	B-2 (mg) / NIA (mg)	B-6 (mg) / B-12 (mcg)	FOL (mcg) / PANT (mg)	Na (mg) / K (mg)	Ca (mg) / P (mg)	Mg (mg) / Fe (mg)	Zn (mg) / Cu (mg)	Mn (mg) / RFF
Chicken Helper, stir-fried chicken, prep,	270		18.0	30.0	1.0	1.0		0	.17			810	60			
Betty Crocker—1 cup	234	9.0	2.0			110	300	.12	5.0			210		.72		I
corkscrew pasta w/ 4 cheese sce, dry	268	6.7	9.2	45.0	5.0	2.1		0	.27	.09	11	773	89	33	.94	
mix, Pasta Roni—2.5 oz	70	6.1	1.9	3.4	0.6	4	32	.47	3.0	.10	.42	244	267	1.71	.210	I
corkscrew pasta w/ creamy garlic sce, dry	212	5.2	6.6	37.2	4.8	1.7		0	.22	.08	9	762	79	28	.78	
mix, Pasta Roni—2 oz	56	4.5	1.2	2.8	0.5	1	431	.37	2.4	.08	.38	169	165	1.39	.150	I
egg noodles w/ cheddar cheese, from	430		12.0	46.0	8.0	1.0		0	.43			780	150	40		
mix, Kraft—1 cup	229	21.0	6.0			70	1000	.30	2.0			310	350	2.70		I
egg noodles w/ chicken, from mix, Kraft	330		10.0	45.0	5.0	1.0		0	.26			1430	40	32		
1 cup	260	12.0	3.5			60	100	.30	2.0			180	150	2.70		I
fettuccini w/ alfredo sce, dry mix, Pasta	273	6.6	9.1	45.4	4.0	2.0		0	.24	.09	12	913	55	30	.88	
Roni—2.5 oz	70	6.6	1.9	3.9	0.6	2	285	.49	3.1	.07	.34	177	128	1.75	.230	I
Hamburger Helper prep w/ ground beef																
beef pasta, Betty Crocker	270		20.0	26.0	2.0	1.0	0	0	.26			910	40			
1 cup	191	10.0	4.0			50	0	.23	4.0			300		1.80		I
beef romanoff, Betty Crocker	290		20.0	28.0	4.0	1.0	0	0	.34			930	60			
1 cup	220	11.0	4.0			50	0	.30	4.0			340		1.80		I
beef stew, Betty Crocker	250		18.0	26.0	3.0	2.0		0	.14			750	20			
1 cup	184	10.0	3.5			50	500	.06	4.0			480		1.80		I
beef taco, Betty Crocker	310		20.0	30.0	3.0	1.0		0	.26			920	40			
1 cup	245	11.0	4.0			50	500	.30	4.0			350		2.70		I
beef teriyaki, Betty Crocker	290		18.0	34.0	5.0	2.0		0	.10			990	60			
1 cup	248	10.0	3.5			50	500	.15	5.0			300		2.70		I
cheddar 'n bacon, Betty Crocker	350		24.0	28.0	5.0	1.0		0	.34			890	100			
1 cup	220	16.0	6.0			65	100	.30	5.0			400		1.80		I
cheddar melt, Betty Crocker	310		20.0	31.0	4.0	1.0	0	0	.34			900	80			
1 cup	227	12.0	4.5			55	0	.30	4.0			330		1.80		I
cheddar primavera, Betty Crocker	320		21.0	27.0	5.0	1.0		0	.34			650	100			
1 cup	217	14.0	5.0			60	500	.23	4.0			720		1.80		I
cheeseburger macaroni, Betty Crocker	360		23.0	31.0	6.0	1.0	0	0	.17			1000	40			
1 cup	227	16.0	6.0			65	0	.23	2.0			440		.72		I
cheesy italian, Betty Crocker	330		22.0	29.0	6.0	1.0		0	.34			920	100			
1 cup	200	14.0				60	300	.30	5.0			400		2.70		I
cheesy shells, Betty Crocker	340		22.0	30.0	5.0	1.0		0	.34			850	100			
1 cup	241	14.0	5.0			60	100	.30	5.0			400				I
chili macaroni, Betty Crocker	290		19.0	30.0	4.0	1.0		0	.26			870	20			
1 cup	212	10.0	4.0			55	1000	.30	5.0			400		2.70		I
fettuccini alfredo, Betty Crocker	310		20.0	26.0	5.0	1.0	0	0	.34			850	80			
1 cup	205	13.0	5.0			55	0	.30	4.0			330		1.80		I
hamburger stew, Betty Crocker	250		19.0	22.0	3.0	3.0		0	.17			920	20			
1 cup	155	10.0	4.0			55	1000	.06	4.0			520		1.80		I
italian rigatoni, Betty Crocker	180		19.0	29.0	6.0	1.0		0	.26			870	20			
1 cup	212	10.0	4.0			50	300	.30	5.0			340		2.70		I
lasagna, Betty Crocker	280		19.0	30.0	7.0	0.0	0	0	.26			950	20			
1 cup	220	10.0	4.0			50	0	.23	5.0			350		2.70		I
meat loaf, Betty Crocker	280		25.0	11.0	3.0	0.0	0	0	.26			600	40			
⅙ loaf	85	15.0	6.0			110	0	.09	4.0			390		2.70		I
mushrooms & wild rice, Betty Crocker	310		20.0	30.0	4.0	2.0		0	.26			880	100			
1 cup	234	12.0	4.5			55	100	.23	5.0			400		2.70		I
nacho cheese, Betty Crocker	320		22.0	30.0	5.0	1.0	0	0	.34			930	100			
1 cup	212	13.0	5.0			55	0	.30	5.0			420		1.80		I
pizza pasta w/cheese topping, Betty	290		19.0	31.0	5.0	1.0		0	.26			700	40			
Crocker—1 cup	238	10.0	4.0			50	300	.30	4.0			390		1.80		I
pizzabake, Betty Crocker	270		17.0	28.0	4.0	1.0		0	.17			720	40			
⅙ pan of pizza	234	10.0	3.5			45	200	.15	4.0			320		2.70		I
potatoes au gratin, Betty Crocker	290		18.0	24.0	5.0	2.0		0	.17			820	60			
1 cup	184	14.0	5.0			55	100	.06	4.0			500		1.80		I
red sodium, italian herb, Betty Crocker	270		19.0	29.0	6.0	2.0		0	.26			650	20			
1 cup	218	10.0	3.5			50	500	.30	5.0			570				I
red sodium, southwestern beef, Betty	300		21.0	32.0	6.0	2.0		0	.26			650	20			
Crocker—1 cup	228	10.0	4.0			50	500	.30	5.0			610		2.70		I

	KCAL / WT (g)	H₂O (g) / FAT (g)	PRO (g) / SFA (g)	CHO (g) / MUFA (g)	SUGR (g) / PUFA (g)	DFIB (g) / CHOL (mg)	A (RE) / A (IU)	C (mg) / B-1 (mg)	B-2 (mg) / NIA (mg)	B-6 (mg) / B-12 (mcg)	FOL (mcg) / PANT (mg)	Na (mg) / K (mg)	Ca (mg) / P (mg)	Mg (mg) / Fe (mg)	Zn (mg) / Cu (mg)	Mn (mg) / REF
rice oriental, Betty Crocker	310		19.0	35.0	4.0	0.0	0	0	.14			1050	0			
1 cup	227	10.0	4.0			55	0	.15	4.0			300		1.80		I
salisbury, Betty Crocker	270		19.0	26.0	2.0	1.0		0	.26			790	40			
1 cup	205	10.0	4.0			50	300	.23	4.0			290		1.80		I
spaghetti, Betty Crocker	300		21.0	29.0	6.0	1.0		0	.26			940	20			
1 cup	212	11.0	4.0			55	500	.38	5.0			430		2.70		I
stroganoff, Betty Crocker	320		21.0	30.0	7.0	0.0		0	.34			830	100			
1 cup	227	13.0	5.0			55	100	.23	5.0			370		2.70		I
swedish meatball, Betty Crocker	300		19.0	24.0	2.0	1.0		0	.26			780	20			
1 cup	203	14.0	5.0			55	400	.23	4.0			320		1.80		I
three cheese, Betty Crocker	340		21.0	32.0	5.0	1.0		0	.34			830	80			
1 cup	241	15.0	5.0			55	100	.30	5.0			350		1.80		I
zesty italian, Betty Crocker	320		21.0	34.0	8.0	1.0		0	.34			890	20			
1 cup	234	11.0	4.0			55	300	.38	6.0			470		2.70		I
zesty mexican, Betty Crocker	300		19.0	32.0	5.0	1.0		0	.26			730	60			
1 cup	235	11.0	4.0			50	750	.23	4.0			400		2.70		I
lasagna w/ tomato & garden veg, dry,	146	4.0	5.4	30.6	4.3	2.1		16	.17	.09	12	314	23	24	.57	
mix, Pasta Roni—*1.5 oz*	42	0.7	0.2	0.1	0.4	0	598	.31	2.3	.00	.32	18	74	1.42	.190	I
linguine w/ chicken & broccoli sce, dry,	251	6.8	10.1	47.6	2.5	3.2		2	.27	.13	24	780	38	39	.91	
mix, Pasta Roni—*2.5 oz*	70	3.1	0.7	1.8	0.4	0	78	.49	3.5	.00	.37	296	106	2.11	.220	I
linguine w/ creamy chicken parmesan	258	6.7	9.9	45.9	2.5	2.8		0	.25	.11	12	906	24	29	.78	
sce, dry, mix, Pasta Roni—*2.5 oz*	70	4.7	1.2	2.4	0.8	2	4	.48	3.6	.01	.36	328	109	1.89	.210	I
macaroni & cheese																
dry mix, Golden Grain	200	5.4	7.4	39.4	6.1	1.7		0	.29	.06	9	498	49	32	.74	
2 oz	56	1.9	0.6	0.7	0.5	3	9	.41	2.6	.13	.20	210	166	1.43	.160	I
from mix, Kraft Deluxe Original	320		14.0	44.0	4.0	1.0		0	.26			730	200	40		
1 cup	175	10.0	6.0			25	500	.30	2.0			190	450	2.70		I
from mix, Kraft Original	390		11.0	48.0	8.0	1.0		0	.43			730	100	40		
1 cup[1]	196	17.0	4.0			10	750	.38	2.0			290	250	2.70		I
from mix, Kraft Thick 'n Creamy	320		12.0	50.0	9.0	2.0		0	.43			730	150	40		
1 cup	175	10.0	6.0			25	750	.38	3.0			190	300	2.70		I
Manwich, dry mix	22		0.2	5.3	0.0	0.3	12	0				355	8			
.25 oz	7	0.1	0.0			0								.14		I
noodles																
chicken & broccoli w/ sce, Lipton	230		9.0	41.0	1.0	2.0		9	.34		100	740	20			
⅔ cup	59	1.5				65	100	.60	4.0					2.70		I
w/ alfredo broccoli sce, Lipton	260		10.0	39.0	2.0	2.0		2				880	80			
⅔ cup	63	7.0	4.0			75	100							2.70		I
w/ alfredo sce, Lipton	250		10.0	39.0	2.0	2.0		0	.25		100	940	80			
⅔ cup	62	7.0	4.0			75	100	.60	4.0					2.70		I
w/ beef sce, Lipton	230		8.0	43.0	2.0	2.0		0	.25			840				
⅔ cup	60	3.5				60	200	.60	4.0					2.70		I
w/ butter & herb sce, Lipton	250		9.0	41.0	4.0	2.0		0	.59		100	710	20			
⅔ cup	62	7.0	3.5			65	0	.60	4.0					2.70		I
w/ butter sce, Lipton	260		9.0	41.0	4.0	2.0			.25		100	810	20			
⅔ cup	63	8.0	4.5				200	.60	4.0					2.70		I
w/ chicken flavor sce, Lipton	240		8.0	42.0	2.0	2.0		1	.34		100	760				
⅔ cup	60	4.5	2.0			65	300	.67	5.0					2.70		I
w/ chicken tetrazzini sce, Lipton	220		8.0	38.0	1.0	2.0						850				
⅔ cup	56	4.5	2.0			65	100							2.70		I
w/ creamy chicken sce, Lipton	240		9.0	39.0	2.0	2.0		1	.25		100	710				
⅔ cup	59	6.0	3.0			70	1000	.60	4.0					2.70		I
w/ parmesan sce, Lipton	250		10.0	37.0	2.0	2.0		1	.25		100	750	60			
⅔ cup	60	8.0	4.0			70	0	.60	4.0					1.80		I
w/ sour cream & chive sce, Lipton	260		8.0	41.0	4.0	2.0			.25		100	800	20			
⅔ cup	63	8.0	4.0			70	100	.60	4.0					1.80		I
w/ stroganoff sce, Lipton	220		9.0	37.0	2.0	2.0		0	.34		100	850				
⅔ cup	56	4.0	2.0			65	100	.60	4.0					2.70		I

	KCAL	H_2O (g)	PRO (g)	CHO (g)	SUGR (g)	DFIB (g)	Vitamins A (RE)	C (mg)	B-2 (mg)	B-6 (mg)	FOL (mcg)	Minerals Na (mg)	Ca (mg)	Mg (mg)	Zn (mg)	Mn (mg)
	WT (g)	FAT (g)	SFA (g)	MUFA (g)	PUFA (g)	CHOL (mg)	A (IU)	B-1 (mg)	NIA (mg)	B-12 (mcg)	PANT (mg)	K (mg)	P (mg)	Fe (mg)	Cu (mg)	REF
Pasta & Sce																
alfredo broccoli, Lipton	250		7.0	43.0	1.0	1.0		6	.10		100	890	60			
½ cup	62	5.0	3.0			10	100	.60	4.0					2.70		I
cheddar broccoli, Lipton	260		9.0	46.0	3.0	1.0		4	.25		120	870	80			
⅔ cup	68	3.5	1.5			10	200	.75	5.0					2.70		I
cheddar cheese, Lipton	210		8.0	38.0	1.0	1.0			.17		100	830	60			
¾ cup	59	3.0	1.5			5	100	.67	4.0					1.80		I
chicken herb parmesan, Lipton	230		8.0	43.0	3.0	2.0			.25		100	840	40			
½ cup	62	2.5	1.0			5	200	.67	4.0					1.80		I
chicken primavera w/ bow ties, Lipton	230		8.0	37.0	2.0	2.0			.17		100	790	60			
¾ cup	58	5.0	2.5			10	100	.60	3.0					1.80		I
chicken stir fry, Lipton	220		8.0	43.0	3.0	2.0		1			100	830	20			
½ cup	62	1.5	0.0			0	400	.67						1.80		I
garlic & butter, Lipton	210		7.0	40.0	3.0	2.0			.17		100	780	20			
⅓ cup	58	3.0	1.0			5	100	.60	3.0					1.80		I
herb & garlic, Lipton	230		8.0	42.0	3.0	2.0			.25		100	820	20			
½ cup	61	3.0	1.5			5	100	.67	4.0					1.80		I
italian cheese w/ bow ties, Lipton	230		8.0	37.0	2.0	2.0			.17		100	790	60			
¾ cup	58	5.0	2.5			10	100	.60	3.0					1.80		I
rotini primavera, Lipton	240		8.0	42.0	1.0	2.0		2	.25		100	880				
¾ cup	63	5.0	3.0			10	500	.67	4.0				40	1.80		I
three cheese rotini, Lipton	240		9.0	41.0	2.0	1.0		0	.25		100	870	60			
¾ cup	63	5.0	3.0			10	0	.67	4.0					1.80		I
pasta, broccoli au gratin, dry mix, Pasta	205	5.3	7.3	37.2	3.9	2.0		2	.24	.10	18	780	84	36	.78	
Roni—*2 oz*	56	3.5	1.0	1.9	0.4	1	80	.39	2.6	.07	.37	237	146	1.56	.170	I
pasta, chicken, dry mix, Pasta Roni	203	4.7	8.4	37.7	2.1	1.9		0	.19	.07	10	883	15	31	.71	
2 oz	56	2.6	0.6	0.5	0.6	1	11	.38	2.8	.00	.24	253	107	1.51	.170	I
pasta, mild cheddar, dry mix, Pasta Roni	207	5.3	7.1	37.3	4.2	1.6		0	.22	.08	9	803	73	28	.79	
2 oz	56	3.6	1.1	2.0	0.4	1	28	.39	2.5	.08	.35	220	148	1.41	.160	I
pasta, oriental stir fry, dry mix, Pasta	195	5.6	6.9	38.4	3.5	2.0		1	.18	.08	12	891	20	28	.79	
Roni—*2 oz*	56	2.0	0.3	0.8	0.9	0	179	.36	2.5	.00	.23	176	91	1.59	.160	I
pasta, parmesano, dry mix, Pasta Roni	256	6.9	9.7	46.2	3.6	2.2		1	.26	.08	13	780	75	42	.93	
2.5 oz	70	4.2	1.2	2.1	0.8	2	266	.52	3.2	.09	.35	212	173	1.82	.230	I
pasta, romanoff, dry mix, Pasta Roni	273	6.4	9.0	44.6	5.9	1.9		0	.26	.08	12	910	48	32	.95	
2.5 oz	70	6.9	2.2	3.4	0.5	5	53	.43	2.9	.14	.31	244	171	1.61	.200	I
pasta salad																
caesar, from mix, Suddenly Salad, Betty	220		5.0	30.0	4.0	1.0	0	0	.17			580	20			
Crocker—*¾ cup*	206	9.0	1.5			0	0	.30	2.0			130		1.44		I
classic, from mix, Suddenly Salad, Betty	220		5.0	34.0	3.0	1.0	0	0	.17			830	0			
Crocker—*¾ cup*	220	7.0	1.0			0	0	.30	2.0			150		1.44		I
classic ranch w/ bacon, from mix, Kraft	360		7.0	30.0	3.0	2.0		0	.26			500	20	32		
¾ cup	135	23.0	4.0			15	300	.60	3.0			170	100	1.80		I
creamy caesar, from mix, Kraft	350		7.0	30.0	5.0	2.0		1	.10			650	60	40		
¾ cup	137	22.0	4.0			15	100	.15	1.6			310	150	1.80		I
garden italian, from mix, Suddenly Salad,	140		5.0	29.0	4.0	2.0		0	.17			540	20			
Betty Crocker—*¾ cup*	191	1.0	0.0			0	750	.38	2.0			130		1.44		I
garden primavera, from mix, Kraft	280		8.0	34.0	4.0	2.0		1	.17			730	80	32		
¾ cup	142	12.0	2.5			5	200	.15	2.0			200	150	1.80		I
light italian, from mix, Kraft	190		8.0	34.0	5.0	2.0		1	.17			660	80	32		
¾ cup	142	2.0	1.0			5	200	.15	2.0			220	150	1.80		I
parmesan peppercorn, from mix, Kraft	360		8.0	28.0	3.0	2.0		0	.14			610	80	24		
¾ cup	140	25.0	4.5			20	300	.15	1.6			150	150	1.80		I
ranch & bacon, from mix, Suddenly	320		7.0	31.0	3.0	1.0		0	.17			490	20			
Salad, Betty Crocker—*¾ cup*	212	19.0	3.0			15	750	.38	2.0			210		1.44		I
pasta shapes & cheese, from mix, Kraft	390		12.0	48.0	8.0	1.0		0	.43			770	150	40		
1 cup[2]	193	17.0	4.5			10	750	.38	2.0			310	300	2.70		I
pasta, stroganoff, dry mix, Pasta Roni	272	6.5	9.0	44.4	4.6	2.0		0	.27	.09	12	913	72	32	.92	
2.5 oz	70	6.9	1.6	2.8	0.5	2	44	.46	3.1	.10	.47	193	153	1.73	.210	I
pasta w/ broccoli & mushrooms, dry	258	6.7	8.7	46.8	4.0	2.4		1	.28	.11	19	884	71	49	.94	
mix, Pasta Roni—*2.5 oz*	70	4.7	1.2	2.9	0.7	0	153	.49	3.4	.06	.47	226	183	1.94	.241	I

	KCAL	H₂O (g)	PRO (g)	CHO (g)	SUGR (g)	DFIB (g)	A (RE)	C (mg)	B-2 (mg)	B-6 (mg)	FOL (mcg)	Na (mg)	Ca (mg)	Mg (mg)	Zn (mg)	Mn (mg)
	WT (g)	FAT (g)	SFA (g)	MUFA (g)	PUFA (g)	CHOL (mg)	A (IU)	B-1 (mg)	NIA (mg)	B-12 (mcg)	PANT (mg)	K (mg)	P (mg)	Fe (mg)	Cu (mg)	REF
pasta w/ broccoli, dry mix, Pasta Roni	202	6.6	7.3	36.3	6.0	1.7		12	.18	.07	10	751	32	27	.72	
2 oz	56	3.4	0.7	1.5	0.5	1	198	.39	2.5	.03	.25	182	159	1.50	.160	I
pasta w/ creamy garlic sce, Lipton	270		8.0	47.0	2.0			0	.34		100	880				
⅔ cup	69	6.0	3.0			10	200	.75	5.0					2.70		I
penne pasta, w/ herb & butter sce, dry mix, Pasta Roni—2 oz	199	6.6	6.7	37.9	3.1	1.7	1	.20	.10	11	630	46	23	.66		
	56	2.8	0.7	1.4	0.7	1	544	.40	2.7	.18	.29	138	130	1.49	.200	I
pizza mix, reg/thin crust, Appian Way	250		7.0	48.0	4.0	2.0		0				740	40			
⅓ pizza	118	3.0	1.0			0	100							1.80		I
pizza mix, thick crust, Appian Way	290		10.0	51.0	4.0	2.0		0				830	100			
⅕ pizza	119	5.0	2.0			10	100							2.70		I
potato stroganoff, Betty Crocker	270		18.0	25.0	2.0	2.0	0	0	.17			870	60			
1 cup	177	12.0	4.5			55	0	.06	4.0			510		1.80		I
rigatoni w/ tomato basil sce, dry mix, Pasta Roni—1.5 oz	149	4.2	5.2	30.3	2.9	1.5	2	.14	.05	9	286	17	20	.52		
	42	1.2	0.2	0.2	0.4	0	194	.31	2.1	.00	.19	108	66	1.25	.150	I
rigatoni w/ white cheddar & broccoli sce, dry mix, Pasta Roni—2 oz	214	5.2	7.5	36.0	4.4	2.0	2	.24	.10	18	672	82	35	.79		
	56	4.9	1.6	2.3	0.7	4	103	.36	2.4	.10	.39	192	237	1.50	.170	I
rotini & cheese, broccoli, from mix, Kraft Velvetta—1 cup	400		18.0	46.0	3.0	2.0		2	.26			1240	300	60		
	205	16.0	10.0			45	750	.38	2.0			270	700	1.20		I
shells & cheese																
bacon, from mix, Kraft Velvetta	360		17.0	43.0	4.0	1.0		0	.26			1140	250	40		
1 cup	195	14.0	8.0			40	500	.30	2.0			230	600	2.70		I
from mix, Kraft Velveeta	360		16.0	44.0	4.0	1.0		0	.26			1030	250	40		
1 cup	188	13.0	8.0			40	500	.30	2.0			210	600	2.70		I
salsa, from mix, Kraft Velveeta	380		17.0	47.0	5.0	2.0		0	.26			1180	250	60		
1 cup	214	14.0	9.0			40	750	.38	2.0			300	600	1.20		I
shells w/ white cheddar, dry mix, Pasta Roni—2.5 oz	270	6.4	9.3	45.0	6.1	2.0		0	.29	.10	12	892	98	34	1.03	
	70	6.3	2.3	3.1	0.8	7	60	.44	2.9	.15	.48	222	320	1.67	.200	I
spaghetti, mild american, from mix, Kraft	270		9.0	48.0	5.0	3.0		9	.17			690	40	40		
1 cup	230	4.5	1.0			5	750	.30	3.0			410	150	2.70		I
spaghetti, tangy italian, from mix, Kraft	270		10.0	46.0	4.0	3.0		9	.26			780	80	32		
1 cup	226	4.5	1.0			5	750	.53	4.0			410	150	2.70		I
spaghetti w/ meat sce, from mix, Kraft	330		12.0	46.0	8.0	3.0		1	.26			830	100	60		
1 cup	235	11.0	4.0			15	500	.60	5.0			410	150	3.60		I
Tuna Helper, prep w/ cnd tuna																
au gratin, Betty Crocker	310		14.0	36.0	5.0	1.0		0	.26			930	100			
1 cup	262	12.0	3.0			20	400	.30	5.0			270		1.44		I
cheesy pasta, Betty Crocker	280		14.0	32.0	5.0	1.0		0	.26			890	100			
1 cup	220	11.0	3.0			20	400	.30	5.0			270		1.44		I
creamy broccoli, Betty Crocker	310		14.0	35.0	6.0	1.0		0	.26			880	80			
1 cup	255	12.0	3.0			20	400	.30	5.0			290		1.44		I
creamy pasta, Betty Crocker	300		14.0	31.0	4.0	1.0		0	.26			910	80			
1 cup	234	13.0	3.5			20	500	.30	5.0			290		1.44		I
fettuccine alfredo, Betty Crocker	310		14.0	32.0	6.0	1.0		0	.26			950	80			
1 cup	227	14.0	3.5			15	400	.30	5.0			260		1.44		I
garden cheddar, Betty Crocker	310		16.0	35.0	5.0	1.0		0	.26			1040	100			
1 cup	262	12.0	3.0			20	500	.30	5.0			290		1.44		I
pasta salad, Betty Crocker	380		10.0	26.0	4.0	1.0		0	.14			730	20			
¾ cup	234	27.0	3.0			10	100	.23	4.0			160		1.44		I
tetrazzini, Betty Crocker	310		17.0	33.0	3.0	1.0		0	.26			1010	60			
1 cup	198	12.0	2.0			20	400	.38	6.0			250		1.80		I
tuna pot pie, Betty Crocker	440		18.0	40.0	9.0	1.0		0	.34			1080	150			
1 cup	333	24.0	7.0			110	1250	.23	5.0			390		1.80		I
tuna romanoff, Betty Crocker	280		15.0	38.0	3.0	1.0		0	.26			800	40			
1 cup	262	8.0	1.5			20	200	.30	6.0			270		1.44		I
vermicelli w/ garlic & olive oil, dry mix, Pasta Roni—2.5 oz	254	7.0	8.8	47.7	2.5	2.2	1	.21	.08	12	876	16	29	.80		
	70	3.7	0.6	0.9	0.6	0	206	.49	3.3	.00	.27	137	107	1.83	.210	I

10.2 CANNED & SHELF STABLE ENTREES

	KCAL	H₂O (g)	PRO (g)	CHO (g)	SUGR (g)	DFIB (g)	A (RE)	C (mg)	B-2 (mg)	B-6 (mg)	FOL (mcg)	Na (mg)	Ca (mg)	Mg (mg)	Zn (mg)	Mn (mg)
beef & veg stew	194	202.1	14.2	17.4				7	.12			1007	29			
1 cup	245	7.6					2380	.07	2.5			426	110	2.20		456

	KCAL	H₂O (g)	PRO (g)	CHO (g)	SUGR (g)	DFIB (g)	A (RE)	C (mg)	B-2 (mg)	B-6 (mg)	FOL (mcg)	Na (mg)	Ca (mg)	Mg (mg)	Zn (mg)	Mn (mg)
	WT (g)	FAT (g)	SFA (g)	MUFA (g)	PUFA (g)	CHOL (mg)	A (IU)	B-1 (mg)	NIA (mg)	B-12 (mcg)	PAN (mg)	K (mg)	P (mg)	Fe (mg)	Cu (mg)	REF
beef & veg stew, Armour Star	220		8.0	21.0	0.0	2.0		0				1250	20			
1 cup	244	12.0	5.0			30	400							1.08		I
beef chow mein, LaChoy Bi-Pack	78		8.4	10.9	3.0	3.0	11	14				718	32			
1 cup	246	0.8	0.4			6								4.12		I
beef oriental w/ noodles, LaChoy Bi-Pack	156		17.5	17.5	1.6	3.9	25	25				896	29			
1 cup	250	2.7	1.2			17								2.05		I
beef pepper oriental, LaChoy Bi-Pack	98		9.8	13.1	0.0	2.5	25	20				865	26			
1 cup	252	1.6	0.7			14								.63		I
beef stew, Hunt Homestyle	155		14.1	19.6	5.5	5.0	124	21				1140	33			
1 cup	248	4.4	1.9			21								1.26		I
beef stew, Lunch Bucket	170		6.0	17.0	0.0	2.0		0				810	20			
7.5 oz container	213	9.0	4.0			25	500							.72		I
chicken a la king, Swanson Main Dish	320		15.0	17.0	2.0	0.0	0	0				1080	80			
1 cup	245	22.0	8.0			60	0							1.08		I
chicken & dumplings, Swanson Main Dish—1 cup	260		11.0	22.0	1.0	0.0		0				1120	40			
	247	14.0	5.0			65	400							1.08		I
chicken & mushrooms, Hunt Homestyle	199		9.7	31.8	3.1	3.7	17	27				908	31			
1 cup	247	4.3	1.9			25								1.01		I
chicken fiesta, Lunch Bucket	160		13.0	30.0	6.0	5.0		0				530	20			
7.5 oz container	213	2.0	0.5			5	200							1.80		I
chicken, oriental w/ noodles, LaChoy Bi-Pack—1 cup	154		13.6	17.6	2.8	2.5	47	21				1100	20			
	247	3.8	1.4			23								1.16		I
chicken stew, Swanson Main Dish	180		11.0	17.0	2.0	2.0		2				1110	40			
1 cup	245	8.0	3.0			35	3500							1.08		I
chicken teriyaki, LaChoy Bi-Pack	109		7.8	15.0	5.2	2.9	23	15				1230	27			
1 cup	244	3.0	1.2			20								.72		I
chili w/ beans	286	192.6	14.6	30.4		11.2	87	4	.27	.34	58	1331	120	115	5.10	.342
1 cup	255	14.0	6.0	5.9	0.9	43	859	.12	0.9	.00	3.62	931	393	8.75	.298	816
Gebhardt	322		15.4	31.7	0.1	14.5	101	0				673				
1 cup	168	14.9	5.7			29										I
Just Rite	379		17.6	30.6	0.0	13.0		4				51	101			
1 cup	257	26.5	12.5			35								1.21		I
Libby's	420		16.0	29.0	1.0	4.0		0				1210	60			
1 cup	255	27.0	13.0			50	750							3.60		I
Longhorn	215		6.6	19.0	2.3	5.2	45	5				630	54			
½ cup	126	14.5	6.4			25								.57		I
Lunch Bucket	260		12.0	25.0	1.0	8.0		6				1040	60			
7.5 oz container	213	12.0	5.0			25	750							1.80		I
reg/hot, Armour Star	370		13.0	33.0	2.0	10.0		0				1220	80			
1 cup	247	21.0	9.0			50	750							3.60		I
reg/hot, Ultimate	320		18.0	25.0	4.0	9.0		0				920	80			
1 cup	247	16.0	7.0			50	2000							2.70		I
Ryans	281		17.1	25.3	7.2	10.3		9				1291	111			
1 cup	257	16.0	7.3			26	51							2.41		I
western style, Armour Star	370		14.0	29.0	4.0	9.0		0				1130	60			
1 cup	252	22.0	10.0			60	500							2.70		I
chili w/o beans																
Armour Star	390		14.0	18.0	0.0	0.0		0				1200	40			
1 cup	249	29.0	13.0			70	1250							1.80		I
Gebhardt	232		7.3	11.1	0.0	3.2	66	6				737	36			
½ cup	123	18.6	7.6			42								1.23		I
hot, Ultimate	420		20.0	18.0	4.0	5.0		0				1420	60			
1 cup	249	30.0	13.0			85	1750							2.70		I
Libby's	480		21.0	16.0	2.0	1.0		0				1580	80			
1 cup	253	37.0	17.0			75	1250							3.60		I
Open Range	353		17.5	18.8	6.3	5.6	100	12				1216	63			
1 cup	251	25.6	11.5			48								.53		I
chow mein																
chicken, LaChoy	80		7.9	5.7	2.5	2.9	21	1				1325	87			
1 cup	265	3.5	1.0			9								.71		I

	KCAL	H₂O (g)	PRO (g)	CHO (g)	SUGR (g)	DFIB (g)	A (RE)	C (mg)	B-2 (mg)	B-6 (mg)	FOL (mcg)	Na (mg)	Ca (mg)	Mg (mg)	Zn (mg)	Mn (mg)
	WT (g)	FAT (g)	SFA (g)	MUFA (g)	PUFA (g)	CHOL (mg)	A (IU)	B-1 (mg)	NIA (mg)	B-12 (mcg)	PANT (mg)	K (mg)	P (mg)	Fe (mg)	Cu (mg)	REF
chicken, LaChoy Bi-Pack	98		8.0	10.7	2.3	2.5	10	13				1123	24			
1 cup	250	3.1	0.9			6								1.20		I
shrimp, LaChoy Bi-Pack	52		3.7	9.1	0.0	3.0	14	19				965	30			
1 cup	246	0.7	0.3			4								1.07		I
Circuso's w/ meatballs, Franco-American	205		9.2	25.1				4	.18			944	29			
7.4 oz	209	7.5					520	.18	3.1			316		2.20		I
Circuso's w/ tomato & cheese sce,	166		5.2	32.7				0	.16			883	29			
Franco-American—7.5 oz	213	1.6					696	.23	2.5			233		1.60		I
corned beef & bacon hash w/ onions,	440		19.0	23.0	1.0	2.0		0				990	20			
Armour Star—1 cup	236	30.0	14.0			100	100							1.80		I
corned beef hash																
Armour Star	440		19.0	23.0	1.0	2.0		0				840	20			
1 cup	236	30.0	14.0			100	100							1.80		I
Libby's	470		21.0	25.0	1.0	8.0	0	0				1200	20			
1 cup	252	35.0	16.0			90	0							1.80		I
w/ peppers & onions, Armour Star	440		19.0	23.0	2.0	3.0		0				1220	20			
1 cup	236	30.0	14.0			100	100							1.80		I
cowpeas w/ pork	199	186.2	6.6	39.7		7.9	0	0	.12	.11	122	840	41	103	2.50	.941
1 cup	240	3.8	1.5	1.6	0.5	17	0	.15	1.0	.00	.46	427	230	3.41	.408	816
dumplings 'n chicken, Lunch Bucket	140		5.0	21.0	2.0	1.0	0	0				780	20			
7.5 oz container	213	5.0	1.5			10	0							1.08		I
enchiladas, Gebhardt	258		4.5	20.4	0.0	3.3	40	2				687	28			
2 enchiladas	162	19.1	8.9			25								.92		I
lasagna, Lunch Bucket	160		5.0	29.0	9.0	2.0		0				850	20			
7.5 oz container	213	3.0	1.5			5	300							1.44		I
macaroni 'n beef, Lunch Bucket	180		6.0	29.0	8.0	2.0	0	0				820	20			
7.5 oz container	213	4.5	2.0			10	0							1.44		I
macaroni & cheese	228	192.5	9.4	25.7				0	.24			730	199			
1 cup	240	9.6	4.2				260	.12	1.0			139	182	1.00		456
macaroni & cheese, Franco-American	167		6.5	23.1				0	.23			934	95			
7.5 oz	213	5.4					867	.24	2.1			114		1.50		I
macaroni & cheese, Lunch Bucket	190		7.0	24.0	0.0	2.0	0	0				930	150			
7.5 oz container	213	7.0	4.5			20	0							.36		I
macaroni w/ beef in tomato sce,	191		9.0	30.1				7	.17			792	43			
Hearty Franco-American—7.5 oz	213	3.8					963	.18	3.2			333		2.20		I
Morning Classics, Libby's	240		8.0	22.0	0.0	1.0	0	9				967	20			
1 cup[3]	172	13.0	6.0			20	0					0				I
noodles & beef, Hunt Homestyle	151		10.0	21.7	2.2	5.3	19	33				1241	22			
1 cup	247	3.9	1.7			17								1.63		I
noodles & chicken, Hunt Homestyle	176		11.7	21.1	3.1	2.2	17	36				1283	33			
1 cup	247	5.9	2.0			37								1.29		I
pasta 'n chicken, Lunch Bucket	150		5.0	22.0	1.0	2.0		0				810	20			
7.5 oz container	213	5.0	1.5			20	200							1.08		I
pasta italian style w/ chicken, Lunch	130		5.0	24.0	7.0	2.0		0				610	20			
Bucket—7.5 oz container	213	1.5	0.5			10	100							1.08		I
potatoes, scalloped, w/ ham chunks,	170		2.0	24.0	0.0	3.0	0	0				660	20			
Lunch Bucket—7.5 oz container	213	7.0	2.5			10	0							.36		I
ravioli & meat sce, Hunt Homestyle	221		10.4	31.5	16.9	3.8	34	21				1116	56			
1 cup	252	7.7	2.8			13								2.68		I
ravioli, beef, Lunch Bucket	180		5.0	32.0	8.0	3.0	0	0				740	40			
7.5 oz container	213	3.5	1.5			5	0							1.44		I
Raviolio's, beef, Franco-American	247		10.3	36.0				7	.19			950	37			
7.8 oz	220	6.9					566	.24	3.4			402		2.40		I
roast beef hash, Armour Star	400		20.0	23.0	0.0	3.0	0	0				1460	40			
1 cup	240	25.0	12.0			95	0							2.70		I
roast beef hash, Libby's	460		19.0	23.0	0.9	3.0	0	0				1390	20			
1 cup	234	33.0	13.0			80	0							1.80		I
roast beef in gravy, Armour Star	150		25.0	3.0	0.0	0.0	0	0				640	0			
½ cup	131	4.0	2.0			75	0							2.70		I
spaghetti & meatballs w/ tomato sce,	216		9.6	27.5				4	.19			863	29			
Franco-American—7.4 oz	209	7.4					566	.18	3.2			336		2.30		I

	KCAL / WT (g)	H₂O (g) / FAT (g)	PRO (g) / SFA (g)	CHO (g) / MUFA (g)	SUGR (g) / PUFA (g)	DFIB (g) / CHOL (mg)	A (RE) / A (IU)	C (mg) / B 1 (mg)	B-2 (mg) / NIA (mg)	B-6 (mg) / B-12 (mcg)	FOL (mcg) / PANT (mg)	Na (mg) / K (mg)	Ca (mg) / P (mg)	Mg (mg) / Fe (mg)	Zn (mg) / Cu (mg)	Mn (mg) / REF
spaghetti & meatballs w/ tomato sce	258	195.0	12.3	28.5				5	.18			1220	53			
1 cup	250	10.3	2.2				1000	.15	2.3			245	113	3.30		456
spaghetti 'n beef, Franco-American	217		9.0	26.1				5	.19			1088	32			
7.5 oz	213	8.5					833	.19	3.2			373		2.20		I
spaghetti 'n meat sce, Lunch Bucket	160		5.0	29.0	9.0	2.0		0				850	20			
7.5 oz container	213	3.0	1.5			5	300							1.44		I
spaghetti w/ meat sce, Franco-American	211		8.5	26.2				5	.21			1101	28			
7.5 oz	213	8.1					928	.22	3.5			391		2.20		I
spaghetti w/ tomato & cheese sce	190	200.3	5.5	38.5				10	.28			955	40			
1 cup	250	1.5					930	.35	4.5			303	88	2.80		456
spaghetti w/ tomato & cheese sce,	181		5.4	36.9				0	.19			883	30			
Franco-American—*7.8 oz*	220	1.3					753	.28	2.8			234		1.60		I
Spaghettio's w/ franks, Franco-American	210		7.6	26.1				4	.18			989	32			
7.4 oz	209	8.4					511	.20	3.2			300		2.20		I
Spaghettio's w/ meatballs,	202		9.0	24.8				4	.18			930	29			
Franco-American—*7.3 oz*	206	7.4					512	.18	3.0			311		2.20		I
Spaghettio's w/ tomato & cheese sce,	166		5.2	32.7				0	.16			883	29			
Franco-American—*7.5 oz*	213	1.6					696	.23	2.5			233		1.60		I
Sportyo's w/ meatballs, Franco-American	205		9.2	25.1				4	.18			944	29			
7.4 oz	209	7.5					520	.18	3.1			316		2.20		I
Sportyo's w/ tomato & cheese sce,	166		5.2	32.7				0	.16			883	29			
Franco-American—*7.5 oz*	213	1.6					696	.23	2.5			233		1.60		I
sweet & sour, chicken, LaChoy Bi-Pack	161		6.8	28.6	25.8	2.8	37	12				687	32			
1 cup	253	2.2	0.8			25								.90		I
tamales																
beef, Derby	253		7.3	20.8	0.0	4.0		7				1034	30			
3 tamales	186	17.4	8.2			23								.65		I
Gebhardt	268		4.6	18.6	0.6	2.6	51	2				770	27			
2 tamales	163	20.7	9.5			28								.80		I
jumbo, Gebhardt	332		5.6	24.0	0.0	3.2	55	2				930	36			
2 tamales	197	25.2	11.6			34								.73		I
Teddyo's w/ meatballs, Franco-American	205		9.2	25.1				4	.18			944	29			
7.4 oz	209	7.5					520	.18	3.1			316		2.20		I
Teddyo's w/ tomato & cheese sce,	166		5.2	32.7				0	.16			883	29			
Franco-American—*7.5 oz*	213	1.6					696	.23	2.5			233		1.60		I
turkey chili w/ beans, Ultimate	260		17.0	28.0	4.0	9.0		0				930	10			
1 cup	247	9.0	3.0			50	2000							3.60		I
vienna sausage & chili, Armour Star	410		14.0	27.0	4.0	15.0		2				1270	100			
1 cup	247	27.0	11.0			80	2000							3.60		I

10.3 FROZEN BREAKFASTS

	KCAL / WT (g)	H₂O (g) / FAT (g)	PRO (g) / SFA (g)	CHO (g) / MUFA (g)	SUGR (g) / PUFA (g)	DFIB (g) / CHOL (mg)	A (RE) / A (IU)	C (mg) / B 1 (mg)	B-2 (mg) / NIA (mg)	B-6 (mg) / B-12 (mcg)	FOL (mcg) / PANT (mg)	Na (mg) / K (mg)	Ca (mg) / P (mg)	Mg (mg) / Fe (mg)	Zn (mg) / Cu (mg)	Mn (mg) / REF
burrito																
bacon & scrambled eggs, Swanson	250		10.0	27.0	3.0	1.0		1				540	80			
Great Starts—*3.5 oz entree*	99	11.0	4.0			90	100							1.80		I
ham & cheese, Swanson Great Starts	210		9.0	30.0	2.0	0.0	0	1				500	60			
3.5 oz entree	99	6.0	2.0			100	0							2.70		I
hot & spicy, Swanson Great Starts	220		9.0	30.0	3.0	3.0		1				490	80			
3.5 oz entree	99	7.0	3.0			55	100							2.70		I
sausage, Swanson Great Starts	240		9.0	24.0	2.0	1.0		1				500	60			
3.5 oz entree	99	12.0	4.0			90	100							1.44		I
scrambled eggs, Swanson Great Starts	200		8.0	25.0	2.0	2.0		2				510	80			
3.5 oz entree	99	8.0	3.0			60	100							1.44		I
egg & cheese sandwich, Swanson Great	350		12.0	30.0	4.0	1.0	0	0				890	150			
Starts—*4.2 oz entree*	119	20.0	8.0			110	0							1.80		I
egg & silver dollar pancakes, Swanson	250		9.0	22.0	6.0	1.0	0	0				540	60			
Great Starts—*4.2 oz entree*	120	14.0	6.0			290	0							1.44		I

	KCAL	H$_2$O (g)	PRO (g)	CHO (g)	SUGR (g)	DFIB (g)	A (RE)	C (mg)	B-2 (mg)	B-6 (mg)	FOL (mcg)	Na (mg)	Ca (mg)	Mg (mg)	Zn (mg)	Mn (mg)
	WT (g)	FAT (g)	SFA (g)	MUFA (g)	PUFA (g)	CHOL (mg)	A (IU)	B-1 (mg)	NIA (mg)	B-12 (mcg)	PANT (mg)	K (mg)	P (mg)	Fe (mg)	Cu (mg)	REF
egg substitute																
& canadian bacon, Swanson Great Starts	240		14.0	33.0	2.0	2.0	0	2				720	200			
4.2 oz entree	120	6.0	2.5			25	0							1.80		I
& pancakes, Swanson Great Starts	220		10.0	30.0	7.0	1.0		1				520	40			
5 oz entree	142	7.0	1.5			50	500							1.08		I
sausage & home fries, Swanson Great	240		12.0	18.0	2.0	2.0		5				620	40			
Starts—6 oz entree	170	13.0	3.0			40	750							.72		I
french toast																
& sausage, Swanson Great Starts	410		13.0	33.0	8.0	3.0		0				580	100			
5.5 oz entree	156	26.0	9.0			110	400							1.80		I
cinn swirl, Swanson Great Starts	440		14.0	34.0	11.0	2.0		0				580	80			
5.5 oz entree	156	28.0	12.0			150	300							1.80		I
sticks w/ syrup, Swanson Great Starts	320		7.0	50.0	16.0	2.0		0				260	80			
4.2 oz entree	120	10.0	5.0			25	0							.72		I
muffin w/ egg, bacon, & cheese,	290		14.0	25.0	2.0	2.0		0				750	150			
Swanson Great Starts—4.1 oz entree	116	15.0	6.0			95	0							1.80		I
pancakes & bacon, Swanson Great Starts	400		12.0	42.0	13.0	1.0		0				1030	60			
4.5 oz entree	128	20.0	7.0			100	0							1.08		I
pancakes & sausage, Swanson Great	490		14.0	52.0	15.0	3.0		0				950	80			
Starts—6 oz entree	170	25.0	11.0			90	0							1.80		I
pancakes, silver dollar & sausage,	340		9.0	36.0	11.0	1.0		0				670	60			
Swanson Great Starts—3.7 oz entree	106	18.0				70	0							1.44		I
scrambled eggs																
& bacon, Swanson Great Starts	290		11.0	17.0	2.0	1.0		0				700	60			
5.3 oz entree	149	19.0	9.0			240	0							1.44		I
& home fries, Swanson Great Starts	200		7.0	15.0	2.0	2.0		1				390	40			
4.4 oz entree	124	12.0	8.0			190	0							1.44		I
& sausage, Swanson Great Starts	360		12.0	21.0	2.0	3.0		0				800	60			
6.2 oz entree	177	26.0	10.0			280	0							1.80		I

10.4 FROZEN DINNERS

	KCAL	H$_2$O (g)	PRO (g)	CHO (g)	SUGR (g)	DFIB (g)	A (RE)	C (mg)	B-2 (mg)	B-6 (mg)	FOL (mcg)	Na (mg)	Ca (mg)	Mg (mg)	Zn (mg)	Mn (mg)
angel hair pasta																
w/ sausage & breadstick, Marie	460		18.0	60.0	9.0	5.0		0				740	100			
Callender's—1 cup & 2 oz breadstick	227	16.0	4.5			10	750							3.60		I
beans & frankfurters, Swanson	439		13.8	53.3				10	.18			898	148			
10.5 oz meal	298	18.9					308	.13	2.6			562		3.70		I
beef																
chopped, Swanson Hungry-Man	602		38.4	44.1				10	.38			1578	71			
16.75 oz meal	475	30.2					432	.17	8.5			752		6.50		I
mesquite w/ bbq sce, Healthy Choice	310		21.0	38.0	14.0	6.0		18				490	80			
11 oz meal	312	8.0	2.5				2500							3.60		I
sliced, Banquet	240		26.0	19.0	12.0	4.0		6				660	20			
9 oz meal	255	7.0	3.0			70	200							3.60		I
sliced, Swanson Hungry-Man	454		37.8	50.0				7	.36			1003	43			
15.2 oz meal	432	11.3					526	.16	7.7			772		5.90		I
Swanson	334		27.9	37.9				6	.25			775	43			
11.25 oz meal	319	7.9					422	.18	5.4			539		4.80		I
w/ bbq sce, Swanson	460		29.7	50.6				4	.34			863	75			
11 oz meal	312	15.4					1687	.18	3.8			552		4.60		I
beef & peppers cantonese, Healthy	270		22.0	32.0	4.0	5.0		36				480	40			
Choice—11.5 oz meal	326	6.0	2.5			55	1500							1.80		I
beef broccoli beijing, Healthy Choice	300		21.0	45.0	11.0	6.0		36				420	40			
12 oz meal	340	4.5	1.5			25	3000							2.70		I
beef oriental, Le Menu Lightstyle	222		18.8	24.5				9	.54			560	39			
10 oz meal	284	5.4	1.5		0.9	39	1449	.07	3.4			362		3.40		I

	KCAL / WT (g)	H₂O (g) / FAT (g)	PRO (g) / SFA (g)	CHO (g) / MUFA (g)	SUGR (g) / PUFA (g)	DFIB (g) / CHOL (mg)	A (RE) / A (IU)	C (mg) / B-1 (mg)	B-2 (mg) / NIA (mg)	B-6 (mg) / B-12 (mcg)	FOL (mcg) / PANT (mg)	Na (mg) / K (mg)	Ca (mg) / P (mg)	Mg (mg) / Fe (mg)	Zn (mg) / Cu (mg)	Mn (mg) / REF
beef patty																
charbroiled w/ gravy, Morton	290		11.0	26.0	3.0	6.0		2				1210	40			
9 oz meal	255	16.0	7.0			25	0							1.80		I
western style, Banquet	350		14.0	28.0	4.0	5.0		2				1400	40			
9.5 oz meal	269	20.0	9.0			30	0							1.80		I
w/ country veg, Banquet	300		11.0	21.0	2.0	3.0		4				1060	40			
9.5 oz meal	269	20.0	8.0			35	300							1.80		I
beef pepper steak, Le Menu	354		25.8	34.7		3.9		14	.26			1008	53			
11.5 oz meal	326	12.5					1462	.09	4.0			368		4.20		I
beef steak, chicken fried																
& gravy, Marie Callender's	650		23.0	69.0	9.0	7.0		24				2260	150			
15 oz meal	425	31.0	10.0			50	750							2.70		I
Banquet	400		15.0	39.0	9.0	4.0		0				1180	100			
10 oz meal	284	20.0	6.0			30	100							1.80		I
Banquet Extra Helping	800		29.0	73.0	14.0	6.0		0				2050	250			
18.65 oz meal	529	44.0	14.0			55	0							2.70		I
beef stroganoff, Healthy Choice	310		21.0	44.0	19.0	3.0		0				440	40			
11 oz meal	312	6.0	2.5			60	750							1.80		I
beef stroganoff, Le Menu	384		26.5	23.8				1	.31			867	107			
10 oz meal	284	20.3					1103	.13	5.1			469		4.30		I
beef tips, Healthy Choice	260		20.0	32.0	18.0	6.0		42				390	20			
11.25 oz meal	319	6.0	3.0			40	3000							1.80		I
cannelloni, chicken, Le Menu Lightstyle	262		14.9	39.2				9	.41			621	93			
10.3 oz meal	291	5.0	1.6		1.8	38	1753	.57	3.2			368		3.10		I
chicken a la king, Le Menu	307		23.1	28.1		3.8		7	.27			829	81			
10.2 oz meal	290	11.2					716	.16	6.7			366		1.70		I
chicken & dumplings w/gravy, Banquet	260		13.0	35.0	16.0	3.0		0				780	40			
10 oz meal	284	8.0	2.5			35	2000							1.08		I
chicken, bbq, potatoes & veg, Tyson	358	227.1	18.3	49.0	17.2	5.5		5				588	45			
11 oz meal	308	9.8	2.7	2.8	0.5	32	614							1.44		I
chicken, bbq style, Banquet	320		18.0	36.0	15.0	3.0		6				800	60			
9 oz meal	255	12.0	2.5			60	300							1.80		I
chicken, bbq tabasco, potatoes, & green beans, Tyson—9 oz meal	266	189.1	16.0	38.3	14.0	5.7		9				495	52			
	252	5.4	1.3	1.8	0.5	29	530							1.02		I
chicken, blackened, spanish rice & corn, Tyson—9 oz meal	262	190.2	17.8	36.2	4.6	3.6		6				473	55			
	252	5.1	1.2	1.3	1.4	33	356							1.09		I
chicken, boneless, Swanson Hungry-Man	668		44.0	65.5				7	.49			1420	84			
17.7 oz meal	503	25.6					691	.42	12.8			653		5.50		I
chicken, breaded parmigiana, Marie Callender's—16 oz meal	620		31.0	63.0	9.0	9.0		9				730	20			
	454	27.0	8.0			50	1000							3.60		I
chicken breast, glazed, Le Menu Lightstyle—10 oz meal	267		25.6	29.4				5	.29			651	58			
	284	5.2	1.4		1.4	51	2346	.10	8.2			457		1.90		I
chicken breast w/ wine sce, Le Menu	277		26.1	27.1				4	.16			675	72			
10 oz meal	284	7.1					4938	.17	8.0			424		2.40		I
chicken broccoli alfredo, Healthy Choice	300		25.0	38.0	0.0	4.0		0				530	150			
11.5 oz meal	326	6.0	2.5			40	200							1.80		I
chicken, broccoli & cheese sce, carrots, & pasta, Tyson—9 oz meal	259	196.9	19.0	21.4	5.3	3.5		1				632	110			
	252	10.8	4.8	3.2	1.8	38	19023							.95		I
chicken cacciatore																
Healthy Choice	250		21.0	36.0	4.0	6.0		12				550	40			
12.5 oz meal	354	2.5	0.5			25	200							1.80		I
Le Menu Lightstyle	260		21.4	27.0		6.2		17	.30			652	90			
10 oz meal	284	7.4	2.6		1.7	66	5077	.14	4.8			481		2.50		I
linguini w/marinara sce, Tyson	563	290.4	21.8	63.7	8.9	11.0		0				1592	247			
15 oz meal	420	24.6	6.2	7.7	6.5	57	1239							3.23		I
chicken cantonese, Healthy Choice	260		25.0	35.0	6.0	4.0		12				430	60			
10.75 oz meal	305	2.0	1.0			40	5000							1.80		I
chicken cordon bleu, Le Menu	458		23.3	47.5		5.5		4	.21			841	133			
11 oz meal	312	19.5					7283	.16	8.8			458		1.80		I

						Vitamins					Minerals				
KCAL	H₂O (g)	PRO (g)	CHO (g)	SUGR (g)	DFIB (g)	A (RE)	C (mg)	B-2 (mg)	B-6 (mg)	FOL (mcg)	Na (mg)	Ca (mg)	Mg (mg)	Zn (mg)	Mn (mg)
WT (g)	FAT (g)	SFA (g)	MUFA (g)	PUFA (g)	CHOL (mg)	A (IU)	B-1 (mg)	NIA (mg)	B-12 (mcg)	PANT (mg)	K (mg)	P (mg)	Fe (mg)	Cu (mg)	REF
chicken cordon bleu, Marie Callender's															
590		33.0	58.0	0.0	7.0		36				1920	250			
13 oz meal															
369	25.0	8.0			55	2250							2.70		I
chicken, country breaded, Healthy Choice—*10.25 oz meal*															
360		18.0	53.0	20.0	5.0		0				480	60			
291	9.0	2.0			45	500							1.44		I
chicken, country fried & gravy, Marie Callender's—*16 oz meal*															
610		25.0	67.0	9.0	6.0		9				1680	20			
454	27.0	8.0			55	300							.36		I
chicken, country herb, Healthy Choice *12.15 oz meal*															
310		20.0	49.0	21.0	4.0		0				540	40			
344	4.0	1.5			45	2500							1.80		I
chicken, dark meat w/ bbq sce, Swanson Hungry-Man—*16.5 oz meal*															
605		39.2	70.7				17	.50			1081	86			
468	18.4					1750	.16	7.0			836		4.20		I
chicken dijon, Healthy Choice *11 oz meal*															
270		23.0	33.0	6.0	6.0		18				470	80			
312	5.0	2.0			40	4500							1.44		I
chicken drumlet, Swanson *10 oz meal*															
518		24.6	43.9				5	.26			697	53			
284	27.1					467	.20	5.6			480		2.90		I
chicken francesca, Healthy Choice *12.5 oz meal*															
330		23.0	46.0	0.0	5.0		15				600	100			
354	6.0	2.5			30	100							1.80		I
chicken francis, red potatoes, & green beans, Tyson—*9 oz meal*															
258	196.2	19.2	23.0	4.8	6.3		18				794	166			
252	9.9	3.0	3.5	1.9	46	0							1.23		I
chicken, fried															
Banquet															
470		21.0	35.0	1.0	6.0		5				980	80			
9 oz meal															
255	27.0	9.0			105	0							1.08		I
Banquet Extra Helping															
790		37.0	72.0	14.0	8.0		0				1820	150			
18 oz meal															
510	39.0	9.0			110	0							1.80		I
bbq flavor, Swanson															
544		25.1	61.0				3	.26			1163	80			
10 oz meal															
284	22.2					703	.28	5.8			498		3.50		I
dark meat, Swanson															
559		22.3	55.2				3	.29			1127	55			
9.7 oz meal															
276	27.6					139	.26	5.2			434		3.20		I
dark meat, Swanson Hungry-Man															
832		35.4	76.7				5	.45			1709	70			
14.25 oz meal															
404	42.6					61	.39	10.2			727		4.90		I
gravy, mashed potatoes, & corn, Tyson															
356	233.7	16.1	39.3	4.1	3.9		5				840	60			
11 oz meal															
312	14.9	2.9	5.3	3.9	32	207							1.27		I
Morton															
420		20.0	30.0	4.0	4.0		9				1000	60			
9 oz meal															
255	25.0	8.0			85	2250							1.08		I
platter, Swanson Budget															
402		15.7	37.5				2	.25			919	55			
7.8 oz meal															
220	21.0					5738	.20	6.0			387		2.80		I
white meat, Banquet															
470		22.0	33.0	2.0	6.0		5				1100	40			
8.75 oz meal															
248	28.0	11.0			100	0							1.44		I
white meat, Banquet Extra Helping															
820		40.0	72.0	13.0	8.0		0				1890	150			
18 oz meal															
510	41.0	9.0			95	0							1.80		I
white meat, Swanson															
549		22.5	60.1				3	.26			1420	68			
10.3 oz meal															
291	24.3					140	.27	6.9			459		3.00		I
white meat, Swanson Hungry-Man															
840		35.4	77.4				5	.43			2149	90			
14.25 oz meal															
404	43.2					44	.43	12.8			749		4.60		I
chicken, ginger hunan, Healthy Choice *12.6 oz meal*															
350		24.0	59.0	11.0	5.0		0				430	60			
357	2.5	0.5			25	750							2.70		I
chicken, glazed, rice pilaf, broccoli, & carrots, Tyson—*9.25 oz meal*															
236	203.6	16.1	29.7	3.6	2.5		9				450	40			
259	5.8	1.3	1.6	1.1	30	6278							.66		I
chicken, grilled, corn o'brien, & ranch beans, Tyson—*9 oz meal*															
234	193.5	19.4	30.2	3.9	6.9		6				589	36			
252	3.9	0.9	1.3	1.3	28	657							1.21		I
chicken, grilled w/ mushroom sce, Marie Callender's—*14 oz meal*															
480		33.0	54.0	0.0	7.0		54				1030	80			
397	15.0	6.0			65	500							2.70		I
chicken, herb roasted															
& mashed potatoes, Marie Callender's															
670		43.0	32.0	7.0	7.0		60				2100	100			
14 oz meal															
397	31.0	15.0			205	750							1.80		I
Le Menu Lightstyle															
220		23.6	19.1				8	.20			531	60			
9.2 oz meal															
262	5.4	1.8		1.2	48	645	.10	7.5			557		1.90		I
pasta & veg, Tyson															
286	253.9	21.2	39.0	3.4	5.4		1				696	37			
11.5 oz meal															
322	5.0	1.3	1.6	1.2	30	415							1.60		I
chicken, honey dijon, pasta & peas, Tyson															
346	238.7	20.5	51.8	5.2	6.5		3				786	87			
11.5 oz meal															
322	6.3	1.3	2.1	2.1	27	294							3.28		I

	KCAL / WT (g)	H₂O (g) / FAT (g)	PRO (g) / SFA (g)	CHO (g) / MUFA (g)	SUGR (g) / PUFA (g)	DFIB (g) / CHOL (mg)	A (RE) / A (IU)	C (mg) / B-1 (mg)	B-2 (mg) / NIA (mg)	B-6 (mg) / B-12 (mcg)	FOL (mcg) / PANT (mg)	Na (mg) / K (mg)	Ca (mg) / P (mg)	Mg (mg) / Fe (mg)	Zn (mg) / Cu (mg)	Mn (mg) / RFF
chicken, italian style, pasta primavera, & veg medley, Tyson—9 oz meal	193	205.3	20.9	19.2	3.3	2.9		2				436	74			
	252	3.7	1.3	0.6	0.3	32	2638							1.18		I
chicken kiev, rice pilaf, broccoli, & carrots, Tyson—9.25 oz meal	443	177.0	17.7	36.4	3.9	2.2		8				683	42			
	259	25.2	11.4	7.9	2.6	84	7026							.49		I
chicken marsala, Marie Callender's 14 oz meal	450		33.0	42.0	5.0	6.0		33				1260	60			
	397	17.0	7.0			70	400							2.70		I
chicken marsala, red potatoes & carrots, Tyson—9 oz meal	180	208.8	14.9	18.8	6.3	4.5		1				521	41			
	252	5.0	1.3	2.1	1.2	29	3342							1.20		I
chicken mesquite																
au gratin potatoes, corn, & peas, Tyson 9 oz meal	308	180.5	22.9	38.1	13.3	5.6		11				593	66			
	252	7.1	2.0	2.6	0.6	40	723							1.26		I
bbq, Healthy Choice 10.5 oz meal	270		19.0	44.0	13.0	6.0		9				490	40			
	298	2.5	1.0			60	2500							1.80		I
Le Menu 10 oz meal	330		28.4	36.1				6	.26			678	23			
	284	8.0					417	.18	10.0			517		2.30		I
chicken, mushroom sce, rice pilaf, & candied carrots, Tyson—9 oz meal	218	200.1	15.1	27.5	8.4	2.1		4				473	69			
	252	5.3	1.1	1.9	1.6	27	3896							1.03		I
chicken nuggets																
Banquet 6.75 oz meal	410		18.0	38.0	11.0	4.0		6				650	20			
	191	21.0	5.0			45	0							1.80		I
Morton 7 oz meal	320		13.0	30.0	12.0	3.0		2				460	40			
	198	17.0	4.0			30	2000							1.44		I
platter, Swanson 8.75 oz meal	473		19.3	46.9				3	.22			651	30			
	248	23.1					130	.19	4.6			497		2.40		I
Swanson Hungry-Man 13 oz meal	596		23.4	68.4				10	.23			695	41			
	369	25.5					188	.20	8.5			400		2.60		I
chicken oriental, Le Menu 10.5 oz meal	321		21.6	41.8				10	.20			860	66			
	298	7.6					3089	.15	7.8			357		1.60		I
chicken, oriental style w/ egg rolls, Banquet—9 oz meal	260		12.0	34.0	16.0	4.0		18				610	40			
	255	9.0	2.5			40	1250							1.08		I
chicken parmigiana																
Banquet 9.5 oz meal	290		14.0	27.0	3.0	3.0		60				900	60			
	269	15.0	4.0			50	300							1.80		I
Banquet Extra Helping 19 oz meal	650		24.0	64.0	9.0	9.0		108				1770	150			
	539	33.0	8.0			65	200							2.70		I
Healthy Choice 11.5 oz meal	300		20.0	47.0	13.0	5.0		18				490	100			
	326	4.0	2.0			35	3500							1.44		I
Le Menu 11.7 oz meal	397		26.3	29.6		5.9		13	.26			1030	163			
	333	19.2					680	.19	8.2			450	313	3.30		I
chicken pasta primavera, Banquet 9.5 oz meal	300		11.0	36.0	9.0	6.0		12				840	60			
	269	12.0	5.0			25	2500							1.80		I
chicken patty, breaded, Morton 6.75 oz meal	280		11.0	24.0	12.0	4.0		0				840	40			
	191	15.0	3.0			20	3000							1.08		I
chicken picante, Healthy choice 10.75 oz meal	260		21.0	30.0	3.0	4.0		30				550	100			
	305	6.0	2.5			45	750							1.80		I
chicken picatta, new potatoes, & broccoli, Tyson—9 oz meal	181	208.9	14.8	19.2	2.1	5.4		10				456	34			
	252	5.1	1.9	1.7	1.0	32	1130							1.15		I
chicken primavera, pasta & veg, Tyson 11.5 oz meal	328	244.8	23.9	43.1	3.4	4.7		26				664	136			
	322	6.7	2.1	2.0	1.5	37	476							1.00		I
chicken, roasted, garlic sce, pasta, & veg medley, Tyson—9 oz meal	206	205.0	16.7	19.8	2.3	3.4		16				462	38			
	252	6.6	1.3	2.3	2.1	27	764							1.53		I
chicken, roasted, Healthy Choice 11 oz meal	220		23.0	27.0	9.0	6.0		15				470	20			
	312	3.0	1.0			35	4500							1.44		I
chicken, sesame shanghai, Healthy Choice—12 oz meal	310		23.0	47.0	0.0	7.0		18				550	40			
	340	2.5	0.0			25	1750							1.80		I
chicken, southern fried, Banquet 8.75 oz meal	520		26.0	32.0	1.0	4.0		6				1410	60			
	248	31.0	7.0			100	0							1.80		I
chicken, southern fried, Banquet Extra Helping—17.5 oz meal	750		38.0	67.0	14.0	9.0		0				2140	150			
	496	37.0	9.0			120	0							2.70		I

	KCAL / WT (g)	H₂O (g) / FAT (g)	PRO (g) / SFA (g)	CHO (g) / MUFA (g)	SUGR (g) / PUFA (g)	DFIB (g) / CHOL (mg)	A (RE) / A (IU)	C (mg) / B-1 (mg)	B-2 (mg) / NIA (mg)	B-6 (mg) / B-12 (mcg)	FOL (mcg) / PANT (mg)	Na (mg) / K (mg)	Ca (mg) / P (mg)	Mg (mg) / Fe (mg)	Zn (mg) / Cu (mg)	Mn (mg) / REF
chicken, southwestern grilled,	200		21.0	23.0	1.0	4.0		42				450	40			
Healthy Choice—10.2 oz meal	289	3.0	1.0			40	750							1.08		I
chicken, sweet & sour																
Healthy Choice	330		20.0	53.0	30.0	5.0		30				210	40			
11 oz meal	312	5.0	1.5			45	2000							1.08		I
Le Menu	381		18.8	41.0				5	.24			1020	80			
10.5 oz meal	298	15.7					1648	.14	5.5			400		2.10		I
Marie Callender's	530		25.0	86.0	36.0	7.0		27				700	60			
14 oz meal	397	9.0	2.0			35	5000							2.70		I
Swanson	381		21.4	47.4				10	.32			534	96			
12 oz meal	340	11.6					1056	.11	4.0			331		2.00		
chicken teriyaki, Healthy Choice	230		19.0	32.0	8.0	4.0		36				580	20			
11 oz meal	312	3.0	1.5			45	1000							1.08		
chicken w/ bbq sce, Swanson	464		29.2	56.3				7	.35			992	70			
11.75 oz meal	333	13.6					974	.22	4.6			638		3.80		I
chimichanga, Banquet	470		13.0	56.0	9.0	9.0		6				1180	60			
9.6 oz meal	269	23.0	7.0			15	400							2.70		I
chow mein, chicken & white rice,	249		17.5	33.6	5.4			5	.33			754	58			
Le Menu Lightstyle—10 oz meal	284	4.9	1.6		1.2	41	556	.18	4.7			304		1.70		I
chow mein, chicken w/ egg rolls, Banquet	210		9.0	28.0	3.0	3.0		9				850	20			
9 oz meal	255	7.0	2.0			30	500							.72		I
enchilada																
beef & cheese w/ chili & beans, Patio	250		12.0	35.0	2.0	9.0		4				1130	150			
15.5 oz dinner	439	6.0	2.5			20	750							1.80		I
beef & tamale combo, Banquet	400		14.0	56.0	7.0			0				1520	150			
11 oz meal	312	13.0	5.0			15	750							2.70		I
beef, Banquet	380		15.0	54.0	7.0	10.0		0				1330	150			
11 oz meal	312	12.0	5.0			15	750							2.70		I
beef, Patio	350		12.0	52.0	2.0	9.0		4				1700	150			
12 oz meal	340	10.0	4.0			15	500							1.80		I
beef, Swanson	475		17.2	55.4				4	.21			1349	210			
13.8 oz meal	390	20.5					1569	.22	2.8			524		3.40		I
beef, tamale, & chili gravy, Morton	260		8.0	40.0	3.0	8.0		6				1000	80			
10 oz meal	284	7.0	3.0			5	500							1.80		I
beef w/ chili & beans, Patio	250		12.0	35.0	2.0	8.0		0				1350	100			
15.5 oz meal	439	7.0	2.5			15	1000							1.80		I
cheese, Banquet	340		15.0	56.0	7.0	9.0		4				1500	200			
11 oz meal	312	6.0	2.5			15	750							2.70		I
cheese, Patio	330		13.0	52.0	7.0	10.0		5				1570	200			
12 oz meal	340	8.0	3.0			15	500							1.80		I
chicken, Banquet	360		15.0	54.0	7.0	9.0		0				1580	150			
11 oz meal	312	10.0	3.0			20	750							2.70		I
chicken suprema, Healthy Choice	270		14.0	45.0	2.0	6.0		30				560	100			
11.3 oz meal	320	4.0	2.0			20	1000							1.08		I
chicken w/ red chili sce, Swanson	269		9.7	41.3				6	.16			1235	103			
9 oz meal	255	7.2					1105	.20	2.1			487		2.50		I
combo, Banquet	350		15.0	53.0	3.0	10.0		0				1640	200			
11 oz meal	312	9.0	3.5			35	750							2.70		I
fettuccine alfredo, Banquet	330		11.0	36.0	5.0	4.0		18				850	150			
9.5 oz meal	269	16.0	7.0			25	200							1.08		I
fiesta, Patio	340		13.0	51.0	5.0	11.0		4				1760	750			
12 oz meal	340	9.0	4.0			15	400							1.80		I
fillet of sole, Le Menu	354		17.9	43.5	3.7			2	.29			956	105			
10 oz meal	284	12.1					2079	.20	2.4			341		2.00		I
fish 'n chips, Swanson	497		19.8	59.9				4	.18			963	68			
10 oz meal	284	19.8					382	.28	3.5			548		2.70		I
fish, herb baked, Healthy Choice	340		16.0	54.0	11.0	5.0		0				480	40			
10.9 oz meal	309	7.0	1.5			35	3000							.72		I
fish, lemon pepper, Healthy Choice	290		14.0	47.0	20.0	7.0		30				360	20			
10.7 oz meal	303	5.0	1.0			25	500							1.08		I

	KCAL	H₂O (g)	PRO (g)	CHO (g)	SUGR (g)	DFIB (g)	A (RE)	C (mg)	B-2 (mg)	B-6 (mg)	FOL (mcg)	Na (mg)	Ca (mg)	Mg (mg)	Zn (mg)	Mn (mg)
	WT (g)	FAT (g)	SFA (g)	MUFA (g)	PUFA (g)	CHOL (mg)	A (IU)	B-1 (mg)	NIA (mg)	B-12 (mcg)	PANT (mg)	K (mg)	P (mg)	Fe (mg)	Cu (mg)	REF
fish nuggets, Swanson	400		17.5	44.8				3	.18			897	49			
9.5 oz meal	269	16.8					1516	.17	3.1			407		2.40		I
ham steak, Le Menu	288		18.3	31.0				31	.29			1486	67			
10 oz meal	284	10.1					7397	.58	4.5			426		2.20		I
ham w/ macaroni & cheese, Marie Callender's—14 oz meal	450		29.0	63.0	32.0	6.0		30				2200	40			
	397	9.0	4.0			60	3500							1.08		I
lasagna w/ meat sce, Banquet	260		12.0	35.0	10.0	6.0		60				820	150			
9.5 oz meal	269	8.0	2.0			10	750							1.80		I
macaroni & beef, Marie Callender's 14 oz meal	590		28.0	80.0	16.0	9.0		0				1230	150			
	397	18.0	5.0			30	1500							5.40		I
macaroni & beef, Swanson Budget 12 oz meal	369		12.6	48.4				11	.23			925	126			
	340	13.9					595	.12	3.2			353		2.90		I
macaroni & cheese, Banquet 9.5 oz meal	320		12.0	43.0	6.0	4.0		24				970	150			
	269	11.0	3.5			20	1250							1.44		I
macaroni & cheese, Swanson 12.2 oz meal	373		12.9	47.9				6	.22			1014	239			
	347	14.4					3605	.18	1.8			177		2.70		I
meatloaf																
Banquet 9.5 oz meal	280		13.0	22.0	3.0	3.0		6				1020	40			
	269	16.0	6.0			80	200							1.80		I
Banquet Extra Helping 19 oz meal	650		29.0	49.0	13.0	10.0		102				2100	100			
	539	38.0	16.0			85	4500							3.60		I
Healthy Choice 12 oz meal	320		15.0	52.0	17.0	6.0		54				460	40			
	340	5.0	2.5			35	750							1.80		I
Le Menu 10 oz meal	300		17.8	27.3				5	.31			860	97			
	284	13.3					4672	.23	4.3			626		4.00		I
Swanson 10.8 oz meal	414		17.7	42.1				11	.20			1014	93			
	305	19.4					457	.19	4.0			574		3.80		I
w/ tomato sce, Morton 9 oz meal	250		9.0	24.0	17.0	5.0		0	.17			1110	40			
	255	13.0	4.0			20	2500	.19	1.7					1.44		I
w/ tomato sce, Swanson Hungry-Man 16.5 oz meal	639		29.0	57.3				29	.17			1817	179			
	468	32.6					834	.27	5.9			1026		5.90		I
mexican style																
Banquet Extra Helping 22 oz meal	820		28.0	100.0	35.0	20.0		6				2060	300			
	624	34.0	14.0			50	1500							6.30		I
combination, Swanson 14.25 oz meal	521		18.5	60.0				4	.21			1593	184			
	404	23.0					1554	.25	3.7			669		4.50		I
Patio 13.25 oz meal	430		15.0	59.0	3.0	13.0		6				1840	100			
	376	15.0	6.0			20	500							2.70		I
noodles & chicken, Swanson Budget 10.5 oz meal	280		7.3	45.2				3	.27			741	77			
	298	7.7					4102	.15	3.3			213		1.60		I
pasta shells marinara, Healthy Choice 12 oz meal	380		25.0	55.0	10.0	5.0		0				390	400			
	340	6.0	3.5			25	500							1.80		I
pasta w/ beef & broccoli, Marie Callender's—15 oz meal	570		35.0	73.0	32.0	6.0		15				1160	40			
	425	15.0	4.0			70	400							4.50		I
pasta w/ italian sausage & peppers, Banquet—9.5 oz meal	300		10.0	39.0	9.0	6.0		60				760	60			
	269	12.0	3.5			10	500							1.80		I
pork chop, country fried, Marie Callender's—15 oz meal	550		26.0	50.0	16.0	9.0		9				2240	150			
	425	27.0	9.0			65	5000							2.70		I
pork cutlet, Banquet 10.25 oz meal	410		11.0	39.0	21.0	4.0		9				1060	80			
	291	24.0	7.0			25	200							1.44		I
pork loin, Swanson 10.8 oz meal	282		20.4	26.2				6	.15			790	40			
	305	10.6					5315	.47	5.3			433		1.70		I
pork patty, grilled, glazed, Healthy Choice—9.6 oz meal	280		16.0	46.0	28.0	6.0		30				380	40			
	272	4.0	1.5			20	2250							1.80		I
pork riblet, Banquet 10 oz meal	400		18.0	39.0	18.0	7.0		2				1070	100			
	284	19.0	8.0			40	400							1.80		I
pork w/ apple glaze, Le Menu 10 oz meal	298		19.3	34.2				115	.20			789	51			
	284	9.4					5453	.49	5.1			477		2.20		I
pot roast, Swanson Hungry-Man 16 oz meal	406		30.1	48.0				9	.49			955	81			
	454	10.4					1794	.19	7.8			949		5.60		I

	KCAL / WT (g)	H₂O (g) / FAT (g)	PRO (g) / SFA (g)	CHO (g) / MUFA (g)	SUGR (g) / PUFA (g)	DFIB (g) / CHOL (mg)	Vitamins A (RE) / A (IU)	C (mg) / B-1 (mg)	B-2 (mg) / NIA (mg)	B-6 (mg) / B-12 (mcg)	FOL (mcg) / PANT (mg)	Minerals Na (mg) / K (mg)	Ca (mg) / P (mg)	Mg (mg) / Fe (mg)	Zn (mg) / Cu (mg)	Mn (mg) / REF
ranchera, Patio	470		13.0	55.0	1.0	14.0		6				2400	100			
13 oz meal	369	15.0	6.0			25	500							2.70		I
ravioli, beef, Swanson Hungry-Man	489		16.1	68.3				25	.28			975	162			
16.5 oz meal	468	16.8					983	.34	4.2			275		4.40		I
salisbury con queso, Patio	390		18.0	33.0	7.0	10.0		4				1570	100			
11 oz meal	312	20.0	11.0			40	300							2.70		I
salisbury steak																
& gravy, Marie Callender's	550		30.0	51.0	14.0	6.0		12				1680	250			
14 oz meal	397	25.0	11.0			85	1500							3.60		I
Banquet	340		15.0	28.0	4.0	4.0		0				1040	40			
9.5 oz meal	269	19.0	7.0			60	0							1.80		I
Banquet Extra Helping	740		31.0	52.0	3.0	11.0		6				1860	100			
19 oz meal	539	46.0	19.0			75	100							3.60		I
Healthy Choice	320		18.0	48.0	20.0	7.0		60				470	40			
11.5 oz meal	326	6.0	3.0			45	1500							1.80		I
Le Menu	360		20.3	27.3				2	.26			864	120			
10.5 oz meal	298	18.9					731	.17	4.4			735		3.60		I
Le Menu Lightstyle	234		19.9	23.4				0	.31			785	91			
10.5 oz meal	298	6.8	3.2		0.9	33	455	.18	4.5			611		3.50		I
Morton	210		9.0	23.0	7.0	3.0		2				950	40			
9 oz meal	255	9.0	4.0			20	2000							1.44		I
Swanson	409		18.9	43.2				5	.19			899	71			
10.8 oz meal	305	17.9					214	.15	4.6			531		3.80		I
Swanson Hungry-Man	622		36.8	42.2				5	.46			1670	219			
16.5 oz meal	468	34.0					508	.23	7.1			814		5.80		I
shrimp & veg maria, Healthy Choice	270		15.0	46.0	1.0	5.0		21				540	40			
12.5 oz meal	354	3.0	1.0			35	500							2.70		I
sirloin, chopped, Le Menu	420		25.9	27.5				9	.32			999	154			
12.2 oz meal	347	23.0					201	.13	5.6			567		4.40		I
sirloin, chopped, Swanson	356		21.1	27.9				5	.24			805	87			
10.76 oz meal	305	17.8					5650	.12	5.1			549		3.60		I
sirloin tips, Le Menu	383		29.5	26.7		5.5		28	.38			736	99			
11.5 oz meal	326	17.5					681	.16	5.2			686	333	4.60		I
sirloin tips, Swanson Hungry-Man	450		30.5	50.2				8	.50			1190	92			
15.8 oz meal	447	14.1					2381	.25	5.6			728		6.90		I
spaghetti & meatballs, Swanson Budget	374		13.5	46.0				14	.23			1097	113			
12.5 oz meal	354	15.1					1212	.21	3.4			411		3.10		I
spaghetti w/ meat sce, Morton	170		6.0	30.0	13.0	4.0		0				600	20			
8.5 oz meal	241	3.0	1.0			5	2500							1.80		I
steak patty, charbroiled, Healthy Choice	280		16.0	41.0	4.0	7.0		30				550	20			
11 oz meal	312	6.0	3.0			25	2500							1.80		I
stuffed shells, 3 cheeses, Le Menu Lightstyle—10 oz meal	270		17.3	33.5				34	.13			686	241			
	284	7.3	3.3		1.2	20	1341	.11	2.0			315		2.70		I
swiss steak, Swanson	347		26.2	37.0				11	.22			701	49			
10 oz meal	284	10.5					563	.20	4.6			483		4.40		I
tamales, beef, Swanson Budget	352		13.4	45.5				11	.18			1204	122			
10 oz meal	284	12.9					1605	.27	3.0			563		2.90		I
tamales, chicken, Swanson Budget	325		7.9	45.2				5	.26			1201	134			
9.7 oz meal	276	12.5					1447	.25	2.0			264		1.50		I
tortellini, cheese, Le Menu Lightstyle	225		10.2	34.1				45	.43			455	134			
10 oz meal	284	5.3	1.7		1.4	13	295	.26	2.8			418		2.70		I
turkey & gravy w/ dressing, Banquet Extra Helping—18.8 oz meal	560		32.0	63.0	26.0	7.0		0				1910	100			
	533	20.0	5.0			75	0							3.60		I
turkey & gravy w/ dressing, Morton	230		14.0	27.0	5.0	5.0		0				1090	40			
9 oz meal	255	8.0	3.0			35	2500							1.80		I
turkey breast, Healthy Choice	280		22.0	40.0	20.0	7.0		60				460	20			
10.5 oz meal	298	3.0	1.0			45	400							1.44		I
turkey, country roast, Healthy Choice	280		16.0	46.0	28.0	6.0		30				380	40			
10 oz meal	284	4.0	1.5			20	2250							1.80		I
turkey divan, Le Menu Lightstyle	267		22.7	25.6				22	.21			817	116			
10 oz meal	284	8.2	2.5		1.4	43	663	.11	6.0			492		1.70		I

	KCAL	H₂O (g)	PRO (g)	CHO (g)	SUGR (g)	DFIB (g)	A (RE)	C (mg)	B-2 (mg)	B-6 (mg)	FOL (mcg)	Na (mg)	Ca (mg)	Mg (mg)	Zn (mg)	Mn (mg)
	WT (g)	FAT (g)	SFA (g)	MUFA (g)	PUFA (g)	CHOL (mg)	A (IU)	B-1 (mg)	NIA (mg)	B-12 (mcg)	PANT (mg)	K (mg)	P (mg)	Fe (mg)	Cu (mg)	REF
turkey, light meat, Le Menu Lightstyle	199		19.2	20.8				11	.29			639	44			
8.25 oz meal	234	4.3	1.0		1.6	26	1584	.37	6.6			410		2.60		I
turkey, Swanson	350		20.1	42.5				6	.24			1047	52			
11.5 oz meal	326	11.1					284	.22	6.6			415		2.70		I
turkey, Swanson Hungry-Man	537		36.3	61.8				11	.41			1721	84			
17 oz meal	482	16.1					594	.34	12.4			799				I
turkey, white meat, Banquet	290		17.0	34.0	7.0	5.0		6				1060	40			
9.25 oz meal	262	10.0	2.5			55	100							1.80		I
turkey, white meat, Le Menu	325		28.0	24.0				17	.29			831	54			
10.5 oz meal	298	13.0					2693	.16	7.8			625				I
veal marsala, Le Menu Lightstyle	250		25.3	25.4				3	.53			728	33			
10 oz meal	284	5.2	1.0		1.0	112	1216	.18	7.4			492		1.80		I
veal parmigiana																
Banquet	320		13.0	35.0	14.0	7.0		27				960	60			
9 oz meal	255	14.0	5.0			25	300							1.80		I
Swanson	441		21.9	42.7				9	.30			1106	162			
12.2 oz meal	347	20.3					669	.27	5.8			412		3.70		I
w/ rotini alfredo, Le Menu	383		24.6	32.4				18	.35			819	265			
11.5 oz meal	326	17.2					1441	.25	4.9			476		3.20		I
w/ spaghetti, Swanson Hungry-Man	574		32.7	56.3				22	.54			1784	231			
18.2 oz meal	517	24.2					1449	.36	8.9			768		5.50		I
w/ tomato sce, Morton	280		9.0	30.0	8.0	4.0		18				950	40			
8.75 oz meal	248	13.0	4.0			20	2250							1.80		I
western style, Swanson	428		21.8	42.6				14	.21			1061	74			
11.5 oz meal	326	18.9					624	.16	4.3			480		4.50		I
white cheddar & broccoli, Banquet	320		11.0	43.0	4.0	5.0		60				810	150			
9.5 oz meal	269	11.0	4.0			15	1000							1.80		I
yankee pot roast, Healthy Choice	280		19.0	38.0	20.0	5.0		42				460	40			
11 oz meal	312	5.0	2.0			45	3000							1.80		I
yankee pot roast, Le Menu	316		25.6	26.5		4.8	17	9	.26			697	47			
10 oz meal	284	12.0					7206	.13	5.4			644	196	4.10		
ziti w/ meat sce, Swanson Hungry-Man	558		28.4	58.4				38	.45			1689	255			
17.6 oz meal	489	23.5					2381	.37	6.6			1027		7.50		I

10.5 FROZEN ENTREES[4]

	KCAL	H₂O (g)	PRO (g)	CHO (g)	SUGR (g)	DFIB (g)	A (RE)	C (mg)	B-2 (mg)	B-6 (mg)	FOL (mcg)	Na (mg)	Ca (mg)	Mg (mg)	Zn (mg)	Mn (mg)
	WT (g)	FAT (g)	SFA (g)	MUFA (g)	PUFA (g)	CHOL (mg)	A (IU)	B-1 (mg)	NIA (mg)	B-12 (mcg)	PANT (mg)	K (mg)	P (mg)	Fe (mg)	Cu (mg)	REF
beef burgundy, Le Menu	316		25.1	12.3				2	.26			640	37			
7.5 oz entree	213	18.5					1037	.14	3.6			231				I
beef casserole, Pillsbury Microwave	163	69.0	6.1	13.0		1.1		1	.10			417	15			
Classic—3.5 oz	100	9.6					517	.08	1.4			117	70	1.30		I
beef, chipped & creamed, Stouffers	162	84.8	8.7	5.9				1	.23			644	90			
4 oz entree	113	11.5				43	45	.05	1.5			226		.79		I
beef, chipped & creamed, Swanson	288		17.3	14.0				3	.37			1051	177			
9 oz entree	255	18.1					93	.09	2.9			394		2.20		I
beef, creamed, Banquet	100		9.0	8.0	1.0	0.0		0				700	80			
4 oz entree	113	3.0	1.5			25	0							.72		I
beef macaroni, Healthy Choice	210		14.0	34.0	9.0	5.0		54				450	40			
8.5 oz entree	241	2.0	0.5			15	500							2.70		I
beef oriental, Lean Cuisine	270		20.0	30.0				0	.10			700	20			
8.6 oz entree	244	8.0	2.0		0.0	45	750	.12	3.0			250		1.44		I
beef patties w/ mushroom gravy, Banquet	180		15.0	7.0	0.0	2.0		0	0			640	20			
Family—1 patty w/ gravy (4.7 oz)	132	13.0	6.0			25	0							1.08		I
beef patties w/ onion gravy, Banquet	180		8.0	7.0	5.0	2.0		0	0			630	20			
Family—1 patty w/ gravy (4.7 oz)	132	14.0	6.0			20	0							1.08		I
beef pepper steak oriental, Healthy	250		19.0	34.0	0.0	3.0		9				470	20			
Choice—9.5 oz entree	269	4.0	2.0			35	200							1.08		I
beef pot roast & gravy, Marie Callender's	250		17.0	31.0	5.0	3.0		1				790	20			
1 cup (7.5 oz)	213	6.0	2.5			45	1750							1.80		I
beef, sliced w/ brown gravy, Banquet	100		13.0	7.0	2.0	1.0		0				850	0			
Family—2 slices (5.6 oz)	159	3.0	1.5			40	0							1.80		I
beef, sliced w/ gravy, Banquet	70		8.0	5.0	1.0	0.0		0				440	0			
4 oz entree	113	2.0	1.0			25	0							1.08		I

	KCAL	H2O (g)	PRO (g)	CHO (g)	SUGR (g)	DFIB (g)	A (RE)	C (mg)	B-2 (mg)	B-6 (mg)	FOL (mcg)	Na (mg)	Ca (mg)	Mg (mg)	Zn (mg)	Mn (mg)
	WT (g)	FAT (g)	SFA (g)	MUFA (g)	PUFA (g)	CHOL (mg)	A (IU)	B-1 (mg)	NIA (mg)	B-12 (mcg)	PANT (mg)	K (mg)	P (mg)	Fe (mg)	Cu (mg)	REF
beef steak ranchero, Lean Cuisine	270		16.0	30.0				9	.26			950	40			
9.2 oz entree	262	9.0	3.0		1.0	45	300	.09	3.0			450		1.44		I
beef stew, hearty, Banquet Family	160		14.0	17.0	3.0	4.0		9				1120	20			
1 cup (8.7 oz)	246	4.0	2.0			25	500							1.44		I
beef stew, Stouffers	129	116.4	9.7	7.2				3	.13			540	14			
5 oz entree	142	6.8				28	1065	.06	1.4			213		1.28		I
beef stroganoff, Stouffers	159	83.6	12.4	4.6				0	.20			633	27			
4 oz entree	113	10.2				45	34	.05	2.1			215		1.13		I
beef stroganoff w/ noodles, Marie Callender's—*1 cup (6.5 oz)*	440		24.0	23.0	4.0	3.0		6				780	20			
	184	27.0	11.0			40	100							1.44		I
beef szechuan, Green Giant	121		11.0	12.0				23	.11			457	29			
5 oz[5]	142	4.0	0.8		1.0	25	1115	.04	1.7			306	157	1.50		I
beef szechuan, Lean Cuisine	280		20.0	25.0				12	.34			720	40			
9.2 oz entree	262	11.0	3.0		2.0	95	1250	.15	4.0			320		1.80		I
beef tips francis, Healthy Choice	280		20.0	40.0	1.0	4.0		0				520	20			
9.5 oz entree	269	5.0	1.5			30	0							1.80		I
britos																
beef & bean, Patio	420		11.0	51.0	2.0	7.0		2				800	40			
10 britos (6 oz)	170	19.0	7.0			20	500							1.44		I
beef nacho, Patio	410		13.0	48.0	3.0	5.0		1				1050	60			
10 britos (6 oz)	170	18.0	18.0			20	100							1.44		I
cheese nacho, Patio	360		10.0	52.0	8.0	3.0		2				500	150			
10 britos (6 oz)	170	13.0	4.0			15	0							1.08		I
chicken spicy, Patio	400		13.0	52.0	2.0	3.0		0				640	100			
10 britos (6 oz)	170	16.0	4.0			25	0							1.80		I
burrito																
beef & bean, Patio	280		10.0	45.0	5.0	7.0		1				860	0			
5 oz burrito	142	7.0	3.0			15	300							.00		I
beef & cheese, Patio	270		9.0	46.0	2.0	7.0		4				530	60			
5 oz burrito	142	5.0	2.5			5	200							1.08		I
beef, bean & green chili, Patio	270		10.0	42.0	3.0	4.0		1				870	20			
5 oz burrito	142	7.0	3.5			10	0							.72		I
beef, bean & red chili, Patio	260		11.0	42.0	3.0	7.0		5				640	20			
5 oz burrito	142	5.0	2.0			10	200							1.80		I
beef, bean & red chili peppers, Patio	270		11.0	42.0	4.0	6.0		4				850	20			
5 oz burito	142	6.0	2.0			10	400							2.70		I
chicken con queso, Healthy Choice	360		16.0	66.0	11.0	8.0		15				590	100			
10.55 oz entree	299	3.0	1.0			15	1500							2.70		I
chicken, Patio	260		12.0	44.0	5.0	3.0		1				740	60			
5 oz burrito	142	4.0	1.5			15	0							.72		I
cabbage, stuffed																
w/ beef, rice & sce, Stouffers	218	172.2	11.3	19.8				13	.15			1177	120			
7.7 oz entree	218	10.2				26	371	.13	2.6			371		1.74		I
w/ beef, Stouffers	97	51.1	6.0	8.5				1	.07			369	18			
2.5 oz entree	71	4.3				14	0	.06	1.1			107		.99		I
w/ meat & sce, Lean Cuisine	220		15.0	20.0				6	.14			930	80			
10.7 oz entree	304	9.0	2.0		0.0	40	1250	.15	3.0			530		1.80		I
cajun seasoned stew, Stouffers	97	93.8	5.8	5.3				7	.08			463	24			
4 oz entree[6]	113	5.9				25	418	.07	1.6			283		.68		I
cannelloni																
beef & pork, Lean Cuisine	270		19.0	25.0				0	.34			940	200			
9.6 oz entree	273	10.0	4.0		1.0	45	2000	.15	2.0			400		1.44		I
cheese, Stouffers	172	121.7	10.1	13.7				17	.19			608	218			
5.5 oz entree	156	8.3				20	780	.06	0.9			218		.62		I
cheese w/ tomato, Lean Cuisine	270		22.0	24.0				6	.26			900	300			
9.1 oz entree	258	10.0	5.0		1.0	30	750	.12	1.2			330		.72		I
cheese stuffed shells, Stouffers	268	215.3	14.9	33.3	5.2			5	.30			572	303			
9.7 oz entree[7]	275	8.5				24	762	.25	3.0			517		2.23		I

	KCAL / WT (g)	H₂O (g) / FAT (g)	PRO (g) / SFA (g)	CHO (g) / MUFA (g)	SUGR (g) / PUFA (g)	DFIB (g) / CHOL (mg)	A (RE) / A (IU)	C (mg) / B-1 (mg)	B-2 (mg) / NIA (mg)	B-6 (mg) / B-12 (mcg)	FOL (mcg) / PANT (mg)	Na (mg) / K (mg)	Ca (mg) / P (mg)	Mg (mg) / Fe (mg)	Zn (mg) / Cu (mg)	Mn (mg) / REF
chicken a l'orange, Lean Cuisine	270		26.0	31.0				9	.10			400	20			
8 oz entree	226	5.0	1.0		1.0	50	500	.12	8.0			420		.72		I
chicken a la king, Le Menu Lightstyle	241		17.9	31.0				1	.32			659	91			
8.25 oz entree	234	5.0	1.1		1.3	29	105	.08	5.7			328		1.20		I
chicken a la king w/ rice, Swanson	275		14.4	32.1				2	.26			859	64			
9 oz entree	255	9.9					583	.09	5.0			217		.90		I
chicken almond, Green Giant	150		11.0	10.0				5	.06			585	34			
5 oz[8]	142	8.0	1.0		2.0	22	3336	.01	4.0			265	116	1.00		I
chicken & cheese casserole, Pillsbury Microwave Classic—3.5 oz	181	66.0	8.0	12.6		1.0		4	.15			358	75			
	100	11.0					495	.11	2.2			147	92	.97		I
chicken & dumplings, Banquet Family	290		12.0	30.0	2.0	2.0		0				1270	40			
1 cup (7 oz)	198	14.0	5.0			40	0							1.44		I
chicken & dumplings, Marie Callender's	260		17.0	22.0	8.0	3.0		0				1030	60			
1 cup (7 oz)	198	12.0	5.0			90	2500							1.44		I
chicken & noodles																
escalloped, Stouffers	247	125.8	12.8	14.6				0	.24			663	65			
6 oz entree[9]	170	15.1				56	68	.14	2.4			153		1.02		I
homestyle, Stouffers	254	174.8	18.2	17.5				0	.36			931	148			
8 oz entree[10]	227	12.5				54	1362	.20	3.4			318		1.14		I
w/ veg, Swanson	305		14.0	30.3				0	.27			990	78			
9 oz entree	255	14.2					731	.17	3.4			216		1.60		I
chicken & veg																
Lean Cuisine	270		23.0	29.0				30	.17			1120	100			
11.7 oz entree	333	7.0	2.0		2.0	45	500	.12	4.0			400		1.44		I
marsala, Healthy Choice	230		22.0	32.0	1.0	3.0		4				440	60			
11.5 oz entree	326	1.5	0.5			30	500							1.80		I
oriental, Stouffers	88	94.9	6.0	5.9				6	.11			429	16			
4 oz entree[11]	113	4.5				18	565	.03	1.6			147		.40		I
chicken breast, fried & whipped potatoes, Stouffers—7.1 oz entree	350		17.0	30.0								900				
	202	18.0														I
chicken breast, grilled sandwich, Tyson	205	52.3	12.7	24.9	3.7	2.5	0	0				460	41			
3.5 oz sandwich	98	6.1	1.5			23	0							.98		I
chicken breast w/ gravy & veg medley, Stouffers—7.4 oz entree	190		22.0	11.0								560				
	209	6.0														I
chicken cacciatore, Lean Cuisine	280		23.0	25.0				12	.17			950	40			
10.9 oz entree	308	10.0	1.0		2.0	45	500	.12	5.0			440		1.80		I
chicken casserole, Pillsbury Microwave Classic—3.5 oz	152	70.0	8.0	11.0		1.0		3	.10			338	35			
	100	8.3					677	.09	2.6			130	83	1.25		I
chicken classica, Stouffers	179	185.9	14.5	18.4		4.3		19	.32			665	113			
8 oz entree[12]	227	5.2				43	205	.18	4.1			397		1.07		I
chicken, country fried & gravy w/ mashed potatoes, Marie Callender's—12 oz	520		21.0	57.0	3.0	5.0		0				1550	100			
	340	22.0	6.0			70	0							1.08		I
chicken, creamed, Stouffers	186	81.4	11.3	4.6				0	.15			452	45			
4 oz entree	113	13.6				51	40	.03	2.0			141		.45		I
chicken croquettes, breaded w/gravy, Weaver—2 croquettes & ½ cup gravy	342	98.6	13.5	26.2	5.4	2.1		0				743	98			
	162	20.3	5.5	9.9	3.4	50	0							.74		I
chicken dijon, Le Menu Lightstyle	229		20.5	22.1				4	.18			523	89			
8.5 oz entree	241	6.6	1.7		1.3	36	1394	.06	5.4			352		1.80		I
chicken, empress, Le Menu	208		16.5	24.8				10	.17			664	32			
8.25 oz entree	234	4.8	1.0		1.6	30	1471	.14	5.1			394		1.30		I
chicken fettuccini alfredo, Healthy Choice—8.5 oz entree	260		22.0	35.0	3.0	3.0		0				410	100			
	241	4.5	2.0			40	0							1.44		I
chicken, fiesta, Lean Cuisine	250		21.0	29.0				12	.17			880	20			
8.5 oz entree	241	6.0	1.0		2.0	45	750	.23	4.0			410		1.08		I
chicken, fried & whipped potatoes, Swanson—7 oz entree	384		18.3	31.8				5	.22			1080	47			
	198	20.4					15	.18	6.6			409		2.70		I
chicken, garlic milano, Healthy Choice	240		18.0	34.0	4.0	3.0		18				510	100			
9.5 oz entree	269	4.0	2.0			35	500							1.08		I

Vitamins columns: A (RE), C (mg), B-2 (mg), B-6 (mg), FOL (mcg) / A (IU), B-1 (mg), NIA (mg), B-12 (mcg), PANT (mg). Minerals columns: Na (mg), Ca (mg), Mg (mg), Zn (mg), Mn (mg) / K (mg), P (mg), Fe (mg), Cu (mg), REF.

	KCAL / WT (g)	H2O / FAT (g)	PRO / SFA (g)	CHO / MUFA (g)	SUGR / PUFA (g)	DFIB / CHOL (mg)	A (RE) / A (IU)	C / B-1 (mg)	B-2 / NIA (mg)	B-6 / B-12	FOL / PANT	Na / K (mg)	Ca / P (mg)	Mg / Fe (mg)	Zn / Cu (mg)	Mn / REF
chicken, glazed Healthy Choice	210		17.0	30.0	1.0	3.0	0					480	20			
8.5 oz entree	241	2.0	0.0			30	0							.36		I
Lean Cuisine	270		26.0	23.0				2	.10			710	20			
8.5 oz entree	241	8.0	1.0		4.0	60	100	.12	8.0			390		.72		I
Stouffers	102	91.5	12.8	3.1				1	.08			407	5			
4 oz entree[13]	113	4.3				32	23	.79	4.2			192		.23		I
chicken, grilled sonoma, Healthy Choice	240		19.0	34.0	2.0	6.0		24				540	40		1.80	
9 oz entree	255	2.5	0.5			40	3000									I
chicken grilled w/ mashed potatoes,	170		18.0	18.0	0.0	3.0		5				600	0			
Healthy Choice—8 oz entree	227	3.5	1.5			40	200							.72		I
chicken, honey mustard, Healthy Choice	260		21.0	40.0	4.0	4.0		0				550	20			
9.5 oz entree	269	2.0	0.0			30	1500							.36		I
chicken imperial, Healthy Choice	230		17.0	31.0	2.0	3.0		9				470	20			
9 oz entree	255	4.0	1.0			50	750							1.44		I
chicken in herb sce, Lean Cuisine	260		23.0	19.0				2	.34			840	100			
9.5 oz entree	269	10.0	3.0		2.0	80	1250	.15	8.0			460		1.08		I
chicken italienne, Stouffers	85	93.8	9.3	4.4				8	.10			452	25			
4 oz entree[14]	113	3.4				23	294	.05	1.9			215		.68		I
chicken kiev, Le Menu	491		18.1	33.6				2	.16			777	44			
8 oz entree	227	31.6					1611	.15	7.3			236		1.20		I
chicken king pao, Green Giant	161		11.0	12.0				10	.03			253	24			
5 oz[15]	142	7.0	1.0		2.0	22	3210	.04	4.7			240	144	.80		I
chicken, mandarin, Healthy Choice	280		20.0	44.0	9.0	4.0		15				520	20			
10 oz entree	284	2.5	0.0			35	1500							.72		I
chicken marsala, Lean Cuisine	190		25.0	11.0				9	.17			850	20			
8.1 oz entree	230	5.0	1.0		1.0	75	1500	.15	8.0			400		1.08		I
chicken mexicali, Stouffers	119	144.5	8.3	10.7		2.0		41	.15			289	69			
6 oz entree[16]	170	4.9	0.8	1.3	0.9	29	1722	.10	3.4			410		1.07		I
chicken nibbles & french fried	324		11.2	27.6				3	.12			719	28			
potatoes, Swanson—4.3 oz entree	121	18.8					0	.14	3.5			316		1.70		I
chicken nuggets & french fried	291		12.9	29.6				0	.10			555	21			
potatoes, Swanson—4.8 oz entree	135	13.4					39	.15	4.9			384		1.50		I
chicken oriental, Lean Cuisine	240		23.0	23.0				15	.26			1050	60			
9.4 oz entree	266	6.0	1.0		2.0	100	200	.15	8.0			400		1.80		I
chicken parmesan, Lean Cuisine	250		25.0	19.0				6	.26			850	150			
10 oz entree	283	8.0	2.0		2.0	70	500	.23	7.0			750		1.44		I
chicken parmigiana & pasta alfredo,	360		31.0	24.0								750				
Stouffers—9.8 oz entree	279	15.0										990				I
chicken parmigiana, pasta, & veg w/	434	298.9	19.2	54.5	6.3	6.3		13				908	93			
cheese sce, Tyson—14 oz entree	392	15.4	3.6	5.0	4.3	26	1706							2.00		I
chicken primavera, Stouffers	66	98.3	6.7	4.6				8	.09			452	17			
4 oz entree[17]	113	2.3				17	1017	.05	1.2			158		.57		I
chicken, sesame, Healthy Choice	240		16.0	38.0	9.0	3.0		12				600	20			
9.75 oz entree	276	3.0	0.5			30	1750							.72		I
chicken, sweet & sour, Green Giant	180		8.0	30.0				14	.03			235	15			
5 oz[18]	142	3.0	0.6		1.0	21	553	.03	3.5			178	80	.60		I
chili & cornbread, Marie Callender's	350		14.0	45.0	13.0	5.0		4				1380	60			
1 cup &1.5 oz cornbread	227	13.0	6.0			30	0							1.08		I
chili, chopped beef, Stouffers	111	63.8	7.7	5.2				7	.10			357	16			
3 oz entree	85	6.6				26	425	.03	1.5			230		1.11		I
chili con carne w/ beans, Stouffers	259	170.9	20.7	21.8				18	.27			897	93			
8 oz entree	227	9.8				50	738	.16	3.2			704		3.41		I
chili, three bean (meatless), Stouffers	125	139.6	6.1	18.9		5.1		8	.19			517	89			
6 oz entree	170	2.7	0.6	0.8	1.0	3	675	.10	1.5			536		2.04		I
chow mein, chicken, Lean Cuisine	250		14.0	36.0				15	.17			1030	40			
11.3 oz entree	319	5.0	1.0		1.0	30	100	.15	4.0			270		1.08		I
chow mein, veg, Stouffers	51	101.7	1.2	5.9				15	.06			576	16			
4 oz[19]	113	2.5					113	.01	0.3			90		.23		I
corn fritters, Mrs. Paul's	273		5.7	32.6				0	.12			512	27			
2 fritters	113	13.3				9	106	.16	1.4			98		1.40		I

	KCAL / WT (g)	H_2O (g) / FAT (g)	PRO (g) / SFA (g)	CHO (g) / MUFA (g)	SUGR (g) / PUFA (g)	DFIB (g) / CHOL (mg)	A (RE) / A (IU)	C (mg) / B-1 (mg)	B-2 (mg) / NIA (mg)	B-6 (mg) / B-12 (mcg)	FOL (mcg) / PANT (mg)	Na (mg) / K (mg)	Ca (mg) / P (mg)	Mg (mg) / Fe (mg)	Zn (mg) / Cu (mg)	Mn (mg) / REF
egg rolls																
chicken, Chun King	170		7.0	25.0	4.0	4.0	1					450	20			
3 oz egg roll	85	5.0	2.5			10	1000							1.08		I
chicken, Jeno's Snacks	217	50.0	5.5	25.0				7	.20			416	17			
3.5 oz	100	10.4					155	.30	2.8			135	76	2.50		I
chicken, LaChoy	170		7.0	25.0	4.0	4.0	1					450	20			
3 oz egg roll	85	5.0	2.5			10	1000							1.08		I
chicken, mini, Chun King	170		6.0	22.0	2.0	2.0	0					570	20			
5 egg rolls (2.9 oz)	82	6.0	1.5			10	750							1.08		I
chicken, mini, LaChoy	180		7.0	26.0	2.0	3.0	1					550	20			
6 egg rolls (2.9 oz)	82	5.0	1.5			10	750							1.08		I
chinese veg & lobster, mini, LaChoy	410		13.0	65.0	6.0	9.0	4					690	40			
14 egg rolls (7.25 oz)	206	11.0	2.5			0	100							1.80		I
meat & shrimp, Jeno's Snacks	240	54.0	6.3	25.0				3	.12			494	20			
3.5 oz	100	12.6					65	.20	2.0			145	65	1.60		I
pork & shrimp, bite size, LaChoy	240		8.0	31.0	2.0	3.0	4					350	20			
15 egg rolls (3.75 oz)	106	9.0	2.0			10	100							1.08		I
pork & shrimp, mini, Chun King	420		11.0	56.0	3.0	6.0	6					500	40			
12 egg rolls (7.25 oz)	206	16.0	4.0			25	200							1.08		I
pork & shrimp, mini, LaChoy	430		15.0	65.0	10.0	7.0	0					890	40			
14 egg rolls (7.25 oz)	206	12.0	3.0			15	200							2.70		I
pork & shrimp, mini, LaChoy	160		6.0	26.0	2.0	3.0	0					580	20			
5 egg rolls (2.9 oz)	82	3.5	1.0			5	750							1.08		I
pork, Chun King	170		6.0	23.0	6.0	3.0	0					390	20			
3 oz egg roll	85	6.0	1.5			5	400							1.44		I
pork, LaChoy	170		6.0	23.0	6.0	3.0	0					390	20			
3 oz egg roll	85	6.0	1.5			5	250							1.44		I
shrimp & cheese, Jeno's Snacks	221	55.0	7.8	26.0				9	.12			346	53			
3.5 oz	100	9.5					321	.18	2.1			183	100	1.80		I
shrimp, Chun King	150		6.0	24.0	6.0	3.0	0					420	40			
3 oz egg roll	85	4.0	0.5			10	200							1.44		I
shrimp, LaChoy	150		6.0	24.0	6.0	3.0	0					420	40			
3 oz egg roll	85	4.0	0.5			10	200							1.44		I
shrimp, mini, LaChoy	170		6.0	28.0	2.0	2.0	0					530	20			
6 egg rolls (2.9 oz)	82	3.5	1.0			5	750							1.08		I
sweet & sour chicken, LaChoy	180		6.0	29.0	10.0	3.0	2					300	20			
3 oz egg roll	85	4.0	1.0			5	100							1.44		I
enchanada, beef & bean, Lean Cuisine	280		15.0	32.0				6	.34			890	150			
9.2 oz entree[20]	262	10.0	2.0		1.0	60	1000	.23	3.0			420		2.70		I
enchanada, chicken, Lean Cuisine	270		17.0	31.0				6	.34			850	150			
9.9 oz[21]	280	9.0	2.0		2.0	65	1250	.23	3.0			410		2.70		I
enchiladas																
beef, Patio	200		5.0	31.0	1.0	5.0	1					740	100			
2 w/ sce (5.7 oz)	161	6.0	3.0			10	250							1.44		I
cheese, Patio	170		6.0	26.0	3.0	4.0	1					880	100			
2 enchiladas (5.7 oz)	161	4.0	2.0			10	400							.72		I
chicken, Le Menu Lightstyle	268		19.1	33.2				11	.38			537	215			
8.25 oz entree	234	6.6	2.0		1.9	33	344	.11	3.2			624		1.80		I
chicken suiza, Healthy Choice	270		14.0	43.0	4.0	5.0	2					440	150			
10 oz entree	284	4.0	2.0			25	300							1.08		I
fajita, chicken fiesta, Healthy Choice	260		21.0	36.0	6.0	5.0	36					410	20			
7 oz entree	198	4.0	1.0			30	750							1.80		I
fettucini																
alfredo, Healthy Choice	250		11.0	39.0	4.0	3.0	0					480	150			
8 oz entree	227	5.0	2.0			15	0							1.44		I
primavera, Garden Gourmet Microwave	258	209.8	16.7	25.0		5.7		41	.30			635	269			
9.5 oz	269	12.9					1154	.12	1.6			280	412	2.88		I
primavera w/ tortellini, Marie	310		10.0	25.0	2.0	2.0	15					380	80			
Callender's—1 cup (7 oz)	198	19.0	8.0			50	300							.72		I

	KCAL / WT (g)	H₂O (g) / FAT (g)	PRO (g) / SFA (g)	CHO (g) / MUFA (g)	SUGR (g) / PUFA (g)	DFIB (g) / CHOL (mg)	A (RE) / A (IU)	C (mg) / B-1 (mg)	B-2 (mg) / NIA (mg)	B-6 (mg) / B-12 (mcg)	FOL (mcg) / PANT (mg)	Na (mg) / K (mg)	Ca (mg) / P (mg)	Mg (mg) / Fe (mg)	Zn (mg) / Cu (mg)	Mn (mg) / REF
w/ broccoli & chicken, Marie Callender's	410		18.0	32.0	0.0	4.0		9				550	150			
1 cup (6.5 oz)	184	24.0	10.0			45	300							1.44		I
fettucini alfredo & garlic bread, Marie	460		14.0	39.0	2.0	2.0		2				590	150			
Callender's—1 cup & 1 oz bread	198	27.0	10.0			45	750							1.80		I
fillet of fish																
divan, Lean Cuisine	270		31.0	17.0				30	.34			700	200			
12.3 oz entree	350	9.0	2.0		1.0	90	750	.23	2.0			850		1.08		I
florentine, Lean Cuisine	240		27.0	13.0				0	.26			700	150			
9 oz entree	255	9.0	2.0		2.0	100	750	.15	2.0			600		1.08		I
jardiniere, Lean Cuisine	280		30.0	18.0				0	.26			840	200			
11.2 oz entree	318	10.0	4.0		0.0	100	1000	.09	2.0			850		.36		I
fish 'n chips, Swanson	363		14.0	39.4				5	.15			694	35			
6.5 oz entree	184	16.5				0		.18	2.8			539		2.10		I
green pepper steak, beef, Stouffers	86	67.2	7.7	3.8				7	.09			527	14			
3 oz entree[22]	85	4.4				19	136	.04	1.5			170		.85		I
green pepper, stuffed w/ beef, rice,	192	181.2	10.2	18.6				13	.15			1072	33			
& sce, Stouffers—7.8 oz	221	8.6				22	398	.13	2.7			398		1.55		I
green pepper, stuffed w/ beef, Stouffers	114	84.2	7.5	10.2				43	.11			497	16			
3.8 oz entree	108	4.9				24	97	.11	1.8			184		1.40		I
ham & cheese casserole, Pillsbury	179	66.3	6.8	12.9		1.0		7	.17			494	75			
Microwave Classic—3.5 oz	100	11.0					710	.19	1.6			156	103	1.10		I
Heartland Medley, Stouffers	132	195.2	11.4	14.3		2.3		4	.16			194	41			
8 oz entree[23]	227	3.4	0.6	0.8	0.7	26	2238	.11	2.3			479		1.43		I
lasagna																
extra cheese, Marie Callender's	330		15.0	32.0	8.0	4.0		1				770	200			
1 cup (7.5 oz)	213	16.0	8.0			32	300							.72		I
garden veg, Le Menu Lightstyle	252		12.4	34.0				44	.39			462	174			
10.5 oz entree	298	7.4	2.7		1.5	24	1838	.23	2.8			531		2.80		I
primavera, Marie Callender's	260		17.0	22.0	8.0	3.0		0				1030	60			
1 cup (6.5 oz)	184	12.0	5.0			90	2500							1.44		I
roma, Healthy Choice	390		26.0	60.0	11.0	9.0		6				580	150			
13.5 oz entree	383	5.0	2.0			15	500							3.60		I
tuna, Lean Cuisine	280		19.0	28.0				4	.34			990	250			
9.7 oz entree	276	10.0	2.0		2.0	25	3000	.15	4.0			440		1.44		I
veg, Stouffers	338	158.9	19.3	28.1				2	.39			658	454			
8 oz entree	227	16.6				39	2270	.14	0.9			250		.91		I
verde, Stouffers	336	161.2	21.1	21.1					.36			1044	363			
8 oz entree[24]	227	18.6				45	1135	.11	3.6			295		.91		I
w/ meat sce, Banquet Family	230		12.0	29.0	1.0	3.0		60				530	150			
1 cup (7 oz)	198	8.0	4.0			35	100							1.44		I
w/ meat sce, Le Menu Lightstyle	288		18.6	36.1				19	.29			506	168			
10 oz entree	284	7.7	2.3		1.1	30	1309	.19	5.0			624		3.60		I
w/ meat sce, Lean Cuisine	280		27.0	24.0				5	.43			1000	250			
10.3 oz entree	291	8.0	3.0		0.0	70	2000	.90	4.0			540		1.44		I
w/ meat sce, Marie Callender's	370		17.0	34.0	8.0	4.0		4				740	300			
1 cup (7.5 oz)	213	18.0	9.0			35	500							2.70		I
w/ meat sce, Stouffers	302	163.4	22.2	27.2				5	.30			885	272			
8 oz entree	227	11.8				34	409	.11	2.0			363		1.36		I
w/ meat sce, Swanson	395		25.9	39.3				8	.33			1074	498			
10.5 oz entree	298	15.0					1024	.26	2.8			479		3.00		I
zucchini, Healthy Choice	330		20.0	58.0	11.0	11.0		0				310	200			
13.5 oz entree	383	1.5	1.0			10	1250							2.70		I
zucchini, Lean Cuisine	260		21.0	28.0				6	.26			975	300			
11 oz entree	311	7.0	2.0		0.0	20	2500	.12	2.0			600		1.80		I
linguini w/ clam sce, Lean Cuisine	260		16.0	32.0				0	.10			800	20			
9.6 oz entree	272	7.0	1.0		2.0	30	0	.06	1.2			100		1.80		I
linguini w/ shrimp & clams, Mrs. Paul's	288		13.6	39.6				9	.12			603	34			
Light—10 oz entree	284	8.3					94	.12	1.7			94		3.00		I
macaroni & beef w/ cheese topping,	265		19.8	25.6				33	.29			1114	165			
Swanson—9 oz entree	255	9.2					296	.11	5.2			517		2.90		I

Item	KCAL / WT (g)	H₂O (g) / FAT (g)	PRO (g) / SFA (g)	CHO (g) / MUFA (g)	SUGR (g) / PUFA (g)	DFIB (g) / CHOL (mg)	A (RE) / A (IU)	C (mg) / B-1 (mg)	B-2 (mg) / NIA (mg)	B-6 (mg) / B-12 (mcg)	FOL (mcg) / PANT (mg)	Na (mg) / K (mg)	Ca (mg) / P (mg)	Mg (mg) / Fe (mg)	Zn (mg) / Cu (mg)	Mn (mg) / REF
macaroni & beef w/ tomato sce, Stouffers	187	130.9	10.4	16.2				14	.15			918	32			
6 oz entree	170	9.0				26	408	.01	2.6			315		1.70		I
macaroni & cheese																
Banquet Family	210		8.0	33.0	7.0	4.0		0				1290	100			
1 cup (7 oz)	198	5.0	2.0			10	100							1.08		I
Healthy Choice	290		15.0	45.0	13.0	4.0		0				580	300			
9 oz entree	255	5.0	2.0			15	0							1.08		I
Morton	230		9.0	40.0	1.0	3.0		0				1000	100			
1 cup (8 oz)	227	4.0	2.0			5	500							1.44		I
Pillsbury	230		9.0	28.0								590				
5.75 oz entree	163	9.0	4.0			25						170				I
Stouffers	258	119.0	11.4	23.8				0	.34			714	241			
6 oz	170	13.1				24	119	.17	1.0			128		.85		I
Swanson Homestyle	388		17.2	37.3				1	.29			1119	456			
10 oz entree	284	18.9					140	.23	1.0			136		2.10		I
Swanson Microwavable	188		7.9	23.1				1	.20			739	151			
6 oz entree	170	7.1					382	.11	1.1			102		1.60		I
manicotti, 3 cheese w/ tomato sce,	394		20.0	44.3				17	.38			871	493			
Le Menu—11.7 oz entree	333	15.2					110	.28	4.0			401		3.10		I
manicotti w/ 3 cheeses, Healthy Choice	260		16.0	40.0	7.0	5.0		0				450	350			
11 oz entree	312	4.5	2.0			25	750							1.80		I
meatball stew, Lean Cuisine	250		21.0	20.0				4	.34			1120	40			
10 oz entree	283	10.0	3.0		1.0	75	1500	.30	4.0			440		2.70		I
meatballs																
italian style, Swanson	483		24.5	60.4				16	.39			935	148			
13 oz entree	369	15.9					1679	.33	4.9			645		5.70		I
swedish, Healthy Choice	280		22.0	35.0	4.0	4.0		0				590	100			
9.1 oz entree	258	9.0	2.5			60	0							2.70		I
swedish, Le Menu Lightstyle	264		18.3	31.2				0	.27			682	93			
8.5 oz entree	241	7.3	2.8		1.8	40	1045	.25	4.4			438		3.20		I
swedish & noodles, Swanson	346		18.3	25.3				1	.17			764	84			
8.5 oz entree	241	19.0					420	.16	4.1			459		3.10		I
meatloaf & gravy w/ mashed potatoes,	540		23.0	44.0	9.0	7.0		5				1230	40			
Marie Callender's—14 oz	397	30.0	11.0			80	200							1.08		I
meatloaf, beef, Stouffers	155	53.6	14.5	6.5				0	.17			578	20			
3 oz entree	85	7.8				44	68	.09	2.3			204		1.96		I
meatloaf w/ gravy & whipped	360		20.0	26.0								970				
potatoes, Stouffers—9.8 oz entree	279	20.0														I
meatloaf w/ gravy, Banquet	160		10.0	8.0	1.0	1.0		0				620	0			
1 patty (4.7 oz)	132	10.0	4.5			35	0							1.08		I
noodles & beef w/ brown gravy, Banquet	290		12.0	30.0	2.0	2.0		0				1270	40			
Family—1 cup (7 oz)	198	14.0	4.0			40	0							1.20		I
noodles, escalloped & chicken, Marie	270		10.0	22.0	2.0	1.0		2				670	40			
Callender's—1 cup (6.5 oz)	184	16.0	6.0			20	300							.72		I
noodles romanoff, Stouffers	130	59.5	5.4	11.1				0	.14			544	70			
3 oz entree[25]	85	7.1				14	102	.08	0.5			77		.51		I
pasta																
Callender's Deluxe, Marie Callender's	450		15.0	35.0	1.0	4.0		0				680	150			
1 cup (6.5 oz)	184	27.0	12.0			80	200							1.80		I
dijon, Garden Gourmet Microwave	296	215.2	7.0	23.9	2.7			58	.16			568	72			
9.5 oz	269	20.2					516	.13	1.8			285	116	1.08		I
florentine, Garden Gourmet Microwave	230		14.0	27.0								840				
9.5 oz	269	9.0	5.0		1.0	25						290				I
marinara, Pillsbury	180		5.0	29.0								730				
6 oz entree	170	5.0			1.0	0						340				I
parmesan w/ sweet peas, Pillsbury	170		9.0	24.0								510				
5.5 oz entree	156	5.0	2.0		0.0	10						160				I
penne w/ pork & tomato sce, Healthy	230		9.0	36.0	3.0	5.0		0				490	40			
Choice—8 oz entree	227	5.0	1.0			10	500							1.80		I

	KCAL	H₂O (g)	PRO (g)	CHO (g)	SUGR (g)	DFIB (g)	A (RE)	C (mg)	B-2 (mg)	B-6 (mg)	FOL (mcg)	Na (mg)	Ca (mg)	Mg (mg)	Zn (mg)	Mn (mg)
	WT (g)	FAT (g)	SFA (g)	MUFA (g)	PUFA (g)	CHOL (mg)	A (IU)	B-1 (mg)	NIA (mg)	B-12 (mcg)	PANT (mg)	K (mg)	P (mg)	Fe (mg)	Cu (mg)	REF
primavera w/ chicken, Marie Callender's	340		12.0	27.0	3.0	3.0		21				520	100			
1 cup (7.5 oz)	213	20.0	8.0			40	3000							1.80		I
roma, Stouffers	204	180.5	12.7	24.7		10.2		11	.30			627	103			
8 oz entree[26]	227	5.9				24	692		3.6			477		2.72		I
w/ cheddar cheese seasoning, Pasta Accents—½ cup	95	55.2	3.6	11.3		1.5		13	.10			245	80			
	76	4.6	2.0			5	1417	.08	1.0			125	114	.68		I
w/ garlic seasoning, Pasta Accents ½ cup	99	54.1	2.4	14.0		1.5		15	.07			217	35			
	76	4.3	2.0			5	1352	.06	0.9			124	49	1.14		I
w/ lemon butter seasoning, Pasta Accents—½ cup	76	57.9	2.4	11.8		1.7		20	.08			201	25			
	76	2.8					1293	.11	1.2			112	40	.52		I
w/ parmesan cheese, Pasta Accents ½ cup	94	54.7	3.3	12.7		1.6		7	.11			220	55			
	76	4.0					285	.09	1.0			99	55	.68		I
w/ sour cream & herb seasoning, Pasta Accents—½ cup	111	53.2	3.0	12.5		1.1		11	.12			263	65			
	76	5.9					1071	.10	1.1			144	61	.61		I
w/ southwestern seasoning, Pasta Accents—½ cup	86	59.6	2.2	8.0		0.8		22	.08			111	38			
	76	5.3					368	.05	0.9			144	48	.53		I
peppercorn steak patty, grilled, Healthy Choice—9 oz entree	220		16.0	26.0	1.0	5.0		27				470	60			
	255	6.0	2.5			30	200							1.80		I
pot pie, beef																
Banquet	330		9.0	38.0	2.0	3.0		0				1000	20			
7 oz pie	198	15.0	7.0			25	750							1.08		I
Swanson	364		12.1	36.0				2	.24			708	25			
7 oz pie	198	19.0					1445	.28	3.5			203		2.80		I
Swanson Chunky	575		20.1	58.1				2	.40			932	30			
10 oz pie	284	29.2					3242	.39	6.0			248		4.20		I
Swanson Hungry-Man	610		24.3	58.7				5	.49			1363	40			
14 oz pie	397	30.9					3009	.49	6.6			428		5.30		I
pot pie, chicken																
& broccoli, Marie Callender's	780		18.0	88.0	13.0	3.0		2				1030	80			
10 oz pie	284	48.0	16.0			20	200							3.60		I
au gratin, Marie Callender's	720		19.0	53.0	5.0	4.0		2				1040	150			
10 oz pie	284	48.0	13.0			25	200							2.70		I
Banquet	350		10.0	36.0	2.0	3.0		0				950	200			
7 oz pie	198	18.0	7.0			40	1000							1.08		I
broccoli & cheese, Tyson	591	145.4	17.4	47.5	1.7	2.1		3				1269	14			
9 oz pie	252	36.8	9.8	12.8	3.3	30	247							3.36		I
Marie Callender's	680		1.0	54.0	5.0	3.0		2				920	40			
10 oz pie	284	44.0	9.0			30	100							1.80		I
Swanson	379		11.1	34.9				2	.24			737	32			
7 oz pie	198	21.7					2035	.28	3.7			161		2.20		I
Swanson Chunky	596		19.5	56.7				1	.34			945	44			
10 oz pie	284	32.4					4324	.41	6.2			209		3.20		I
Swanson Deluxe	412		15.2	40.4				4	.30			1023	50			
9 oz pie	255	21.0					1914	.28	5.6			251		2.70		I
Swanson Hungry-Man	637		23.5	57.2				1	.42			1455	64			
14 oz pie	397	34.9					3812	.45	7.5			333		4.10		I
Tyson	567	152.7	13.6	45.8	2.1	1.5		1				856	42			
9 oz pie	252	36.6	8.3	13.0	4.2	23	1233							2.73		I
pot pie, macaroni & cheese, Banquet	200		7.0	35.0	2.0	2.0		0				600	100			
6.5 oz pie	184	3.0	1.5			10	0							1.08		I
pot pie, macaroni & cheese, Morton	200		7.0	35.0	2.0	2.0		0				600	100			
6.5 oz pie	184	3.0	1.5			10	0							1.08		I
pot pie, turkey																
Banquet	370		10.0	38.0	3.0	3.0		0				850	40			
7 oz pie	198	20.0	8.0			45	750							1.08		I
Marie Callender's	710		17.0	57.0		4.0		2				770	40			
10 oz pie	284	46.0	10.0			20	100							1.80		I
Swanson	381		10.9	36.1				2	.24			719	29			
7 oz pie	198	21.4					1967	.29	3.1			138		2.40		I

| | KCAL | H_2O (g) | PRO (g) | CHO (g) | SUGR (g) | DFIB (g) | A (RE) | C (mg) | B-2 (mg) | B-6 (mg) | FOL (mcg) | Na (mg) | Ca (mg) | Mg (mg) | Zn (mg) | Mn (mg) |
	WT (g)	FAT (g)	SFA (g)	MUFA (g)	PUFA (g)	CHOL (mg)	A (IU)	B-1 (mg)	NIA (mg)	B-12 (mcg)	PANT (mg)	K (mg)	P (mg)	Fe (mg)	Cu (mg)	REF
Swanson Chunky	589		19.5	54.6				1	.37			1011	39			
10 oz pie	284	32.5					4374	.41	5.4			186		3.20		I
Swanson Hungry-Man	649		23.9	57.0				4	.41			1454	57			
14 oz pie	397	36.2					3621	.43	6.5			295		4.30		I
Tyson	552	151.6	14.9	49.2	5.7	4.0	0					784	45			
9 oz pie	252	32.9	8.0	12.2	4.5	22	559							1.39		I
pot pie, veg																
cheese, Banquet	390		8.0	49.0	2.0	3.0	0					1000	80			
7 oz pie	198	18.0	8.0			15	1250							1.08		I
w/ beef, Morton	320		7.0	34.0	2.0	2.0	0					1380	20			
7 oz pie	198	17.0	8.0			15	500							1.08		I
w/ chicken, Morton	320		8.0	32.0	2.0	3.0	0					1020	40			
7 oz pie	198	18.0	7.0			25	500							1.08		I
w/ turkey, Morton	300		8.0	29.0	2.0	2.0	0					1060	40			
7 oz pie	198	18.0	9.0			25	500							1.08		I
pot pie, yankee, Marie Callender's	690		16.0	57.0	4.0	3.0		5				1390	40			
10 oz pie	284	44.0	10.0			25	100							1.80		I
ravioli, cheese																
Le Menu Lightstyle	259		13.5	37.6					.40			639	133			
8.75 oz entree	248	6.1	2.6		1.0	12	553	.33	3.3			505		2.50		I
Parmigiano, Healthy Choice	260		11.0	44.0	14.0	6.0	0					290	150			
9 oz entree	255	5.0	2.5			20	750							1.80		I
w/ tomato sce, Swanson	273		12.8	38.7				9	.24			1017	219			
8.75 oz entree	248	7.5					997	.23	3.4			354		2.40		I
ravioli, cheese in marinara sce																
w/ spirals & garlic sce, Marie Callender's	370		14.0	47.0	3.0	4.0		1				520	100			
1 cup & 1 oz bread	227	14.0	5.0			35	200							1.08		I
rigatoni parmigiana																
w/ soft breadstick, Marie Callender's	300		12.0	32.0	7.0	3.0	0					650	250			
1 cup & 1 oz breadstick	213	14.0	6.0			25	0							1.08		I
rigatoni w/ beef sce, Stouffers	180	130.9	11.7	17.0				9	.17			510	170			
6 oz entree	170	7.1				22	425	.15	2.2			357		1.70		I
rigatoni w/ meat sce, Lean Cuisine	260		18.0	25.0				6	.34			1040	250			
9.7 oz entree[27]	276	10.0	3.0		1.0	35	1250	.15	3.0			470		2.70		I
rotini cheddar, Garden Gourmet	282	215.2	10.0	33.1		2.7		37	.24			557	172			
Microwave—9.5 oz pkg	269	13.2					6375	.19	1.4			317	210	1.08		I
salisbury steak																
w/ brown gravy, Banquet Family	200		12.0	7.0	0.0	2.0	0					610	20			
1 patty w/ gravy (4.7 oz)	132	14.0	6.0			25	0							1.08		I
w/ gravy & macaroni & cheese, Stouffers	350		25.0	22.0								950				
8.6 oz entree	244	18.0														I
w/ gravy & mashed potatoes, Swanson	319		20.8	22.4				0	.30			980	53			
9 oz entree	255	16.2					0	.07	5.4			716		3.40		I
w/ gravy, Banquet	220		9.0	8.0	1.0	2.0		1				790	20			
5 oz entree	142	16.0	7.0			25	0							1.08		I
w/ gravy, Stouffers	241	124.1	17.0	10.2				0	.22			884	26			
6 oz entree	170	14.6				73	77	.12	2.9			255		2.38		I
w/ scalloped potatoes, Lean Cuisine	260		22.0	22.0				2	.34			800	100			
9.5 oz entree	269	9.0	2.0		0.0	85	500	.15	5.0					2.70		I
w/ sce & vegetables, Lean Cuisine	270		25.0	14.0				6	.26			700	150			
9.5 oz entree	269	13.0	5.0		1.0	95	500	.15	5.0			680		2.70		I
seafood casserole, Pillsbury	166	67.0	5.7	14.4		1.0		4	.10			372	103			
3.5 oz	100	9.2					497	.10	1.0			131	66	.90		I
shrimp & chicken cantonese, Lean Cuisine—10.1 oz entree	260		23.0	22.0				4	.26			970	60			
	287	9.0	1.0		3.0	105	750	.15	6.0			300		1.80		I
shrimp, breaded w/ angel hair pasta, Marie Callender's—1 cup (7.5 oz)	300		11.0	37.0	5.0	3.0		9				470	80			
	213	12.0	2.0			30	100							1.80		I

	KCAL	H₂O (g)	PRO (g)	CHO (g)	SUGR (g)	DFIB (g)	A (RE)	C (mg)	B-2 (mg)	B-6 (mg)	FOL (mcg)	Na (mg)	Ca (mg)	Mg (mg)	Zn (mg)	Mn (mg)
	WT (g)	FAT (g)	SFA (g)	MUFA (g)	PUFA (g)	CHOL (mg)	A (IU)	B-1 (mg)	NIA (mg)	B-12 (mcg)	PANT (mg)	K (mg)	P (mg)	Fe (mg)	Cu (mg)	REF
sirloin tips w/ noodles, Swanson	258		18.9	22.6				1	.25			567	30			
7 oz entree	198	10.2					739	.20	3.1			191		3.40		I
spaghetti & meat sce w/ garlic bread, Marie	260		11.0	32.0	5.0	3.0		4				570	60			
Callender's—*1 cup & 1 oz bread*	193	10.0	3.0			5	100							1.08		I
spaghetti, beef & mushrooms, Lean	280		15.0	38.0				6	.17			1140	60			
Cuisine—*11.5 oz entree*	326	7.0	2.0		1.0	25	500	.15	4.0			590		2.70		I
spaghetti marinara w/ cheese garlic bread,	270		10.0	35.0	5.0	3.0		15				540	80			
Marie Callender's—*1 cup & 1.4 oz bread*	227	10.0	3.0			10	300							1.08		I
spaghetti w/ beef sce, Healthy Choice	260		14.0	43.0	7.0	5.0		15				470	40			
10 oz entree	284	3.0	1.0			15	500							3.60		I
spaghetti w/ meat sce, Le Menu	284		12.6	44.6				32	.30			406	45			
Lightstyle—*9.5 oz entree*	269	6.1	1.2		1.3	14	732	.20	3.0			494		3.90		I
steak, chicken fried & gravy w/ mashed pota-	480		21.0	46.0	2.0	4.0		0				1960	100			
toes, Marie Callender's—*12 oz entree*	340	23.0	8.0			75	0							2.70		I
tortellini																
beef w/ egg pasta, Stouffers	238	78.1	15.4	25.6				1	.19			282	70			
4.5 oz entree	128	8.3				83	32	.10	2.2			147		1.66		I
beef w/ spinach pasta, Stouffers	252	75.5	16.6	25.6				1	.24			320	96			
4.5 oz entree	128	9.2				90	83	.10	2.3			192		1.66		I
cheese marinara, Pillsbury	260			8.0	37.0							930				
5.5 oz entree	156	9.0										310				I
cheese, Stouffers	268	73.0	15.4	26.9				1	.20			326	243			
4.5 oz entree	128	10.9				77	38	.09	1.2			95		1.02		I
cheese w/ spinach pasta, Stouffers	258	71.7	15.4	26.9				1	.27			396	294			
4.5 oz entree	128	11.8				90	115	.09	1.2			128		1.02		I
chicken, Stouffers	241	75.5	15.4	28.2				1	.22			282	36			
4.5 oz entree	128	7.4				81	448	.20	3.7			173		1.54		I
provencale, Garden Gourmet Microwave	210			7.0	36.0							720				
9.5 oz	269	5.0	1.0		1.0	15						550				I
w/ meat & cheese, Le Menu Lightstyle	256		12.8	35.5				37	.31			474	110			
8.25 oz entree	234	7.0	2.8		1.2	14	461	.26	3.2			532		2.60		I
tuna noodle casserole, Stouffers	194	130.9	11.4	15.8				0	.26			731	102			
6 oz entree[28]	170	9.4				27	68	.10	3.4			238		1.02		I
tuna noodle casserole, Swanson	259		13.4	33.5				1	.23			1043	113			
9 oz entree	255	7.9					297	.15	3.3			198		1.90		I
turkey																
& gravy w/ dressing, Marie Callender's	530		33.0	51.0	4.0	2.0		54				2030	100			
14 oz entree	397	17.0	7.0			85	400							3.60		I
& gravy w/ mashed potatoes, Marie Callen-	280		25.0	25.0	4.0	3.0		0				1080	60			
der's—*2 pieces turkey & ½ cup potatoes*	262	9.0	3.5			65	0							.36		I
breast w/ gravy & stuffing, Stouffers	300		22.0	24.0								990				
7.9 oz entree	223	13.0														I
casserole, Pillsbury Microwave Classic	168	67.0	8.1	12.3		1.0		3	.12			345	39			
3.5 oz	100	9.6					600	.08	2.3			160	91	1.40		I
country roast w/ mushrooms, Healthy	220		19.0	28.0	0.0	3.0		0				440	20			
Choice—*8.5 oz entree*	241	4.0	1.0			25	750							.72		I
dijon, Lean Cuisine	280		26.0	21.0				1	.26			820	100			
9.5 oz entree	269	10.0	3.0		1.0	65	4500	.15	6.0			470		1.08		I
dijon, Stouffers	190	130.9	16.0	11.9				2	.24			697	102			
6 oz entree[29]	170	8.7				39	1020	.12	4.1			306		.85		I
glazed, Le Menu Lightstyle	248		18.9	32.3				3	.24			605	23			
8.25 oz entree	234	4.7	0.9		2.0	29	300	.09	5.9			341		1.50		I
sliced w/ gravy, Banquet	140		8.0	6.0	0.0	9.0		0				670	20			
5 oz entree	142	9.0	4.0			30	0							.36		I
sliced w/ gravy, Banquet Family	150		12.0	8.0				2	.14			1010	31			
8 oz	227	8.0					45	.01	2.9					1.00		I
tetrazzini, Stouffers	238	125.8	11.9	15.5				0	.27			663	77			
6 oz entree[30]	170	14.3				43	51	.14	2.0			170		1.02		I
white meat w/ gravy & veg, Le Menu	203		21.5	19.6				40	.14			538	64			
10 oz entree	284	4.3	1.0		1.0	29	3703	.14	6.2			573		1.30		I

							Vitamins					Minerals				
	KCAL	H_2O (g)	PRO (g)	CHO (g)	SUGR (g)	DFIB (g)	A (RE)	C (mg)	B-2 (mg)	B-6 (mg)	FOL (mcg)	Na (mg)	Ca (mg)	Mg (mg)	Zn (mg)	Mn (mg)
	WT (g)	FAT (g)	SFA (g)	MUFA (g)	PUFA (g)	CHOL (mg)	A (IU)	B-1 (mg)	NIA (mg)	B-12 (mcg)	PANT (mg)	K (mg)	P (mg)	Fe (mg)	Cu (mg)	REF
w/ gravy	95	120.8	8.3	6.5		0.0	18	0	.18	.14	6	787	20	11	.99	.007
5 oz entree	142	3.7	1.2	1.4	0.7	26	60	.03	2.6	.34	.30	87	115	1.32	.031	805
w/ gravy & dressing, Lean Cuisine	240		20.0	26.0				0	.26			720	40			
7.8 oz entree	222	6.0	1.0		1.0	45	0	.23	8.0					1.44		I
w/ gravy, dressing, & potatoes, Swanson	279		17.8	29.0				4	.20			995	46			
9 oz entree	255	10.2					19	.15	6.9			444		2.20		I
w/ mushroom sce, Lean Cuisine	220		24.0	20.0				2	.26			750	20			
8 oz entree	226	5.0	2.0		1.0	50	500	.09	8.0			350		.72		I
veal parmigiana																
& pasta alfredo, Stouffers	350		28.0	26.0								1060				
9.2 oz entree	262	15.0														I
& spaghetti in tomato sce, Swanson	322		19.0	33.5				9	.27			963	104			
10 oz entree	284	12.4					568	.22	5.3			386		3.20		I
Le Menu Lightstyle	174		21.9	9.0					.40			636	79			
8.25 oz entree	234	5.5	2.7		0.6	97	335	.11	5.3			615		3.20		I
patties w/ tomato sce, Banquet Family	230		9.0	19.0	2.0	2.0		54				740	40			
1 patty w/ sce (4 oz)	113	14.0	4.0			20	200							.60		I

10.6 FROZEN MEALS FOR CHILDREN

	KCAL	H_2O (g)	PRO (g)	CHO (g)	SUGR (g)	DFIB (g)	A (RE)	C (mg)	B-2 (mg)	B-6 (mg)	FOL (mcg)	Na (mg)	Ca (mg)	Mg (mg)	Zn (mg)	Mn (mg)
Big League hamburger pizza, Kid Cuisine—8.3 oz meal	400		14.0	61.0	28.0	6.0		6				530	100			
	235	11.0	3.5			25	200							1.80		I
Buckaroo beef patty & cheese sandwich, Kid Cuisine—8.5 oz meal	410		12.0	58.0	27.0	4.0		0				540	150			
	241	15.0	5.0			15	100							1.80		I
Circus Show corn dog, Kid Cuisine 8.8 oz meal	450		8.0	70.0	46.0	5.0		12				750	80			
	249	15.0	4.5			20	0							1.80		I
Cosmic chicken nuggets, Kid Cuisine 9.1 oz meal	440		18.0	54.0	12.0	5.0		0				1070	100			
	258	16.0	4.5			30	0							1.80		I
Funtastic fish nuggets, Kid Cuisine 8.25 oz meal	370		11.0	55.0	21.0	4.0		0				550	60			
	234	12.0	2.5			15	0							1.44		I
High Flying fried chicken, Kid Cuisine 10.1 oz meal	440		18.0	49.0	12.0	5.0		0				940	80			
	286	19.0	4.5			40	0							1.44		I
Magical macaroni & cheese, Kid Cuisine 10.6 oz meal	410		10.0	63.0	27.0	5.0		0				840	100			
	301	13.0	5.0			15	500							1.08		I
Pirate cheese pizza, Kid Cuisine 8 oz meal	430		12.0	71.0	34.0	5.0		0				440	150			
	227	11.0	3.0			20	100							1.80		I
Raptor cheese ravioli, Kid Cuisine 9.82 oz meal	310		7.0	59.0	30.0	5.0		6				730	40			
	278	5.0	2.0			2	500							1.08		I
Rip-Roaring macaroni & beef, Kid Cuisine—9.6 oz meal	370		12.0	58.0	23.0	5.0		0				900	100			
	272	9.0	4.0			30	100							1.44		I

10.7 FROZEN PIZZA

	KCAL	H_2O (g)	PRO (g)	CHO (g)	SUGR (g)	DFIB (g)	A (RE)	C (mg)	B-2 (mg)	B-6 (mg)	FOL (mcg)	Na (mg)	Ca (mg)	Mg (mg)	Zn (mg)	Mn (mg)
bacon, Totino's Party	371	70.3	10.5	34.6				4	.27			1035	217			
5 oz (½ pizza)	142	19.9					403	.37	3.6			223	317	2.56		I
canadian bacon																
Jeno's Crisp 'n Tasty	253	57.0	10.9	27.3				5	.19			876	168			
3.85 oz (½ pizza)	109	11.3					239	.33	1.4			149	256	1.96		I
Top Frost	171	60.0	9.2	23.0				5	.17			688	154			
3.5 oz	100	4.5					209	.27	2.5			226	181	1.70		I
Totino's Party	315	79.8	13.1	34.8				4	.23			1154	203			
5.1 oz (½ pizza)	145	13.9					341	.36	3.2			220	280	2.46		I
cheese																
extra cheese, Lean Cuisine	350		21.0	39.0				15	.43			850	500			
5.5 oz	155	12.0	4.0		2.0	20	200	.45	3.0					3.60		I
Jeno's Crisp 'n Tasty	272	51.5	9.9	27.6				3	.21			770	196			
3.7 oz (½ pizza)	105	13.7					442	.21	2.1			141	277	1.58		I
Jeno's Snack Size	163	30.9	5.9	16.6				2	.13			462	118			
2.2 oz (¼ pkg)	63	8.3					265	.13	1.3			84	166	1.13		I

Food / Serving	KCAL / WT (g)	H₂O (g) / FAT (g)	PRO (g) / SFA (g)	CHO (g) / MUFA (g)	SUGR (g) / PUFA (g)	DFIB (g) / CHOL (mg)	A (RE) / A (IU)	C (mg) / B-1 (mg)	B-2 (mg) / NIA (mg)	B-6 (mg) / B-12 (mcg)	FOL (mcg) / PANT (mg)	Na (mg) / K (mg)	Ca (mg) / P (mg)	Mg (mg) / Fe (mg)	Zn (mg) / Cu (mg)	Mn (mg) / REF
Jeno's Snack Tray	243	52.0	8.8	21.0				5	.15			820	137			
3.5 oz	100	13.8					402	.20	2.3			228	155	1.80		I
John's	249	50.0	9.7	26.2				2	.17			630	212			
3.5 oz	100	12.0					222	.20	1.9			94	266	1.80		I
Lean Cuisine	310		17.0	39.0				6	.43			830	350			
5.1 oz	145	9.0	3.0		2.0	10	300	.45	3.0			300		3.60		I
Pillsbury Heat 'n Eat	269	54.2	12.8	31.3				5	.22			667	241			
4.1 oz	116	10.4					537	.16	1.7			202	204	1.16		I
Pillsbury Microwave	242	52.0	10.4	27.9				4	.16			539	194			
3.55 oz (½ pizza)	102	9.8					395	.13	1.5			157	162	1.33		I
three cheese, Totino's Pan Pizza	286	44.4	15.0	33.3				3	.20			505	286			
3.92 oz (⅙ pizza)	111	10.0					502	.14	1.7			174	242	1.44		I
Top Frost	197	56.3	8.8	24.2				3	.20			693	201			
3.5 oz	100	7.2					394	.19	1.8			217	224	1.70		I
Totino's Classic	205	45.2	9.6	22.2				3	.17			412	198			
3.12 oz (⅙ pizza)	87	8.9					330	.17	1.7			127	192	1.57		I
Totino's Crisp Crust Microwave	253	49.0	9.0	29.0				4	.19			685	150			
3.5 oz	100	11.2					446	.14	1.6			158	189	1.40		I
Totino's Extra	251	44.7	11.3	24.4				3	.19			461	229			
3.33 oz (¼ pizza)	94	12.2					451	.12	1.3			115	182	1.03		I
Totino's Microwave	250	55.0	10.6	33.7				1	.22			758	218			
3.9 oz	110	8.0					116	.33	2.6			308	231	2.31		I
Totino's Party	345	70.9	12.9	34.5				4	.28			1005	264			
4.9 oz (½ pizza)	139	17.5					595	.28	2.6			190	346	2.50		I
Totino's Slices	173	36.4	7.3	20.2				2	.13			351	127			
2.55 oz (⅙ pizza)	72	6.9					272	.11	1.1			88	112	.79		I

combination

Food / Serving	KCAL / WT (g)	H₂O (g) / FAT (g)	PRO (g) / SFA (g)	CHO (g) / MUFA (g)	SUGR (g) / PUFA (g)	DFIB (g) / CHOL (mg)	A (RE) / A (IU)	C (mg) / B-1 (mg)	B-2 (mg) / NIA (mg)	B-6 (mg) / B-12 (mcg)	FOL (mcg) / PANT (mg)	Na (mg) / K (mg)	Ca (mg) / P (mg)	Mg (mg) / Fe (mg)	Zn (mg) / Cu (mg)	Mn (mg) / REF
Jeno's Extra Topping	211	56.0	10.0	20.8				7	.18			709	155			
3.5 oz	100	9.7					400	.20	2.3			277	164	1.90		I
Jeno's Snack Size	180	33.0	7.1	16.9				1	.12			467	105			
2.4 oz (¼ pkg)	68	9.4					162	.14	1.6			108	157	1.43		I
Mr. P's	260	51.0	9.8	25.5				2	.17			641	122			
3.6 oz (½ pizza)	102	13.2					171	.26	2.4			148	202	2.14		I
Pappalo's Pan Pizza	336	51.7	16.6	33.8				3	.23			699	242			
4.42 oz (⅙ pizza)	126	14.5					481	.23	2.5			214	243	1.76		I
Pappalo's Thin Crust Pizza	258	43.1	12.9	28.1				4	.10			573	220			
3.67 oz (⅙ pizza)	104	10.2					433	.10	1.5			185	188	.94		I
Pillsbury Microwave	308	66.6	14.0	29.4				9	.23			781	196			
4.5 oz (½ pizza)	128	15.0					439	.24	2.4			200	205	1.66		I
Top Frost	200	56.0	9.7	22.8				5	.16			636	152			
3.5 oz	100	7.7					244	.20	2.2			234	178	2.00		I
Totino's Classic Deluxe	235	46.4	11.3	20.0				3	.18			539	177			
3.75 oz (⅙ pizza)	91	12.2					329	.27	2.0			177	196	1.55		I
Totino's Crisp Crust Microwave	263	49.0	10.2	25.0				3	.17			716	149			
3.5 oz	100	13.5					282	.21	1.9			158	194	1.50		I
Totino's Extra	269	34.8	10.1	23.0				3	.19			738	149			
3.33 oz (¼ pizza)	94	15.0					468	.19	1.9			185	170	1.50		I
Totino's Party	383	69.3	13.7	35.3				4	.10			1232	219			
5.25 oz (½ pizza)	149	20.9					408	.12	1.5			224	316	1.34		I

croissant crust pizza

Food / Serving	KCAL / WT (g)	H₂O (g) / FAT (g)	PRO (g) / SFA (g)	CHO (g) / MUFA (g)	SUGR (g) / PUFA (g)	DFIB (g) / CHOL (mg)	A (RE) / A (IU)	C (mg) / B-1 (mg)	B-2 (mg) / NIA (mg)	B-6 (mg) / B-12 (mcg)	FOL (mcg) / PANT (mg)	Na (mg) / K (mg)	Ca (mg) / P (mg)	Mg (mg) / Fe (mg)	Zn (mg) / Cu (mg)	Mn (mg) / REF
cheese, Pepperidge Farm	430		14.8	40.5				2	.24			639	330			
4.4 oz	125	23.2					337	.05	2.4			187		2.10		I
deluxe, Pepperidge Farm	438		15.8	43.2				1	.20			787	298			
5 oz[31]	142	22.4					182	.21	2.7			168		2.70		I
pepperoni, Pepperidge Farm	423		14.3	42.7				4	.23			689	256			
4.5 oz	128	21.7					309	.27	3.1			199		2.20		I
sausage, Pepperidge Farm	428		13.9	41.7				5	.23			718	268			
4.7 oz	135	22.9					215	.11	2.8			204		2.20		I
deluxe, Lean Cuisine	340		19.0	40.0				6	.43			1080	300			
6.1 oz	173	12.0	3.0		2.0	30	400	.53	5.0			370		3.60		I

	KCAL	H₂O (g)	PRO (g)	CHO (g)	SUGR (g)	DFIB (g)	A (RE)	C (mg)	B-2 (mg)	B-6 (mg)	FOL (mcg)	Na (mg)	Ca (mg)	Mg (mg)	Zn (mg)	Mn (mg)
	WT (g)	FAT (g)	SFA (g)	MUFA (g)	PUFA (g)	CHOL (mg)	A (IU)	B-1 (mg)	NIA (mg)	B 12 (mcg)	PANT (mg)	K (mg)	P (mg)	Fe (mg)	Cu (mg)	REF
french bread pizza																
cheese, Healthy Choice	320		22.0	51.0	4.0	7.0		0				410	400			
6 oz entree	170	3.0	1.0			5	200							4.50		I
cheese, Pappalo's	364	85.3	16.1	40.3				5	.29			832	325			
5.7 oz pizza	161	15.3					564	.32	2.9			198	237	1.93		I
cheese, Pillsbury Microwave	390	79.5	18.5	43.0				1	.21			708	309			
5.7 oz pizza	161	15.8					167	.40	2.7			274	250	2.21		I
cheese, Stouffers	341	75.0	14.7	41.2				15	.41			853	243			
5.2 oz pizza	147	13.1				18	441	.47	3.4			265		2.65		I
combination, Pappalo's	431	97.5	19.0	41.2				6	.29			1121	289			
6.5 oz pizza	184	20.6					569	.37	3.9			296	247	2.39		I
pepperoni, Healthy Choice	340		24.0	49.0	5.0	6.0		0				510	300			
6 oz entree	170	5.0	1.5			20	300							5.40		I
pepperoni, Pappalo's	411	86.7	16.5	40.8				5	.29			1134	241			
6 oz pizza	170	20.0					502	.34	3.7			255	201	2.21		I
pepperoni, Pillsbury Microwave	435	79.9	19.2	45.9				1	.24			944	253			
6 oz pizza	170	19.2					243	.46	5.4			342	218	2.89		I
pepperoni, Stouffers	407	77.9	17.5	41.3				16	.43			1113	215			
5.6 oz pizza	159	19.1				35	477	.52	4.5			318		2.86		I
sausage & pepperoni, Pillsbury	453	92.0	19.0	46.6				3	.24			955	243			
Microwave—6.5 oz pizza	184	21.0					232	.48	6.3			370	230	3.31		I
sausage, Healthy Choice	300		21.0	48.0	5.0	5.0		0				500	150			
6 oz pizza	170	3.0	1.0			25	200							2.70		I
sausage, Pillsbury Microwave	406	90.8	18.2	48.1				0	.36			1024	246			
6.3 oz pizza	178	15.7					206	.43	4.8			390	224	4.27		I
supreme, Healthy Choice	310		21.0	51.0	5.0	6.0		0				500	150			
6.35 oz entree	180	3.0	1.0			20	400							3.60		I
veg, Healthy Choice	270		17.0	45.0	5.0	5.0		0				370	300			
6 oz pizza	170	2.5	1.0			10	200							2.70		I
golden topping, Fox Deluxe	239	48.0	9.3	25.2				1	.16			605	204			
3.4 oz (½ pizza)	96	11.5					213	.19	1.8			90	255	1.73		I
golden topping, Mr. P's	239	48.0	9.3	25.2				1	.16			605	204			
3.4 oz (½ pizza)	96	11.5					213	.19	1.8			90	255	.77		I
ground beef/hamburger																
Fox Deluxe	264	55.1	11.4	26.5				2	.17			705	123			
3.8 oz (½ pizza)	108	12.4					150	.22	2.8			136	198	2.16		I
Jeno's Crisp 'n Tasty	296	57.5	11.8	27.6				2	.16			811	170			
4.05 oz (12 pizza)	115	15.4					239	.21	2.8			163	245	1.84		I
Jeno's Snack Size	180	35.2	8.0	17.0				1	.12			502	105			
2.5 oz (¼ pkg)	71	8.9					148	.13	1.8			100	152	1.42		I
Mr. P's	264	55.1	11.4	26.5				2	.17			705	123			
3.8 oz (½ pizza)	108	12.4					150	.22	2.8			136	198	2.16		I
Pappalo's Pan Pizza	312	52.7	17.4	33.5				3	.20			584	243			
4.38 oz (⅙ pizza)	124	11.7					481	.12	2.4			226	237	1.86		I
Pappalo's Thin Crust Pizza	241	52.0	13.5	28.1				4	.10			475	214			
3.67 oz (⅙ pizza)	104	8.1					413	.04	1.5			198	179	1.25		I
Top Frost	194	57.0	9.8	22.3				3	.16			646	145			
3.5 oz	100	7.0					207	.17	2.2			185	170	1.90		I
Totino's Crisp Crust Microwave	240	51.2	10.5	24.4				3	.16			712	134			
3.5 oz	100	11.0					266	.14	2.4			178	190	1.70		I
Totino's Party	372	79.5	14.7	35.3				4	.26			1056	201			
5.3 oz (½ pizza)	150	19.5					345	.30	3.6			221	300	3.00		I
mexican style, Totino's Party	381	64.2	13.1	35.5				10	.26			973	213			
5.1 oz (½ pizza)	145	20.3					421	.36	3.3			270	296	3.33		I
pepperoni																
Fox Deluxe	248	50.5	8.2	25.5				2	.16			636	121			
3.5 oz (½ pizza)	99	12.7					185	.27	2.3			116	187	1.98		I
Jeno's Crisp 'n Tasty	284	52.9	10.0	27.5				2	.18			759	172			
3.8 oz (½ pizza)	108	15.1					275	.22	2.5			144	243	2.16		I

	KCAL / WT (g)	H₂O (g) / FAT (g)	PRO (g) / SFA (g)	CHO (g) / MUFA (g)	SUGR (g) / PUFA (g)	DFIB (g) / CHOL (mg)	A (RE) / A (IU)	C (mg) / B-1 (mg)	B-2 (mg) / NIA (mg)	B-6 (mg) / B-12 (mcg)	FOL (mcg) / PANT (mg)	Na (mg) / K (mg)	Ca (mg) / P (mg)	Mg (mg) / Fe (mg)	Zn (mg) / Cu (mg)	Mn (mg) / REF
Jeno's Extra Topping	218	55.0	9.7	21.8				5	.19			811	160			
3.5 oz	100	10.3					370	.20	2.5			267	153	1.80		I
Jeno's Snack Size	170	31.9	6.0	16.6				1	.11			457	103			
2.3 oz (¼ pkg)	65	9.0					166	.13	1.5			86	146	1.30		I
Lean Cuisine	340		18.0	40.0				6	.43			970	250			
5.2 oz	148	12.0	4.0		2.0	25	300	.53	4.0			340		3.60		I
Mr. P's	248	50.5	8.2	25.5				2	.16			636	121			
3.5 oz (½ pizza)	99	12.7					185	.27	2.3			116	187	1.98		I
Pappalo's Pan Pizza	331	46.4	16.2	33.3				3	.21			706	240			
4.2 oz (⅙ pizza)	119	14.3					480	.17	2.3			219	225	1.67		I
Pappalo's Thin Crust Pizza	370		17.0	31.0		1.0						770				
3.67 oz (⅙ pizza)	104	20.0														I
Pillsbury Heat 'n Eat	346	58.1	13.4	31.2				5	.29			1070	217			
4.6 oz	130	18.2					673	.20	2.5			226	228	1.69		I
Pillsbury Microwave	302	60.2	13.4	29.0				9	.20			790	194			
4.24 oz (½ pizza)	120	14.4					439	.18	2.3			205	184	1.56		I
Top Frost	205	56.0	8.8	23.7				3	.17			736	159			
3.5 oz	100	8.3					262	.25	2.3			204	178	1.90		I
Totino's Classic Deluxe	263	49.0	12.0	23.2				4	.20			632	206			
3.52 oz (⅙ pizza)	100	13.5					341	.20	2.1			167	211	1.70		I
Totino's Crisp Crust Microwave	269	47.0	10.4	26.3				3	.16			788	151			
3.5 oz	100	13.7					290	.16	1.9			161	189	1.40		I
Totino's Extra	260	40.0	10.2	24.1				4	.19			686	159			
3.33 oz (¼ pizza)	94	13.7					507	.15	1.9			169	175	1.50		I
Totino's Microwave	283	54.5	10.2	33.6				5	.23			881	130			
4 oz	113	11.9					571	.23	2.5			315	163	1.70		I
Totino's Pan Pizza	352	49.1	17.1	35.7				3	.23			769	253			
4.43 oz (⅙ pizza)	126	15.1					491	.18	2.4			227	238	1.64		I
Totino's Party	371	72.5	13.2	35.4				4	.25			1311	209			
5.1 oz (½ pizza)	145	19.7					464	.29	3.3			181	306	2.90		I
Totino's Slices	193	37.2	6.8	20.3				3	.15			533	85			
2.63 oz (⅙ pizza)	75	9.3					317	.15	1.5			88	107	1.13		I
pizza rolls																
cheese, Jeno's	237	40.4	8.2	22.5				2	.26			347	162			
6 rolls (3 oz)	85	12.3					300	.26	2.6			94	179	2.38		I
hamburger, Jeno's	239	40.8	8.5	20.8				1	.23			275	60			
6 rolls (3 oz)	85	13.2					120	.30	3.0			74	119	2.47		I
pepperoni & cheese, Jeno's	232	41.7	6.6	21.8				6	.17			394	53			
6 rolls (3 oz)	85	12.8					275	.34	3.1			119	102	2.55		I
pepperoni & cheese, Jeno's Microwave	239	40.0	6.9	22.5				7	.26			435	54			
6 rolls (3 oz)	85	13.2					303	.34	3.1			132	110	2.64		I
sausage & cheese, Jeno's Microwave	246	38.3	7.8	23.6				7	.26			440	61			
6 rolls (3 oz)	85	13.1					314	.34	3.1			176	117	2.55		I
sausage & pepperoni, Jeno's	230	42.5	6.6	21.8				4	.17			378	42			
6 rolls (3 oz)	85	12.8					164	.34	3.1			111	88	2.72		I
sausage																
Fox Deluxe	259	51.0	10.2	25.7				2	.17			628	123			
3.6 oz (½ pizza)	102	13.0					165	.26	2.4			154	205	2.24		I
Jeno's Crisp 'n Tasty	300	47.1	10.7	27.8				3	.19			857	174			
3.8 oz (½ pizza)	111	16.3					255	.22	2.3			172	248	2.11		I
Jeno's Extra Topping	216	55.0	10.8	20.6				4	.18			707	172			
3.5 oz	100	10.0					373	.20	2.3			281	185	2.00		I
Jeno's Snack Size	180	32.6	7.3	16.9				1	.12			460	106			
2.4 oz (¼ pkg)	68	9.3					156	.14	1.6			113	160	1.50		I
Jeno's Snack Tray	236	53.0	9.0	21.0				5	.15			699	112			
3.5 oz	100	13.0					360	.20	2.2			247	129	1.70		I
John's	254	50.0	10.0	25.2				2	.17			616	121			
3.5 oz	100	12.7					162	.25	2.4			151	201	2.20		I
Lean Cuisine	330		21.0	40.0				6	.43			1040	300			
6 oz	170	10.0	3.0		1.0	30	300	.53	5.0			390		3.60		I

	KCAL	H_2O (g)	PRO (g)	CHO (g)	SUGR (g)	DFIB (g)	Vitamins A (RE)	C (mg)	B-2 (mg)	B-6 (mg)	FOL (mcg)	Minerals Na (mg)	Ca (mg)	Mg (mg)	Zn (mg)	Mn (mg)
	WT (g)	FAT (g)	SFA (g)	MUFA (g)	PUFA (g)	CHOL (mg)	A (IU)	B-1 (mg)	NIA (mg)	B-12 (mcg)	PANT (mg)	K (mg)	P (mg)	Fe (mg)	Cu (mg)	REF
Mr. P's	259	51.0	10.2	25.7				2	.17			628	123			
3.6 oz (½ pizza)	102	13.0					165	.26	2.4			154	205	2.24		I
Pappalo's Pan Pizza	357	49.0	13.9	33.5				3	.21			547	184			
4.38 oz (1/ 6 pizza)	124	18.4					414	.25	2.4			186	206	1.61		I
Pappalo's Thin Crust Pizza	251	44.5	12.7	28.9				4	.13			502	224			
3.67 oz (⅙ pizza)	106	9.1					461	.13	1.4			186	192	1.06		I
Pillsbury Heat 'n Eat	360	53.0	13.3	31.3				5	.27			1127	219			
4.8 oz	136	19.7					681	.26	2.3			262	241	1.90		I
Pillsbury Microwave	286	65.7	13.0	29.0				9	.22			689	193			
4.38 oz (½ pizza)	124	13.0					435	.25	2.2			182	201	1.61		I
Top Frost	197	57.0	9.5	23.0				3	.17			638	153			
3.5 oz	100	7.4					220	.20	2.2			243	180	2.00		I
Totino's Crisp Crust Microwave	257	49.4	9.8	25.0				3	.17			669	145			
3.5 oz	100	13.0					280	.20	1.9			157	192	1.50		I
Totino's Extra	279	34.1	9.8	24.3				4	.20			767	141			
3.45 oz (¼ pizza)	98	15.5					472	.20	2.0			202	166	1.57		I
Totino's Microwave	318	56.4	11.1	32.6				5	.24			870	132			
4.2 oz	119	15.9					534	.24	2.3			340	162	1.67		I
Totino's Pan Pizza	317	52.1	15.7	34.0				3	.22			629	242			
4.38 oz (⅙ pizza)	124	12.8					467	.24	1.9			193	244	1.74		I
Totino's Party	387	66.5	13.5	35.4				4	.26			1179	210			
5.3 oz (½ pizza)	150	21.5					365	.38	3.3			246	202	2.85		I
Totino's Slices	195	33.4	6.9	19.8				3	.15			543	84			
2.67 oz (16 pizza)	76	9.9					275	.15	1.4			118	104	1.06		I
sausage & pepperoni																
Fox Deluxe	260	51.0	9.8	25.5				2	.17			641	122			
3.6 oz (½ pizza)	102	13.2					171	.26	2.4			148	202	2.14		I
Jeno's Crisp 'n Tasty	297	48.8	10.5	27.8				3	.19			842	173			
3.9 oz (½ pizza)	111	16.1					263	.22	2.4			168	246	2.22		I
Pillsbury Heat 'n Eat	378	55.0	13.9	31.3				5	.28			1202	218			
4.9 oz	139	21.3					678	.25	2.6			270	243	1.95		I
Totino's Microwave	311	57.4	11.9	31.1				5	.23			971	140			
4.2 oz	119	15.5					562	.24	2.4			352	171	1.74		I
Totino's Pan Pizza	319	48.8	15.7	28.6				3	.21			685	228			
4.2 oz (⅙ pizza)	119	13.7					441	.21	2.3			198	230	1.67		I
Totino's Slices	195	35.9	6.8	19.8					.15	.14		629	90			
2.67 oz (⅙ pizza)	76	9.7					299	.14	1.4			106	109	1.14		I
vegetable, Totino's Party	304	88.5	10.6	36.0				13	.26			909	210			
5.35 oz (½ pizza)	152	13.4					523	.27	2.9			205	284	2.58		I

10.8 HOMEMADE ENTREES

	KCAL / WT	H_2O / FAT	PRO / SFA	CHO / MUFA	SUGR / PUFA	DFIB / CHOL	A (RE) / A (IU)	C / B-1	B-2 / NIA	B-6 / B-12	FOL / PANT	Na / K	Ca / P	Mg / Fe	Zn / Cu	Mn / REF
beef & veg stew	221	201.0	22.0	20.0		1.0		14	.25	.33	25	461	32	39	5.70	.265
1 cup[32]	252	5.2	1.8	2.1	0.3	60	6626	.18	3.6	1.53	.52	527	223	3.15	.263	806
beef, dried, chipped, ckd, creamed	377	176.4	20.1	17.4				1	.47			1754	257			
1 cup	245	25.2	13.7				880	.15	1.5			375	343	2.00		456
brunswick stew	232	191.7	26.6	17.3		1.0		14	.19	.39	21	438	39	43	2.09	.252
1 cup[33]	243	6.2	1.6	2.1	1.5	71	433	.13	6.6	.18	.90	509	183	1.97	.183	806
chicken a la king	468	167.1	27.4	12.3				12	.42			760	127			
1 cup	245	34.3	12.7				1130	.10	5.4			404	358	2.50		456
chicken & noodles	367	170.6	22.3	25.7				0	.17			600	26			
1 cup	240	18.5	5.9				430	.05	4.3			149	247	2.20		456
chicken fricassee	386	171.1	36.7	7.4					.17			370	14			
1 cup	240	22.3	7.2				170	.05	5.8			336	271	2.20		456
chop suey	300	188.5	26.0	12.8				33	.38			1053	60			
1 cup	250	17.0	8.5				600	.28	5.0			425	248	4.80		456
chow mein	255	195.0	31.0	10.0				10	.23			718	58			
1 cup	250	10.0	2.4				280	.08	4.3			473	293	2.50		456
clam fritter	124	16.1	4.6	12.4					.05				30			
1 fritter	40	6.0						.01	0.4			59	78	1.40		456

	KCAL / WT (g)	H_2O (g) / FAT (g)	PRO (g) / SFA (g)	CHO (g) / MUFA (g)	SUGR (g) / PUFA (g)	DFIB (g) / CHOL (mg)	A (RE) / A (IU)	C (mg) / B-1 (mg)	B-2 (mg) / NIA (mg)	B-6 (mg) / B-12 (mcg)	FOL (mcg) / PANT (mg)	Na (mg) / K (mg)	Ca (mg) / P (mg)	Mg (mg) / Fe (mg)	Zn (mg) / Cu (mg)	Mn (mg) / REF
corn fritter	132	10.2	2.7	13.9				1	.07			167	22			
1 fritter	35	7.5	2.0				140	.06	0.6			47	54	.60		456
crab, deviled	451	151.9	27.4	31.9				14	.26			2081	113			
1 cup[34]	240	22.6						.19	3.5			398	329	2.90		456
crab, imperial	323	158.2	32.1	8.6				11	.26			1602	132			
1 cup[35]	220	16.7						.13	2.4			288	365	2.00		456
fish cake, fried	103	39.6	8.8	5.6												
1 piece[36]	60	4.8														456
fish loaf, ckd	186	108.3	21.2	11.0												
1 slice[37]	150	5.6														456
green pepper stuffed w/ beef & crumbs	315	116.7	24.1	31.1				74	.81			581	78			
1 stuffed	185	10.2	4.8				520	.17	4.6			477	224	3.90		456
ham croquette	163	35.1	10.6	7.6				0	.14			222	45			
1 croquette	65	9.8	3.9				170	.18	1.6			54	104	1.40		456
lobster newburg	485	160.0	46.3	12.8					.28			573	218			
1 cup[38]	250	26.5						.18				428	480	2.30		456
lobster thermidor	405		28.5	14.8	0.5			0	.51				290			
5.5 oz	157	26.6					984	.15	4.8				451	1.90		456
macaroni & cheese	430	116.4	16.8	40.2				0	.40			1086	362			
1 cup	200	22.2	11.9				860	.20	1.8			240	322	1.80		456
oyster stew	233	196.8	12.5	10.8					.43			812	274			
1 cup[39]	240	15.4					820	.14	2.2			319	266	4.60		456
pizza, cheese	153	31.4	7.8	18.4				5	.13			456	144			
1 slice	65	5.4	2.1				410	.04	0.7			85	127	.70		456
pizza, sausage	157	33.9	5.2	19.8				6	.08			488	11			
1 slice	67	6.2	1.8				380	.06	1.0			113	62	.80		456
pot pie																
beef	517	115.7	21.2	39.5				6	.25			596	29			
⅓ of 9" pie	210	30.5	8.4				1720	.23	4.2			334	149	3.80		456
chicken	545	131.3	23.4	42.5				5	.26			594	70			
⅓ of 9" pie	232	31.3	10.9				3090	.26	4.2			343	232	3.00		456
turkey	550	130.4	24.1	42.9				5	.30			633	63			
⅓ of 9" pie	232	31.3	10.5				3090	.26	5.8			459	234	3.20		456
salmon patty	239		15.8	16.1	0.8			4	.22	.07	13	96	78	34	.84	
3.5 oz	100	12.4				64	66	.12	4.0	3.00	.66	89	104	1.24		456
salmon rice loaf	212	129.5	20.9	12.7												
1 slice	174	7.8														456
spaghetti & meatballs w/ tomato sce	332	173.8	18.6	38.7				22	.30			1009	124			
1 cup	248	11.7	3.3				1590	.25	4.0			665	236	3.70		456
spaghetti w/ tomato sce	260	192.5	8.8	37.0				13	.18			955	80			
1 cup	250	8.8	2.0				1080	.25	2.3			408	135	2.30		456
spanish rice	213	192.3	4.4	40.7				37	.07			774	34			
1 cup	245	4.2					1620	.10	1.7			566	96	1.50		456
tuna patty	209		19.8	7.4				1	.16			154	56	25		
3.5 oz	100	10.6			0.7	47	78	.08	7.4			64	173	1.70		456
welsh rarebit	415	162.9	18.8	14.6				0	.53			770	582			
1 cup	232	31.6	17.3				1230	.09	0.2			320	432	.70		456

1. Values for mild white cheddar cheese are similar.
2. Includes values for Dianosaurs, Santa Mac, Spirals, Super Mario Brothers, TeddyBears, and Flintstones shapes.
3. A potato and beef entree. Values are averages for original flavor, sausage flavor, and smoke flavor.
4. Frozen entrees contain one or two food items; they constitute part of a meal, but not the entire meal.
5. Beef, water chestnuts, red peppers, and broccoli in sauce.
6. Dark chicken meat, smoked sausage, yellow, red, and green pepper strips, celery, and onions in a cajun tomato sauce.
7. Pasta shells filled with ricotta, mozzarella, and parmesan cheese in tomato sauce.
8. Chicken, bamboo shoots, straw mushrooms, and water chestnuts in sauce with almonds.
9. Chicken, egg noodles, mushrooms, and celery in cream sauce topped with bread crumbs.

10. Chicken, wide egg noodles, carrots, and celery in chicken cream sauce.
11. Chicken, baby corn, cauliflower, green beans, red pepper, water chestnuts, and carrots in a ginger, soy, red pepper sauce.
12. Chicken, carrots, broccoli, red bell pepper, onions and corkscrew pasta in herb cream sauce.
13. Broiled chicken and mushrooms in light tarragon sauce.
14. Chicken, sliced mushrooms, onions, and green peppers in tomato sauce.
15. Chicken, baby corn, straw mushrooms, water chestnuts, and peanuts in peanut sauce.
16. Chicken, bell peppers, tomatoes, and green chilies in sauce.
17. Light and dark chicken, broccoli, carrots, zucchini, peas, cauliflower, onions, mushrooms, and tomatoes in an herb sauce.
18. Chicken, pineapple, bamboo shoots, red and green peppers and water chestnuts in sweet and sour sauce.
19. Bean sprouts, celery, onions, mushrooms, green peppers, and water chestnuts in soy flavored sauce.
20. Corn pasta filled with beef, beans, red pepper and topped with tomato sauce and monterey jack cheese.
21. Corn pasta with chicken filling in a sour cream sauce with onion, green chilies, topped with monterey jack cheese.
22. Flank steak and green pepper strips in tomato-soy sauce.
23. Beef, potatoes, green beans, carrots and onions in beef gravy.
24. Spinach lasagna noodles with tuna, yellow squash, red peppers, carrots, and mozzarella and parmesan cheeses in a white cream sauce topped with parmesan bread crumbs.

25. Egg noodles in sauce with parmesan cheese, cottage cheese, and sour cream.
26. Pasta and meatballs in tomato sauce.
27. Rigatoni and ground beef in tomato sauce topped with mozzarella and parmesan cheeses.
28. Tuna, celery, mushrooms, and egg noodles in cream sauce topped with bread crumbs.
29. Turkey slices, carrots, zucchini, and yellow squash in dijon mustard sauce topped with bread crumbs.
30. Turkey, mushrooms, celery, and spaghetti in sherry cream sauce topped with parmesan cheese and bread crumbs.
31. Pepperoni, sausage, and mushroom.
32. Contains beef, potatoes, carrots, onions, tomatoes, peas, flour, and salt.
33. Contains chicken, water, tomatoes, corn, lima beans, potatoes, onion, flour, salt, and pepper.
34. Prepared with bread crumbs, butter or margarine, parsley, eggs, lemon jce, and catsup.
35. Prepared with butter or margarine, flour, milk, onion, green pepper, eggs, and lemon jce.
36. Prepared with canned flaked fish, potato, and egg.
37. Prepared with canned flaked fish, bread cubes, egg, tomatoes, onions, and butter or margarine.
38. Prepared with butter or margarine, egg yolks, sherry, and cream.
39. Approximately 6 medium oysters per cup of stew.

	KCAL	H₂O (g)	PRO (g)	CHO (g)	SUGR (g)	DFIB (g)	A (RE)	C (mg)	B-2 (mg)	B-6 (mg)	FOL (mcg)	Na (mg)	Ca (mg)	Mg (mg)	Zn (mg)	Mn (mg)
	WT (g)	FAT (g)	SFA (g)	MUFA (g)	PUFA (g)	CHOL (mg)	A (IU)	B-1 (mg)	NIA (mg)	B-12 (mcg)	PANT (mg)	K (mg)	P (mg)	Fe (mg)	Cu (mg)	REF

11. FAST FOODS
11.1 GENERIC

biscuit

w/ egg	316	69.5	11.1	24.2			178	0	.34	.08	30	654	154	20	1.10	.299
1 biscuit	136	20.2	6.2	8.2	4.2	233	649	.34	0.7	.75	1.05	160	185	3.13	.084	821
w/ egg & bacon	458	70.0	17.0	28.6		0.8	53	3	.22	.14	30	999	189	24	1.64	.279
1 biscuit	150	31.1	7.9	13.4	7.5	353	191	.14	2.4	1.03	1.22	251	239	3.74	.112	821
w/ egg & ham	442	104.9	20.4	30.3		0.8	240	0	.60	.27	33	1382	221	31	2.23	.305
1 biscuit	192	27.0	5.9	11.0	7.7	300	874	.67	2.0	1.19	1.67	319	317	4.55	.138	821
w/ egg & sausage	581	77.2	19.2	41.1		0.9	164	0	.45	.20	40	1141	155	25	2.16	.315
1 biscuit	180	38.7	15.0	16.4	4.4	302	635	.50	3.6	1.37	1.53	320	490	3.96	.104	821
w/ egg & steak	410	77.7	17.9	21.3			191	0	.52	.18	28	888	138	25	2.80	.244
1 biscuit	148	28.4	8.6	11.7	5.8	272	704	.36	3.1	1.41	1.08	306	225	5.30	.107	821
w/ egg, cheese, & bacon	477	59.3	16.3	33.4			166	2	.43	.10	37	1260	164	20	1.54	.255
1 biscuit	144	31.4	11.4	14.2	3.5	261	648	.30	2.3	1.05	1.18	230	459	2.55	.075	821
w/ ham	386	32.1	13.4	43.8		0.8	34	0	.32	.14	8	1433	160	23	1.65	.362
1 biscuit	113	18.4	11.4	4.8	1.0	25	133	.51	3.5	.03	.41	197	554	2.72	.036	821
w/ sausage	485	36.3	12.1	40.0		1.4	14	0	.29	.11	9	1071	128	20	1.55	.360
1 biscuit	124	31.8	14.2	12.8	3.0	35	56	.40	3.3	.51	.36	198	446	2.58	.050	821
w/ steak	455	46.2	13.1	44.4			16	0	.39	.16	11	795	116	27	2.66	.422
1 biscuit	141	26.0	6.9	11.1	6.4	25	65	.35	4.2	.94	.41	234	204	4.30	.118	821

burritos

w/ beans	447	114.0	14.1	71.4			33	2	.61	.30	117	985	113	87	1.52	.868
2 burritos	217	13.5	6.9	4.7	1.2	4	332	.63	4.1	1.08	2.00	653	98	4.51	.378	821
w/ beans & cheese	378	100.3	15.1	55.0			238	2	.71	.24	82	1166	214	80	1.64	.432
2 burritos	186	11.7	6.8	2.5	1.8	28	1250	.22	3.6	.89	1.60	497	180	2.27	.352	821
w/ beans & chili peppers	412	110.9	16.4	58.1			20	1	.71	.29	118	1044	100	71	3.41	.783
2 burritos	204	14.7	7.6	5.4	1.0	33	204	.45	4.4	1.16	1.88	579	114	4.55	.333	821
w/ beans & meat	508	119.9	22.5	66.0			65	2	.83	.37	74	1335	106	83	3.83	.832
2 burritos	231	17.8	8.3	7.0	1.2	49	635	.53	5.4	1.73	2.24	656	141	4.90	.377	821

	KCAL / WT (g)	H₂O (g) / FAT (g)	PRO (g) / SFA (g)	CHO (g) / MUFA (g)	SUGR (g) / PUFA (g)	DFIB (g) / CHOL (mg)	A (RE) / A (IU)	C (mg) / B-1 (mg)	B-2 (mg) / NIA (mg)	B-6 (mg) / B-12 (mcg)	FOL (mcg) / PANT (mg)	Na (mg) / K (mg)	Ca (mg) / P (mg)	Mg (mg) / Fe (mg)	Zn (mg) / Cu (mg)	Mn (mg) / REF
w/ beans, cheese, & beef	331	131.8	14.6	39.7			150	5	.71	.22	61	991	130	51	2.35	.396
2 burritos	203	13.3	7.1	4.5	1.0	124	800	.30	3.9	1.10	1.66	410	140	3.74	.329	821
w/ beans, cheese, & chili peppers	662	187.4	33.3	85.2			383	7	1.21	.40	144	2060	289	97	6.08	.813
2 burritos	336	23.0	11.2	8.5	1.3	158	1596	.54	7.7	1.98	2.89	810	286	7.69	.588	821
w/ beef	524	109.1	26.6	58.5			29	1	.92	.31	40	1492	84	81	4.73	.785
2 burritos	220	20.8	10.5	7.4	0.9	64	277	.24	6.4	1.96	2.99	739	174	6.09	.409	821
w/ beef & chili peppers	426	109.4	21.5	49.4			46	2	.80	.30	36	1116	86	60	4.32	.746
2 burritos	201	16.5	8.0	6.1	1.0	54	462	.40	5.1	1.29	1.87	498	141	4.44	.316	821
w/ beef, cheese, & chili peppers	632	167.8	40.9	63.7			112	4	1.25	.36	58	2092	222	70	7.90	.608
2 burritos	304	24.8	10.4	9.9	2.2	170	973	.61	8.3	2.07	3.01	666	316	7.81	.362	821
w/ fruit (apple/cherry)	484	55.2	5.2	73.3			78	2	.37	.16	8	443	33	16	.84	.271
1 large	155	19.9	9.6	7.2	2.2	8	849	.36	3.9	1.07	1.98	219	31	2.25	.171	821
w/ fruit (apple/cherry)	231	26.4	2.5	35.0			37	1	.18	.07	4	212	16	7	.40	.130
1 small	74	9.5	4.6	3.4	1.1	4	406	.17	1.9	.51	.95	104	15	1.07	.081	821
cheeseburger																
large	609	71.5	30.1	47.4			148	0	.57	.28	39	1589	91	39	5.55	.309
1 sandwich	185	33.0	14.8	12.7	2.4	96	616	.48	11.2	2.53	.74	644	422	5.46	.157	821
large w/ bacon	608	85.0	32.0	37.1			80	2	.41	.31	33	1043	162	45	6.83	.332
1 sandwich	195	36.8	16.2	14.5	2.7	111	406	.31	6.6	2.34	.35	332	400	4.74	.158	821
large w/ double meat, lettuce, & tomato	704	131.8	38.0	39.7			54	1	.49	.41	49	1148	240	52	6.68	.317
1 sandwich	258	43.7	17.7	17.4	4.7	142	348	.36	7.2	3.41	.85	596	395	5.91	.206	821
large w/ ham, lettuce, & tomato	744	127.1	39.5	37.7			104	7	.56	.38	51	1712	302	51	6.63	.373
1 sandwich	254	48.2	21.1	18.9	3.9	122	505	.53	9.2	2.87	1.04	538	531	5.03	.246	821
large w/ lettuce & tomato	563	115.0	28.2	38.4			129	8	.46	.28	28	1108	206	44	4.60	.311
1 sandwich	219	32.9	15.0	12.6	2.0	88	613	.39	7.4	2.56	.72	445	311	4.66	.186	821
large w/ triple meat	796	164.5	56.1	26.7			85	3	.64	.61	52	1213	283	61	10.88	.353
1 sandwich	304	51.0	21.7	21.5	3.2	161	359	.61	11.5	5.90	1.16	821	541	8.30	.258	821
reg	319	38.0	14.8	31.8	5.2		37	0	.40	.09	27	500	141	21	2.37	.225
1 sandwich	102	15.1	6.5	5.8	1.5	50	153	.40	3.7	.97	.43	164	196	2.44	.094	821
reg w/ double meat	457	65.7	27.7	22.1			79	0	.37	.25	29	636	233	33	4.96	.234
1 sandwich	155	28.5	13.0	11.0	1.9	110	332	.25	6.0	2.31	.62	308	374	3.41	.130	821
reg w/ double meat & double-decker bun	461	69.4	22.1	44.3			66	0	.38	.22	37	891	224	34	4.35	.304
1 sandwich	160	21.6	9.5	8.3	1.8	80	277	.34	6.0	1.92	.66	285	338	3.70	.141	821
reg w/ double meat, double-decker bun, lettuce, & tomato—*1 sandwich*	650	106.2	29.7	53.1			84	3	.43	.27	34	921	169	36	4.13	.274
	228	35.3	12.8	12.6	6.4	93	372	.57	8.3	2.07	.64	390	349	4.72	.162	821
reg w/ double meat, lettuce, & tomato	417	85.0	21.2	35.2			65	2	.28	.18	23	1051	171	30	3.49	.299
1 sandwich	166	21.1	8.7	7.8	2.7	60	398	.35	8.1	1.93	.43	335	242	3.42	.149	821
reg w/ lettuce & tomato	359	85.0	17.8	28.1			71	2	.23	.15	22	976	182	26	2.62	.293
1 sandwich	154	19.8	9.2	7.2	1.5	52	431	.32	6.4	1.23	.34	229	216	2.65	.123	821
chicken, breaded & fried, boneless pieces	290	50.3	16.9	15.5		0.4	31	0	.14	.32	11	543	16	20	1.06	.129
6 pieces	102	17.7	5.5	8.7	2.2	61	102	.09	6.9	.31	.91	251	204	1.27	.169	821
w/ barbecue sce	330	67.4	17.1	25.0			47	1	.16	.34	27	829	21	25	1.12	.163
6 pieces	130	18.0	5.6	8.8	2.4	61	342	.10	7.0	.30	.96	319	215	1.46	.173	821
w/ honey sce	329	52.2	16.8	26.9			30	0	.15	.31	12	537	17	20	1.08	.138
6 pieces	115	17.5	5.5	8.6	2.2	61	101	.09	6.8	.30	.91	255	202	1.32	.172	821
w/ mustard sce	322	70.5	17.4	20.9			33	0	.16	.31	12	790	25	26	1.14	.165
6 pieces	130	18.9	5.7	9.0	2.9	61	109	.12	6.9	.31	.92	280	218	1.48	.168	821
w/ sweet & sour sce	346	64.0	17.0	29.0			73	1	.20	.33	12	677	21	23	1.09	.151
6 pieces	130	18.0	5.5	8.6	2.2	61	242	.10	6.9	.36	.92	277	211	1.48	.170	821
chicken, breaded & fried, dark meat	431	72.5	30.1	15.7			67	0	.43	.33	9	755	36	37	3.24	.127
drumstick & thigh	148	26.7	7.0	10.9	6.3	166	222	.13	7.2	.83	2.46	445	240	1.60	.118	821
chicken, breaded & fried, light meat	494	74.5	35.7	19.6			59	0	.29	.57	8	975	60	37	1.55	.155
side breast & wing	163	29.5	7.8	12.2	6.8	148	192	.15	12.0	.67	2.59	566	306	1.48	.101	821
chicken fillet sandwich	515	86.1	24.1	38.7			31	9	.24	.20	29	957	60	35	1.87	.473
1 sandwich	182	29.4	8.5	10.4	8.4	60	100	.33	6.8	.38	.60	353	233	4.68	.231	821
chicken fillet sandwich w/ cheese	632	104.9	29.4	41.6			128	3	.46	.41	46	1238	258	43	2.90	.381
1 sandwich	228	38.8	12.4	13.7	9.9	78	620	.41	9.1	.46	1.35	333	406	3.63	.171	821
chili con carne	256	194.1	24.6	21.9			167	2	1.14	.33	30	1007	68	46	3.57	.397
1 cup	253	8.3	3.4	3.4	0.5	134	1662	.13	2.5	1.14	3.59	691	197	5.19	.595	821

	KCAL	H₂O (g)	PRO (g)	CHO (g)	SUGR (g)	DFIB (g)	A (RE)	C (mg)	B-2 (mg)	B-6 (mg)	FOL (mcg)	Na (mg)	Ca (mg)	Mg (mg)	Zn (mg)	Mn (mg)
	WT (g)	FAT (g)	SFA (g)	MUFA (g)	PUFA (g)	CHOL (mg)	A (IU)	B-1 (mg)	NIA (mg)	B-12 (mcg)	PANT (mg)	K (mg)	P (mg)	Fe (mg)	Cu (mg)	REF
chimichanga																
beef	425	88.2	19.6	42.8			16	5	.64	.28	31	910	63	63	4.96	.557
1 chimichanga	174	19.7	8.5	8.1	1.1	9	146	.49	5.8	1.51	2.05	586	124	4.54	.423	821
beef & cheese	443	96.4	20.1	39.3			126	3	.86	.22	33	957	238	60	3.37	.489
1 chimichanga	183	23.4	11.2	9.4	0.7	51	540	.38	4.7	1.30	1.79	203	187	3.84	.351	821
beef & red chili peppers	424	103.1	18.1	45.8			27	0	.66	.23	34	1169	70	65	3.02	.616
1 chimichanga	190	19.1	8.3	7.8	1.1	10	262	.28	5.3	1.08	2.18	614	112	4.18	.275	821
beef, cheese, & red chili peppers	364	106.5	14.7	38.3			99	2	.95	.16	32	895	218	41	4.63	.391
1 chimichanga	180	17.6	8.4	7.1	0.5	50	702	.23	3.5	1.28	1.48	329	146	3.15	.563	821
clams, breaded & fried	451	33.6	12.8	38.8			37	0	.26	.03	9	834	21	31	1.63	.308
¾ cup	115	26.4	6.6	11.4	6.8	87	122	.21	2.9	1.10	.30	266	238	3.05	.095	821
coleslaw	147	73.3	1.5	12.8			50	8	.03	.11	39	267	34	9	.20	.124
¾ cup	99	11.0	1.6	2.4	6.4	5	338	.04	0.1	.18	.15	177	36	.72	.042	821
cookies, animal crackers	299	2.5	4.1	50.5			8	1	.24	.02	22	273	11	11	.30	.326
1 box	67	9.0	3.5	3.8	1.0	11	27	.25	2.5	.05	.21	56	64	1.47	.051	821
cookies, choc chip	233	2.9	2.9	36.2			15	1	.19	.03	16	188	20	17	.34	.237
1 box	55	12.1	5.3	5.1	1.0	12	52	.09	1.4	.10	.14	82	52	1.47	.184	821
corn-on-the-cob w/ butter	155	105.2	4.5	31.9			96	7	.10	.32	44	29	4	41	.91	.000
1 ear	146	3.4	1.6	1.0	0.6	6	391	.25	2.2	.00	.36	359	108	.88	.000	821
corndog (frank w/ corn flour coating)	460	81.7	16.8	55.8			37	0	.70	.09	60	973	102	18	1.31	.193
1 corndog	175	18.9	5.2	9.1	3.5	79	207	.28	4.2	.44	1.35	263	166	6.18	.245	821
crab, baked	160	71.6	28.5	4.2		0.0	23	3	.16	.46	21	549	415	82	7.02	.785
1 crab (3.8 oz meat)	109	2.3	0.4	0.6	0.8	184	77	.28	4.5	15.75	.41	597	337	1.38	1.079	821
crab cake	160	32.0	11.3	5.1		0.2	82	0	.07	.15	10	491	202	25	2.12	.282
2.1 oz cake	60	10.3	2.2	4.3	3.1	82	313	.06	1.2	4.40	.27	162	227	1.12	.366	821
crab, soft shell, fried	334	62.3	11.0	31.2			4	1	.07	.15	20	1118	55	25	1.06	.313
1 crab (4.4 oz meat)	125	17.9	4.4	7.7	4.9	45	15	.10	1.8	4.47	.47	163	131	1.81	.188	821
croissant w/ egg																
& cheese	368	57.7	12.8	24.3			255	0	.38	.10	37	551	244	22	1.75	.226
1 croissant	127	24.7	14.1	7.5	1.4	216	1001	.19	1.5	.77	1.05	174	348	2.20	.091	821
cheese & bacon	413	56.7	16.2	23.6			120	2	.34	.12	35	889	151	23	1.90	.222
1 croissant	129	28.4	15.4	9.2	1.8	215	472	.35	2.2	.86	1.07	201	276	2.19	.099	821
cheese & ham	474	77.7	18.9	24.2			117	11	.30	.23	36	1081	144	26	2.17	.220
1 croissant	152	33.6	17.5	11.4	2.4	213	451	.52	3.2	1.00	1.25	272	336	2.13	.126	821
cheese & sausage	523	73.4	20.3	24.7			109	0	.32	.11	38	1115	144	24	2.14	.253
1 croissant	160	38.2	18.2	14.3	3.0	216	422	.99	4.0	.90	1.31	283	290	3.04	.109	821
danish pastry																
cheese	353	30.8	5.8	28.7			43	3	.21	.05	15	319	70	15	.63	.350
3.2 oz pastry	91	24.6	5.1	15.6	2.4	20	155	.26	2.5	.23	.57	116	80	1.85	.086	821
cinn	349	18.4	4.8	46.9			5	3	.19	.05	14	326	37	14	.48	.370
3.1 oz pastry	88	16.7	3.5	10.6	1.6	27	18	.26	2.2	.22	.55	96	74	1.80	.075	821
fruit	335	27.3	4.8	45.1			24	2	.21	.06	15	333	22	14	.48	.193
3.3 oz pastry	94	15.9	3.3	10.1	1.6	19	86	.29	1.8	.23	.59	110	69	1.40	.055	821
egg & cheese sandwich	340	82.2	15.6	25.9			181	1	.57	.13	37	804	225	22	1.65	.219
1 sandwich	146	19.4	6.6	8.3	2.6	291	669	.26	2.1	1.14	.88	188	302	2.98	.110	821
egg, scrambled	199	62.7	13.0	2.0	0.8	0.0	252	3	.49	.18	53	211	54	13	1.56	.040
2 eggs	94	15.2	5.8	5.5	1.9	400	836	.08	0.2	.95	.88	138	227	2.43	.063	821
enchilada w/ cheese & beef	323	128.4	11.9	30.5			142	1	.40	.27	192	1319	228	83	2.69	.584
1 enchilada	192	17.6	9.0	6.1	1.4	40	1135	.10	2.5	1.02	1.44	574	167	3.07	.518	821
enchilada w/ cheese & sour cream	319	103.1	9.6	28.5			186	1	.42	.39	34	784	324	51	2.51	.240
1 enchilada	163	18.8	10.6	6.3	0.8	44	1161	.08	1.9	.75	1.52	240	134	1.32	.259	821
enchirito w/ cheese, beef, & beans	344	121.0	17.9	33.8			133	5	.69	.21	253	1251	218	71	2.76	.384
1 enchirito	193	16.1	7.9	6.5	0.3	50	1015	.17	3.0	1.62	1.83	560	224	2.39	.270	821
english muffin																
w/ butter	189	20.6	4.9	30.4			33	1	.32	.04	17	386	103	13	.42	.209
1 muffin	63	5.8	2.4	1.5	1.3	13	136	.25	2.6	.02	.14	69	85	1.59	.064	821
w/ cheese & sausage	393	43.4	15.3	29.2		1.5	86	1	.25	.15	18	1036	168	24	1.68	.220
1 sandwich	115	24.3	9.9	10.1	2.7	59	379	.70	4.1	.68	.53	215	186	2.25	.076	821

							Vitamins					Minerals				
	KCAL	H_2O (g)	PRO (g)	CHO (g)	SUGR (g)	DFIB (g)	A (RE)	C (mg)	B-2 (mg)	B-6 (mg)	FOL (mcg)	Na (mg)	Ca (mg)	Mg (mg)	Zn (mg)	Mn (mg)
	WT (g)	FAT (g)	SFA (g)	MUFA (g)	PUFA (g)	CHOL (mg)	A (IU)	B-1 (mg)	NIA (mg)	B-12 (mcg)	PANT (mg)	K (mg)	P (mg)	Fe (mg)	Cu (mg)	REF
w/ egg, cheese, & canadian bacon	383	71.5	19.8	31.4	2.9		158	1	.53	.16	44	784	207	34	1.81	.264
1 sandwich	146	19.8	9.1	6.8	2.1	234	594	.48	3.9	.80	.89	213	320	3.29	.131	821
w/ egg, cheese, & sausage	487	78.2	21.7	31.0			172	1	.49	.20	54	1135	196	30	2.36	.299
1 sandwich	165	30.9	12.4	12.7	3.3	274	660	.84	4.5	1.37	1.40	294	287	3.46	.119	821
fish fillet, battered/breaded & fried	211	48.7	13.3	15.4		0.5	11	0	.10	.09	12	484	16	22	.40	.168
3.2 oz fillet	91	11.2	2.6	2.3	5.7	31	35	.10	1.9	1.01	.18	291	156	1.92	.041	821
fish sandwich w/ tartar sce	431	74.8	16.9	41.0	5.2		30	3	.22	.11	44	615	84	33	1.00	.365
1 sandwich	158	22.8	5.2	7.7	8.2	55	109	.33	3.4	1.07	.58	340	212	2.61	.191	821
fish sandwich w/ tartar sce & cheese	523	82.7	20.6	47.6			97	3	.42	.11	31	939	185	37	1.17	.362
1 sandwich	183	28.6	8.1	8.9	9.4	68	432	.46	4.2	1.08	.44	353	311	3.50	.119	821
french fries, fried in veg oil																
french fries, fried in veg oil	235	30.0	3.0	29.3		2.4	2	4	.03	.20	25	124	12	25	.40	.194
20-25 fries	76	12.2	3.8	6.0	1.9	0	22	.11	1.7	.09	.33	541	101	1.03	.104	821
french fries, fried in veg oil	355	45.4	4.6	44.4		3.7	3	6	.05	.30	38	187	18	38	.60	.293
30-40 fries	115	18.5	5.7	9.1	2.8	0	33	.16	2.6	.14	.49	819	153	1.55	.158	821
french toast sticks	513	42.2	8.3	57.9		2.7	13	0	.25	.25	134	499	78	27	.93	.219
5 sticks	141	29.0	4.7	12.6	9.9	75	45	.23	3.0	.07	.56	127	123	2.96	.271	821
french toast w/ butter	356	68.5	10.3	36.0			146	0	.50	.05	30	513	73	16	.59	.209
2 slices	135	18.8	7.7	7.1	2.4	116	473	.58	3.9	.36	.54	177	146	1.89	.065	821
frijoles w/ cheese	225	115.4	11.4	28.7			70	2	.33	.20	112	882	189	85	1.74	.503
1 cup	167	7.8	4.1	2.6	0.7	37	456	.13	1.5	.68	1.10	605	175	2.24	.341	821
ham & cheese sandwich	352	74.2	20.7	33.3			76	3	.48	.20	72	771	130	16	1.37	.139
1 sandwich	146	15.5	6.4	6.7	1.4	58	320	.31	2.7	.54	1.04	291	152	3.24	.182	821
ham, egg, & cheese sandwich	347	73.1	19.2	30.9			149	3	.56	.16	43	1005	212	26	1.99	.243
1 sandwich	143	16.3	7.4	5.7	1.7	246	562	.43	4.2	1.23	.94	210	346	3.10	.122	821
hamburger																
large	426	57.7	22.6	31.7			0	0	.29	.23	32	474	74	27	4.11	.244
1 sandwich	137	22.9	8.4	9.9	2.1	71	0	.29	6.2	2.06	.53	267	175	3.58	.130	821
large w/ double meat, lettuce, & tomato	540	121.5	34.3	40.3			11	1	.38	.54	27	791	102	50	5.67	.249
1 sandwich	226	26.6	10.5	10.3	2.8	122	102	.36	7.6	4.07	.54	570	314	5.85	.219	821
large w/ lettuce & tomato	512	121.4	25.8	40.0			33	3	.37	.33	37	824	96	44	4.88	.349
1 sandwich	218	27.4	10.4	11.4	2.2	87	312	.41	7.3	2.38	.72	480	233	4.93	.198	821
large w/ triple meat	692	135.6	50.0	28.6			16	1	.54	.62	31	712	65	54	10.75	.233
1 sandwich	259	41.5	15.9	18.2	2.7	142	158	.31	11.0	4.92	.67	785	394	8.31	.197	821
reg	231	41.0	11.4	27.5	4.1		11	2	.27	.11	14	474	43	19	1.73	.177
1 sandwich	90	8.6	3.0	3.1	1.5	36	106	.22	4.0	.70	.32	181	93	2.07	.104	821
reg w/ double meat	472	88.9	26.0	31.7			4	1	.33	.30	37	607	76	37	4.75	.266
1 sandwich	176	26.6	9.8	11.6	2.3	84	44	.28	5.5	2.73	.63	431	232	4.54	.158	821
reg w/ lettuce & tomato	554	107.7	25.6	54.1			17	3	.39	.24	37	998	124	44	4.08	.501
1 sandwich	218	26.7	8.2	10.5	5.1	52	164	.46	7.3	1.74	.59	449	246	5.21	.203	821
hash brown potatoes	151	43.3	1.9	16.1			3	5	.01	.17	8	290	7	16	.22	.110
½ cup	72	9.2	4.3	3.9	0.5	9	18	.08	1.1	.01	.34	267	69	.48	.070	821
hot dog	242	52.9	10.4	18.0			0	0	.27	.05	29	670	24	13	1.98	.091
1 hot dog	98	14.5	5.1	6.9	1.7	44	0	.24	3.6	.51	.51	143	97	2.31	.076	821
hot dog w/ chili	296	54.5	13.5	31.3			6	3	.40	.05	50	480	19	10	.78	.114
1 hot dog	114	13.4	4.9	6.6	1.2	51	58	.22	3.7	.30	.55	166	192	3.28	.103	821
hush puppies	257	25.2	4.9	34.9			27	0	.02	.10	21	965	69	16	.43	.267
5 pieces	78	11.6	2.7	7.8	0.4	135	94	.00	2.0	.17	.22	188	190	1.43	.204	821
ice milk, vanilla, soft serve w/ cone	164	67.4	3.9	24.1		0.1	52	1	.26	.06	5	92	153	15	.57	.021
1 cone	103	6.1	3.5	1.8	0.4	28	211	.05	0.3	.21	.27	169	139	.15	.019	821
nachos																
w/ cheese	346	45.7	9.1	36.3			92	1	.37	.20	10	816	272	55	1.79	.224
6-8 nachos	113	19.0	7.8	8.0	2.2	18	559	.19	1.5	.82	1.31	172	276	1.28	.140	821
w/ cheese & jalapeno peppers	608	87.1	16.8	60.1			471	1	.49	.37	18	1736	620	108	2.90	.439
6-8 nachos	204	34.1	14.0	14.4	4.0	84	4062	.12	2.8	1.02	2.45	294	394	2.45	.173	821
w/ cheese, beans, ground beef, & peppers	569	142.7	19.8	55.8			469	5	.69	.41	38	1800	385	97	3.65	.423
6-8 nachos	255	30.7	12.5	11.0	5.7	20	3402	.23	3.3	1.02	2.52	451	388	2.78	.745	821
w/ cinn & sugar	592	1.1	7.2	63.4			11	8	.45	.17	8	439	85	20	.59	.493
6-8 nachos	109	36.0	18.2	11.8	4.1	39	108	.19	3.9	1.72	1.90	78	33	2.89	.156	821

	KCAL / WT (g)	H₂O (g) / FAT (g)	PRO (g) / SFA (g)	CHO (g) / MUFA (g)	SUGR (g) / PUFA (g)	DFIB (g) / CHOL (mg)	A (RE) / A (IU)	C (mg) / B-1 (mg)	B-2 (mg) / NIA (mg)	B-6 (mg) / B-12 (mcg)	FOL (mcg) / PANT (mg)	Na (mg) / K (mg)	Ca (mg) / P (mg)	Mg (mg) / Fe (mg)	Zn (mg) / Cu (mg)	Mn (mg) / REF
onion rings	276	30.8	3.7	31.3			1	1	.10	.06	12	430	73	16	.35	.296
8-9 rings	83	15.5	7.0	6.7	0.7	14	8	.08	0.9	.12	.20	129	86	.85	.069	821
oysters, battered/breaded & fried	368	66.7	12.5	39.9			108	4	.35	.03	13	677	28	24	15.64	.424
6 oysters	139	17.9	4.6	6.9	4.6	108	363	.31	4.4	1.01	1.06	182	196	4.46	.796	821
pancakes w/ butter & syrup	520	115.4	8.3	90.9			70	3	.56	.12	35	1104	128	49	1.02	.322
3 pancakes	232	14.0	5.9	5.3	2.0	58	281	.39	3.4	.23	.67	251	476	2.62	.151	821
pie, fruit (apple/cherry/lemon), fried	266	34.1	2.4	33.0			33	1	.08	.03	4	325	13	8	.17	.173
1 pie	85	14.4	6.5	5.8	1.2	13	149	.10	1.0	.08	.15	51	37	.88	.043	821
pizza																
cheese	140	30.1	7.7	20.5			74	1	.16	.04	59	336	117	16	.81	.232
⅛ of 12" pizza	63	3.2	1.5	1.0	0.5	9	382	.18	2.5	.33	.22	110	113	.58	.081	821
cheese, meat, & veg	184	37.7	13.0	21.3			101	2	.17	.09	27	382	101	18	1.11	.118
⅛ of 12" pizza	79	5.4	1.5	2.5	0.9	21	524	.21	2.0	.36	.83	179	131	1.53	.118	821
pepperoni	181	33.0	10.1	19.9			55	2	.23	.06	53	267	65	9	.52	.099
⅛ of 12" pizza	71	7.0	2.2	3.1	1.2	14	282	.13	3.0	.18	.25	153	75	.94	.064	821
potato, baked																
w/ cheese sce	474	194.6	14.6	46.5			228	26	.21	.71	27	382	311	65	1.89	.515
1 potato	296	28.7	10.6	10.7	6.0	18	835	.24	3.3	.18	1.30	1166	320	3.02	.630	821
w/ cheese sce & bacon	451	194.4	18.4	44.4			173	29	.24	.75	30	972	308	69	2.15	.505
1 potato	299	25.9	10.1	9.7	4.8	30	628	.27	4.0	.33	1.29	1178	347	3.14	.646	821
w/ cheese sce & broccoli	403	237.4	13.7	46.6			278	48	.27	.78	61	485	336	78	2.03	.803
1 potato	339	21.4	8.5	7.7	4.2	20	1695	.27	3.6	.34	1.42	1441	346	3.32	.647	821
w/ cheese sce & chili	482	276.8	23.2	55.9			174	32	.36	.95	51	699	411	111	3.79	.675
1 potato	395	21.8	13.0	6.8	0.9	32	766	.28	4.2	.24	2.57	1572	498	6.12	.826	821
w/ sour cream & chives	393	209.7	6.7	50.0			278	34	.18	.79	33	181	106	69	.91	.580
1 potato	302	22.3	10.0	7.9	3.3	24	1347	.27	3.7	.21	1.48	1383	184	3.11	.686	821
potato salad	108	74.8	1.5	12.9			16	1	.10	.14	24	312	13	8	.19	.070
⅓ cup	95	5.7	1.0	1.6	2.9	57	95	.07	0.3	.11	.35	257	53	.69	.075	821
potatoes, mashed	66	63.4	1.8	12.9			8	0	.04	.18	6	182	17	14	.26	.094
⅓ cup	80	1.0	0.4	0.3	0.2	2	33	.07	1.0	.04	.38	235	44	.38	.078	821
roast beef sandwich	346	67.6	21.5	33.4			21	2	.31	.26	40	792	54	31	3.39	.125
1 sandwich	139	13.8	3.6	6.8	1.7	51	210	.38	5.9	1.22	.83	316	239	4.23	.097	821
roast beef sandwich w/ cheese	473	76.6	32.2	45.4			46	0	46	.33	40	1633	183	40	5.37	.312
1 sandwich	176	18.0	9.0	3.7	3.5	77	194	.39	5.9	2.06	.69	345	401	5.05	.199	821
roast beef submarine sandwich	410	127.4	28.6	44.3			50	6	.41	.32	45	845	41	67	4.38	.432
1 sub	216	13.0	7.1	1.8	2.6	73	413	.41	6.0	1.81	.78	330	192	2.81	.361	821
salad, vegetable w/o dressing	33	197.7	2.6	6.7			236	48	.10	.17	77	54	27	23	.43	.304
1 ½ cups	207	0.1	0.0	0.0	0.1	0	2352	.06	1.1	.00	.25	356	81	1.30	.103	821
w/ cheese & egg	102	196.3	8.8	4.8			115	10	.17	.11	85	119	100	24	1.00	.273
1 ½ cups	217	5.8	3.0	1.8	0.5	98	822	.09	1.0	.30	.52	371	132	.67	.089	821
w/ chicken	105	189.8	17.4	3.7			96	17	.13	.44	68	209	37	33	.89	.249
1 ½ cups	218	2.2	0.6	0.7	0.6	72	935	.11	5.9	.20	.59	447	170	1.09	.094	821
w/ pasta & seafood	379	335.1	16.4	32.0			638	38	.21	.33	100	1572	71	50	1.67	.667
1 ½ cups	417	20.9	2.6	4.8	9.1	50	6247	.29	3.5	1.71	.38	600	204	3.17	.363	821
w/ shrimp	106	210.3	14.5	6.6			78	9	.17	.14	87	489	59	38	1.27	.142
1 ½ cup	236	2.5	0.7	0.8	0.5	179	791	.12	1.2	3.78	.50	404	160	.90	.160	821
w/ turkey, ham, & cheese	267	268.8	26.0	4.7			137	16	.39	.42	101	743	235	49	3.13	.359
1 ½ cups	326	16.1	8.2	5.2	1.4	140	1053	.39	6.0	.85	.91	401	401	1.96	.166	821
scallops, breaded & fried	386	69.1	15.8	38.5			42	0	.85	.07	40	919	19	32	1.08	.298
6 scallops	144	19.4	4.9	12.6	0.6	108	138	.20	0.0	.43	.50	294	292	2.04	.216	821
shake																
choc	359	202.3	9.6	58.0		2.3	65	1	.69	.14	10	275	320	48	1.16	.110
10 fl oz	283	10.5	6.5	3.0	0.4	37	263	.16	0.5	.96	1.10	566	289	.88	.184	814
strawberry	320	209.7	9.6	53.5		1.1	82	2	.55	.12	8	235	320	37	1.02	.042
10 fl oz	283	7.9	4.9			31	340	.13	0.5	.88	1.39	515	283	.31	.062	814
van	314	211.4	9.9	50.7		1.1	91	2	.52	.15	9	232	345	34	1.02	.040
10 fl oz	283	8.5	5.3	2.4	0.3	31	368	.13	0.5	1.02	1.18	492	289	.25	.144	814
shrimp, breaded & fried	454	78.4	18.9	40.0			36	0	.90	.07	48	1446	84	39	1.21	.333
6-8 shrimp	164	24.9	5.4	17.4	0.6	200	120	.21	0.0	.15	.48	184	344	2.95	.144	821

	KCAL	H_2O (g)	PRO (g)	CHO (g)	SUGR (g)	DFIB (g)	A (RE)	C (mg)	B-2 (mg)	B-6 (mg)	FOL (mcg)	Na (mg)	Ca (mg)	Mg (mg)	Zn (mg)	Mn (mg)
	WT (g)	**FAT (g)**	**SFA (g)**	**MUFA (g)**	**PUFA (g)**	**CHOL (mg)**	**A (IU)**	**B-1 (mg)**	**NIA (mg)**	**B-12 (mcg)**	**PANT (mg)**	**K (mg)**	**P (mg)**	**Fe (mg)**	**Cu (mg)**	**REF**
steak sandwich w/ lettuce, tomato,	459	104.2	30.3	52.0			45	6	.37	.37	90	798	92	49	4.53	.367
& mayonnaise—*1 sandwich*	204	14.1	3.8	5.3	3.3	73	367	.41	7.3	1.57	.92	524	298	5.16	.220	821
submarine sandwich	456	131.8	21.8	51.0			80	12	.80	.14	55	1651	189	68	2.58	.531
1 sub[1]	228	18.6	6.8	8.2	2.3	36	424	1.00	5.5	1.09	.89	394	287	2.51	.303	821
sundae																
caramel	304	87.6	7.3	49.3	38.8	0.0	68	3	.29	.05	12	195	189	28	.82	.093
1 sundae	155	9.3	4.5	3.0	1.0	25	264	.06	0.9	.60	.37	318	217	.22	.082	821
hot fudge	284	94.3	5.6	47.7	40.1	0.0	57	2	.30	.13	9	182	207	33	.95	.126
1 sundae	158	8.6	5.0	2.3	0.8	21	221	.06	1.1	.65	.33	395	228	.58	.130	821
strawberry	268	93.2	6.3	44.6	41.6	0.0	58	2	.28	.08	18	92	161	24	.66	.168
1 sundae	153	7.8	3.7	2.7	1.0	21	222	.06	0.9	.64	.44	271	155	.32	.077	821
taco, large	568	153.6	31.8	41.1			226	3	.68	.37	37	1233	339	108	6.05	.676
9.3 oz	263	31.6	17.5	10.1	1.5	87	1315	.24	4.9	1.60	2.60	729	313	3.71	.316	821
taco salad	279	143.3	13.2	23.6			77	4	.36	.22	40	762	192	51	2.69	.331
1 ½ cup	198	14.8	6.8	5.2	1.7	44	588	.10	2.5	.63	1.35	416	143	2.28	.224	821
taco salad w/ chili con carne	290	200.4	17.4	26.6			214	3	.50	.52	63	885	245	52	3.29	.337
1 ½ cups	261	13.1	6.0	4.5	1.5	5	1574	.16	2.5	.73	1.44	392	154	2.66	.300	821
taco, small	369	99.9	20.7	26.7			147	2	.44	.24	24	802	221	70	3.93	.439
6 oz	171	20.6	11.4	6.6	1.0	56	855	.15	3.2	1.04	1.69	474	203	2.41	.205	821
tostada																
beans & cheese	223	95.4	9.6	26.5			85	1	.33	.16	75	543	210	59	1.90	.367
1 tostada	144	9.9	5.4	3.1	0.7	30	622	.10	1.3	.69	1.14	403	117	1.89	.206	821
beans, beef, & cheese	333	158.5	16.1	29.7			173	4	.49	.25	97	871	189	68	3.17	.360
1 tostada	225	16.9	11.5	3.5	0.6	74	1276	.09	2.9	1.13	1.87	491	173	2.45	.315	821
beef & cheese	315	101.1	19.0	22.8			96	3	.55	.23	15	896	217	64	3.68	.504
1 tostada	163	16.3	10.4	3.3	1.0	41	712	.10	3.1	1.17	1.89	572	179	2.87	.264	821
w/ guacamole	360	189.3	12.5	32.0			217	4	.57	.26	110	799	423	73	4.07	.352
2 tostadas	261	23.3	9.9	8.5	3.1	39	1751	.13	2.0	.99	2.01	650	232	1.62	.253	821
tuna salad submarine sandwich	584	139.0	29.7	55.4			41	4	.33	.23	56	1293	74	79	1.87	.512
9 oz sandwich	256	28.0	5.3	13.4	7.3	49	187	.46	11.3	1.61	1.87	335	220	2.64	.428	821

11.2 BURGER KING

	KCAL	H_2O (g)	PRO (g)	CHO (g)	SUGR (g)	DFIB (g)	A (RE)	C (mg)	B-2 (mg)	B-6 (mg)	FOL (mcg)	Na (mg)	Ca (mg)	Mg (mg)	Zn (mg)	Mn (mg)
biscuit w/ bacon, egg, & cheese	510		19.0	39.0	3.0	1.0	0					1530	150			
1 biscuit	171	31.0	10.0			225	400							2.70		I
biscuit w/ sausage	590		16.0	41.0	2.0	1.0	0					1390	60			
1 biscuit	151	40.0	13.0			45	0							3.60		I
cheeseburger	380		23.0	28.0	5.0	1.0	0					770	100			
1 sandwich	138	19.0	9.0			65	300							2.70		I
double	600		41.0	28.0	5.0	1.0	0					1060	200			
1 sandwich	210	36.0	17.0			135	400							4.50		I
double w/ bacon	640		44.0	28.0	5.0	1.0	0					1240	200			
1 sandwich	218	39.0	18.0			145	400							4.50		I
chicken sandwich	710		26.0	54.0	4.0	2.0	0					1400	100			
1 sandwich	229	43.0	9.0			60	0							3.60		I
chicken sandwich, broiler	550		30.0	41.0	4.0	2.0		6				480	60			
1 sandwich	248	29.0	6.0			80	300							5.40		I
Chicken Tenders	310		21.0	19.0	0.0	3.0	0					710	0			
8 pieces	117	17.0	4.0			50	100							1.08		I
Croissandwich w/ sausage, egg, & cheese	600		22.0	25.0	3.0	1.0	0					1140	150			
1 croissandwich	176	46.0	16.0			260	400							3.60		I
fish sandwich	700		26.0	56.0	4.0	3.0		1				980	60			
1 sandwich	255	41.0	6.0			90	100							2.70		I
french fries	370		5.0	43.0	0.0	3.0		4				240	0			
1 med serving	116	20.0	5.0			0	0							1.08		I
french fries, coated	340		0.0	43.0	0.0	3.0		6				680	0			
1 med serving	102	17.0	5.0			0	0							1.08		I
french toast sticks	500		4.0	60.0	11.0	1.0	0					490	60			
1 serving	141	27.0	7.0			0	0							2.70		I

	KCAL / WT (g)	H₂O (g) / FAT (g)	PRO (g) / SFA (g)	CHO (g) / MUFA (g)	SUGR (g) / PUFA (g)	DFIB (g) / CHOL (mg)	A (RE) / A (IU)	C (mg) / B-1 (mg)	B-2 (mg) / NIA (mg)	B-6 (mg) / B-12 (mcg)	FOL (mcg) / PANT (mg)	Na (mg) / K (mg)	Ca (mg) / P (mg)	Mg (mg) / Fe (mg)	Zn (mg) / Cu (mg)	Mn (mg) / REF
hamburger	330		20.0	28.0	4.0	1.0		0				530				
1 sandwich	126	15.0	6.0			55	100							2.70		I
hash browns	220		2.0	25.0	0.0	2.0		5				320				
1 serving	71	12.0	3.0			0	500							1.44		I
onion rings	310		4.0	41.0	6.0	6.0		0				810	100			
1 reg serving	124	14.0	2.0			0	0							1.44		I
pie, apple	300		3.0	39.0	22.0	2.0		6				230				
1 snack pie	113	15.0	3.0			0	0							1.44		I
salad dressing																
bleu cheese	160		2.0	1.0	0.0	0.0						260				
1 serving	30	16.0	4.0			30										I
french	140		0.0	11.0	9.0	0.0						190				
1 serving	30	10.0	2.0			0										I
italian, red cal	15		0.0	3.0	2.0	0.0						50				
1 serving	30	0.5	0.0			0										I
ranch	180		0.0	2.0	0.0	0.0						170				
1 serving	30	19.0	4.0			10										I
thousand island	140		0.0	7.0	5.0	0.0						190				
1 serving	30	12.0	3.0			15										I
salad w/o dressing																
chicken, broiled	200		21.0	7.0	4.0	3.0		15				110	150			
1 salad	302	10.0	4.0			60	5000							3.60		I
garden	100		6.0	7.0	4.0	3.0		30				110	150			
1 salad	215	5.0	3.0			15	5500							1.08		I
side	60		3.0	4.0	2.0	2.0		12				55	80			
1 salad	133	3.0	2.0			5	2500							.72		I
sauce																
barbecue dipping sce	35		0.0	9.0	7.0	0.0						400				
1 serving	28	0.0	0.0	0.0	0.0	0										I
barbecue sce, Bull's Eye	20		0.0	5.0	5.0	0.0						140				
1 serving	14	0.0	0.0	0.0	0.0	0										I
Burger King AM Express dip	80		0.0	21.0	14.0	0.0						20				
1 serving	28	0.0	0.0	0.0	0.0	0										I
honey dipping sce	90		0.0	23.0	23.0	0.0						10				
1 serving	28	0.0	0.0	0.0	0.0	0										I
ranch dipping sce	170		0.0	2.0	1.0	0.0						200				
1 serving	28	17.0				0										I
sweet & sour dipping sce	45		0.0	11.0	10.0	0.0						50				
1 serving	28	0.0	0.0	0.0	0.0	0										I
tartar sce	180		0.0	0.0	0.0	0.0						220				
1 serving	28	19.0	3.0			15										I
shake																
choc	320		9.0	54.0	48.0	3.0		0				230	200			
1 med	284	7.0	4.0			20	300							1.80		I
choc w/ added syrup	440		10.0	84.0	78.0	2.0		4				430	300			
1 med	341	7.0	4.0			20	300							1.08		I
strawberry w/ added syrup	420		9.0	83.0	78.0	1.0		4				260	300			
1 med	341	6.0	4.0			20	300							.00		I
van	300		9.0	53.0	47.0	1.0		4				230	300			
1 med	284	6.0	4.0			20	300							.00		I
Whopper sandwich	640		27.0	45.0	8.0	3.0		9				870	80			
1 sandwich	270	39.0	11.0			90	500							4.50		I
double	870		46.0	45.0	8.0	3.0		8				940	80			
1 sandwich	351	56.0	19.0			170	500							7.20		I
double w/ cheese	960		52.0	46.0		3.0		9				1420	250			
1 sandwich	375	63.0	24.0			195	750							7.20		I
Jr.	420		21.0	29.0	5.0	2.0		2				530	60			
1 sandwich	164	24.0	8.0			60	200							3.60		I

	KCAL / WT (g)	H₂O (g) / FAT (g)	PRO (g) / SFA (g)	CHO (g) / MUFA (g)	SUGR (g) / PUFA (g)	DFIB (g) / CHOL (mg)	A (RE) / A (IU)	C (mg) / B-1 (mg)	B-2 (mg) / NIA (mg)	B-6 (mg) / B-12 (mcg)	FOL (mcg) / PANT (mg)	Na (mg) / K (mg)	Ca (mg) / P (mg)	Mg (mg) / Fe (mg)	Zn (mg) / Cu (mg)	Mn (mg) / REF
Jr. w/ cheese	460		23.0	29.0	5.0	2.0		5				770	150			
1 sandwich	177	28.0	10.0			75	400							3.60		I
w/ cheese	730		33.0	46.0	8.0	3.0		9				1350	250			
1 sandwich	294	46.0	16.0			115	750							4.50		I

11.3 HARDEE'S

	KCAL / WT (g)	H₂O (g) / FAT (g)	PRO (g) / SFA (g)	CHO (g) / MUFA (g)	SUGR (g) / PUFA (g)	DFIB (g) / CHOL (mg)	A (RE) / A (IU)	C (mg) / B-1 (mg)	B-2 (mg) / NIA (mg)	B-6 (mg) / B-12 (mcg)	FOL (mcg) / PANT (mg)	Na (mg) / K (mg)	Ca (mg) / P (mg)	Mg (mg) / Fe (mg)	Zn (mg) / Cu (mg)	Mn (mg) / REF
baked beans	170		8.0	32.0								600				
5 oz	142	1.0	0.0			0										I
big cookie	280		4.0	41.0								150				
2 oz	57	12.0	4.0			15										I
Big Country Breakfast w/ bacon	820		33.0	62.0								1870				
1 breakfast	267	49.0	15.0			535										I
Big Country Breakfast w/ sausage	1000		41.0	62.0								2310				
1 breakfast	324	66.0	38.0			570										I
biscuit																
apple	200		2.0	30.0								350				
1 biscuit	61	8.0	2.0			0										I
bacon & egg	570		22.0	45.0								1400				
1 biscuit	158	33.0	11.0			275										I
bacon, egg, & cheese	610		24.0	45.0								1630				
1 biscuit	189	37.0	13.0			260										I
country ham	430		15.0	45.0								1830				
1 biscuit	108	22.0	6.0			25										I
ham	400		9.0	47.0								1340				
1 biscuit	114	20.0	6.0			15										I
ham, egg, & cheese	540		20.0	48.0								1660				
1 biscuit	185	30.0	11.0			285										I
jelly	440		6.0	57.0								1000				
1 biscuit	100	21.0	6.0			0										I
'n gravy	510		10.0	55.0								1500				
1 biscuit	221	28.0	9.0			15										I
Rise 'n Shine	390		6.0	44.0								1000				
1 biscuit	83	21.0	6.0			0										I
sausage	510		14.0	44.0								1360				
1 biscuit	118	31.0	10.0			25										I
sausage & egg	630		23.0	45.0								1480				
1 biscuit	179	40.0	22.0			285										I
Ultimate Omelet	570		22.0	45.0								1370				
1 biscuit	164	33.0	12.0			290										I
burger																
Frisco	720		33.0	43.0								1340				
1 sandwich	232	46.0	16.0			95										I
The Boss	570		27.0	42.0								810				
1 sandwich	199	33.0	12.0			85										I
The Works	530		25.0	41.0								1030				
1 sandwich	231	30.0	12.0			80										I
cheeseburger	310		16.0	30.0								890				
1 sandwich	123	14.0	6.0			40										I
Cravin Bacon	690		30.0	38.0								1160				
1 sandwich	231	46.0	16.0			95										I
mesquite bacon	370		19.0	32.0								870				
1 sandwich	129	18.0	7.0			45										I
Quarter-Pound Double	470		27.0	31.0								1290				
1 sandwich	171	27.0	11.0			80										I
chicken fillet sandwich	480		26.0	54.0								1280				
1 sandwich	215	18.0	9.0			55										I

	KCAL	H₂O (g)	PRO (g)	CHO (g)	SUGR (g)	DFIB (g)	A (RE)	C (mg)	B-2 (mg)	B-6 (mg)	FOL (mcg)	Na (mg)	Ca (mg)	Mg (mg)	Zn (mg)	Mn (mg)
	WT (g)	FAT (g)	SFA (g)	MUFA (g)	PUFA (g)	CHOL (mg)	A (IU)	B-1 (mg)	NIA (mg)	B-12 (mcg)	PANT (mg)	K (mg)	P (mg)	Fe (mg)	Cu (mg)	REF
chicken, fried																
breast	370		29.0	29.0								1190				
1 piece	148	15.0	4.0			75										I
leg	170		13.0	15.0								570				
1 piece	68	7.0	2.0			45										I
thigh	330		19.0	30.0								1000				
1 piece	121	15.0	4.0			60										I
wing	200		10.0	23.0								740				
1 piece	86	6.0	2.0			30										I
chicken, grilled sandwich	350		25.0	38.0								960				
1 sandwich	203	11.0	2.0			65										I
coleslaw	240		2.0	13.0								340				
4 oz	113	20.0	3.0			10										I
cone																
choc	180		5.0	34.0								110				
1 cone	118	2.0	1.0			15										I
van	170		4.0	34.0								130				
1 cone	116	2.0	1.0			10										I
van-choc, Cool Twist	180		4.0	34.0								120				
1 cone	116	1.0	1.0			10										I
Fisherman's Fillet sandwich	560		26.0	54.0								1330				
1 sandwich	237	27.0	7.0			65										I
french fries																
large	430		6.0	58.0								180				
6.1 oz	173	18.0	8.0			0										I
medium	350		5.0	48.0								160				
5 oz	142	15.0	4.0			0										I
small	240		4.0	33.0								100				
3.4 oz	96	10.0	3.0			0										I
Frisco Breakfast Sandwich, ham	500		24.0	46.0								1370				
1 sandwich	210	25.0	9.0			290										I
gravy	20		0.0	3.0								260				
1.5 oz	43	0.0	0.0	0.0	0.0	0										I
hamburger	270		14.0	29.0								670				
1 sandwich	110	11.0	3.0			35										I
Hash Rounds	230		3.0	24.0								560				
1 serving	79	14.0	3.0			0										I
hot ham 'n cheese sandwich	310		18.0	34.0								1410				
1 sandwich	148	12.0	6.0			50										I
mashed potatoes	70		2.0	14.0								330				
4 oz	113	0.0	0.0	0.0	0.0	0										I
mushroom 'n swiss burger	490		28.0	39.0								1100				
1 sandwich	193	25.0	12.0			80										I
pancakes	280		8.0	56.0								890				
3 pancakes	137	2.0	1.0			15										I
peach cobbler	310		2.0	60.0								380				
6.3 oz cobbler	178	7.0	1.0			0										I
roast beef sandwich	320		17.0	26.0								820				
1 sandwich	123	18.0	8.0			48										I
roast beef sandwich, big	460		26.0	35.0								1230				
1 sandwich	184	24.0	8.0			70										I
salad dressing																
french, fat-free	70		0.0	17.0								580				
2 oz	57	0.0	0.0	0.0	0.0	0										I
ranch	290		1.0	6.0								510				
2 oz	57	29.0	4.0			25										I
thousand island	250		1.0	9.0								540				
2 oz	57	23.0	3.0			35										I

	KCAL	H₂O (g)	PRO (g)	CHO (g)	SUGR (g)	DFIB (g)	A (RE)	C (mg)	B-2 (mg)	B-6 (mg)	FOL (mcg)	Na (mg)	Ca (mg)	Mg (mg)	Zn (mg)	Mn (mg)
	WT (g)	FAT (g)	SFA (g)	MUFA (g)	PUFA (g)	CHOL (mg)	A (IU)	B-1 (mg)	NIA (mg)	B-12 (mcg)	PANT (mg)	K (mg)	P (mg)	Fe (mg)	Cu (mg)	REF
salad w/o dressing																
garden	220		12.0	11.0								350				
1 salad	309	13.0	9.0			40										I
grilled chicken	150		20.0	11.0								810				
1 salad	329	3.0	1.0			60										I
side	25		1.0	4.0								45				
1 salad	131	0.0	0.0	0.0	0.0	0										I
shake																
choc	370		13.0	67.0								270				
1 shake	349	5.0	3.0			30										I
peach	390		10.0	77.0								290				
1 shake	345	4.0	3.0			25										I
strawberry	420		11.0	83.0								270				
1 shake	369	4.0	3.0			20										I
vanilla	350		12.0	65.0								300				
1 shake	349	5.0	3.0			20										I
sundae, hot fudge	290		7.0	51.0								310				
1 sundae	156	6.0	3.0			20										I
sundae, strawberry	210		5.0	43.0								140				
1 sundae	164	2.0	1.0			10										I

11.4 JACK-IN-THE-BOX

	KCAL	H₂O (g)	PRO (g)	CHO (g)	SUGR (g)	DFIB (g)	A (RE)	C (mg)	B-2 (mg)	B-6 (mg)	FOL (mcg)	Na (mg)	Ca (mg)	Mg (mg)	Zn (mg)	Mn (mg)
	WT (g)	FAT (g)	SFA (g)	MUFA (g)	PUFA (g)	CHOL (mg)	A (IU)	B-1 (mg)	NIA (mg)	B-12 (mcg)	PANT (mg)	K (mg)	P (mg)	Fe (mg)	Cu (mg)	REF
Breakfast Jack	300		18.0	30.0	5.0	0.0		9				890	200			
1 sandwich	121	12.0	5.0			185	400					220		2.70		I
burger, ¼ lb	510		26.0	39.0	8.0	0.0		0				1080	150			
1 sandwich	172	27.0	10.0			65	300					300		3.60		I
cake, carrot	370		3.0	58.0	39.0	1.0		0				310	20			
3.5 oz piece	99	15.0	3.0			30	7500					150		1.80		I
cheeseburger	320		16.0	32.0	5.0	0.0		1				670	150			
1 sandwich	110	15.0	6.0			35	300					210		2.70		I
double	450		24.0	35.0	6.0	0.0		0				970	250			
1 sandwich	152	24.0	12.0			75	500					320		3.60		I
ultimate	1030		50.0	30.0	6.0	0.0		1				1200	300			
1 sandwich	278	79.0	26.0			205	500					520		6.30		I
cheesecake	310		8.0	29.0	22.0	2.0						210				
1 serving	99	18.0	9.0			65						15				I
cheesecake, choc chip cookie dough	360		7.0	44.0	29.0	1.0		0				200	150			
3.6 oz piece	102	18.0	8.0			45	300					240		1.08		I
Chicken Caesar sandwich	520		27.0	44.0	5.0	4.0		2				1050	250			
1 sandwich	237	26.0	6.0			55	400					490		2.70		I
chicken fajita pita	290		24.0	29.0	3.0			6				700	250			
1 sandwich	189	8.0	3.0			35	500					430		2.70		I
chicken fillet, grilled sandwich	430		29.0	36.0	7.0	0.0		6				1070	150			
1 sandwich	211	19.0	5.0			65	300					540		6.30		I
chicken sandwich	400		20.0	38.0	0.0			0				1290	150			
1 sandwich	160	18.0	4.0			45	200					180		1.80		I
chicken sandwich, spicy crispy	560		24.0	55.0	5.0	0.0		5				1020	100			
1 sandwich	224	27.0	5.0			50	200					470		2.70		I
chicken strips, breaded																
chicken strips, breaded	290		25.0	18.0	0.0	0.0	0	0				700	0			
4 pieces	112	13.0	3.0			50	0					390		.72		I
chicken strips, breaded	450		39.0	28.0	0.0	0	0					1100	0			
6 pieces	177	20.0	5.0			80	0					600		1.08		I
Chicken Supreme sandwich	620		25.0	48.0	5.0	0.0		2				1520	200			
1 sandwich	245	36.0	11.0			75	500					190		2.70		I
chicken teriyaki bowl	580		28.0	115.0	20.0	6.0		9				1220	100			
1 bowl	440	1.5				30	5500					380		1.80		I
croutons	50		1.0	8.0	0.0	0.0	0	0				105	0	0		
.4 oz	11	2.0	0.5			0	0					20				I

	KCAL / WT (g)	H₂O (g) / FAT (g)	PRO (g) / SFA (g)	CHO (g) / MUFA (g)	SUGR (g) / PUFA (g)	DFIB (g) / CHOL (mg)	A (RE) / A (IU)	C (mg) / B-1 (mg)	B-2 (mg) / NIA (mg)	B-6 (mg) / B-12 (mcg)	FOL (mcg) / PANT (mg)	Na (mg) / K (mg)	Ca (mg) / P (mg)	Mg (mg) / Fe (mg)	Zn (mg) / Cu (mg)	Mn (mg) / REF
curley fries, seasoned	360		5.0	39.0	0.0	4.0	0	5				1070	20			
1 serving	109	20.0	5.0			0	0					560		1.44		I
egg rolls																
egg rolls	440		3.0	54.0		4.0		4				960	80			
3 pieces	165	24.0	7.0			30	0					510		2.70		I
egg rolls	750		5.0	92.0	10.0	7.0		6				1640	150			
5 pieces	285	41.0	12.0			50	0					870		3.60		
french fries																
jumbo	400		5.0	51.0	0.0	4.0	0	27				220	0			
4.3 oz	123	19.0	5.0			0	0					780		1.44		I
regular	350		4.0	45.0		4.0	0	24				190	0			
3.8 oz	109	17.0	4.0			0	0					690		1.08		I
small	220		3.0	28.0	0.0	3.0	0	18				120	0			
2.4 oz	68	11.0	2.5			0	0					500		.72		I
super scoop	590		8.0	76.0	6.0	0	42					330	20			
6.5 oz	184	29.0	7.0			0	0					1170		1.80		I
grilled sourdough burger	670		32.0	39.0	4.0	0.0		6				1180	200			
1 sandwich	223	43.0	16.0			110	750					510		4.50		I
hamburger	280		13.0	31.0	5.0	0.0		1				470	100			
1 sandwich	97	11.0	4.0			25	100					190		2.70		I
hash browns	160		1.0	14.0	0.0	1.0	0	6				310	0			
2 oz	57	11.0	2.5			0	0					190		.36		I
jalapenos, stuffed																
jalapenos, stuffed	420		15.0	29.0	3.0	3.0		9				1620	350			
7 pieces	136	27.0	12.0			55	750					170		.72		I
jalapenos, stuffed	600		22.0	41.0	4.0	4.0		12				2320	500			
10 pieces	195	39.0	16.0			75	1000					240		.72		I
Jumbo Jack	560		26.0	41.0	6.0	0.0		6				740	100			
1 sandwich	229	32.0	10.0			65	200					450		4.50		I
Jumbo Jack w/ cheese	650		31.0	42.0	6.0	0.0		6				1150	250			
1 sandwich	242	40.0	14.0			90	500					480		4.50		I
onion rings	380		5.0	38.0	4.0	0.0	0	2				450	20			
1 serving	103	23.0	6.0			0	0					130		1.80		I
pancake platter	400		13.0	59.0	12.0	3.0	0	0				980	80			
1 platter	160	12.0	3.0			30	0					280		1.80		I
potato wedges, bacon, & cheddar	800		20.0	49.0	2.0	4.0		12				1470	350			
9.35 oz	265	58.0	16.0			55	500					960		1.80		I
salad dressing																
blue cheese	210		1.0	11.0	3.0	0.0	0	0				750	0			
2 oz	57	18.0	3.5			15	0					35		.00		I
buttermilk house	290		1.0	6.0	2.0	0.0		4				560	20			
2 oz	57	30.0	11.0			20	100					70		.72		I
italian, low cal	25		0.0	2.0	2.0	0.0	0	0				670	0			
2 oz	57	1.5	0.0			0	0					40		.00		I
thousand island	250		1.0	10.0	8.0	0.0	0	0				570	0			
2 oz	57	24.0	4.0			20	0					65		.00		I
salad w/o dressing, garden chicken	200		23.0	8.0	4.0	3.0		12				420	200			
1 salad	253	9.0	4.0			65	3500					560		.72		I
salad w/o dressing, side	70		4.0	3.0	1.0	2.0		0				80	100			
1 salad	110	4.0	2.5			10	1250					190		.36		I
sauce																
barbecue dipping	45		1.0	11.0	7.0	0.0	0	0				300	0			
1 oz	28	0.0	0.0	0.0	0.0	0	0					75		.00		I
buttermilk house dipping	130		3.0	0	1							240	0			
.9 oz	25	13.0	5.0			10	0					30		.00		I
hot	5		1.0	0.0	0	0						110	0			
.5 oz	13	0.0	0.0	0.0	0.0	0	0					40		.00		I

	KCAL	H$_2$O (g)	PRO (g)	CHO (g)	SUGR (g)	DFIB (g)	A (RE)	C (mg)	B-2 (mg)	B-6 (mg)	FOL (mcg)	Na (mg)	Ca (mg)	Mg (mg)	Zn (mg)	Mn (mg)
	WT (g)	FAT (g)	SFA (g)	MUFA (g)	PUFA (g)	CHOL (mg)	A (IU)	B-1 (mg)	NIA (mg)	B-12 (mcg)	PANT (mg)	K (mg)	P (mg)	Fe (mg)	Cu (mg)	REF
salsa	10		0.0	2.0	1.0	0.0		0				200	0			
1 oz	28	0.0	0.0	0.0	0.0	0	100					70		.00		I
sweet & sour dipping	40		11.0	10.0	0.0	0		0				160	0			
1 oz	28	0.0	0.0	0.0	0.0	0	0					10		.00		I
tartar dipping	150		0.0	2.0	2.0	0	0	0				200	0			
1 oz	28	15.0	1.0			10	0					25		.00		I
sausage croissant	670		21.0	39.0	4.0	2.0		1				940	150			
1 croissant	182	48.0	19.0			250	1000					180		3.60		I
scrambled egg pocket	430		29.0	31.0	0.0		0					1060	200			
1 pocket	183	21.0	8.0			355	1000					340		3.60		I
shake																
cappuccino	630		11.0	80.0	58.0	0.0		0				320	350			
1 shake	306	29.0	17.0			90	750					710		.00		I
choc	630		11.0	85.0	67.0			0				330	350			
1 shake	310	27.0	16.0			85	750					715		.36		I
strawberry	640		10.0	85.0	67.0	0.0		0				300	350			
1 shake	299	28.0	15.0			85	750					620		.00		I
van	610		12.0	73.0	12.0	0.0		0				320	400			
1 shake	306	31.0	18.0			95	750					730		.00		I
sourdough breakfast sandwich	380		21.0	31.0	2.0	0.0		9				1120	250			
1 sandwich	147	20.0	7.0			235	750					260		3.60		I
Supreme Croissant	570		21.0	39.0	4.0	2.0		12				1240	100			
1 sandwich	172	36.0	15.0			245	750					300		3.60		I
taco	190		7.0	15.0	0.0	2.0	0	0				410	100			
1 taco	78	11.0	4.0			20						240		1.08		I
taco, monster	283		12.0	22.0	1.0	3.0	0	2				760	150			
1 taco	130	17.0	6.0			30	0					360		1.80		I
turnover, hot apple	310		8.0	29.0	22.0	2.0	0	0				210	100			
1 turnover	110	18.0	9.0			65	0					15		.36		I
Ultimate Breakfast sandwich	620		36.0	39.0	4.0			9				1800	250			
1 sandwich	242	35.0	11.0			455	750					450		4.50		I

11.5 KENTUCKY FRIED CHICKEN

	KCAL	H$_2$O (g)	PRO (g)	CHO (g)	SUGR (g)	DFIB (g)	A (RE)	C (mg)	B-2 (mg)	B-6 (mg)	FOL (mcg)	Na (mg)	Ca (mg)	Mg (mg)	Zn (mg)	Mn (mg)
	WT (g)	FAT (g)	SFA (g)	MUFA (g)	PUFA (g)	CHOL (mg)	A (IU)	B-1 (mg)	NIA (mg)	B-12 (mcg)	PANT (mg)	K (mg)	P (mg)	Fe (mg)	Cu (mg)	REF
bbq baked beans	190		6.0	33.0	13.0	6.0		0				760	80			
5.5 oz	156	3.0	1.0			5	400							1.80		I
biscuit	180		4.0	20.0	2.0	0	0					560	20			
2 oz biscuit	56	10.0	2.5			0	0							1.08		I
chicken, Extra Tasty Crispy																
breast	470		31.0	25.0	0.0	1.0	0	0				930	40			
5.9 oz	168	28.0	7.0			80	0							1.08		I
drumstick	190		13.0	8.0	0.0	0	0					260	0			
2.4 oz	67	11.0	3.0			60	0							.72		I
thigh	370		19.0	18.0	0.0	2.0						540	20			
4.2 oz	118	25.0	6.0			70								1.08		I
wing	200		10.0	10.0	0.0	0	0					290	0			
1.9 oz	55	13.0	4.0			45	0							.36		I
chicken, Hot & Spicy																
breast	530		32.0	23.0	0.0	2.0	0	0				1110	40			
6.5 oz	180	35.0	8.0			110	0							1.08		I
drumstick	190		13.0	10.0	0.0	0	0					300	0			
2.3 oz	64	11.0	3.0			50	0							.72		I
thigh	370		18.0	13.0	0.0	1.0	0	0				570	0			
3.8 oz	107	27.0	7.0			90	0							1.08		I
wing	210		10.0	9.0	0.0	0	0					340	40			
1.9 oz	55	15.0	4.0			50	0							.36		I

	KCAL	H₂O (g)	PRO (g)	CHO (g)	SUGR (g)	DFIB (g)	A (RE)	C (mg)	B-2 (mg)	B-6 (mg)	FOL (mcg)	Na (mg)	Ca (mg)	Mg (mg)	Zn (mg)	Mn (mg)
	WT (g)	FAT (g)	SFA (g)	MUFA (g)	PUFA (g)	CHOL (mg)	A (IU)	B-1 (mg)	NIA (mg)	B-12 (mcg)	PANT (mg)	K (mg)	P (mg)	Fe (mg)	Cu (mg)	REF
chicken, Original Recipe																
breast	400		29.0	16.0	0.0	1.0	0	0				1116	40			
5.4 oz	153	24.0	6.0			135	0							1.08		I
drumstick	140		13.0	4.0	0.0	0.0	0	0				422	0			
2.2 oz	61	9.0	2.0			75	0							.72		I
thigh	250		16.0	6.0	0.0	1.0	0	0				747	20			
3.2 oz	91	18.0	4.5			95	0							.72		I
wing	140		9.0	5.0	0.0	0.0	0	0				414	0			
1.6 oz	47	10.0	2.5			55	0							.36		I
chicken sandwich, bbq	256		17.0	28.0	18.0	2.0	0	4				782	60			
5.3 oz sandwich	149	8.0	1.0			57	0							4.14		I
chicken sandwich, Original Recipe	497		28.6	45.5	2.0	3.0	0	0				1213	10			
7.3 oz sandwich	206	22.3	4.8			52	0							2.70		I
chicken, Tender Roast																
breast w/o skin	169		31.4	1.0	0.0	0.0	0	0				797	0			
4.2 oz	118	4.3	1.2			112	0							.00		I
breast w/ skin	251		37.0	1.0	0.0	0	0					830	0				
4.9 oz	139	10.8	3.0			151	0							.00		I
drumstick w/o skin	67		11.0	0.0	0.0	0	0					259	0				
1.2 oz	38	2.4	0.7			63	0							.00		I
drumstick w/ skin	97		14.5	0.0	0	0						271	0				
1.9 oz	55	4.3	1.2			85	0							.00		I
thigh w/o skin	106		12.9	0.0	0	0						312	0				
2.1 oz	59	5.5	1.7			84	0							.00		I
thigh w/ skin	207		18.4	0.0	0	0						504	0				
3.2 oz	90	12.0	3.8			120	0							.00		I
wing w/ skin	121		12.2	1.0	0.0	0	0					331	0				
1.8 oz	50	7.7	2.1			74	0							.00		I
chunky chicken pot pie	770		29.0	69.0	8.0	5.0		1				2160	10			
13 oz	368	42.0	13.0			70	4000							1.80		I
coleslaw	180		2.0	21.0	20.0	3.0	0	36				280	40			
5 oz serving	142	9.0	1.5			5	0							.72		I
Colonel's Crispy Strips	261		19.8	10.0	0.0	3.0	0	0				658	0			
3 strips	92	15.8	3.7			40	0							.54		I
corn-on-the-cob	190		5.0	34.0	2.0	4.0		6				20	0			
5 oz ear	143	3.0	0.5			0	1250							.72		I
cornbread	228		3.0	25.0	10.0	1.0	0	0				194	60			
2 oz piece	56	13.0	2.0			42	0							.72		I
garden rice	120		3.0	23.0	2.0	1.0		9				890	20			
4.4 oz	125	1.5	0.0			0	500							.00		I
green beans	45		1.0	7.0	3.0	3.0		2				730	40			
4.7 oz	132	1.5	0.5			5	200							.72		I
Hot Wings	471		27.0	18.0	0.0	2.0	0	0				1230	40			
6 pieces (4.8 oz)	135	33.0	8.0			150	0							1.44		I
Kentucky Nuggets	284		16.0	15.0	0.0	0	0					865	20				
3.4 oz	95	18.0	4.0			66	0							.72		I
macaroni & cheese	180		7.0	21.0	2.0	2.0		0				860	150			
5.4 oz	153	8.0	3.0			10	1000							.00		I
Mean Greens	70		4.0	11.0	1.0	5.0		6				650	200			
5.4 oz	152	3.0	1.0			10	3000							1.80		I
potato salad	230		4.0	23.0	9.0	3.0		0				540	20			
5.6 oz	160	14.0	2.0			15	500							2.70		I
potato wedges	280		5.0	28.0	1.0	5.0	0	1				750	20			
4.8 oz	135	13.0	4.0			5	0							.00		I
potatoes, mashed w/ gravy	120		1.0	17.0	0.0	2.0	0	0				440	0			
4.8 oz	136	6.0	1.0			0								.00	I	
red beans & rice	130		5.0	21.0	2.0	3.0	0	0				360	20			
4.5 oz	128	3.0	1.0			5	0							.72		I

	KCAL	H₂O (g)	PRO (g)	CHO (g)	SUGR (g)	DFIB (g)	A (RE)	C (mg)	B-2 (mg)	B-6 (mg)	FOL (mcg)	Na (mg)	Ca (mg)	Mg (mg)	Zn (mg)	Mn (mg)
	WT (g)	FAT (g)	SFA (g)	MUFA (g)	PUFA (g)	CHOL (mg)	A (IU)	B-1 (mg)	NIA (mg)	B-12 (mcg)	PANT (mg)	K (mg)	P (mg)	Fe (mg)	Cu (mg)	REF

11.6 MCDONALD'S

	KCAL/WT	H₂O/FAT	PRO/SFA	CHO/MUFA	SUGR/PUFA	DFIB/CHOL	A(RE)/A(IU)	C/B-1	B-2/NIA	B-6/B-12	FOL/PANT	Na/K	Ca/P	Mg/Fe	Zn/Cu	Mn/REF
Big Mac	560		25.2	42.5				2	.41			950	256			
1 sandwich	215	32.4	10.1	20.9	1.5	103	352	.48	6.8					4.00		I
biscuit	260		4.6	31.9				0	.11			730	75			
1 biscuit	75	12.7	3.4	8.6	0.6	1	0	.23	1.7					1.31		I
w/ bacon, egg, & cheese	440		17.5	33.3				0	.33			1230	185			
1 biscuit	156	26.4	8.2	16.1	2.0	253	534	.36	2.5					2.56		I
w/ sausage	440		13.0	31.9				0	.21			1080	83			
1 biscuit	123	29.0	9.3	17.2	2.5	49	0	.49	4.0					1.98		I
w/ sausage & egg	520		19.9	32.6				0	.35			1250	116			
1 biscuit	180	34.5	11.2	20.0	3.4	275	294	.53	4.0					3.16		I
cheeseburger	310		15.0	31.2				2	.21			750	199			
1 sandwich	116	13.8	5.2	7.7	0.9	53	392	.29	3.9					2.30		I
Chicken McNugget Sce																
barbecue	50		0.3	12.1				2	.01			340	13			
1 container	32	0.5	0.1	0.2	0.2	0	153	.01	0.2					.31		I
honey	45		0.0	11.5				0	.01			0	1			
1 container	14	0.0	0.0	0.0	0.0	0	0	.00	0.0					.07		I
hot mustard	70		0.5	8.2				0	.01			250	15			
1 container	30	3.6	0.5	1.2	1.9	5	16	.01	0.2					.22		I
sweet & sour	60		0.2	13.8				1	.01			190	11			
1 container	32	0.2	0.0	0.1	0.1	0	324	.00	0.1					.17		I
Chicken McNuggets	290		19.0	16.5				0	.12			520	13			
1 serving	113	16.3	4.1	10.4	1.8	65	0	.11	9.0					1.00		I
cookies, Chocolaty Chip	330		4.2	41.9				0	.21			280	24			
1 box	62	15.6	5.0	10.2	0.4	4	0	.18	2.5					2.18		I
cookies, McDonaldland	290		4.2	47.1				0	.18			300	9			
1 box	60	9.2	1.9	6.8	0.5	10	0	.25	2.5					2.07		I
danish																
apple	390		5.8	51.2				16	.20			370	14			
1 danish	115	17.9	3.5	10.8	2.0	25	115	.28	2.2					1.37		I
cheese, iced	390		7.4	42.3				1	.23			420	33			
1 danish	110	21.8	6.0	12.1	1.8	47	188	.29	2.1					1.42		I
cinnamon	440		6.4	57.5				3	.24			430	35			
1 danish	110	21.0	4.2	13.0	1.6	34	110	.33	2.8					1.81		I
raspberry	410		6.1	61.5				3	.31			310	14			
1 danish	117	15.9	3.1	10.2	1.1	26	117	.33	2.1					1.47		I
Egg McMuffin	290		18.2	28.1				0	.33			740	256			
1 McMuffin	138	11.2	3.8	6.1	1.3	226	499	.47	3.7					2.77		I
english muffin w/ butter	170		5.4	26.7				0	.14			270	151			
1 muffin	59	4.6	2.4	1.7	0.5	9	122	.33	2.5					1.61		I
Fillet-O-Fish sandwich	440		13.8	37.9				0	.15			1030	165			
1 sandwich	142	26.1	5.2	10.2	10.8	50	146	.30	2.7					1.83		I
french fries																
large	400		5.6	45.9				15	.00			200	18			
4.3 oz	122	21.6	9.1	11.6	0.9	16	0	.24	3.3					.93		I
medium	320		4.4	36.3				12	.00			150	14			
3.4 oz	97	17.1	7.2	9.2	0.7	12	0	.19	2.6					.73		I
small	220		3.1	25.6				8	.00			110	10			
2.4 oz	68	12.0	5.1	6.5	0.5	9	0	.14	1.8					.52		I
frzn yogurt, lowfat																
hot caramel sundae	270		6.6	59.3				0	.35			180	222			
1 sundae	174	2.8	1.5	1.2	0.1	13	291	.08	0.3					.08		I
hot fudge sundae	240		7.3	50.5				0	.35			170	235			
1 sundae	169	3.2	2.4	0.8	0.1	6	214	.08	0.3					.48		I

	KCAL / WT (g)	H₂O (g) / FAT (g)	PRO (g) / SFA (g)	CHO (g) / MUFA (g)	SUGR (g) / PUFA (g)	DFIB (g) / CHOL (mg)	A (RE) / A (IU)	C (mg) / B-1 (mg)	B-2 (mg) / NIA (mg)	B-6 (mg) / B-12 (mcg)	FOL (mcg) / PANT (mg)	Na (mg) / K (mg)	Ca (mg) / P (mg)	Mg (mg) / Fe (mg)	Zn (mg) / Cu (mg)	Mn (mg) / REF
strawberry sundae	210		5.7	49.2				1	.29			95	190			
1 sundae	171	1.1	0.6	0.4	0.0	5	214	.07	0.3					.16		I
van cone	100		4.0	22.0				0	.18			80	112			
1 cone	86	0.8	0.4	0.3	0.1	3	128	.04	0.4					.23		I
hamburger	260		12.2	30.6				2	.16			500	122			
1 sandwich	102	9.5	3.6	5.1	0.8	37	152	.28	3.8					2.29		I
hash brown potatoes	130		1.4	14.9				2	.02			330	6			
1 serving	53	7.3	3.2	3.7	0.4	9	0	.06	0.9					.27		I
hotcakes w/ butter & syrup	410		8.2	74.4				0	.33			640	114			
1 serving	176	9.2	3.7	3.1	2.5	21	173	.32	2.8					2.08		I
McChicken	490		19.2	39.8				2	.21			780	143			
6.7 oz sandwich	190	28.6	5.4	11.5	11.6	43	104	.96	8.9					2.61		I
McDLT	580		26.3	36.0				7	.36			990	225			
1 sandwich	234	36.8	11.5	16.7	8.5	109	754	.39	6.9					3.91		I
muffin, apple bran	190		5.0	46.0				1	.08			230	31			
1 muffin	85	0.0	0.0	0.0	0.0	0	7	.02	0.4					.60		I
pie, apple	260		2.2	30.0				11	.02			240	11			
1 snack pie	83	14.8	4.8	9.1	0.9	6	0	.06	0.3					.71		I
Quarter Pounder	410		23.1	34.0				3	.29			660	142			
1 sandwich	166	20.7	8.1	11.4	1.2	86	223	.36	6.7					3.68		I
Quarter Pounder w/ cheese	520		28.5	35.1				3	.39			1150	295			
1 sandwich	194	29.2	11.2	16.5	1.5	118	703	.37	6.7					3.72		I
salad dressing/topping																
bacon bits	16		1.3	0.1				0	.00			95	0			
.1 oz	3	1.2	0.0	1.2	0.0	0	0	.00	0.0					.00		I
blue cheese	70		0.5	1.2				0	.02			150	15			
.5 oz	14	6.9	1.3	1.8	3.8	6	18	.00	0.0					.03		I
croutons	50		1.4	6.8				0	.03			140	6			
.4 oz	11	2.2	0.5	1.3	0.1	0	0	.05	0.4					.35		I
peppercorn	80		0.2	0.5				0	.00			85	3			
.5 oz	14	8.7	1.4	2.2	5.2	7	9	.00	0.0					.05		I
ranch	83		0.2	1.3				0	.02			130	7			
.5 oz	14	8.6	1.4	2.2	5.1	5	11	.01	0.0					.04		I
red french, red cal	40		0.1	5.2				1	.00			110	3			
.5 oz	14	1.9	0.3	0.5	1.1	0	74	.00	0.1					.10		I
thousand island	78		0.2	2.4				0	.00			100	3			
.5 oz	14	7.5	1.2	1.9	4.4	8	49	.00	0.0					.08		I
vinaigrette, lite	15		0.2	2.0				0	.00			75	3			
.5 oz	14	0.5	0.1	0.1	0.3	0	92	.00	0.0					.04		I
salad w/o dressing																
chef	230		20.5	7.5				14	.29			490	256			
1 salad	283	13.3	5.9	6.5	0.9	128	4114	.31	3.6					1.51		I
chunky chicken	140		23.1	5.3				20	.17			230	34			
1 salad	250	3.4	0.9	2.0	0.5	78	3660	.22	8.5					1.02		I
garden	110		7.1	6.2				13	.16			160	149			
1 salad	213	6.6	2.9	3.2	0.5	83	3915	.10	0.6					1.26		I
side	60		3.7	3.3				7	.08			85	76			
1 salad	115	3.3	1.5	1.6	0.3	41	2173	.05	0.3					.67		I
sausage	180		8.4	0.0	0.0			0	.10			350	8			
1 serving	48	16.3	5.9	8.5	1.9	48	0	.27	2.3					.67		I
sausage McMuffin	370		16.5	27.3				0	.29			830	235			
1 McMuffin	117	21.9	7.8	11.7	2.4	64	240	.60	4.8					2.30		I
sausage McMuffin w/ egg	440		22.6	27.9				0	.42			980	263			
1 McMuffin	167	26.8	9.5	14.2	3.2	263	499	.64	4.8					3.34		I
scrambled eggs	140		12.4	1.2				0	.26			290	57			
1 serving	100	9.8	3.3	5.0	1.4	399	518	.07	0.1					2.08		I
shake, lowfat																
choc	320		11.6	66.0				0	.50			240	332			
1 shake	293	1.7	0.8	0.9	0.1	10	306	.13	0.4					.84		I

	KCAL / WT (g)	H₂O (g) / FAT (g)	PRO (g) / SFA (g)	CHO (g) / MUFA (g)	SUGR (g) / PUFA (g)	DFIB (g) / CHOL (mg)	A (RE) / A (IU)	C (mg) / B-1 (mg)	B-2 (mg) / NIA (mg)	B-6 (mg) / B-12 (mcg)	FOL (mcg) / PANT (mg)	Na (mg) / K (mg)	Ca (mg) / P (mg)	Mg (mg) / Fe (mg)	Zn (mg) / Cu (mg)	Mn (mg) / REF
strawberry	320		10.7	67.0				0	.48			170	327			
1 shake	239	1.3	0.6	0.6	0.1	10	306	.13	0.3					.09		I
van	290		10.8	60.0				0	.48			170	327			
1 shake	239	1.3	0.6	0.7	0.1	10	306	.13	0.3					.10		I

11.7 PIZZA HUT

Bigfoot Pizza

	KCAL / WT (g)	H₂O (g) / FAT (g)	PRO (g) / SFA (g)	CHO (g) / MUFA (g)	SUGR (g) / PUFA (g)	DFIB (g) / CHOL (mg)	A (RE) / A (IU)	C (mg) / B-1 (mg)	B-2 (mg) / NIA (mg)	B-6 (mg) / B-12 (mcg)	FOL (mcg) / PANT (mg)	Na (mg) / K (mg)	Ca (mg) / P (mg)	Mg (mg) / Fe (mg)	Zn (mg) / Cu (mg)	Mn (mg) / REF
cheese	186		10.0	25.0		2.0						525	104			
2.7 oz slice	76	6.0	3.0			16	348							1.60		I
pepperoni	205		10.0	25.0		2.0						589	105			
2.8 oz slice	79	7.0	3.0			20	369							1.60		I
pepperoni, mushroom, & italian sausage	214		11.0	25.0		2.0						665	106			
3.2 oz slice	90	8.0	4.0			21	366							1.70		I

Hand Tossed Pizza

	KCAL / WT (g)	H₂O (g) / FAT (g)	PRO (g) / SFA (g)	CHO (g) / MUFA (g)	SUGR (g) / PUFA (g)	DFIB (g) / CHOL (mg)	A (RE) / A (IU)	C (mg) / B-1 (mg)	B-2 (mg) / NIA (mg)	B-6 (mg) / B-12 (mcg)	FOL (mcg) / PANT (mg)	Na (mg) / K (mg)	Ca (mg) / P (mg)	Mg (mg) / Fe (mg)	Zn (mg) / Cu (mg)	Mn (mg) / REF
beef	260		15.0	29.0		2.0						797	113			
4.2 oz slice	120	9.0	4.0			26	438							2.10		I
cheese	235		13.0	29.0		2.0						621	142			
3.8 oz slice	108	7.0	4.0			25	496							1.50		I
ham	213		12.0	29.0		2.0						657	100			
3.7 oz slice	105	5.0	3.0			21	425							1.60		I
italian sausage	267		13.0	29.0		2.0						737	104			
4.1 oz slice	116	11.0	5.0			31	432							1.07		I
Meat Lover's	314		17.0	29.0		2.0						958	110			
4.6 oz slice	130	11.0	6.0			38	463							2.10		I
pepperoni	238		12.0	29.0		2.0						689	101			
3.7 oz slice	104	8.0	4.0			24	467							1.60		I
Pepperoni Lover's	306		16.0	30.0		2.0						897	145			
4.3 oz slice	123	14.0	6.0			40	615							1.80		I
pork topping	268		14.0	29.0		2.0						797	115			
4.25 oz slice	121	10.0	5.0			26	448							2.10		I
Super Supreme	296		16.0	30.0		3.0						946	116			
5.05 oz slice	143	13.0	5.0			34	496							2.20		I
Supreme	284		16.0	30.0		3.0						884	116			
4.8 oz slice	136	12.0	5.0			30	480							2.30		I
Veggie Lover's	216		11.0	30.0		3.0						632	108			
4.8 oz slice	133	6.0	3.0			17	474							1.80		I

Pan Pizza

	KCAL / WT (g)	H₂O (g) / FAT (g)	PRO (g) / SFA (g)	CHO (g) / MUFA (g)	SUGR (g) / PUFA (g)	DFIB (g) / CHOL (mg)	A (RE) / A (IU)	C (mg) / B-1 (mg)	B-2 (mg) / NIA (mg)	B-6 (mg) / B-12 (mcg)	FOL (mcg) / PANT (mg)	Na (mg) / K (mg)	Ca (mg) / P (mg)	Mg (mg) / Fe (mg)	Zn (mg) / Cu (mg)	Mn (mg) / REF
beef	286		14.0	28.0		2.0						677	116			
4.2 oz slice	120	13.0	5.0			26	458							1.60		I
cheese	261		12.0	28.0		2.0						501	144			
3.8 oz slice	108	11.0	5.0			25	528							1.50		I
ham	239		11.0	28.0		2.0						537	101			
3.7 oz slice	105	9.0	3.0			21	432							1.60		I
Meat Lover's	340		16.0	28.0		2.0						838	111			
4.6 oz slice	130	18.0	7.0			38	471							2.10		I
pepperoni	265		11.0	28.0		2.0						569	103			
3.7 oz slice	104	12.0	4.0			24	475							1.60		I
Pepperoni Lover's	332		15.0	28.0		2.0						777	147			
4.3 oz slice	123	17.0	7.0			40	622							1.80		I
pork topping	294		13.0	28.0		2.0						677	116			
4.25 oz slice	121	14.0	5.0			26	456							2.10		I
sausage	293		12.0	27.0		2.0						617	105			
4.1 oz slice	116	15.0	5.0			31	439							1.70		I
Super Supreme	323		15.0	28.0		3.0						826	118			
5.1 oz slice	143	17.0	6.0			34	503							2.20		I
Supreme	311		15.0	28.0		3.0						764	117			
4.8 oz slice	136	15.0	6.0			30	488							2.30		I

	KCAL / WT (g)	H₂O (g) / FAT (g)	PRO (g) / SFA (g)	CHO (g) / MUFA (g)	SUGR (g) / PUFA (g)	DFIB (g) / CHOL (mg)	A (RE) / A (IU)	C (mg) / B-1 (mg)	B-2 (mg) / NIA (mg)	B-6 (mg) / B-12 (mcg)	FOL (mcg) / PANT (mg)	Na (mg) / K (mg)	Ca (mg) / P (mg)	Mg (mg) / Fe (mg)	Zn (mg) / Cu (mg)	Mn (mg) / REF
Veggie Lover's	243		10.0	29.0		3.0						512	109			
4.8 oz slice	133	10.0	3.0			17	482							1.80		I
Personal Pan Pizza, pepperoni	637		27.0	69.0		5.0						1340	250			
9 oz pizza	255	28.0	10.0			55	1165							4.00		I
Personal Pan Pizza, Supreme	722		33.0	70.0		6.0						1760	276			
11.5 oz pizza	327	34.0	12.0			66	1200							5.20		I
Thin 'n Crispy Pizza																
beef	229		13.0	21.0		2.0						709	116			
3.5 oz slice	99	11.0	5.0			26	458							1.60		I
cheese	205		11.0	21.0		2.0						534	145			
3 oz slice	87	8.0	4.0			25	541							1.03		I
ham	184		10.0	21.0		1.0						591	103			
3 oz slice	85	7.0	3.0			22	446							1.10		I
italian sausage	236		11.0	21.0		2.0						650	107			
3.3 oz slice	94	12.0	5.0			31	452							1.20		I
Meat Lover's	288		15.0	21.0		2.0						892	113			
3.9 oz slice	110	13.0	6.0			39	488							1.60		I
pepperoni	215		11.0	21.0		1.0						627	104			
3 oz slice	84	10.0	4.0			25	496							1.10		I
Pepperoni Lover's	289		15.0	22.0		2.0						862	149			
3.7 oz slice	105	16.0	7.0			42	652							1.30		I
pork topping	237		12.0	21.0		2.0						709	118			
3.5 oz slice	99	12.0	5.0			26	468							1.60		I
Super Supreme	270		14.0	22.0		2.0						880	119			
4.3 oz slice	123	14.0	6.0			35	520							1.70		I
Supreme	257		14.0	21.0		2.0						795	119			
4.1 oz slice	116	13.0	5.0			31	493							1.80		I
Veggie Lover's	186		9.0	22.0		2.0						545	111			
3.9 oz slice	112	7.0	3.0			17	494							1.30		I

11.8 TACO BELL

	KCAL / WT (g)	H₂O (g) / FAT (g)	PRO (g) / SFA (g)	CHO (g) / MUFA (g)	SUGR (g) / PUFA (g)	DFIB (g) / CHOL (mg)	A (RE) / A (IU)	C (mg) / B-1 (mg)	B-2 (mg) / NIA (mg)	B-6 (mg) / B-12 (mcg)	FOL (mcg) / PANT (mg)	Na (mg) / K (mg)	Ca (mg) / P (mg)	Mg (mg) / Fe (mg)	Zn (mg) / Cu (mg)	Mn (mg) / REF
burrito																
bean	373		13.1	54.6	2.2	12.0	281		.10	.01	1	1139	139	33	.76	.350
1 burrito	199	12.0	3.7	2.4	0.5	8		.09	0.0	.09		363	133	2.28	.166	I
chili cheese	326		14.3	37.1	1.5	4.3	607	0	.11			874	173		.33	
1 burrito	142	13.4	5.6	1.8	0.1	34		.06	0.8	.17		100	69	1.27		I
light chicken	309		18.3	41.0	3.0	2.5	395	2	.01	.01	9	985	190	2	.05	.031
1 burrito	177	7.9				27		.04	0.1		.01	56	5	.94	.008	I
seven layers	530		16.2	64.8	3.7	13.9	113	5	.16	.15	10	1306	193	42	.97	.415
1 burrito	284	23.5	8.6	7.4	1.3	25		.19	1.1	.33		487	171	2.94	.232	I
Burrito Supreme	449		18.6	50.2			295					1217	151	30	1.73	.272
1 burrito	255	18.4	7.8	4.4	0.6	43						422	173	2.22	.142	I
big beef	534		25.8	51.6	3.4	8.0	295		.28	.17	15	1451	157	39	2.86	.328
1 burrito	291	22.9	10.0	6.2	0.8	68		.17	3.8	1.58	.39	546	234	2.88	.184	I
light chicken	425		25.4	51.8	4.4	2.7	327	6	.05			1415	166	3	.10	
1 burrito	248	12.9	3.1	3.5	0.8	54		.06	0.4	.18	.25	54	42	1.41	.002	I
cinnamon twists	139		1.2	19.7			41	1	.05			189	12			
1 twist	28	6.1	3.0		1.0	0		.01	0.3			27		.41		I
fajita																
chicken	461		17.8	49.3	3.5	2.6	32	4	.01	.01	2	1214	137	2	.02	.015
1 fajita	220	21.2				44		.05	0.4		.04	34	10	1.19	.012	I
steak	465		19.9	47.7	2.4	2.6	32	3	.01	.01	2	1128	129	2	.02	.015
1 fajita	220	21.3				37		.05	0.4		.04	34	10	1.77	.012	I
Supreme, chicken	505		18.6	51.2	4.7	2.8	41	7	.05	.03	4	1227	157	5	.13	.030
1 fajita	255	25.1				55		.09	0.6	.07	.13	96	33	1.26	.024	I
Supreme, steak	510		20.7	49.6	3.6	2.8	41	6	.05	.03	4	1141	150	5	.13	.030
1 fajita	255	25.2				47		.09	0.6	.07	.13	96	33	1.84	.024	I
Supreme, veg	466		11.4	52.6	3.6	2.8	88		.05	.03	4	934	152	5	.13	.030
1 fajita	255	23.1				29		.09	0.6	.07	.13	96	33	1.15	.024	I

	KCAL / WT (g)	H₂O (g) / FAT (g)	PRO (g) / SFA (g)	CHO (g) / MUFA (g)	SUGR (g) / PUFA (g)	DFIB (g) / CHOL (mg)	A (RE) / A (IU)	C (mg) / B-1 (mg)	B-2 (mg) / NIA (mg)	B-6 (mg) / B-12 (mcg)	FOL (mcg) / PANT (mg)	Na (mg) / K (mg)	Ca (mg) / P (mg)	Mg (mg) / Fe (mg)	Zn (mg) / Cu (mg)	Mn (mg) / REF
veg	421		10.6	50.7	2.4	2.6	80	3	.01	.01	2	921	132	2	.02	.015
1 fajita	220	19.2				18		.05	0.4		.04	34	10	1.08	.012	I
mexican pizza	565		20.9	40.9	0.7	5.6	470	4	.33	.09		1047	234		1.77	.247
1 serving	216	36.3	11.4	13.3	9.8	52		.35	3.8	.89	.18	351	184	3.72	.136	I
mexican rice	191		5.8	19.6	0.1	0.4	325	1	.07	.00	2	508	117	1	.35	.006
1 serving	131	10.0	4.1	4.4	0.4	14		.13	0.8	.17	.00	50	84	.78	.007	I
nachos	322		2.4	34.3	1.8	3.2	51	0	.07	.00	0	538	102	5	.08	
1 serving	99	18.1	3.6	5.1	1.9	3		.01	0.0	.02		137	184	.07	.003	I
Bell Grande	774		15.6	83.2	3.7	16.8	61	4	.23	.09	6	1198	217	50	1.91	.471
1 serving	308	38.8	10.4	9.7	2.7	40		.18	2.0	.80	.24	568	366	2.59	.221	I
Supreme, big beef	453		11.8	43.4	2.5	8.8	36	4	.18	.09	6	723	123	31	1.58	.247
1 serving	195	23.5	7.5	6.3	1.5	38		.13	2.0	.79	.24	382	226	1.69	.139	I
pintos 'n cheese w/ red sauce	179		9.1	18.2	0.5	9.8	305	1				693	147	32	.91	.340
1 serving	128	8.4	3.8	3.0	0.6	15						358	166	1.78	.162	I
sauce																
green sce	4		0.1	0.8	0.1		21	0				129	4			
1 serving	28	0.0	0.0	0.0	0.0	0						10		.04		I
guacamole	36		0.4	2.0	0.3	1.4	8	2	.02	.13		144	4	5	.07	.038
1 serving	21	2.9	0.7	1.8	0.4	1		.01	0.5	.18	.17	94	8	.21	.053	I
nacho cheese	115		2.4	4.5	1.6	0.1	51	0	.07	.00	0	465	49	5	.08	
1 serving	57	9.6	2.3	5.1	1.9	3		.01	0.0	.02		76	184	.07	.003	I
pico de gallo	7		0.2	1.1	0.7	0.3	128	4				67	3			
1 serving	21	0.2	0.0	0.0	0.0	1						0		.11		I
red sce	10		0.3	2.3			257	1	.03			261	11			
1 serving	28	0.0	0.0	0.0	0.0	0						45				I
salsa	24		0.9	5.0	3.1		1347	10				492	34			
1 serving	85	0.0	0.0	0.0	0.0	0						376		.33		I
sour cream	42		0.7	1.2	0.8		0	0	.03	.00		12	19	2	.09	
1 serving	21	3.8	2.3	1.1	0.1	11		.03	0.0	.07	.06	31	20	.01	.001	I
taco sce, mild	2			0.0	0.0		6					75				
1 serving	11	0.0	0.0	0.0	0.0	0						13				I
soft taco	226		11.9	20.0	1.2	1.8	33	3	.11	.08	4	527	78	10	1.30	.071
1 taco	99	9.7	4.3	2.5	0.2	32		.05	1.9	.80	.18	162	99	1.00	.053	I
light chicken	183		13.0	21.4	2.8	1.5	189	5	.00	.01	8	660	102	1	.03	.021
1 taco	99	5.1				27		.01	0.0		.01	22	3	.68	.004	I
steak	197		14.5	18.3	1.0	1.3	29	1	.03	.01	8	502	78	1	.19	.021
1 taco	99	7.3				26		.01	0.0	.09	.01	29	38	1.18	.004	I
Supreme	270		12.8	21.6	2.2	1.9	37	3	.15	.09	12	540	100	13	1.43	.092
1 taco	135	13.5	6.6	3.6	0.4	43		.09	2.0	.87	.25	215	122	1.08	.057	I
taco	183		10.2	11.1	0.4	1.5	44	1	.11	.08	9	281	69	10	1.32	.078
1 taco	78	9.7	4.1	2.5	0.2	32		.05	1.9	.80	.15	153	99		.046	I
Double Decker	350		15.7	36.9	1.4	7.5	44	1	.13	.08	9	698	107	26	1.62	.248
1 taco	156	14.5	5.2	3.3	0.5	32		.09	1.9	.80	.15	303	147	2.00	.127	I
Supreme	228		11.0	13.0	1.6	1.7	53	3	.15	.09	12	295	89		1.43	.092
1 taco	113	13.5	6.4	3.6	0.4	43		.09	2.0	.87	.25	215	122	.95	.057	I
Supreme, Double Decker	395		16.5	38.8	2.6	7.7	53	4	.17	.09	12	711	127	30	1.72	.262
1 taco	191	18.4	7.6	4.4	0.6	43		.13	2.0	.87	.25	365	170	2.07	.138	I
taco salad w/ salsa	431		26.4	29.3	7.8	12.6	1460	22	.35	.22	89	1419	232	68	3.61	.702
1 salad	464	21.5	10.6	7.7	1.2	76		.28	4.2	1.66	.48	889	344	4.34	.309	I
taco salad w/ salsa & shell	856		32.1	62.4	7.8	13.2	1460		.47	.22	89	1674	265	68	3.61	.702
1 salad	535	51.8	14.8	23.0	11.6	76		.53	5.8	1.66	.48	889	344	6.33	.309	I
tostada w/ red sce	292		10.8	31.2	1.2	11.4	339	2	.13	.01	16	696	166	35	1.25	.383
1 tostada	177	14.4	4.8	3.0	0.6	15		.10	0.1	.17	.01	403	173	2.05	.169	I

11.9 WENDY'S

	KCAL / WT (g)	H₂O (g) / FAT (g)	PRO (g) / SFA (g)	CHO (g) / MUFA (g)	SUGR (g) / PUFA (g)	DFIB (g) / CHOL (mg)	A (RE) / A (IU)	C (mg) / B-1 (mg)	B-2 (mg) / NIA (mg)	B-6 (mg) / B-12 (mcg)	FOL (mcg) / PANT (mg)	Na (mg) / K (mg)	Ca (mg) / P (mg)	Mg (mg) / Fe (mg)	Zn (mg) / Cu (mg)	Mn (mg) / REF
breadstick, soft	130		4.0	24.0		1.0	0	0				250	40			
1.6 oz breadstick	44	3.0	0.5			5	0							1.44		I
cheeseburger																
Jr	320		17.0	34.0	7.0	2.0		1				770	150			
4.1 oz sandwich	129	13.0	6.0			45	300							3.60		I

	KCAL	H₂O (g)	PRO (g)	CHO (g)	SUGR (g)	DFIB (g)	A (RE)	C (mg)	B-2 (mg)	B-6 (mg)	FOL (mcg)	Na (mg)	Ca (mg)	Mg (mg)	Zn (mg)	Mn (mg)
	WT (g)	FAT (g)	SFA (g)	MUFA (g)	PUFA (g)	CHOL (mg)	A (IU)	B-1 (mg)	NIA (mg)	B-12 (mcg)	PANT (mg)	K (mg)	P (mg)	Fe (mg)	Cu (mg)	REF
Jr, bacon	380		21.0	34.0	7.0	2.0		6				790	150			
5.9 oz sandwich	166	19.0	7.0			60	400							3.60		I
Jr, Deluxe	360		18.0	36.0	9.0	3.0		6				840	150			
6.3 oz sandwich	179	16.0	6.0			45	500							3.60		I
Kid's Meal	270		15.0	33.0	7.0	2.0		0				560	100			
4.3 oz sandwich	111	10.0	3.0			30	100							3.60		I
chicken																
breaded sandwich	440		28.0	44.0	6.0	2.0		6				840	100			
7.3 oz sandwich	208	18.0	3.0			60	200							2.70		I
club sandwich	470		31.0	44.0	7.0	2.0		6				980	100			
7.6 oz sandwich	216	20.0	4.0			70	200							2.70		I
grilled sandwich	310		27.0	35.0	8.0	2.0		6				780	100			
6.7 oz sandwich	189	8.0	1.5			65	200							2.70		I
spicy sandwich	410		28.0	43.0	6.0	2.0		6				1280	100			
7.5 oz sandwich	213	15.0	2.5			65	200							2.70		I
chicken nugget sce																
barbecue	50		1.0	11.0				0				100	0			
1 oz pkt	28	0.0	0.0	0.0	0.0	0	300							.72		I
honey	130		0.0	6.0	5.0	0.0	0	0				220	0			
1 oz pkt	28	12.0	2.0			10	0							.00		I
spicy buffalo wing	25		0.0	12.0	10.0	0.0	0	2				210	0			
1 oz pkt	28	1.0	0.0			0	0							.00		I
sweet & sour	50		0.0	12.0	10.0	0.0	0	2				120	0			
1 oz pkt	28	0.0	0.0	0.0	0.0	0	0							.00		I
chicken nuggets	210		14.0	7.0	0.0	0.0	0	1				460	20			
5 pieces	75	14.0	3.0			45	0							.36		I
chili, large	310		23.0	32.0	8.0	7.0		6				1190	100			
12 oz	340	10.0	4.0			45	500							4.50		I
chili, small	210		15.0	21.0	5.0	5.0		4				800	80			
8 oz	227	7.0	2.5			30	400							2.70		I
coleslaw	45		0.0	5.0	4.0	1.0	0	27				65	20			
2 T	36	3.0	0.0			5	0							.36		I
cookie, choc chip	270		4.0	38.0	23.0	3.0	0	0				150	60			
2 oz cookie	57	11.0	8.0			15	0							.72		I
french fries																
Biggie	460		6.0	58.0	0.0	6.0	0	9				150	20			
5.6 oz	159	23.0	5.0			0	0							1.44		I
med	380		5.0	47.0	0.0	5.0	0	6				120	20			
4.6 oz	130	19.0	4.0			0	0							1.08		I
small	260		3.0	33.0	0.0	3.0	0	5				85	20			
3.2 oz	91	13.0	2.5			0	0							.72		I
Frosty Dairy Dessert																
large	570		15.0	95.0	79.0	5.0		0				330	500			
20 fl oz	405	17.0	9.0			70	500							1.44		I
med	460		12.0	76.0	63.0	4.0		0				260	400			
16 fl oz	324	13.0	7.0			55	500							1.08		I
small	340		9.0	57.0	47.0	3.0		0				200	300			
12 fl oz	243	10.0	5.0			40	400							1.08		I
hamburger																
Big Bacon Classic	570		34.0	46.0	11.0	3.0		15				1320	250			
9.9 oz sandwich	280	29.0	12.0			100	750							5.40		I
Jr	270		15.0	34.0	7.0	2.0		1				560	100			
4.1 oz sandwich	117	10.0	3.0			30	100							3.60		I
Kid's Meal	270		15.0	33.0	7.0	2.0		0				560	100			
3.9 oz sandwich	111	10.0	3.0			30	100							3.60		I
single	360		25.0	31.0	5.0	2.0	0	0				460	100			
4.7 oz	133	16.0	6.0			65	0							4.50		I

	KCAL	H₂O (g)	PRO (g)	CHO (g)	SUGR (g)	DFIB (g)	A (RE)	C (mg)	B-2 (mg)	B-6 (mg)	FOL (mcg)	Na (mg)	Ca (mg)	Mg (mg)	Zn (mg)	Mn (mg)
	WT (g)	FAT (g)	SFA (g)	MUFA (g)	PUFA (g)	CHOL (mg)	A (IU)	B-1 (mg)	NIA (mg)	B-12 (mcg)	PANT (mg)	K (mg)	P (mg)	Fe (mg)	Cu (mg)	REF
single w/ everything	420		26.0	37.0	9.0	3.0		6				810	100			
7.7 oz	219	20.0	7.0			70	300							5.40		I
hot choc	80		1.0	15.0	14.0	0.0		0				135	20			
6 fl oz	170	3.0	0.0			0	0							.00		I
pasta salad	25		1.0	3.0	0.0	1.0		0				75	0			
2 T	35	0.0	0.0	0.0	0.0	0	1000							.00		I
potato, baked	310		7.0	71.0	5.0	7.0	0	36				25	20			
10 oz potato	284	0.0	0.0			0	0							3.60		I
w/ bacon & cheese	540		17.0	78.0	5.0	7.0		36				1430	200			
1 potato	380	18.0	4.0			20	500							4.50		I
w/ broccoli & cheese	470		9.0	80.0	6.0	9.0		72				470	200			
1 potato	411	14.0	3.0			5	1750							4.50		I
w/ cheese	570		14.0	78.0	5.0	7.0		36				640	400			
1 potato	383	23.0	9.0			30	750							4.50		I
w/ chili & cheese	620		20.0	83.0	7.0	9.0		36				780	350			
1 potato	439	24.0	9.0			40	1000							5.40		I
w/ sour cream & chives	380		8.0	74.0	6.0	8.0		48				40	80			
1 potato	314	6.0	4.0			15	1500							4.50		I
potato salad	80		0.0	5.0	0.0	0.0	0	4				180	0			
2 T	36	7.0	2.5			5	0							.00		I
pudding, choc/van	70		0.0	10.0	8.5	0.0	0	0				60	100			
¼ cup	50	3.0	0.5			0	0							.36		I
salad																
caesar side	110		8.0	8.0	0.0	2.0		15				660	40			
1 salad	89	5.0	2.0			10	1750							1.08		I
chicken	70		4.0	2.0		0.0	0	1				135	0			
2 T	35	5.0	1.0			0	0							.36		I
chicken, grilled, caesar	260		28.0	17.0	2.0	4.0		36				1210	80			
9.2 oz salad	262	10.0	3.0			60	4000							2.70		I
deluxe garden	110		7.0	10.0	5.0	4.0		36				320	200			
1 salad	271	6.0	1.0			0	5500							1.44		I
grilled chicken	200		25.0	10.0	5.0	4.0		36				690	200			
11.9 oz salad	338	8.0	1.5			50	5500							1.80		I
side	60		4.0	5.0	2.0	2.0		18				160	100			
5.5 oz salad	155	3.0	0.5			0	2500							.72		I
taco	590		29.0	53.0	8.0	10.0		24				1230	400			
1 salad	510	30.0	11.0			65	1750							4.50		I
salad dressing																
blue cheese	170		0.0	0.0	0.0	0.0	0	0				190	20			
2 T	28	19.0	3.0			15	0							.00		I
french	120		0.0	6.0	5.0	0.0		1				330	0			
2 T	28	10.0	1.5			0	100							.00		I
french, fat-free	30		0.0	8.0	6.0	0.0	0	1				150	0			
2 T	28	0.0	0.0			0	0							.00		I
french, sweet red	130		0.0	9.0	8.0	0.0		1				230	0			
2 T	28	10.0	1.5			0	100							.00		I
Hidden Valley Italian red fat, red cal	40		0.0	2.0	2.0	0.0	0	1				340	0			
2 T	28	3.0	0.0			0	0							.36		I
Hidden Valley Ranch	90		0.0	1.0	1.0	0.0	0	0				240	20			
2 T	28	10.0	1.5			10	0							.00		I
Hidden Valley Ranch red fat, red cal	60		0.0	2.0	1.0	0.0	0	0				240	20			
2 T	28	5.0	1.0			10	0							.00		I
italian caesar	150		1.0	1.0	0.0	0.0	0	0				250	20			
2 T	28	16.0	2.5			20	0							.00		I
thousand island	130		0.0	3.0	3.0	0.0		1				170	0			
2 T	28	13.0	2.0			10	100							.00		I
seafood salad	70		3.0	5.0	0.0	0.0	0	1				300	150			
¼ cup	37	4.0	0.5			0	0							.36		I

	KCAL	H₂O (g)	PRO (g)	CHO (g)	SUGR (g)	DFIB (g)	A (RE)	C (mg)	B-2 (mg)	B-6 (mg)	FOL (mcg)	Na (mg)	Ca (mg)	Mg (mg)	Zn (mg)	Mn (mg)
	WT (g)	FAT (g)	SFA (g)	MUFA (g)	PUFA (g)	CHOL (mg)	A (IU)	B-1 (mg)	NIA (mg)	B-12 (mcg)	PANT (mg)	K (mg)	P (mg)	Fe (mg)	Cu (mg)	REF
Stuffed Pita																
chicken caesar	490		36.0	46.0	5.0	4.0		12				1300	200			
8.4 oz sandwich[2]	237	17.0	5.0			65	2500							1.08		I
classic Greek	430		17.0	49.0	7.0	4.0		18				1070	200			
8.25 oz sandwich[3]	234	19.0	7.0			35	2500							1.08		I
garden ranch chicken	480		32.0	49.0	6.0	5.0		48				1170	60			
10 oz sandwich[4]	283	17.0	4.0			70	3000							1.44		I
garden veggie	390		13.0	51.0	7.0	6.0		54				780	60			
9.07 oz sandwich[5]	257	15.0	3.0			20	3000							1.08		I

1. Contains cheese, salami, ham, lettuce, tomato, onion, and oil.
2. Contains chunks of chicken breast and shredded parmesan cheese with reduced calorie caesar vinaigrette dressing.
3. Contains feta cheese, tomatoes, cucumber, and red onion with reduced fat, reduced calorie vinaigrette dressing.
4. Contains chunks of chicken breast, broccoli, red cabbage, and carrots with reduced fat, reduced calorie garden ranch dressing.
5. Contains broccoli, red cabbage, carrots, tomatoes, cucumber, and red onion with reduced fat, reduced calorie garden ranch dressing.

12. FATS, OILS, & SHORTENINGS
12.1 ANIMAL FATS

	KCAL	H₂O (g)	PRO (g)	CHO (g)	SUGR (g)	DFIB (g)	A (RE)	C (mg)	B-2 (mg)	B-6 (mg)	FOL (mcg)	Na (mg)	Ca (mg)	Mg (mg)	Zn (mg)	Mn (mg)
	WT (g)	FAT (g)	SFA (g)	MUFA (g)	PUFA (g)	CHOL (mg)	A (IU)	B-1 (mg)	NIA (mg)	B-12 (mcg)	PANT (mg)	K (mg)	P (mg)	Fe (mg)	Cu (mg)	REF
beef separable fat, ckd	193	5.3	3.0	0.0	0.0	0.0	0	0	.03	.04	1	12	4	2	.40	.002
1 oz	28	19.9	8.1	8.6	0.8	27	0	.01	0.4	.46	.04	34	22	.30	.013	813
beef suet, raw	242	1.1	0.4	0.0	0.0	0.0	0	0	.00	.01	0	2	1	0	.06	.000
1 oz	28	26.6	14.8	8.9	0.9	19	0	.00	0.1	.08	.01	5	4	.05	.002	813
beef tallow, raw	116	0.0	0.0	0.0		0.0						0				
1 T	13	12.8	6.4	5.4	0.5	14						0				813
chicken fat, raw	117	0.0	0.0	0.0	0.0	0.0	0	0	.00	.00	0	0	0	0	.00	
1 T	13	13.0	3.9	5.8	2.7	11	0	.00	0.0	.00	.00	0	0	.00	.000	805
duck fat, raw	117	0.0	0.0	0.0	0.0	0.0	0	0	.00	.00	0	0	0	0	.00	
1 T	13	13.0	4.3	6.4	1.7	13	0	.00	0.0	.00	.00	0	0	.00	.000	804
goose fat, raw	117	0.0	0.0	0.0	0.0	0.0	0	0	.00	.00	0	0	0	0	.00	
1 T	13	13.0	3.6	7.4	1.4	13	0	.00	0.0	.00	.00	0	0	.00		804
lamb fat, ckd	166	7.4	3.4	0.0	0.0	0.0	0	0	.05	.01	1	16	7	4	.49	.001
1 oz	28	16.8	7.7	6.9	1.3	32	0	.02	2.2	.67	.16	55	32	.37	.025	817
lard (pork fat), raw	117	0.0	0.0	0.0	0.0	0.0	0	0	.00	.00	0	0	0	0	.01	.000
1 T	13	13.0	5.1	5.9	1.5	12	0	.00	0.0	.00	.00	0	0	.00	.000	804
mutton tallow, raw	117	0.0	0.0	0.0	0.0	0.0	0	0	.00	.00	0	0	0	0	.00	
1 T	13	13.0	6.1	5.3	1.0	13	0	.00	0.0	.00	.00	0	0	.00	.000	810
pork separable fat, ckd	178	6.6	3.5	0.0	0.0	0.0	1	0	.03	.04	1	10	15	2	.36	.001
1 oz	28	18.1	6.9	7.8	1.8	26	4	.09	0.7	.13	.09	67	46	.10	.015	810
salt pork, raw	212	3.1	1.4	0.0	0.0	0.0	0	0	.02	.02	0	404	2	2	.26	.001
1 oz	28	22.8	8.3	10.8	2.7	24	0	.06	0.5	.08	.06	19	15	.12	.014	810
turkey fat, raw	117	0.0	0.0	0.0	0.0	0.0	0	0	.00	.00	0	0	0	0	.00	
1 T	13	13.0	3.8	5.6	3.0	13	0	.00	0.0	.00	.00	0	0	.00	.000	804

12.2 FISH OILS

	KCAL	H₂O (g)	PRO (g)	CHO (g)	SUGR (g)	DFIB (g)	A (RE)	C (mg)	B-2 (mg)	B-6 (mg)	FOL (mcg)	Na (mg)	Ca (mg)	Mg (mg)	Zn (mg)	Mn (mg)
	WT (g)	FAT (g)	SFA (g)	MUFA (g)	PUFA (g)	CHOL (mg)	A (IU)	B-1 (mg)	NIA (mg)	B-12 (mcg)	PANT (mg)	K (mg)	P (mg)	Fe (mg)	Cu (mg)	REF
cod liver oil	126	0.0	0.0	0.0	0.0	0.0	4200	0	.00	.00	0	0	0	0	.00	.000
1 T	14	14.0	3.2	6.5	3.2	80	14000		0.0	.00	.00	0	0	.00	.000	804
herring oil	126	0.0	0.0	0.0	0.0	0.0	0	0	.00	.00	0	0	0	0	.00	.000
1 T	14	14.0	3.0	7.9	2.2	107	0	.00	0.0	.00	.00	0	0	.00	.000	804
menhaden oil	126	0.0	0.0	0.0	0.0	0.0	0	0	.00	.00	0	0	0	0	.00	.000
1 T	14	14.0	4.3	3.7	4.8	73	0	.00	0.0	.00	.00	0	0	.00	.000	804
menhaden oil, fully hydg	117	0.0	0.0	0.0	0.0	0.0	0	0	.00	.00	0	0	0	0	.00	.000
1 T	13	13.0	12.4	0.0	0.0	65	0	.00	0.0	.00	.00	0	0	.00	.000	804
salmon oil	126	0.0	0.0	0.0	0.0	0.0	0	0	.00	.00	0	0	0	0	.00	.000
1 T	14	14.0	2.8	4.1	5.6	68	0	.00	0.0	.00	.00	0	0	.00	.000	804

	KCAL	H₂O (g)	PRO (g)	CHO (g)	SUGR (g)	DFIB (g)	A (RE)	C (mg)	B-2 (mg)	B-6 (mg)	FOL (mcg)	Na (mg)	Ca (mg)	Mg (mg)	Zn (mg)	Mn (mg)
	WT (g)	FAT (g)	SFA (g)	MUFA (g)	PUFA (g)	CHOL (mg)	A (IU)	B-1 (mg)	NIA (mg)	B-12 (mcg)	PANT (mg)	K (mg)	P (mg)	Fe (mg)	Cu (mg)	REF
sardine oil	126	0.0	0.0	0.0	0.0	0.0	0	0	.00	.00	0	0	0	0	.00	.000
1 T	14	14.0	4.2	4.7	4.5	99	0	.00	0.0	.00	.00	0	0	.00	.000	804

12.3 SHORTENINGS

	KCAL	H₂O (g)	PRO (g)	CHO (g)	SUGR (g)	DFIB (g)	A (RE)	C (mg)	B-2 (mg)	B-6 (mg)	FOL (mcg)	Na (mg)	Ca (mg)	Mg (mg)	Zn (mg)	Mn (mg)
	WT (g)	FAT (g)	SFA (g)	MUFA (g)	PUFA (g)	CHOL (mg)	A (IU)	B-1 (mg)	NIA (mg)	B-12 (mcg)	PANT (mg)	K (mg)	P (mg)	Fe (mg)	Cu (mg)	REF
beef tallow & cottonseed (for frying)	117	0.0	0.0	0.0	0.0	0.0	0	0	.00	.00	0	0	0	0	.00	
1 T	13	13.0	5.8	5.0	1.1	13	0	.00	0.0	.00	.00	0	0	.00		804
Crisco, reg/butter flavor	110	0.0	0.0	0.0	0.0	0.0	0	0	.00			0	0			
1 T	12	12.0	3.0	4.0	3.0	0	0	.00	0.0			0		.00		I
Harvest Blend, Fleichman's	122	0.0	0.0	0.0	0.0	0.0	0	0	.00			0	0			
1 T	14	13.6	1.2	7.0	4.8	0	0	.00	0.0					.00		I
hydg coconut & palm kernel (for confectionery)—1 T	115	0.0	0.0	0.0	0.0	0.0	0	0	.00	.00	0	0	0	0	.00	
	13	13.0	11.9	0.3	0.1	0	0	.00	0.0	.00	.00	0	0	.00	.000	804
hydg palm (for confectionery)	124	0.0	0.0	0.0	0.0	0.0	0	0	.00	.00	0	0	0	0	.00	
1 T	14	14.0	9.2	4.1	0.1	0	0	.00	0.0	.00	.00	0	0	.00		804
hydg soybean, 1% linoleic acid (for heavy duty frying)—1 T	115	0.0	0.0	0.0	0.0	0.0	0	0	.00	.00	0	0	0	0	.00	
	13	13.0	2.7	9.6	0.1	0	0	.00	0.0	.00	.00	0	0	.00		804
hydg soybean, 30% linoleic acid (for heavy duty frying)—1 T	115	0.0	0.0	0.0	0.0	0.0	0	0	.00	.00	0	0	0	0	.00	
	13	13.0	2.4	5.7	4.4	0	0	.00	0.0	.00	.00	0	0	.00		804
hydg soybean & cottonseed	115	0.0	0.0	0.0	0.0	0.0	0	0	.00	.00	0	0	0	0	.00	
1 T	13	13.0	3.3	5.8	3.4	0	0	.00	0.0	.00	.00	0	0	.00	.000	804
hydg soybean & cottonseed (for bread)	115	0.0	0.0	0.0	0.0	0.0	0	0	.00	.00	0	0	0	0	.00	.000
1 T	13	13.0	2.9	4.3	5.3	0	0	.00	0.0	.00	.00	0	0	.00	.000	804
hydg soybean & cottonseed (for frying)	115	0.0	0.0	0.0	0.0	0.0	0	0	.00	.00	0	0	0	0	.00	
1 T	13	13.0	2.0	7.6	2.9	0	0	.00	0.0	.00	.00	0	0	.00		804
hydg soybean & palm (household)	115	0.0	0.0	0.0	0.0	0.0	0	0	.00	.00	0	0	0	0	.00	.000
1 T	13	13.0	3.3	5.5	3.5	0	0	.00	0.0	.00	.00	0	0	.00	.000	804
hydg soybean (for cakes & frostings)	115	0.0	0.0	0.0	0.0	0.0	0	0	.00	.00	0	0	0	0	.00	.000
1 T	13	13.0	2.6	4.8	4.9	0	0	.00	0.0	.00	.00	0	0	.00	.000	804
hydg soybean, palm & cottonseed (for baking)—1 T	115	0.0	0.0	0.0	0.0	0.0	0	0	.00	.00	0	0	0	0	.00	.000
	13	13.0	3.7	3.8	4.8	0	0	.00	0.0	.00	.00	0	0	.00	.000	804
lard & veg oil	117	0.0	0.0	0.0	0.0	0.0	0	0	.00	.00	0	0	0	0	.00	
1 T	13	13.0	5.2	5.8	1.4	7	0	.00	0.0	.00	.00	0	0	.00	.000	804

12.4 VEGETABLE OILS & SPRAYS

	KCAL	H₂O (g)	PRO (g)	CHO (g)	SUGR (g)	DFIB (g)	A (RE)	C (mg)	B-2 (mg)	B-6 (mg)	FOL (mcg)	Na (mg)	Ca (mg)	Mg (mg)	Zn (mg)	Mn (mg)
	WT (g)	FAT (g)	SFA (g)	MUFA (g)	PUFA (g)	CHOL (mg)	A (IU)	B-1 (mg)	NIA (mg)	B-12 (mcg)	PANT (mg)	K (mg)	P (mg)	Fe (mg)	Cu (mg)	REF
almond oil	124	0.0	0.0	0.0	0.0	0.0	0	0	.00	.00	0	0	0	0	.00	
1 T	14	14.0	1.1	9.8	2.4	0	0	.00	0.0	.00	.00	0	0	.00	.000	804
apricot kernel oil	124	0.0	0.0	0.0	0.0	0.0	0	0	.00	.00	0	0	0	0	.00	
1 T	14	14.0	0.9	8.4	4.1	0	0	.00	0.0	.00	.00	0	0	.00		804
avocado oil	124	0.0	0.0	0.0	0.0	0.0	0	0	.00	.00	0	0	0	0	.00	.000
1 T	14	14.0	1.6	9.9	1.9	0	0	.00	0.0	.00	.00	0	0	.00	.000	804
babassu oil	124	0.0	0.0	0.0	0.0	0.0	0	0	.00	.00	0	0	0	0	.00	
1 T	14	14.0	11.4	1.6	0.2	0	0	.00	0.0	.00	.00	0	0	.00		804
Baker's Joy baking spray	5		0.0	0.0	0.0	0.0	0	0				0	0			
½ second spray	0.8	0.0	0.0	0.0	0.0	0	0							.00		I
Best Blend Oil, Wesson	122		0.0	0.0	0.0	0.0	0	0	.00			0	0			
1 T	14	13.6	1.2	6.9	4.8	0	0	.00	0.0			0		.00		I
Buttery Flavor Oil, Wesson	122		0.0	0.0	0.0	0.0	0	0	.00			0	0			
1 T	14	13.6	2.0	3.1	7.7	0	0	.00	0.0					.00		I
canola oil	124	0.0	0.0	0.0	0.0	0.0	0	0	.00	.00	0	0	0	0	.00	.000
1 T	14	14.0	1.0	8.2	4.1	0	0	.00	0.0	.00	.00	0	0	.00	.000	804
canola oil, Wesson	122	0.0	0.0	0.0	0.0	0.0	0	0	.00			0	0			
1 T	14	13.6	1.0	7.9	4.1	0	0	.00	0.0			0		.00		I
canola/olive oil, Wesson	122	0.0	0.0	0.0	0.0	0.0	0	0	.00			0	0			
1 T	14	13.6	1.2	8.0	3.5	0	0	.00	0.0			0		.00		I
cocoa (cacao) oil	124	0.0	0.0	0.0	0.0	0.0	0	0	.00	.00	0	0	0	0	.00	.000
1 T	14	14.0	8.4	4.6	0.4	0	0	.00	0.0	.00	.00	0	0	.00	.000	804
coconut oil	121	0.0	0.0	0.0	0.0	0.0	0	0	.00	.00	0	0	0	0	.00	.000
1 T	14	14.0	12.1	0.8	0.3	0	0	.00	0.0	.00	.00	0	0	.01	.000	804
corn oil	124	0.0	0.0	0.0	0.0	0.0	0	0	.00	.00	0	0	0	0	.00	
1 T	14	14.0	1.8	3.4	8.2	0	0	.00	0.0	.00	.00	0	0	.00	.000	804

	KCAL / WT (g)	H₂O (g) / FAT (g)	PRO (g) / SFA (g)	CHO (g) / MUFA (g)	SUGR (g) / PUFA (g)	DFIB (g) / CHOL (mg)	A (RE) / A (IU)	C (mg) / B 1 (mg)	B-2 (mg) / NIA (mg)	B-6 (mg) / B 12 (mcg)	FOL (mcg) / PANT (mg)	Na (mg) / K (mg)	Ca (mg) / P (mg)	Mg (mg) / Fe (mg)	Zn (mg) / Cu (mg)	Mn (mg) / RFF
Crisco	120	0.0	0.0	0.0	0.0	0.0	0	0	.00			0	0			
1 T	14	14.0	1.5	6.0	6.0	0	0	.00	0.0			0		.00		I
Mazola	125	0.0	0.0	0.0	0.0							0				
1 T	14	14.0	1.8	3.6	8.4	0										I
Wesson	122		0.0	0.0	0.0	0.0						0	0			
1 T	14	13.6	1.8	3.6	7.7	0						0		.00		I
cottonseed oil	124	0.0	0.0	0.0	0.0	0.0	0	0	.00	.00	0	0	0	0	.00	
1 T	14	14.0	3.6	2.5	7.3	0	0	.00	0.0	.00	.00	0	0	.00	.000	804
Crisco oil	120	0.0	0.0	0.0	0.0	0.0	0	0	.00			0	0			
1 T	14	14.0	1.5	6.0	6.0	0	0	.00	0.0			0		.00		I
hazelnut oil	124	0.0	0.0	0.0	0.0	0.0	0	0	.00	.00	0	0	0	0	.00	
1 T	14	14.0	1.0	10.9	1.4	0	0	.00	0.0	.00	.00	0	0	.00		804
Mazola No Stick	2	0.0	0.0	0.0	0.0							0				
2.5 sec spray	0.2	0.2	0.0	0.0	0.1	0										I
mustard oil	124	0.0	0.0	0.0	0.0	0.0	0	0	.00	.00	0	0	0	0	.00	.000
1 T	14	14.0	1.6	8.3	3.0	0	0	.00	0.0	.00	.00	0	0	.00	.000	804
No-stick cooking spray, Wesson	2	0.0	0.0	0.0	0.0	0	0	.00				0	0			
1 spray	0.3	0.2	0.0	0.1	0.1	0	0	.00						.00		I
nutmeg oil	124	0.0	0.0	0.0	0.0	0.0	0	0	.00	.00		0	0	0	.00	
1 T	14	14.0	12.6	0.7	0.0	0	0	.00	0.0	.00	.00	0	0	.00		804
oat oil	124	0.0	0.0	0.0	0.0	0.0	0	0	.00	.00	0	0	0	0	.00	.000
1 T	14	14.0	2.7	4.9	5.7	0	0	.00	.00	.00	.00	0	0	.00	.000	804
olive oil	124	0.0	0.0	0.0	0.0	0.0	0	0	.00	.00	0	0	0	0	.01	
1 T	14	14.0	1.9	10.3	1.2	0	0	.00	0.0	.00	.00	0	0	.05	.000	804
palm kernel oil	121	0.0	0.0	0.0	0.0	0.0	0	0	.00	.00	0	0	0	0	.00	.000
1 T	14	14.0	11.4	1.6	0.2	0	0	.00	0.0	.00	.00	0	0	.00	.000	804
palm oil	124	0.0	0.0	0.0	0.0	0.0	0	0	.00	.00	0	0	0	0	.00	
1 T	14	14.0	6.9	5.2	1.3	0	0	.00	0.0	.00	.00	0	0	.00	.000	804
peanut oil	124	0.0	0.0	0.0	0.0	0.0	0	0	.00	.00	0	0	0	0	.00	
1 T	14	14.0	2.4	6.5	4.5	0	0	.00	0.0	.00	.00	0	0	.00	.000	804
peanut oil, Wesson	122		0.0	0.0	0.0	0.0	0	0	.00			0	0			
1 T	14	13.6	2.5	6.8	4.2	0	0	.00	0.0			0		.00		I
poppyseed oil	124	0.0	0.0	0.0	0.0	0.0	0	0	.00	.00	0	0	0	0	.00	
1 T	14	14.0	1.9	2.8	8.7	0	0	.00	0.0	.00	.00	0	0	.00		804
Puritan oil	120	0.0	0.0	0.0	0.0	0.0	0	0	.00			0	0			
1 T	14	14.0	1.0	8.0	4.0	0	0	.00	0.0			0		.00		I
rice bran oil	124	0.0	0.0	0.0	0.0	0.0	0	0	.00	.00	0	0	0	0	.00	
1 T	14	14.0	2.8	5.5	4.9	0	0	.00	0.0	.00	.00	0	0	.01		804
safflower oil, commercial, 70% & over linoleic acid—1 T	124	0.0	0.0	0.0	0.0	0.0	0	0	.00	.00	0	0	0	0	.00	
	14	14.0	1.3	1.7	10.4	0	0	.00	0.0	.00	.00	0	0	.00	.000	804
sesame oil	124	0.0	0.0	0.0	0.0	0.0	0	0	.00	.00	0	0	0	0	.00	
1 T	14	14.0	2.0	5.6	5.8	0	0	.00	0.0	.00	.00	0	0	.00	.000	804
sheanut oil	124	0.0	0.0	0.0	0.0	0.0	0	0	.00	.00	0	0	0	0	.00	
1 T	14	14.0	6.5	6.2	0.7	0	0	.00	0.0	.00	.00	0	0	.00		804
soybean (hydg) & cottonseed oil	124	0.0	0.0	0.0	0.0	0.0	0	0	.00	.00	0	0	0	0	.00	
1 T	14	14.0	2.5	4.1	6.7	0	0	.00	0.0	.00	.00	0	0	.00	.000	804
soybean lecithin	107	0.0	0.0	0.0	0.0	0.0	0	0	.00	.00	0	0	0	0	.00	.000
1 T[1]	14	14.0	2.1	1.5	6.3	0	0	.00	0.0	.00	.00	0	0	.00	.000	804
soybean oil	124	0.0	0.0	0.0	0.0	0.0	0	0	.00	.00	0	0	0	0	.00	
1 T	14	14.0	2.0	3.3	8.1	0	0	.00	0.0	.00	.00	0	0	.00	.000	804
soybean oil, hydg	124	0.0	0.0	0.0	0.0	0.0	0	0	.00	.00	0	0	0	0	.00	
1 T	14	14.0	2.1	6.0	5.3	0	0	.00	0.0	.00	.00	0	0	.00	.000	804
stir fry oil, Wesson	122		0.0	0.0	0.0	0.0	0	0	.00			0	0			
1 T	14	13.6	1.2	7.5	4.7	0	0	.00	0.0			0		.00		I
sunflower oil																
60% & over linoleic acid	124	0.0	0.0	0.0	0.0	0.0	0	0	.00	.00	0	0	0	0	.00	
1 T	14	14.0	1.4	2.7	9.2	0	0	.00	0.0	.00	.00	0	0	.00	.000	804
70% & over oleic acid	124	0.0	0.0	0.0	0.0	0.0	0	0	.00	.00	0	0	0	0	.00	.000
1 T	14	14.0	1.4	11.7	0.5	0	0	.00	0.0	.00	.00	0	0	.00	.000	804
hydg	124	0.0	0.0	0.0	0.0	0.0	0	0	.00	.00	0	0	0	0	.00	.000
1 T	14	14.0	1.8	6.5	5.1	0	0	.00	0.0	.00	.00	0	0	.00	.000	804

							Vitamins					Minerals			
KCAL	H₂O (g)	PRO (g)	CHO (g)	SUGR (g)	DFIB (g)	A (RE)	C (mg)	B-2 (mg)	B-6 (mg)	FOL (mcg)	Na (mg)	Ca (mg)	Mg (mg)	Zn (mg)	Mn (mg)
WT (g)	FAT (g)	SFA (g)	MUFA (g)	PUFA (g)	CHOL (mg)	A (IU)	B-1 (mg)	NIA (mg)	B-12 (mcg)	PANT (mg)	K (mg)	P (mg)	Fe (mg)	Cu (mg)	REF
southern crops (60%															
linoleic acid) 1 T															
124	0.0	0.0	0.0	0.0	0.0	0	0	.00	.00	0	0	0	0	.00	
14	14.0	1.4	6.4	5.6	0	0	.00	0.0	.00	.00	0	0	.00		804
Wesson															
122		0.0	0.0	0.0	0.0	0	0	.00			0	0			
1 T															
14	13.6	1.7	1.9	9.1	0	0	.00	0.0			0		.00		I
vegetable oil, Wesson															
122		0.0	0.0	0.0	0.0	0	0	.00			0	0			
1 T															
14	13.6	2.0	3.1	7.7	0	0	.00	0.0			0		.00		I
walnut oil															
124	0.0	0.0	0.0	0.0	0.0	0	0	.00	.00	0	0	0	0	.00	
1 T															
14	14.0	1.3	3.2	8.9	0	0	.00	0.0	.00	.00	0	0	.00	.000	804
wheat germ oil															
124	0.0	0.0	0.0	0.0	0.0	0	0	.00	.00	0	0	0	0	.00	
1 T															
14	14.0	2.6	2.1	8.6	0	0	.00	0.0	.00	.00	0	0	.00	.000	804

13. FISH, SHELLFISH, & CRUSTACEA

							Vitamins					Minerals			
abalone, fried															
161	51.1	16.7	9.4		0.0	2	2	.11	.13	5	503	31	48	.81	.060
3 oz[1]															
85	5.8	1.4	2.3	1.4	80	4	.19	1.6	.59	2.44	242	185	3.23	.194	815
abalone, raw															
89	63.4	14.5	5.1		0.0	2	2	.09	.13	4	256	26	41	.70	.034
3 oz															
85	0.6	0.1	0.1	0.1	72	4	.16	1.3	.62	2.55	213	162	2.71	.167	815
alewife, cnd															
127	79.4	19.4	0.0		0.0							218			
3.5 oz															
100	4.9														B&C
alewife, raw															
141	73.0	16.2	0.0		0.0										
3.5 oz															
100	8.0														B&C
anchovy, cnd in olive oil															
42	10.1	5.8	0.0	0.0	0.0	4	0	.07	.04	3	734	46	14	.49	.020
5 anchovies															
20	1.9	0.4	0.8	0.5	17	14	.02	4.0	.18	.18	109	50	.93	.068	815
anchovy paste															
14		1.4	0.3		0.0										
1 t															
7	0.8			0.5											B&C
anchovy, raw															
111	62.4	17.3	0.0	0.0	0.0	13	0	.22	.12	7	88	125	35	1.46	.060
3 oz															
85	4.1	1.1	1.0	1.4	51	43	.05	11.9	.53	.55	326	148	2.76	.179	815
barracuda, pacific, raw															
113	75.4	21.0	0.0		0.0										
3.5 oz															
100	2.6														B&C
bass, black															
baked, fat added															
287		23.6	3.0		0.0		0	.16	3.50		68	96			
4 oz															
113	19.4					97	.07				256	269	1.20		B&C
raw															
93	79.3	19.2	0.0		0.0						68				
3.5 oz															
100	1.2										256				B&C
stuffed, baked															
259	52.9	16.2	11.4		0.0										
3.5 oz[2]															
100	15.8														B&C
bass, freshwater, ckd by dry heat															
124	58.5	20.6	0.0	0.0	0.0	30	2	.08	.12	14	77	88	32	.71	.969
3 oz															
85	4.0	0.9	1.6	1.2	74	98	.07	1.3	1.96	.74	388	218	1.62	.101	815
bass, freshwater, raw															
97	64.3	16.0	0.0	0.0	0.0	26	2	.06	.10	13	60	68	26	.55	.756
3 oz															
85	3.1	0.7	1.2	0.9	58	85	.06	1.1	1.70	.64	303	170	1.27	.079	815
bass, striped, ckd by dry heat															
105	62.4	19.3	0.0	0.0	0.0	26	0	.03	.29	9	75	16	43	.43	.016
3 oz															
85	2.5	0.6	0.7	0.9	88	88	.10	2.2	3.75	.74	279	216	.92	.034	815
bass, striped, raw															
82	67.4	15.1	0.0	0.0	0.0	23	0	.03	.26	8	59	13	34	.34	.013
3 oz															
85	2.0	0.4	0.6	0.7	68	77	.09	1.8	3.25	.64	218	168	.71	.026	815
bluefish, ckd by dry heat															
135	53.3	21.8	0.0	0.0	0.0	117	0	.08	.39	2	65	8	36	.88	.023
3 oz															
85	4.6	1.0	2.0	1.2	65	390	.06	6.2	5.29	.81	406	247	.53	.058	815
bluefish, raw															
105	60.3	17.0	0.0	0.0	0.0	101	0	.07	.34	1	51	6	28	.69	.018
3 oz															
85	3.6	0.8	1.5	0.9	50	338	.05	5.1	4.58	.70	316	193	.41	.045	815
bonito, cnd															
257		19.8	0.0		0.0			.09			514	8	28		
3.5 oz															
100	19.1						.01	9.8			302	193	1.00		B&C
bullhead, black, raw															
84	81.3	16.3	0.0		0.0										
3.5 oz															
100	1.6														B&C
burbot, ckd by dry heat															
98	62.4	21.1	0.0	0.0	0.0	4	0	.15	.29	1	105	54	35	.82	.763
3 oz															
85	0.9	0.2	0.1	0.3	65	14	.36	1.7	.78	.15	441	218	.98	.218	815

	KCAL	H2O (g)	PRO (g)	CHO (g)	SUGR (g)	DFIB (g)	A (RE)	C (mg)	B-2 (mg)	B-6 (mg)	FOL (mcg)	Na (mg)	Ca (mg)	Mg (mg)	Zn (mg)	Mn (mg)
	WT (g)	FAT (g)	SFA (g)	MUFA (g)	PUFA (g)	CHOL (mg)	A (IU)	B-1 (mg)	NIA (mg)	B-12 (mcg)	PANT (mg)	K (mg)	P (mg)	Fe (mg)	Cu (mg)	RFF
burbot, raw	77	67.4	16.4	0.0	0.0	0.0	3	0	.12	.26	1	82	43	27	.65	.595
3 oz	85	0.7	0.1	0.1	0.3	51	13	.32	1.4	.68	.13	344	170	.77	.170	815
butterfish, ckd by dry heat	159	56.8	18.8	0.0	0.0	0.0	28	0	.16	.29	14	97	24	27	.84	.016
3 oz	85	8.7				71	93	.12	4.9	1.56	.74	409	262	.54	.059	815
butterfish, raw	124	63.0	14.7	0.0	0.0	0.0	26	0	.13	.26	13	76	19	21	.65	.013
3 oz	85	6.8	2.9	2.9	0.5	55	85	.10	3.8	1.62	.64	319	204	.43	.046	815
carp, ckd by dry heat	138	59.2	19.4	0.0	0.0	0.0	8	1	.06	.19	15	54	44	32	1.62	.043
3 oz	85	6.1	1.2	2.5	1.6	71	27	.12	1.8	1.25	.74	363	452	1.35	.062	815
carp, raw	108	64.9	15.2	0.0	0.0	0.0	8	1	.05	.16	13	42	35	25	1.26	.036
3 oz	85	4.8	0.9	2.0	1.2	56	25	.10	1.4	1.30	.64	283	353	1.05	.048	815
catfish, channel																
breaded & fried	195	50.0	15.4	6.8		0.6	7	0	.11	.16	14	238	37	23	.73	.034
3 oz[3]	85	11.3	2.8	4.8	2.8	69	24	.06	1.9	1.62	.62	289	184	1.22	.086	815
farmed, cooked by dry heat	129	60.9	15.9	0.0	0.0	0.0	13	1	.06	.14	6	68	8	22	.89	.017
3 oz	85	6.8	1.5	3.5	1.2	54	43	.36	2.1	2.38	.52	273	208	.70	.104	815
farmed, raw	115	64.1	13.2	0.0	0.0	0.0	13	1	.06	.16	9	45	8	20	.63	.015
3 oz	85	6.5	1.5	3.0	1.3	40	43	.31	2.0	2.10	.51	254	172	.43	.086	815
wild, ckd by dry heat	89	66.1	15.7	0.0	0.0	0.0	13	1	.06	.09	9	43	9	24	.52	.023
3 oz	85	2.4	0.6	0.9	0.5	61	43	.19	2.0	2.47	.77	356	259	.30	.033	815
wild, raw	81	68.3	13.9	0.0	0.0	0.0	13	1	.06	.10	9	37	12	20	.43	.021
3 oz	85	2.4	0.6	0.7	0.7	49	43	.18	1.6	1.90	.65	304	178	.26	.029	815
catfish fillets, frzn, Mrs. Paul's Light	280		15.7	19.2				0	.10			405	26			
4.5 oz	128	15.6	3.4		3.3	64	0	.09	1.7			295		1.20		I
catfish strips, frzn, Mrs. Pauls	246		12.4	18.9				0	.11			283	15			
4.0 oz	113	13.4					0	.31	1.8			272		.70		I
caviar, black & red, granular	40	7.6	3.9	0.6		0.0	90	0	.10	.05	8	240	44	48	.15	.008
1 T	16	2.9	0.6	0.7	1.2	94	299	.03	0.0	3.20	.56	29	57	1.90	.018	815
cisco, raw	83	67.1	16.2	0.0	0.0	0.0	26	0	.09	.26	13	47	10	14	.31	.057
3 oz	85	1.6	0.4	0.4	0.5	43	85	.07	2.1	.85	.64	301	129	.34	.061	815
cisco, smoked	151	59.4	13.9	0.0	0.0	0.0	241	0	.14	.23	2	409	22	14	.26	.018
3 oz	85	10.1	1.5	4.7	1.9	27	802	.04	2.0	3.62	.26	249	128	.42	.183	815
clam liquid, cnd	5	234.5	1.0	0.2		0.0	22	2	.05	.02	5	516	31	26	.24	.178
1 cup	240	0.0	0.0	0.0	0.0	7	72	.02	0.4	12.00	.10	358	274	.72	.934	815
clams																
breaded & fried	172	52.3	12.1	8.8			77	9	.21	.05	15	310	54	12	1.24	.459
3 oz (9 small)[4]	85	9.5	2.3	3.9	2.4	52	257	.09	1.8	34.25	.37	277	160	11.83	.303	815
ckd by moist heat	126	54.1	21.7	4.4		0.0	145	19	.36	.09	24	95	78	15	2.32	.850
3 oz (19 small)[5]	85	1.7	0.2	0.1	0.5	57	485	.13	2.9	84.10	.58	534	287	23.78	.585	815
cnd, drained	126	54.1	21.7	4.4		0.0	145	19	.36	.09	24	95	78	15	2.32	.850
3 oz	85	1.7	0.2	0.1	0.5	57	485	.13	2.9	84.05	.58	534	287	23.77	.585	815
fried, frzn, Mrs. Paul's	233		7.2	23.3				0	.07			380	21			
2.5 oz	71	12.4				6	22	.14	1.4			114		1.20		I
raw	63	69.6	10.9	2.2		0.0	77	11	.18	.05	14	48	39	8	1.17	.425
3 oz (4 large or 9 small)	85	0.8	0.1	0.1	0.2	29	255	.07	1.5	42.05	.31	267	144	11.89	.293	815
cod, atlantic																
ckd by dry heat	89	64.6	19.4	0.0	0.0	0.0	12	1	.07	.24	7	66	12	36	.49	.017
3 oz	85	0.7	0.1	0.1	0.2	47	39	.07	2.1	.89	.15	208	117	.42	.031	815
cnd	89	64.3	19.4	0.0	0.0	0.0	12	1	.07	.24	7	185	18	35	.49	.017
3 oz	85	0.7	0.1	0.1	0.2	47	39	.07	2.1	.89	.14	449	221	.42	.031	815
dried & salted	247	13.7	53.4	0.0	0.0	0.0	36	3	.20	.73	21	5976	136	113	1.35	.043
3 oz	85	2.0	0.4	0.3	0.7	129	120	.23	6.4	8.50	1.42	1240	808	2.13	.150	815
fillets, frzn, Mrs. Paul's Light	268		15.3	26.5				0	.15			503	26			
4.5 oz	128	11.2	2.9		4.8	42	0	.12	1.6			347		1.00		I
raw	70	69.1	15.1	0.0	0.0	0.0	10	1	.06	.21	6	46	14	27	.38	.013
3 oz	85	0.6	0.1	0.1	0.2	37	34	.06	1.8	.77	.13	351	173	.32	.024	815
cod, pacific, ckd by dry heat	89	64.6	19.5	0.0	0.0	0.0	9	3	.04	.39	7	77	8	26	.43	.013
3 oz	85	0.7	0.1	0.1	0.3	40	27	.02	2.1	.88	.14	440	190	.28	.028	815
cod, pacific, raw	70	69.1	15.2	0.0	0.0	0.0	7	2	.04	.34	6	60	6	20	.34	.010
3 oz	85	0.5	0.1	0.1	0.2	31	24	.02	1.7	.77	.12	343	148	.22	.022	815

	KCAL / WT (g)	H₂O (g) / FAT (g)	PRO (g) / SFA (g)	CHO (g) / MUFA (g)	SUGR (g) / PUFA (g)	DFIB (g) / CHOL (mg)	A (RE) / A (IU)	C (mg) / B-1 (mg)	B-2 (mg) / NIA (mg)	B-6 (mg) / B-12 (mcg)	FOL (mcg) / PANT (mg)	Na (mg) / K (mg)	Ca (mg) / P (mg)	Mg (mg) / Fe (mg)	Zn (mg) / Cu (mg)	Mn (mg) / REF
crab, alaska king																
ckd by moist heat	82	66.0	16.5	0.0	0.0	0.0	8	6	.05	.15	43	912	50	54	6.48	.034
3 oz	85	1.3	0.1	0.2	0.5	45	25	.05	1.1	9.78	.34	223	238	.65	1.005	815
imitation, made from surimi	87	62.7	10.2	8.7		0.0	17	0	.02	.03	1	715	11	37	.28	.009
3 oz	85	1.1	0.2	0.2	0.6	17	56	.03	0.2	1.36	.06	77	240	.33	.027	815
raw	71	67.7	15.6	0.0	0.0	0.0	6	6	.04	.13	37	711	39	42	5.06	.030
3 oz	85	0.5	0.1	0.1	0.1	36	20	.04	0.9	7.65	.30	174	186	.50	.784	815
crab, blue																
ckd by moist heat	87	65.9	17.2	0.0	0.0	0.0	2	3	.04	.15	43	237	88	28	3.59	.162
3 oz	85	1.5	0.2	0.2	0.6	85	5	.09	2.8	6.21	.37	276	175	.77	.549	815
cnd	84	64.8	17.5	0.0	0.0	0.0	2	2	.07	.13	36	283	86	33	3.42	.162
3 oz	85	1.0	0.2	0.2	0.4	76	4	.07	1.2	.39	.31	318	221	.71	.646	815
raw	74	67.2	15.4	0.0		0.0	2	3	.03	.13	37	249	76	29	3.01	.128
3 oz	85	0.9	0.2	0.2	0.3	66	4	.07	2.3	7.65	.30	280	195	.63	.569	815
crab cake	93	42.6	12.1	0.3		0.0	49	2	.05	.10	25	198	63	20	2.45	.114
1 cake[6]	60	4.5	0.9	1.7	1.4	90	151	.05	1.7	3.56	.30	194	128	.65	.366	815
crab, deviled, frzn, Mrs. Paul's	186		7.7	19.4				0	.11			432	87			
3 oz	85	8.7				33	59	.12	0.8			118		1.10		I
crab, deviled mineatures, frzn, Mrs. Paul's—3.5 oz	249		8.5	28.3				0	.31			475	116			
	99	11.3					0	.16	1.4			185		1.60		I
crab, dungeness, ckd by moist heat	94	62.4	19.0	0.8		0.0	26	3	.17	.15	36	321	50	49	4.65	.082
3 oz	85	1.1	0.1	0.2	0.3	65	88	.05	3.1	8.83	.34	347	149	.37	.624	815
crab, dungeness, raw	73	67.3	14.8	0.6		0.0	23	3	.14	.13	37	251	39	38	3.63	.068
3 oz	85	0.8	0.1	0.1	0.3	50	77	.04	2.7	7.65	.30	301	155	.31	.573	815
crab, queen, ckd by moist heat	98	63.9	20.2	0.0	0.0	0.0	44	6	.21	.15	36	588	28	54	3.05	.031
3 oz	85	1.3	0.2	0.3	0.5	60	147	.08	2.5	8.83	.34	170	109	2.45	.528	815
crab, queen, raw	77	68.5	15.7	0.0	0.0	0.0	38	6	.17	.13	37	458	22	42	2.38	.026
3 oz	85	1.0	0.1	0.2	0.4	47	128	.07	2.1	7.65	.30	147	113	2.13	.485	815
crayfish																
farmed, ckd by moist heat	74	68.7	14.9	0.0	0.0	0.0	13	0	.07	.11	9	82	43	28	1.26	.185
3 oz	85	1.1	0.2	0.2	0.4	117	43	.04	1.4	2.64	.44	202	205	.94	.493	815
farmed, raw	61	71.5	12.6	0.0	0.0	0.0	13	0	.03	.06	26	53	21	26	.86	.124
3 oz	85	0.8	0.1	0.2	0.3	91	43	.04	1.6	1.79	.48	222	185	.47	.202	815
wild, ckd by moist heat	75	67.5	14.3	0.0	0.0	0.0	13	1	.07	.06	37	80	51	28	1.50	.444
3 oz	85	1.0	0.2	0.2	0.3	113	43	.04	1.9	1.83	.49	252	230	.71	.583	815
wild, raw	65	69.9	13.6	0.0	0.0	0.0	14	1	.03	.09	31	49	23	23	1.11	.192
3 oz	85	0.8	0.1	0.1	0.2	97	44	.06	1.9	1.70	.46	257	218	.71	.356	815
croaker, atlantic, breaded & fried	188	50.8	15.5	6.4		0.4	19	0	.11	.22	15	296	27	36	.44	.068
3 oz[4]	85	10.8	3.0	4.5	2.5	71	64	.08	3.7	1.79	.63	289	185	.73	.055	815
croaker, atlantic, raw	88	66.4	15.1	0.0	0.0	0.0	15	0	.08	.26	13	48	13	34	.36	.021
3 oz	85	2.7	0.9	1.0	0.4	52	51	.06	3.6	2.13	.64	293	179	.31	.036	815
cusk, ckd by dry heat	95	59.3	20.7	0.0	0.0	0.0	18	0	.14	.38	2	34	11	34	.42	.016
3 oz	85	0.7				45	59	.04	2.8	1.02	.27	428	223	.90	.020	815
cusk, raw	74	64.9	16.2	0.0	0.0	0.0	15	0	.11	.33	2	26	9	26	.32	.013
3 oz	85	0.6	0.1	0.1	0.2	35	51	.04	2.3	.89	.24	333	174	.71	.015	815
cuttlefish, ckd by moist heat	134	52.0	27.6	1.4		0.0	173	7	1.47	.23	20	633	153	51	2.94	.178
3 oz	85	1.2	0.2	0.1	0.2	191	574	.01	1.9	4.59	.77	542	493	9.22	.849	815
cuttlefish, raw	67	68.5	13.8	0.7		0.0	95	5	.77	.13	14	316	77	26	1.47	.094
3 oz	85	0.6	0.1	0.1	0.1	95	319	.01	1.0	2.55	.43	301	329	5.12	.499	815
dolphinfish, ckd by dry heat	93	60.6	20.2	0.0	0.0	0.0	53	0	.07	.39	5	96	16	32	.50	.016
3 oz	85	0.8	0.2	0.1	0.2	80	177	.02	6.3	.59	.74	453	156	1.23	.045	815
dolphinfish, raw	72	66.0	15.7	0.0	0.0	0.0	46	0	.06	.34	4	75	13	26	.39	.013
3 oz	85	0.6	0.1	0.1	0.1	62	153	.02	5.2	.51	.64	354	122	.96	.035	815
drum, freshwater, ckd by dry heat	130	60.3	19.1	0.0	0.0	0.0	50	1	.18	.29	14	82	65	32	.72	.763
3 oz	85	5.4	1.2	2.4	1.3	70	167	.07	2.4	1.96	.74	300	196	.98	.253	815
drum, freshwater, raw	101	65.8	14.9	0.0	0.0	0.0	43	1	.14	.26	13	64	51	26	.56	.595
3 oz	85	4.2	1.0	1.9	1.0	54	145	.06	2.0	1.70	.64	234	153	.77	.197	815
fish cakes, frzn, Mrs. Paul's	241		11.0	25.9				0	.25			783	75			
4 oz	113	10.3					0	.16	1.5			230		1.50		I

Each food item occupies two rows. The first row of each pair uses the upper header labels (KCAL, H₂O, PRO, CHO, SUGR, DFIB, A(RE), C, B-2, B-6, FOL, Na, Ca, Mg, Zn, Mn); the second row uses the lower header labels (WT, FAT, SFA, MUFA, PUFA, CHOL, A(IU), B-1, NIA, B-12, PANT, K, P, Fe, Cu, REF).

Item	KCAL / WT (g)	H₂O (g) / FAT (g)	PRO (g) / SFA (g)	CHO (g) / MUFA (g)	SUGR (g) / PUFA (g)	DFIB (g) / CHOL (mg)	A (RE) / A (IU)	C (mg) / B-1 (mg)	B-2 (mg) / NIA (mg)	B-6 (mg) / B-12 (mcg)	FOL (mcg) / PANT (mg)	Na (mg) / K (mg)	Ca (mg) / P (mg)	Mg (mg) / Fe (mg)	Zn (mg) / Cu (mg)	Mn (mg) / REF
fish dijon, frzn, Mrs. Paul's Light	232		20.7	14.7				2	.20			682	112			
8.5 oz entree	241	10.1					807	.08	2.4			304		1.20		I
fish fillets																
batter-dipped, frzn, Mrs. Paul's	447		15.9	37.6				0	.12			789	50			
6 oz	170	25.8	5.3		8.4	41	0	.12	2.4			151		1.00		I
buttered, frzn, Mrs. Paul's	163		20.3	1.9				0	.07			406	26			
5 oz	142	8.2					0	.03	2.2			286		.70		I
crispy crunchy, frzn, Mrs. Paul's	275		10.9	25.4				0	.12			487	32			
4 oz	113	14.4	5.2		5.9	31	0	.11	1.5			188		1.40		I
lightly battered, crunchy, frzn, Mrs. Paul's—4.5 oz	301		12.2	27.3				1	.13			803	33			
	128	15.9	3.2		4.4	30	0	.12	1.4			166		1.20		I
lightly battered, frzn, Mrs. Paul's Supreme—3.35 oz	199		9.3	16.8				0	.07			437	20			
	95	10.5					0	.07	1.1			130		.70		I
fish florentine, frzn, Mrs. Paul's Light	263		27.2	11.0				2	.24			739	262			
9 oz entree	255	12.2					1556	.09	2.3			561		1.70		I
fish mornay, frzn, Mrs. Paul's Light	274		25.5	16.1				17	.26			915	270			
10 oz entree	283	12.0					359	.16	2.3			515		1.20		I
fish pieces, frzn, reheated	155	26.4	8.9	13.5		0.0	18	0	.10	.03	10	332	11	14	.38	.135
1 piece (4" x 2' x ½")[7]	57	7.0	1.8	2.9	1.8	64	60	.07	1.2	1.02	.19	149	103	.42	.058	815
fish sticks																
frzn	77	13.1	4.4	6.7		0.0	9	0	.05	.02	5	165	6	7	.19	.067
1 stick (4" x 2" x ½")[7]	28	3.5	0.9	1.4	0.9	32	30	.04	0.6	.51	.09	74	51	.21	.029	815
frzn, crispy crunchy, Mrs. Paul's	201		8.6	18.5				0	.09			368	23			
3 oz	85	10.3				32	0	.09	0.8			108		.90		I
lightly battered, frzn, crunchy, Mrs. Paul's—3.5 oz	238		7.8	24.4				0	.13			597	21			
	99	12.2				19	0	.08	0.8			187		.70		I
minced, crunchy, frzn, Mrs. Paul's	208		10.2	16.4				0	.09			358	26			
3 oz	85	11.3				20	0	.10	0.9			158		1.20		I
fish thins, frzn, Mrs. Paul's	298		14.4	28.0				1	.23			1116	77			
5 oz	142	14.3					0	.22	2.4			257		1.30		I
flatfish (flounder/sole)																
ckd by dry heat	100	62.2	20.5	0.0	0.0	0.0	9	0	.10	.20	8	89	15	49	.54	.017
3 oz	85	1.3	0.3	0.2	0.5	58	32	.07	1.9	2.13	.49	293	246	.29	.022	815
crispy crunchy, frzn, Mrs. Paul's	277		11.6	24.3				0	.15			472	32			
4 oz	113	14.9	3.0		4.9	32	0	.10	1.7			180		1.30		I
fillets, au natural, frzn, Mrs. Paul's	101		21.3	0.7				0	.12			175	31			
5 oz	142	1.5					0	.32	2.9			165		.80		I
raw	77	67.2	16.0	0.0	0.0	0.0	9	1	.06	.18	7	69	15	26	.38	.014
3 oz	85	1.0	0.2	0.2	0.3	41	28	.08	2.5	1.29	.43	307	156	.31	.027	815
gefiltefish w/ broth, sweet	35	33.7	3.8	3.1		0.0	11	0	.02	.03	1	220	10	4	.34	.031
1 piece	42	0.7	0.2	0.3	0.1	13	37	.03	0.4	.35	.08	38	31	1.04	.082	815
grouper, ckd by dry heat	100	62.4	21.1	0.0	0.0	0.0	43	0	.01	.30	9	45	18	31	.43	.010
3 oz	85	1.1	0.3	0.2	0.3	40	140	.07	0.3	.59	.74	404	122	.97	.038	815
grouper, raw	78	67.4	16.5	0.0	0.0	0.0	37	0	.00	.26	7	45	23	26	.41	.012
3 oz	85	0.9	0.2	0.2	0.3	31	122	.06	0.3	.51	.64	411	138	.76	.017	815
haddock																
ckd by dry heat	95	63.1	20.6	0.0	0.0	0.0	16	0	.04	.29	11	74	36	43	.41	.026
3 oz	85	0.8	0.1	0.1	0.3	63	54	.03	3.9	1.18	.13	339	205	1.15	.028	815
fillets, crispy crunchy, frzn, Mrs. Paul's	284		13.5	25.6				1	.14			460	28			
4.2 oz	120	14.2					0	.12	3.0			259		1.00		I
lightly battered, crunchy, frzn, Mrs. Paul's—4.5 oz	316		11.3	31.4				0	.10			711	26			
	128	16.2					0	.10	1.8			267		.60		I
raw	74	68.0	16.1	0.0	0.0	0.0	14	0	.03	.26	10	58	28	33	.31	.021
3 oz	85	0.6	0.1	0.1	0.2	48	47	.03	3.2	1.02	.11	265	160	.89	.022	815
smoked	99	60.8	21.5	0.0	0.0	0.0	19	0	.04	.34	13	649	42	46	.43	.026
3 oz	85	0.8	0.1	0.1	0.3	65	62	.04	4.3	1.36	.14	353	213	1.19	.036	815
halibut, atlantic & pacific, ckd by dry heat—3 oz	119	61.0	22.7	0.0	0.0	0.0	46	0	.08	.34	12	59	51	91	.45	.017
	85	2.5	0.4	0.8	0.8	35	152	.06	6.1	1.16	.32	490	242	.91	.030	815

	KCAL / WT (g)	H₂O (g) / FAT (g)	PRO (g) / SFA (g)	CHO (g) / MUFA (g)	SUGR (g) / PUFA (g)	DFIB (g) / CHOL (mg)	A (RE) / A (IU)	C (mg) / B-1 (mg)	B-2 (mg) / NIA (mg)	B-6 (mg) / B-12 (mcg)	FOL (mcg) / PANT (mg)	Na (mg) / K (mg)	Ca (mg) / P (mg)	Mg (mg) / Fe (mg)	Zn (mg) / Cu (mg)	Mn (mg) / REF
halibut, atlantic & pacific, raw	94	66.3	17.7	0.0	0.0	0.0	40	0	.06	.29	10	46	40	71	.36	.013
3 oz	85	1.9	0.3	0.6	0.6	27	132	.05	5.0	1.01	.28	383	189	.71	.023	815
halibut, greenland, ckd by dry heat	203	52.6	15.7	0.0	0.0	0.0	15	0	.09	.41	1	88	3	28	.43	.013
3 oz	85	15.1	2.6	9.1	1.5	50	51	.06	1.6	.82	.24	293	179	.72	.032	815
halibut, greenland, raw	158	59.8	12.2	0.0	0.0	0.0	14	0	.07	.36	1	68	3	22	.34	.010
3 oz	85	11.8	2.1	7.1	1.2	39	47	.05	1.3	.85	.21	228	139	.56	.026	815
herring, atlantic																
ckd by dry heat	173	54.6	19.6	0.0	0.0		26	1	.25	.30	10	98	63	35	1.08	.034
3 oz	85	9.9	2.2	4.1	2.3	65	87	.10	3.5	11.18	.63	356	258	1.20	.100	815
kippered	87	23.9	9.8	0.0	0.0	0.0	16	0	.13	.17	5	367	34	18	.54	.020
1 piece (4 ⅜" x 1 ¾" x ¼")	40	4.9	1.1	2.0	1.2	33	51	.05	1.8	7.48	.35	179	130	.60	.054	815
pickled	39	8.3	2.1	1.4		0.0	39	0	.02	.03	0	131	12	1	.08	.006
1 piece (1 ¾" x ⅞" x ½")	15	2.7	0.4	1.8	0.3	2	129	.01	0.5	.64	.01	10	13	.18	.016	815
raw	134	61.3	15.3	0.0	0.0	0.0	24	1	.20	.26	9	77	48	27	.84	.030
3 oz	85	7.7	1.7	3.2	1.8	51	80	.08	2.7	11.62	.55	278	201	.94	.078	815
herring, pacific, ckd by dry heat	213	54.0	17.9	0.0	0.0	0.0	30	0	.22	.44	5	81	90	35	.58	.049
3 oz	85	15.1	3.5	7.5	2.6	84	99	.06	2.4	8.18	.98	461	248	1.22	.085	815
herring, pacific, raw	166	60.8	13.9	0.0	0.0	0.0	27	0	.17	.38	4	63	71	27	.45	.038
3 oz	85	11.8	2.8	5.8	2.1	65	90	.05	1.9	8.50	.85	360	194	.95	.066	815
inconnu, raw	146	72.0	19.9	0.0												B&C
3.5 oz	100	6.8														
kingfish, breaded, ckd w/ fat	255		22.3	11.7		0.0		0	.13			101	80	56		
3.5 oz	100	13.4					93	.11	2.9			293	287	1.90		B&C
kingfish, raw	105	77.3	18.3	0.0		0.0						83				
3.5 oz	100	3.0										250				B&C
ling, ckd by dry heat	94	62.8	20.7	0.0	0.0	0.0	30	0	.20	.30	7	147	37	69	.85	.032
3 oz	85	0.7				43	98	.11	2.4	.55	.31	413	216	.71	.120	815
ling, raw	74	67.7	16.2	0.0	0.0	0.0	26	0	.16	.26	6	115	29	54	.66	.026
3 oz	85	0.5	0.1	0.1	0.2	34	85	.09	2.0	.48	.27	322	168	.55	.094	815
lingcod, ckd by dry heat	93	64.4	19.3	0.0	0.0	0.0	14	0	.12	.29	9	65	15	28	.49	.022
3 oz	85	1.2	0.2	0.4	0.3	57	49	.03	2.0	3.53	.74	476	219	.35	.030	815
lingcod, raw	72	68.9	15.0	0.0	0.0	0.0	13	0	.10	.26	8	50	12	22	.38	.017
3 oz	85	0.9	0.2	0.3	0.3	44	43	.03	1.6	3.06	.64	372	171	.27	.023	815
lobster, northern, ckd by moist heat	83	64.7	17.4	1.1		0.0	22	0	.06	.07	9	323	52	30	2.48	.052
3 oz	85	0.5	0.1	0.1	0.1	61	74	.01	0.9	2.65	.24	299	157	.33	1.650	815
lobster, northern, raw	77	65.3	16.0	0.4		0.0	18	0	.04	.05	8	252	41	23	2.57	.047
3 oz	85	0.8	0.2	0.2	0.1	81	60	.01	1.2	.79	1.39	234	122	.26	1.414	815
lobster paste	13	4.3	1.5	0.1							.02		5			
1 t	7	0.7						.01					13		.10	B&C
lobster salad	110	80.3	10.1	2.3				18	.80			124	36			
3.5 oz[8]	100	6.4			0.9			.09				264	95	.90		B&C
mackerel, atlantic, ckd by dry heat	223	45.3	20.3	0.0	0.0	0.0	46	0	.35	.39	1	71	13	82	.80	.017
3 oz	85	15.1	3.6	6.0	3.7	64	153	.14	5.8	16.16	.84	341	236	1.34	.080	815
mackerel, atlantic, raw	174	54.0	15.8	0.0	0.0	0.0	43	0	.27	.34	1	77	10	65	.54	.013
3 oz	85	11.8	2.8	4.6	2.8	60	140	.15	7.7	7.41	.73	267	185	1.39	.062	815
mackerel, jack, cnd	296	131.4	44.1	0.0	0.0	0.0	247	2	.40	.40	10	720	458	70	1.94	.076
1 cup	190	12.0	3.5	4.2	3.1	150	825	.08	11.7	13.19	.58	369	572	3.88	.279	815
mackerel, king, ckd by dry heat	114	58.7	22.1	0.0	0.0	0.0	214	1	.49	.43	8	173	34	35	.61	.005
3 oz	85	2.2	0.4	0.8	0.5	58	714	.10	8.9	15.31	.82	475	270	1.94	.028	815
mackerel, king, raw	89	64.5	17.2	0.0	0.0	0.0	185	1	.40	.38	6	134	26	27	.48	.004
3 oz	85	1.7	0.3	0.6	0.4	45	618	.09	7.3	13.27	.71	370	211	1.51	.022	815
mackerel, pacific, and jack, ckd by dry heat—3 oz	171	52.5	21.9	0.0	0.0	0.0	12	2	.46	.32	2	94	25	31	.73	.016
	85	8.6	2.4	2.9	2.1	51	40	.11	9.1	3.60	.31	443	136	1.27	.101	815
mackerel, pacific, and jack, raw	134	59.7	17.1	0.0	0.0	0.0	11	2	.36	.28	2	73	20	24	.57	.013
3 oz	85	6.7	1.9	2.2	1.6	40	37	.09	7.1	3.74	.27	345	106	.99	.079	815
mackerel, spanish, ckd by dry heat	134	58.2	20.1	0.0	0.0	0.0	28	1	.18	.39	1	56	11	32	.53	.010
3 oz	85	5.4	1.5	1.8	1.5	62	93	.11	4.3	5.95	.74	471	230	.63	.055	815
mackerel, spanish, raw	118	61.0	16.4	0.0	0.0	0.0	26	1	.14	.34	1	50	9	28	.42	.012
3 oz	85	5.4	1.6	1.3	1.5	65	85	.11	2.0	2.04	.64	379	174	.37	.047	815
menhaden, atlantic, cnd	172	67.9	18.7	0.0	0.0											
3.5 oz	100	10.2														B&C

	KCAL / WT (g)	H₂O (g) / FAT (g)	PRO (g) / SFA (g)	CHO (g) / MUFA (g)	SUGR (g) / PUFA (g)	DFIB (g) / CHOL (mg)	A (RE) / A (IU)	C (mg) / B-1 (mg)	B-2 (mg) / NIA (mg)	B-6 (mg) / B-12 (mcg)	FOL (mcg) / PANT (mg)	Na (mg) / K (mg)	Ca (mg) / P (mg)	Mg (mg) / Fe (mg)	Zn (mg) / Cu (mg)	Mn (mg) / REF
milkfish, ckd by dry heat	162	53.3	22.4	0.0	0.0	0.0	28	0	.06	.42	15	78	55	32	.89	.022
3 oz	85	7.3				57	93	.01	7.0	2.78	.74	318	177	.35	.037	815
milkfish, raw	126	60.3	17.5	0.0	0.0	0.0	26	0	.05	.36	14	61	43	26	.70	.017
3 oz	85	5.7	1.4	2.2	1.6	44	85	.01	5.5	2.89	.64	248	138	.27	.029	815
monkfish, ckd by dry heat	82	66.8	15.8	0.0	0.0	0.0	12	1	.06	.24	7	20	9	23	.45	.026
3 oz	85	1.7				27	39	.02	2.2	.88	.15	436	218	.35	.031	815
monkfish, raw	65	70.8	12.3	0.0	0.0	0.0	10	1	.05	.20	6	15	7	18	.35	.020
3 oz	85	1.3	0.3	0.2	0.5	21	34	.02	1.8	.77	.13	340	170	.27	.024	815
mullet, striped, ckd by dry heat	128	60.0	21.1	0.0	0.0	0.0	36	1	.09	.42	8	60	26	28	.75	.019
3 oz	85	4.1	1.2	1.2	0.8	54	120	.09	5.4	.21	.75	390	208	1.20	.120	815
mullet, striped, raw	100	65.5	16.5	0.0	0.0	0.0	31	1	.07	.36	7	55	35	25	.44	.014
3 oz	85	3.2	0.9	0.9	0.6	42	104	.08	4.4	.19	.65	304	188	.87	.043	815
mussels, blue, ckd by moist heat	146	52.0	20.2	6.3		0.0	77	12	.36	.09	64	314	28	31	2.27	5.783
3 oz	85	3.8	0.7	0.9	1.0	48	259	.26	2.6	20.41	.81	228	242	5.72	.127	815
mussels, blue, raw	73	68.5	10.1	3.1		0.0	41	7	.18	.04	36	243	22	29	1.36	2.892
3 oz	85	1.9	0.4	0.4	0.5	24	136	.14	1.4	10.21	.43	272	168	3.36	.080	815
ocean perch, atlantic, ckd by dry heat	103	61.8	20.3	0.0	0.0	0.0	12	1	.11	.23	9	82	117	33	.52	.017
3 oz	85	1.8	0.3	0.7	0.5	46	39	.11	2.1	.98	.36	298	236	1.00	.028	815
ocean perch, atlantic, raw	80	66.9	15.8	0.0	0.0	0.0	10	1	.09	.20	8	64	91	26	.41	.013
3 oz	85	1.4	0.2	0.5	0.4	36	34	.09	1.7	.85	.31	232	184	.78	.022	815
octopus, ckd by moist heat	139	51.5	25.4	3.7		0.0	69	7	.06	.55	20	391	90	51	2.86	.040
3 oz	85	1.8	0.4	0.3	0.4	82	230	.05	3.2	30.62	.77	536	237	8.11	.629	815
octopus, raw	70	68.3	12.7	1.9		0.0	38	4	.03	.31	14	196	45	26	1.43	.021
3 oz	85	0.9	0.2	0.1	0.2	41	128	.03	1.8	17.01	.43	298	158	4.51	.370	815
orange roughy, ckd by dry heat	76	58.8	16.0	0.0	0.0	0.0	20	0	.16	.29	7	69	32	32	.82	.016
3 oz	85	0.8	0.0	0.5	0.0	22	69	.10	3.1	1.96	.54	327	218	.20	.152	815
orange roughy, raw	59	64.6	12.5	0.0	0.0	0.0	18	0	.13	.26	6	54	26	26	.64	.013
3 oz	85	0.6	0.0	0.4	0.0	17	60	.09	2.6	1.70	.47	255	170	.15	.119	815
oysters, eastern																
breaded & fried	168	55.0	7.5	9.9			77	3	.17	.05	12	355	53	49	74.10	.417
3 oz (about 6 med)[4]	85	10.7	2.7	4.0	2.8	69	257	.13	1.4	13.29	.23	208	135	5.91	3.652	815
cnd	59	72.4	6.0	3.3		0.0	77	4	.14	.08	8	95	38	46	77.35	.383
3 oz	85	2.1	0.5	0.2	0.6	47	255	.13	1.1	16.27	.15	195	118	5.70	3.794	815
farmed, ckd by dry heat	47	48.4	4.1	4.3		0.0	11	4	.03	.04	14	90	33	19	26.64	.251
6 med	59	1.3	0.4	0.1	0.4	22	37	.08	1.1	14.34	.12	150	37	4.58	.846	815
farmed, raw	50	72.4	4.4	4.6		0.0	7	4	.05	.05	15	150	37	28	31.85	.331
6 med	84	1.3	0.4	0.1	0.5	21	21	.09	1.1	13.61	.13	104	78	4.86	.620	815
wild, ckd by dry heat	42	49.1	4.9	2.8		0.0	0	2	.05	.06	11	144	27	27	43.42	.170
6 med	59	1.1	0.3	0.1	0.5	29	0	.05	1.0	16.40	.13	99	80	2.55	2.038	815
wild, ckd by moist heat	58	29.5	5.9	3.3		0.0	23	3	.08	.05	6	177	38	40	76.28	.293
6 med	42	2.1	0.6	0.3	0.8	44	76	.08	1.0	14.71	.15	118	85	5.04	3.179	815
wild, raw	57	71.5	5.9	3.3		0.0	25	3	.08	.05	8	177	38	39	76.28	.308
6 med	84	2.1	0.6	0.3	0.8	45	84	.08	1.2	16.35	.16	131	113	5.59	3.740	815
oysters, pacific, ckd by moist heat	139	54.5	16.1	8.4		0.0	124	11	.38	.08	13	180	14	37	28.27	1.039
3 oz	85	3.9	0.9	0.6	1.5	85	413	.11	3.1	24.49	.77	257	207	7.82	2.278	815
oysters, pacific, raw	69	69.8	8.0	4.2		0.0	69	7	.20	.04	9	90	7	19	14.14	.547
3 oz	85	2.0	0.4	0.3	0.8	43	230	.06	1.7	13.61	.43	143	138	4.35	1.340	815
perch																
ckd by dry heat	100	62.3	21.1	0.0	0.0	0.0	9	1	.10	.12	5	67	87	32	1.22	.765
3 oz	85	1.0	0.2	0.2	0.4	98	27	.07	1.6	1.87	.74	293	219	.99	.163	815
fillet, crispy crunchy, frzn, Mrs. Paul's	315		13.1	22.6				1	.11			469	35			
4.2 oz	120	19.1					0	.11	1.5			190		1.60		I
fillet, frzn, Mrs. Paul's	270		16.3	21.5				0	.23			514	29			
4.5 oz	128	13.2	3.0		4.0	39	0	.12	1.4			331		1.20		I
raw	77	67.3	16.5	0.0	0.0	0.0	8	1	.09	.10	4	53	68	26	.94	.595
3 oz	85	0.8	0.2	0.1	0.3	77	24	.06	1.3	1.62	.64	229	170	.77	.128	815
pike, northern, ckd by dry heat	96	62.1	21.0	0.0	0.0	0.0	20	3	.07	.11	15	42	62	34	.73	.264
3 oz	85	0.7	0.1	0.2	0.2	43	69	.06	2.4	1.96	.74	282	240	.60	.055	815
pike, northern, raw	75	67.1	16.4	0.0	0.0	0.0	18	3	.05	.10	13	33	48	26	.57	.204
3 oz	85	0.6	0.1	0.1	0.2	33	60	.05	2.0	1.70	.64	220	187	.47	.043	815

	KCAL / WT (g)	H₂O (g) / FAT (g)	PRO (g) / SFA (g)	CHO (g) / MUFA (g)	SUGR (g) / PUFA (g)	DFIB (g) / CHOL (mg)	A (RE) / A (IU)	C (mg) / B-1 (mg)	B-2 (mg) / NIA (mg)	B-6 (mg) / B-12 (mcg)	FOL (mcg) / PANT (mg)	Na (mg) / K (mg)	Ca (mg) / P (mg)	Mg (mg) / Fe (mg)	Zn (mg) / Cu (mg)	Mn (mg) / REF
pike, walleye, ckd by dry heat	101	62.5	20.9	0.0	0.0	0.0	20	0	.17	.12	14	55	120	32	.67	.873
3 oz	85	1.3	0.3	0.3	0.5	94	69	.27	2.4	1.96	.74	424	229	1.42	.194	815
pike, walleye, raw	79	67.5	16.3	0.0	0.0	0.0	18	0	.14	.10	13	43	94	26	.53	.680
3 oz	85	1.0	0.2	0.3	0.4	73	60	.23	2.0	1.70	.64	331	179	1.11	.151	815
pollock, atlantic, ckd by dry heat	100	61.3	21.2	0.0	0.0	0.0	10	0	.19	.28	3	94	65	73	.51	.016
3 oz	85	1.1	0.1	0.1	0.5	77	34	.05	3.4	3.13	.35	388	241	.50	.054	815
pollock, atlantic, raw	78	66.5	16.5	0.0	0.0	0.0	9	0	.16	.24	3	73	51	57	.40	.013
3 oz	85	0.8	0.1	0.1	0.4	60	30	.04	2.8	2.71	.30	303	188	.39	.043	815
pollock, ckd, creamed	128	74.7	13.9	4.0		0.0		0	.13			11				
3.5 oz	100	5.9						.03	0.7			238				B&C
pollock, walleye, ckd by dry heat	96	63.0	20.0	0.0	0.0	0.0	20	0	.06	.06	3	99	5	62	.51	.017
3 oz	85	1.0	0.2	0.1	0.4	82	65	.06	1.4	3.57	.14	329	410	.24	.047	815
pollock, walleye, raw	69	69.4	14.6	0.0	0.0	0.0	17	0	.05	.05	3	84	4	48	.37	.013
3 oz	85	0.7	0.1	0.1	0.4	60	56	.06	1.1	2.64	.12	277	320	.20	.037	815
pompano, florida, ckd by dry heat	179	53.6	20.1	0.0	0.0	0.0	31	0	.13	.20	15	65	37	26	.59	.021
3 oz	85	10.3	3.8	2.8	1.2	54	102	.58	3.2	1.02	.74	541	290	.57	.066	815
pompano, florida, raw	139	60.5	15.7	0.0	0.0	0.0	28	0	.10	.17	13	55	19	23	.61	.011
3 oz	85	8.1	3.0	2.2	1.0	43	94	.48	2.6	1.11	.64	324	166	.51	.032	815
pout, ocean, ckd by dry heat	87	64.7	18.1	0.0	0.0	0.0	12	0	.06	.24	7	66	11	14	1.12	.016
3 oz	85	1.0	0.3	0.4	0.0	57	39	.08	2.2	.88	.15	436	218	.31	.035	815
pout, ocean, raw	67	69.2	14.2	0.0	0.0	0.0	10	0	.05	.20	6	52	9	11	.88	.013
3 oz	85	0.8	0.3	0.3	0.0	44	34	.07	1.8	.77	.13	340	170	.24	.027	815
rockfish, pacific, ckd by dry heat	103	62.4	20.4	0.0	0.0	0.0	56	0	.07	.23	9	65	10	29	.45	.017
3 oz	85	1.7	0.4	0.4	0.5	37	186	.04	3.3	1.02	.74	442	194	.45	.031	815
rockfish, pacific, raw	80	67.4	15.9	0.0	0.0	0.0	48	0	.06	.20	8	51	8	22	.35	.014
3 oz	85	1.3	0.3	0.3	0.4	30	162	.03	2.7	.85	.64	344	151	.35	.025	815
roe, mixed species, ckd by dry heat	58	16.6	8.1	0.5		0.0	26	5	.27	.05	26	33	8	7	.36	.004
1 oz	28	2.3	0.5	0.6	1.0	136	86	.08	0.6	3.27	.33	80	146	.22	.036	815
roe, mixed species, raw	40	19.2	6.3	0.4		0.0	22	5	.21	.05	23	26	6	6	.28	.003
1 oz	28	1.8	0.4	0.5	0.8	106	75	.07	0.5	2.84	.28	63	114	.17	.028	815
sablefish																
ckd by dry heat	213	53.5	14.6	0.0	0.0	0.0	86	0	.10	.29	14	61	38	60	.35	.016
3 oz	85	16.7	3.5	8.8	2.2	54	287	.10	4.4	1.22	.74	390	183	1.39	.024	815
raw	166	60.4	11.4	0.0	0.0	0.0	79	0	.08	.26	13	48	30	47	.27	.013
3 oz	85	13.0	2.7	6.9	1.7	42	264	.09	3.4	1.28	.64	304	143	1.09	.019	815
smoked	219	51.1	15.0	0.0	0.0	0.0	104	0	.10	.33	17	627	43	63	.37	.017
3 oz	85	17.1	3.6	9.0	2.3	54	347	.11	4.5	1.70	.84	401	189	1.44	.031	815
salmon, atlantic																
farmed, ckd by dry heat	175	55.1	18.8	0.0	0.0	0.0	13	3	.11	.55	29	52	13	26	.37	.014
3 oz	85	10.5	2.1	3.8	3.8	54	43	.29	6.8	2.38	1.25	327	214	.29	.042	815
farmed, raw	156	58.6	16.9	0.0	0.0	0.0	13	3	.10	.54	22	50	10	24	.34	.013
3 oz	85	9.2	1.9	3.3	3.3	50	43	.29	6.4	2.38	1.17	308	198	.31	.042	815
wild, ckd by dry heat	155	50.7	21.6	0.0	0.0	0.0	11	0	.41	.80	25	48	13	31	.70	.018
3 oz	85	6.9	1.1	2.3	2.8	60	37	.23	8.6	2.59	1.63	534	218	.88	.273	815
wild, raw	121	58.3	16.9	0.0	0.0	0.0	10	0	.32	.70	21	37	10	25	.54	.014
3 oz	85	5.4	0.8	1.8	2.2	47	34	.19	6.7	2.70	1.42	417	170	.68	.213	815
salmon, chinook																
ckd by dry heat	196	55.8	21.9	0.0	0.0	0.0	127	3	.13	.39	30	51	24	104	.48	.016
3 oz	85	11.4	2.7	4.9	2.3	72	422	.04	8.5	2.44	.74	430	316	.77	.045	815
raw	153	62.2	17.1	0.0	0.0	0.0	116	3	.10	.34	26	40	19	81	.37	.013
3 oz	85	8.9	2.1	3.8	1.8	56	387	.03	6.7	2.54	.64	335	246	.60	.035	815
smoked	100	61.2	15.5	0.0	0.0	0.0	22	0	.09	.24	2	667	9	15	.26	.014
3 oz	85	3.7	0.8	1.7	0.8	20	75	.02	4.0	2.77	.74	149	139	.72	.196	815
salmon, chum																
ckd by dry heat	131	58.2	22.0	0.0	0.0	0.0	29	0	.19	.39	4	54	12	24	.51	.016
3 oz	85	4.1	0.9	1.7	1.0	81	97	.08	7.3	2.94	.74	468	309	.60	.060	815
cnd w/ bone	120	60.2	18.2	0.0	0.0	0.0	15	0	.14	.32	17	414	212	26	.85	.017
3 oz	85	4.7	1.3	1.6	1.3	33	52	.02	6.0	3.74	.48	255	301	.60	.085	815

						Vitamins					Minerals				
KCAL	H₂O (g)	PRO (g)	CHO (g)	SUGR (g)	DFIB (g)	A (RE)	C (mg)	B-2 (mg)	B-6 (mg)	FOL (mcg)	Na (mg)	Ca (mg)	Mg (mg)	Zn (mg)	Mn (mg)
WT (g)	FAT (g)	SFA (g)	MUFA (g)	PUFA (g)	CHOL (mg)	A (IU)	B-1 (mg)	NIA (mg)	B-12 (mcg)	PANT (mg)	K (mg)	P (mg)	Fe (mg)	Cu (mg)	REF
raw															
102	64.1	17.1	0.0	0.0	0.0	26	0	.15	.34	3	43	9	19	.40	.013
85	3.2	0.7	1.3	0.8	63	84	.07	6.0	2.55	.64	365	241	.47	.047	815
salmon, coho															
farmed, ckd by dry heat															
151	57.0	20.7	0.0	0.0	0.0	50	1	.10	.48	12	44	10	29	.40	.018
85	7.0	1.7	3.1	1.7	54	168	.09	6.3	2.70	1.08	391	282	.33	.076	815
farmed, raw															
136	59.9	18.1	0.0	0.0	0.0	48	1	.09	.56	11	40	10	26	.37	.010
85	6.5	1.5	2.8	1.6	43	160	.08	5.8	2.27	.97	383	248	.29	.041	815
wild, ckd by dry heat															
118	60.8	19.9	0.0	0.0	0.0	33	1	.12	.48	11	49	38	28	.48	.016
85	3.7	0.9	1.3	1.1	47	111	.06	6.8	4.25	.69	369	274	.52	.060	815
wild, ckd, moist heat															
156	55.6	23.3	0.0	0.0	0.0	27	1	.14	.47	8	45	39	30	.44	.015
85	6.4	1.4	2.3	2.1	48	92	.10	6.6	3.81	.71	387	253	.60	.055	815
wild, raw															
124	61.8	18.4	0.0	0.0	0.0	26	1	.12	.47	8	39	31	26	.35	.012
85	5.0	1.1	1.8	1.7	38	85	.10	6.1	3.54	.70	360	223	.48	.043	815
salmon, pink															
boneless, cnd, Libby's															
70		14.0	0.0	0.0	0.0	0	0				190	0			
⅓ cup	56	2.0	0.0			40	0							.40		I
ckd by dry heat															
127	59.3	21.7	0.0	0.0	0.0	35	0	.06	.20	4	73	14	28	.60	.016
85	3.8	0.6	1.0	1.5	57	116	.17	7.3	2.94	.74	352	251	.84	.084	815
cnd, Libby's															
90		12.0	0.0	0.0	0.0	0	0				270	100			
¼ cup	63	5.0	1.0			40	0							.40		I
cnd w/ bone															
118	58.5	16.8	0.0	0.0	0.0	14	0	.16	.26	13	471	181	29	.78	.017
85	5.1	1.3	1.5	1.7	47	47	.02	5.6	3.74	.47	277	280	.71	.087	815
raw															
99	64.9	17.0	0.0	0.0	0.0	30	0	.05	.17	3	57	11	22	.47	.013
85	2.9	0.5	0.8	1.2	44	100	.14	6.0	2.55	.64	275	196	.65	.065	815
salmon, red, cnd, Libby's															
110		13.0	0.0	0.0	0.0		0				270	100			
¼ cup	63	7.0	1.5			0	100							.40		I
salmon, sockeye															
ckd by dry heat															
184	52.6	23.2	0.0	0.0	0.0	54	0	.15	.19	4	56	6	26	.43	.017
85	9.3	1.6	4.5	2.0	74	178	.18	5.7	4.93	.60	319	235	.47	.057	815
cnd w/ bone															
130	58.4	17.4	0.0	0.0	0.0	45	0	.16	.26	8	458	203	25	.87	.026
85	6.2	1.4	2.7	1.6	37	150	.01	4.7	.26	.47	321	277	.90	.071	815
raw															
143	59.7	18.1	0.0	0.0	0.0	49	0	.13	.16	3	40	5	20	.46	.012
85	7.3	1.3	3.5	1.6	53	163	.17	4.9	4.25	.52	333	183	.40	.044	815
sardines, cnd, atlantic w/ soybean oil															
50	14.3	5.9	0.0	0.0	0.0	16	0	.05	.04	3	121	92	9	.31	.026
2 sardines	24	2.7	0.4	0.9	1.2	34	54	.02	1.3	2.15	.15	95	118	.70	.045	815
sardines, cnd, pacific w/ tomato sce															
68	26.0	6.2	0.0	0.0	0.0	27	0	.09	.05	9	157	91	13	.53	.078
1 sardine	38	4.6	1.2	2.1	0.9	23	139	.02	1.6	3.42	.28	130	139	.87	.103	815
scallops															
bay, raw															
88	78.8	15.9	2.9								170	5	23	.80	
3.5 oz	100	1.0	0.2	0.1	0.4	37						126	107	.10	.000	I
breaded & fried															
67	18.1	5.6	3.1			7	1	.03	.04	6	144	13	18	.33	.043
2 large[4]	31	3.4	0.8	1.4	0.9	19	23	.01	0.5	.41	.06	103	73	.25	.024	815
french fried, frzn, Mrs. Paul's															
203		12.5	20.2				0	.17			363	50			
3.5 oz	99	8.0					0	.07	1.5			234		1.20		I
imitation, made from surimi															
84	62.8	10.9	9.0		0.0	17	0	.01	.03	1	676	7	37	.28	.009
85	0.3	0.1	0.1	0.2	19	56	.01	0.3	1.36	.06	88	240	.26	.027	815
mixed species, raw															
75	66.8	14.3	2.0		0.0	13	3	.06	.13	14	137	20	48	.81	.077
3 oz (6 large)	85	0.6	0.1	0.0	0.2	28	43	.01	1.0	1.30	.12	274	186	.25	.045	815
sea, raw															
59	86.2	10.6	1.6								39	3	13	.40	.300
3.5 oz	100	0.7	0.1	0.0	0.3	27						98	74	.10	.200	I
scup, ckd by dry heat															
115	58.2	20.6	0.0	0.0	0.0	26	0	.10	.29	14	46	43	25	.53	.038
85	3.0				57	88	.11	4.2	1.38	.74	313	202	.58	.055	815
scup, raw															
89	64.1	16.1	0.0	0.0	0.0	23	0	.09	.26	13	36	34	20	.41	.030
85	2.3	0.5	0.5	0.9	44	77	.09	3.5	1.19	.64	244	157	.45	.043	815
sea bass, ckd by dry heat															
105	61.4	20.1	0.0	0.0	0.0	54	0	.13	.39	5	74	11	45	.44	.017
85	2.2	0.6	0.5	0.8	45	181	.11	1.6	.26	.74	279	211	.31	.020	815
sea bass, raw															
82	66.6	15.7	0.0	0.0	0.0	47	0	.10	.34	4	58	9	35	.34	.013
85	1.7	0.4	0.4	0.6	35	156	.09	1.4	.26	.64	218	165	.25	.016	815

	KCAL / WT (g)	H₂O (g) / FAT (g)	PRO (g) / SFA (g)	CHO (g) / MUFA (g)	SUGR (g) / PUFA (g)	DFIB (g) / CHOL (mg)	A (RE) / A (IU)	C (mg) / B-1 (mg)	B-2 (mg) / NIA (mg)	B-6 (mg) / B-12 (mcg)	FOL (mcg) / PANT (mg)	Na (mg) / K (mg)	Ca (mg) / P (mg)	Mg (mg) / Fe (mg)	Zn (mg) / Cu (mg)	Mn (mg) / REF
seafood platter combo, fried, frzn, Mrs. Paul's—9 oz	588		20.8	56.1				1	.38			1221	102			
	255	31.2					0	.06	4.1			426		2.50		I
seatrout, ckd by dry heat	113	61.2	18.3	0.0	0.0	0.0	30	0	.18	.39	5	63	19	34	.49	.016
3 oz	85	3.9	1.1	1.0	0.8	90	98	.06	2.5	2.94	.74	372	273	.30	.032	815
seatrout, raw	88	66.4	14.2	0.0	0.0	0.0	26	0	.14	.34	4	49	14	26	.38	.013
3 oz	85	3.1	0.9	0.8	0.6	71	85	.05	2.0	2.55	.64	290	213	.23	.026	815
shad, american, ckd by dry heat	214	50.4	18.5	0.0	0.0	0.0	31	0	.26	.39	14	55	51	32	.40	.046
3 oz	85	15.0				82	102	.16	9.2	.12	.74	418	297	1.05	.070	815
shad, american, raw	168	58.0	14.4	0.0	0.0	0.0	28	0	.20	.34	13	43	40	26	.31	.036
3 oz	85	11.7	2.7	4.9	2.8	64	94	.13	7.1	.13	.64	327	231	.82	.054	815
shark, batter-dipped & fried	194	51.1	15.8	5.4		0.0	46	0	.08	.26	4	104	43	37	.41	.043
3 oz	85	11.8	2.7	5.0	3.1	50	153	.06	2.4	1.03	.53	132	165	.94	.036	815
shark, raw	111	62.6	17.8	0.0	0.0	0.0	60	0	.05	.34	3	67	29	42	.37	.013
3 oz	85	3.8	0.8	1.5	1.0	43	198	.04	2.5	1.27	.59	136	179	.71	.028	815
sheepshead, ckd by dry heat	107	58.7	22.1	0.0	0.0	0.0	30	0	.04	.30	15	62	31	30	.54	.018
3 oz	85	1.4	0.3	0.3	0.3	54	98	.01	1.5	1.96	.74	435	298	.57	.104	815
sheepshead, raw	92	66.3	17.2	0.0	0.0	0.0	26	0	.03	.26	13	60	18	27	.33	.011
3 oz	85	2.0	0.5	0.6	0.4	43	85	.01	1.3	1.70	.64	344	266	.39	.026	815
shrimp																
breaded & fried	206	45.0	18.2	9.8		0.3	48	1	.12	.08	7	293	57	34	1.17	.085
3 oz (11 large)[4]	85	10.4	1.8	3.2	4.3	151	161	.11	2.6	1.59	.30	191	185	1.07	.233	815
cajun style, frzn, Mrs. Paul's	206		8.7	30.1				10	.31			822	77			
9 oz entree	255	5.7					700	.08	6.4			168		1.20		I
ckd by moist heat	84	65.7	17.8	0.0	0.0	0.0	56	2	.03	.11	3	191	33	29	1.33	.029
3 oz (15 ½ large)	85	0.9	0.2	0.2	0.4	166	186	.03	2.2	1.27	.29	155	117	2.63	.164	815
cnd	102	61.7	19.6	0.9		0.0	15	2	.03	.09	2	144	50	35	1.07	.051
3 oz	85	1.7	0.3	0.2	0.6	147	51	.02	2.3	.95	.19	179	198	2.33	.255	815
fried, frzn, Mrs. Paul's	197		8.9	16.0				1	.07			394	44			
3 oz	85	10.8					0	.12	1.4			33		1.20		I
imitation, made from surimi	86	63.7	10.5	7.8		0.0	17	0	.03	.03	1	600	16	37	.28	.009
3 oz	85	1.3	0.2	0.2	0.6	31	56	.02	0.1	1.36	.06	76	240	.51	.027	815
primavera, frzn, Mrs. Paul's Light	282		15.4	35.8				14	.30			885	80			
11 oz entree	312	8.6					2986	.25	3.1			130		3.60		I
raw	90	64.5	17.3	0.8		0.0	46	2	.03	.09	3	126	44	31	.94	.043
3 oz (12 large)	85	1.5	0.3	0.2	0.6	129	153	.02	2.2	.99	.23	157	174	2.05	.225	815
shrimp paste	180	61.3	20.8	1.5											.26	
3.5 oz	100	9.4														B&C
skate (rajah fish), raw	98	77.8	21.5	0.0		0.0										
3.5 oz	100	0.7						.02								B&C
smelt, rainbow, ckd by dry heat	105	61.9	19.2	0.0	0.0	0.0	14	0	.12	.14	4	65	65	32	1.80	.765
3 oz	85	2.6	0.5	0.7	1.0	77	49	.01	1.5	3.38	.63	316	251	.98	.151	815
smelt, rainbow, raw	82	67.0	15.0	0.0	0.0	0.0	13	0	.10	.13	3	51	51	26	1.40	.595
3 oz	85	2.1	0.4	0.5	0.8	60	43	.01	1.2	2.93	.54	247	196	.77	.118	815
snapper, ckd by dry heat	109	59.8	22.4	0.0	0.0	0.0	30	1	.00	.39	5	48	34	31	.37	.014
3 oz	85	1.5	0.3	0.3	0.5	40	98	.05	0.3	2.98	.74	444	171	.20	.039	815
snapper, raw	85	65.4	17.4	0.0	0.0	0.0	26	1	.00	.34	4	54	27	27	.31	.011
3 oz	85	1.1	0.2	0.2	0.4	31	85	.04	0.2	2.55	.64	355	168	.15	.024	815
spiny lobster, ckd by dry heat	122	56.8	22.5	2.7		0.0	5	2	.05	.15	1	193	54	43	6.18	.015
3 oz	85	1.6	0.3	0.3	0.6	77	17	.01	4.2	3.44	.34	177	195	1.20	.353	815
spiny lobster, raw	95	63.0	17.5	2.1		0.0	4	2	.04	.13	1	151	42	34	4.82	.013
3 oz	85	1.3	0.2	0.2	0.5	60	14	.01	3.6	2.98	.30	153	202	1.04	.324	815
spot, ckd by dry heat	134	58.8	20.2	0.0	0.0	0.0	30	0	.23	.39	5	31	15	46	.55	.038
3 oz	85	5.3	1.6	1.5	1.2	65	98	.16	7.3	2.94	.74	541	202	.35	.050	815
spot, raw	105	64.6	15.7	0.0	0.0	0.0	26	0	.19	.34	4	25	12	36	.43	.030
3 oz	85	4.2	1.2	1.1	0.9	51	85	.14	6.0	2.55	.64	422	158	.27	.039	815
squid, fried	149	54.9	15.3	6.6		0.0	9	4	.39	.05	5	260	33	32	1.48	.060
3 oz[1]	85	6.4	1.6	2.3	1.8	221	30	.05	2.2	1.04	.43	237	213	.86	1.798	815
squid, raw	78	66.8	13.3	2.6		0.0	9	4	.35	.05	4	37	27	28	1.30	.030
3 oz	85	1.2	0.3	0.1	0.4	198	28	.02	1.8	1.10	.43	209	188	.58	1.608	815

	KCAL / WT (g)	H₂O (g) / FAT (g)	PRO (g) / SFA (g)	CHO (g) / MUFA (g)	SUGR (g) / PUFA (g)	DFIB (g) / CHOL (mg)	A (RE) / A (IU)	C (mg) / B-1 (mg)	B-2 (mg) / NIA (mg)	B-6 (mg) / B-12 (mcg)	FOL (mcg) / PANT (mg)	Na (mg) / K (mg)	Ca (mg) / P (mg)	Mg (mg) / Fe (mg)	Zn (mg) / Cu (mg)	Mn (mg) / REF
sturgeon																
ckd by dry heat	115	59.5	17.6	0.0	0.0	0.0	206	0	.08	.20	15	59	14	38	.46	.026
3 oz	85	4.4	1.0	2.1	0.8	65	687	.07	8.6	2.13	.74	310	230	.77	.045	815
raw	89	65.1	13.7	0.0	0.0	0.0	179	0	.06	.17	13	46	11	30	.36	.021
3 oz	85	3.4	0.8	1.6	0.6	51	595	.06	7.1	1.87	.64	242	179	.60	.035	815
smoked	147	53.2	26.5	0.0	0.0	0.0	238	0	.08	.23	17	629	14	40	.48	.026
3 oz	85	3.7	0.9	2.0	0.4	68	794	.08	9.4	2.47	.85	322	239	.79	.043	815
sucker, white, ckd by dry heat	101	62.9	18.3	0.0	0.0	0.0	50	0	.07	.20	14	43	77	32	.82	.654
3 oz	85	2.5	0.5	0.8	0.9	45	167	.01	1.2	1.96	.74	414	229	1.42	.213	815
sucker, white, raw	78	67.8	14.3	0.0	0.0	0.0	43	0	.06	.17	13	34	60	26	.64	.510
3 oz	85	2.0	0.4	0.6	0.7	35	145	.01	1.0	1.70	.64	323	179	1.11	.166	815
sunfish, pumpkinseed, ckd by dry heat	97	62.7	21.2	0.0	0.0	0.0	14	1	.07	.12	14	88	88	32	1.69	.763
3 oz	85	0.8	0.2	0.1	0.3	73	49	.08	1.2	1.96	.74	382	196	1.31	.327	815
sunfish, pumpkinseed, raw	76	67.6	16.5	0.0	0.0	0.0	13	1	.06	.10	13	68	68	26	1.32	.595
3 oz	85	0.6	0.1	0.1	0.2	57	43	.07	1.0	1.70	.64	298	153	1.02	.255	815
surimi	84	64.9	12.9	5.8		0.0	17	0	.02	.03	1	122	8	37	.28	.009
3 oz[9]	85	0.8	0.2	0.1	0.4	26	56	.02	0.2	1.36	.06	95	240	.22	.027	815
chunk style, frzn, Crab Delight, Tyson	76		8.4	10.1	8.4	0.4		0				563	42			
3 oz[10]	84	0.0	0.0	0.0		13	273							.25		I
chunk style, frzn, Lobster Delight, Tyson	77		8.1	10.9	6.3	0.7		0				655	25			
3 oz	84	0.1	0.0			10	5							.21		I
Scallop Delight, Tyson	84		9.2	11.0	3.2	0.0		0				561	9			
½ cup	85	0.3	0.1	0.0	0.0	7	0							.17		I
swordfish, ckd by dry heat	132	58.5	21.6	0.0	0.0	0.0	35	1	.10	.32	2	98	5	29	1.25	.017
3 oz	85	4.4	1.2	1.7	1.0	43	117	.04	10.0	1.72	.32	314	287	.88	.138	815
swordfish, raw	103	64.3	16.8	0.0	0.0	0.0	31	1	.08	.28	2	77	3	23	.98	.016
3 oz	85	3.4	0.9	1.3	0.8	33	101	.03	8.2	1.49	.35	245	224	.69	.107	815
tautog (blackfish), raw	89	79.3	18.6	0.0		0.0							227			B&C
3.5 oz	100	1.1														
tilefish, ckd by dry heat	125	59.7	20.8	0.0	0.0	0.0	18	0	.16	.26	15	50	22	28	.45	.013
3 oz	85	4.0	0.7	1.1	1.1	54	59	.12	3.0	2.13	.74	435	201	.26	.044	815
tilefish, raw	82	67.1	14.9	0.0	0.0	0.0	15	0	.14	.22	13	45	22	24	.31	.009
3 oz	85	2.0	0.4	0.5	0.5	43	51	.10	2.5	1.87	.64	368	159	.21	.035	815
tomcod, atlantic, raw	77	81.5	17.2	0.0		0.0			.17							B&C
3.5 oz	100	0.4														
trout, Dolly Varden, raw	144	73.1	19.9	0.0		0.0			.06							B&C
3.5 oz	100	6.5						.06								
trout, mixed species, ckd by dry heat	162	53.9	22.6	0.0	0.0	0.0	16	0	.36	.20	13	57	47	24	.72	.928
3 oz	85	7.2	1.3	3.5	1.6	63	54	.36	4.9	6.37	1.90	394	267	1.63	.205	815
trout, mixed species, raw	126	60.7	17.7	0.0	0.0	0.0	14	0	.28	.17	11	44	37	19	.56	.724
3 oz	85	5.6	1.0	2.8	1.3	49	49	.30	3.8	6.63	1.65	307	208	1.28	.160	815
trout, rainbow																
farmed, ckd by dry heat	144	57.4	20.6	0.0	0.0	0.0	73	3	.07	.34	20	36	73	27	.42	.017
3 oz	85	6.1	1.8	1.8	2.0	58	244	.20	7.5	4.23	1.11	375	226	.28	.052	815
farmed, raw	117	61.9	17.7	0.0	0.0	0.0	71	2	.06	.53	9	30	57	27	.35	.015
3 oz	85	4.6	1.3	1.3	1.5	50	236	.17	7.0	3.21	1.22	384	240	.23	.039	815
wild, ckd by dry heat	128	60.0	19.5	0.0	0.0	0.0	13	2	.08	.29	16	48	73	26	.43	.018
3 oz	85	4.9	1.4	1.5	1.6	59	43	.13	4.9	5.36	.91	381	229	.32	.049	815
wild, raw	101	61.1	17.4	0.0	0.0	0.0	16	2	.09	.35	10	26	57	26	.92	.134
3 oz	85	2.9	0.6	1.0	1.1	50	53	.10	4.6	3.78	.79	409	230	.60	.093	815
tuna, bluefin, ckd by dry heat	156	50.3	25.4	0.0	0.0	0.0	643	0	.26	.45	2	43	9	54	.65	.017
3 oz	85	5.3	1.4	1.7	1.6	42	2143	.24	9.0	9.25	1.17	275	277	1.11	.094	815
tuna, bluefin, raw	122	57.9	19.8	0.0	0.0	0.0	557	0	.21	.39	2	33	7	43	.51	.013
3 oz	85	4.2	1.1	1.4	1.2	32	1857	.20	7.4	8.02	.90	214	216	.87	.073	815
tuna, cnd in oil, light, drained	168	50.9	24.8	0.0	0.0	0.0	20	0	.10	.09	5	301	11	26	.77	.013
3 oz	85	7.0	1.3	2.5	2.5	15	66	.03	10.5	1.87	.31	176	265	1.18	.060	815
tuna, cnd in oil, white, drained	158	54.4	22.6	0.0	0.0	0.0	20	0	.07	.37	4	337	3	29	.40	.014
3 oz	85	6.9	1.4	2.1	2.9	26	68	.01	9.9	1.87	.31	283	227	.55	.111	815
tuna, cnd in water, light, drained	99	63.4	21.7	0.0	0.0	0.0	14	0	.06	.30	3	287	9	23	.65	.009
3 oz	85	0.7	0.2	0.1	0.3	26	48	.03	11.3	2.54	.18	202	139	1.30	.043	815

	KCAL	H_2O (g)	PRO (g)	CHO (g)	SUGR (g)	DFIB (g)	A (RE)	C (mg)	B-2 (mg)	B-6 (mg)	FOL (mcg)	Na (mg)	Ca (mg)	Mg (mg)	Zn (mg)	Mn (mg)
	WT (g)	FAT (g)	SFA (g)	MUFA (g)	PUFA (g)	CHOL (mg)	A (IU)	B-1 (mg)	NIA (mg)	B-12 (mcg)	PANT (mg)	K (mg)	P (mg)	Fe (mg)	Cu (mg)	REF
tuna, cnd in water, white, drained	109	62.2	20.1	0.0	0.0	0.0	5	0	.04	.18	2	321	12	28	.41	.016
3 oz	85	2.5	0.7	0.7	0.9	36	16	.01	4.9	1.00	.11	202	185	.82	.033	815
tuna salad	383	129.5	32.9	19.3		0.0	55	5	.14	.17	15	824	35	39	1.15	.082
½ cup[11]	205	19.0	3.2	5.9	8.5	27	199	.06	13.7	2.46	.53	365	365	2.05	.297	815
tuna, skipjack, ckd by dry heat	112	53.0	24.0	0.0	0.0	0.0	15	1	.10	.83	9	40	31	37	.89	.016
3 oz	85	1.1	0.4	0.2	0.3	51	51	.03	16.0	1.86	.41	444	242	1.36	.094	815
tuna, skipjack, raw	88	60.0	18.7	0.0	0.0	0.0	14	1	.09	.72	8	31	25	29	.70	.013
3 oz	85	0.9	0.3	0.2	0.3	40	44	.03	13.1	1.62	.36	346	189	1.06	.073	815
tuna, yellowfin, ckd by dry heat	118	53.4	25.5	0.0	0.0	0.0	17	1	.05	.88	2	40	18	54	.57	.016
3 oz	85	1.0	0.3	0.2	0.3	49	58	.43	10.2	.51	.74	484	208	.80	.070	815
tuna, yellowfin, raw	92	60.4	19.9	0.0	0.0	0.0	15	1	.04	.77	2	31	14	43	.44	.013
3 oz	85	0.8	0.2	0.1	0.2	38	50	.37	8.3	.44	.64	378	162	.62	.054	815
turbot, european, ckd by dry heat	104	59.9	17.5	0.0	0.0	0.0	10	1	.08	.21	8	163	20	55	.24	.019
3 oz	85	3.2				53	34	.06	2.3	2.16	.56	259	140	.39	.040	815
turbot, european, raw	81	65.4	13.7	0.0	0.0	0.0	9	1	.07	.18	7	128	15	43	.19	.014
3 oz	85	2.5	0.6	0.5	0.7	41	30	.06	1.9	1.87	.48	202	110	.31	.031	815
whelk (sea snail), ckd by moist heat	234	27.2	40.6	13.2		0.0	42	6	.18	.55	10	350	96	146	2.77	.757
3 oz	85	0.7	0.1	0.0	0.0	111	138	.04	1.7	15.43	.34	590	240	8.56	1.752	815
whelk (sea snail), raw	117	56.1	20.3	6.6		0.0	22	3	.09	.29	5	175	48	73	1.39	.380
3 oz	85	0.3	0.0	0.0	0.0	55	72	.02	0.9	7.71	.18	295	120	4.28	.876	815
white perch, fried fillet	98		12.5	0.0		0.0		0	.05				9			
2.3 oz	65	5.3					0	.04	2.7				113	.70		B&C
white perch, raw	118	75.7	19.3	0.0		0.0										
3.5 oz	100	4.0										192				B&C
whitefish																
baked, stuffed	215	63.2	15.2	58.0				0	.11			195				
3.5 oz[12]	100	5.8						.11	2.3			291	246	.50		B&C
ckd by dry heat	146	55.4	20.8	0.0	0.0	0.0	33	0	.13	.29	14	55	28	36	1.08	.073
3 oz	85	6.4	1.0	2.2	2.3	65	111	.15	3.3	.82	.74	345	294	.40	.078	815
raw	114	61.9	16.2	0.0	0.0	0.0	31	0	.10	.26	13	43	22	28	.84	.057
3 oz	85	5.0	0.8	1.7	1.8	51	102	.12	2.6	.85	.64	270	230	.31	.061	815
smoked	92	60.2	19.9	0.0	0.0	0.0	48	0	.09	.33	6	867	15	20	.42	.029
3 oz	85	0.8	0.2	0.2	0.2	28	162	.03	2.0	2.77	.09	360	112	.43	.268	815
whiting, ckd by dry heat	99	63.5	20.0	0.0	0.0	0.0	29	0	.05	.15	13	112	53	23	.45	.111
3 oz	85	1.4	0.3	0.4	0.5	71	97	.06	1.4	2.21	.21	369	242	.36	.034	815
whiting, raw	77	68.3	15.6	0.0	0.0	0.0	26	0	.04	.13	11	61	41	18	.75	.088
3 oz	85	1.1	0.2	0.2	0.4	57	84	.05	1.1	1.96	.18	212	189	.29	.026	815
wolffish, atlantic, ckd by dry heat	105	63.1	19.1	0.0	0.0	0.0	111	0	.08	.39	5	93	7	32	.85	.016
3 oz	85	2.6	0.4	0.9	0.9	50	368	.18	2.2	2.00	.56	327	218	.10	.031	815
wolffish, atlantic, raw	82	68.0	14.9	0.0	0.0	0.0	96	0	.07	.34	4	72	5	26	.66	.013
3 oz	85	2.0	0.3	0.7	0.7	39	319	.15	1.8	1.73	.48	255	170	.08	.025	815
yellowtail, ckd by dry heat	159	57.3	25.2	0.0	0.0	0.0	26	2	.04	.16	3	43	25	32	.57	.016
3 oz	85	5.7				60	88	.15	7.4	1.06	.58	458	171	.54	.049	815
yellowtail, raw	124	63.4	19.7	0.0	0.0	0.0	25	2	.03	.14	3	33	20	26	.44	.013
3 oz	85	4.5	1.1	1.7	1.2	47	81	.12	5.8	1.11	.50	357	134	.42	.038	815

1. Dipped in flour and salt before frying.
2. Stuffed with bacon, butter, celery, onion, and bread cubes.
3. Breading consists of cornmeal, egg, milk, and salt.
4. Breading consists of bread crumbs, egg, milk, and salt.
5. These values also apply to canned clams.
6. Prepared with crab meat, egg, onion, and margarine.
7. Prepared from walleye pollock, bread crumbs, egg, milk, and salt.
8. Prepared with onion, sweet pickel, celery, egg, mayonnaise, and tomato.
9. Prepared from walleye pollock.
10. Alaskan pollock surimi that resembles King Crab meat.
11. Prepared with light tuna canned in oil, pickle relish, salad dressing, onion, and celery.
12. Stuffed with bacon, onion, celery, and bread crumbs.

	KCAL	H₂O (g)	PRO (g)	CHO (g)	SUGR (g)	DFIB (g)	A (RE)	C (mg)	B-2 (mg)	B-6 (mg)	FOL (mcg)	Na (mg)	Ca (mg)	Mg (mg)	Zn (mg)	Mn (mg)
	WT (g)	FAT (g)	SFA (g)	MUFA (g)	PUFA (g)	CHOL (mg)	A (IU)	B-1 (mg)	NIA (mg)	B-12 (mcg)	PANT (mg)	K (mg)	P (mg)	Fe (mg)	Cu (mg)	REF

14. FRUIT & VEGETABLE JUICES

	KCAL	H₂O	PRO	CHO	SUGR	DFIB	A	C	B-2	B-6	FOL	Na	Ca	Mg	Zn	Mn
acerola jce, fresh	51	228.2	1.0	11.6		0.7	123	3872	.15	.01	34	7	24	29	.24	
8 fl oz	242	0.7	0.2	0.2	0.2	0	1232	.05	1.0	.00	.50	235	22	1.21	.208	809
apple cranberry jce, cnd, Mott's	120		0.0	30.0	24.0	0.0						20				
8 fl oz	249	0.0	0.0	0.0	0.0							300				I
apple grape jce, cnd, Mott's	130		0.0	33.0	31.0							15				
8.5 fl oz	240	0.0	0.0	0.0	0.0											I
apple jce, cnd/bottled	117	218.1	0.1	29.0	27.0	0.2	0	2	.04	.07	0	7	17	7	.07	.280
8 fl oz	248	0.3	0.0	0.0	0.1	0	2	.05	0.2	.00	.16	295	17	.92	.055	809
apple jce, from frzn conc	112	210.1	0.3	27.6		0.2	0	1	.04	.08	1	17	14	12	.10	.151
8 fl oz	239	0.2	0.0	0.0	0.1	0	0	.01	0.1	.00	.15	301	17	.62	.033	809
apple raspberry jce, cnd, Mott's	120		0.0	31.0	28.0							15				
8.5 fl oz	262	0.0	0.0	0.0	0.0											I
apricot nectar, cnd	141	213.0	0.9	36.1		1.5	331	2	.04	.06	3	8	18	13	.23	.080
8 fl oz	251	0.2	0.0	0.1	0.0	0	3303	.02	0.7	.00	.24	286	23	.95	.183	809
Beefamato, cnd, Mott's	90		0.0	20.0	12.0	0.0						840				
8 fl oz	249	0.0	0.0	0.0	0.0											I
carrot jce, cnd	74	163.5	1.7	17.1		1.5	4738	16	.10	.40	7	53	44	26	.33	.239
6 fl oz	184	0.3	0.0	0.0	0.1	0	47382	.17	0.7	.00	.42	537	77	.85	.085	811
clam & tomato jce, cnd	76	145.3	1.0	18.1		0.3	37	7	.05	.14	26	664	20	37	1.79	.124
5.5 fl oz	166	0.2	0.0	0.0	0.0	0	357	.07	0.3	50.80	.42	149	129	1.00	.578	814
Clamato, cnd, Mott's	110		1.0	24.0	15.0							900				
8 fl oz	249	0.0	0.0	0.0	0.0											I
grape jce, cnd/bottled	154	212.8	1.4	37.8		0.3	3	0	.09	.16	7	8	23	25	.13	.911
8 fl oz	253	0.2	0.1	0.0	0.1	0	20	.07	0.7	.00	.10	334	28	.61	.071	809
grape jce, from frzn conc, sweetened	128	217.3	0.5	31.9		0.3	3	60	.07	.11	3	5	10	10	.10	.443
8 fl oz	250	0.2	0.1	0.0	0.1	0	20	.04	0.3	.00	.06	53	10	.25	.033	809
grapefruit jce																
Citrus Hill Plus Calcium	70		0.0	19.0				60				10	200			
6 fl oz	185	0.0						.03				140	15			I
cnd	94	222.5	1.3	22.1	18.5	0.2	2	72	.05	.05	26	2	17	25	.22	.049
8 fl oz	247	0.2	0.0	0.0	0.1	0	17	.10	0.6	.00	.32	378	27	.49	.094	809
cnd, sweetened	115	218.4	1.4	27.8		0.3	0	67	.06	.05	26	5	20	25	.15	.050
8 fl oz	250	0.2	0.0	0.0	0.1	0	0	.10	0.8	.00	.33	405	28	.90	.120	809
fresh	96	222.3	1.2	22.7		0.2	2	94	.05	.11	25	2	22	30	.12	.049
8 fl oz	247	0.2	0.0	0.0	0.1	0	25	.10	0.5	.00	.47	400	37	.49	.082	809
from frzn conc	101	220.6	1.4	24.0	25.9	0.2	2	83	.05	.11	9	2	20	27	.12	.049
8 fl oz	247	0.3	0.0	0.0	0.1	0	22	.10	0.5	.00	.47	336	35	.35	.082	809
lemon jce																
cnd/bottled	3	13.9	0.1	1.0		0.1	0	4	.00	.01	2	3	2	1	.01	.003
1 T	15	0.0	0.0	0.0	0.0	0	2	.01	0.0	.00	.01	15	1	.02	.006	809
fresh	4	13.6	0.1	1.3		0.1	0	7	.00	.01	2	0	1	1	.01	.001
1 T	15	0.0	0.0	0.0	0.0	0	3	.00	0.0	.00	.02	19	1	.00	.004	809
fresh	61	221.4	0.9	21.1		1.0	5	112	.02	.12	31	2	17	15	.12	.020
8 fl oz	244	0.0	0.0	0.0	0.0	0	49	.07	0.2	.00	.25	303	15	.07	.071	809
frzn, single-strength	3	13.9	0.1	1.0		0.1	0	5	.00	.01	1	0	1	1	.01	.004
1 T	15	0.0	0.0	0.0	0.0	0	2	.01	0.0	.00	.02	13	1	.02	.004	809
lime jce,																
cnd/bottled	3	13.9	0.0	1.0		0.1	0	1	.00	.00	1	2	2	1	.01	.001
1 T	15	0.0	0.0	0.0	0.0	0	2	.00	0.0	.00	.01	11	2	.03	.004	809
fresh	4	13.5	0.1	1.4	0.4	0.1	0	4	.00	.01	1	0	1	1	.01	.001
1 T	15	0.0	0.0	0.0	0.0	0	2	.00	0.0	.00	.02	16	1	.00	.004	809
fresh	66	221.9	1.1	22.2	5.9	1.0	2	72	.02	.11	20	2	22	15	.15	.020
8 fl oz	246	0.2	0.0	0.0	0.1	0	25	.05	0.2	.00	.34	268	17	.07	.074	809
orange grapefruit jce, cnd	106	218.9	1.5	25.4		0.2	30	72	.07	.06	35	7	20	25	.17	.042
8 fl oz	247	0.2	0.0	0.0	0.0	0	294	.14	0.8	.00	.35	390	35	1.14	.188	809

	KCAL	H_2O (g)	PRO (g)	CHO (g)	SUGR (g)	DFIB (g)	A (RE)	C (mg)	B-2 (mg)	B-6 (mg)	FOL (mcg)	Na (mg)	Ca (mg)	Mg (mg)	Zn (mg)	Mn (mg)
	WT (g)	FAT (g)	SFA (g)	MUFA (g)	PUFA (g)	CHOL (mg)	A (IU)	B-1 (mg)	NIA (mg)	B-12 (mcg)	PANT (mg)	K (mg)	P (mg)	Fe (mg)	Cu (mg)	REF
orange jce																
Citrus Hill Plus Calcium	90		0.0	20.0				72				10	200			
6 fl oz	185	0.0						.12				350	25			I
cnd	105	221.6	1.5	24.5		0.5	45	86	.07	.22	45	5	20	27	.17	.035
8 fl oz	249	0.3	0.0	0.1	0.1	0	436	.15	0.8	.00	.37	436	35	1.10	.142	809
fresh	112	219.0	1.7	25.8	25.3	0.5	50	124	.07	.10	75	2	27	27	.12	.035
8 fl oz	248	0.5	0.1	0.1	0.1	0	496	.22	1.0	.00	.47	496	42	.50	.109	809
from frzn conc	112	219.4	1.7	26.8	26.4	0.5	20	97	.04	.11	109	2	22	25	.12	.035
8 fl oz	249	0.1	0.0	0.0	0.0	0	194	.20	0.5	.00	.39	473	40	.25	.110	809
orange, pineapple, banana jce, Land	100		1.0	24.0									0			
O'Lakes—*6 fl oz*	186	0.0	0.0	0.0	0.0	0						360				I
papaya nectar, cnd	143	212.5	0.4	36.3		1.5	28	8	.01	.02	5	13	25	8	.38	.033
8 fl oz	250	0.4	0.1	0.1	0.1	0	278	.01	0.4	.00	.14	78	0	.85	.033	809
passion fruit jce, purple, fresh	126	211.5	1.0	33.6		0.5	178	74	.32	.12	17	15	10	42	.12	
8 fl oz	247	0.1	0.0	0.0	0.1	0	1771	.00	3.6	.00		687	32	.59	.131	809
passion fruit jce, yellow, fresh	148	208.0	1.7	35.7		0.5	595	45	.25	.15	20	15	10	42	.15	
8 fl oz	247	0.4	0.0	0.1	0.3	0	5953	.00	5.5	.00		687	62	.89	.124	809
peach nectar, cnd	134	213.2	0.7	34.7		1.5	65	13	.03	.02	3	17	12	10	.20	.047
8 fl oz	249	0.0	0.0	0.0	0.0	0	642	.01	0.7	.00	.17	100	15	.47	.172	809
pear nectar, cnd	150	210.0	0.3	39.4		1.5	0	3	.03	.04	3	10	13	8	.18	.075
8 fl oz	250	0.0	0.0	0.0	0.0	0	3	.01	0.3	.00	.05	33	8	.65	.168	809
pineapple jce, cnd	140	213.8	0.8	34.4	31.3	0.5	0	27	.05	.24	58	3	43	33	.28	2.475
8 fl oz	250	0.2	0.0	0.0	0.1	0	13	.14	0.6	.00	.25	335	20	.65	.225	809
pineapple jce, from frzn conc	130	216.3	1.0	31.9		0.5	3	30	.05	.18	27	3	28	23	.28	2.475
8 fl oz	250	0.1	0.0	0.0	0.0	0	25	.18	0.5	.00	.31	340	20	.75	.225	809
prune jce, cnd	182	208.0	1.6	44.7	34.3	2.6	0	10	.18	.56	1	10	31	36	.54	.387
8 fl oz	256	0.1	0.0	0.1	0.0	0	8	.04	2.0	.00	.27	707	64	3.02	.174	809
tangerine jce																
cnd, sweetened	125	216.6	1.2	29.9		0.5	105	55	.05	.08	11	2	45	20	.07	.092
8 fl oz	249	0.5	0.0	0.0	0.1	0	1046	.15	0.2	.00	.31	443	35	.50	.062	809
fresh	106	219.6	1.2	24.9		0.5	104	77	.05	.10	11	2	44	20	.07	.091
8 fl oz	247	0.5	0.1	0.1	0.1	0	1037	.15	0.2	.00	.31	440	35	.49	.062	809
from frzn conc, sweetened	111	212.3	1.0	26.7			137	58	.05	.10	11	2	19	19	.07	.089
8 fl oz	241	0.3	0.0	0.0	0.0	0	1381	.13	0.2	.00	.30	272	19	.24	.060	809
tomato & chili cocktail, cnd, Snap-E-Tom	40		2.0	8.0	4.0	1.0		12				500	0			
6 fl oz	177 ml	0.0	0.0	0.0	0.0	0	2500							1.08		I
tomato jce	31	170.9	1.4	7.7	5.3	0.7	102	33	.06	.20	36	657	16	20	.25	.140
6 fl oz	182	0.1	0.0	0.0	0.0	0	1012	.09	1.2	.00	.46	400	35	1.06	.184	811
Campbell's	50		2.0	9.0	7.0	1.0		24				860	20			
8 fl oz	243	0.0	0.0	0.0	0.0	0	1000							1.44		I
Hunt	22		0.1	5.0	4.4	1.2	12	15				452	13			
5.2 fl oz	165	0.2	0.0			0								.51		I
w/ enchanced tomato flavor, low Na,	50		2.0	10.0	8.0	1.0		60				140	40			
Campbell's—*8 fl oz*	243	0.0	0.0	0.0	0.0	0	750							.36		I
veg jce cocktail																
cnd	35	170.2	1.1	8.3	6.0	1.5	213	50	.05	.25	38	491	20	20	.36	.182
6 fl oz	182	0.2	0.0	0.0	0.1	0	2129	.08	1.3	.00	.48	351	31	.76	.364	811
Hunt	36		2.0	7.0	3.0	2.0	50	48				630	2			
5.5 fl oz	177	0.0	0.0			0								.36		I
V-8, Campbell's	50		1.0	10.0	8.0	1.0		60				620	40			
8 fl oz[1]	243	0.0	0.0	0.0	0.0	0	2000							1.08		I
V-8 Lightly Tangy, Campbell's	60		2.0	11.0	9.0	1.0		60				340	40			
8 fl oz	243	0.0	0.0	0.0	0.0	0	3000							1.08		I
V-8 Picante, Campbell's	50		2.0	10.0	7.0	1.0		60				680	40			
8 fl oz	243	0.0	0.0	0.0	0.0	0	2000							1.08		I
V-8 Plus, Campbell's	50		1.0	11.0	8.0	1.0		60				460	40			
8 fl oz	243	0.0	0.0	0.0	0.0	0	5000							1.08		I
V-8, Spicy Hot, Campbell's	50		2.0	10.0	7.0	1.0		36				780	20			
8 fl oz	243	0.0	0.0	0.0	0.0	0	2000							.72		I

1. Low sodium product contains 140 mg sodium per 1 fluid ounce.

	KCAL / WT (g)	H₂O (g) / FAT (g)	PRO (g) / SFA (g)	CHO (g) / MUFA (g)	SUGR (g) / PUFA (g)	DFIB (g) / CHOL (mg)	A (RE) / A (IU)	C (mg) / B-1 (mg)	B-2 (mg) / NIA (mg)	B-6 (mg) / B-12 (mcg)	FOL (mcg) / PANT (mg)	Na (mg) / K (mg)	Ca (mg) / P (mg)	Mg (mg) / Fe (mg)	Zn (mg) / Cu (mg)	Mn (mg) / REF

15. FRUITS

Item	KCAL / WT	H₂O / FAT	PRO / SFA	CHO / MUFA	SUGR / PUFA	DFIB / CHOL	A(RE) / A(IU)	C / B-1	B-2 / NIA	B-6 / B-12	FOL / PANT	Na / K	Ca / P	Mg / Fe	Zn / Cu	Mn / REF
acerola, raw	31	89.6	0.4	7.5		1.1	75	1644	.06	.01	14	7	12	18	.10	
1 cup	98	0.3	0.1	0.1	0.1	0	752	.02	0.4	.00	.30	143	11	.20	.084	809
apple																
boiled, w/o skin	91	146.2	0.4	23.3		4.1	7	0	.02	.08	1	2	9	5	.07	.202
1 cup	171	0.6	0.1	0.0	0.2	0	75	.03	0.2	.00	.08	150	14	.32	.060	809
cnd, sliced, sweetened	68	84.0	0.2	17.0		1.7	5	0	.01	.04	0	3	4	2	.03	.156
½ cup	102	0.5	0.1	0.0	0.1	0	52	.01	0.1	.00	.03	69	5	.23	.054	809
dried, sulfured	156	20.3	0.6	42.2		5.6	0	2	.10	.08	0	56	9	10	.13	.058
10 rings	64	0.2	0.0	0.0	0.1	0	0	.00	0.6	.00	.16	288	24	.90	.122	809
escalloped, frzn, Stouffers	94	62.9	0.3	20.0				72	.00			26	3			
3 oz	85	1.3					85	.02	0.6			60		.09		I
micro ckd w/o skin	95	143.9	0.5	24.5		4.8	7	1	.02	.08	1	2	9	5	.07	.241
1 cup	170	0.7	0.1	0.0	0.2	0	68	.03	0.1	.00	.08	158	14	.29	.078	809
raw, w/o skin	73	108.1	0.2	19.0		2.4	5	5	.01	.06	1	0	5	4	.05	.029
1 med	128	0.4	0.1	0.0	0.1	0	56	.02	0.1	.00	.07	145	9	.09	.040	809
raw, w/ skin	81	115.8	0.3	21.0	18.4	3.7	7	8	.02	.07	4	0	10	7	.06	.062
1 med	138	0.5	0.1	0.0	0.1	0	73	.02	0.1	.00	.08	159	10	.25	.057	809
applesauce, cnd																
chunky, Mott's	90		0.0	23.0	20.0	2.0	2					0				
½ cup	123	0.0	0.0	0.0	0.0							90				I
cinn, Mott's	110		0.0	28.0	26.0	1.0						0				
4 oz	129	0.0	0.0	0.0	0.0	0						80				I
strawberry fruit pak, Mott's	80		0.0	19.0	15.0		6					5				
3.9 oz	111	0.0	0.0	0.0	0.0							70				I
sweetened	97	101.9	0.2	25.5	21.1	1.5	1	2	.04	.03	1	4	5	4	.05	.096
½ cup	128	0.2	0.0	0.0	0.1	0	14	.02	0.2	.00	.07	78	9	.45	.055	809
unsweetened	52	107.8	0.2	13.8		1.5	4	1	.03	.03	1	2	4	4	.04	.091
½ cup	122	0.1	0.0	0.0	0.0	0	35	.02	0.2	.00	.12	92	9	.15	.032	809
apricots																
cnd, heavy syrup	75	69.8	0.5	19.3		1.4	111	3	.02	.05	2	4	8	6	.10	.046
4 halves	90	0.1	0.0	0.0	0.0	0	1107	.02	0.3	.00	.08	126	11	.27	.070	809
cnd, jce pack	40	72.8	0.5	10.4		1.3	142	4	.02	.05	1	3	10	8	.09	.044
3 halves	84	0.0	0.0	0.0	0.0	0	1420	.02	0.3	.00	.08	139	17	.25	.045	809
cnd, light syrup	54	70.2	0.5	14.0		1.4	112	2	.02	.05	1	3	9	7	.09	.044
3 halves	85	0.0	0.0	0.0	0.0	0	1124	.01	0.3	.00	.08	117	11	.33	.067	809
cnd, water pack	24	83.1	0.6	5.8		1.4	116	3	.02	.05	2	3	7	6	.10	.048
4 halves	90	0.1	0.0	0.1	0.0	0	1164	.02	0.4	.00	.08	173	12	.29	.074	809
dried, sulfured	83	10.9	1.3	21.6	13.6	3.1	253	1	.05	.05	4	4	16	16	.26	.096
10 halves	35	0.2	0.0	0.1	0.0	0	2534	.00	1.0	.00	.26	482	41	1.65	.150	809
frzn, sweetened	119	88.7	0.8	30.4		2.7	203	11	.05	.07	2	5	12	11	.12	.060
½ cup	121	0.1	0.0	0.1	0.0	0	2033	.02	1.0	.00	.24	277	23	1.09	.077	809
raw	51	91.5	1.5	11.8	9.0	2.5	277	11	.04	.06	9	1	15	8	.28	.084
3 med	106	0.4	0.0	0.2	0.1	0	2769	.03	0.6	.00	.25	314	20	.57	.094	809
avocado, raw, calif	306	125.5	3.7	12.0		8.5	106	14	.21	.48	113	21	19	71	.73	.422
1 med	173	30.0	4.5	19.4	3.5	0	1059	.19	3.3	.00	1.68	1097	73	2.04	.460	809
avocado, raw, florida	340	242.4	4.8	27.1		16.1	185	24	.37	.85	162	15	33	103	1.28	.517
1 med	304	27.0	5.3	14.8	4.5	0	1860	.33	5.8	.00	2.95	1484	119	1.61	.763	809
banana, raw	105	84.7	1.2	26.7	17.8	2.7	9	10	.11	.66	22	1	7	33	.18	.173
1 med	114	0.5	0.2	0.0	0.1	0	92	.05	0.6	.00	.30	451	23	.35	.119	809
blackberries																
cnd, heavy syrup	118	96.1	1.7	29.6		4.4	28	4	.05	.05	34	4	27	22	.23	.892
½ cup	128	0.2	0.0	0.0	0.1	0	280	.03	0.4	.00	.19	127	18	.83	.170	809
frzn, unsweetened	97	124.1	1.8	23.7		7.5	17	5	.07	.09	51	2	44	33	.38	1.847
1 cup	151	0.6	0.0	0.1	0.4	0	172	.04	1.8	.00	.23	211	45	1.21	.181	809

	KCAL	H₂O (g)	PRO (g)	CHO (g)	SUGR (g)	DFIB (g)	Vitamins A (RE)	C (mg)	B-2 (mg)	B-6 (mg)	FOL (mcg)	Minerals Na (mg)	Ca (mg)	Mg (mg)	Zn (mg)	Mn (mg)
	WT (g)	FAT (g)	SFA (g)	MUFA (g)	PUFA (g)	CHOL (mg)	A (IU)	B-1 (mg)	NIA (mg)	B-12 (mcg)	PANT (mg)	K (mg)	P (mg)	Fe (mg)	Cu (mg)	REF
raw	37	61.7	0.5	9.2		3.8	12	15	.03	.04	24	0	23	14	.19	.930
½ cup	72	0.3	0.0	0.0	0.2	0	119	.02	0.3	.00	.17	141	15	.41	.101	809
blueberries																
cnd, heavy syrup	113	98.3	0.8	28.2		1.9	8	1	.07	.05	2	4	6	5	.09	.260
½ cup	128	0.4	0.0	0.1	0.2	0	82	.04	0.1	.00	.11	51	13	.42	.068	809
frzn, sweetened	186	178.0	0.9	50.5		4.8	9	2	.12	.14	15	2	14	5	.14	.603
1 cup	230	0.3	0.0	0.0	0.1	0	101	.05	0.6	.00	.29	138	16	.90	.090	809
raw	81	122.7	1.0	20.5	10.6	3.9	15	19	.07	.05	9	9	9	7	.16	.409
1 cup	145	0.6	0.0	0.1	0.2	0	145	.07	0.5	.00	.13	129	15	.25	.088	809
boysenberries, cnd, heavy syrup	113	97.6	1.3	28.6		3.3	5	8	.04	.05	44	4	23	14	.24	.320
½ cup	128	0.2	0.0	0.0	0.1	0	51	.03	0.3	.00	.17	115	13	.55	.090	809
boysenberries, frzn, unsweetened	66	113.4	1.5	16.1		5.1	9	4	.05	.07	84	1	36	21	.29	.722
1 cup	132	0.3	0.0	0.0	0.2	0	88	.07	1.0	.00	.33	183	36	1.12	.106	809
breadfruit, raw	99	67.8	1.0	26.0		4.7	4	28	.03	.10	13	2	16	24	.12	.058
¼ small	96	0.2	0.0	0.0	0.1	0	38	.11	0.9	.00	.44	470	29	.52	.081	809
cantaloupe, raw	56	143.6	1.4	13.4	13.9	1.3	515	68	.03	.18	27	14	18	18	.26	.075
1 cup pieces	160	0.4	0.1	0.0	0.2	0	5158	.06	0.9	.00	.20	494	27	.34	.067	809
carambola, raw	42	115.5	0.7	9.9		3.4	62	27	.03	.13	18	3	5	11	.14	.104
1 med	127	0.4	0.0	0.0	0.2	0	626	.04	0.5	.00		207	20	.33	.152	809
carissa, raw	12	16.8	0.1	2.7			1	8	.01			1	2	3		
1 med	20	0.3				0	8	.01	0.0	.00		52	1	.26	.042	809
casaba melon, raw	44	156.4	1.5	10.5		1.4	5	27	.03	.20	29	20	9	14	.27	
1 cup pieces	170	0.2	0.0	0.0	0.1	0	51	.10	0.7	.00		357	12	.68	.068	809
cherimoya, raw	514	402.0	7.1	131.3		13.1	5	49	.60				126			
1 med	547	2.2				0	55	.55	7.1	.00			219	2.73		809
cherries, sour																
cnd, heavy syrup	116	96.8	0.9	29.8		1.4	91	3	.05	.06	10	9	13	8	.08	.092
½ cup	128	0.1	0.0	0.0	0.0	0	914	.02	0.2	.00	.13	119	13	1.66	.084	809
cnd, water pack	44	109.7	0.9	10.9		1.3	92	3	.05	.05	10	9	13	7	.09	.093
½ cup	122	0.1	0.0	0.0	0.0	0	920	.02	0.2	.00	.13	120	12	1.67	.085	809
raw	34	58.6	0.7	8.3	9.9	1.1	87	7	.03	.03	5	2	11	6	.07	.076
10 cherries	68	0.2	0.0	0.1	0.1	0	872	.02	0.3	.00	.10	118	10	.22	.071	809
cherries, sweet																
cnd, heavy syrup	107	100.1	0.8	27.4		1.9	19	5	.05	.04	5	4	12	12	.13	.076
½ cup	129	0.2	0.0	0.1	0.1	0	199	.03	0.5	.00	.16	187	23	.45	.183	809
cnd, jce pack	68	106.2	1.1	17.3		1.9	16	3	.03	.04	5	4	18	15	.13	.076
½ cup	125	0.0	0.0	0.0	0.0	0	156	.02	0.5	.00	.16	164	28	.72	.091	809
cnd, water pack	57	107.9	1.0	14.6		1.9	20	3	.05	.04	5	1	14	11	.10	.077
½ cup	124	0.2	0.0	0.0	0.0	0	198	.03	0.5	.00	.16	162	19	.45	.093	809
frzn, sweetened	231	195.6	3.0	57.9		5.4	49	3	.12	.09	11	3	31	26	.10	.282
1 cup	259	0.3	0.1	0.1	0.1	0	490	.07	0.5	.00	.33	515	41	.91	.062	809
raw	49	54.9	0.8	11.3		1.6	14	5	.04	.02	3	0	10	7	.04	.063
10 cherries	68	0.7	0.1	0.2	0.2	0	146	.03	0.3	.00	.09	152	13	.27	.065	809
crabapples, raw	84	86.8	0.4	21.9			4	9	.02			1	20	8		.127
1 cup slices	110	0.3	0.1	0.0	0.0	0	44	.03	0.1	.00		213	17	.40	.074	809
cranberries, raw	47	82.2	0.4	12.0		4.0	5	13	.02	.06	2	1	7	5	.12	.149
1 cup whole	95	0.2	0.0	0.0	0.1	0	44	.03	0.1	.00	.21	67	9	.19	.055	809
cranberry orange relish, cnd	246	73.4	0.4	63.8		0.0	10	25	.03			44	15	6		
½ cup	138	0.1	0.0			0	97	.04	0.1	.00		52	11	.28	.055	809
cranberry sce, jelled, cnd	208	83.7	0.3	53.7		1.4	3	3	.03	.02	1	40	6	4	.07	.083
½ cup	138	0.2	0.0	0.0	0.1	0	28	.02	0.1	.00		36	8	.30	.028	809
currants																
european black, raw	35	45.9	0.8	8.6			13	101	.03	.04		1	31	13	.15	.143
½ cup	56	0.2	0.0	0.0	0.1	0	129	.03	0.2	.00	.22	180	33	.86	.048	809
red & white, raw	31	47.0	0.8	7.7		2.4	7	23	.03	.04	4	1	18	7	.13	.104
½ cup	56	0.1	0.0	0.0	0.0	0	67	.02	0.1	.00	.04	154	25	.56	.060	809
zante, dried	204	13.8	2.9	53.3		4.9	5	3	.10	.21	7	6	62	30	.48	.338
½ cup[1]	72	0.2	0.0	0.0	0.1	0	53	.12	1.2	.00	.03	642	90	2.35	.337	809

	KCAL	H₂O (g)	PRO (g)	CHO (g)	SUGR (g)	DFIB (g)	A (RE)	C (mg)	B-2 (mg)	B-6 (mg)	FOL (mcg)	Na (mg)	Ca (mg)	Mg (mg)	Zn (mg)	Mn (mg)
	WT (g)	FAT (g)	SFA (g)	MUFA (g)	PUFA (g)	CHOL (mg)	A (IU)	B-1 (mg)	NIA (mg)	B-12 (mcg)	PANT (mg)	K (mg)	P (mg)	Fe (mg)	Cu (mg)	REF
custard apple, raw	100	70.9	1.7	25.0			3	19	.10	.22		4	30	18		
3.5 oz	99	0.6				0	33	.08	0.5	.00	.13	379	21	.70		809
dates, dried	228	18.7	1.6	61.0	53.3	6.2	4	0	.08	.16	10	2	27	29	.24	.247
10 dates	83	0.4	0.2	0.1	0.0	0	42	.07	1.8	.00	.65	541	33	.95	.239	809
elderberries, raw	106	115.7	1.0	26.7		10.2	87	52	.09	.33	9	9	55	7	.16	
1 cup	145	0.7	0.0	0.1	0.4	0	870	.10	0.7	.00	.20	406	57	2.32	.088	809
feijoa, raw	25	43.3	0.6	5.3			0	10	.02	.03	19	2	9	5	.02	.043
1 feijoa	50	0.4				0	0	.00	0.1	.00	.11	78	10	.04	.028	809
figs																
cnd, heavy syrup	75	64.9	0.3	19.5		1.9	3	1	.03	.06	2	1	23	9	.09	.071
3 figs	85	0.1	0.0	0.0	0.0	0	31	.02	0.4	.00	.06	84	9	.24	.090	809
dried	477	53.2	5.7	122.2	124.4	17.4	24	1	.16	.42	14	21	269	110	.95	.726
10 figs	187	2.2	0.4	0.5	1.0	0	249	.13	1.3	.00	.81	1331	127	4.17	.585	809
raw	37	39.6	0.4	9.6		1.6	7	1	.03	.06	3	1	18	9	.07	.064
1 med	50	0.1	0.0	0.0	0.1	0	71	.03	0.2	.00	.15	116	7	.18	.035	809
fruit cocktail																
cnd, heavy syrup	93	102.9	0.5	24.2		1.3	26	2	.02	.06	3	8	8	6	.10	.184
½ cup²	128	0.1	0.0	0.0	0.0	0	262	.02	0.5	.00	.08	113	14	.37	.088	809
cnd, jce pack	57	108.4	0.6	14.7	19.0	1.2	38	3	.02	.06	3	5	10	9	.11	.181
½ cup	124	0.0	0.0	0.0	0.0	0	378	.01	0.5	.00	.08	118	17	.26	.077	809
cnd, water pack	39	110.7	0.5	10.4		1.2	31	3	.01	.06	3	5	6	9	.11	.183
½ cup	122	0.1	0.0	0.0	0.0	0	305	.02	0.4	.00	.08	115	13	.30	.087	809
fruit salad																
cnd, heavy syrup	93	102.7	0.4	24.5		1.3	64	3	.03	.04	3	8	8	6	.09	.186
½ cup³	128	0.1	0.0	0.0	0.0	0	645	.02	0.4	.00	.07	102	12	.36	.082	809
cnd, jce pack	62	106.8	0.6	16.2		1.2	74	4	.02	.03	3	6	14	10	.17	.187
½ cup³	124	0.0	0.0	0.0	0.0	0	744	.01	0.4	.00	.07	144	17	.31	.062	809
cnd, tropical, heavy syrup	110	98.3	0.5	28.6		1.7	17	22	.06	.15	12	3	17	17	.14	
½ cup⁴	128	0.1	0.0	0.0	0.0	0	163	.07	0.7	.00		168	9	.67	.102	809
fruit snack																
fruit bar	81	3.2	0.4	18.1		0.8	3	16	.01	.07	1	18	7	5	.04	.042
.81 oz bar	23	1.2	0.9	0.1	0.0	0	27	.01	0.0	.00	.02	32	13	.18	.039	819
fruit bar w/ cream	89	2.9	0.2	18.7		0.9	3	15	.01	.07	1	23	5	3	.04	.021
.85 oz bar	24	2.0	0.6	1.0	0.2	1	13	.01	0.0	.01	.02	51	7	.20	.023	819
Fruit by the Foot, Betty Crocker	80		0.0	17.0	10.0	0.0		18				45	0			
1 roll⁵	21	1.5	0.5			0	0							.00		I
Fruit Jammers, Christmas, Sunbelt	208	5.1	0.2	47.5	30.5	0.3		1	.02			58	4			
1.9 oz pkg	55	2.0	0.5			0	2	.01	0.1							I
Fruit Jammers, Sunbelt	106	2.6	0.1	24.2	15.5	0.1		0	.01			30	2			
1 oz pkg	28	1.0	0.3			0	1	.01	0.0							I
fruit pieces	97	3.5	0.3	22.2		1.0	3	16	.03	.09	4	114	5	4	.05	.052
1 oz	28	2.0	0.3	0.9	0.8	0	33	.01	0.0	.00	.09	46	7	.21	.048	819
fruit roll	74	2.3	0.2	17.7		0.8	3	1	.00	.06	2	13	7	4	.04	.039
1 large roll (.74 oz)	21	0.6	0.1	0.3	0.1	0	24	.01	0.0	.00	.07	62	7	.21	.036	819
fruit roll, Lipton	75		0.2	18.2				1	.00			15	7	4	.00	.030
1 roll	21	0.1				0	24	.00	0.0			68	7	.30	.000	I
Fruit Roll-Up Pouch, Betty Crocker	50		0.0	12.0	5.0	0.0	0	10				54	0			
1 roll⁶	14	0.0				0	0							.00		I
Fruit Roll-Ups, Betty Crocker	110		0.0	24.0	10.0	0.0		23				106	0			
2 rolls⁷	28	1.0	0.1			0	0							.00		I
Fruit String Thing, Betty Crocker	80		0.0	17.0	9.0	0.0		15				45	0			
1 pouch⁸	21	1.0	0.0			0	0							.00		I
Fun Snacks, Betty Crocker	90		0.0	21.0	12.3	0.0	0	8				23	0			
1 pouch⁹	25	1.0	0.0			0	0							.00		I
Gushers, all flavors, Betty Crocker	90		0.0	20.0	12.0	0.0		15				45	0			
1 pouch	25	1.0	0.0			0	0							.00		I
Squeezit, Betty Crocker	102		0.0	25.5	23.1	0.0	0	0				14	0			
1 bottle¹⁰	200 ml	0.0	0.0			0	0							.18		I

	KCAL	H₂O (g)	PRO (g)	CHO (g)	SUGR (g)	DFIB (g)	Vitamins A (RE)	C (mg)	B-2 (mg)	B-6 (mg)	FOL (mcg)	Minerals Na (mg)	Ca (mg)	Mg (mg)	Zn (mg)	Mn (mg)
	WT (g)	FAT (g)	SFA (g)	MUFA (g)	PUFA (g)	CHOL (mg)	A (IU)	B-1 (mg)	NIA (mg)	B-12 (mcg)	PANT (mg)	K (mg)	P (mg)	Fe (mg)	Cu (mg)	REF
gooseberries, cnd, light syrup	92	100.9	0.8	23.6		3.0	18	13	.07	.02	4	3	20	8	.14	.223
½ cup	126	0.3	0.0	0.0	0.1	0	174	.03	0.2	.00	.17	97	9	.42	.273	809
gooseberries, raw	66	131.8	1.3	15.3		6.4	44	42	.04	.12	9	2	38	15	.18	.216
1 cup	150	0.9	0.1	0.1	0.5	0	435	.06	0.4	.00	.43	297	41	.46	.105	809
grapefruit																
cnd, jce pack	46	111.2	0.9	11.4		0.5	0	42	.02	.02	11	9	19	14	.10	.009
½ cup	124	0.1	0.0	0.0	0.0	0	0	.04	0.3	.00	.15	210	15	.26	.046	809
cnd, light syrup	76	106.2	0.7	19.6		0.5	0	27	.03	.03	11	3	18	13	.10	.009
½ cup	127	0.1	0.0	0.0	0.0	0	0	.05	0.3	.00	.15	164	13	.51	.084	809
raw, pink & red	39	111.8	0.8	9.9		1.4	15	42	.02	.05	13	0	15	10	.09	.015
½ med	123	0.1	0.0	0.0	0.0	0	153	.04	0.3	.00	.35	171	10	.11	.058	809
raw, white	39	106.8	0.8	9.9	7.3	1.3	1	39	.02	.05	12	0	14	11	.08	.015
½ med	118	0.0	0.0	0.0	0.0	0	12	.04	0.3	.00	.33	175	9	.07	.059	809
grapes																
american (slip skin), raw	58	74.8	0.6	15.8	15.1	0.9	9	4	.05	.10	4	2	13	5	.04	.661
1 cup	92	0.3	0.1	0.0	0.1	0	92	.08	0.3	.00	.02	176	9	.27	.037	809
european (adherent skin), raw	114	128.9	1.1	28.4		1.6	11	17	.09	.18	6	3	18	10	.08	.093
1 cup	160	0.9	0.3	0.0	0.3	0	117	.15	0.5	.00	.04	296	21	.42	.144	809
thompson seedless, cnd, heavy syrup	93	101.8	0.6	25.2		0.5	8	1	.03	.08	3	6	13	8	.06	.049
½ cup	128	0.1	0.0	0.0	0.0	0	82	.04	0.2	.00	.05	132	22	1.20	.069	809
groundcherries, raw	74	119.6	2.7	15.7			101	15	.06				13			
1 cup[11]	140	1.0				0	1008	.15	3.9	.00			56	1.40		809
guava, raw	46	77.5	0.7	10.7		4.9	71	165	.05	.13	13	3	18	9	.21	.130
1 med	90	0.5	0.2	0.0	0.2	0	713	.05	1.1	.00	.14	256	23	.28	.093	809
guava, strawberry, raw	168	196.8	1.4	42.4			22	90	.07				90	51	41	
1 cup	244	1.5	0.4	0.1	0.6	0	220	.07	1.5	.00		712	66	.54		809
honeydew melon, raw	60	152.4	0.8	15.6		1.0	7	42	.03	.10	10	17	10	12	.12	.031
1 cup cubed pieces	170	0.2	0.0	0.0	0.1	0	68	.13	1.0	.00	.35	461	17	.12	.070	809
jackfruit, raw	93	72.7	1.5	23.8		1.6	30	7	.11	.11	14	3	34	37	.42	.195
3.5 oz	99	0.3	0.1	0.0	0.1	0	295	.03	0.4	.00		301	36	.60	.186	809
java plum, raw	81	112.2	1.0	21.0			0	19	.02	.05		19	26	20		
1 cup	135	0.3				0	4	.01	0.4	.00		107	23	.26		809
jujube, dried	285	19.5	3.7	73.0				13	.36			9	78	37	.19	.303
3.5 oz	99	1.1				0		.21	0.5	.00		527	99	1.79	.263	809
jujube, raw	78	77.3	1.2	20.1			4	68	.04	.08		3	21	10	.05	.083
3.5 oz	99	0.2				0	40	.02	0.9	.00		248	23	.48	.072	809
kiwifruit, raw	46	63.1	0.8	11.3	8.0	2.6	14	74	.04	.07	29	4	20	23	.13	
1 med	76	0.3	0.0	0.0	0.2	0	133	.02	0.4	.00		252	30	.31	.119	809
kumquats, raw	12	15.5	0.2	3.1		1.3	6	7	.02	.01	3	1	8	2	.02	.016
1 med	19	0.0	0.0	0.0	0.0	0	57	.02	0.1	.00		37	4	.07	.020	809
lemon peel	3	4.9	0.1	1.0		0.6	0	8	.00	.01	1	0	8	1	.01	
1 T	6	0.0	0.0	0.0	0.0	0	3	.00	0.0	.00	.02	10	1	.05	.006	809
lemon, raw	17	51.6	0.6	5.4	1.4	1.6	2	31	.01	.05	6	1	15	5	.03	.017
1 med	58	0.2	0.0	0.0	0.1	0	17	.02	0.1	.00	.11	80	9	.35	.021	809
lime, raw	20	59.1	0.5	7.1	0.3	1.9	1	19	.01	.03	5	1	22	4	.07	.005
1 med	67	0.1	0.0	0.0	0.0	0	7	.02	0.1	.00	.15	68	12	.40	.044	809
loganberries, frzn	81	124.4	2.2	19.1		7.2	6	22	.05	.10	38	1	38	31	.50	1.833
1 cup	147	0.5	0.0	0.0	0.3	0	51	.07	1.2	.00	.36	213	38	.94	.172	809
longans, dried	284	17.5	4.9	73.4			0	28	.50			48	45	46	.22	.246
3.5 oz	99	0.4				0	0	.04	1.0	.00		653	194	5.36	.801	809
longans, raw	60	82.8	1.3	15.1		1.1		84	.14			0	1	10	.05	.052
31 fruits	100	0.1				0		.03	0.3	.00		266	21	.13	.169	809
loquats, raw	47	86.7	0.4	12.1		1.7	153	1	.02	.10	14	1	16	13	.05	.148
6 med	100	0.2	0.0	0.0	0.1	0	1528	.02	0.2	.00		266	27	.28	.040	809
!ychees, dried	275	22.1	3.8	70.2		4.6	0	182	.57	.09	12	3	33	42	.28	.232
3.5 oz	99	1.2	0.3	0.3	0.4	0	0	.01	3.1	.00		1101	180	1.69	.626	809
lychees, raw	66	81.8	0.8	16.5		1.3	0	72	.07	.10	14	1	5	10	.07	.055
10 med	100	0.4	0.1	0.1	0.1	0	0	.01	0.6	.00		171	31	.31	.148	809
mammy apple, raw	51	86.2	0.5	12.5		3.0	23	14	.04	.10	14	15	11	16	.10	
⅛ med	100	0.5	0.1	0.2	0.1	0	230	.02	0.4	.00	.10	47	11	.70	.086	809

	KCAL / WT (g)	H₂O (g) / FAT (g)	PRO (g) / SFA (g)	CHO (g) / MUFA (g)	SUGR (g) / PUFA (g)	DFIB (g) / CHOL (mg)	A (RE) / A (IU)	C (mg) / B-1 (mg)	B-2 (mg) / NIA (mg)	B-6 (mg) / B-12 (mcg)	FOL (mcg) / PANT (mg)	Na (mg) / K (mg)	Ca (mg) / P (mg)	Mg (mg) / Fe (mg)	Zn (mg) / Cu (mg)	Mn (mg) / REF
mandarin oranges, cnd, jce pack	46	111.0	0.8	11.9		0.9	105	42	.04	.05	6	6	14	14	.63	.040
½ cup	124	0.0	0.0	0.0	0.0	0	1056	.10	0.6	.00	.15	165	12	.33	.041	809
mandarin oranges, cnd, light syrup	77	104.7	0.6	20.4		0.9	106	25	.06	.05	6	8	9	10	.30	.040
½ cup	126	0.1	0.0	0.0	0.0	0	1058	.07	0.6	.00	.16	98	13	.47	.055	809
mango, raw	135	169.1	1.1	35.2		3.7	805	57	.12	.28	29	4	21	19	.08	.056
1 med	207	0.6	0.1	0.2	0.1	0	8061	.12	1.2	.00	.33	323	23	.27	.228	809
melon balls (cantaloupe & honeydew),	57	156.1	1.5	13.7		1.2	306	11	.04	.18	44	54	17	24	.29	.069
frzn—1 cup	173	0.4	0.1	0.0	0.2	0	3069	.29	1.1	.00	.28	484	21	.50	.104	809
mincemeat, cnd, S&W	180		0.0	43.0	37.0	4.0		6				210	40			
¼ cup	95	2.5	1.5			0	0					190		4.50		I
mixed fruit																
cnd, heavy syrup	92	103.1	0.5	24.0		1.3	24	88	.05	.05	4	5	1	6	.09	.494
½ cup[12]	128	0.1	0.0	0.0	0.1	0	248	.02	0.8	.00	.07	108	13	.46	.074	809
dried	241	30.9	2.4	63.6		7.7	242	4	.16	.16	4	18	38	39	.50	.225
3.5 oz	99	0.5	0.0	0.2	0.1	0	2423	.04	1.9	.00	.44	790	76	2.69	.382	809
dried, diced, Del Monte	110		30.0	17.0	5.0		1				50	0				
⅓ cup	40	0.0	0.0	0.0	0.0	0	1250							1.08		I
frzn, in syrup, Birds Eye	123	109.2	0.8	31.0				27	.05	.03	8	4	9	8	.09	
½ cup[13]	142	0.4	0.1		0.1	0	348	.03	0.6	.00	.14	161	14	.42	.058	I
frzn, sweetened	139	104.7	2.0	34.4		2.7	45	107	.05	.04	11	4	10	9	.07	.091
1 cup[13]	142	0.3	0.0	0.0	0.1	0	457	.02	0.6	.00	.13	186	17	.40	.048	809
mulberries, raw	60	122.8	2.0	13.7		2.4	4	51	.14	.07	8	14	55	25	.17	
1 cup	140	0.5		0.1	0.3		35	.04	0.9	.00		272	53	2.59	.084	809
nectarine, raw	67	117.3	1.3	16.0	12.1	2.2	101	7	.06	.03	5	0	7	11	.12	.060
1 med	136	0.6	0.1	0.2	0.3	0	1001	.02	1.3	.00	.21	288	22	.20	.099	809
oheloberries, raw	39	129.2	0.5	9.6			116	8	.05			1	10	8		
1 cup	140	0.3				0	1162	.02	0.4	.00		53	14	.13		809
orange, navel, raw	60	113.7	1.3	15.2		3.1	24	75	.05	.09	44	1	52	13	.08	.035
1 fruit	131	0.1	0.0	0.0	0.0	0	240	.11	0.4	.00	.33	233	25	.16	.073	809
orange peel	6	4.3	0.1	1.5		0.6	3	8	.01	.01	2	0	10	1	.01	
1 T	6	0.0	0.0	0.0	0.0	0	25	.01	0.1	.00	.03	13	1	.05	.006	809
orange, valencia, raw	59	104.5	1.3	14.4		3.0	28	59	.05	.08	47	0	48	12	.07	.028
1 med	121	0.4	0.0	0.1	0.1	0	278	.11	0.3	.00	.30	217	21	.11	.045	809
papaya, raw	119	270.0	1.9	29.8		5.5	85	188	.10	.06	116	9	73	30	.21	.033
1 med	304	0.4	0.1	0.1	0.1	0	863	.08	1.0	.00	.66	781	15	.30	.049	809
passion fruit (grandilla), purple, raw	17	13.1	0.4	4.2		1.9	13	5	.02	.02	3	5	2	5	.02	
1 med	18	0.1	0.0	0.0	0.1	0	126	.00	0.3	.00		63	12	.29	.015	809
peach																
cnd, heavy syrup	189	203.0	1.2	51.0		3.3	84	7	.06	.05	8	15	8	13	.23	.115
1 cup	256	0.3	0.0	0.1	0.1	0	850	.03	1.6	.00	.13	236	28	.69	.131	809
cnd, heavy syrup, spiced	66	69.7	0.4	17.7		1.1	28	5	.03	.02	3	4	5	6	.07	
1 med	88	0.1	0.0	0.0	0.0	0	279	.01	0.5	.00	.04	75	8	.25	.086	809
cnd, jce pack	109	217.0	1.6	28.7	43.2	3.2	94	9	.04	.05	8	10	15	17	.27	.119
1 cup	248	0.1	0.0	0.0	0.0	0	945	.02	1.4	.00	.12	317	42	.67	.124	809
cnd, light syrup	136	212.6	1.1	36.5		3.3	88	6	.06	.05	8	13	8	13	.23	.115
1 cup	251	0.1	0.0	0.0	0.0	0	889	.02	1.5	.00	.13	243	28	.90	.131	809
cnd, water pack	59	227.2	1.1	14.9		3.2	129	7	.05	.05	8	7	5	12	.22	.117
1 cup	244	0.1	0.0	0.1	0.1	0	1298	.02	1.3	.00	.12	242	24	.78	.132	809
dried, sulfured	311	41.3	4.7	79.7	58.0	10.7	281	6	.28	.09	0	9	36	55	.74	.397
10 halves	130	1.0	0.1	0.4	0.5	0	2812	.00	5.7	.00	.73	1295	155	5.28	.473	809
frzn, sweetened	235	186.8	1.6	60.0		4.5	70	236	.09	.04	8	15	8	13	.13	.073
1 cup	250	0.3	0.0	0.1	0.2	0	710	.03	1.6	.00	.33	325	28	.93	.060	809
raw	37	76.3	0.6	9.7	7.6	1.7	47	6	.04	.02	3	0	4	6	.12	.041
1 med	87	0.1	0.0	0.0	0.0	0	465	.01	0.9	.00	.15	171	10	.10	.059	809
pear																
cnd, heavy pack	189	204.9	0.5	48.9	38.8	4.1	0	3	.06	.04	3	13	13	10	.20	.082
1 cup	255	0.3	0.0	0.1	0.1	0	0	.03	0.6	.00	.06	166	18	.56	.125	809
cnd, jce pack	124	214.4	0.8	32.1	24.1	4.0	2	4	.03	.03	3	10	22	17	.22	.084
1 cup	248	0.2	0.0	0.0	0.0	0	15	.03	0.5	.00	.05	238	30	.72	.131	809

	KCAL / WT (g)	H₂O (g) / FAT (g)	PRO (g) / SFA (g)	CHO (g) / MUFA (g)	SUGR (g) / PUFA (g)	DFIB (g) / CHOL (mg)	A (RE) / A (IU)	C (mg) / B-1 (mg)	B-2 (mg) / NIA (mg)	B-6 (mg) / B-12 (mcg)	FOL (mcg) / PANT (mg)	Na (mg) / K (mg)	Ca (mg) / P (mg)	Mg (mg) / Fe (mg)	Zn (mg) / Cu (mg)	Mn (mg) / REF
cnd, light syrup	143	212.0	0.5	38.1		4.0	0	2	.04	.04	3	13	13	10	.20	.083
1 cup	251	0.1	0.0	0.0	0.0	0	0	.03	0.4	.00	.06	166	18	.70	.123	809
cnd, water pack	71	224.0	0.5	19.1	14.9	3.9	0	2	.02	.03	3	5	10	10	.22	.083
1 cup	244	0.1	0.0	0.0	0.0	0	0	.02	0.1	.00	.05	129	17	.51	.124	809
dried, sulfured	459	46.7	3.3	122.0		13.1	0	12	.25	.13	0	11	60	58	.68	.572
10 halves	175	1.1	0.1	0.2	0.3	0	5	.01	2.4	.00	.27	933	103	3.68	.649	809
raw	98	139.1	0.6	25.1	17.4	4.0	3	7	.07	.03	12	0	18	10	.20	.126
1 med	166	0.7	0.0	0.1	0.2	0	33	.03	0.2	.00	.12	208	18	.41	.188	809
pear, asian, raw																
1 pear (2 ½" high, 2 ½" dia)	51	107.7	0.6	13.0		4.4	0	5	.01	.03	10	0	5	10	.02	.073
	122	0.3	0.0	0.1	0.1	0	0	.01	0.3	.00	.09	148	13	.00	.061	809
persimmon, japanese, dried	93	7.8	0.5	25.0		4.9	19	0	.01			1	9	11	.14	.473
1 med	34	0.2				0	190		0.1	.00		273	28	.25	.150	809
persimmon, japanese, raw	118	134.9	1.0	31.2		6.0	365	13	.03	.17	13	2	13	15	.18	.596
1 med	168	0.3	0.0	0.1	0.1	0	3641	.05	0.2	.00		270	29	.25	.190	809
persimmon, raw	32	16.1	0.2	8.4				17				0	7			
1 med	25	0.1				0				.00		78	7	.63		809
pineapple																
cnd, heavy syrup	199	201.4	0.9	51.5		2.0	3	19	.06	.19	12	3	36	41	.31	2.754
1 cup pieces	255	0.3	0.0	0.0	0.1	0	36	.23	0.7	.00	.26	265	18	.97	.258	809
cnd, jce pack	150	208.8	1.1	39.3	35.5	2.0	10	24	.05	.18	12	3	35	35	.25	2.803
1 cup pieces	250	0.2	0.0	0.0	0.1	0	95	.24	0.7	.00	.25	305	15	.70	.215	809
raw	76	134.1	0.6	19.2	18.4	1.9	3	24	.06	.13	16	2	11	22	.12	2.556
1 cup pieces	155	0.7	0.0	0.1	0.2	0	36	.14	0.7	.00	.25	175	11	.57	.171	809
pitanga, raw	57	157.1	1.4	13.0			260	45	.07			5	16	21		
1 cup	173	0.7				0	2595	.05	0.5	.00		178	19	.35		809
plantain, ckd	179	103.6	1.2	48.0		3.5	140	17	.08	.37	40	8	3	49	.20	
1 cup slices	154	0.3	0.1	0.0	0.1	0	1400	.07	1.2	.00	.36	716	43	.89	.102	809
plums																
cnd, heavy syrup	118	101.2	0.5	30.9		1.3	35	1	.05	.04	3	25	12	7	.09	.041
3 plums	133	0.1	0.0	0.1	0.0	0	344	.02	0.4	.00	.10	121	17	1.12	.049	809
cnd, jce pack	55	79.8	0.5	14.4		0.9	96	3	.06	.03	2	1	10	8	.10	.031
3 plums	95	0.0	0.0	0.0	0.0	0	959	.02	0.4	.00	.07	146	14	.32	.051	809
raw	36	56.2	0.5	8.6	5.0	1.0	21	6	.06	.05	1	0	3	5	.07	.032
1 med	66	0.4	0.0	0.3	0.1	0	213	.03	0.3	.00	.12	114	7	.07	.028	809
pomegranate, raw	105	124.7	1.5	26.4		0.9	0	9	.05	.16	9	5	5	5	.18	
1 med	154	0.5	0.1	0.1	0.1	0	0	.05	0.5	.00	.92	399	12	.46	.108	809
pricklypear, raw	42	90.2	0.8	9.9		3.7	5	14	.06	.06	6	5	58	88	.12	
1 med	103	0.5	0.1	0.1	0.2	0	53	.01	0.5	.00		227	25	.31	.082	809
prunes																
cnd, heavy syrup	90	60.8	0.7	23.9		3.3	69	2	.10	.17	0	3	15	13	.16	.084
5 prunes	86	0.2	0.0	0.1	0.0	0	685	.03	0.7	.00	.09	194	22	.35	.101	809
dried	201	27.2	2.2	52.7		6.0	167	3	.14	.22	3	3	43	38	.45	.185
10 prunes	84	0.4	0.0	0.3	0.1	0	1669	.07	1.6	.00	.39	626	66	2.08	.361	809
dried, ckd	113	73.9	1.2	29.8		7.0	33	3	.11	.23	0	2	24	21	.25	.104
½ cup	106	0.2	0.0	0.2	0.1	0	324	.03	0.8	.00	.11	354	37	1.18	.205	809
pummelo, raw	72	169.3	1.4	18.3		1.9	0	116	.05	.07		2	8	11	.15	.032
1 cup pieces	190	0.1				0	0	.06	0.4	.00		410	32	.21	.091	809
quince, raw	52	77.1	0.4	14.1		1.7	4	14	.03	.04	3	4	10	7	.04	
1 med	92	0.1	0.0	0.0	0.0	0	37	.02	0.2	.00	.07	181	16	.64	.120	809
raisins																
golden seedless	302	15.0	3.4	79.5		4.0	4	3	.19	.32	3	12	53	35	.32	.308
⅔ cup	100	0.5	0.2	0.0	0.1	0	44	.01	1.1	.00	.14	746	115	1.79	.363	809
seeded	296	16.6	2.5	78.5		6.8	0	5	.18	.19	3	28	28	30	.18	.267
⅔ cup	100	0.5	0.2	0.0	0.2	0	0	.11	1.1	.00	.04	825	75	2.59	.302	809
seedless	300	15.4	3.2	79.1		4.0	1	3	.09	.25	3	12	49	33	.27	.308
⅔ cup	100	0.5	0.1	0.0	0.1	0	8	.16	0.8	.00	.04	751	97	2.08	.309	809
w/ van yogurt coating, Del Monte	110		2.0	20.0	17.0	0	0				25	40				
.9 oz bag	26	3.0	2.5			0	0							.00		I

	KCAL	H₂O (g)	PRO (g)	CHO (g)	SUGR (g)	DFIB (g)	A (RE)	C (mg)	B-2 (mg)	B-6 (mg)	FOL (mcg)	Na (mg)	Ca (mg)	Mg (mg)	Zn (mg)	Mn (mg)
	WT (g)	FAT (g)	SFA (g)	MUFA (g)	PUFA (g)	CHOL (mg)	A (IU)	B-1 (mg)	NIA (mg)	B-12 (mcg)	PANT (mg)	K (mg)	P (mg)	Fe (mg)	Cu (mg)	REF
raspberries																
cnd, heavy syrup	116	96.4	1.1	29.9		4.2	4	11	.04	.05	13	4	14	15	.20	.298
½ cup	128	0.2	0.0	0.0	0.1	0	42	.03	0.6	.00	.31	120	12	.54	.073	809
frzn, in lite syrup, Birds Eye	99	115.7	0.8	24.6		4.3		23	.08	.05	24	0	20	17	.43	
½ cup	142	0.5	0.0		0.3	0	120	.03	0.8	.00	.22	141	11	.54	.071	I
frzn, sweetened	103	72.8	0.7	26.2		4.4	6	17	.04	.03	26	1	15	13	.18	.650
⅖ cup	100	0.2	0.0	0.0	0.1	0	60	.02	0.2	.00	.15	114	17	.65	.105	809
raw	60	106.5	1.1	14.2		8.4	16	31	.11	.07	32	0	27	22	.57	1.246
1 cup	123	0.7	0.0	0.1	0.4	0	160	.04	1.1	.00	.30	187	15	.70	.091	809
rose apple, raw	25	92.3	0.6	5.7			34	22	.03			0	29	5	.06	.029
3.5 oz	99	0.3				0	336	.02	0.8	.00		122	8	.07	.016	809
roselle, raw	28	49.4	0.5	6.4			17	7	.02			3	123	29		
1 cup	57	0.4				0	164	.01	0.2	.00		119	21	.84		809
sapodilla, raw	141	132.6	0.7	33.9		9.0	10	25	.03	.06	24	20	36	20	.17	
1 med	170	1.9	0.3	0.9	0.0	0	102	.00	0.3	.00	.43	328	20	1.36	.146	809
sapote, raw	302	140.5	4.8	76.0		5.9	92	45	.04			23	88	68		
1 med	225	1.3				0	923	.02	4.0	.00		774	63	2.25		809
soursop, raw	149	182.6	2.3	37.9		7.4	0	46	.11	.13	32	32	32	47	.23	
1 cup	225	0.7	0.1	0.2	0.2	0	5	.16	2.0	.00	.57	626	61	1.35	.193	809
strawberries																
frzn, in lite syrup, Birds Eye	87	118.8	0.7	21.6		2.2		64	.07	.07	20	1	16	11	.15	
½ cup	142	0.4	0.2		0.2	0	31	.02	0.3	.00	.39	189	22	.44	.058	I
frzn, sweetened	199	199.0	1.3	53.5		4.8	8	101	.20	.07	10	3	28	15	.13	.635
1 cup	255	0.4	0.0	0.0	0.2	0	69	.04	0.7	.00	.28	250	31	1.20	.048	809
frzn, unsweetened	52	134.1	0.6	13.6		3.1	6	61	.06	.04	25	3	24	16	.19	.432
1 cup	149	0.2	0.0	0.0	0.1	0	67	.03	0.7	.00	.16	221	19	1.12	.073	809
raw	45	136.4	0.9	10.5	8.6	3.4	4	84	.10	.09	26	1	21	15	.19	.432
1 cup	149	0.6	0.0	0.1	0.3	0	40	.03	0.3	.00	.51	247	28	.57	.073	809
sugar apple, raw	146	113.5	3.2	36.6		6.8	2	56	.18	.31	22	14	37	33	.16	
1 med	155	0.4	0.1	0.2	0.1	0	9	.17	1.4	.00	.35	383	50	.93	.133	809
tamarind, raw	287	37.7	3.4	75.0		6.1	4	4	.18	.08	17	34	89	110	.12	
1 cup	120	0.7	0.3	0.2	0.1	0	36	.51	2.3	.00	.17	754	136	3.36	.103	809
tangerine, raw	37	73.6	0.5	9.4		1.9	77	26	.02	.06	17	1	12	10	.20	.027
1 med	84	0.2	0.0	0.0	0.0	0	773	.09	0.1	.00	.17	132	8	.08	.024	809
watermelon, raw	51	146.4	1.0	11.5	14.4	0.8	59	15	.03	.23	4	3	13	18	.11	.059
1 cup	160	0.7	0.1	0.2	0.2	0	586	.13	0.3	.00	.34	186	14	.27	.051	809

1. Dried black corinth grapes; not related to European black, red, or white currants.
2. Peaches, pears, grapes, pineapples, and cherries.
3. Peaches, pears, apricots, pineapples, and cherries.
4. Pineapples, papayas, pineapple juice, bananas, guava puree, cherries, and passion fruit juice.
5. Values are averages for cherry, grape, rainbow punch, strawberry, and watermelon.
6. Values are averages for cherry, Crazy Colors, grape, Hot Colors, Peel 'n Build, raspberry, Secret Pictures, strawberry, and Webslinger Blue.
7. Values are averages for cherry, Crazy Colors, grape, Hot Colors, Peel 'n Build, raspberry, Secret Pictures, and strawberry.
8. Includes Berry 'n Blue, cherry, strawberry, and Stripes.
9. Values are averages for Bugs Bunny & Friends assorted fruit, Kids Cash, Rollerblade assorted fruit, Shark Bite assorted fruit, Tazmanian Devil assorted fruit, and X-men.
10. Values are averages for apple, berry, blue raspberry, cherry, color changing, grape, orange, punch, red punch, strawberry, tropical lemonade, tropical punch, and watermelon.
11. Roundish yellow berries ¾ inches across, sweet and slightly acid; native to eastern and central North America.
12. Peaches, pears, and pineapple.
13. Peaches, sweet cherries, red sour cherries, red raspberries, boysenberries, and grapes.

	KCAL	H₂O (g)	PRO (g)	CHO (g)	SUGR (g)	DFIB (g)	A (RE)	C (mg)	B-2 (mg)	B-6 (mg)	FOL (mcg)	Na (mg)	Ca (mg)	Mg (mg)	Zn (mg)	Mn (mg)
	WT (g)	FAT (g)	SFA (g)	MUFA (g)	PUFA (g)	CHOL (mg)	A (IU)	B-1 (mg)	NIA (mg)	B-12 (mcg)	PANT (mg)	K (mg)	P (mg)	Fe (mg)	Cu (mg)	REF

16. GRAIN FRACTIONS

Food	KCAL / WT	H₂O / FAT	PRO / SFA	CHO / MUFA	SUGR / PUFA	DFIB / CHOL	A(RE) / A(IU)	C / B-1	B-2 / NIA	B-6 / B-12	FOL / PANT	Na / K	Ca / P	Mg / Fe	Zn / Cu	Mn / REF
amaranth	729	19.2	28.2	129.0		29.6	0	8	.41	.43	96	41	298	519	6.20	4.407
1 cup	195	12.7	3.2	2.8	5.6	0	0	.16	2.5	.00	2.04	714	887	14.80	1.515	820
arrowroot flour	457	14.6	0.4	112.8		4.4	0	0	.00	.01	9	3	51	4	.09	.602
1 cup	128	0.1	0.0	0.0	0.1	0	0	.00	0.0	.00	.17	14	6	.42	.051	820
barley, pearled, med/quick, Scotch Brand	166	4.6	5.2	36.7	0.3	5.0		0	.04	.13	11	3	13	29	.70	
¼ cup	48	1.1	0.2	0.1	0.5	0	11	.12	2.2	.00	.14	125	101	.96	.180	I
Bisquick Mix, General Mills	170		3.0	25.0	1.0	1.0	0	0	.10			490	40			
⅓ cup	40	6.0	1.5			0	0	.15	1.6			50		1.08		I
Bisquick Mix, red fat, General Millls	150		3.0	28.0	2.0	1.0	0	0	.10			460	40			
⅓ cup	40	2.5	0.5			0	0	.15	1.6			30		1.44		I
buckwheat flour, whole groat	402	13.4	15.1	84.7		12.0	0	0	.23	.70	65	13	49	301	3.74	2.436
1 cup	120	3.7	0.8	1.1	1.1	0	0	.50	7.4	.00	.53	692	404	4.87	.618	820
carob (St. Johnsbread) flour	185	3.7	4.8	91.5		41.0	1	0	.47	.38	30	36	358	56	.95	.523
1 cup	103	0.7	0.1	0.2	0.2	0	14	.05	2.0	.00	.05	852	81	3.03	.588	816
corn bran	56	1.2	2.1	21.4		21.4	2	0	.03	.04	1	2	11	16	.39	.035
⅓ cup	25	0.2	0.0	0.1	0.1	0	18	.00	0.7	.00	.16	11	18	.70	.062	820
corn flake crumbs, Kellogg's	40	0.3	0.8	9.0	1.0	0.0		5	.14	.16	32	120	0			
2 T	11	0.0	0.0	0.0	0.0	0	0	.12	1.6			10		2.70		I
corn flour, masa harina																
enr	416	10.3	10.6	86.9		10.9	0	0	.86	.42	27	6	161	125	2.03	.552
1 cup	114	4.3	0.6	1.1	2.0	0	0	1.63	11.2	.00	.75	340	254	8.22	.193	820
enr, Quaker	114	1.9	2.8	24.6	0.4	2.3		0	.17	.12	5	3	54	30	.58	
¼ cup	31	1.2	0.2	0.3	0.6	0	4	.38	2.6	.00	.12	91	87	2.11	.060	I
yellow, unenr, Quaker	111	2.7	2.8	23.6	0.5	2.6		0	.04	.12	5	2	57	30	.58	
¼ cup	31	1.4	0.2	0.3	0.7	0	5	.09	0.7	.00	.12	96	87	.82	.060	I
corn flour, whole grain	422	12.8	8.1	89.9		15.7	55	0	.09	.43	29	6	8	109	2.02	.538
1 cup	117	4.5	0.6	1.2	2.1	0	549	.29	2.2	.00	.77	369	318	2.78	.269	820
cornmeal mix																
white, bolted, Aunt Jemima	84	2.5	2.0	18.6	0.3	1.1	0	0	.14	.06	2	339	76	11	.22	
3 T	25	0.6	0.1	0.1	0.2	0	0	.24	1.9	.00	.08	57	158	2.03	.030	I
white, buttermilk, self-rising, Aunt Jemima—3 T	83	2.5	2.1	18.4	0.6	1.2	0	0	.18	.11	9	437	76	22	.51	
	25	0.6	0.1	0.1	0.3	0	0	.32	2.3	.13	.09	68	168	2.28	.050	I
yellow, self-rising, Aunt Jemima	82	2.7	2.0	18.8	0.3	1.2		0	.16	.05	9	314	76	8	.19	
3 T	25	0.4	0.1	0.1	0.2	0	72	.29	2.3	.00	.08	47	140	1.91	.020	I
cornmeal, white																
bolted, enr, self-rising	407	15.4	10.1	85.7		8.2	57	0	.49	.66	70	1521	440	105	2.44	.608
1 cup	122	4.1	0.6	1.1	1.9	0	572	.81	6.5	.00	.52	311	981	7.03	.183	820
bolted, enr, self-rising, Aunt Jemima	91	2.7	2.1	20.2	0.3	1.1	0	0	.11	.08	8	356	96	12	.28	
3 T	27	0.6	0.1	0.1	0.2	0	0	.20	1.5	.00	.08	63	186	1.73	.040	I
bolted, enr, self-rising, wheat flour added	592	17.6	14.3	124.8		10.7	49	0	.74	.65	112	2242	508	92	2.36	.877
1 cup	170	4.8	0.7	1.3	2.2	0	488	1.21	8.8	.00	.65	352	1107	8.42	.236	820
degermed, enr	505	16.0	11.7	107.2		10.2	57	0	.56	.35	66	4	7	55	.99	.145
1 cup	138	2.3	0.3	0.6	1.0	0	570	.99	6.9	.00	.43	224	116	5.70	.108	820
degermed, enr, Quaker	94	3.0	2.2	21.1	0.3	1.3	0	0	.09	.07	3	1	1	13	.25	
3 T	27	0.5	0.1	0.2	0.2	0	0	.16	1.2	.00	.08	45	45	1.23	.030	I
degermed, enr, self-rising	490	14.0	11.6	103.2		9.8	57	0	.53	.54	43	1860	483	68	1.38	.145
1 cup	138	2.4	0.3	0.6	1.0	0	570	.94	6.3	.00	.43	235	860	6.53	.179	820
degermed, enr, self-rising, Aunt Jemima	91	2.7	2.1	20.2	0.3	1.1	0	0	.11	.08	8	356	96	12	.28	
3 T	27	0.6	0.1	0.1	0.2	0	0	.20	1.5	.00	.08	63	186	1.73	.040	I
degermed, unenr, Quaker	94	3.0	2.2	21.1	0.3	1.3	0	0	.01	.07	3	1	1	13	.25	
3 T	27	0.5	0.1	0.2	0.2	0	0	.04	0.3	.00	.08	45	45	.30	.030	I
cornmeal, white/yellow, Alber's	110		2.0	25.5	0.0	0.7	0	0	.10			0	0			
3 T	30	0.0	0.0	0.0	0.0	0	0	.15	1.2					1.08		I
cornmeal, whole grain	442	12.5	9.9	93.8		8.9	57	0	.25	.37	31	43	7	155	2.22	.608
1 cup	122	4.4	0.6	1.2	2.0	0	572	.47	4.4	.00	.52	350	294	4.21	.235	820

	KCAL / WT (g)	H₂O (g) / FAT (g)	PRO (g) / SFA (g)	CHO (g) / MUFA (g)	SUGR (g) / PUFA (g)	DFIB (g) / CHOL (mg)	A (RE) / A (IU)	C (mg) / B-1 (mg)	B-2 (mg) / NIA (mg)	B-6 (mg) / B-12 (mcg)	FOL (mcg) / PANT (mg)	Na (mg) / K (mg)	Ca (mg) / P (mg)	Mg (mg) / Fe (mg)	Zn (mg) / Cu (mg)	Mn (mg) / REF
cornmeal, yellow, degermed, enr, Quaker	92	3.0	2.1	21.3	0.3	1.5		0	.09	.07	13	1	1	11	.19	
3 T	27	0.5	0.1	0.2	0.2	0	110	.15	1.4	.00	.08	43	33	.98	.020	I
cracker meal	440	8.7	10.7	93.0		2.9	0	0	.54	.04	25	32	26	28	.79	1.086
1 cup	115	2.0	0.3	0.2	0.8	0	0	.80	6.6	.00	.35	132	120	5.34	.259	818
graham cracker crumbs, Keebler	179	20.1	4.4	28.7		1.3	0	0	.34	.38	6	615	154	14	.31	.280
½ cup	59	5.8	1.4	1.9	0.5	7	0	.32	3.4	1.44	.28	88	248	4.22	.060	I
La Pina flour, General Mills	100		2.0	23.0	1.0	1.0	0	0	.10			0	0			
¼ cup	30	0.0	0.0	0.0	0.0	0	0	.15	1.6			35		1.08		I
oat bran																
ckd	44	92.4	3.5	12.6		2.9	0	0	.04	.03	7	1	11	44	.58	1.060
½ cup	110	0.9	0.2	0.3	0.4	0	0	.18	0.2	.00	.24	101	131	.97	.073	820
dry, Quaker	146	3.6	6.8	25.2	0.6	5.7	0	0	.12	.04	15	2	32	96	1.68	
½ cup	40	3.2	0.6	1.0	1.2	0	40	.39	0.3	.00	.34	232	278	3.23	.120	I
raw	76	2.0	5.4	20.5		4.8	0	0	.07	.05	16	1	18	73	.96	1.745
⅓ cup	31	2.2	0.4	0.7	0.9	0	0	.36	0.3	.00	.46	175	228	1.68	.125	820
oats, reg/quick/inst, dry	104	2.4	4.3	18.1		2.9	3	0	.04	.03	9	1	14	40	.83	.980
⅓ cup (.95 oz)	27	1.7	0.3	0.5	0.6	0	27	.20	0.2	.00	.34	95	128	1.13	.093	808
potato flour	316	6.8	7.2	71.9		5.5	0	17	.13	.01	46	31	30	79	1.47	.987
½ cup	90	0.7	0.2	0.0	0.3	0	0	.38	3.1	.00	1.35	1429	160	15.48	.972	811
quinoa	318	7.9	11.1	58.6		5.0	0	0	.34	.19	42	18	51	179	2.80	1.921
½ cup	85	4.9	0.5	1.3	2.0	0	0	.17	2.5	.00	.89	629	349	7.86	.697	820
rice bran	90	1.7	3.8	14.1		6.0	0	0	.08	1.15	18	1	16	221	1.71	4.029
1 oz	28	5.9	1.2	2.1	2.1	0	0	.78	9.6	.00	2.10	421	475	5.26	.206	820
rice flour, brown	574	18.9	11.4	120.8		7.3	0	0	.13	1.16	25	13	17	177	3.87	6.341
1 cup	158	4.4	0.9	1.6	1.6	0	0	.70	10.0	.00	2.51	457	532	3.13	.363	820
rice flour, white	597	19.4	9.7	130.6		3.9	0	0	.03	.71	7	0	16	57	1.30	1.956
1 cup	163	2.3	0.6	0.7	0.6	0	0	.22	4.2	.00	1.33	124	160	.57	.212	820
rye & wheat flour, bohemian style, Pillsbury—1 cup	400	12.9	12.3	84.4			0	0	.29			2	24			
	112	1.5					0	.56	4.4			167	196	4.03		I
rye flour																
dark	415	14.2	18.0	88.0		28.9	0	0	.32	.57	77	1	72	317	7.19	8.614
1 cup	128	3.4	0.4	0.4	1.5	0	0	.40	5.5	.00	1.86	934	809	8.26	.960	820
light	374	9.0	8.6	81.8		14.9	0	0	.09	.24	22	2	21	71	1.79	2.009
1 cup	102	1.4	0.1	0.2	0.6	0	0	.34	0.8	.00	.68	238	198	1.84	.255	820
medium	361	10.0	9.6	79.0		14.9	0	0	.12	.27	19	3	24	77	2.03	5.569
1 cup	102	1.8	0.2	0.2	0.8	0	0	.29	1.8	.00	.50	347	211	2.16	.293	820
seasoning/coating mix																
extra crispy recipe for chicken, Oven Fry	60		2.0	10.0	2.0	0.0	0	0				420				
⅛ pkt[2]	15	1.0	0.0			0	0					30		.36		I
extra crispy recipe for pork, Oven Fry	60		2.0	11.0	2.0	0.0	0	0				340	0			
⅛ pkt[3]	15	1.5	0.0			0	0					20		.00		I
glaze, Shake 'n Bake	43		0.0	9.0	5.3	0.0	0	0				308	0			
⅛ pkt[4]	12	0.8	0.0			0	125					34		.00		I
homestyle flour recipe for chicken, Oven Fry—⅛ pkt[2]	40		1.0	7.0	0.0	0.0	0	0				470	0			
	11	1.0	0.0			0	0					15		.00		I
hot & spicy for chicken, Shake & Bake	40		1.0	7.0	1.0	0.0	0	0				190	0			
⅛ pkt[3]	10	1.0	0.0			0	0					20		.36		I
hot & spicy for pork, Shake & Bake	45		1.0	8.0	1.0	0.0	0	0				220	0			
⅛ pkt[3]	11	0.5	0.0			0	0					25		.00		I
italian herb recipe, Shake 'n Bake	40		1.0	7.0	1.0	0.0	0	0				300	0			
⅛ pkt[2]	10	0.5	0.0			0	0					25		.00		I
meat/poultry, Mrs. Dash Crispy Coating Mix—2 T	70		2.0	14.0	1.0	0.0		0				0	0			
	18	1.0				0	100					25		.32		I
orig country mild recipe, Shake 'n Bake	35		0.0	5.0	0.0	0.0		0				240	0			
⅛ pkt[2]	8	2.0	1.0			0	100					10		.00		I
orig recipe for chicken, Shake 'n Bake	40		1.0	7.0	1.0	0.0		0				230	0			
⅛ pkt[2]	10	1.0	0.0			0	100					20		.36		I
orig recipe for fish, Shake 'n Bake	70		1.0	14.0	1.0	1.0	0	0				420	0			
¼ pkt[5]	19	1.5	0.0			0	0					25		.00		I

	KCAL	H₂O (g)	PRO (g)	CHO (g)	SUGR (g)	DFIB (g)	A (RE)	C (mg)	B-2 (mg)	B-6 (mg)	FOL (mcg)	Na (mg)	Ca (mg)	Mg (mg)	Zn (mg)	Mn (mg)
	WT (g)	FAT (g)	SFA (g)	MUFA (g)	PUFA (g)	CHOL (mg)	A (IU)	B-1 (mg)	NIA (mg)	B-12 (mcg)	PANT (mg)	K (mg)	P (mg)	Fe (mg)	Cu (mg)	REF
orig recipe for pork, Shake 'n Bake	40		1.0	9.0	1.0	0.0	0	0				320	0			
⅛ pkt³	11	0.0	0.0	0.0	0.0	0	0					15		.00		I
semolina, enr	302	10.6	10.7	61.2		3.3	0	0	.48	.09	60	1	14	39	.88	.520
½ cup	84	0.9	0.1	0.1	0.4	0	0	.68	5.0	.00	.49	156	114	3.66	.159	820
sorghum	325	8.8	10.8	71.6			0	0	.14			6	27			
½ cup	96	3.2	0.4	1.0	1.3	0	0	.23	2.8	.00		336	276	4.22		820
soy flour																
defatted	280	6.2	40.0	32.6		14.9	3	0	.22	.49	260	17	205	247	2.09	2.565
1 cup	85	1.0	0.1	0.2	0.5	0	34	.59	2.2	.00	1.70	2026	573	7.85	3.455	816
full fat	371	4.4	29.4	29.9		8.2	10	0	.99	.39	293	11	175	365	3.33	1.934
1 cup	85	17.6	2.5	3.9	9.9	0	102	.49	3.7	.00	1.35	2138	420	5.41	2.482	816
full fat, roasted	375	3.2	29.6	28.6		8.2	9	0	.80	.30	193	10	160	314	3.04	1.765
1 cup	85	18.6	2.7	4.1	10.5	0	94	.35	2.8	.00	1.03	1735	405	4.95	1.888	816
low fat	287	2.4	40.9	33.4		9.0	4	0	.25	.46	361	16	165	202	1.04	2.710
1 cup	88	5.9	0.9	1.3	3.3	0	35	.33	1.9	.00	1.60	2262	522	5.27	4.470	816
soy meal, defatted, raw	414	8.5	54.8	49.0			5	0	.31	.69	369	4	298	37	6.17	4.636
1 cup	122	2.9	0.3	0.5	1.3	0	49	.84	3.2	.00	2.41	3038	855	16.71	2.440	820
triticale flour, whole grain	439	13.0	17.1	95.1		19.0	0	0	.17	.52	96	3	46	199	3.46	5.441
1 cup	130	2.4	0.4	0.2	1.0	0	0	.49	3.7	.00	2.82	606	417	3.37	.727	820
wheat bran	65	3.0	4.7	19.4	0.7	12.8	0	0	.17	.39	24	1	22	183	2.18	3.450
½ cup	30	1.3	0.2	0.2	0.7	0	0	.16	4.1	.00	.65	355	304	3.17	.299	820
toasted, Kretschmer	32	1.9	2.8	9.5	0.4	6.6	0	0	.07	.11	31	1	11	97	1.80	
¼ cup (.56 oz)	16	0.8	0.1	0.1	0.4	0	0	.18	3.3	.04	.47	205	210	2.22	.170	I
unprocessed, Quaker	30	1.7	2.7	11.1	0.4	7.8	0	0	.08	.10	23	1	15	93	1.55	
⅓ cup	17	0.5	0.1	0.1	0.1	0	0	.09	4.1	.45		253	221	2.42	.210	I
wheat flour, white																
all purpose, enr	455	14.9	12.9	95.4	2.1	3.4	0	0	.62	.05	33	3	19	28	.88	.853
1 cup	125	1.2	0.2	0.1	0.5	0	0	.98	7.4	.00	.55	134	135	5.80	.180	820
bread, enr	495	18.3	16.4	99.4		3.3	0	0	.70	.05	40	3	21	34	1.16	1.085
1 cup	137	2.3	0.3	0.2	1.0	0	0	1.11	10.3	.00	.60	137	133	6.04	.249	820
cake, enr	395	13.6	8.9	85.1		1.9	0	0	.47	.04	21	2	15	17	.68	.691
1 cup	109	0.9	0.1	0.1	0.4	0	0	.97	7.4	.00	.50	114	93	7.98	.152	820
enr, General Mills	100		3.0	22.0	1.0	1.0	0	0	.10			0	0			
¼ cup⁶	30	0.0	0.0	0.0	0	0	0	.15	1.6			40		1.08		I
enr, Gold Medal Better for Bread Wheat	110		4.0	21.0	0.0	1.0	0	0	.10			0	0			
Blend—¼ cup	30	0.5	0.0			0	0	.15	1.6			70		1.08		I
enr, Gold Metal Better for Bread	100		4.0	22.0	1.0	1.0	0	0	.10			0				
¼ cup	30	0.0	0.0	0.0	0.0	0	0	.15	1.6			35		1.08		I
enr, self-rising, General Mills	100		3.0	22.0	1.0	1.0	0	0	.10			400	60			
¼ cup⁷	30	0.0	0.0	0.0	0.0	0	0	.15	1.6			35		1.08		I
enr, Softasilk Velvet Cake, Betty Crocker	100		2.0	23.0	1.0	1.0	0	0	.10			0	0			
¼ cup	30	0.0	0.0	0.0	0.0	0	0	.15	1.6			35		1.08		I
enr, Supreme Hygluten	100		4.0	22.0	1.0	1.0	0	0	.10			0	0			
¼ cup	30	0.0	0.0	0.0	0.0	0	0	.15	1.6			30		1.08		I
gluten (45% gluten & 55% all-purpose)	529	11.9	58.0	66.1				0				3	56			
1 cup	140	2.7						0				84	196			456
Sauce'n Gravy, Pillsbury's Best	50	1.5	1.5	10.8				0	.05			1	30			
2 T	14	0.1						.08	0.7			12	14	.41		I
self-rising, enr	443	13.2	12.4	92.8		3.4	0	0	.52	.06	53	1588	423	24	.78	1.250
1 cup	125	1.2	0.2	0.1	0.5	0	0	.84	7.3	.00	.55	155	744	5.84	.140	820
self-rising, enr, Aunt Jemima	92	2.9	2.8	20.0	0.4	0.8	0	0	.12	.01	11	307	85	7	.15	
3 T	27	0.3	0.0	0.0	0.1	0	0	.22	1.5	.00	.09	35	155	1.37	.020	I
tortilla mix	450	11.2	10.7	74.5			0	0	.55	.04	26	751	228	23	.71	.682
1 cup⁸	111	11.8	4.6	5.0	1.7	0	0	.82	6.5	.00	.44	111	233	7.83	.111	820
wheat flour, whole wheat	407	12.3	16.4	87.1	2.4	14.6	0	0	.26	.41	53	6	41	166	3.52	4.559
1 cup	120	2.2	0.4	0.3	0.9	0	0	.54	7.6	.00	1.21	486	415	4.66	.458	820
wheat flour, whole wheat, Gold Medal	90		4.0	21.0	1.0	3.0	0	0	.30			0	0			
¼ cup	30	0.5	0.0			0	0	.12	1.2			110		1.08		I

	KCAL / WT (g)	H₂O (g) / FAT (g)	PRO (g) / SFA (g)	CHO (g) / MUFA (g)	SUGR (g) / PUFA (g)	DFIB (g) / CHOL (mg)	A (RE) / A (IU)	C (mg) / B-1 (mg)	B-2 (mg) / NIA (mg)	B-6 (mg) / B-12 (mcg)	FOL (mcg) / PANT (mg)	Na (mg) / K (mg)	Ca (mg) / P (mg)	Mg (mg) / Fe (mg)	Zn (mg) / Cu (mg)	Mn (mg) / REF
wheat germ																
crude	104	3.2	6.7	15.0	3.5	3.8	0	0	.14	.38	81	3	11	69	3.56	3.857
¼ cup	29	2.8	0.5	0.4	1.7	0	0	.55	2.0	.00	.65	259	244	1.82	.231	
Honey Crunch, Kretschmer	52	0.5	3.7	8.1	3.5	1.4		0	.10	.07	47	2	7	38	1.94	
1 ⅔ T	14	1.1	0.2	0.2	0.7	0	13	.19	0.7	.00	.15	135	142	1.13	.100	I
toasted	111	1.6	8.4	14.4		3.7	0	2	.24	.28	102	1	13	93	4.83	5.787
¼ cup	29	3.1	0.5	0.4	1.9	0	0	.48	1.6	.00	.40	275	332	2.64	.180	820
toasted, Kretschmer	48	0.6	4.1	6.4	1.4	1.6		1	.10	.08	51	1	7	41	2.08	
2 T	13	1.2	0.0	0.2	0.8	0	17	.26	0.7	.03	.18	143	147	1.08	.080	I
Zesty Meal, Keebler																
Zesty Meal, Keebler	189		4.1	30.5					.17			520	8			
½ cup	43	5.2	1.3		0.4	0		.17	2.3			56		1.89		I

1. Includes potato flour soybean flour and meal.
2. Serving size coats 1 to 2 pieces of chicken.
3. Serving size coats 1 pork chop.
4. Values are averages for barbecue chicken, barbecue pork, honey mustard, and tangy honey. Serving size coats 1-2 pieces of chicken or 1 pork chop.
5. Serving size coats ¼ lb fish fillets.
6. Values apply to Gold Medal All Purpose, Gold Medal Wondra, Gold Metal unbleached, Red Band All Purpose, Robin Hood All Purpose, and Robin Hood unbleached flours.
7. Includes Gold Medal, Red Band, and Robin Hood brands.
8. Contains enriched wheat flour, lard, salt, leavening agents, and calcium carbonate.

17. GRAIN PRODUCTS
17.1 BAGELS

	KCAL / WT (g)	H₂O (g) / FAT (g)	PRO (g) / SFA (g)	CHO (g) / MUFA (g)	SUGR (g) / PUFA (g)	DFIB (g) / CHOL (mg)	A (RE) / A (IU)	C (mg) / B-1 (mg)	B-2 (mg) / NIA (mg)	B-6 (mg) / B-12 (mcg)	FOL (mcg) / PANT (mg)	Na (mg) / K (mg)	Ca (mg) / P (mg)	Mg (mg) / Fe (mg)	Zn (mg) / Cu (mg)	Mn (mg) / REF
cinn raisin	195	22.7	7.0	39.2		1.6	6	0	.20	.04	15	229	13	15	.53	.217
1 bagel (3 ½")	71	1.2	0.2	0.1	0.5	0	52	.27	2.2	.00	.05	108	55	2.70	.106	818
cinn raisin/egg/multigrain/onion/	154		6.2	33.2	4.8	2.2	0	0				268	60			
plain, Thomas'—1 bagel	61	1.0	0.0			0	0							1.80		I
egg	197	23.2	7.5	37.6		1.6	23	0	.17	.06	16	359	9	18	.55	.291
1 bagel (3 ½")	71	1.5	0.3	0.3	0.5	17	77	.38	2.4	.11	.48	48	60	2.83	.064	818
oat bran	181	23.4	7.6	37.8		2.6	0	0	.24	.14	33	360	9	40	1.48	.091
1 bagel (3 ½")	71	0.9	0.1	0.2	0.3	0	3	.24	2.1	.00	.13	145	117	2.19	.084	818
plain/onion/poppy seed/sesame seed	195	23.1	7.5	37.9		1.6	0	0	.22	.04	16	379	53	21	.62	.383
1 bagel (3 ½")	71	1.1	0.2	0.1	0.5	0	0	.38	3.2	.00	.26	72	68	2.53	.116	818

17.2 BISCUITS

	KCAL / WT (g)	H₂O (g) / FAT (g)	PRO (g) / SFA (g)	CHO (g) / MUFA (g)	SUGR (g) / PUFA (g)	DFIB (g) / CHOL (mg)	A (RE) / A (IU)	C (mg) / B-1 (mg)	B-2 (mg) / NIA (mg)	B-6 (mg) / B-12 (mcg)	FOL (mcg) / PANT (mg)	Na (mg) / K (mg)	Ca (mg) / P (mg)	Mg (mg) / Fe (mg)	Zn (mg) / Cu (mg)	Mn (mg) / REF
baking powder, refrig dough, 1869 Brand	102	10.8	1.9	12.3				0	.09			303	12			
1.1 oz biscuit	31	5.1					1	.10	0.9			29	131	.75		I
baking powder, refrig dough, Pillsbury	56	6.5	1.0	7.2				0	.04			171	3			
Tenderflake—.63 oz biscuit	18	2.7					0	.05	0.5			10	72	.40		I
biscuit mix, Gold Medal	180		4.0	27.0	3.0	0	0	0	.14			480	80			
amt for 2 bisquits	40	6.0	2.5			0	0	.23	1.2			70		1.08		I
butter, refrig dough, Pillsbury	49	8.4	1.3	9.7				0	.05			177	5			
.74 oz biscuit	21	0.7					0	.07	0.7			102	96	.57		I
Butter Tastin', refrig dough, Big Country	94	13.4	1.8	13.5				0	.08			324	6			
1.2 oz biscuit	34	3.9					0	.13	1.0			91	145	.63		I

	KCAL	H₂O (g)	PRO (g)	CHO (g)	SUGR (g)	DFIB (g)	A (RE)	C (mg)	B-2 (mg)	B-6 (mg)	FOL (mcg)	Na (mg)	Ca (mg)	Mg (mg)	Zn (mg)	Mn (mg)
	WT (g)	FAT (g)	SFA (g)	MUFA (g)	PUFA (g)	CHOL (mg)	A (IU)	B-1 (mg)	NIA (mg)	B-12 (mcg)	PANT (mg)	K (mg)	P (mg)	Fe (mg)	Cu (mg)	REF
Butter Tastin', refrig dough, Hungry Jack	88	9.8	1.5	11.4				0	.06			277	4			
1 oz biscuit	28	4.2					0	.08	0.8			16	118	.63		I
butterflake, refrig dough, Pillsbury	138	17.0	3.1	20.0				0	.10			520	11			
1.7 oz roll	47	4.9					0	.15	1.4			29	216	1.23		I
buttermilk																
extra rich, refrig dough, Hungry Jack	53	8.3	1.2	9.3				0	.05			172	5			
.74 oz biscuit	21	1.3					0	.07	0.6			100	93	.54		I
flaky, refrig dough, Butter Tastin'/1869	103	10.6	1.8	12.6				0	.08			292	11			
Brand—*1.1 oz biscuit*	31	5.1					2	.09	0.8			28	126	.67		I
flaky, refrig dough, Pillsbury Extra Lights	53	7.8	1.2	8.4				0	.05			158	5			
.72 oz biscuit	20	1.8					0	.07	0.6			91	85	.38		I
fluffy, refrig dough, Hungry Jack	84	10.1	1.5	11.7				0	.06			294	4			
1 oz biscuit	28	3.6					0	.09	0.8			16	122	.68		I
refrig dough	56	8.2	1.2	8.9				0	.05			169	5			
.74 oz biscuit	21	1.8					0	.07	0.7			97	91	.54		I
refrig dough, Ballard Ovenready	48	8.6	1.3	9.7				0	.05			176	5			
.74 oz biscuit	21	0.6					0	.07	0.6			102	95	.53		I
refrig dough, Big Country	102	12.2	2.2	14.7				0	.05			322	7			
1.2 oz biscuit	34	3.8					0	.16	0.6			89	154	1.05		I
refrig dough, Heat 'n Eat, Pillsbury	170	14.5	3.9	26.7				0	.14			532	25			
1.8 oz biscuit	52	5.3					3	.19	1.6			55	237	1.03		I
refrig dough, Hungry Jack	86	10.0	1.5	11.4				0	.06			281	4			
1 oz biscuit	28	4.0					0	.09	0.8			16	117	.68		I
refrig dough, Pillsbury	49	8.4	1.3	9.7				0	.05			177	5			
.74 oz biscuit	21	0.7					0	.08	0.7			102	96	.56		I
refrig dough, Pillsbury Tenderflake	66	7.5	1.2	8.5				0	.04			199	3			
.74 oz biscuit	21	3.2					0	.06	0.6			12	84	.47		I
country, refrig dough, Pillsbury	50	8.4	1.3	9.7				0	.05			177	5			
.74 oz biscuit	21	0.7					0	.08	0.7			102	96	.56		I
flaky, refrig dough, Hungry Jack	84	10.1	1.5	11.6				0	.06			294	4			
1 oz biscuit	28	3.6					0	.09	0.8			16	122	.68		I
Good 'n Buttery, refrig dough, Pillsbury	89	9.9	1.4	10.5				0	.06			363	6			
1 oz biscuit	28	4.8					0	.09	0.8			71	119	.67		I
Heat 'n Eat Big Premium, refrig dough,	277	16.8	4.6	32.2				0	.31			606	36			
Pillsbury—*2.5 oz biscuit*	71	14.6					5	.19	1.7			76	225	1.42		I
mixed grain, refrig dough	125	11.4	2.9	22.6		1.1	0	0	.09	.02	4	319	8	14	.30	.318
1 biscuit (3" x 1")	41	2.7	0.7	1.4	0.4	0	0	.15	1.5	.00	.10	217	158	1.31	.057	818
old fashioned, Arnold	130		3.0	18.0	4.0		0	0	.10			250	40			
2 biscuits	38	5.0	1.0			0	0	.12	1.2					.00		I
Ovenready, refrig dough, Ballard	48	8.6	1.3	9.7				0	.05			177	5			
.74 oz biscuit	21	0.6					0	.08	0.7			102	96	.57		I
plain/buttermilk	127	9.3	2.2	17.0		0.5	0	0	.10	.02	2	368	17	6	.17	.137
1 biscuit (2 ½" x 1")	35	5.8	0.9	2.4	2.2	0	1	.15	1.2	.05	.10	78	151	1.15	.029	818
from mix	191	16.5	4.2	27.6	2.5	1.0	15	0	.20	.04	3	544	105	14	.35	.142
1 biscuit (3" x 1 ½")	57	6.9	1.6	2.4	2.5	2	54	.20	1.7	.12	.31	107	268	1.17	.066	818
from refrig dough (12 -28% fat)	93	7.5	1.8	12.8		0.4	0	0	.06	.01	1	325	5	4	.10	.068
1 biscuit (2 ½" x 1")	27	4.0	1.0	2.2	0.5	0	0	.09	0.8	.00	.10	42	104	.70	.020	818
from refrig dough (2 -12% fat)	63	5.8	1.6	11.6		0.4	0	0	.05	.01	1	305	4	4	.10	.073
1 biscuit (2 ¼" x 1")	21	1.1	0.3	0.6	0.2	0	0	.09	0.7	.00	.06	39	98	.65	.019	818
homemade	212	17.3	4.2	26.8		0.9	14	0	.19	.02	7	348	141	11	.32	.227
1 biscuit (2 ½" x 1 ½")	60	9.8	2.6	4.2	2.5	2	49	.21	1.8	.05	.17	73	98	1.74	.049	818
Southern Style, refrig dough, Big	98	12.7	1.9	14.1				0	.08			324	6			
Country—*1.2 oz biscuit*	34	4.0					0	.12	1.1			91	151	.87		I

17.3 BREADS, QUICK

	KCAL	H₂O (g)	PRO (g)	CHO (g)	SUGR (g)	DFIB (g)	A (RE)	C (mg)	B-2 (mg)	B-6 (mg)	FOL (mcg)	Na (mg)	Ca (mg)	Mg (mg)	Zn (mg)	Mn (mg)
apple cinn, Elfin Loaves	180		2.7	31.2					.12			261	18			
2.1 oz slice	60	4.8	1.2		0.6	21		.06	1.0			87		1.02		I
banana																
Elfin Loaves	192		2.9	29.4					.18			258	16			
2.1 oz slice	60	7.2	1.2		1.2	0		.06	1.6			54		1.14		I

							Vitamins					Minerals				
	KCAL	H_2O (g)	PRO (g)	CHO (g)	SUGR (g)	DFIB (g)	A (RE)	C (mg)	B-2 (mg)	B-6 (mg)	FOL (mcg)	Na (mg)	Ca (mg)	Mg (mg)	Zn (mg)	Mn (mg)
	WT (g)	FAT (g)	SFA (g)	MUFA (g)	PUFA (g)	CHOL (mg)	A (IU)	B-1 (mg)	NIA (mg)	B-12 (mcg)	PANT (mg)	K (mg)	P (mg)	Fe (mg)	Cu (mg)	REF
homemade w/ marg	196	17.5	2.6	32.8		0.7	72	1	.12	.09	7	181	13	8	.21	.125
1 slice (4 3/8" x 2 ½" x ½")	60	6.3	1.3	2.7	1.9	26	278	.10	0.9	.06	.16	80	35	.84	.043	818
homemade w/ veg shortening	203	16.7	2.6	33.1			14	1	.12	.09	7	119	11	8	.22	.127
1 slice (4 3/8" x 2 ½" x ½")	60	7.1	1.8	3.0	1.8	26	55	.10	0.9	.05	.16	79	34	.84	.044	818
blueberry, Elfin Loaves	168		2.9	30.2					.22			218	15			
2 oz slice	56	3.9	0.6			14		.06	1.3			50		1.01		I
boston brown, cnd	88	21.2	2.3	19.5		2.1	5	0	.05	.04	3	284	32	28	.23	.459
1 slice (3 1/" x 2")	45	0.7	0.1	0.1	0.3	0	39	.01	0.5	.00	.25	143	50	.95	.036	818
carrot, Elfin Loaves	210		2.9	27.6					.24			174	16			
2.1 oz slice	60	10.2	1.8		2.4	24		.06	1.3			72		1.14		I
corn pone w/ white whole ground corn	122	31.1	2.7	21.7				0	.03			238	37			
meal—*1 piece*[1]	60	3.2	0.6				0	.09	0.5			37	98	.70		456
cornbread easy mix, dry, Aunt Jemima	147	3.3	2.4	25.9	6.2	1.0		0	.13	.04	6	448	6	11	.23	
⅓ cup	37	4.0	1.0	1.1	0.5	0	44	.19	1.9	.09	.14	42	202	1.30	.050	I
cornbread, from mix	188	19.1	4.3	28.9		1.4	26	0	.16	.06	7	467	44	12	.38	.130
1 slice (3 ¾" x 2 ½" x 4/4")	60	6.0	1.6	3.1	0.7	37	123	.15	1.2	.10	.26	77	226	1.14	.037	818
cornbread, homemade w/ low fat milk	173	25.4	4.4	28.3			35	0	.19	.07	12	428	162	16	.39	.077
1 slice (2 ½" x 1 ½")	65	4.6	1.0	1.2	2.1	26	180	.19	1.5	.10	.22	96	110	1.63	.033	818
cornbread, homemade w/ whole milk	176	25.1	4.4	28.3		2.3	28	0	.19	.07	12	428	161	16	.38	.077
1 piece (2 ½" x 1 ½")	65	5.0	1.3	1.3	2.1	28	158	.19	1.5	.10	.22	95	109	1.63	.033	818
cornbread w/ honey butter, frzn, Marie	200		2.0	29.0	10.0	2.0		2				340	60			
Callender's—*2 oz piece w/ 1 T butter*	65	8.0	3.0			10	100							1.08		I
date nut loaf, Thomas'	80		1.0	16.0	5.0	1.0	0	0				135	0			
1 oz	28	2.0	0.0			0							.72		I	
hush puppy, homemade	74	6.4	1.7	10.1		0.6	9	0	.07	.02	4	147	61	5	.15	.048
1 hush puppy (2 ¼" x 1 ¼")	22	3.0	0.5	0.7	1.6	10	31	.08	0.6	.04	.08	32	42	.67	.015	818
pumpkin, homemade	199	18.5	2.4	30.7			334	1	.10	.02	7	188	11	8	.20	.142
1 slice	60	7.7	1.2	1.9	4.1	26	3259	.09	0.8	.05	.17	55	32	.99	.046	818

17.4 BREADS, YEAST & UNLEAVENED[2]

bran, country, Bakery Light	80		4.0	21.0	3.0	5.0	0	0				180	40			
2 slices	43	1.0	0.0			0	0							.72		I
Bran'ola Original	90		4.0	18.0	3.0	3.0	0	0				125	0			
1 slice	38	2.0	0.0			0	0							1.08		I
bread crumbs																
dry, grated	427	6.7	13.5	78.3		2.6	0	0	.47	.11	27	931	245	50	1.32	.883
1 cup	108	5.8	1.4	2.3	1.7	0	1	.83	7.4	.02	.33	239	159	6.61	.179	818
dry, grated, seasoned	440	6.7	17.0	84.5		5.0	4	0	.20	.16	24	3180	119	46	1.09	.925
1 cup	120	3.1	0.9	1.2	0.8	2	17	.19	3.3	.04	.26	324	160	3.82	.186	818
dry, seasoned, Contadina	100		3.0	19.0	1.0	1.0	0	0				700	60			
¼ cup	28	1.5	0.0			0	0							1.40		I
buttermilk, country, Arnold	100		4.0	18.0	3.0	1.0	0	0	.10			170	20			
1 slice	38	2.0	0.0			0	0	.15	0.8					1.08		I
cinn, apple & walnut, Pepperidge Farms	76		1.9	11.5				0	.08			92	9			
.9 oz slice	25	2.5					0	.08	0.9			33		.70		I
cinn, Pepperidge Farms	91		2.2	15.0				0	.06			112	11			
1 oz slice	28	2.5					0	.11	0.9			28		.70		I
corn & molasses, Pepperidge Farms	72		1.8	14.4				0	.08			136	16			
.9 oz slice	25	0.8					0	.09	0.8			47		.90		I
cracked wheat	65	8.9	2.2	12.4		1.4	0	0	.06	.08	10	135	11	13	.31	.343
1 slice	25	1.0	0.2	0.5	0.2	0	0	.09	0.9	.01	.13	44	38	.70	.056	818
cracked wheat, Pepperidge Farms	73		2.3	13.2				0	.06			146	7			
.9 oz slice	25	1.2					0	.09	0.9			42		.80		I
cranberry, Arnold	70		2.0	14.0	3.0	1.0	0	0				80	0			
1 slice	25	1.0	0.0			0	0							.72		I
croissant, petite all butter, Pepperidge	117		2.6	13.4				0	.08			166	25			
Farms—*1 oz croissant*	30	5.9					0	.14	0.9			35		.90		I
date walnut, Pepperidge Farms	96		2.3	14.3				0	.08			106	9			
1 oz slice	28	3.3					0	.08	0.8			48		.70		I

	KCAL	H₂O (g)	PRO (g)	CHO (g)	SUGR (g)	DFIB (g)	A (RE)	C (mg)	B-2 (mg)	B-6 (mg)	FOL (mcg)	Na (mg)	Ca (mg)	Mg (mg)	Zn (mg)	Mn (mg)
	WT (g)	FAT (g)	SFA (g)	MUFA (g)	PUFA (g)	CHOL (mg)	A (IU)	B-1 (mg)	NIA (mg)	B-12 (mcg)	PANT (mg)	K (mg)	P (mg)	Fe (mg)	Cu (mg)	REF
egg	115	13.9	3.8	19.1		0.9	9	0	.17	.03	28	197	37	8	.32	.200
1 slice (5″ x 3″ x ½″)	40	2.4	0.6	1.1	0.4	20	30	.18	1.9	.04	.11	46	42	1.22	.065	818
french	81	8.3	2.7	14.8		0.6			.07	.01	9	163	22	6	.24	.154
1 slice	28	1.1						.11	1.2		.12 •	32	30	.92	.056	I
for french toast, Pepperidge Farms	154		4.5	28.3				0	.13			275	52			
2 oz slice	57	2.6					0	.18	2.2			53		1.90		I
for toast, Pepperidge Farms	157		5.1	29.3				0	.17			279	69			
2 oz slice	57	2.2					0	.26	2.3			52		2.10		
fully baked, enr, Pepperidge Farms	76		2.5	14.6				0	.10			142	27			
1 oz slice	28	0.8					0	.12	1.3			32		1.10		I
loaf, from refrig dough, crusty, Pillsbury	56	9.8	2.4	10.6				0	.07			119	4			
1″ slice	24	0.3					0	.11	0.9			15	14	.78		I
stick, Francisco	70		3.0	14.0	1.0	0	0					150	20			
1 oz	28	1.0	0.0			0	0							.72		I
twin, Pepperidge Farms	76		2.5	14.5				0	.09			158	24			
1 oz slice	28	1.0					0	.13	1.2			30		.90		I
french/vienna/sourdough	69	8.6	2.2	13.0		0.8	0	0	.08	.01	8	152	19	7	.22	.127
1 med slice (4 ¾″ x 4″ x ½″)	25	0.8	0.2	0.3	0.2	0	0	.13	1.2	.00	.10	28	26	.63	.048	818
garlic bread, frzn, Marie Callender's	190		4.0	25.0	5.0	2.0	0					290	100			
2 oz piece	57	8.0	2.0			0	100							1.80		I
garlic bread w/ parmesan & romano, frzn, Marie Callender's—2 oz piece	200		5.0	23.0	2.0	2.0	•	0				430	200			
	57	10.0	3.0			5	300							1.44		I
honey & oat bran, Roman Meal	71		3.0	12.7		0.9			.12			140	19			
1 oz slice	28	1.1				0		.18	1.1					1.00		I
honey bran, Pepperidge Farms	92		2.9	17.9				0	.09			161	10			
1.2 oz slice	34	1.0					0	.14	1.4			57		1.30		I
honey nut & oat bran, Roman Meal	72		3.3	12.1		1.0			.12			130	21			
1 oz slice	28	1.6				0		.18	1.1					1.00		I
honey wheat berry																
Arnold	70		3.0	16.0	2.0	3.0	0	0				160	0			
1 slice	32	1.0	0.0			0	0							.72		I
Bran'ola	90		3.0	19.0	3.0	3.0	0	0				150	0			
1 slice	38	1.5	0.0			0	0							1.08		I
Pepperidge Farms	71		2.1	13.6				0	.06			143	7			
.9 oz slice	25	0.9					0	.08	0.8			42		.80		I
Roman Meal	64		3.4	12.7		1.6			.10			141	19			
1 oz slice	28	0.7				0		.20	1.2					1.10		I
indian (navajo) fry	296	23.9	6.4	48.0		1.6	0	0	.27	.02	12	626	210	14	.45	.423
5″ dia	90	8.6	1.7	2.8	3.6	0	0	.39	3.3	.00	.18	67	141	3.24	.092	818
irish soda, homemade	174	18.1	4.0	33.6		1.6	30	0	.16	.05	6	239	49	14	.34	.213
1 slice	60	3.0	0.7	1.2	0.9	11	116	.18	1.4	.03	.15	160	68	1.61	.078	818
italian	81	10.7	2.6	15.0		0.8	0	0	.09	.01	9	175	23	8	.26	.139
1 slice (4 ½″ x 3 ¼″ x ¾″)	30	1.1	0.3	0.2	0.4	0	0	.14	1.3	.00	.11	33	31	.88	.057	818
Bakery Light	80		4.0	21.0	3.0	5.0	0	0				200	40			
2 slices	43	1.0	0.0			0	0							.72		I
brown & serve, enr, Pepperidge Farms	75		2.4	13.9				0	.09			154	25			
1 oz slice	28	1.2					0	.14	1.3			31		.80		I
Francisco	110		4.0	23.0	0.0	1.0	0	0				240	60			
2 slices	48	1.0	0.0			0	0							1.44		I
Savoni's	60		2.0	13.0	0	0						125	20			
1 slice	27	0.5	0.0			0	0							.72		I
Francisco	70		3.0	14.0	0.0	1.0	0	0				135	20			
1 oz	28	1.0	0.0			0	0							1.08		I
mixed grain/whole grain/7-grain	65	9.8	2.6	12.1		1.7	0	0	.09	.09	12	127	24	14	.33	.386
1 slice	26	1.0	0.2	0.4	0.2	0	0	.11	1.1	.02	.13	53	46	.90	.066	818
multi-grain, Roman Meal Sun Grain	71		3.1	12.6		1.6			.09			140	20			
1 oz slice	28	1.6				0		.23	1.0					1.00		I
multi-grain, very thin sliced, Pepperidge Farms—.56 oz slice	43		1.4	7.6				0	.04			89	7			
	16	0.7					0	.06	0.7			29		.60		I
Nutty Grains, Bran'ola	90		4.0	18.0	3.0	3.0	0	0				95	0			
1 slice	38	2.5	0.0			0	0							1.08		I

	KCAL / WT (g)	H₂O / FAT (g)	PRO / SFA (g)	CHO / MUFA (g)	SUGR / PUFA (g)	DFIB / CHOL	A (RE) / A (IU)	C / B-1 (mg)	B-2 / NIA	B-6 / B-12	FOL / PANT	Na / K	Ca / P	Mg / Fe	Zn / Cu	Mn / REF
oat & honey, Pepperidge Farms	74		2.6	11.1				0	.06			107	5			
.8 oz slice	23	2.2					0	.08	0.7			24		.80		I
oat bran	71	13.2	3.1	11.9		1.3	0	0	.10	.01	8	122	20	9	.28	.207
1 slice	30	1.3	0.2	0.5	0.5	0	2	.15	1.4	.00	.05	34	32	.94	.035	818
oat bran, split top, Roman Meal	68		2.9	12.9		1.1			.10			136	25			
1 oz slice	28	0.9				0		.12	1.3					1.10		I
oat, Bran'ola	90		4.0	18.0	3.0	3.0	0	0				115	0			
1 slice	38	2.5	0.5			0	0							1.08		I
oat, Roman Meal	71		2.6	13.6		0.7			.10			141	16			
1 oz slice	28	1.0				0		.20	1.1					1.00		I
oatmeal	73	9.9	2.3	13.1		1.1	1	0	.06	.02	7	162	18	10	.28	.254
1 slice	27	1.2	0.2	0.4	0.5	0	4	.11	0.8	.01	.09	38	34	.73	.056	818
Bakery Light	80		4.0	20.0	3.0	4.0	0	0				200	40			
2 slices	43	1.0	0.0			0	0							.72		I
Pepperidge Farms	94		2.9	17.5				0	.07			198	17			
1.2 oz slice	34	1.4						.11	1.2			36		1.00		I
very thin sliced, low cal, Pepperidge Farms—*.6 oz slice*	43		1.4	7.9				0	.04			81	13			
	16	0.6						.05	0.6			20		.60		I
w/ raisins, Pepperidge Farms	80		2.7	14.3				0	.07			93	12			
1 oz slice	28	1.3						.09	1.0			67		.90		I
onion rye, August Bros	80		3.0	16.0		1.0	0	0				140	40			
1 slice	32	1.0	0.0			0	0							.72		I
orange & raisin, Pepperidge Farms	75		1.7	13.3				0	.05			72	8			
.9 oz slice	25	1.7					0	.10	0.6			39		.80		I
pita																
oat bran, Sahara	130		6.0	30.0	3.0	3.0	0	0				300	100			
2 oz pita	57	1.0	0.0			0	0							1.80		I
white	165	19.3	5.5	33.4		1.3	0	0	.20	.02	14	322	52	16	.50	.289
1 pita (6 ½" dia)	60	0.7	0.1	0.1	0.3	0	0	.36	2.8	.00	.24	72	58	1.57	.101	818
white, large, Sahara/Middle Eastern	215		8.0	46.0	3.0	1.0	0	0	.07			390	8			
1 large pita[3]	85	1.0	0.3			0		.12	1.2					1.71		I
white, mini, Sahara/Middle Eastern	70		3.0	15.0	0	0	.00					128	20			
1 mini pita[3]	28	0.0	0.0			0	0	.03	0.0					.36		I
white, Sahara/Middle Eastern	145		5.5	30.0	2.5	1.0	0	0	.07			260	60			
2 oz pita[4]	57	0.8	0.0			0		.06	0.8					1.26		I
whole wheat	170	19.6	6.3	35.2		4.7	0	0	.05	.15	22	340	10	44	.97	1.114
1 pita (6 ½" dia)	64	1.7	0.3	0.2	0.7	0	0	.22	1.8	.00	.35	109	115	1.85	.180	818
whole wheat, large, Middle Eastern	200		9.0	42.0	3.0	5.0	0	0	.07			350	0			
1 large pita	85	1.5	1.0			0		.30	2.0					1.44		I
whole wheat, mini, Sahara/Middle Eastern—*1 mini pita[3]*	65		3.0	13.0	2.0	0	0	0	.00			128	20			
	28	0.2	0.0			0	0	.09	0.8					.54		I
whole wheat, Sahara/Middle Eastern	135		6.5	28.5	2.0	4.0	0	0				270	50			
2 oz pita[5]	57	1.0	0.0			0	0							1.08		I
potato, Arnold Country	100		3.0	18.0	4.0	1.0	0	0	.07			150	0			
1 slice	38	2.0	0.0			0	0	.08	0.8					1.08		I
protein/gluten	47	7.6	2.3	8.3		0.6	0	0	.07	.01	7	104	24	10	.20	.137
1 slice	19	0.4	0.1	0.0	0.2	0	0	.07	0.8	.00	.08	60	33	.79	.098	818
pumpernickel	80	12.1	2.8	15.2		2.1	0	0	.10	.04	11	215	22	17	.47	.418
1 slice (5" x 4" x ⅜")	32	1.0	0.1	0.3	0.4	0	0	.10	1.0	.00	.13	67	57	.92	.092	818
Arnold/August Bros/Levy's	80		3.0	16.0	1.0	1.0	0	0				150	27			
1 slice[6]	32	0.8	0.0			0	0							.72		I
family, Pepperidge Farms	83		3.2	15.2				0	.08			231	24			
1.1 oz slice	32	1.0					0	.12	1.0			56		1.10		I
party slices, Pepperidge Farms	65		2.3	12.0				0	.07			164	18			
.8 oz slice	24	0.9						.09	0.8			37		.80		I
raisin	71	8.7	2.1	13.6		1.1	0	0	.10	.02	9	101	17	7	.19	.130
1 slice	26	1.1	0.3	0.6	0.2	0	1	.09	0.9	.00	.10	59	28	.75	.051	818
raisin & cinn, Arnold	70		2.0	14.0	3.0	0.0	0	0				90	0			
1 slice	27	1.0	0.0			0								.72		I
raisin, Sunmaid	70		2.0	14.0	3.0	0.0	0	0				85	0			
1 slice	27	1.0	0.0			0								.72		I

	KCAL / WT (g)	H₂O (g) / FAT (g)	PRO (g) / SFA (g)	CHO (g) / MUFA (g)	SUGR (g) / PUFA (g)	DFIB (g) / CHOL (mg)	A (RE) / A (IU)	C (mg) / B-1 (mg)	B-2 (mg) / NIA (mg)	B-6 (mg) / B-12 (mcg)	FOL (mcg) / PANT (mg)	Na (mg) / K (mg)	Ca (mg) / P (mg)	Mg (mg) / Fe (mg)	Zn (mg) / Cu (mg)	Mn (mg) / REF
raisin w/ cinn, Pepperidge Farms	86		2.1	15.6				0	.08			99	12			
1 oz slice	28	1.7					0	.10	1.0			54		.80		I
rice bran	66	11.1	2.4	11.7		1.3	0	0	.08	.06	8	119	19	19	.34	.378
1 slice	27	1.2	0.2	0.4	0.5	0	1	.18	1.8	.00	.10	53	43	.97	.045	818
Roman Meal Round Top	69		2.9	13.4		1.2			.10			140	25			
1 oz slice	28	0.9				0		.10	1.3					1.10		I
rye																
american	83	11.9	2.7	15.5		1.9	0	0	.11	.02	16	211	23	13	.36	.264
1 slice (5" x 4" x ½")	32	1.1	0.2	0.4	0.3	0	1	.14	1.2	.00	.14	53	40	.91	.060	818
& pumpernickel, August Bros	90		3.0	18.0	1.0	1.0	0	0				170	40			
1 slice	38	1.0	0.0			0	0							1.08		I
deli, Arnold	80		3.0	16.0	0	0						150	20			
1 slice	32	0.5	0.0			0	0							.72		I
dijon, Arnold	80		3.0	16.0	1.0	0						200	20			
1 slice	32	1.0	0.0			0	0							.72		I
dijon, Pepperidge Farms	55		2.4	9.6				0	.07			180	17			
.8 oz slice	22	0.8					0	.60	0.8			32		.60		I
dijon, thick sliced, Pepperidge Farms	85		3.3	14.9				0	.09			255	23			
1.1 oz slice	32	1.4					0	.12	1.2			51		1.10		I
dill, Arnold	80		3.0	16.0	2.0	0						160	40			
1 slice	32	1.0	0.0			0	0							.72		I
family, Pepperidge Farms	84		3.1	15.7				0	.10			215	26			
1.1 oz slice	32	1.0					0	.14	1.2			46		1.00		I
party slices, Pepperidge Farms	65		2.3	12.2				0	.08			248	24			
.8 oz slice	24	0.7					0	.12	1.0			56		1.10		I
seedless, Pepperidge Farms	84		3.1	15.5				0	.09			209	24			
1.1 oz slice	32	1.0					0	.14	1.2			46		1.10		I
soft, Arnold/Bakery Light	80		3.0	15.0	1.0	0						170	20			
1 slice	30	1.0	0.0			0	0							.72		I
thin, Arnold/August Bros/Levy's	90		3.0	19.0	1.0	1.3	0	0				183	33			
2 slices[6]	39	1.0	0.0			0	0							1.08		I
w/o seeds, Arnold/August Bros/Levy's	73		3.0	16.0	1.0	0						150	20			
1 slice[6]	32	0.8	0.0			0	0							.72		I
w/ seeds, Arnold/August Bros/Levy's	73		3.0	16.0	1.0	0						147	33			
1 slice[6]	32	1.0	0.0			0	0							.72		I
seven grain, Bran'ola	90		4.0	18.0	3.0	3.0	0	0				120	0			
1 slice	38	2.0	0.0			0	0							.72		I
seven grain, Roman Meal	66		3.4	12.9		1.2			.10			140	21			
1 oz slice	28	0.7				0		.20	1.0					1.10		I
sourdough, Arnold/August Bros/Francisco—1 slice[6]	93		3.7	20.7	1.7	1.0	0	0				230	27			
	42	0.8	0.0			0	0							1.08		I
sourdough, brown 'n serve, Francisco	70		2.0	14.0	0.0	1.0	0	0				240	40			
1 slice	28	0.5	0.0			0	0							1.08		I
spoon bread w/ white whole ground corn-meal—1 cup[7]	468	151.2	16.1	40.6				1	.43			1157	230			
	240	27.4	8.7				700	.22	1.0			317	394	2.40		456
sprouted wheat, Pepperidge Farms	69		2.6	11.0				0	.04			104	9			
.9 oz slice	25	1.6					0	.08	0.8			58		.80		I
texas toast, August Bros	150		5.0	28.0	3.0	1.0	0	0				260	60			
1 slice	57	3.0	0.5			0	0							1.80		I
Toast-R-Cakes, Thomas'	103		1.7	17.1	8.8	1.0	0					173				
1 cake[8]	33	3.7	0.5			0								.59	I	
twelve grain, Bran'ola	90		4.0	18.0	3.0	3.0	0	0				135	0			
1 slice	38	2.0	0.0			0	0							1.08		I
vienna, Pepperidge Farms	73		2.5	12.8				0	.08			126	18			
.9 oz slice	25	1.3					7	.10	1.2			27		.90		I
wheat																
Arnold Country	90		4.0	18.0	4.0	1.0	0	0	.07			170	0			
1 slice	38	1.5	0.0			0	0	.12	0.8					.72		I
Brick Oven	110		5.0	21.0	2.0	3.0	0	0				170	0			
2 slices	48	3.0	0.5			0	0							.72		I

	KCAL / WT (g)	H₂O (g) / FAT (g)	PRO (g) / SFA (g)	CHO (g) / MUFA (g)	SUGR (g) / PUFA (g)	DFIB (g) / CHOL (mg)	A (RE) / A (IU)	C (mg) / B-1 (mg)	B-2 (mg) / NIA (mg)	B-6 (mg) / B-12 (mcg)	FOL (mcg) / PANT (mg)	Na (mg) / K (mg)	Ca (mg) / P (mg)	Mg (mg) / Fe (mg)	Zn (mg) / Cu (mg)	Mn (mg) / REF
dark, Bran'ola	90		4.0	16.0	3.0	3.0	0	0				130	0			
1 slice	38	2.0	0.0			0	0							.72		I
family, Pepperidge Farms	71		2.3	13.0				0	.06			129	24			
1 oz slice	27	1.1					0	.11	0.9			42		.80		I
golden, Bakery Light	80		4.0	20.0	3.0	5.0	0	0				180	40			
2 slices	43	0.5	0.0			0	0							.72		I
hearty, Bran'ola	90		4.0	16.0	2.0	3.0	0	0				130				
1 slice	38	3.0	0.5			0	0							.72		I
lite, Thomas'	40		2.0	6.0		2.0						75	100			
1 slice	19	1.0				0								.36		I
loaf, from dough, Pipin' Hot Pillsbury	73	11.0	2.6	11.9				0	.06			167	5			
1" slice	28	1.5					0	.59	0.9			19	24	.80		I
Pepperidge Farms	97		3.0	17.9				0	.07			189	10			
1.2 oz slice	34	1.5					0	.12	1.2			55		1.00		I
Sunny Valley	100		4.0	20.0	3.0	2.0	0	0	.07			220	0			
2 slices	43	1.5	0.0			0	0	.12	1.2					1.08		I
very thin sliced, Pepperidge Farms	42		1.5	7.4				0	.02			78	16			
.6 oz slice	16	0.7					0	.04	0.5			30		.50		I
wheat bran	89	13.6	3.2	17.2		1.4	0	0	.10	.06	9	175	27	29	.49	.600
1 slice	36	1.2	0.3	0.6	0.2	0	0	.14	1.6	.00	.19	82	67	1.11	.080	818
wheat germ	73	10.4	2.7	13.5		0.6	0	0	.11	.03	15	155	25	10	.38	.325
1 slice	28	0.8	0.2	0.4	0.2	0	0	.10	1.3	.02	.09	71	45	.97	.052	818
wheat germ, Pepperidge Farms	66		2.6	12.0				0	.09			137	22			
.9 oz slice	25	0.8					0	.09	1.0			47		.90		I
wheat/wheat berry	65	9.3	2.3	11.8		1.1	0	0	.07	.02	10	133	26	12	.26	.256
1 slice	25	1.0	0.2	0.4	0.2	0	0	.10	1.0	.00	.11	50	38	.83	.053	818
white	67	9.2	2.0	12.4	0.9	0.6	0	0	.09	.02	9	135	27	6	.15	.096
1 slice	25	0.9	0.2	0.4	0.2	0	0	.12	1.0	.01	.10	30	24	.76	.032	818
Arnold Country	100		3.0	19.0	4.0		0	0	.07			190	0			
1 slice	38	1.5	0.0			0	0	.15	0.8					1.08		I
Bakery Light	80		4.0	21.0	3.0	4.0	0	0				200	40			
2 slices	43	0.5	0.0			0	0							.72		I
Brick Oven	130		3.0	24.0	4.0	1.0	0	0	.10			250	40			
2 slices	48	2.5	0.0			0	0	.15	1.2					1.44		I
loaf, from dough, Pipin' Hot Pillsbury	74	11.0	2.6	12.0				0	.07			167	5			
1" slice	28	1.5					0	.58	0.9			17	21	.79		I
Pepperidge Farms	200		5.8	36.6				0	.16			358	22			
2.4 oz slice	68	3.4					0	.27	2.1			50		2.70		I
Rich's, from dough, baked	116	16.5	3.9	22.7					.14			300	110	11	.30	
2 slices	46	1.1				0		.18	1.7			51	55	2.10	.070	I
sandwich, enr, Pepperidge Farms	129		3.7	23.6				0	.13			258	38			
1.6 oz slice	45	2.2					0	.21	1.8			41		1.30		I
Sunny Valley	100		4.0	21.0	2.0	1.0	0	0	.10			210	0			
2 slices	43	1.5	0.0			0	0	.15	1.2					1.08		I
thin sliced, enr, Pepperidge Farms	64		1.8	11.6				0	.06			119	23			
.8 oz slice	23	1.2					0	.09	0.7			24		.70		I
Toasting, enr, Pepperidge Farms	87		2.8	16.3				0	.12			202	30			
1.1 oz slice	32	1.1					0	.14	1.2			42		1.00		I
very thin sliced, enr, Pepperidge Farms	42		1.3	8.2				0	.05			82	14			
.6 oz slice	16	0.5					0	.06	0.6			15		.50		I
whole wheat	69	10.6	2.7	12.9	1.1	1.9	0	0	.06	.05	14	148	20	24	.54	.651
1 slice	28	1.2	0.3	0.5	0.3	0	0	.10	1.1	.00	.15	71	64	.92	.080	818
100%, Roman Meal	67		3.3	11.1		1.6			.10			139	27			
1 oz slice	28	0.9				0		.14	1.4					1.30		I
100%, Roman Meal Harvest Recipe	63		3.0	12.1		1.5			.10			138	28			
1 oz slice	28	0.8				0		.10	1.2					.90		I
homemade	128	15.0	3.9	23.6		2.8	0	0	.10	.09	22	159	15	37	.69	.865
1 slice	46	2.5	0.4	0.5	1.4		0	.14	1.8	.00	.22	144	86	1.43	.116	818
stoneground 100%, Arnold	60		3.0	12.0	2.0	2.0	0	0				115	0			
1 slice	27	1.0	0.0			0	0							.36		I
thin sliced, Pepperidge Farms	68		2.4	11.9				0	.04			119	22			
.9 oz slice	25	1.1					0	.08	0.8			56		.80		I

							Vitamins						Minerals				
KCAL	H₂O (g)	PRO (g)	CHO (g)	SUGR (g)	DFIB (g)		A (RE)	C (mg)	B-2 (mg)	B-6 (mg)	FOL (mcg)		Na (mg)	Ca (mg)	Mg (mg)	Zn (mg)	Mn (mg)
WT (g)	FAT (g)	SFA (g)	MUFA (g)	PUFA (g)	CHOL (mg)		A (IU)	B-1 (mg)	NIA (mg)	B-12 (mcg)	PANT (mg)		K (mg)	P (mg)	Fe (mg)	Cu (mg)	REF

17.5 BREADSTICKS

KCAL/WT	H₂O/FAT	PRO/SFA	CHO/MUFA	SUGR/PUFA	DFIB/CHOL	A(RE)/A(IU)	C/B-1	B-2/NIA	B-6/B-12	FOL/PANT	Na/K	Ca/P	Mg/Fe	Zn/Cu	Mn/REF
cracked pepper, Stella D'Oro															
70		2.0	11.0								290				
4 breadsticks — 16	2.0	0.0	0.0	1.0	0										I
fat-free, Stella D'Oro															
70		2.0	15.0	1.0	1.0						150				
2 breadsticks — 19	0.0	0.0	0.0	0.0	0										I
garlic, Lance															
109	1.1	3.5	20.7				0	.17			236	6			
2 breadsticks — 28	1.0	0.3	0.4	0.3	0	0	.18	1.2			28		1.60		I
garlic, Stella D'Oro															
40		1.0	7.0	0.0							60				
1 breadstick — 10	1.0	0.0	0.0	0.5	0										I
plain															
82	1.2	2.4	13.7		0.6	0	0	.11	.01	6	131	4	6	.18	.111
2 breadsticks — 20	1.9	0.3	0.7	0.7	0	0	.12	1.1	.00	.11	25	24	.86	.038	818
Keebler — 32		1.2	5.8			0	0	.03			17	2			
2 breadsticks[9] — 8	0.4	0.1		0.1	0	0	.05	0.6			15		.34		I
Lance — 109	1.1	3.5	20.7				0	.30			201	48			
2 breadsticks — 28	1.1	0.3	0.3	0.3	0	0	.19	1.6			28		1.42		I
Stella D'Oro — 40		1.0	7.0	0.0							40				
1 breadstick — 9	1.0	0.0	0.0	0.5	0										I
potato onion, Stella D'Oro															
70		2.0	11.0	0.0							300				
4 breadsticks — 16	2.0	0.0	0.0	1.0	0										I
sesame, Lance															
120	1.1	3.5	20.7				0	.22			202	72			
2 breadsticks — 28	2.6	0.3	1.2	1.1	0	0	.18	1.0			42		1.42		I
sesame, Stella D'Oro															
50		1.0	7.0								45				
1 breadstick — 11	2.5	0.0	0.5	1.0	0										I
soft, from refrig dough, Pillsbury															
101	15.4	3.3	16.6				1	.10			234	7			
1.4 oz breadstick — 39	2.3					0	1.51	1.2			24	29	1.05		I

17.6 CRACKERS & CROUTONS

KCAL/WT	H₂O/FAT	PRO/SFA	CHO/MUFA	SUGR/PUFA	DFIB/CHOL	A(RE)/A(IU)	C/B-1	B-2/NIA	B-6/B-12	FOL/PANT	Na/K	Ca/P	Mg/Fe	Zn/Cu	Mn/REF
bacon flavored thins, Nabisco															
160		3.0	19.0	2.0							460				
15 crackers — 31	8.0	1.5	3.0	0.5	0										I
Better Cheddars, Nabisco															
150		4.0	17.0								290				
22 crackers[10] — 30	8.0	2.0													I
Better Cheddars, red fat, Nabisco															
140		3.0	19.0								350				
24 crackers — 30	6.0	1.5	2.0	0.0											I
Big Town, Lance															
237	6.6	2.7	38.6					.11			141	55			
2 oz — 57	7.9						.05	0.6			291		1.05		I
Bonnie, Lance															
156	1.0	2.1	23.5				2	.19			175	14			
1.2 oz — 34	6.5	2.0	3.6	0.9	5	83	.12	1.3			40		1.08		I
Captain's Wafer															
Lance — 32	0.2	0.6	4.6					.02			58	10			
2 crackers — 7	1.0	0.2	0.6	0.1	0		.03	0.2			5		.18		I
low sodium, Lance — 32	0.2	0.5	4.8					.02			25	8			
2 crackers — 7	1.0	0.2	0.6	0.1	0		.03	0.2			9		.36		I
w/ cream cheese & chives, Lance — 174	1.1	3.7	22.9					.15			260	63			
1.3 oz — 37	9.0	2.0	5.6	1.4	2	16	.16	1.5			61				I
cheese															
71	0.4	1.4	8.2		0.3	4	0	.06	.08	4	141	21	5	.16	.089
14 1" sq crackers — 14	3.6	1.3	1.3	0.7	2	23	.08	0.7	.07	.07	21	31	.68	.030	818
Cheese Nips															
Air Crisps, Nabisco — 130		3.0	22.0	0.0							290				
32 crackers — 30	4.0	1.0	1.5	0.0											I
Nabisco — 150		3.0	18.0	0.0							310				
29 crackers — 30	6.0	1.5	2.5	0.5	0										I
red fat, Nabisco — 130		3.0	21.0	0.0							310				
31 crackers — 30	3.5	1.0	1.0	0.0	0										I
Cheese-On-Wheat, Lance															
181	0.7	4.1	22.3					.10			252	60			
1.3 oz — 37	9.0	1.9	5.2	1.9	2		.15	1.1			61		1.02		I

	KCAL / WT (g)	H₂O (g) / FAT (g)	PRO (g) / SFA (g)	CHO (g) / MUFA (g)	SUGR (g) / PUFA (g)	DFIB (g) / CHOL (mg)	A (RE) / A (IU)	C (mg) / B-1 (mg)	B-2 (mg) / NIA (mg)	B-6 (mg) / B-12 (mcg)	FOL (mcg) / PANT (mg)	Na (mg) / K (mg)	Ca (mg) / P (mg)	Mg (mg) / Fe (mg)	Zn (mg) / Cu (mg)	Mn (mg) / REF
Cheese Tidbit, Nabisco	150		2.0	17.0								420				
32 crackers	30	8.0	1.5			0										I
cheese w/ cheese filling, Little Debbie	199	1.1	5.4	22.5	2.9	1.2		0	.20			364	16			
1.4 oz pkg	40	9.7	2.2			0	18	.18	3.4					1.56		I
cheese w/ peanut butter filling	34	0.3	0.9	4.0		0.2	2	0	.02	.10	2	69	6	4	.08	.053
1 sandwich	7	1.6	0.4	0.8	0.3	0	22	.03	0.5	.00	.04	17	23	.20	.016	818
cheese w/ peanut butter filling, Little Debbie—.9 oz	131	0.9	3.1	14.5	1.3	1.0		0	.05			210	10			
	26	6.7	1.1			0	3	.09	1.5					.99		I
Chicken in a Biskit, Nabisco	160		2.0	17.0	2.0							270				
14 crackers	30	9.0	1.5			0										I
Classic Golden, reduced fat, Snackwell's	60		1.0	11.0	2.0	0.0						140				
6 crackers	14	1.0	0.0	0.0	0.0	0										I
Club, Keebler	34		0.5	4.2					.03			78				
2 crackers	7	1.4	0.3		0.1	0		.04	0.0			9		.22		I
cracker pepper, Snackwell's	60		2.0	13.0	1.0							150				
7 crackers	15	0.0	0.0	0.0	0.0	0										I
croutons	122	1.6	3.6	22.1		1.5	0	0	.08	.01	7	209	23	9	.27	.150
1 cup	30	2.0	0.5	1.0	0.3	0	0	.19	1.6	.00	.13	37	35	1.22	.049	818
crispy, Arnold	30		1.0	5.0	0.0	0.0	0	0				65	0			
2 T¹¹	7	1.0	0.0			0	0							.36		I
seasoned	186	1.4	4.3	25.4		2.0	2	0	.17	.03	16	495	38	17	.38	.206
1 cup	40	7.3	2.0	3.8	1.0	1	8	.20	1.9	.03	.33	72	56	1.13	.067	818
french onion, reduced fat, Snackwell's	120		2.0	24.0	2.0	1.0						290				
32 crackers	30	2.0	0.0	0.0	1.0	0										I
Gold-N-Chee, Lance	179	1.0	1.7	22.9					.11			410	28			
1.4 oz	39	9.0	2.3	4.9	1.8	4		.24	1.2			40		1.19		I
Harvest Crisps, 5 grain, Nabisco	130		3.0	23.0	4.0	1.0						300				
13 crackers	31	3.5	0.5			0										I
Lanchee & Salsa, Lance	168	3.0	2.7	21.2	3.6	0.6		1	.19			327	96			
1.25 oz	35	8.0	1.2			3	53	.36	0.8			216	142	1.10		I
Lanchee, Lance	184	1.1	5.0	19.4					.15			108	20			
1.2 oz	35	11.0	2.1	5.7	3.2	2		.11	1.9					.93		I
malt, Lance	187	1.0	5.3	16.4					.13			126	68			
1.2 oz	35	11.0	2.1	5.9	3.0	0		.11	1.1			43		.72		I
matzo	112	1.2	2.8	23.7		0.9	0	0	.08	.03	4	1	4	7	.19	.184
1 matzo (1 oz)	28	0.4	0.1	0.0	0.2	0	0	.11	1.1	.00	.13	32	25	.90	.017	818
egg	111	1.8	3.5	22.3		0.8	4	0	.18	.02	8	6	11	7	.21	.170
1 matzo (1 oz)	28	0.6	0.2	0.2	0.1	25	12	.18	1.4	.14	.12	43	45	.77	.045	818
egg & onion	111	2.0	2.8	21.9		1.4	5	0	.12	.03	3	81	10	9	.21	.233
1 matzo (1 oz)	28	1.1	0.3	0.3	0.3	15	17	.16	1.4	.06	.16	24	25	1.24	.023	818
whole wheat	100	1.4	3.7	22.4		3.3	0	0	.08	.05	10	1	7	38	.74	.992
1 matzo (1 oz)	28	0.4	0.1	0.1	0.2	0	0	.10	1.5	.00	.35	90	86	1.32	.099	818
melba toast	20	0.3	0.6	3.8		0.3	0	0	.01	.00	1	41	5	3	.10	.056
1 toast	5	0.2	0.0	0.0	0.1	0	0	.02	0.2	.00	.03	10	10	.19	.014	818
Keebler	25		1.0	4.0					.03			33	2			
2 pieces⁹	5	0.1	0.0		0.0	0		.03	0.4			9		.30		I
oblong, Lance	37	0.6	1.5	7.4								8				
2 pieces	9	0.2	0.0	0.0	0.0	0						14				I
round, Lance	20		0.9	3.7				0	.04			32	7			
.2 oz	5	0.1	0.0	0.0	0.1	0	10	.03	0.4			10		.30		I
rye/pumpernickel	74	0.9	2.2	14.7		1.5	0	0	.05	.02	4	171	15	7	.26	.140
1 toast	19	0.6	0.1	0.2	0.3	0	0	.09	0.9	.00	.09	37	35	.70	.076	818
wheat	19	0.3	0.6	3.8		0.4	0	0	.01	.01	1	42	2	3	.08	.053
1 toast	5	0.1	0.0	0.0	0.0	0	0	.02	0.3	.00	.03	7	8	.23	.013	818
milk	55	0.6	0.9	8.4		0.2	1	0	.05	.00	2	71	21	3	.08	.066
1 cracker	12	1.9	0.4	1.0	0.3	2	4	.06	0.5	.01	.04	14	36	.43	.027	818
multigrain, Lance	69	0.5	1.7	9.6	1.3	0.7			.09			104	22			
4 crackers	15	2.7	0.6			0		.09	0.7			32				I
multigrain thins, Nabisco	130		2.0	21.0	4.0	2.0						290				
17 crackers	30	4.0	0.5	1.5	0.0	0										I
Nip-Chee, Lance	178	1.0	4.4	20.6				0	.18			315	72			
1.3 oz	37	9.0	2.6	5.3	1.2	2		.16	2.0			41		1.00		I

	KCAL	H₂O (g)	PRO (g)	CHO (g)	SUGR (g)	DFIB (g)	A (RE)	C (mg)	B-2 (mg)	B-6 (mg)	FOL (mcg)	Na (mg)	Ca (mg)	Mg (mg)	Zn (mg)	Mn (mg)
	WT (g)	FAT (g)	SFA (g)	MUFA (g)	PUFA (g)	CHOL (mg)	A (IU)	B-1 (mg)	NIA (mg)	B-12 (mcg)	PANT (mg)	K (mg)	P (mg)	Fe (mg)	Cu (mg)	REF
Nut-O-Lunch, Lance	136	0.4	3.5	18.1					.27			106				
1 oz	28	5.9	1.5	3.1	1.3	0		.07	1.7			70			.92	I
oat thins, Nabisco	140		3.0	20.0	2.0	2.0						190				
18 crackers	30	6.0	1.0	2.0	0.5	0										I
oyster & soup																
Keebler	79		1.7	12.8					.07			176	3			
50 small	18	2.2	0.5		0.2	0		.07	1.0			23			.79	I
Lance	65	0.4	1.5	9.8					.07			163	4			
.5 oz	14	1.9	0.5	1.0	0.4	0		.09	0.5			16			.52	I
Nabisco	60		1.0	11.0	0.0							230				
23 crackers	15	1.5	0.0	0.5	0.0	0										I
peanut butter & jelly, Little Debbie	134	3.2	1.6	21.6	12.5	0.6		0	.04			103	7			
1.1 oz	32	5.0	1.0			2	2	.09	0.6						.70	I
peanut butter Combos	258		7.6	23.6				0	.12			351	53			
1.7 oz	48	14.8					5	.09	3.2					1.57		I
peanut butter Ritz Bits, Nabisco	150		3.0	18.0	3.0	1.0						200				
14 pieces	31	8.0	1.5	3.0	1.5	0										I
peanut butter wheat, Lance	192	1.1	6.3	18.1					.10			208	37			
1.3 oz	37	11.0	2.1	6.3	2.6			.15	1.1			67				
Ritz Air Crisps, Nabisco	140		2.0	22.0	3.0							240				
24 crackers	30	5.0	1.0	1.5	0.0	0										I
Ritz Bits, Nabisco	160		2.0	18.0	3.0	1.0						250				
48 crackers	30	9.0	1.5	3.0	0.5	0										I
Ritz, Nabisco	80		1.0	10.0	1.0							135				
5 crackers[12]	16	4.0	0.5	1.5	0.0	0										I
Ritz, red fat, Nabisco	70		1.0	11.0	2.0	0.0						140				
5 crackers	15	2.0				0										I
Ritz sour cream & onion Air Crisps,	140		2.0	22.0	3.0							310				
Nabisco—*23 crackers*	30	5.0	1.0	1.5	0.0	0										I
round	15	0.1	0.2	1.8		0.0	0	0	.01	.00	0	25	4	1	.02	.017
1 cracker	3	0.8	0.1	0.3	0.2	0	0	.01	0.1	.00	.01	4	7	.11	.006	818
Royal Lunch, Nabisco	50		8.0	0.0								65				
1 cracker	11	2.0	0.0	1.0	0.0	0										I
rusk	41	0.6	1.4	7.2			1	0	.04	.00	6	25	3	4	.11	.044
1 rusk	10	0.7	0.2	0.4	0.1	3	5	.04	0.5	.01	.04	25	15	.27	.025	818
Rye-Chee, Lance	193	1.6	4.4	22.4					.15			313	60			
1.4 oz	41	9.0	2.1	5.3	1.6	4		.17	1.7			38			1.19	I
rye, crispbread	37	0.6	0.8	8.2		1.7	0	0	.01	.02	2	26	3	8	.24	.248
1 cracker	10	0.1	0.0	0.0	0.1	0	0	.02	0.1	.00	.07	32	27	.24	.026	818
Rye Twins, Lance	32	0.2	0.7	4.5					.03			62				
2 crackers	7	1.0	0.2	0.6	0.2	0		.03	0.2			9			.22	I
rye wafers	84	1.3	2.4	20.1	0.8	5.7	1	0	.07	.07	11	199	10	30	.70	.629
1 triple cracker	25	0.2	0.0	0.0	0.1	0	6	.11	0.4	.00	.14	124	84	1.49	.115	818
rye wafers, seasoned	84	0.9	2.0	16.2		4.6	0	0	.05	.04	11	195	10	23	.56	.506
1 triple cracker	22	2.0	0.3	1.1	0.4	0	5	.07	0.5	.00	.12	100	68	.67	.109	818
rye w/ cheese filling	5	0.0	0.1	0.6		0.0	0	0	.00	.00	0	10	2	0	.01	.006
1 sandwich	1.0	0.2	0.1	0.1	0.0	0	0	.01	0.0	.00	.00	3	3	.02	.001	818
saltines	13	0.1	0.3	2.1		0.1	0	0	.01	.00	1	39	4	1	.02	.021
1 saltine	3	0.4	0.1	0.2	0.1	0	0	.02	0.2	.00	.01	4	3	.16	.006	818
fat-free, low-sodium	59	0.5	1.6	12.3		0.4	0	0	.09	.01	2	95	3	4	.14	.096
3 crackers	15	0.2	0.0	0.0	0.1	0	0	.08	0.9	.00	.06	17	17	1.16	.022	818
fat-free, Nabisco	60		2.0	12.0	0.0	0.0						180				
5 crackers	15	0.0	0.0	0.0	0.0	0										I
Lance	49	0.2	1.2	7.8					.05			130	3			
2 crackers	11	1.5	0.4	0.8	0.3	0		.07	0.4			13			.41	I
multigrain, Nabisco	60		1.0	10.0	0.0	1.0						150				
5 crackers	14	1.5	0.0	0.5	0.0	0										I
Nabisco	60		1.0	10.0	0.0							180				
5 crackers[13]	14	1.5	0.0	0.5	0.0	0										I
Zesta	26		0.6	4.3					.02			73	1			
2 crackers	6	0.7	0.2		0.1	0		.02	0.3			21			.26	I

							Vitamins					Minerals				
	KCAL	H₂O (g)	PRO (g)	CHO (g)	SUGR (g)	DFIB (g)	A (RE)	C (mg)	B-2 (mg)	B-6 (mg)	FOL (mcg)	Na (mg)	Ca (mg)	Mg (mg)	Zn (mg)	Mn (mg)
	WT (g)	FAT (g)	SFA (g)	MUFA (g)	PUFA (g)	CHOL (mg)	A (IU)	B-1 (mg)	NIA (mg)	B-12 (mcg)	PANT (mg)	K (mg)	P (mg)	Fe (mg)	Cu (mg)	REF
sandwich w/ cheese filling	33	0.3	0.7	4.3		0.1	0	0	.05	.00	1	98	18	3	.04	.020
1 sandwich	7	1.5	0.4	0.8	0.2	0	2	.03	0.3	.00	.03	30	28	.17	.006	818
sandwich w/ peanut butter filling	34	0.2	0.8	4.1		0.2	0	0	.02	.01	2	66	7	4	.07	.054
1 sandwich	7	1.7	0.4	0.9	0.3	0	0	.03	0.4	.00	.04	16	17	.21	.018	818
Sesame Twins, Lance	47	0.2	1.3	7.7	0.5	0.5			.04			79	16			
4 crackers	11	1.2	0.3	0.5	0.2	0	66	.05	0.3			7		.49		I
Sociables, Nabisco	80		1.0	9.0								150				
7 crackers	15	4.0	0.5	1.5	0.5	0										I
sour dough w/ cheddar, Lance	236	1.5	3.6	22.5	3.6	1.3			.14			423	79			
1.56 oz	44	14.6	4.1	8.7	1.8	6	66	.13	1.2			91		.66		I
swiss cheese, Nabisco	140		2.0	18.0	2.0							350				
15 crackers	29	7.0	1.5			0										I
Toastchee, Lance	198	1.0	5.6	19.1					.14			263	10			
1.4 oz	39	11.0	2.1	6.0	2.8	2		.15	0.9			71		1.04		I
Toasted Snacks, Keebler	29		0.5	3.9					.02			54	2			
2 crackers[14]	6	1.3	0.2		0.2	0		.02	0.3			9		.24		I
Toasty, Lance	180	1.1	4.9	17.5					.13			151				
1.2 oz	35	10.0	1.9	5.7	2.4	0		.13	1.2			64		.97		I
Toasty w/ peanut butter, Little Debbie	130	0.8	2.8	15.0	4.3	0.6		0	.11			242	7			
.9 oz pkg	26	6.5	1.4			0	3	.13	1.8					.81		I
Townhouse, Keebler	31		0.4	3.6					.02			51	1			
2 crackers	6	1.7	0.3		0.2	0		.02	0.3			6		.20		I
Triscuits																
Nabisco	140		3.0	21.0	0.0	4.0						170				
7 crackers[10]	31	5.0	1.0	1.5	0.5	0										I
red fat, Nabisco	130		3.0	24.0	0.0	4.0						180				
8 wafers	32	3.0	0.5	1.0	0.0	0										I
whole wheat n' rye, Nabisco	140		3.0	22.0	0.0	4.0						180				
7 wafers	32	5.0	1.0	1.5	0.5	0										I
Twigs sesame & cheese sticks, Nabisco	150		4.0	17.0	1.0							300				
15 pieces	30	7.0	1.5	3.0	1.0	0										I
Uneeda, Nabisco	60		1.0	11.0	0.0	1.0						110				
2 crackers	15	1.5	0.0	0.5	0.0	0										I
vegetable thins, Nabisco	160		2.0	19.0	2.0	1.0						310				
14 crackers	31	9.0	1.5			0										I
wafers w/ cheese filling, Lance	183	3.0	3.2	21.3	3.7	0.5		0	.11			450	75			
1.3 oz	37	9.5	2.1			4	45	.16	0.8			110		.94		I
wafers w/ honey peanut butter, Lance	187	3.0	5.1	20.2	0.6	1.1			.06			165	39			
1.3 oz	37	9.6	1.8			0		.13	4.7			105	113	.94		I
Waverly, Nabisco	70		1.0	10.0	0.0	0.0						135				
5 crackers	15	3.5	1.0	1.0	0.0	0										I
wheat	66	0.4	1.2	9.1		0.6	0	0	.05	.02	3	111	7	9	.22	.249
7 crackers	14	2.9	0.5	1.6	0.4	0	0	.07	0.7	.00	.07	26	31	.62	.045	818
wheat, Snackwell's	60		2.0	12.0	2.0	1.0						170				
5 crackers	15	0.0	0.0	0.0	0.0	0										I
wheat thins																
air crisps, Nabisco	130		2.0	21.0	3.0	1.0						290				
24 crackers	29	4.5	1.0	1.5	0.0	0										I
air crisps, ranch, Nabisco	140		2.0	21.0	3.0	1.0						290				
23 crackers	30	4.5	1.0	1.5	0.0	0										I
Nabisco	140		2.0	19.0	2.0	2.0						170				
16 crackers[10]	29	6.0	1.0	2.5	0.5	0										I
red fat, Nabisco	120		2.0	21.0	3.0	2.0						220				
18 crackers	29	4.0	0.5	1.5	0.0	0										I
Wheat Twins, Lance	32	0.2	0.6	4.7					.02			66				
2 crackers	7	1.0	0.2	0.6	0.2	0		.02	0.3			10		.34		I
wheat w/ cheddar cheese, Little Debbie	129	1.0	2.2	15.4	3.7	0.6		0	.21			252	29			
.9 oz pkg	26	6.6	1.6			3	16	.11	1.1					.65		I
wheat w/ cheese filling	35	0.2	0.7	4.1		0.2	1	0	.03	.02	1	64	14	4	.06	.062
1 sandwich	7	1.8	0.5	0.9	0.2	0	5	.03	0.2	.01	.03	21	27	.18	.011	818

	KCAL / WT (g)	H₂O (g) / FAT (g)	PRO (g) / SFA (g)	CHO (g) / MUFA (g)	SUGR (g) / PUFA (g)	DFIB (g) / CHOL (mg)	A (RE) / A (IU)	C (mg) / B-1 (mg)	B-2 (mg) / NIA (mg)	B-6 (mg) / B-12 (mcg)	FOL (mcg) / PANT (mg)	Na (mg) / K (mg)	Ca (mg) / P (mg)	Mg (mg) / Fe (mg)	Zn (mg) / Cu (mg)	Mn (mg) / REF
wheat w/ peanut butter filling	35	0.2	0.9	3.8		0.3	0	0	.02	.01	3	56	12	3	.06	.049
1 sandwich	7	1.9	0.4	1.0	0.4	0	0	.03	0.4	.00	.04	21	24	.19	.004	818
Wheatsworth stoneground, Nabisco	80		2.0	10.0	0.0	1.0						170				
5 crackers	16	3.0	0.5	1.0	0.0	0										I
whole grain wheat, Keebler	33		0.6	4.5					.02			66	2			
2 crackers	7	1.4	0.3		0.2	0		.04	0.4			11		.30		I
whole wheat	18	0.1	0.4	2.7		0.4	0	0	.00	.01	1	26	2	4	.09	.090
1 sq cracker	4	0.7	0.1	0.4	0.1	0		.01	0.2	.00	.03	12	12	.12	.018	818
Zesty Cheese, red fat, Snackwell's	120		3.0	23.0	2.0	1.0						330				
32 crackers	30	2.0	0.5	0.0	1.0	0										I
Zwieback, Nabisco	35		1.0	6.0	1.0	0.0						10				
1 piece	8	1.0				0										I

17.7 ENGLISH MUFFINS

	KCAL / WT (g)	H₂O (g) / FAT (g)	PRO (g) / SFA (g)	CHO (g) / MUFA (g)	SUGR (g) / PUFA (g)	DFIB (g) / CHOL (mg)	A (RE) / A (IU)	C (mg) / B-1 (mg)	B-2 (mg) / NIA (mg)	B-6 (mg) / B-12 (mcg)	FOL (mcg) / PANT (mg)	Na (mg) / K (mg)	Ca (mg) / P (mg)	Mg (mg) / Fe (mg)	Zn (mg) / Cu (mg)	Mn (mg) / REF
bran nut, Thomas'	140		5.0	23.0	4.0		0	0				200	60			
1 muffin	57	3.0	0.0			0	0							1.08		I
Bran'ola	130		6.0	29.0	5.0	3.0	0	0				160	60			
1 muffin	66	1.5	0.0			0	0							1.80		I
cinn apple, Pepperidge Farms	137		3.9	27.3				0	.15			211	31			
2 oz muffin	57	1.3					0	.21	1.7			94		1.50		I
cinn chip, Pepperidge Farms	157		4.3	28.3				0	.14			184	27			
2 oz muffin	57	3.0					0	.26	1.9			70		1.60		I
cinn raisin, Pepperidge Farms	149		4.2	29.3				0	.15			196	29			
2 oz muffin	57	1.7					0	.24	1.8			100		1.60		I
extra crisp, Arnold	120		4.0	25.0	2.0	1.0	0	0				190	60			
2 oz muffin	57	1.0	0.0			0	0							1.44		I
honey & oat bran, Roman Meal	149		5.7	27.1		1.8			.20			282	72			
1 muffin	62	2.5	0.3			0		.24	2.5					1.44		I
honey wheat, Thomas'	110		5.0	24.0	2.0	3.0	0	0				190	80			
1 muffin	57	1.0	0.0			0	0							1.08		I
mixed grain/granola	155	26.5	6.0	30.6		1.8	1	0	.21	.06	23	275	129	29	.64	.500
1 muffin	66	1.2	0.2	0.5	0.4	0	4	.28	2.4	.00	.30	103	98	1.99	.154	818
oat bran, Thomas'	120		4.0	26.0	2.0	2.0	0	0				210	80			
2 oz muffin	57	1.0	0.5			0	0							1.44		I
plain	134	24.0	4.4	26.2		1.5	0	0	.16	.02	21	264	99	12	.40	.203
1 muffin	57	1.0	0.1	0.2	0.5	0	0	.25	2.2	.02	.25	75	76	1.42	.074	818
Pepperidge Farms	142		3.8	28.0				0	.11				28			
2 oz muffin	57	1.7					0	.19	1.8			112		1.50		I
Thomas'	138		4.0	30.0	6.3	1.8	0	0				193	50			
1 muffin[15]	61	1.0	0.0			0	0							1.53		I
Thomas'	120		4.0	25.0	1.0	1.0	0	0				200	80			
2 oz muffin	57	1.0	0.0			0	0							1.44		I
raisin, Arnold	150		5.0	32.0	10.0	1.0	0	0				160	60			
1 muffin	66	1.0	0.0			0	0							1.44		I
raisin cinn/apple cinn	139	22.0	4.3	27.8		1.7	0	0	.17	.04	18	255	84	9	.57	.278
1 muffin	57	1.5	0.2	0.3	0.8	0	1	.22	2.0	.00	.14	119	44	1.38	.077	818
Roman Meal	148		5.8	29.8		2.7			.18			346	93			
2.3 oz muffin	66	0.8				0		.26	2.7					2.10		I
rye, Thomas'	120		5.0	24.0		3.0	0	0				210	60			
1 muffin	57	1.0				0	0							1.08		I
sandwich size, Thomas'	188		7.3	39.5	1.8	2.5	0	0				290	113			
1 large muffin[16]	92	1.8	0.0			0	0							2.48		I
sourdough, Pepperidge Farms	135		4.4	27.1				0	.17			259	25			
2 oz muffin	57	0.9					0	.25	1.9			102		1.90		I
sourdough, Thomas'	120		4.0	25.0	2.0	1.0	0	0				190	80			
1 muffin	57	1.0	0.0			0	0							1.80		I
wheat	127	24.1	5.0	25.5		2.6	0	0	.17	.05	22	218	101	22	.64	.587
1 muffin	57	1.1	0.2	0.2	0.5	0	1	.25	1.9	.00	.17	106	66	1.64	.085	818
whole wheat	134	30.2	5.8	26.7		4.4	0	0	.09	.11	32	420	175	47	1.06	1.181
1 muffin	66	1.4	0.2	0.3	0.6	0	0	.20	2.3	.00	.46	139	186	1.62	.136	818

						Vitamins					Minerals				
KCAL	H₂O (g)	PRO (g)	CHO (g)	SUGR (g)	DFIB (g)	A (RE)	C (mg)	B-2 (mg)	B-6 (mg)	FOL (mcg)	Na (mg)	Ca (mg)	Mg (mg)	Zn (mg)	Mn (mg)
WT (g)	FAT (g)	SFA (g)	MUFA (g)	PUFA (g)	CHOL (mg)	A (IU)	B-1 (mg)	NIA (mg)	B-12 (mcg)	PANT (mg)	K (mg)	P (mg)	Fe (mg)	Cu (mg)	REF

17.8 FRENCH TOAST

frzn															
126	31.0	4.4	18.9		0.7	32	0	.22	.29	14	292	63	10	.45	.145
1 slice															
59	3.6	1.1	1.2	0.7	48	110	.16	1.6	.99	.55	79	82	1.30	.050	818
frzn, cinn swirl, Pepperidge Farms															
94		2.5	17.1				0	.08			143	29			
1.1 oz piece															
32	1.8					0	.10	1.1			27		1.10		I
homemade w/ low-fat milk															
149	35.6	5.0	16.3			86	0	.21	.05	15	311	65	11	.44	.122
1 slice															
65	7.0	1.8	2.9	1.7	75	315	.13	1.1	.20	.36	87	76	1.09	.038	818
homemade w/ whole milk															
151	35.4	5.0	16.2			81	0	.21	.05	15	311	64	11	.44	.122
1 slice															
65	7.3	2.0	3.0	1.7	76	298	.13	1.1	.20	.36	86	76	1.09	.038	818

17.9 MUFFINS

apple cinn, fat-free, from mix, Betty Crocker Sweet Rewards—*1 muffin*															
120		2.0	28.0	16.0	0.0	0	0	.07			200	0			
38	0.0	0.0	0.0	0.0	0	0	.09	0.4			35		.72		I
apple cinn, from mix, Robin Hood															
170		3.0	23.0	11.0	0.0	0	0	.10			220	20			
1 muffin															
49	8.0	1.5			35	0	.09	0.8			55		.72		I
apple streusel, from mix, Betty Crocker															
210		2.0	33.0	18.0	0.0	0	0	.07			220	0			
1 muffin															
62	8.0	1.5			20	0	.09	0.8			40		.72		I
banana nut															
from mix, Betty Crocker															
150		2.0	24.0	12.0	0.0	0	0	.07			200	0			
1 muffin															
55	5.0	1.0	2.0	2.0	20	0	.09	0.8			45		.72		I
from mix, Gold Medal/Robin Hood															
170		3.0	22.0	9.0	0.0	0	0	.10			180	20			
⅙ pkg															
48	8.0	1.5			35	0	.09	0.8			75		.72		I
frzn, Pepperidge Farms															
172		3.2	29.7				0	.08			288	33			
2 oz muffin															
58	4.5					0	.05	0.9			84		1.40		I
muffin loaf, Little Debbie															
217	10.8	2.5	30.9	19.2	0.7		2	.11			224	16			
1.9 oz pkg															
55	9.7	1.6			12	81	.14	1.1					1.16		I
blueberry															
158	21.8	3.1	27.4		1.5	5	1	.07	.01	9	255	32	9	.28	.251
1 muffin (2 ½" x 2 ¼")															
57	3.7	0.7	1.4	1.2	17	19	.08	0.6	.33	.19	70	112	.92	.042	818
from mix															
150	17.8	2.5	24.4		0.6	11	1	.16	.04	6	219	13	6	.19	.108
1 muffin															
50	4.4	0.7	1.8	1.5	23	39	.07	1.1	.04	.20	39	95	.56	.035	818
from mix, Robin Hood															
160		3.0	25.0	13.0	0.0	0	0	.10			220	20			
⅙ pkg															
47	6.0	1.5			35	0	.09	0.4			45		.36		I
homemade w/ 2% milk															
162	22.5	3.7	23.2			22	1	.16	.02	7	251	108	9	.31	.178
1 muffin (2 ¾" x 2")															
57	6.2	1.2	1.5	3.1	21	80	.16	1.3	.08	.19	70	83	1.29	.040	818
homemade w/ whole milk															
165	22.2	3.7	23.1			16	1	.16	.02	7	251	107	9	.31	.178
1 muffin (2 ¾" x 2")															
57	6.4	1.4	1.6	3.1	22	63	.16	1.3	.08	.19	70	82	1.29	.041	818
muffin loaf, Little Debbie															
230	11.5	3.2	30.7	19.7	0.5		0	.13			238	19			
2 oz pkg															
57	10.7	3.8			0	233	.12	1.3					.97		I
muffin mix, Duncan Hines															
110	5.7	2.0	21.0					.07			180	10	3	.10	
1/12 pkg															
30	2.0	1.0		1.0	0		.08	1.1			33	63	.40	.020	I
muffin mix, Duncan Hines Bakery Style															
180	10.0	2.0	32.0				1	.08			245	8	7	.20	
1/12 pkg															
50	5.0	2.0	2.0	1.0	0		.10	1.2				120	.70	.050	I
bran w/ raisins, Pepperidge Farms															
183		3.9	30.9		3.9		0	.09			312	66			
2 oz muffin															
58	4.9					0	.05	1.6			224		2.80		I
caramel nut, from mix, Gold Medal/ Robin Hood—*⅙ pkg*															
170		3.0	24.0	11.0	0.0	0	0	.10			230	20			
49	7.0	1.5			35	0	.09	0.8			50		.72		I
cinn streusel mix, Betty Crocker															
170		3.0	22.0	11.0	0.0	0	0	.06			180	40			
¼ cup															
50	7.0	1.5	4.0	1.5	20	0	.09	0.4			70		.72		I
cinn swirl muffin mix, Duncan Hines Bakery Style—*1/12 pkg*															
190	2.5	2.0	32.0					.09			240	15	7	.20	
45	6.0	1.0	4.0	1.0	0		.10	1.4				115	.90	.050	I
corn															
174	18.6	3.4	29.0		1.9	21	0	.19	.05	19	297	42	21	.41	.120
1 muffin (2 ½" x 2 ¼")															
57	4.8	0.9	1.9	1.6	29	119	.16	1.2	.11	.25	39	162	1.60	.035	818
from mix															
161	15.3	3.7	24.6		1.2	23	0	.14	.05	6	398	38	11	.32	.111
1 muffin (2 ¼" x 1 ½")															
50	5.1	1.4	2.6	0.6	31	105	.12	1.1	.08	.23	66	192	.97	.032	818
from mix, Gold Medal															
160		3.0	25.0	6.0	0.0	0	0	.14			270	20			
⅙ pkg															
52	6.0	1.5			35	200	.12	0.4			60		.72		I

							Vitamins					Minerals				
	KCAL	H_2O (g)	PRO (g)	CHO (g)	SUGR (g)	DFIB (g)	A (RE)	C (mg)	B-2 (mg)	B-6 (mg)	FOL (mcg)	Na (mg)	Ca (mg)	Mg (mg)	Zn (mg)	Mn (mg)
	WT (g)	FAT (g)	SFA (g)	MUFA (g)	PUFA (g)	CHOL (mg)	A (IU)	B-1 (mg)	NIA (mg)	B-12 (mcg)	PANT (mg)	K (mg)	P (mg)	Fe (mg)	Cu (mg)	REF
homemade w/ 2% milk	180	18.8	4.0	25.2			29	0	.18	.05	10	333	148	13	.35	.106
1 muffin (2 ¾″ x 2″)	57	7.0	1.3	1.7	3.5	24	137	.17	1.4	.09	.20	83	101	1.49	.034	818
homemade w/ whole milk	183	18.5	4.0	25.2			23	0	.18	.05	10	333	147	13	.35	.106
1 muffin (2 ¾″ x 2″)	57	7.4	1.5	1.8	3.5	26	117	.17	1.4	.09	.20	82	100	1.49	.034	818
muffin mix, Flako	163	3.5	2.9	29.1	8.0	1.0		0	.02	.05	5	383	21	11	.24	
⅓ cup	41	4.3	0.8	0.9	0.5	0	46	.05	0.5	.00	.11	35	114	.40	.050	I
cranberry orange nut muffin mix,	190	7.9	3.0	29.0					.10			210	16	14	.40	
Duncan Hines—*1⁄12 pkg*	54	7.0	1.0	4.0	2.0	0		.20	1.5				125	1.20	.200	I
homemade w/ 2% milk	169	21.5	3.9	23.6		1.5	23	0	.17	.02	7	266	114	10	.32	.169
1 muffin (2 ¾″ x 2″)	57	6.5	1.2	1.6	3.3	22	80	.16	1.3	.09	.20	69	87	1.36	.039	818
homemade w/ whole milk	172	21.2	3.9	23.6		1.5	17	0	.17	.02	7	266	113	9	.32	.169
1 muffin (2 ¾″ x 2″)	57	6.8	1.4	1.7	3.3	24	61	.16	1.3	.09	.20	68	87	1.36	.040	818
lemon poppy seed, from mix, Betty	190		3.0	30.0	16.0	0.0	0	0	.07			220	20			
Crocker—*¼ cup*	55	7.0	1.5	2.0	3.0	20	0	.12	0.8			25		.72		I
oat bran	154	19.9	4.0	27.5		2.6	1	0	.05	.09	10	224	36	89	1.05	1.499
1 muffin (2 ½″ x 2 ¼″)	57	4.2	0.5	0.8	2.6	0	10	.15	0.2	.00	.58	289	214	2.39	.188	818
oat bran w/ apple, Pepperidge Farms	193		3.6	29.8				0	.09			212	40			
2 oz muffin	58	6.6					0	.09	0.9			101		1.20		I
oatmeal w/ apples & walnuts muffin mix,	200		3.0	30.0		4.0						290				
Duncan Hines Hearty Style—*1⁄12 pkg*	50	8.0	1.0	5.0	2.0	0										I
pecan crunch muffin mix, Duncan Hines	210	2.3	3.0	27.0					.10			245	11	15	.50	
1⁄12 pkg	44	10.0	2.0	6.0	2.0	0		.20	1.5			79	145	.90	.090	I
toaster muffin																
apple spice, Pillsbury	139	8.6	1.8	22.7		1.3		0	.05			104	15			
1.4 oz muffin	39	5.1					11	.06	0.5			44	61	.59		I
banana nut, Pillsbury	135	10.5	1.8	19.5		1.2		0	.07			88	8			
1.4 oz muffin	39	5.7					94	.08	0.9			44	30	.66		I
blueberry	103	8.2	1.5	17.6		0.6	20	0	.09	.01	3	158	4	5	.15	.146
1 muffin	31	3.1	0.5	0.7	1.7	2	94	.06	0.6	.00	.06	27	60	.17	.031	818
blueberry, wild Maine, Pillsbury	135	10.3	1.6	24.8		1.2		0	.05			149	21			
1.4 oz muffin	39	3.7					9	.05	0.5			27	61	.51		I
corn	114	5.8	1.7	19.1		0.5	6	0	.11	.01	3	142	6	4	.11	.071
1 muffin	31	3.7	0.6	0.9	1.9	2	29	.08	0.7	.01	.07	30	80	.48	.019	818
corn, old fashioned, Pillsbury	137	8.9	2.3	19.1		1.0		0	.07			235	18			
1.4 oz muffin	39	5.8					37	.08	0.6			46	120	.43		I
raisin bran, Pillsbury	121	11.3	2.7	16.8		2.5		0	.08			225	28			
1.4 oz muffin	39	4.8					16	.03	1.8			102	100	1.05		I
wheat bran raisin	106	9.2	1.9	18.9		2.8	16	0	.10	.02	2	179	13	7	.15	.147
1 muffin	34	3.2	0.5	0.8	1.7	3	58	.07	0.8	.01	.06	60	97	.96	.041	818
Twice the Blueberry Mix, General Mills	140		2.0	25.0	13.0	0.0	0	0	.07			180	0			
¼ cup	52	4.0	1.0	2.0	1.0	20	0	.09	0.8			20		.72		I
wheat bran, from mix	138	17.7	3.3	23.3		2.1	16	0	.12	.09	8	234	16	29	.57	.826
1 muffin (2 ¼″ x 1 ¾″)	50	4.6	1.2	2.3	0.7	34	51	.10	1.4	.07	.22	74	167	1.26	.066	818
wheat bran, homemade w/ 2% milk	161	20.2	4.0	23.9			143	4	.25	.18	30	335	107	44	1.57	.088
1 muffin (2 ¾″ x 2″)	57	7.0	1.3	1.7	3.6	19	478	.19	2.3	.08	.27	181	162	2.39	.023	I
wheat bran, homemade w/ whole milk	164	19.9	4.0	23.8			136	4	.25	.18	30	335	106	44	1.57	.088
1 muffin (2 ¾″ x 2″)	57	7.3	1.5	1.8	3.6	21	459	.19	2.3	.08	.27	181	162	2.39	.023	818
wild blueberry, from mix, fat-free, Betty	120		2.0	27.0	15.0	0.0	0	0	.07			200	0			
Crocker Sweet Rewards—*1 muffin*	36	0.0	0.0	0.0	0.0	0	0	.09	0.4			25		.36		I
wild blueberry muffin mix, Betty Crocker	170		2.0	29.0	15.0	0.0	0	0	.07			220	0			
¼ cup	59	5.0	1.0	2.0	2.0	20	0	.09	0.8			25		.72		I

17.10 PANCAKES

blueberry																
from batter, Bisquick Shake 'n Pour	220		6.0	40.0	8.0	1.0	0	0	.17			640	80			
3 pancakes	110	4.0	1.0			0	0	.15	1.2			80		1.80		I
frzn, Pillsbury Microwave	255	46.7	5.4	49.1				1	.18			545	86			
3 pancakes	108	3.7					22	.27	2.3			85	158	1.30		I

KCAL	H₂O (g)	PRO (g)	CHO (g)	SUGR (g)	DFIB (g)	A (RE)	C (mg)	B-2 (mg)	B-6 (mg)	FOL (mcg)	Na (mg)	Ca (mg)	Mg (mg)	Zn (mg)	Mn (mg)
WT (g)	FAT (g)	SFA (g)	MUFA (g)	PUFA (g)	CHOL (mg)	A (IU)	B-1 (mg)	NIA (mg)	B-12 (mcg)	PANT (mg)	K (mg)	P (mg)	Fe (mg)	Cu (mg)	REF
homemade															
84	20.2	2.3	11.0			19	1	.10	.02	5	157	78	6	.21	.090
4" pancake 38	3.5	0.8	0.9	1.6	21	76	.07	0.6	.08	.15	52	57	.65	.021	818
buckwheat, from incomplete mix 62	16.1	2.4	8.5		0.7	20	0	.08	.04	5	160	77	17	.35	.195
4" pancake[17] 30	2.3	0.6	0.6	0.8	20	70	.05	0.4	.10	.15	70	122	.56	.034	818
buckwheat mix, Aunt Jemima 106	3.0	3.9	24.1	1.3	3.8		0	.09	.06	12	490	153	53	.54	
¼ cup 34	0.9	0.2	0.3	0.4	0	25	.15	1.6	.00	.25	117	313	1.95	.120	I
buttermilk															
from batter, Bisquick Shake 'n Pour 200		7.0	38.0	6.0	1.0	0	0	.17			680	80			
3 pancakes 110	3.0	1.0			0	0	.15	1.6			90		1.80		I
from complete mix, Betty Crocker 200		5.0	39.0	7.0	1.0	0	0	.17			540	80			
3 pancakes 110	2.5	0.5			10	0	.23	1.6			130		1.40		I
from mix, Robin Hood 230		8.0	35.0	6.0	1.0	0	0	.34			560	150			
3 pancakes 110	6.0	2.0			60	200	.23	2.0			160		1.80		I
frzn, Pillsbury Microwave 260	44.3	5.6	51.2				0	.22			592	90			
3 pancakes 108	3.7					26	.22	2.4			85	162	1.30		I
homemade 86	19.9	2.6	10.9			11	0	.11	.02	5	198	60	6	.24	.077
4" pancake 38	3.5	0.7	0.9	1.7	22	40	.08	0.6	.07	.16	55	53	.65	.020	818
mix, complete, Aunt Jemima 162	3.9	5.1	32.3	4.9	1.4		0	.21	.12	12	409	187	18	.52	
⅓ cup 43	1.8	0.5	0.4	0.4	9	42	.24	1.3	.13	.36	151	309	2.22	.040	I
mix, complete, red cal, Aunt Jemima 136	3.4	7.0	28.7	4.1	5.0		0	.48	.16	43	572	320	45	1.23	
⅓ cup 43	1.3	0.4	0.3	0.4	15	34	.62	3.9	.16	1.35	162	432	3.50	.230	I
mix w/ white & yellow corn flour, Aunt Jemima—¼ cup 115	3.6	3.9	24.3	1.7	1.1		0	.16	.06	7	437	130	15	.33	
34	0.6	0.2	0.1	0.3	2	14	.21	1.6	.14	.22	79	239	1.80	.060	I
harvest wheat, frzn, Pillsbury Microwave 240	47.5	6.0	47.5		3.0		1	.18			420	84			
3 pancakes 108	4.1					35	.29	4.2			168	306	1.62		I
plain															
from batter, Bisquick Shake 'n Pour 210		5.0	39.0	9.0	0	0		.10			710	80			
3 pancakes 110	4.0	1.0			0	0	.15	1.2			70		1.40		I
from complete mix 74	20.1	2.0	13.9		0.5	3	0	.08	.03	3	239	48	8	.15	.103
4" pancake 38	0.9	0.2	0.3	0.3	5	12	.08	0.7	.08	.09	67	127	.59	.036	818
from complete mix, Betty Crocker 200		6.0	39.0	9.0	1.0	0	0	.17			540	80			
3 pancakes 110	3.0	1.0			10	0	.23	2.0			120		1.80		I
from incomplete mix 83	20.1	3.0	11.0		0.7	27	0	.12	.04	4	192	82	8	.29	.053
4" pancake[17] 38	2.9	0.8	0.8	1.1	27	95	.08	0.5	.13	.19	76	119	.49	.018	818
frzn 82	16.3	1.9	15.7		0.6	10	0	.17	.02	5	183	22	5	.24	.108
4" pancake 36	1.2	0.3	0.4	0.3	3	36	.14	1.4	.06	.13	26	134	1.25	.014	818
frzn, Pillsbury Microwave 240	48.6	5.5	47.5				0	.19			552	86			
3 pancakes 108	3.6					33	.27	2.3			86	156	1.19		I
homemade 86	20.1	2.4	10.8			21	0	.11	.02	5	167	83	6	.21	.076
4" pancake 38	3.7	0.8	0.9	1.7	22	74	.08	0.6	.08	.15	50	60	.68	.019	818
mix, Aunt Jemima 161	4.4	4.6	35.1	5.0	1.2	0	0	.18	.06	4	645	16	6	.41	
⅓ cup 47	0.6	0.1	0.1	0.3	0	0	.30	2.3	.00	.18	49	324	2.01	.030	I
whole wheat, from incomplete mix 92	23.2	3.7	12.9		1.2	28	0	.23	.05	9	252	110	20	.46	.680
4" pancake[17] 44	2.9	0.8	0.8	1.1	27	99	.09	1.0	.13	.23	123	164	1.37	.035	818
whole wheat mix, Aunt Jemima 124	3.3	5.4	26.3	3.7	3.1		0	.35	.05	19	523	161	46	.91	
¼ cup 38	0.6	0.1	0.1	0.3	0	7	.23	3.2	.00	.31	184	296	3.31	.190	I

17.11 PASTA

KCAL	H₂O (g)	PRO (g)	CHO (g)	SUGR (g)	DFIB (g)	A (RE)	C (mg)	B-2 (mg)	B-6 (mg)	FOL (mcg)	Na (mg)	Ca (mg)	Mg (mg)	Zn (mg)	Mn (mg)
WT (g)	FAT (g)	SFA (g)	MUFA (g)	PUFA (g)	CHOL (mg)	A (IU)	B-1 (mg)	NIA (mg)	B-12 (mcg)	PANT (mg)	K (mg)	P (mg)	Fe (mg)	Cu (mg)	REF
capellini, durum, Fideo 204	6.2	7.7	41.3	1.9	1.9	0	0	.22	.08	12	3	12	27	.73	
⅔ cup dry 57	1.3	0.3	0.2	0.8	0	0	.50	3.4	.00	.28	107	92	1.64	.200	I
corn, ckd 176	95.6	3.7	39.1		6.7	8	0	.03	.08	8	0	1	50	.88	.214
1 cup 140	1.0	0.1	0.3	0.5	0	80	.07	0.8	.00	.18	43	106	.35	.090	820
egg, homemade, ckd 74	39.0	3.0	13.3			10	0	.10	.02	11	47	6	8	.25	.104
2 oz 57	1.0	0.2	0.1	0.3	23	33	.10	0.7	.06	.13	12	29	.66	.032	820
egg, refrig, ckd 74	38.9	2.9	14.1			3	0	.09	.02	4	3	3	10	.32	.127
2 oz 57	0.6	0.1	0.1	0.2	19	11	.12	0.6	.08	.10	14	36	.65	.053	820
elbow macaroni, 100% semolina, Golden Grain—½ cup (2 oz) dry 201	6.1	7.5	40.8	1.9	1.9	0	0	.21	.07	10	3	12	26	.72	
56	1.3	0.3	0.2	0.8	0	0	.49	3.3	.00	.24	105	90	1.61	.190	I

	KCAL / WT (g)	H₂O (g) / FAT (g)	PRO (g) / SFA (g)	CHO (g) / MUFA (g)	SUGR (g) / PUFA (g)	DFIB (g) / CHOL (mg)	A (RE) / A (IU)	C (mg) / B-1 (mg)	B-2 (mg) / NIA (mg)	B-6 (mg) / B-12 (mcg)	FOL (mcg) / PANT (mg)	Na (mg) / K (mg)	Ca (mg) / P (mg)	Mg (mg) / Fe (mg)	Zn (mg) / Cu (mg)	Mn (mg) / REF
fettuccini																
1% egg white, Golden Grain	196	7.3	7.6	39.4	1.8	1.8	0	0	.21	.07	11	9	12	26	.69	
1 ½ cups dry	56	1.3	0.3	0.2	0.8	0	0	.49	3.3	.00	.24	107	88	1.61	.190	I
2% egg white, Golden Grain	191	7.2	7.8	38.4	1.0	1.8	0	0	.22	.07	109	16	12	25	.67	
1 ½ cups dry	55	1.2	0.1			0	0	.48	3.2	.00	.25	110	86	1.57	.180	I
spinach, Golden Grain	193	7.3	7.7	39.0	1.8	2.3	0	0	.21	.10	0	18	31	41	.78	
1 ⅓ cups dry	56	1.3	0.3	0.2	0.8	0	270	.49	3.3	.00	.24	210	95	1.61	.210	I
homemade w/o egg, ckd	70	39.0	2.5	14.2			0	0	.08	.02	10	42	3	8	.21	.109
2 oz	57	0.6	0.1	0.1	0.3	0	0	.10	0.8	.00	.09	11	23	.64	.034	820
lasagne, Mueller's	210	5.2	8.0	41.8					.20			4				
2 oz dry	57	1.3				0		.50	3.0					1.80		I
macaroni																
enr, ckd	197	92.4	6.7	39.7		1.8	0	0	.14	.05	10	1	10	25	.74	.399
1 cup	140	0.9	0.1	0.1	0.4	0	0	.29	2.3	.00	.16	43	76	1.96	.137	820
protein-fortified, ckd	189	68.7	9.3	36.4			0	0	.19	.07	13	6	12	35	.57	.480
1 cup	115	0.2	0.0	0.0	0.1	0	0	.34	2.1	.00	.33	48	57	.83	.097	820
veg, ckd	172	91.6	6.1	35.7		5.8	7	0	.08	.03	8	8	15	25	.59	1.321
1 cup	134	0.1	0.0	0.0	0.1	0	71	.15	1.4	.00	.47	42	67	.66	.123	820
whole wheat, ckd	174	94.0	7.5	37.2		3.9	0	0	.06	.11	7	4	21	42	1.13	1.931
1 cup	140	0.8	0.1	0.1	0.3	0	0	.15	1.0	.00	.59	62	125	1.48	.234	820
Noodle Trio, Mueller's	220	5.9	8.1	40.1					.20			18	20			
2 oz dry	57	2.4				55		.50	3.0					1.80		I
noodles, chow mein	237	0.3	3.8	25.9		1.8	4	0	.19	.05	10	198	9	23	.63	.611
1 cup	45	13.8	2.0	3.5	7.8	0	38	.26	2.7	.00	.24	54	72	2.13	.075	820
noodles, chow mein, LaChoy	148		2.5	16.0	0.0	1.1	0	0				289	6			
½ cup	28	8.3	1.6			0	0							.41		I
noodles, egg																
& spinach, ckd	211	109.6	8.1	38.8		3.7	22	0	.20	.18	34	19	30	38	1.01	.507
1 cup	160	2.5	0.6	0.8	0.6	53	165	.39	2.4	.22	.37	59	91	1.74	.128	820
enr, ckd	213	109.9	7.6	39.7		1.8	10	0	.13	.06	11	11	19	30	.99	.419
1 cup	160	2.4	0.5	0.7	0.7	53	32	.30	2.4	.14	.23	45	110	2.54	.138	820
Golden Grain	208	6.2	7.8	38.7	1.7	1.8	0	0	.21	.09	29	9	21	32	1.26	
1 ¼ cups (2 oz) dry	56	2.8	0.8	0.8	0.9	65	92	.49	3.3	.22	.48	106	121	1.61	.680	I
Mueller's	220	5.9	8.1	39.7					.20			8	20			
2 oz dry	57	2.5				55		.50	3.0					1.80		I
noodles, japanese, soba, ckd	174	128.5	8.9	37.7			0	0	.05	.07	12	106	7	16	.21	.658
1 cup	176	0.2	0.0	0.0	0.1	0	0	.17	0.9	.00	.41	62	44	.84	.014	820
noodles, japanese, somen, ckd	231	119.5	7.0	48.5			0	0	.06	.02	4	283	14	4	.39	.442
1 cup	176	0.3	0.0	0.0	0.1	0	0	.04	0.2	.00	.30	51	48	.92	.044	820
noodles, rice, dry, LaChoy	121		2.3	21.4	0.0	0.4	0	0				378	17			
½ cup	28	3.0	0.6			0	0							.83		I
pasta, 1.5% egg white, Golden Grain	196	7.3	7.8	39.3	1.8	1.8	0	0	.21	.07	11	13	12	26	.69	
1 ¾ cups dry	56	1.2	0.3	0.2	0.8	0	0	.49	3.3	.00	.25	109	87	1.61	.190	I
Rainbow Radiatore, Golden Grain	184	6.9	7.0	37.4	2.0	1.9	0	2	.20	.08	18	7	16	29	.68	
¾ cup dry	53	1.2	0.2	0.2	0.6	0	376	.47	3.2	.00	.24	132	86	1.52	.190	I
spaghetti																
enr, ckd	197	92.4	6.7	39.7		2.4	0	0	.14	.05	10	1	10	25	.74	.399
1 cup	140	0.9	0.1	0.1	0.4	0	0	.29	2.3	.00	.16	43	76	1.96	.137	820
Mueller's	210	5.4	7.6	42.1					.20			3	8			
2 oz dry	57	1.1				0		.50	3.0					1.80		I
protein-fortified, ckd	230	83.6	11.3	44.3		2.4	0	0	.23	.09	15	7	14	42	.70	.584
1 cup	140	0.3	0.0	0.0	0.1	0	0	.42	2.6	.00	.40	59	70	1.01	.118	820
spinach, ckd	182	95.4	6.4	36.6			21	0	.14	.13	17	20	42	87	1.51	2.106
1 cup	140	0.9	0.1	0.1	0.4	0	213	.14	2.1	.00	.26	81	151	1.46	.287	820
whole wheat, ckd	174	94.0	7.5	37.2		6.3	0	0	.06	.11	7	4	21	42	1.13	1.931
1 cup	140	0.8	0.1	0.1	0.3	0	0	.15	1.0	.00	.59	62	125	1.48	.234	820
spinach, refrig, ckd	74	38.9	2.9	14.2			8	0	.08	.06	10	3	10	14	.36	.179
2 oz	57	0.5	0.1	0.2	0.1	19	58	.10	0.6	.08	.13	21	32	.63	.045	820

	KCAL	H₂O (g)	PRO (g)	CHO (g)	SUGR (g)	DFIB (g)	A (RE)	C (mg)	B-2 (mg)	B-6 (mg)	FOL (mcg)	Na (mg)	Ca (mg)	Mg (mg)	Zn (mg)	Mn (mg)
	WT (g)	FAT (g)	SFA (g)	MUFA (g)	PUFA (g)	CHOL (mg)	A (IU)	B-1 (mg)	NIA (mg)	B-12 (mcg)	PANT (mg)	K (mg)	P (mg)	Fe (mg)	Cu (mg)	REF
Super Shapes, Mueller's	210	5.4	7.6	42.1					.20			3	8			
2 oz dry	57	1.1				0		.50	3.0					1.80		I
twists, tricolor, Mueller's	210	5.7	7.9	41.3					.20			10	8			
2 oz dry	57	1.2				0		.50	3.0					1.80		I

17.12 PASTRY CRUST

	KCAL	H₂O (g)	PRO (g)	CHO (g)	SUGR (g)	DFIB (g)	A (RE)	C (mg)	B-2 (mg)	B-6 (mg)	FOL (mcg)	Na (mg)	Ca (mg)	Mg (mg)	Zn (mg)	Mn (mg)
	WT (g)	FAT (g)	SFA (g)	MUFA (g)	PUFA (g)	CHOL (mg)	A (IU)	B-1 (mg)	NIA (mg)	B-12 (mcg)	PANT (mg)	K (mg)	P (mg)	Fe (mg)	Cu (mg)	REF
cream puff shell, homemade	239	26.7	5.9	15.0		0.5	203	0	.24	.05	15	368	24	8	.48	.139
1 shell	66	17.1	3.7	7.3	4.9	129	764	.14	1.0	.26	.41	64	79	1.33	.034	818
pastry pockets, Pillsbury	231	22.0	4.2	24.8				0	.13			550	11			
1 pocket	67	13.2					0	.19	1.7			151	256	1.49		I
phyllo dough	57	6.2	1.3	10.0		0.4	0	0	.06	.01	3	92	2	3	.09	.090
1 sheet (16 ½" x 12")	19	1.1	0.2	0.2	0.6	0	0	.10	0.8	.00	.06	14	14	.61	.019	818
pie crust, choc, Keebler Ready Crust	96		1.2	13.4					.16			107	5			
⅛ of 9" crust	20	4.2	0.6		0.2	0		.06	0.6			62		.62		I
pie crust, choc wafer, homemade	139	1.5	1.4	15.0			60	0	.06	.00	0	185	8	11	.22	.143
⅛ of 9" crust	27	8.6	1.9	4.1	2.1	1	231	.04	0.6	.01	.08	46	29	.83	.095	I
pie crust, deep dish, frzn, Mrs. Smith's	110		1.0	12.0	1.0	0.0						105				
⅛ of 10" crust	27	7.0	1.5	4.0	1.0	0						15				I
pie crust, graham, homemade	148	1.3	1.3	19.6		0.4	61	0	.05	.01	2	171	6	5	.14	.139
⅛ of 9" crust	30	7.5	1.6	3.4	2.1	0	236	.03	0.6	.01	.07	26	20	.65	.037	818
pie crust, graham, Keebler Ready Crust	100		1.0	13.2					.08			124	2			
⅛ of 9" crust	20	4.8	0.8		0.2	0		.02	0.5			27		.50		I
pie crust, plain																
Betty Crocker	110		1.0	9.0	0.0	0.0	0	0	.03			150	0			
⅛ of 9" crust	20	8.0	2.0			0	0	.06	0.4					.36		I
from mix	100	2.1	1.3	10.1		0.4	0	0	.04	.01	2	146	12	3	.08	.061
⅛ of 9" crust	20	6.1	1.5	3.5	0.8	0	0	.06	0.5	.00	.03	12	17	.43	.015	818
frzn	82	1.8	0.7	7.9		0.2	0	0	.06	.01	1	104	3	3	.05	.098
⅛ of 9" crust	16	5.2	1.7	2.5	0.6	0	0	.04	0.4	.00	.03	18	9	.36	.012	818
frzn, Mrs. Smith's	120		1.0	14.0	1.0	0.0						110				
⅛ of 9 ⅝" crust	28	6.0	1.0	4.0	1.0	0						15				I
homemade	121	2.3	1.5	10.9		0.4	0	0	.06	.01	3	125	2	3	.10	.099
⅛ pf 9" crust	23	8.0	2.0	3.5	2.1	0	0	.09	0.8	.00	.04	15	15	.66	.021	818
mix, Flako	128	2.1	1.9	12.6	0.3	0.6	0	0	.08	.01	5	170	13	5	.14	
¼ cup	25	8.0	3.1	3.5	1.0	7	0	.14	1.5	.00	.04	22	29	.80	.030	I
Pillsbury All Ready	236	12.1	1.7	23.8				0	.00			210	4			
⅛ of double crust	53	14.6					31	.00	0.1			31	17	.25		I
red fat, frzn, Mrs. Smith's	100		1.0	13.0	1.0	0.0						95				
⅛ 9" crust	27	5.0	1.0			0						30				I
shallow, frzn, Mrs. Smith's	70		1.0	8.0	1.0	0.0						70				
⅛ of 9" crust	18	4.0	1.0	2.0	1.0	0						15				I
pie crust, van wafer, homemade	119	1.5	0.8	11.3			64	0	.05	.01	2	116	9	2	.06	.040
⅛ of 9" crust	22	8.1	1.7	3.5	2.4	9	248	.04	0.5	.02	.07	18	17	.37	.015	818
pizza crust, Pillsbury All Ready	88	14.5	3.2	15.9				0	.09			172	6			
⅛ crust	35	1.1					0	.13	1.2			21	20	1.05		I
pizza crust, Robin Hood	160		4.0	33.0	1.0	1.0	0	0	.15			340	0			
¼ crust	49	2.0	0.5			0	0	.23	2.0			55		.00		I
puff pastry, frzn	223	3.0	3.0	18.3		0.6	0	0	.10	.01	4	101	4	6	.22	.198
1 pastry	40	15.4	2.2	3.5	8.9	0	0	.13	1.5	.00	.00	25	24	1.04	.046	818
wonton wrappers	23	2.3	0.8	4.6		0.1	0	0	.03	.00	1	46	4	2	.06	.051
1 wrapper (7" sq)	8	0.1	0.0	0.0	0.0	1	1	.04	0.4	.00	.00	7	6	.27	.012	818

17.13 RICE & RICE DISHES

	KCAL	H₂O (g)	PRO (g)	CHO (g)	SUGR (g)	DFIB (g)	A (RE)	C (mg)	B-2 (mg)	B-6 (mg)	FOL (mcg)	Na (mg)	Ca (mg)	Mg (mg)	Zn (mg)	Mn (mg)
	WT (g)	FAT (g)	SFA (g)	MUFA (g)	PUFA (g)	CHOL (mg)	A (IU)	B-1 (mg)	NIA (mg)	B-12 (mcg)	PANT (mg)	K (mg)	P (mg)	Fe (mg)	Cu (mg)	REF
brown rice																
inst, whole grain, Minute	170		4.0	34.0	0.0	2.0	0	0	.00			10	0			
⅔ cup	137	1.5				0	0	.03	1.6			40		.36		I
long grain, ckd	216	142.5	5.0	44.8		3.5	0	0	.05	.28	8	10	20	84	1.23	1.765
1 cup	195	1.8	0.4	0.6	0.6	0	0	.19	3.0	.00	.56	84	162	.82	.195	820

	KCAL / WT (g)	H_2O (g) / FAT (g)	PRO (g) / SFA (g)	CHO (g) / MUFA (g)	SUGR (g) / PUFA (g)	DFIB (g) / CHOL (mg)	A (RE) / A (IU)	C (mg) / B-1 (mg)	B-2 (mg) / NIA (mg)	B-6 (mg) / B-12 (mcg)	FOL (mcg) / PANT (mg)	Na (mg) / K (mg)	Ca (mg) / P (mg)	Mg (mg) / Fe (mg)	Zn (mg) / Cu (mg)	Mn (mg) / REF
med grain, ckd	218	142.3	4.5	45.8		3.5	0	0	.02	.29	8	2	20	86	1.21	2.139
1 cup	195	1.6	0.3	0.6	0.6	0	0	.20	2.6	.00	.76	154	150	1.03	.158	820
rice dish																
chinese fried rice, frzn, LaChoy	236		5.1	53.4	6.2	1.9	0	0				1024	17			
1 cup	139	1.1	0.2			0	0							.83		I
fried rice, cantonese style, frzn, Green Giant—3 oz[18]	107		2.0	18.0				1	.02			287	14			
	85	3.0	0.3		0.8	15	955	.07	0.7			69	34	.70		I
rice & broccoli w/ cheese sce, frzn, Pillsbury—4.5 oz	178	117.8	4.5	25.1				8	.03			697	86			
	156	6.2	2.0		1.0	5	1362	.22	2.2			105	131	.78		I
rice & broccoli w/ cheese sce, frzn, Rice Originals—½ cup	124	85.6	3.5	18.0		0.2		6	.05			505	49			
	113	4.3					986	.23	1.5			72	75	1.47		I
rice & spinach w/ cheese sce, italian blend, frzn, Pillsbury—½ cup	140		4.0	22.0								400				
	113	4.0	3.0			10						105				I
rice & spinach w/ cheese sce, italian blend, frzn, Rice Originals—½ cup	167	78.0	4.1	23.1		1.2		0	.08			399	66			
	113	6.4					591	.21	1.9			99	59	2.15		I
rice confetti, frzn, Stouffers	72	67.2	1.7	13.6				1	.03			383	6			
3 oz entree[19]	85	1.2				2	94	.05	0.6			43		.09		I
rice jubilee, frzn, Rice Originals	150	80.6	2.4	22.2		0.9		0	.03			333	15			
½ cup	112	5.7					1025	.19	2.4			54	34	1.57		I
rice medley, frzn, Rice Originals	121	85.2	2.9	21.2		0.4		0	.03			263	14			
½ cup	113	2.7					440	.33	2.4			53	43	1.81		I
rice, peas, & mushrooms w/ sce, frzn, Pillsbury—5.5 oz	130		4.0	27.0								410				
	156	2.0			0.0	5						85				I
rice pilaf, frzn, Pillsbury	110		2.0	21.0								530				
½ cup	113	1.0			0.0	2						55				I
rice pilaf, frzn, Rice Originals	116	84.8	2.7	22.6		0.1		1	.03			519	11			
½ cup	113	1.6					34	.25	2.5			85	34	1.47		I
rice w/ herb butter sce, frzn, Rice Originals—½ cup	150	86.5	2.9	23.3		0.8		0	.04			406	18			
	119	5.0					206	.24	2.5			49	40	1.79		I
risotto milanese w/ saffron, from mix, Knorr—½ cup	130		2.2	24.2				0	.01			400	18			
	100	3.0					0	.13	1.1					.90		I
risotto tomato, from mix, Knorr	130		2.5	23.4				17	.02			440	22			
½ cup	100	3.0					383	.14	1.2					.90		I
risotto w/ mushrooms, from mix, Knorr	130		2.3	24.1				0	.03			410	18			
½ cup	100	3.0					2	.13	1.4					.30		I
risotto w/ onion, from mix, Knorr	130		2.2	24.3				0	.00			370	18			
½ cup	100	3.0					3	.13	1.0					.80		I
risotto w/ peas & corn, from mix, Knorr	130		2.4	23.6				6	.01			450	19			
½ cup	100	3.0					160	.13	1.1					.90		I
rice mix (not prepared)																
beef & mushroom, Rice-a-Roni	240	7.2	7.3	50.9	2.6	2.3		4	.18	.14	31	1148	51	50	.64	
2.5 oz	70	1.4	0.3	0.5	0.5	1	244	.37	2.9	.00	.42	244	90	2.21	.160	I
beef flavored rice & sce, Lipton	230		5.0	48.0	1.0	1.0		0	.07		80	940	20			
½ cup	62	1.5	0.0			0	100	.53	4.0					2.70		I
beef w/ broccoli, Rice-a-Roni	189	5.8	6.0	40.5	2.7	2.2		4	.14	.12	32	877	50	45	.48	
2 oz	56	0.9	0.1	0.2	0.4	0	301	.29	2.2	.00	.32	147	77	1.80	.130	
broccoli & cheddar rice & sce, Lipton	240		6.0	47.0	1.0	1.0		5	.07		80	930	60			
½ cup	63	3.0	1.5			5	200	.53	4.0					2.70		I
broccoli au gratin, Rice-a-Roni	269	6.8	7.3	46.6	4.5	1.6		2	.18		23	819	68	41	.67	
2.5 oz	70	6.3	1.9	3.8	0.3	4	139	.35	2.7		.35	281	118	2.03	.130	I
broccoli rice, Rice-a-Roni	198	5.4	5.4	40.9	1.4	1.2		12	.10	.14	12	780	28	25	.64	
2 oz	56	1.8	0.7	0.7	0.2	4	249	.28	2.0	.02	.44	164	89	1.65	.120	I
chicken broccoli rice & sce, Lipton	230		7.0	46.0		2.0		6	.14		100	840	40			
½ cup	63	2.5				0	300	.68	0.5					2.70		I
chicken flavor rice & sce, Lipton	230		7.0	46.0	1.0			0	.07		60	890	20			
½ cup	62	2.5	1.0			5	100	.53	4.0					2.70		I
chicken parmesan rissotto rice & sce, Lipton—½ cup	220		6.0	44.0	0.0			1	.10		100	760	0			
	59	2.5	0.5			0	300	.67	4.0					.36		I
creamy chicken rice & sce, Lipton	250		6.0	45.0	2.0	1.0		1	.10		80	760	20			
½ cup	63	5.0	2.0			0	500	.60	4.0					2.70		I

	KCAL	H₂O (g)	PRO (g)	CHO (g)	SUGR (g)	DFIB (g)	A (RE)	C (mg)	B-2 (mg)	B-6 (mg)	FOL (mcg)	Na (mg)	Ca (mg)	Mg (mg)	Zn (mg)	Mn (mg)
	WT (g)	FAT (g)	SFA (g)	MUFA (g)	PUFA (g)	CHOL (mg)	A (IU)	B-1 (mg)	NIA (mg)	B-12 (mcg)	PANT (mg)	K (mg)	P (mg)	Fe (mg)	Cu (mg)	REF
fried rice, Rice-a-Roni	240	7.2	6.4	51.0	4.8	1.8		1	.12	.09	18	1425	26	40	.58	
2.5 oz	70	1.7	0.2	0.8	0.5	0	31	.33	2.5	.00	.33	143	85	1.89	.140	I
medley rice & sce, Lipton	220		7.0	44.0	1.0	2.0		1	.10		80	800	20			
½ cup	60	2.5	0.5			5	400	.60	4.0					2.70		I
mushroom rice & sce, Lipton	220		6.0	46.0	1.0				.10			80	890	20		
½ cup	60	1.5	0.0			0		.52	4.0					2.70		I
rice pilaf, Rice-a-Roni	240	7.1	6.6	52.2	1.2	1.4		0	.12	.18	12	1085	19	24	.76	
2.5 oz	70	0.9	0.2	0.3	0.3	0	8	.40	2.7	.00	.56	106	101	2.00	.161	I
rice pilaf w/ sce, Lipton	220		6.0	45.0	1.0	1.0		0	.06		80	860	20			
½ cup	59	1.5	0.0			0	0	.52	4.0					2.70		I
rice risotto, Rice-a-Roni	238	7.3	6.3	51.3	1.8	1.7		0	.11	.08	14	1442	21	36	.55	
2.5 oz	70	1.3	0.3	0.4	0.5	1	31	.36	2.6	.00	.32	98	82	1.87	.150	I
rice stroganoff, Rice-a-Roni	261	6.8	7.0	48.5	3.4	1.3		1	.16	.09	14	916	71	38	.65	
2.5 oz	70	4.7	1.3	2.0	0.4	2	36	.34	2.4	.09	.46	166	133	1.71	.130	I
rice w/ beef flavor, Rice-a-Roni	238	7.5	6.7	51.9	3.2	1.9		0	.12	.09	18	1068	21	37	.57	
2.5 oz	70	0.9	0.1	0.2	0.4	0	271	.36	2.6	.00	.33	125	83	1.94	.140	I
rice w/ cajun sce, Lipton	230		6.0	48.0	0.0	1.0		4	.14		80	840	20			
½ cup	63	1.0	0.0			0	400	.60	4.0					2.70		I
rice w/ chicken & mushroom, Rice-a-Roni—2.5 oz	241	7.2	6.9	50.2	2.1	1.9		1	.21	.11	19	1329	19	36	.74	
	70	2.0	0.4	1.0	0.5	1	6	.36	3.4	.00	.74	261	99	2.11	.230	I
rice w/ chicken flavor, Rice-a-Roni	240	7.6	6.8	51.7	2.3	1.8		1	.14	.10	16	981	21	37	.63	
2.5 oz	70	1.1	0.2	0.3	0.4	0	31	.37	2.8	.00	.38	206	81	2.02	.150	I
rice w/ herbs & butter, Rice-a-Roni	242	6.8	5.6	53.2	1.9	1.4		2	.09	.18	11	1074	46	22	.68	
2.5 oz	70	1.2	0.5	0.6	0.2	3	408	.31	2.4	.11	.58	113	97	1.92	.140	I
rice w/ herbs & butter sce, Lipton	240		5.0	44.0	1.0			0	.07		80	820		5	.20	.200
½ cup	60	4.5	2.5			10	100	.53	4.0				59	1.60	.100	
rice w/ spanish sce, Lipton	230		6.0	47.0	2.0	2.0		5	.14		80	830				
½ cup	62	1.5	0.0			0	400	.68	4.0					2.70		I
scampi rice & sce, Lipton	220		6.0	44.0	1.0			1	.06		80	840	0			
½ cup	59	2.5	0.1			5	250	.60	4.0					.36		I
spanish rice, Rice-a-Roni	189	5.9	5.4	41.0	1.5	1.8		9	.11	.12	17	938	32	33	.50	
2 oz	56	0.8	0.1	0.2	0.3	0	225	.30	2.1	.00	.29	123	75	1.61	.130	I
white & wild w/ mushrooms & herbs, Lipton—½ cup	240		6.0	49.0	0.0	1.0		1	.14		80	550	20			
	63	2.0	1.0			0	100	.60	4.0					2.70		I
white & wild w/ sce, Original Recipe, Lipton—½ cup	230		7.0	49.0	2.0	2.0		2	.07		60	870	40			
	63	1.5	0.0			0	500	.53	4.0					2.70		I
white cheddar w/ herbs, Rice-a-Roni	263	6.4	7.6	48.3	4.1	1.4		2	.17	.37	13	878	74	26	.85	
2.5 oz	70	4.8	1.8	2.5	0.3	6	141	.34	2.5	.44	.50	155	149	1.78	.230	I
yellow rice, Rice-a-Roni	234	7.8	4.8	53.9	0.8	1.2		3	.05	.09	17	1111	19	41	.32	
2.5 oz	70	0.3	0.0	0.2	0.2	0	11	.26	2.1	.00	.36	59	65	2.04	.080	I

white, long grain & wild rice

	KCAL	H₂O (g)	PRO (g)	CHO (g)	SUGR (g)	DFIB (g)	A (RE)	C (mg)	B-2 (mg)	B-6 (mg)	FOL (mcg)	Na (mg)	Ca (mg)	Mg (mg)	Zn (mg)	Mn (mg)
	WT (g)	FAT (g)	SFA (g)	MUFA (g)	PUFA (g)	CHOL (mg)	A (IU)	B-1 (mg)	NIA (mg)	B-12 (mcg)	PANT (mg)	K (mg)	P (mg)	Fe (mg)	Cu (mg)	REF
ckd, Minute	230		6.0	50.0	2.0	1.0	0	0	.00			960	20			
1 cup	230	0.5	0.0			0	0	.15	2.0			95		1.80		I
frzn, Pillsbury	130		3.0	24.0								540				
½ cup	113	2.0			0.0	0						55				I
frzn, Rice Originals	120	80.7	2.6	22.5		0.2		3	.03			530	14			
½ cup	109	2.1					89	.21	1.3			39	40	1.42		I

white rice

	KCAL	H₂O (g)	PRO (g)	CHO (g)	SUGR (g)	DFIB (g)	A (RE)	C (mg)	B-2 (mg)	B-6 (mg)	FOL (mcg)	Na (mg)	Ca (mg)	Mg (mg)	Zn (mg)	Mn (mg)
	WT (g)	FAT (g)	SFA (g)	MUFA (g)	PUFA (g)	CHOL (mg)	A (IU)	B-1 (mg)	NIA (mg)	B-12 (mcg)	PANT (mg)	K (mg)	P (mg)	Fe (mg)	Cu (mg)	REF
boil-in-bag, ckd, Minute	190		4.0	42.0	0.0	0.0	0	0	.00			10	0			
1 cup	200	0.0	0.0	0.0	0.0	0	0	.23	1.6			15		1.44	.	I
ckd, Minute	170		4.0	37.0	0.0	0.0	0	0	.00			10	0			
¾ cup	140	0.0	0.0	0.0	0.0	0	0	.15	1.2			10		1.08		I
glutinous, ckd	234	184.7	4.9	50.8		2.4	0	0	.03	.06	2	12	5	12	.99	.631
1 cup	241	0.5	0.1	0.2	0.2	0	0	.05	0.7	.00	.52	24	19	.34	.118	820
long grain, ckd, Minute Premium	170		3.0	36.0	0.0	0.0	0	0	.00			10	0			
1 cup	206	0.0	0.0	0.0	0.0	0	0	.15	1.2			20		1.08		I
long grain, enr, ckd	205	108.1	4.3	44.5		0.6	0	0	.02	.15	5	2	16	19	.77	.746
1 cup[20]	158	0.4	0.1	0.1	0.1	0	0	.26	2.3	.00	.62	55	68	1.90	.109	820
long grain, inst, ckd	162	126.1	3.4	35.1		1.0	0	0	.08	.02	7	5	13	8	.40	.388
1 cup	165	0.3	0.1	0.1	0.1	0	0	.12	1.5	.00	.29	7	23	1.04	.107	820

						Vitamins					Minerals				
KCAL	H₂O (g)	PRO (g)	CHO (g)	SUGR (g)	DFIB (g)	A (RE)	C (mg)	B-2 (mg)	B-6 (mg)	FOL (mcg)	Na (mg)	Ca (mg)	Mg (mg)	Zn (mg)	Mn (mg)
WT (g)	FAT (g)	SFA (g)	MUFA (g)	PUFA (g)	CHOL (mg)	A (IU)	B-1 (mg)	NIA (mg)	B-12 (mcg)	PANT (mg)	K (mg)	P (mg)	Fe (mg)	Cu (mg)	REF
long grain, parboiled, ckd															
200	126.9	4.0	43.3		0.7	0	0	.03	.03	7	5	33	21	.54	.455
1 cup															
175	0.5	0.1	0.1	0.1	0	0	.44	2.4	.00	.57	65	74	1.98	.165	820
med grain, enr, ckd															
242	127.6	4.4	53.2		0.6	0	0	.03	.09	4	0	6	24	.78	.701
1 cup²¹															
186	0.4	0.1	0.1	0.1	0	0	.31	3.4	.00	.76	54	69	2.77	.071	820
short grain, enr, ckd															
242	127.5	4.4	53.4			0	0	.03	.11	4	0	2	15	.74	.664
1 cup²¹															
186	0.4	0.1	0.1	0.1	0	0	.31	2.8	.00	.74	48	61	2.72	.134	820
wild rice, ckd															
166	121.2	6.5	35.0		3.0	0	0	.14	.22	43	5	5	52	2.20	.462
1 cup															
164	0.6	0.1	0.1	0.3	0	0	.09	2.1	.00	.25	166	134	.98	.198	820
wild rice, w/ sherry, frzn, Garden															
245	212.5	6.2	39.5		2.7		4	.11			592	48			
Gourmet Microwave—*9.5 oz pkg*															
269	7.8					207	.81	8.3			239	129			I

17.14 ROLLS

Bran'ola															
130		6.0	27.0	5.0	3.0	0	0				210	20			
1 roll															
57	1.5	0.0			0	0							1.80		I
crescent, refrig dough, Pillsbury															
98	8.7	1.7	10.8				0	.06			227	6			
1 oz roll															
28	5.5					0	.08	0.7			62	106	.64		I
dinner															
85	9.0	2.4	14.3		0.9	0	0	.09	.02	9	148	34	7	.22	.132
1 roll															
28	2.1	0.5	1.1	0.3	0	0	.14	1.1	.01	.14	38	33	.89	.043	818
egg															
107	10.6	3.3	18.2		1.3	8	0	.18	.03	19	191	21	9	.32	.183
1 roll (2 ½")															
35	2.2	0.6	1.1	0.4	18	26	.18	1.2	.08	.11	37	35	1.23	.046	818
homemade w/ lowfat milk															
111	10.2	3.0	18.7		0.7	31	0	.14	.02	15	145	21	7	.24	.140
1 roll (2 ½")															
35	2.6	0.6	1.0	0.7	12	118	.14	1.2	.05	.16	53	44	1.04	.040	818
homemade w/ whole milk															
112	10.0	3.0	18.7			28	0	.14	.02	15	145	21	7	.24	.140
1 roll (2 ½")															
35	2.7	0.7	1.1	0.7	13	108	.14	1.2	.05	.16	53	44	1.04	.040	818
potato, Arnold															
110		4.0	21.0	3.0	1.0	0	0				125	20			
2 rolls															
43	1.5	0.0			0	0							1.44		I
white, Arnold's/August Bros															
100		3.0	19.5	2.0	1.0	0	0	.07			170	20			
2 rolls²															
38	1.5	0.0			0	0	.15	0.8					1.08		I
w/ sesame seeds, Arnold															
110		4.0	19.0	4.0	0	0	0	.07			140	20			
2 rolls															
38	2.5	0.5			0	0	.15	0.8					1.08		I
dinner/wheat, August Bros															
100		4.0	19.0	2.0	1.0	0	0				160	40			
1 roll															
38	2.0	0.0			0	0							1.08		I
egg twist, Levy Old Country															
170		5.0	30.0	3.0	1.0	0	0				240	0			
1 roll															
57	4.0	1.0			5	0							1.80		I
Francisco															
90		3.0	18.0	1.0	1.0	0	0				200	20			
1 roll															
34	1.0	0.0			0	0							1.08		I
french															
105	13.2	3.3	19.1		1.2	0	0	.11	.02	13	231	35	8	.29	.191
1 roll															
38	1.6	0.4	0.7	0.3	0	2	.20	1.7	.00	.08	43	32	1.03	.073	818
Francisco															
160		6.0	35.0	3.0	2.0	0	0				320	6			
1 roll															
66	1.5	0.0			0	0							1.80		I
mini, Francisco															
110		4.0	22.0	0.0	0	0	0				200	40			
1 roll															
39	1.0	0.0			0	0							1.44		I
hamburger, Arnold/August Bros															
133		5.0	25.7	3.7	1.3	0	0	.10			223	53			
1 roll²²															
51	2.2	0.2			0	0	.15	1.2					1.44		I
hamburger/hot dog															
123	14.6	3.7	21.6	3.2	1.2	0	0	.13	.02	12	241	60	9	.27	.141
1 roll															
43	2.2	0.5	1.1	0.4	0	0	.21	1.7	.01	.23	61	38	1.36	.049	818
hamburger/hotdog, mixed-grain															
113	16.3	4.1	19.2		1.6	0	0	.13	.04	12	197	41	21	.46	.445
1 roll															
43	2.6	0.6	1.3	0.5	0	0	.20	1.9	.00	.09	65	52	1.70	.067	818
hamburger, Roman Meal															
117		4.8	22.1		2.0			.10			238	44			
1.6 oz roll															
46	1.9				0		.20	2.2					1.70		I
hard/kaiser															
167	17.7	5.6	30.0		1.3	0	0	.19	.03	9	310	54	15	.54	.262
1 roll (3 ½" dia)															
57	2.5	0.3	0.6	1.0	0	0	.27	2.4	.00	.13	62	57	1.87	.093	818
homestyle, from dough, Rich's															
152	20.8	4.5	28.1					.20			335	27	12	.34	
2 rolls															
56	2.4				0		.32	2.1			68	76	2.04	.180	I
hot dog															
Arnold															
110		4.0	21.0	3.0	1.0	0	0	.10			210	20			
1 roll															
43	2.0	0.0			0	0	.15	1.2					1.08		I
Bran'ola															
110		5.0	21.0	3.0	2.0	0	0				170	20			
1 roll															
46	1.5	0.0			0	0							1.44		I
potato, Arnold															
120		4.0	23.0	4.0	1.0	0	0				170	20			
1 roll															
46	2.0	0.0			0	0							1.44		I

	KCAL / WT (g)	H_2O / FAT (g)	PRO / SFA (g)	CHO / MUFA (g)	SUGR / PUFA (g)	DFIB / CHOL (mg)	A (RE) / A (IU)	C / B-1 (mg)	B-2 / NIA (mg)	B-6 / B-12	FOL / PANT	Na / K (mg)	Ca / P (mg)	Mg / Fe (mg)	Zn / Cu (mg)	Mn / REF
Roman Meal	109		4.6	20.7		1.9			.10			222	41			
1.5 oz roll	43	1.8				0		.20	2.0					1.60		I
italian, Savoni	280		10.0	56.0	4.0	3.0	0	0				610	100			
1 roll	113	3.5	0.5			0	0							3.60		I
kaiser, August Bros/Francisco/Levy's Old Country—1 roll[6]	167		5.7	33.7	2.7	1.3	0	0				270	47			
1 roll	60	2.0	0.0			0	0							1.80		I
kaiser w/ sesame	140		5.0	25.0	4.0	1.0	0	0				200	40			
1 roll	50	3.5	0.5			0	0							1.80		I
oat bran	78	14.5	3.1	13.3		1.4	0	0	.10	.01	10	136	28	10	.28	.269
1 roll	33	1.5	0.2	0.5	0.5	0	3	.15	1.6	.00	.08	36	34	1.37	.042	818
onion, Arnold/August Bros/Levy Old Country—1 roll[6]	163		5.7	33.0	3.7	2.3	0	0	.14			233	53			
58	2.3	0.2			2	0	.23	1.6					1.80		I
popover																
from mix	67	18.0	2.6	10.4			17	0	.06	.02	6	143	9	5	.21	.095
1 popover (2" x 2")	33	1.5	0.4	0.6	0.2	37	54	.05	0.4	.08	.14	25	30	.56	.022	818
homemade w/ lowfat milk	88	21.8	3.5	11.2		0.4	34	0	.15	.03	7	82	38	7	.30	.092
1 popover (2 ¾" x 4")	40	3.0	0.8	0.9	1.0	46	117	.09	0.7	.13	.23	65	56	.76	.022	818
homemade w/ whole milk	90	21.5	3.4	11.2			28	0	.15	.03	7	82	37	7	.30	.092
1 popover (2 ¾" x 4")	40	3.4	1.1	1.0	1.0	47	97	.09	0.7	.13	.23	64	56	.76	.022	818
potato/potato sesame, Arnold	150		6.0	27.5	5.0	1.0	0	0				170	40			
1 roll[23]	57	2.5	0.3			0	0							1.80		I
Roman Meal	69		2.9	13.0		1.2			.10			140	25			
1 oz roll	28	1.1				0		.10	1.3					1.00		I
rye	81	8.5	2.9	15.1		1.4	0	0	.08	.02	6	253	9	15	.29	.464
1 roll	28	1.0	0.2	0.4	0.2	0	1	.11	1.1	.00	.04	51	45	.77	.045	818
sandwich, soft/soft w/ sesame seeds, Arnold—1 roll	140		5.0	23.0	4.0	1.0	0	0	.10			190	40			
50	3.5	0.5			0	0	.15	1.2					1.44		I
sesame, August Bros	170		6.0	33.0	4.0	1.0	0	0				240	60			
1 roll	57	2.5	0.0			0	0							1.80		I
sourdough/sourdough brown 'n serve, Francisco—1 roll	90		3.0	17.0	1.0	0	0					180	40			
34	1.0	0.0				0							1.08		I
steak, Arnold/August Bros/Francisco	170		6.0	33.7	2.7	2.0	0	0				347	60			
1 roll[6]	66	2.3	0.0			0	0							1.80		I
sub, August Bros/Francisco/Levy Old Country—1 roll[6]	150		5.0	30.3	0.7	1.7	0	0				310	67			
60	1.7	0.0			0	0							1.68		I
wheat	77	10.5	2.4	13.0		1.1	0	0	.08	.02	4	96	50	12	.29	.342
1 roll	28	1.8	0.4	0.9	0.3	0	0	.12	1.2	.00	.04	38	33	1.01	.043	818
whole wheat	75	9.4	2.5	14.5		2.1	0	0	.04	.06	9	136	30	24	.57	.651
1 roll	28	1.3	0.2	0.3	0.6	0	0	.07	1.0	.00	.14	77	64	.69	.068	818
Wiener Wrap, from dough, Pillsbury	60	7.9	1.5	10.5				0	.05			373	4			
1 wrap	22	1.4						.18	0.8			23	112	.75		I

17.15 STUFFING

	KCAL / WT (g)	H_2O / FAT (g)	PRO / SFA (g)	CHO / MUFA (g)	SUGR / PUFA (g)	DFIB / CHOL (mg)	A (RE) / A (IU)	C / B-1 (mg)	B-2 / NIA (mg)	B-6 / B-12	FOL / PANT	Na / K (mg)	Ca / P (mg)	Mg / Fe (mg)	Zn / Cu (mg)	Mn / REF
apple & raisin stuffing mix, Pepperidge Farms—1 oz	106		2.8	21.0				0	.11			402	29			
28	1.1						.14	1.1			104		1.70		I
bread, from mix	178	64.8	3.2	21.7		2.9	81	0	.11	.04	17	543	32	12	.28	.169
½ cup	100	8.6	1.7	3.8	2.6	0	313	.14	1.5	.01	.08	74	42	1.09	.072	818
bread, homemade	195	75.6	4.4	25.8			80	2	.17	.06	20	535	74	17	.37	.242
½ cup	116	8.4	1.7	3.7	2.4	0	349	.20	1.8	.00	.19	152	57	1.90	.080	818
chicken flavor																
from mix, Stove Top	170		4.0	20.0	3.0			0	.07			510	20			
½ cup[24]	109	9.0	1.5			0	300	.09	0.8			90		1.08		I
from mix Stove Top Flexible Serving	170		3.0	19.0	3.0	0		0	.00			460	20			
½ cup[25]	107	8.0	1.5			0	0	.09	2.0			70		1.08		I
homestyle cornbread, from mix, Stove Top Microwave—½ cup[26]	160		3.5	20.0	3.0	1.0		0	.07			480	10			
106	7.0	1.5			0	200	.08	0.8			70		1.08		I
w/ rice stuffing mix, Rice-a-Roni	101	1.7	3.5	20.1	2.4	1.3	1		.10	.02	2	416	59	2	.08	
1 oz	28	1.2	0.3	0.2	0.8	1	40	.15	1.2	.00	.04	85	32	1.38	.010	I
chicken, frzn, Stuffing Originals	170	61.1	3.6	21.8		0.2		0	.12			684	27			
½ cup	96	7.5					127	.32	1.7			93	42	1.44		I

	KCAL / WT (g)	H₂O (g) / FAT (g)	PRO (g) / SFA (g)	CHO (g) / MUFA (g)	SUGR (g) / PUFA (g)	DFIB (g) / CHOL (mg)	A (RE) / A (IU)	C (mg) / B-1 (mg)	B-2 (mg) / NIA (mg)	B-6 (mg) / B-12 (mcg)	FOL (mcg) / PANT (mg)	Na (mg) / K (mg)	Ca (mg) / P (mg)	Mg (mg) / Fe (mg)	Zn (mg) / Cu (mg)	Mn (mg) / REF
cornbread																
from mix	179	64.9	2.9	21.9		2.9	85	1	.09	.04	8	455	26	13	.23	.114
½ cup	100	8.8	1.8	3.9	2.7	0	353	.12	1.2	.01	.06	62	34	.94	.069	818
from mix, Stove Top	170		3.0	21.0	3.0	1.0		0	.07			580	20			
½ cup25	107	8.0	1.5			0	300	.06	0.8			85		.72		I
from mix, Stove Top Flexible Serving	160		3.0	19.0	3.0	1.0		0	.03			560	0			
½ cup25	100	8.0	1.5			0	300	.06				70		.72		I
frzn, Stuffing Originals	170	58.9	3.3	24.7		0.2		0	.10			662	20			
½ cup	95	6.4					125	.28	1.5			100	40	1.02		I
w/ rice stuffing mix, Rice-a-Roni	101	1.5	3.1	20.8	2.5	0.5		0	.08	.02	4	556	24	4	.11	
1 oz	28	0.7	0.1	0.2	0.4	0	41	.13	1.1	.01	.02	43	33	1.37	.010	I
country garden stuffing mix, Pepperidge Farms—1 oz	121		3.6	17.9				0	.10			299	39			
	28	3.9					0	.15	1.3			144		1.70		I
croutettes stuffing mix, Kellogg's	122		4.8	25.0	0.0	0.0		0	.17			460	40			
1 cup	35	3.3				0	0	.12	1.6			50		1.80		I
flavored, from mix, Stove Top	172		4.0	20.3	3.2	1.0		0	.07			565	20			
½ cup27	108	9.0	1.5			0	440	.09	0.9			94		1.35		I
harvest veg stuffing mix, Pepperidge	113		3.8	18.8				0	.11			246	46			
Farms—1 oz	28	2.5					0	.14	1.2			153		2.60		I
herb & butter stuffing mix, Rice-a-Roni	101	1.7	3.5	20.0	2.4	1.4		2	.10	.01	2	401	63	2	.06	
1 oz	28	1.2	0.3	0.2	0.8	1	306	.15	1.1	.09	.03	84	34	1.42	.010	I
homestyle herb, from mix, Stove Top	170		3.0	19.0	3.0			0	.07			500	20			
Flexible Serving—½ cup25	96	8.0	1.5			0	300	.09	0.8			75		1.20		I
long grain & wild rice, from mix, Stove	180		4.0	22.0	3.0			0	.08			560	20			
Top—½ cup25	109	9.0	1.5			0	300	.09	0.8			75		1.08		I
mushroom, frzn, Stuffing Originals	150	60.7	4.1	18.7		0.3		0	.12			763	25			
½ cup	92	6.4					98	.18	1.7			100	46	1.29		I
stuffing mix, Arnold	246		9.0	48.8	3.0	2.8		0				756	40			
2 cups28	67	3.2	0.6				40							3.06		I
wild rice & mushroom stuffing mix,	126		3.6	16.9				0	.11			308	29			
Pepperidge Farms—1 oz	28	4.9					0	.13	1.3			131		1.50		I
wild rice, frzn, Stuffing Originals	160	47.5	2.9	20.9				1	.10			548	18			
½ cup	100	7.0					70	.14	1.3			95	38	1.14		I
w/ wild rice stuffing mix, Rice-a-Roni	102	1.7	3.5	20.0	2.4	1.3		1	.09	.01	2	486	36	2	.04	
1 oz	28	1.3	0.3	0.2	0.8	1	39	.08	1.1	.00	.02	70	41	1.14	.010	I

17.16 TORTILLAS

	KCAL / WT (g)	H₂O (g) / FAT (g)	PRO (g) / SFA (g)	CHO (g) / MUFA (g)	SUGR (g) / PUFA (g)	DFIB (g) / CHOL (mg)	A (RE) / A (IU)	C (mg) / B-1 (mg)	B-2 (mg) / NIA (mg)	B-6 (mg) / B-12 (mcg)	FOL (mcg) / PANT (mg)	Na (mg) / K (mg)	Ca (mg) / P (mg)	Mg (mg) / Fe (mg)	Zn (mg) / Cu (mg)	Mn (mg) / REF
corn	56	11.0	1.4	11.7	0.1	1.3	6	0	.02	.05	4	40	44	16	.23	.101
1 med (6-7" dia)	25	0.6	0.1	0.2	0.3	0	61	.03	0.4	.00	.05	39	79	.35	.038	818
taco shell	61	0.8	0.9	8.1		1.0	5	0	.01	.05	1	48	21	14	.18	.057
1 med (5" dia)	13	2.9	0.4	1.2	1.1	0	46	.03	0.2	.00	.06	23	32	.33	.016	818
taco shell, Gebhardt	155		2.0	19.3	0.0	2.9	0	0				1	0			
3 shells	32	8.3	2.4			0	0							.03		I
flour																
flour	114	9.4	3.0	19.5		1.2	0	0	.10	.02	4	167	44	9	.25	.162
7-8" dia	35	2.5	0.4	1.0	1.0	0	0	.19	1.3	.00	.20	46	43	1.15	.093	818
large, Tyson	171	16.5	3.9	29.5	0.9	1.7	0	0				407	37			
9 ½" dia	55	4.2	0.9	1.6	0.5	0	0							.52		I
medium, Tyson	124	11.9	2.8	21.3	0.6	1.2	0	0				294	26			
8" dia	40	3.0	0.6	1.2	0.4	0	0							.38		I
small, Tyson	88	8.5	2.0	15.2	0.5	0.9	0	0				209	19			
6 ½" dia	28	2.1	0.4	0.8	0.3	0	0							.27		I
tostada shells, Rosarita	125		2.0	17.2	0.3	0.0	0	0				20	30			
2 shells	28	4.9	0.9			37	0							.37		I

17.17 WAFFLES

	KCAL / WT (g)	H₂O (g) / FAT (g)	PRO (g) / SFA (g)	CHO (g) / MUFA (g)	SUGR (g) / PUFA (g)	DFIB (g) / CHOL (mg)	A (RE) / A (IU)	C (mg) / B-1 (mg)	B-2 (mg) / NIA (mg)	B-6 (mg) / B-12 (mcg)	FOL (mcg) / PANT (mg)	Na (mg) / K (mg)	Ca (mg) / P (mg)	Mg (mg) / Fe (mg)	Zn (mg) / Cu (mg)	Mn (mg) / REF
apple cinn, frzn, Eggo	220	29.6	4.9	33.0	5.0	1.0		0	.34	.40	40	451	40			
2 waffles	78	7.8	1.7	4.1	2.0	22	1000	.30	4.0	1.20		39		3.60		I

	KCAL	H₂O (g)	PRO (g)	CHO (g)	SUGR (g)	DFIB (g)	A (RE)	C (mg)	B-2 (mg)	B-6 (mg)	FOL (mcg)	Na (mg)	Ca (mg)	Mg (mg)	Zn (mg)	Mn (mg)
	WT (g)	FAT (g)	SFA (g)	MUFA (g)	PUFA (g)	CHOL (mg)	A (IU)	B-1 (mg)	NIA (mg)	B-12 (mcg)	PANT (mg)	K (mg)	P (mg)	Fe (mg)	Cu (mg)	REF
blueberry, frzn, Eggo	218	30.3	4.9	32.0	6.0	1.0		0	.34	.40	40	460	40			
2 waffles	78	9.0	1.6	5.3	2.1	22	1000	.30	4.0	1.20		39		3.60		I
blueberry minis, frzn, Eggo	239	32.0	5.5	37.5	7.0	1.8		1	.51	.60	60	520	40			
3 pieces	85	8.0	1.4	4.7	1.9	25	1500	.45	6.0	1.80		119		5.40		I
buttermilk, frzn, Eggo	217	32.5	5.0	31.0	2.8	1.4		1	.34	.40	40	460	40			
2 waffles	78	8.0	1.5	5.5	1.0	24	1000	.30	4.0	1.20		90		3.60		I
buttermilk, homemade	217	31.6	6.2	24.8			26	0	.27	.04	11	451	137	14	.56	.199
1 waffle (7" dia)	75	10.2	1.9	2.5	5.1	50	91	.20	1.5	.16	.36	128	124	1.63	.049	818
cinn toast, frzn, Eggo	291	29.8	5.2	45.3	17.2	2.0		1	.51	.60	40	470	40			
3 pieces	92	9.8	2.0	6.3	1.5	23	1500	.45	6.0	1.80		102		5.40		I
homestyle, frzn, Eggo	218	31.2	5.2	32.0	3.3	1.0		1	.34	.40	40	480	40			
2 waffles	78	7.6	1.6	5.5	0.5	23	1000	.30	4.0	1.20		102		3.60		I
homestyle minis, frzn, Eggo	260	37.2	7.0	38.0	3.0	2.0		2	.51	.60	60	600	60			
3 pieces	93	9.0	2.0			25	1500	.45	6.0	1.80		130		5.40		I
multi-bran, frzn, Nutri-Grain	181	34.2	5.1	32.0	4.0	6.0		2	.34	.40	24	410	40			
2 waffles	78	6.2	0.9	3.5	1.5	0	1000	.30	4.0	1.20		160		3.60		I
nut & honey, frzn, Eggo	240	28.9	6.4	31.0	5.0	2.0		1	.34	.40	40	450	40			
2 waffles	78	9.8	1.9	5.2	1.6	23	1000	.30	4.0	1.20		125		3.60		I
Nutri-Grain frzn, Kellogg's	188	34.4	5.0	30.0	4.2	4.0		0	.34	.40	40	450	40			
2 waffles	78	6.0	1.0	3.5	1.5	0	1000	.30	4.0	1.20		150		1.80		I
oat bran, frzn, Common Sense	196	35.0	5.8	27.0	3.0	2.7		1	.34	.40	40	390	40			
2 waffles	78	7.2	1.5	4.5	1.0	0	1000	.30	4.0	1.20		142		3.60		I
plain																
from complete mix	218	31.9	4.6	26.4		1.0	20	0	.19	.08	9	458	93	15	.35	.197
1 waffle (7" dia)	75	10.3	1.7	2.7	5.2	38	68	.15	1.2	.20	.25	134	252	1.22	.068	818
frzn	87	13.9	2.0	13.4		0.8	120	0	.16	.30	12	260	77	7	.19	.121
1 waffle (4" sq)	33	2.7	0.5	1.1	0.9	8	400	.13	1.5	.83	.13	42	139	1.48	.025	818
homemade	218	31.5	5.9	24.7			49	0	.26	.04	11	383	191	14	.51	.199
1 waffle (7" dia)	75	10.6	2.1	2.6	5.1	52	171	.20	1.6	.19	.36	119	143	1.73	.046	818
raisin & bran, frzn, Nutri-Grain	210	36.0	5.1	36.0	10.0	5.0		1	.34	.40	24	430	40			
2 waffles	82	6.2	1.0	3.5	1.5	0	1000	.30	4.0	1.20		213		3.60		I
Special K, frzn, Kellogg's	140	26.0	5.8	29.0	3.8	1.2		1	.34	.40	40	270	40			
2 waffles	58	0.0	0.0	0.0	0.0	0	1000	.30	4.0	1.20		130		3.60		I
strawberry, frzn, Eggo	220	31.0	5.0	32.1	5.0	1.4		1	.34	.40	40	462	40			
2 waffles	78	7.9	1.6	5.4	0.9	22	1000	.30	4.0	1.20		110		3.60		I

1. Cornbread usually made w/o milk or eggs, shaped in irregular ovals by the palm of the hand and baked or fried on a griddle.
2. Toasted breads have essentially the same nutrient content as untoasted bread of the same variety except that the water content is lower in the toasted bread. The weight of the toast is decreased by the weight of the water lost during toasting.
3. Values are averages for both brands.
4. Values are averages for both brands; values for garlic, onion, salsa, and sourdough are similar.
5. Values pertain to both brands.
6. Values are averages for all three brands.
7. Made with cornmeal, hominy, milk, eggs, shortening, and leavening.
8. Values are averages for banana nut, blueberry, chocolate chip, cinnamon apple, corn, raisin bran, and strawberry.
9. Values are averages for garlic, onion, regular, and sesame.
10. The low sodium product contains 75 mg sodium.
11. Values are averages for cheese garlic, herb, italian, onion & garlic, ranch, and seasoned croutons.
12. The low sodium product contains 35 mg sodium.
13. Low sodium product contains 35 mg sodium. The Unsalted Tops Saltines contain 135 mg sodium.
14. Values are averages for bacon, onion, pumpernickel, rye, sesame, and wheat.
15. Values are averages for blueberry, cranberry, onion, and raisin.
16. Values are averages for regular, onion, sourdough, and wheat.
17. Lowfat milk, egg, and vegetable oil added to mix.
18. Long grain rice in oyster and soy sauce with cooked egg and vegetables.
19. White rice in chicken broth with corn, mushrooms, red peppers, onions, and celery.
20. Unenriched rice contains .32 mg iron, .03 mg thiamin, 0.6 mg niacin, and 604 mg sodium if salt is used.
21. Unenriched rice contains 0.37 mg iron, .04 mg thiamin, and 0.7 mg niacin.
22. Values are averages for wheat and white rolls for both brands.
23. Values are averages for both products.
24. Prepared with margarine and salt. Lower sodium product contains 270 mg sodium.
25. Prepared with margarine and salt.
26. Values are averages for chicken flavor and homestyle cornbread made with margarine and salt.
27. Values are averages for beef, pork, turkey, mushroom & onion, San Francisco style, and savory herbs. Prepared with margarine and salt.
28. Values are averages for cornbread, herb seasoned, sage & onion, seasoned, and unspiced.

						Vitamins					Minerals				
KCAL	H₂O (g)	PRO (g)	CHO (g)	SUGR (g)	DFIB (g)	A (RE)	C (mg)	B-2 (mg)	B-6 (mg)	FOL (mcg)	Na (mg)	Ca (mg)	Mg (mg)	Zn (mg)	Mn (mg)
WT (g)	FAT (g)	SFA (g)	MUFA (g)	PUFA (g)	CHOL (mg)	A (IU)	B-1 (mg)	NIA (mg)	B-12 (mcg)	PANT (mg)	K (mg)	P (mg)	Fe (mg)	Cu (mg)	
TRY (mg)	THR (mg)	ISO (mg)	LEU (mg)	LYS (mg)	MET (mg)	D (IU)	E (IU)	K (mcg)	BIO (mcg)	CHLN (mcg)	CI (mg)	I (mcg)	Mo (mcg)	F (mcg)	
CYS (mg)	PHE (mg)	TYR (mg)	VAL (mg)	ARG (mg)	HIS (mg)	INOS (mg)	E (AT) (mg)								REF

18. INFANT FORMULAS[1]

Advance (cow milk, soy protein isolate; soy and corn oils; corn syrup, lactose) — *1 fl oz*

KCAL	H₂O	PRO	CHO	SUGR	DFIB	A	C	B-2	B-6	FOL	Na	Ca	Mg	Zn	Mn
16	27.2	0.6	1.6				2	.03	.01	3	6	15	1	.14	.001
30	0.8	0.1	0.2	0.4	0	59	.02	0.2	.05	.09	23	12		.29	.018
7	24	27	51	40	13										
5	26		30		15										I

Alimentum, Ross Labs (casein hydrolysate, cystine, tyrosine, tryptophan; MCTs, safflower & soy oils; sucrose, modified tapioca starch) — *1 fl oz*

KCAL	H₂O	PRO	CHO	SUGR	DFIB	A	C	B-2	B-6	FOL	Na	Ca	Mg	Zn	Mn
20	26.6	0.6	2.0				2	.02	.01	3	9	21	2	.15	.006
30	1.1	0.5	0.1	0.4		60	.01	0.3	.09	.15	24	15		.36	.015
10	25	30	51	44	15										
9	28		38		14										I

Enfamil, 20 cal/fl oz, Mead Johnson (reduced mineral whey, nonfat milk; coconut & corn oils; lactose) — *1 fl oz[2]*

KCAL	H₂O	PRO	CHO	SUGR	DFIB	A	C	B-2	B-6	FOL	Na	Ca	Mg	Zn	Mn
20	26.8	0.4	2.1				2	.03	.01	3	5	14	2	.16	.003
30	1.1	0.5	0.2	0.3	0	62	.02	0.3	.05	.09	22	9		.03	.019
7	23	27	46	31	9										
5	17	20	27		9										I

Enfamil, 24 cal/fl oz, Mead Johnson (reduced mineral whey, nonfat milk; coconut & soy oils; lactose) — *1 fl oz[3]*

KCAL	H₂O	PRO	CHO	SUGR	DFIB	A	C	B-2	B-6	FOL	Na	Ca	Mg	Zn	Mn
24	26.2	0.5	2.5				2	.04	.02	4	6	17	2	.19	.004
30	1.3	0.6	0.2	0.4	0	74	.02	0.3	.06	.11	26	11		.04	.023
8	28	32	55	37	10										
6	21		33		10										I

Enfamil Human Milk Fortifier, Mead Johnson (whey protein conc, casein; corn syrup solids) — *4 pkts[4]*

KCAL	H₂O	PRO	CHO	SUGR	DFIB	A	C	B-2	B-6	FOL	Na	Ca	Mg	Zn	Mn
14	0.1	0.7	2.7			290	12	.21	.11	25	8	90	1	.71	.005
4	0.1				0	950	.15	3.0	.18	.73	16	45		.060	
						210	4.6	4	3		18				
							3.10								I

Enfamil Premature Formula, 20 cal/fl oz, Mead Johnson (whey, nonfat milk; coconut & soy oils; lactose) — *1 fl oz[5]*

KCAL	H₂O	PRO	CHO	SUGR	DFIB	A	C	B-2	B-6	FOL	Na	Ca	Mg	Zn	Mn
20	26.6	0.6	2.2				7	.07	.05	7	8	23	2	.20	.003
30	1.0	0.3	0.4	0.2	0	240	.05	0.8	.06	.24	22	12		.05	.032
9	33	35	58	46	14										
6	23	27	36		12										I

i-Soyalac (soy protein isolate, L-methionine; soy oil; sucrose, tapioca dextrin) — *1 fl oz*

KCAL	H₂O	PRO	CHO	SUGR	DFIB	A	C	B-2	B-6	FOL	Na	Ca	Mg	Zn	Mn
20	25.6	0.6	2.0				2	.02	.01	5	8	20	2	.16	.009
30	1.1	0.2	0.3	0.7	0	62	.02	0.2	.06	.09	23	14		.38	.023
6	22	30	48	38	14										
	33		28		16										I

Isomil, 20 cal/fl oz, Ross Labs (soy protein isolate; soy & coconut oils; corn syrup, sucrose) — *1 fl oz*

KCAL	H₂O	PRO	CHO	SUGR	DFIB	A	C	B-2	B-6	FOL	Na	Ca	Mg	Zn	Mn
20	26.6	0.5	2.0			18	2	.02	.01	3	9	21	2	.15	.006
30	1.1	0.5	0.2	0.4	0	60	.01	0.3	.09	.15	22	15		.36	.015
6	20	23	43	31	12										
6	27	19	22	38	12		.40								I

Isomil, SF, 20 cal/fl oz, Ross Labs (soy protein isolate; soy & coconut oils; corn syrup, sucrose) — *1 fl oz*

KCAL	H₂O	PRO	CHO	SUGR	DFIB	A	C	B-2	B-6	FOL	Na	Ca	Mg	Zn	Mn
20	26.6	0.5	2.0			18	2	.02	.01	3	9	21	2	.15	.006
30	1.1	0.5	0.2	0.4	0	60	.01	0.3	.09	.15	22	15		.36	.015
6	20	23	43	31	12										
6	27	21	22	43	12		.40								I

Lofenalac, Mead Johnson (enzymatic digest of casein processed to remove phe; corn oil; corn syrup solids, modified tapioca starch) — *3 ½ oz powder[6]*

KCAL	H₂O	PRO	CHO	SUGR	DFIB	A	C	B-2	B-6	FOL	Na	Ca	Mg	Zn	Mn
460	3.8	15.0	60.0			430	37	.43	.29	72	220	430	50	3.60	.143
100	18.0	2.4	4.6	10.9	2	1430	.36	5.8	1.43	2.20	470	320		8.70	.430
200	780	870	1670	1650	540	290	14.3	72	36	61	320	32			
60	75	800	1380	560	480	22	9.60								I

Low Met Diet, Mead Johnson (soy protein isolate; coconut & corn oil; corn syrup solids) — *3 ½ oz powder[7]*

KCAL	H₂O	PRO	CHO	SUGR	DFIB	A	C	B-2	B-6	FOL	Na	Ca	Mg	Zn	Mn
515	2.3	15.5	51.0			480	42	.48	.32	80	185	540	56	6.20	.129
100	28.0	11.2	10.6	5.3	0	1610	.40	6.4	1.61	2.40	630	430		9.70	.480
186	500	710	1180	930	155	320	16.1	80	40	40	430	52			
140	760	530	710	990	360	24	10.80								I

Low Phe/Tyr Diet, Mead Johnson (specially processed casein hydrolysate; corn oil; corn syrup solids, modified tapioca starch) — *3 ½ oz powder[8]*

KCAL	H₂O	PRO	CHO	SUGR	DFIB	A	C	B-2	B-6	FOL	Na	Ca	Mg	Zn	Mn
460	3.8	15.0	60.0			430	37	.43	.29	72	220	430	50	3.60	.143
100	18.0	2.4	4.6	10.9	2	1430	.36	5.8	1.43	2.20	470	320		8.70	.430
200	780	870	1670	1650	540	290	14.3	72	36	61	320	32			
60	75	41	1380	560	480	22	9.6								I

Mono- and Disaccharide-Free Diet, Mead Johnson (casein enzymically hydrolyzed; MCTs, corn oil; modified tapioca starch) — *3 ½ oz powder[9]*

KCAL	H₂O	PRO	CHO	SUGR	DFIB	A	C	B-2	B-6	FOL	Na	Ca	Mg	Zn	Mn
500	3.0	22.0	33.3			900	92	.74	.49	123	340	740	86	4.90	.250
100	33.0	0.0	1.3	3.0	3	3000	.61	9.8	2.50	3.70	860	490		14.80	.740
350	1080	1320	2200	1890	680	590	30.0	148	61	105	680	55			
350	1060	620	1650	880	660	37	20.00								I

	KCAL	H₂O (g)	PRO (g)	CHO (g)	SUGR (g)	DFIB (g)	A (RE)	C (mg)	B-2 (mg)	B-6 (mg)	FOL (mcg)	Na (mg)	Ca (mg)	Mg (mg)	Zn (mg)	Mn (mg)
	WT (g)	FAT (g)	SFA (g)	MUFA (g)	PUFA (g)	CHOL (mg)	A (IU)	B-1 (mg)	NIA (mg)	B-12 (mcg)	PANT (mg)	K (mg)	P (mg)	Fe (mg)	Cu (mg)	
	TRY (mg)	THR (mg)	ISO (mg)	LEU (mg)	LYS (mg)	MET (mg)	D (IU)	E (IU)	K (mcg)	BIO (mcg)	CHLN (mcg)	CI (mg)	I (mcg)	Mo (mcg)	F (mcg)	
	CYS (mg)	PHE (mg)	TYR (mg)	VAL (mg)	ARG (mg)	HIS (mg)	INOS (mg)	E (AT) (mg)								REF
MSUD Diet, Mead Johnson (casein	470	3.3	8.1	63.0			440	38	.44	.30	74	184	490	52	3.70	.147
enzymically hydrolyzed; corn oil; corn	100	20.0	2.7	5.1	12.1	0	1470	.37	5.9	1.47	2.20	490	260	8.90	.440	
syrup solids, modified tapioca starch)	240	520	0	0	770	220	300	14.7	74	37		370	33			
3 ½ oz powder[10]	186	520	630	0	430	240	22	9.80								I
Nursoy, 20 cal/fl oz, Wyeth (soy protein	20	26.6	0.6	2.0			18	2	.03	.01	2	6	18	2	.16	.006
isolate; oleo, coconut, oleic & soy oils;	30	1.1	0.4	0.4	0.1	0	60	.02	0.2	.06	.09	21	13	.34	.014	
sucrose)	9	25	33	54	36	16										
1 fl oz	9	33	26	32	49	17										I
Nutramigen, Mead Johnson (casein	20	26.8	0.6	2.7				2	.02	.01	3	9	19	2	.16	.006
hydrolysate, cystine, tyrosine,	30	0.8	0.1	0.2	0.5	0	62	.02	0.3	.06	.09	22	12	.38	.019	
tryptophan; corn oil; corn syrup solids,	9	27	34	58	48	17										
modified corn starch)—*1 fl oz*[11]	9	27		42		17										I
Pediasure, Ross Labs (low-lactose whey	30	25.2	0.9	3.3				3	.06	.08	11	11	29	6	.36	.075
protein, sodium caseinate; high-oleic	31	1.5	0.4	0.6	0.4	1	77	.08	0.5	.18	.30	39	24	.42	.030	
safflower & soy oils; MCTs; corn syrup	12	43	43	86	68	25										
solids, sucrose)—*1 fl oz*	8	43		51		22										I
Portagen, 20 cal/fl oz, Mead Johnson	470	3.0	16.5	54.0			1110	38	.89	.99	74	260	440	94	4.40	.590
(sodium caseinate; corn oil, MCTs; corn	100	23.0	0.5	0.8	2.0	2	3700	.74	9.9	3.00	5.00	590	330	8.90	.740	
syrup solids, sucrose)	210	680	940	1650	1410	470	370	14.6	74	37	63	410	33			
3 ½ oz powder[12]	49	910	940	1180	660	520	22	9.80								I
Pregestimil, 20 cal/fl oz, Mead Johnson	20	26.8	0.6	2.1				2	.02	.01	3	9	19	2	.19	.006
(casein hydolysate, cys, tyr, try; MCTs,	30	1.1	0.1	0.2	0.2	0	76	.02	0.3	.06	.09	22	13	.38	.019	
corn & safflower oils; corn syrup solids,	8	27	34	58	48	17										
corn starch, dextrose)—*1 fl oz*[13]	8	27	13	42		17										I
ProSobee, 20 cal/fl oz Mead Johnson (soy	20	26.8	0.6	2.0				2	.02	.01	3	7	19	2	.16	.005
protein isolate; coconut & soy oils; corn	30	1.1	0.5	0.2	0.3	0	62	.02	0.3	.06	.09	24	15	.38	.019	
syrup solids)	7	19	28	46	36	11										
1 fl oz[14]	5	29	20	28		14										I
Protein-Free Diet Powder, Mead Johnson	490	3.0	0.0	72.0			540	47	.54	.36	90	72	540	63	4.50	.180
(corn oil; corn syrup solids, modified	100	23.0	3.1	5.9	14.0	0	1800	.45	7.2	1.80	2.70	340	300	10.80	.540	
tapioca starch)							360	18.0	90	45	77	135	40			
3 ½ oz[15] *powder*							27	12.10								I
RCF (Ross Carbohydrate Free), Ross Labs	12	28.1	0.6	0.0	0.0		18	2	.02	.01	3	9	21	1	.15	.006
(soy protein isolate; soy &	30	1.1	0.5	0.2	0.4	0	60	.01	0.3	.09	.15	22	15	.04	.015	
coconut oils)	6	21	26	47	36	13	12	.6	3	1						
1 fl oz	6	29	21	26	43	14		.40								I
Similac, 13 cal/fl oz, Ross Labs	13	27.7	0.4	1.4			12	1	.02	.01	2	4	12	1	.10	.001
(cow milk; soy & coconut oils;	30	0.7	0.3	0.1	0.2	0	39	.01	0.1	.03	.06	17	9	.03	.012	
lactose)	5	15	17	33	25	10										
1 fl oz[16]	3	17	15	19	11	7		.30								I
Similac, 20 cal/fl oz, Ross Labs	20	26.6	0.4	2.1			18	2	.03	.01	3	6	15	1	.15	.001
(cow milk; soy & coconut oils;	30	1.1	0.5	0.2	0.4	0	60	.02	0.2	.05	.09	22	12	.04	.018	
lactose)	6	19	22	42	32	12		.4								
1 fl oz[17]	4	22	20	24	15	9		.50								I
Similac, 24 cal/fl oz, Ross Labs	24	26.2	0.7	2.5			22	2	.04	.01	4	8	22	2	.18	.001
(cow milk; soy & coconut oils;	30	1.3	0.6	0.2	0.5	0	72	.02	0.3	.06	.11	32	17	.05	.021	
lactose)	8	28	32	61	46	18										
1 fl oz[18]	6	32	29	35	22	13		.50								I
Similac, 27 cal/fl oz, Ross Labs	27	25.7	0.7	2.8		0.0	24	2	.04	.02	4	9	24	2	.20	.001
(cow milk; soy & coconut oils;	30	1.4	0.6	0.2	0.5	0	81	.03	0.3	.07	.12	36	19	.06	.024	
lactose)	9	31	36	69	52	20										
1 fl oz	6	36	34	40	25	15		.50								I

	KCAL	H₂O (g)	PRO (g)	CHO (g)	SUGR (g)	DFIB (g)	A (RE)	C (mg)	B-2 (mg)	B-6 (mg)	FOL (mcg)	Na (mg)	Ca (mg)	Mg (mg)	Zn (mg)	Mn (mg)
	WT (g)	FAT (g)	SFA (g)	MUFA (g)	PUFA (g)	CHOL (mg)	A (IU)	B-1 (mg)	NIA (mg)	B-12 (mcg)	PANT (mg)	K (mg)	P (mg)	Fe (mg)	Cu (mg)	
	TRY (mg)	THR (mg)	ISO (mg)	LEU (mg)	LYS (mg)	MET (mg)	D (IU)	E (IU)	K (mcg)	BIO (mcg)	CHLN (mcg)	CI (mg)	I (mcg)	Mo (mcg)	F (mcg)	REF
	CYS (mg)	PHE (mg)	TYR (mg)	VAL (mg)	ARG (mg)	HIS (mg)	INOS (mg)	E (AT) (mg)								
Similac Natural Care, Human Milk Fortifier, Ross Labs (cow milk, whey; MCTs, soy & coconut oils; lactose, corn syrup solids)—*1 fl oz*	24	26.2	0.7	2.5			49	9	.15	.06	9	10	50	3	.36	.003
	30	1.3	0.7	0.1	0.2	1	163	.06	1.2	.13	.46	31	25	.09	.060	
	7	38	34	64	51	16										I
	10	21	22	35	18	13		.70								
Similac PM 60/40, 20 cal/fl oz, Ross Labs (whey, caseinate; soy & coconut oils; lactose) *1 fl oz*	20	26.8	0.5	2.0			18	2	.03	.01	3	5	11	1	.15	.001
	30	1.1	0.5	0.2	0.4	1	60	.02	0.2	.05	.09	17	6	.04	.018	
	7	29	29	51	40	13										I
	7	17	17	28	14	10		.40								
Similac Special Care, 20 cal/fl oz, Ross Labs (cow milk, whey; MCTs, soy & coconut oils; lactose, corn syrup solids)—*1 fl oz*	20	26.6	0.5	2.1			41	7	.12	.05	7	9	36	2	.30	.002
	30	1.1	0.6	0.1	0.2	1	136	.05	1.0	.11	.38	26	18	.07	.050	
	6	32	29	57	43	13										I
	9	18	19	29	15	11		.50								
Similac Special Care, 24 cal/fl oz, Ross Labs (cow milk, whey; MCTs, soy & coconut oils; lactose, corn syrup solids)—*1 fl oz*[19]	24	26.2	0.7	2.5				9	.15	.06	9	10	43	3	.36	.003
	30	1.3	0.7	0.1	0.2	1	163	.06	1.2	.13	.46	31	22	.09	.060	
	7	38	34	64	51	16										I
	10	21	22	35	18	13		.50								
SMA, 20 cal/fl oz, Wyeth (nonfat milk, demineralized whey; oleo, coconut, oleic & soy oils, lactose) *1 fl oz*[20]	20	26.8	0.4	2.1			18	2	.03	.01	2	4	13	1	.16	.004
	30	1.1	0.4	0.4	0.1	1	60	.02	0.2	.04	.06	17	8	.04	.014	
	7	24	25	44	35	11										
	8	19		27		11										I
SMA, 27 cal/fl oz, Wyeth (nonfat milk, demineralized whey; oleo, coconut, oleic & soy oils, lactose) *1 fl oz*[21]	27	25.9	0.6	2.9				2	.04	.02	2	6	17	2	.22	.006
	31	1.4	0.6	0.6	0.2	1	81	.03	0.2	.05	.09	22	11	.05	.019	
	10	32	33	60	47	15										
	11	25		36		15										I
SMA Preemie, 20 cal/fl oz, Wyeth (nonfat milk, demineralized whey; coconut, oleic, oleo & soy oils; MCTs; lactose, glucose polymers)—*1 fl oz*	20	26.6	0.6	2.1				2	.04	.02	3	9	22	2	.24	.006
	30	1.0	0.5	0.3	0.2		95	.02	0.2	.06	.11	22	11	.09	.021	
	11	43	41	75	63	14										
	11	33		44		15										I
SMA Preemie, 24 cal/fl oz, Wyeth (nonfat milk, demineralized whey; oleo, coconut, oleic & soy oils; lactose) *1 fl oz*	24	25.9	0.6	2.5			21	2	.04	.01	3	10	22	2	.24	.006
	30	1.3	0.6	0.4	0.2		72	.02	0.2	.07	.11	22	12	.09	.021	
	9	42	41	74	62	14										
	11	32	32	44	21	15										I
Soylac (soybean solids, L-methionine; soy oil; corn syrup, sucrose, soybean carbohydrates) *1 fl oz*	20	25.6	0.6	2.0				2	.02	.01	5	9	19	2	.16	.031
	30	1.1	0.2	0.3	0.7	0	62	.02	0.3	.06	.09	23	11	.38	.016	
	6	24	28	48	38	13										
		30		28		16										I

1. The product description lists the protein source(s), fat source(s), and carbohydrate source(s), respectively.
2. Enfamil 20 cal/floz with iron contains .38 mg.
3. Enfamil, 24 cal/fl oz with iron contains .45 mg iron.
4. Nutritional supplement added to mother's milk for premature infants.
5. Product with iron contains .38 mg iron.
6. Low phenylalanine formula for infants and children with phenylketonuria.
7. Formula without added methionine for management of infants with homocystinuria.
8. Formula low in phenylalanine and tyrosine for use in tryosinemia.
9. Protein hydrolysate formula base for use with added carbohydrate.
10. Free of branched chain amino acids for use with maple syrup urine disease.
11. Hypoallergenic formula supplying protein nutrients in hydrolyzed form for infants and children sensitive to the intact proteins of milk and other foods.
12. Nutritionally complete formula for infants, children, and adults who do not efficiently digest conventional food fat or absorb the resulting long chain fatty acids.
13. Formula with readily digestible sources of protein, fat, and carbohydrate in a hypoallergenic, low osmolality form.
14. Milk-free, lactose-free, and sucrose-free formula with soy protein for infants with milk sensitivity.
15. Formula base for use in making diets for infants requiring specific mixtures of amino acids.
16. Similac, 13 cal/fl oz with iron contains .23 mg iron.
17. Similac, 20 cal/fl oz with iron contains .36 mg iron.
18. Similac, 24 cal/fl oz with iron contains .43 mg iron.
19. Similac Special Care, 24 cal/fl oz with iron contains .43 mg iron.
20. SMA, 20 cal/fl oz with iron contains .36 mg iron.
21. SMA, 27 cal/fl oz with iron contains .49 mg iron.

	KCAL	H_2O (g)	PRO (g)	CHO (g)	SUGR (g)	DFIB (g)	A (RE)	C (mg)	B-2 (mg)	B-6 (mg)	FOL (mcg)	Na (mg)	Ca (mg)	Mg (mg)	Zn (mg)	Mn (mg)
	WT (g)	FAT (g)	SFA (g)	MUFA (g)	PUFA (g)	CHOL (mg)	A (IU)	B-1 (mg)	NIA (mg)	B-12 (mcg)	PANT (mg)	K (mg)	P (mg)	Fe (mg)	Cu (mg)	REF

19. INFANT, JUNIOR, & TODDLER FOODS
19.1 BAKED PRODUCTS

animal crackers, Gerber	36		0.5	6.2	2.3	0.4			.02	.01		31	2	3	.10	.070
.3 oz	8	1.0	0.2					.03	0.3			12	14	.30	.010	I
arrowroot cookie	27	0.3	0.5	4.3		0.0		0	.03	.00	1	22	2	1	.03	
.2 oz cookie	6	0.9	0.2	0.5	0.1	0	0	.03	0.3	.00	.03	9	7	.18	.004	803
arrowroot cookie, Gerber Graduates	23		0.4	3.6	1.3	0.2			.01			16	2	2	.00	.020
.2 oz cookie	5	0.8	0.1					.02	0.1			6	6	.20	.000	I
baby cookie	30	0.4	0.8	4.7		0.0	0	0	.23	.41	1	13	7	3	.08	
.2 oz cookie	7	0.9	0.3	0.5	0.1	0	2	.10	1.1	.32	.04	35	13	.29	.005	803
baby pretzel	24	0.2	0.6	4.9		0.1	0	0	.02	.00	1	16	2	2	.05	
.2 oz pretzel	6	0.1	0.0	0.0	0.0	0	0	.03	0.2	.00	.03	8	7	.23	.009	803
banana cookie, Gerber Graduates	35		0.5	5.9	2.3	0.3		0	.03	.02		1	7	3	.10	.040
.3 oz cookie	8	1.0	0.2				189	.03	0.3			34	15	.20	.010	I
biter biscuit, Gerber Graduates	43		1.0	8.5	3.4	0.2		0	.04	.01		28	11	4	.10	.030
.4 oz biscuit	11	0.6						.01	0.3			37	15	.30	.010	I
pretzels, Gerber Graduates	23		0.8	4.8	0.4	0.2			.03	.01		15	2	2	.10	.050
.2 oz	6	0.1						.04	0.3			8	7	.30	.010	I
teething biscuit	43	0.7	1.2	8.4		0.2	1	1	.06	.01	2	40	29	4	.10	
.4 oz biscuit	11	0.5	0.2	0.2	0.1	0	13	.03	0.5	.01	.06	36	18	.39	.016	803
veggie crackers, Gerber Graduates	38		0.5	5.3	0.9	0.5		0	.00	.00		63	4	3	.10	.040
.3 oz	8	1.7	0.4				19	.00	0.0			23	13	.30	.020	I
zwieback toast	30	0.3	0.7	5.2		0.2	0	0	.02	.01	1	16	1	1	.04	
.2 oz piece	7	0.7	0.3	0.3	0.1	1	4	.01	0.1	.00	.04	21	4	.04	.010	803
zwieback toast, Gerber Graduates	30		0.9	4.9	0.9	0.4			.04	.01		14	4	2	.01	.040
.2 oz piece	7	0.8						.05	0.4			10	9	.30	.010	I

19.2 CEREALS

barley, dry	9	0.2	0.3	1.8		0.2	0	0	.06	.01	1	1	19	3	.08	
1 T	2.4	0.1	0.0	0.0	0.0	0	0	.07	0.9	.00	.01	9	11	1.14	.011	803
Beech-Nut Stage 1	52		1.6	10.5					.28			11	119			
.5 oz	14	0.4						.22	3.6					6.72		I
Gerber	57		1.9	11.1	0.9	1.7		9	.27	.06		2	90	19	.30	.210
.5 oz	15	0.5						.23	2.0			51	75	6.80	.060	I
barley, prep w/ whole milk	31	21.2	1.3	4.6					.16	.03	3	14	65	9	.24	
1 oz	28	0.9					30	.14	1.7	.09	.10	54	43	3.50	.024	803
cereal & egg yolks, jr	111	188.9	4.0	15.1		1.9	87	1	.10	.04	7	70	51	6	.62	
1 jar	213	3.8	1.3	1.7	0.6	134	307	.02	0.1	.13	1.87	75	85	1.09	.047	803
cereal & egg yolks, str	65	113.7	2.4	9.0		1.2	51	1	.06	.03	4	42	31	4	.36	
1 jar	128	2.3	0.8	1.0	0.4	81	180	.01	0.1	.09	1.12	50	51	.60	.028	803
cereal, egg yolks, & bacon, str	101	110.0	3.2	7.9		1.2	36	1	.10	.03	5	61	36	6	.35	
1 jar	128	6.4	2.1	2.8	0.8	120	120	.06	0.3	.12	1.41	45	64	.60	.026	803
high protein, dry	9	0.1	0.9	1.1		0.2	0	0	.06	.01	5	1	17	5	.11	
1 T	2.4	0.1	0.0	0.0	0.1	0	0	.06	0.8	.00	.03	32	15	1.14	.031	803
high protein, w/ apple and orange, prep	32	21.1	2.0	3.8			8		.24	.03	8	16	63	10	.22	
w/ whole milk—1 oz	28	1.1						.19	1.1	.10		98	47	4.09	.047	803
high protein w/ apple & orange, dry	9	0.1	0.6	1.4		0.2	0	0	.10	.01	5	2	18	4	.06	
1 T	2.4	0.1	0.0	0.0	0.1	0	1	.09	0.6	.01		32	13	1.14	.023	803
mixed, dry	9	0.2	0.3	1.8		0.2	0	0	.07	.00	1	1	18	2	.06	
1 T	2.4	0.1	0.0	0.0	0.0	0	0	.06	0.8	.00	.03	10	9	1.14	.008	803
Beech-Nut Stage 2	54		1.7	10.2					.28			6	119			
.5 oz	14	0.7						.22	3.6					6.72		I
Gerber	58		1.5	11.4	1.4	0.6		9	.27	.02		1	90	10	.20	.270
.5 oz	15	0.7						.23	2.0			31	75	6.80	.040	I
mixed, prep w/ whole milk	32	21.1	1.4	4.5		0.4	7	0	.16	.02	3	13	62	8	.20	
1 oz	28	1.0	0.5			3	30	.12	1.6	.09	.12	56	40	2.96	.018	803
mixed w/ apples & bananas, Gerber 3rd	133		2.4	28.6	12.1			16	.27	.19		14	12	26	1.50	.580
Foods—6 oz	170	1.0					22	.22	3.6			172	74	4.40	.140	I

	KCAL	H₂O (g)	PRO (g)	CHO (g)	SUGR (g)	DFIB (g)	A (RE)	C (mg)	B-2 (mg)	B-6 (mg)	FOL (mcg)	Na (mg)	Ca (mg)	Mg (mg)	Zn (mg)	Mn (mg)
	WT (g)	FAT (g)	SFA (g)	MUFA (g)	PUFA (g)	CHOL (mg)	A (IU)	B-1 (mg)	NIA (mg)	B-12 (mcg)	PANT (mg)	K (mg)	P (mg)	Fe (mg)	Cu (mg)	REF
mixed w/ applesce & bananas																
Beech-Nut Stage 2	83		2.2	16.1				16	.27				14			
4.5 oz	128	1.2						.23	3.6					6.78		I
Gerber 2nd Foods	95		0.9	22.1	10.0	1.6		16	.27	.18		9	8	14	.10	.370
4 oz	113	0.4					28	.23	3.6			102	34	9.50	.070	I
jr	141	135.3	2.0	31.3		2.0	3	15	.61	.24	6	61	7	12	.37	
1 jar	170	0.7	0.1	0.2	0.3	0	32	.48	6.9	.00	.33	54	49	9.54	.093	803
str	93	90.4	1.4	20.2		1.4	2	29	.40	.15	4	2	7	9	.21	
1 jar	113	0.6	0.1	0.2	0.2	0	20	.32	4.5	.00	.22	46	26	7.48	.061	803
mixed w/ bananas & apple jce, inst dry, Heinz—4 T	50		1.0	12.0				17	.28	.06		2	6		.18	
	14	0.0					10	.24	3.6			80	26	7.00	.040	I
mixed w/ bananas, dry	9	0.1	0.3	1.9		0.2	0	0	.09	.01	0	3	17	2	.03	
1 T	2.4	0.1	0.0	0.0	0.0	0	3	.09	0.5	.01		16	9	1.14	.006	803
mixed w/ bananas, dry, Gerber	59		1.1	12.4	3.7	0.5		9	.27	.10		2	90	10	.20	.180
.5 oz	15	0.5					9	.23	2.0			55	50	6.80	.040	I
mixed w/ bananas, prep w/ whole milk	33	21.1	1.3	4.7		0.4	8	0	.20	.03	2	17	61	7	.16	
1 oz	28	1.0	0.6			3	31	.19	1.0	.10		67	39	3.16	.014	803
mixed w/ honey, prep w/ whole milk	33	21.0	1.4	4.5			7		.17	.02	3	14	83	8	.20	
1 oz	28	1.0						.13	1.8	.09	.13	48	52	3.20	.018	803
oatmeal, dry	10	0.1	0.3	1.7		0.2	0	0	.06	.00	1	1	18	3	.09	
1 T	2.4	0.2	0.0	0.1	0.1	0	0	.07	0.9	.00	.04	11	12	1.14	.013	803
Beech-Nut Stage 1	56		2.2	9.3					.28			8	119			
.5 oz	14	1.1						.22	3.6					6.72		I
Gerber	60		2.3	10.0	1.4	1.4		9	.27	.03		1	90	19	.50	.055
.5 oz	15	1.2						.23	2.0			52	75	6.80	.070	I
oatmeal, prep w/ whole milk	33	21.1	1.4	4.3		0.3	7	0	.16	.02	3	13	62	10	.26	
1 oz	28	1.2	0.6			3	30	.14	1.7	.09	.15	58	45	3.44	.027	803
oatmeal w/ apples & cinn, Gerber 3rd Foods—6 oz	112		1.9	24.2	13.0	2.9		16	.27	.19		17	11	23	1.50	.470
	170	0.9					31	.22	3.6			155	62	4.40	.120	I
oatmeal w/ apples & cinn, inst, Gerber Graduates—1 oz	113		2.8	21.0	6.9	2.1		0	.24	.11		62	80	31	1.60	.740
	28	2.0	0.4					.21	2.7			104	120	4.00	.100	I
oatmeal w/ applesce & bananas																
Beech-Nut Stage 2	88		2.2	18.0				16	.27			7				
4.5 oz	128	0.9						.23	3.6							I
Gerber 2nd Foods	94		1.4	20.8	10.6	2.0		16	.27	.18		9	8	18	1.00	.510
4 oz	113	0.5					16	.23	3.6			100	47	9.60	.080	I
jr	128	139.1	2.2	26.7		1.4	5	32	.82	.41	6	53	10	19	.56	
1 jar	170	1.2	0.2	0.4	0.4	0	48	.41	5.7	.00	.39	82	70	9.37	.128	803
str	82	92.9	1.5	17.4		0.9	3	25	.41	.23	4	2	10	12	.40	
1 jar	113	0.8	0.1	0.2	0.3	0	34	.47	5.7	.00	.26	53	46	6.38	.082	803
oatmeal w/ bananas & apple jce, inst dry, Heinz—4 T	60		1.0	12.0				17	.28	.07		1	12		.25	
	14	0.0					4	.24	3.6			112	38	7.00	.050	I
oatmeal w/ bananas, dry	9	0.1	0.3	1.8		0.1	0	0	.09	.01	0	3	16	3	.05	
1 T	2.4	0.1	0.0	0.0	0.1	0	2	.09	0.5	.01		18	11	1.14	.009	803
Beech-Nut Stage 2	56		1.6	10.6					.21			4	90			
.5 oz	14	0.9					10	.18	2.8					5.18		I
Gerber	61		1.7	11.1	2.7	1.1		9	.27	.09		2	90	17	.50	.440
.5 oz	15	1.1					4	.23	2.0			74	75	6.80	.070	I
oatmeal w/ bananas, prep w/ whole milk	33	21.1	1.3	4.5			8	0	.21	.03	2	17	58	9	.18	
1 oz	28	1.1					28	.18	1.0	.09		70	43	3.18	.020	803
oatmeal w/ honey, dry	9	0.1	0.3	1.7			0	0	.07	.00	1	1	28	4	.09	
1 T	2.4	0.2					1	.07	0.9	.00	.04	6	18	1.61	.013	803
oatmeal w/ honey, prep w/ whole milk	33	21.1	1.4	4.3			7		.17	.02	3	14	82	10	.26	
1 oz	28	1.1						.14	1.7	.09	.15	48	56	3.14	.027	803
oatmeal w/ peaches & van, inst, Gerber Graduates—1 oz	113		3.0	20.6	7.0	2.2		1	.24	.11		62	80	31	1.60	.740
	28	2.0	0.4				28	.21	2.7			104	120	4.00	.100	I
rice, dry	9	0.2	0.2	1.9		0.0	0	0	.05	.01	1	1	20	5	.05	
1 T	2.4	0.1	0.0	0.0	0.0	0	0	.06	0.7	.00		9	14	1.14	.008	803
Beech-Nut Stage 1	53		1.1	11.2					.28			3	119			
.5 oz	14	0.4						.22	3.6					6.72		I

	KCAL / WT (g)	H_2O (g) / FAT (g)	PRO (g) / SFA (g)	CHO (g) / MUFA (g)	SUGR (g) / PUFA (g)	DFIB (g) / CHOL (mg)	A (RE) / A (IU)	C (mg) / B-1 (mg)	B-2 (mg) / NIA (mg)	B-6 (mg) / B-12 (mcg)	FOL (mcg) / PANT (mg)	Na (mg) / K (mg)	Ca (mg) / P (mg)	Mg (mg) / Fe (mg)	Zn (mg) / Cu (mg)	Mn (mg) / REF
Gerber	57		1.2	11.9	0.9	0.2		9	.27	.04		1	90	8	.20	.320
.5 oz	15	0.5						.23	2.0			21	75	6.80	.040	I
rice, prep w/ whole milk	33	21.1	1.1	4.7		0.0	7	0	.14	.03	2	13	68	13	.18	
1 oz	28	1.0	0.7			3	30	.13	1.5	.09		54	50	3.46	.018	803
rice w/ apples, dry, Beech-Nut Stage 2	54		0.9	11.7					.21			2	119			
.5 oz	14	0.3						.18	2.8					5.18		I
rice w/ apples, Gerber 2nd Foods	59		0.8	12.9	3.5	0.3		9	.27			3	90	7	.20	.230
.5 oz	15	0.5						.23	2.0			35	50	6.80	.030	I
rice w/ applesce & bananas, str	89	91.5	1.4	19.3		1.1	2	36	.48	.26	3	32	19	3	.09	
1 jar	113	0.5	0.1	0.1	0.1	0	24	.29	4.5	.00		32	14	7.60	.058	803
rice w/ applesce & bananas, str, Beech-Nut Stage 2—4.5 oz	102		2.0	23.4				16	.27			24	51			
	128	0.0						.23	3.6					6.78		I
rice w/ applesce, Gerber 2nd Foods	98		0.8	23.3	10.5	1.0		16	.27	.18		7	18	7	1.00	.180
4 oz	113	0.1					12	.23	3.6			62	18	8.90	.050	I
rice w/ bananas & apple jce, inst dry, Heinz—4 T	50		1.0	12.0				17	.28	.07		1	5		.16	
	14	0.0					10	.24	3.6			70	20	7.00	.040	I
rice w/ bananas, dry	10	0.1	0.2	1.9		0.0	0	0	.09	.02	0	2	17	3	.04	
1 T	2.4	0.1	0.0	0.0	0.0	0	1	.10	0.6	.01		18	10	1.14	.006	803
Beech-Nut Stage 2	54		1.0	11.8					.21			3	90			
.5 oz	14	0.3					4	.18	2.8					5.18		I
Gerber	58		1.0	12.6	2.8	0.3		9	.27	.10		3	90	10	.20	.290
.5 oz	15	0.4					7	.23	2.0			49	50	6.80	.050	I
rice w/ bananas, prep w/ whole milk	33	21.1	1.2	4.8		0.0	7	0	.22	.04	2	16	60	10	.16	
1 oz	28	1.0	0.6			3	7	.19	1.1	.09		72	41	3.13	.014	803
rice w/ honey, prep w/ whole milk	33	21.1	1.1	4.8			7	0	.17	.03	2	14	82	13	.18	
1 oz	28	0.9					26	.13	1.7	.09		40	51	3.06	.018	803
rice w/ mixed fruit																
dry, Gerber	59		1.1	12.5	2.9	0.4		9	.27	.09		2	90	10	.20	.290
.5 oz	15	0.6					2	.23	2.0			43	50	6.80	.040	I
Gerber 3rd Foods	133		1.6	31.0	15.2	1.1		16	.27	.19		16	30	10	1.50	.260
6 oz	170	0.3					12	.22	3.6			95	36	4.50	.040	I
jr	134	136.7	1.5	31.1		1.0	3	16	.27	.19	2	17	27	9	.24	
1 jar	170	0.3	0.1	0.1	0.1	0	26	.22	3.6	.03	.46	85	36	4.42	.043	803
rice w/ pears & apple jce, inst dry, Heinz	50		1.0	13.0				17	.28	.02		8	8		.17	
4 T	14	0.0					12	.24	3.6			43	22	7.00	.060	I

19.3 DESSERTS

	KCAL / WT (g)	H_2O (g) / FAT (g)	PRO (g) / SFA (g)	CHO (g) / MUFA (g)	SUGR (g) / PUFA (g)	DFIB (g) / CHOL (mg)	A (RE) / A (IU)	C (mg) / B-1 (mg)	B-2 (mg) / NIA (mg)	B-6 (mg) / B-12 (mcg)	FOL (mcg) / PANT (mg)	Na (mg) / K (mg)	Ca (mg) / P (mg)	Mg (mg) / Fe (mg)	Zn (mg) / Cu (mg)	Mn (mg) / REF
banana apple, Gerber 2nd Foods	76		0.3	18.6	9.6	0.6		16	.03	.08		8	4	6		.630
4 oz	113	0.1					18	.01	0.1			79	6	.10	.020	I
banana pineapple, str, Beech-Nut Stage 2	113		0.6	27.3				16	.03			13				
4.5 oz	128	0.0					51	.00	0.2							I
banana pudding, str, Heinz	96		1.0	21.6				15	.04	.14		15	13		.15	
1 jar	128	0.6					59	.01	0.2			99	40	.51	.051	I
banana yogurt, Gerber 2nd Foods	84		1.2	19.1	13.2	0.5		16	.05	.10		18	34	11	.02	.060
4 oz	113	0.4					2	.02	0.2			110	33	.10	.020	I
blueberry buckle, Gerber 3rd Foods	124		0.2	30.6	18.6	0.4		16	.01	.02		45	7	2		.020
6 oz	170							.01	0.1			22	5	.20	.020	I
cherry cobbler, Gerber 3rd Foods	133		0.4	32.5	20.4	0.4		16	.02	.03		82	8	4		.030
6 oz	170	0.2					107	.01	0.1			74	10	.20	.020	I
cherry van pudding																
Gerber 2nd Foods	78		0.3	18.8	11.9	0.2		0	.01			7	6	3		.020
4 oz	113	0.2					18	.01	0.0			49	7	.10	.020	I
jr	117	137.7	0.3	31.3		0.5	34	2	.02	.02	1	26	9	3	.05	
1 jar	170	0.3	0.1	0.1	0.1	17	340	.01	0.1	.02		56	12	.29	.087	803
str	77	92.1	0.2	20.1		0.3	23	1	.01	.01	0	18	6	2	.05	
1 jar	113	0.3	0.1	0.1	0.1	11	226	.01	0.0	.01		38	8	.21	.056	803
cottage cheese w/ pineapple, Beech-Nut Stage 2—4.5 oz	120		2.6	25.2				16	.05				23			
	128	1.0						.04								I

							Vitamins					Minerals				
	KCAL	H₂O (g)	PRO (g)	CHO (g)	SUGR (g)	DFIB (g)	A (RE)	C (mg)	B-2 (mg)	B-6 (mg)	FOL (mcg)	Na (mg)	Ca (mg)	Mg (mg)	Zn (mg)	Mn (mg)
	WT (g)	FAT (g)	SFA (g)	MUFA (g)	PUFA (g)	CHOL (mg)	A (IU)	B-1 (mg)	NIA (mg)	B-12 (mcg)	PANT (mg)	K (mg)	P (mg)	Fe (mg)	Cu (mg)	REF
cottage cheese w/ pineapple, Beech-Nut	165		3.6	34.9				16	.09			15	29			
Stage 3—6 oz	170	1.2						.03								I
dutch apple																
Gerber 2nd Foods	92		0.2	22.5	18.6	1.7		16	.03	.05		3	4	5	.02	.020
4 oz	113	0.1					21	.01	0.1			81	8	.10	.030	I
Gerber 3rd Foods	138		0.3	33.7	27.6	2.5		16	.02	.04		4	6	7	.01	.030
6 oz	170	0.2					25	.02	0.1			122	13	.20	.050	I
jr	117	139.6	0.0	28.6		1.5	9	36	.02	.02	1	27	7	3	.04	
1 jar	170	1.7	1.1	0.4	0.1	0	85	.02	0.1	.00		63	7	.34	.102	803
str	77	92.9	0.0	18.9		1.0	6	24	.01	.01	1	18	6	2	.01	
1 jar	113	1.0	0.7	0.3	0.0	0	55	.01	0.1	.00		37	3	.23	.067	803
fruit dessert																
Beech-Nut Stage 2	83		0.0	20.1				16	.03							
4.5 oz	128	0.0	0.0	0.0	0.0		115	.03	0.3							I
Beech-Nut Stage 3	116		0.0	28.1				16	.07							
6 oz	170	0.0					155	.03	0.4							I
Gerber 2nd Foods	90		0.4	21.7	15.9	0.4		16	.02	.05		8	8	8		.070
4 oz	113	0.2					137	.02	0.4			110	11	.10	.030	
Gerber 3rd Foods	131		0.5	31.8	25.4			16	.03	.08		8	13	9	.10	.170
6 oz	170	0.2					163	.03	0.4			134	11	.30	.040	I
jr	107	139.7	0.5	29.2		1.0	41	5	.02	.06	6	22	15	9	.09	
1 jar	170	0.0	0.0	0.0	0.0	0	406	.04	0.2	.00	.17	162	14	.36	.051	803
str	67	94.2	0.3	18.1		0.7	28	3	.01	.04	4	16	10	6	.05	
1 jar	113	0.0	0.0	0.0	0.0	0	284	.02	0.2	.00	.12	106	8	.25	.034	803
guava tropical fruit dessert, Beech-Nut	97		0.0	23.8				16	.01			6				
Stage 2—4.5 oz	128	0.0					77	.01	0.4							I
hawaiian delight, Gerber	98		1.5	22.5	12.6	0.1		16	.04	.05		19	46	10	.20	.220
4 oz	113	0.2					3	.04	0.1			94	40	.10	.020	I
hawaiian delight, Gerber 2nd Foods	150		2.2	34.9	21.5	0.2		16	.08	.07		29	68	14	.40	.200
6 oz	170	0.2					1	.06	0.2			123	60	.20	.030	I
mango, banana w /tapioca & passion	82		0.3	19.8	11.8	0.3		32	.03	.07		7	5	6	.07	.060
fruit, Gerber 2nd Foods—4 oz	113	0.1					238	.01	0.3			81	6	.10	.030	I
mango tropical fruit, Beech-Nut Stage 2	100		0.0	24.3				16	.03			15				
4.5 oz	128	0.0					589	.01	0.1							I
mixed fruit yogurt, Gerber 2nd Foods	89		1.2	20.1	12.8	0.6		16	.05	.06		17	35	10	.02	.110
4 oz	113	0.4					122	.03	0.3			118	34	.20	.020	I
orange pudding, str	90	90.2	1.2	20.0		0.7	14	10	.06	.03	9	23	36	6	.19	
1 jar	113	1.0	0.6	0.3	0.0	3	130	.05	0.1	.01	.28	97	32	.11	.056	803
papaya tropical fruit, Beech-Nut Stage 2	100		0.0	24.2				16	.04			12				
4.5 oz	128	0.0					115	.01	0.2							I
peach cobbler																
Gerber 2nd Foods	86		0.5	20.7	14.3	0.7		16	.02	.02		8	4	5	.10	.030
4 oz	113	0.2					282	.01	0.5			96	11	.10	.030	I
Gerber 3rd Foods	131		0.9	31.5	19.5	1.1		16	.03	.03		11	7	8	.09	.050
6 oz	170	0.2					176	.01	0.7			145	16	.10	.040	I
jr	114	138.0	0.5	31.1		1.2	24	35	.03	.01	2	15	7	3	.05	
1 jar	170	0.0	0.0	0.0	0.0	0	241	.02	0.4	.00		95	10	.17	.333	803
str	73	92.4	0.3	20.1		0.8	16	23	.02	.01	1	8	5	2	.34	
1 jar	113	0.0	0.0	0.0	0.0	0	160	.01	0.3	.00		61	6	.11	.215	803
peaches & mango w/ tapioca, Gerber	80		0.3	19.3	12.4	0.0		32	.01	.04		5	5	5	.06	.040
2nd Foods—4 oz	113	0.2					356	.01	0.4			78	8	.10	.030	I
pineapple pudding, jr	148	129.4	2.4	36.7		1.4	7	45	.08	.07	10	37	58	15	.32	
1 jar	170	0.7	0.2	0.2	0.1	0	63	.07	0.2	.10	.35	153	51	.32	.041	803
pineapple pudding, str	92	87.7	1.5	22.9		0.8	5	31	.05	.05	6	21	35	10	.23	
1 jar	113	0.3	0.1	0.1	0.0	0	45	.04	0.1	.07	.22	92	35	.20	.026	803
raspberry cobbler, Gerber 3rd Foods	121		0.3	29.8	20.2	0.2		16	.01	.02		68	8	4		.080
6 oz	170	0.1						.01	0.1			32	5	.30	.030	I
tropical fruit dessert, jr	102	141.4	0.3	27.9			3	32	.05	.05	6	12	17	9	.08	
1 jar	170	0.0	0.0	0.0	0.0		34	.02	0.1	.00	.16	99	14	.44	.048	803

							Vitamins					Minerals			
	KCAL	H₂O (g)	PRO (g)	CHO (g)	SUGR (g)	DFIB (g)	A (RE)	C (mg)	B-2 (mg)	B-6 (mg)	FOL (mcg)	Na (mg)	Ca (mg)	Mg (mg)	Zn (mg)	Mn (mg)
	WT (g)	FAT (g)	SFA (g)	MUFA (g)	PUFA (g)	CHOL (mg)	A (IU)	B-1 (mg)	NIA (mg)	B-12 (mcg)	PANT	K (mg)	P (mg)	Fe (mg)	Cu (mg)	REF
tutti frutti, jr, Heinz	149		0.9	34.3				15	.04	.04		36	32		.40	
1 jar	213	0.9					430	.06	0.2			92	34	.64	.426	I
tutti frutti, str, Heinz	88		0.5	20.6				16	.03	.03		19	15		.10	
1 jar	128	0.4					166	.03	0.1			51	15	.26	.026	I
van custard pudding																
Beech-Nut Stage 2	128		2.7	21.5					.15			56	86			
4.5 oz	128	3.5					51	.03	0.1							I
Beech-Nut Stage 3	172		3.4	29.1					.17			71	114			
6 oz	170	4.6					60	.03								I
Gerber 2nd Foods	109		2.5	20.3	13.2	0.0		1	.11	.04		36	67	7	.50	
4 oz	113	2.0						.02	0.1			79	80	.40	.020	I
Gerber 3rd Foods	151		2.9	31.4	19.6	0.1			.09	.05		44	90	9	.42	.020
6 oz	170	1.5					5	.02	0.1			113	91	.30	.010	I
jr	151	135.0	2.7	27.5		0.0	7	1	.13	.03	11	49	95	9	.47	
1 jar	170	3.9	2.0	1.3	0.3	23	61	.02	0.1	.02	.43	105	77	.44	.087	803
str	96	90.3	1.8	18.2		0.0	7	1	.09	.02	7	32	62	6	.32	
1 jar	113	2.3	1.1	0.8	0.2	9	72	.01	0.0	.01	.28	75	51	.27	.056	803

19.4 DINNERS

	KCAL	H₂O (g)	PRO (g)	CHO (g)	SUGR (g)	DFIB (g)	A (RE)	C (mg)	B-2 (mg)	B-6 (mg)	FOL (mcg)	Na (mg)	Ca (mg)	Mg (mg)	Zn (mg)	Mn (mg)
	WT (g)	FAT (g)	SFA (g)	MUFA (g)	PUFA (g)	CHOL (mg)	A (IU)	B-1 (mg)	NIA (mg)	B-12 (mcg)	PANT	K (mg)	P (mg)	Fe (mg)	Cu (mg)	REF
apples & chicken, Gerber Simple Recipe	70		2.8	12.0	9.5	2.3		0	.08	.07		15	2	7	.50	.030
4 oz	113	1.5					19	.02	0.7			108	40	.40	.050	I
apples & ham, Gerber Simple Recipe	79		3.3	11.2	9.8	2.0		0	.07	.08		11	5	8	.50	.020
4 oz	113	2.0					12	.07	0.8			129	39	.30	.050	I
apples & turkey, Gerber Simple Recipe	79		3.4	11.1	9.0	2.2		0	.09	.08		15	12	8	.50	.030
4 oz	113	2.1					15	.02	0.9			126	46	.40	.070	I
au gratin potatoes & ham, Gerber Graduates—*6 oz*	131		6.3	19.6	1.4	2.0		0	.19	.25		392	87	23	1.00	.090
	170	3.3	1.9			11	4	.08	1.9			239	177	.70	.100	I
beef & egg noodles																
Beech-Nut Stage 2	87		2.8	10.4					.05			20	18			
4.5 oz	128	3.6					4301	.03	0.8					.51		I
Beech-Nut Stage 3	112		4.3	13.4					.09			41	31			
6 oz	170	4.8					4369	.05	1.1					.85		I
Gerber 2nd Foods	72		3.0	10.2	1.4	1.3		1	.04	.04		14	8	9	.70	.140
4 oz	113	2.1					753	.04	0.7			86	42	.40	.050	I
Gerber 3rd Foods	105		4.2	14.2	1.8	2.2		0	.09	.09		170	16	15	.90	.110
6 oz	170	3.5					3655	.06	1.1			158	56	.70	.030	I
jr	121	187.0	5.3	15.8		2.3	187	3	.08	.07	12	36	17	15	.85	
1 jar	213	4.0	1.6	1.8	0.2	17	1397	.06	1.2	.21	.49	98	64	.92	.068	803
str	68	113.4	2.9	9.0		1.4	141	2	.05	.06	7	37	12	9	.48	
1 jar	128	2.2	0.9	0.9	0.1	9	1053	.04	0.9	.12	.27	60	37	.52	.038	803
beef & rice, toddler	145	145.0	8.8	15.6			140	7	.12	.25	11	632	19	14	1.62	
1 jar	177	5.1					889	.03	2.4	.90		212	62	1.22	.096	803
beef lasagna, toddler	136	145.7	7.4	17.7			276	3	.16	.13	11	804	71	19	1.24	
1 jar	177	3.7					2059	.13	2.4	.90		216	71	1.54	.172	803
beef stew, Beech-Nut Table Time	136		10.7	13.8					.14			311	43			
6 oz	170	4.4					3213	.03	2.0					1.36		I
beef stew, toddler	90	153.8	9.0	9.7		1.9	443	5	.12	.13	11	611	16	19	1.54	
1 jar	177	2.1	1.0	0.8	0.2	22	2919	.02	2.3	.90		251	78	1.27	.127	803
beef supreme, Beech-Nut Stage 2	119		3.7	12.5					.08			32	18			
4.5 oz	128	5.9					2496	.01	1.4					.51		I
broccoli & chicken, Gerber Simple Recipe—*4 oz*	48		4.3	3.5	1.2	2.7		28	.09	.09		22	49	13	.60	.150
	113	1.8					550	.02	0.8			182	67	.70	.050	I
carrots & beef, Gerber Simple Recipe *4 oz*	67		3.9	7.0	3.9	2.9		1	.07	.12		65	25	12	.90	.160
	113	2.9					8220	.03	1.1			239	54	.60	.060	I
carrots & white turkey, diced, Gerber Graduates—*2.1 oz*	34		4.3	2.2		0.8		0	.00	.04		158	12	7	.80	.030
	60	0.9					5839	.00	0.6			58	28	.20	.080	I
carrots, broccoli, & cheese w/ rice, Gerber Veggie Recipes—*4 oz*	71		3.1	10.4	3.1	1.2			.11	.06		72	88	14	.40	.140
	113	1.9					885	.03	0.3			163	83	.30	.030	I
carrots, zucchini, & egg noodles, Gerber Veggie Recipes—*4 oz*	78		3.1	11.9	4.3	3.0		0	.12	.07		28	56	20	.50	.190
	113	2.0					2345	.07	0.5			218	73	.80	.070	I

	KCAL / WT (g)	H₂O (g) / FAT (g)	PRO (g) / SFA (g)	CHO (g) / MUFA (g)	SUGR (g) / PUFA (g)	DFIB (g) / CHOL (mg)	A (RE) / A (IU)	C (mg) / B-1 (mg)	B-2 (mg) / NIA (mg)	B-6 (mg) / B-12 (mcg)	FOL (mcg) / PANT (mg)	Na (mg) / K (mg)	Ca (mg) / P (mg)	Mg (mg) / Fe (mg)	Zn (mg) / Cu (mg)	Mn (mg) / REF
cheese ravioli w/ tomato sce, Gerber Graduates—6 oz	165		6.6	29.0	7.6	3.1		0	.29	.18		230	91	38	.90	.240
	170	2.5	1.2			8	454	.15	2.7			427	121	1.40	.200	I
chicken & noodles																
Beech-Nut Stage 2	82		2.9	11.6				1	.08			24	32			
4.5 oz	128	2.7					3200	.04	1.1					.64		I
Beech-Nut Stage 3	97		3.9	13.4					.07			43	43			
6 oz	170	2.9					3145	.05	1.2					1.02		I
Gerber 2nd Foods	79		3.4	11.3	2.7	2.6		0	.08	.08		27	33	17	.60	.190
4 oz	113	2.2					6298	.05	0.8			172	59	.80	.080	I
Gerber 3rd Foods	94		4.0	15.8	1.9	1.4		0	.08			176	30	15	.70	.180
6 oz	170	1.6					3492	.05	1.2			148	66	.70	.050	I
inst dry, Heinz	60		4.0	7.0				0	.06	.07		35	24		.40	
6 T	14	2.0					150	.08	1.1			161	70	.90	.080	I
jr	109	188.9	4.0	16.0		2.3	228	3	.07	.06	11	36	36	19	.63	
1 jar	213	3.0	0.8	1.2	0.7	36	1906	.06	1.1	.28	.48	75	51	.83	.083	803
str	67	113.3	2.7	9.6		1.4	143	1	.07	.04	7	20	28	12	.38	
1 jar	128	1.9	0.8	0.6	0.3	23	1158	.04	0.6	.17	.29	50	31	.58	.051	803
chicken & rice, Beech-Nut Stage 2	77		2.4	10.5					.04			35	28			
4.5 oz	128	2.8					2330	.03	0.9					.64		I
chicken soup, hearty w/ stars, Beech-Nut Table Time—6 oz	150		4.9	18.5					.10			287	49			
	170	5.8					3128	.03	1.1					.85		I
chicken soup, str	64	114.0	2.0	9.2		1.4	220	1	.04	.05	7	20	47	6	.28	
1 jar	128	2.2	0.4	0.5	1.2	5	1772	.02	0.4	.15		84	31	.35	.357	803
chicken stew, toddler	133	141.6	8.8	10.9		1.0	206	3	.13	.08	2	340	61	17	.70	
1 jar	170	6.3	1.9	2.9	1.3	49	1717	.05	2.0	.24		156	87	1.12	.034	803
chicken stew w/ noodles, Gerber Graduates—6 oz	116		7.4	14.6	1.5	1.8		1	.15	.20		395	23	23	.80	.130
	170	3.2	1.0			18	2301	.08	3.6			179	107	1.20	.130	I
chicken w/ broccoli in cheese sce, Gerber Graduates—6 oz	105		6.7	11.0	2.5	1.4		5	.16	.14		322	89	17	.08	.050
	170	3.7	2.1			14	573	.02	2.2			204	147	.40	.070	I
corn & chicken, diced, Gerber Graduates 2.5 oz	72		4.7	9.0	0.3	0.7		1	.06	.07		157	5	10	.40	.030
	71	1.9					15	.00	1.2			80	46	.20	.070	I
garden veg & pasta, Gerber Veggie Recipes—4 oz	78		3.1	11.9	4.3	3.0		0	.12	.07		28	56	20	.50	.190
	113	2.0					2345	.07	0.5			218	73	.80	.070	I
green beans & turkey, Gerber Simple Recipe—4 oz	71		4.8	5.7	1.7	2.6		2	.11	.08		14	40	24	.70	.300
	113	2.4					420	.03	1.3			195	63	.90	.070	I
green beans & white turkey, diced, Gerber Graduates—2.3 oz	38		4.7	2.5	0.4	1.0		1	.00	.04		167	19	9	.70	.060
	65	0.9					186	.00	0.7			60	31	.20	.060	I
harvest veg stew, Gerber Veggie Recipes 4 oz	75		2.7	11.6	3.5	1.6		0	.10	.04		37	63	21	.40	.210
	113	1.9					1459	.03	0.4			194	74	.40	.040	I
italian spaghetti in tomato sce w/ beef, Gerber 3rd Foods—6 oz	121		4.6	21.5	5.2	1.7		0	.13	.11		168	22	19	.80	.200
	170	1.8					1628	.09	1.8			216	62	.80	.050	I
lasagna w/ meat sce, Gerber 3rd Foods 6 oz	101		3.4	15.2	4.3	1.8		1	.08	.10		165	16	16	.60	.080
	170	3.0					1063	.04	1.0			171	48	.70	.030	I
macaroni & beef																
Beech-Nut Stage 2	93		3.2	11.3				1	.08			40	32			
4.5 oz	128	3.8					3763	.04	0.9					.64		I
Beech-Nut Stage 3	119		4.1	14.8					.12			54	39			
6 oz	170	4.9					5559	.05	1.1					.85		I
in sce, Gerber Graduates	137		8.3	18.6	5.0	2.3		1	.25	.22		320	27	30	1.50	.150
6 oz	170	3.3	1.3			14	269	.08	3.0			246	106	1.40	.140	I
macaroni & cheese																
Gerber 2nd Foods	72		3.1	10.0	1.5	0.7		1	.06	.04		103	65	9	.40	.110
4 oz	113	2.2					7	.04	0.6			65	95	.30	.040	I
jr	130	184.2	5.5	17.5		0.6	6	3	.14	.03	3	162	109	15	.68	
1 jar	213	4.3	2.5	1.1	0.3	13	28	.12	1.2	.06		94	126	.64	.045	803
str	76	111.5	3.3	9.6		0.4	6	2	.09	.02	2	93	69	10	.44	
1 jar	128	2.7	1.6	0.7	0.2	9	35	.07	0.6	.04		59	73	.40	.026	803

	KCAL / WT (g)	H₂O (g) / FAT (g)	PRO (g) / SFA (g)	CHO (g) / MUFA (g)	SUGR (g) / PUFA (g)	DFIB (g) / CHOL (mg)	A (RE) / A (IU)	C (mg) / B-1 (mg)	B-2 (mg) / NIA (mg)	B-6 (mg) / B-12 (mcg)	FOL (mcg) / PANT (mg)	Na (mg) / K (mg)	Ca (mg) / P (mg)	Mg (mg) / Fe (mg)	Zn (mg) / Cu (mg)	Mn (mg) / REF
macaroni, tomato, & beef																
Gerber 2nd Foods	66		2.9	10.9	2.2	1.2		0	.05	.07		39	20	12	.50	.150
4 oz	113	1.2					1312	.03	0.8			138	45	.40	.060	I
jr	126	184.7	5.3	20.0		2.3	232	3	.12	.10	14	36	30	15	.77	
1 jar	213	2.3	0.9	1.0	0.2	9	1472	.10	1.6	.51		153	94	.77	.083	803
str	70	111.7	2.8	11.3		1.4	115	2	.08	.06	26	22	20	12	.40	
1 jar	128	1.4	0.6	0.6	0.1	5	680	.09	1.0	.29		123	54	.63	.051	803
mixed veg dinner, jr	70	193.0	2.1	16.8			520	7	.05	.16	14	19	36	21	.51	
1 jar	213	0.0	0.0	0.0	0.0		5206	.03	0.9	.00	.49	239	47	.66	.077	803
mixed veg dinner, str	52	113.5	1.5	12.2			349	4	.04	.10	10	10	28	14	.21	
1 jar	128	0.1					3492	.02	0.6	.00	.35	155	31	.42	.056	803
pasta shells & cheese, Gerber Graduates	137		5.9	18.7	1.4	1.5			.17	.13		402	150	19	1.00	.120
6 oz	170	4.4	2.8			9	8	.07	1.4			71	212	1.00	.140	I
pears & chicken, Gerber 2nd Foods	75		3.0	12.4	9.8			0	.08	.05		18	35	11	.60	.040
4 oz	113	1.5					7	.01	0.9			136	47	.50	.120	I
peas & chicken, diced, Gerber Graduates	57		5.4	4.9	0.5	2.1		2	.09	.06		132	14	12	.70	.150
2.3 oz	65	1.7					241	.03	0.8			62	50	.70	.090	I
spaghetti rings in meat sce, Beech-Nut Table Time—6 oz	156		8.0	21.4					.14			354	46			
	170	4.9					1632	.05	2.0					1.19		I
spaghetti, tomato, & beef, Beech-Nut Stage 3—6 oz	121		3.7	15.8					.10			53	34			
	170	4.8					3961	.05	1.1					.85		I
spaghetti, tomato, & beef, jr	134	182.1	5.3	21.5		2.3	283	5	.15	.13	15	43	38	17	.89	
1 jar	213	2.8	1.1	1.2	0.2	11	1476	.14	2.3	.02	.38	230	79	1.17	.089	803
spaghetti, tomato, & meat, toddler	133	144.4	9.4	19.1			150	7	.18	.15	11	634	39	27	.85	
1 jar	177	1.8					784	.11	2.8	.41		289	80	1.59	.035	803
spaghetti w/ mini meatballs & sce, Gerber Graduates—6 oz	151		8.2	21.3	6.2	2.7		0	.23	.20		270	29	29	1.40	.190
	170	3.7	1.8			12	227	.10	2.7			349	112	1.20	.130	I
sweet potatoes & turkey, Gerber Simple Recipe—4 oz	90		4.4	13.1	7.5	1.9		2	.07	.09		22	29	18	.80	.230
	113	2.3					8344	.02	0.9			275	61	.60	.100	I
turkey & rice																
Beech-Nut Stage 2	72		2.6	10.6					.04			29	28			
4.5 oz	128	2.0					1395	.01	0.8					.51		I
Beech-Nut Stage 3	83		3.2	12.8					.05			44	39			
6 oz	170	2.2					3366	.02	1.0					.51		I
Gerber 2nd Foods	58		2.9	8.9	1.6	0.7		1	.04	.07		17	12	10	.50	.140
4 oz	113	1.2					1393	.02	0.8			100	40	.30	.030	I
jr	104	190.2	3.8	15.3		2.3	315	3	.06	.06	7	32	49	17	.52	
1 jar	213	3.0	0.9	1.2	0.7	21	2256	.02	0.6	.21	.44	72	36	.62	.051	803
str	63	114.0	2.4	9.3		1.4	122	2	.03	.04	4	22	27	10	.32	
1 jar	128	1.7	0.5	0.7	0.4	13	782	.01	0.4	.13	.27	52	26	.33	.032	803
turkey stew, Beech-Nut Table Time	182		8.7	12.6					.12			320	58			
6 oz	170	10.9					2066	.02	1.4					1.02		I
turkey stew (white) w/ rice, Gerber Graduates—6 oz	105		6.9	13.3	1.2	1.7		0	.17	.24		327	19	24	1.10	
	170	2.6	0.7			14	3373	.04	3.6			184	100	1.10	.120	I
turkey supreme, Beech-Nut Stage 2	106		4.5	10.2					.06			26	49			
4.5 oz	128	5.5					1306	.01	1.3					.64		I
turkey w/ garden veg & rice, Gerber 3rd Foods—6 oz	99		4.4	14.4	2.3	1.8		1	.08	.11		183	35	15	.80	.210
	170	3.0					3234	.03	1.2			177	66	.60	.050	I
veg & bacon																
Gerber 2nd Foods	85		2.3	10.5	2.0	1.8		1	.03	.07		56	14	11	.30	.160
4 oz	113	3.6					2663	.03	0.5			137	33	.40	.050	I
Gerber 3rd Foods	128		3.8	16.0	2.9				.05	.09		147	27	18	.50	.150
6 oz	170	5.5					4530	.06	0.8			224	63	.60	.070	I
jr	151	183.6	3.8	16.2		2.3	464	2	.06	.14	19	96	23	17	.56	
1 jar	213	8.3	3.0	4.0	0.9	6	3357	.11	1.2	.21		183	81	.87	.079	803
str	88	110.0	2.0	11.0		1.4	381	2	.04	.10	12	55	18	9	.32	
1 jar	128	4.2	1.5	2.0	0.5	4	3409	.04	0.7	.13		114	40	.46	.049	803

	KCAL / WT (g)	H₂O (g) / FAT (g)	PRO (g) / SFA (g)	CHO (g) / MUFA (g)	SUGR (g) / PUFA (g)	DFIB (g) / CHOL (mg)	A (RE) / A (IU)	C (mg) / B-1 (mg)	B-2 (mg) / NIA (mg)	B-6 (mg) / B-12 (mcg)	FOL (mcg) / PANT (mg)	Na (mg) / K (mg)	Ca (mg) / P (mg)	Mg (mg) / Fe (mg)	Zn (mg) / Cu (mg)	Mn (mg) / REF
veg & beef																
Beech-Nut Stage 2	84		2.3	10.2					.04			31	17			
4.5 oz	128	3.7					4070	.03	0.8					.51		I
Beech-Nut Stage 3	119		3.2	15.5					.05			43	26			
6 oz	170	4.9					6290	.03	1.0					.68		I
Gerber 2nd Foods	73		3.3	9.7	2.4	2.8		0	.05	.09		19	19	17	.70	.210
4 oz	113	2.3					3984	.04	0.9			211	54	.70	.090	I
Gerber 3rd Foods	106		4.3	16.4	2.8	2.4			.06	.12		173	17	20	.09	.240
6 oz	170	2.6					3713	.05	1.0			234	66	.70	.060	I
inst dry, Heinz	60		3.0	7.0				0	.04	.05		25	12		.51	
5 T	14	2.0					354	.04	0.8			142	47	.90	.070	I
jr	113	187.2	5.1	15.8		2.3	409	3	.07	.14	10	51	21	13	.88	
1 jar	213	3.6	1.5	1.6	0.2	11	3012	.07	1.4	.55	.27	224	92	1.00	.083	803
str	68	113.3	2.6	9.0		1.4	219	2	.04	.07	6	27	15	6	.42	
1 jar	128	2.6	1.0	1.1	0.1	6	1521	.03	0.6	.32	.15	129	52	.49	.013	803
veg & chicken																
Beech-Nut Stage 2	87		3.8	12.0					.10			41	77			
4.5 oz	128	2.6					2445	.03	0.8					.38		I
Beech-Nut Stage 3	100		3.7	13.8					.10			58	95			
6 oz	170	3.4					6001	.03	1.2					.68		I
Gerber 2nd Foods	70		3.1	10.6	1.9	2.7		0	.07	.09		28	31	16	.60	.170
4 oz	113	1.8					6138	.04	0.8			204	57	.70	.080	I
Gerber 3rd Foods	84		3.4	14.5	2.3				.06	.09		170	43	13	.60	.180
6 oz	170	1.3					4596	.03	1.0			145	55	.50	.040	I
inst dry, Heinz	60		3.0	8.0				0	.02	.06		30	24		.36	
6 T dry	14	2.0					424	.05	1.1			130	58	.90	.060	I
jr	107	187.9	4.0	18.1		2.3	315	3	.04	.08	8	19	30	19	.66	
1 jar	213	2.3	0.7	0.9	0.5	21	2545	.03	0.7	.21	.50	55	55	.64	.087	803
str	55	115.2	2.4	8.4		1.4	175	1	.02	.03	4	14	18	10	.33	
1 jar	128	1.4	0.4	0.5	0.3	17	1416	.02	0.2	.13	.26	38	32	.35	.045	803
veg & ham																
Beech-Nut Stage 2	78		3.1	11.4					.05			35	18			
4.5 oz	128	2.3					4339	.05	0.9					.51		I
Gerber 2nd Foods	73		2.3	9.9	1.5	1.9		1	.02	.06		16	18	14	.40	.150
4 oz	113	2.7					3517	.04	0.6			170	37	.40	.090	I
Gerber 3rd Foods	106		3.4	15.0	1.8	1.5			.06	.09		175	22	13	.40	.120
6 oz	170	3.6					2485	.06	0.9			175	56	.40	.050	I
inst dry, Heinz	60		4.0	7.0				1	.04	.05		30	12		.47	
6 T	14	2.0					300	.08	0.6			86	47	.60	.060	I
jr	111	188.3	5.1	14.9		2.3	173	3	.05	.07	11	38	17	11	.47	
1 jar	213	3.6	1.3	1.6	0.4	11	1310	.08	0.7	.11		196	55	.47	.066	803
str	61	114.2	2.3	8.8		1.4	122	2	.04	.04	6	15	10	6	.25	
1 jar	128	2.2	0.8	1.0	0.3	6	873	.04	0.5	.05		109	29	.38	.037	803
veg & lamb																
Beech-Nut Stage 2	88		2.4	11.9					.05			28	18			
4.5 oz	128	3.3					3571	.03	1.0					.51		I
jr	109	188.7	4.5	15.1		2.3	424	4	.07	.09	8	28	28	15	.47	
1 jar	213	3.6	1.5	1.5	0.3	11	3159	.04	1.2	.34	.34	202	104	.72	.062	803
str	67	113.4	2.6	8.8		1.4	362	2	.04	.06	5	26	15	9	.28	
1 jar	128	2.6	1.1	1.1	0.2	8	2554	.02	0.7	.20	.20	120	63	.45	.037	803
veg & turkey																
Gerber 2nd Foods	54		2.8	9.1	1.7	1.9		1	.02	.05		21	31	15	.80	.160
4 oz	113	0.7					5861	.02	0.6			130	53	.40	.110	I
Gerber 3rd Foods	90		3.0	13.3	2.3	1.4		0	.05	.11		180	23	15	.60	.100
6 oz	170	1.8					2506	.04	1.0			184	56	.60	.040	I
inst dry, Heinz	60		4.0	8.0				0	.02	.03		25	12		.42	
6 T	14	2.0					450	.05	1.1			140	57	.90	.070	I

	KCAL / WT (g)	H₂O (g) / FAT (g)	PRO (g) / SFA (g)	CHO (g) / MUFA (g)	SUGR (g) / PUFA (g)	DFIB (g) / CHOL (mg)	A (RE) / A (IU)	C (mg) / B-1 (mg)	B-2 (mg) / NIA (mg)	B-6 (mg) / B-12 (mcg)	FOL (mcg) / PANT (mg)	Na (mg) / K (mg)	Ca (mg) / P (mg)	Mg (mg) / Fe (mg)	Zn (mg) / Cu (mg)	Mn (mg) / REF
jr	100	189.6	3.6	16.4		2.3	245	2	.04	.05	6	36	28	19	.54	
1 jar	213	2.6	0.6	1.0	0.6	21	1908	.03	0.5	.19	.45	53	40	.68	.055	803
str	54	115.3	2.2	8.4		1.4	143	1	.02	.04	3	17	20	10	.29	
1 jar	128	1.5	0.4	0.6	0.4	13	1068	.01	0.4	.12	.24	56	24	.35	.029	803
toddler	142	145.7	8.5	14.2			476	6	.16	.11	5	591	81	28	.57	
1 jar	177	6.0					3715	.04	1.0	.78		294	101	1.06	.074	803
veg, dumplings, & beef, jr	102	188.7	4.5	17.0			190	2	.08	.10	16	111	30	15	.70	
1 jar	213	1.7					1406	.08	1.0	.19	.46	100	62	1.00	.064	803
veg, dumplings, & beef, str	61	113.8	2.6	9.9			72	1	.05	.06	9	63	18	8	.51	
1 jar	128	1.2					532	.06	0.7	.12	.27	59	36	.50	.037	803
veg, noodles, & chicken, jr	136	183.6	3.6	19.4		2.3	277	2	.08	.05	7	55	55	23	.68	
1 jar	213	4.7					2239	.09	1.4	.19	.43	126	70	1.04	.124	803
veg, noodles, & chicken, str	81	111.6	2.6	10.1		1.4	224	1	.06	.03	4	26	36	13	.32	
1 jar	128	3.2					1814	.04	0.5	.10	.24	70	40	.45	.069	803
veg, noodles, & turkey, jr	111	188.9	3.8	16.2		2.3	283	2	.09	.04	6	36	62	19	.64	
1 jar	213	3.2					2117	.05	0.6	.26	.46	155	62	.55	.055	803
veg, noodles, & turkey, str	56	115.6	1.5	8.7		1.4	170	1	.06	.02	3	27	41	10	.35	
1 jar	128	1.5					1268	.02	0.3	.13	.24	81	32	.24	.028	803
veg pasta, Gerber 3rd Foods	101		3.7	17.9	4.0	1.8			.15	.09		203	78	25	.60	.380
6 oz	170	1.8					2415	.06	0.9			210	95	.70	.070	I
veg stew w/ beef, Gerber Graduates	126		9.5	17.2	2.2	3.3		0	.30	.22		347	22	25	1.30	.120
6 oz	170	2.2	1.0			12	2469	.05	2.3			299	86	1.10	.100	I
veg stew w/ chicken, Beech-Nut Table Time—6 oz	168		5.4	20.1					.12			296	61			
	170	7.3					3791	.05	1.5					.85		I

19.5 FRUIT JUICES

	KCAL / WT (g)	H₂O (g) / FAT (g)	PRO (g) / SFA (g)	CHO (g) / MUFA (g)	SUGR (g) / PUFA (g)	DFIB (g) / CHOL (mg)	A (RE) / A (IU)	C (mg) / B-1 (mg)	B-2 (mg) / NIA (mg)	B-6 (mg) / B-12 (mcg)	FOL (mcg) / PANT (mg)	Na (mg) / K (mg)	Ca (mg) / P (mg)	Mg (mg) / Fe (mg)	Zn (mg) / Cu (mg)	Mn (mg) / REF
apple																
Beech-Nut Stage 1	54		0.0	12.9			43					9				
4.2 fl oz	128	0.0												.64		I
Gerber 1st Foods	58		0.1	14.3	13.5	0.1	35	.02	.04			3	4	5	.10	.260
4 fl oz	127	0.1					2	.01	0.1			119	8	.10	.010	I
Gerber Graduates	85		0.1	20.9	20.1		40	.02	.05			6	161	11		.550
6 oz	189	0.2					3		0.1			173	16	.40	.030	I
str	61	114.4	0.0	15.2		0.1	3	75	.02	.04	0	4	5	4	.04	
1 jar	130	0.1	0.0	0.0	0.0	0	23	.01	0.1	.00	.15	118	7	.74	.052	803
w/ yogurt, Gerber 2nd Foods	96		2.4	18.4	12.7	1.2	35	.09	.03			48	95	14	.30	.080
4 fl oz	124	1.4						.03	0.1			204	79	.30	.020	I
apple apricot, str, Heinz	61		0.1	14.7			42	.01	.04			8	14		.09	
1 jar	130	0.3					553	.03	0.2			148	14	.65	.039	I
apple banana, Gerber 2nd Foods	65		0.2	15.6		0.2	35	.02	.07			5	8	8		.150
4 fl oz	127	0.1					11	.01	0.2			157	10	.20	.020	I
apple banana, Gerber Graduates	96		0.2	23.5		0.4	40	.04	.08			11	161	14	.10	.170
6 oz	189	0.1					3		0.2			211	17	.05	.040	I
apple carrot, Gerber 3rd Foods	54		0.2	12.8	11.6	0.7	35	.01	.04			13	15	8	.03	.100
4 fl oz	125	0.2					3705	.01	0.1			129	13	.40	.020	I
apple cherry																
Beech-Nut Stage 2	56		0.0	13.6			42	.01				6				
4.2 fl oz	128	0.0												.90		I
Gerber 2nd Foods	60		0.2	14.6	12.2		35	.03	.03			6	9	7	.04	.130
4 fl oz	127	0.1					2	.01	0.1			143	10	.40	.010	I
str	53	116.4	0.1	12.9		0.1	1	76	.02	.04	0	4	7	4	.04	
1 jar	130	0.3	0.0	0.0	0.1	0	7	.01	0.1	.00	.13	127	8	.86	.056	803
apple cranberry, Beech-Nut Stage 2	55		0.0	13.3			42	.01				8				
4.2 fl oz	128	0.0												.64		I
apple cranberry, Gerber 2nd Foods	57			14.4		0.3	35	.01	.02			13	6	6	.10	.250
4 fl oz	127						1	.00	0.1			128	8	.20	.030	I

	KCAL / WT (g)	H₂O (g) / FAT (g)	PRO (g) / SFA (g)	CHO (g) / MUFA (g)	SUGR (g) / PUFA (g)	DFIB (g) / CHOL (mg)	A (RE) / A (IU)	C (mg) / B-1 (mg)	B-2 (mg) / NIA (mg)	B-6 (mg) / B-12 (mcg)	FOL (mcg) / PANT (mg)	Na (mg) / K (mg)	Ca (mg) / P (mg)	Mg (mg) / Fe (mg)	Zn (mg) / Cu (mg)	Mn (mg) / REF
apple grape Beech-Nut Stage 2	64		0.0	15.2				42	.03			9				
4.2 fl oz	128	0.0												.64		I
Gerber 2nd Foods	61		0.1	14.8		0.1		35	.03	.04		7	9	6	.10	.090
4 fl oz	127	0.1					4	.01	0.1			12	9	.30	.010	I
Gerber Graduates	89		0.2	21.9		0.2		40	.05	.05		9	161	11	.05	.080
6 fl oz	189	0.1						.01	0.2			164	16	.40	.030	I
str	60	114.5	0.1	14.8		0.1	1	70	.03	.04	0	4	8	4	.05	
1 jar	130	0.3	0.1	0.0	0.1	0	8	.01	0.1	.00	.10	117	7	.51	.101	803
apple peach, Gerber 2nd Foods	60		0.2	14.3		0.4		35	.02	.03		5	9	7	.04	.050
4 oz	127	0.2					57	.01	0.3			144	10	.30	.020	I
apple peach, str	55	115.7	0.3	13.7		0.1	8	76	.01	.03	2	1	4	4	.03	
1 jar	130	0.1	0.0	0.0	0.0	0	82	.01	0.3	.00	.11	126	5	.73	.048	803
apple pineapple, str, Heinz	61		0.3	14.6				42	.01	.06		7	16		.07	
1 jar	130	0.3					21	.03	0.1			108	10	.39	.026	I
apple plum, str	64	113.5	0.1	16.0		0.1	5	76	.02	.04	0	1	7	4	.04	
1 jar	130	0.0	0.0	0.0	0.0	0	56	.03	0.3	.00	.16	131	4	.81	.055	803
apple prune, Gerber 2nd Foods	67		0.0	16.3	14.8	0.4		35	.11	.05		4	11	9	.10	.110
4 oz	127	0.0					18	.01	0.3			170	13	.30	.010	I
apple prune, str	95	105.7	0.3	23.4		0.1	3	88	.00	.05	0	7	12	9	.06	
1 jar	130	0.1	0.0	0.0	0.0	0	21	.01	0.4	.00	.24	192	20	1.23	.081	803
apple sweet potato, Gerber 3rd Foods	63		0.4	14.9	13.3	0.6		35	.03	.08		9	17	12	.20	.140
4 fl oz	125	0.1					2850	.02	0.2			183	18	.30	.040	I
banana medley w/ yogurt, Gerber 2nd Foods—4 fl oz	112		2.9	21.5	15.7	1.2		35	.10	.10		47	103	23	.40	.140
	124	1.7					37	.04	0.3			219	88	.03	.050	I
berry punch, Gerber Graduates	95		0.3	23.1	20.5	0.7		40	.06	.09		11	161	15		.180
6 fl oz	189							.02	0.2			168	26	.40	.040	I
fruit punch, Gerber Graduates	87		0.3	21.4	21.1	0.7		40	.03	.08		9	161	12	.10	.180
6 fl oz	189	0.1					2	.01	0.2			158	21	.50	.030	I
guava w/ tapioca, Gerber	79		0.1	19.3	14.3	1.1		32	.03	.02		3	5	4		.040
4 oz	113	0.1					311	.02	0.4			85	5	.20	.030	I
Juice Plus, Beech-Nut Stage 2	80		0.0	19.6				36	.03			6				
4 fl oz	129	0.0												2.71		I
mango & mixed fruit, Gerber	72		0.3	17.3		0.3		35	.04	.05		5	15	11	.10	.100
4 fl oz	127	0.1					110	.01	0.2			123	17	.30	.030	I
mixed fruit Beech-Nut Stage 2	60		0.0	14.7				42	.03			6				
4.2 fl oz	128	0.0					192	.03	0.2					.38		I
Gerber 2nd Foods	61		0.3	14.6		0.2		35	.02	.07		6	11	10		.270
4 fl oz	127	0.2					44	.04	0.2			148	11	.20	.030	I
str	61	114.3	0.1	15.1		0.1	5	83	.02	.06	9	5	10	7	.04	
1 jar	130	0.1	0.0	0.0	0.1	0	55	.03	0.2	.00	.15	131	7	.44	.052	803
w/ yogurt, Gerber 2nd Foods	97		2.6	18.5	13.6	1.2		35	.11	.04		48	103	18	.40	.090
4 fl oz	124	1.4					18	.05	0.2			179	84	.30	.040	I
mixed tropical fruit, Gerber	71		0.6	16.8	15.6	0.4		35	.06	.15		7	14	22	.20	.280
4 fl oz	127	0.1					35	.05	0.4			163	14	.20	.040	I
orange	57	115.0	0.8	13.3		0.1	8	81	.04	.07	34	1	16	12	.07	
1 jar	130	0.4	0.0	0.1	0.1	0	72	.06	0.3	.00	.18	239	14	.22	.060	803
Beech-Nut Stage 3	59		0.8	13.1				42	.03				15			
4.2 fl oz	128	0.0					102	.05	0.3							I
Gerber 2nd Foods	59		0.8	13.4	12.8	0.2		35	.04	.06		4	16	15	.04	.030
4 fl oz	127	0.3					15	.09	0.3			234	20	.10	.050	I
orange apple	56	115.6	0.5	13.1			9	100	.04	.05	16	4	13	7	.03	
1 jar	130	0.3					95	.05	0.2	.00	.16	179	9	.26	.052	803
orange apple-banana	61	113.9	0.5	15.0		0.1	4	42	.04	.08	13	5	7	8	.03	
1 jar	130	0.1	0.0	0.0	0.0	0	35	.06	0.3	.00	.17	174	10	.45	.057	803
orange apricot	60	114.1	1.0	14.2		0.1	29	112	.04	.07	26	8	8	9	.05	
1 jar	130	0.1	0.0	0.0	0.0	0	281	.08	0.3	.00	.12	259	16	.49	.109	803
orange banana	65	113.0	0.9	15.5			7	44	.05	.07	32	4	22	18	.11	
1 jar	130	0.1					60	.07	0.2	.00	.19	260	17	.14	.055	803

	KCAL	H₂O (g)	PRO (g)	CHO (g)	SUGR (g)	DFIB (g)	A (RE)	C (mg)	B-2 (mg)	B-6 (mg)	FOL (mcg)	Na (mg)	Ca (mg)	Mg (mg)	Zn (mg)	Mn (mg)
	WT (g)	FAT (g)	SFA (g)	MUFA (g)	PUFA (g)	CHOL (mg)	A (IU)	B-1 (mg)	NIA (mg)	B-12 (mcg)	PANT (mg)	K (mg)	P (mg)	Fe (mg)	Cu (mg)	REF
orange banana pineapple, Gerber	70		0.8	16.5	14.1	0.5		35	.07	.14		7	12	20	.10	.130
4 fl oz	127	0.1					17	.05	0.4			240	23	.20	.060	I
orange carrot, Gerber 3rd Foods	53		0.7	12.1	10.9	0.7		35	.05	.07		11	18	14	.20	.050
4 fl oz	125	0.2					2660	.06	0.3			215	24	.30	.050	I
orange pineapple	62	113.5	0.7	15.2		0.1	4	69	.03	.08	24	3	10	12	.05	
1 jar	130	0.1	0.0	0.0	0.0	0	40	.07	0.3	.00	.08	183	12	.55	.057	803
papaya w/ mixed tropical fruit, Gerber 3rd Foods—4 fl oz	66		0.4	15.9		0.7		35	.04	.04		7	16	18	.10	.100
	127	0.2					37	.01	0.3			136	18		.040	I
pear, Beech-Nut Stage 1	60		0.0	14.3				43	.04							
4.2 fl oz	128	0.0							0.5							I
pear, Gerber 1st Foods	59		0.2	14.3	13.1	0.3		35	.02	.03		5	12	9	.10	.340
4 oz	127	0.1					8	.01	0.2			156	12	.20	.030	I
pineapple carrot, Gerber 3rd Foods	57		0.5	13.4	12.8	0.6		35	.03	.09		12	18	14	.30	.270
4 fl oz	125	0.1					1675	.07	0.2			135	14	.20	.040	I
prune orange	91	106.5	0.8	21.8			17	83	.16	.08	17	3	16	10	.05	
1 jar	130	0.4					170	.06	0.5	.00	.18	235	13	1.13	.060	803
tropical blend, Beech-Nut Stage 2	72		0.7	17.0				40	.01				21			
4 fl oz	122	0.0					49	.01	0.2							I
white grape, Beech-Nut Stage 1	81		0.0	19.6				43	.03			8	17			
4.2 fl oz	128	0.0							0.4					.38		I
white grape, Gerber 1st Foods	82		0.4	19.8	20.1	0.1		35	.01	.07		8	18	11		.100
4 fl oz	127	0.1					3	.01	0.1			53	22	.20	.020	I

19.6 FRUITS

	KCAL	H₂O (g)	PRO (g)	CHO (g)	SUGR (g)	DFIB (g)	A (RE)	C (mg)	B-2 (mg)	B-6 (mg)	FOL (mcg)	Na (mg)	Ca (mg)	Mg (mg)	Zn (mg)	Mn (mg)
	WT (g)	FAT (g)	SFA (g)	MUFA (g)	PUFA (g)	CHOL (mg)	A (IU)	B-1 (mg)	NIA (mg)	B-12 (mcg)	PANT (mg)	K (mg)	P (mg)	Fe (mg)	Cu (mg)	REF
apple banana, Gerber 3rd Foods	125		0.7	30.1	13.9	2.8		16	.06	.10		2	6	19	.01	.170
6 oz	170	0.2					34	.02	0.4			244	20	.20	.080	I
apple blueberry																
Gerber 2nd Foods	57		0.2	13.6	11.4	1.9		16	.04	.04		1	5	5		.090
4 oz	113	0.2					38	.02	0.1			98	9	.10	.040	I
jr	105	140.8	0.3	28.2		3.1	7	24	.07	.07	6	22	9	5	.06	
1 jar	170	0.3	0.0	0.0	0.1	0	71	.03	0.2	.00	.28	111	12	.68	.097	803
str	69	93.9	0.2	18.4		2.0	2	31	.04	.04	4	2	5	3	.04	
1 jar	113	0.2	0.0	0.0	0.0	0	23	.02	0.1	.00	.18	78	9	.23	.063	803
apple cinn fruit bar, Gerber Graduates	37		0.5	6.6	3.7	0.4			.02	.01		7	4	2		.030
.3 oz	9	0.9	0.2					.03	0.2			12	9	.20	.010	I
apple raspberry, jr	99	142.8	0.3	26.3		3.6	5	49	.05	.06	6	3	9	7	.05	
1 jar	170	0.3	0.1	0.0	0.1	0	51	.02	0.2	.00	.15	122	14	.37	.090	803
apple raspberry, str	66	94.7	0.2	17.7		2.4	2	30	.03	.04	4	2	6	5	.04	
1 jar	113	0.2	0.0	0.0	0.1	0	25	.02	0.1	.00	.10	90	9	.25	.061	803
apple strawberry, Beech-Nut Stage 2	90		0.0	21.8				16	.05							
4.5 oz	128	0.0	0.0	0.0	0.0			.01	0.3							I
apples & apricots																
inst dry, Heinz	50		0.0	13.0				17	.02	.04		2	11		.06	
3 T	14	1.0					566	.02	0.2			160	10		.040	I
jr, Heinz	115		0.9	26.6				15	.04	.11		4	17		.15	
1 jar	213	0.6					694	.09	0.3			217	34	.43	.192	I
str, Heinz	69		0.5	16.0				16	.03	.06		3	19		.09	
1 jar	128	0.4					417	.05	0.2			131	20	.26	.115	I
apples & bananas, inst dry, Heinz	50		0.0	13.0				17	.01	.04		3	0		.04	
4 T	14	0.0					28	.02	0.1			143	7	.20	.010	I
apples & cranberries w/ tapioca, jr, Heinz	179		0.2	43.0				6	.02	.04		19	13		.06	
1 jar	213	0.6					60	.02	0.2			38	13	.43	.085	I
apples & cranberries w/ tapioca, str, Heinz—1 jar	108		0.1	25.9				4	.01	.03		7	8		.04	
	128	0.4					36	.01	0.1			23	8	.26	.051	I
apples & peaches, inst dry, Heinz	50		0.0	13.0				17	.02	.04		7	8		.06	
3 T	14	0.0					212	.02	0.2			128	10	.30	.030	I
apples & pears																
inst dry, Heinz	50		0.0	13.0				17	.01	.02		2	9		.05	
3 T	14	1.0					28	.01	0.1			107	8	.20	.050	I

	KCAL	H₂O (g)	PRO (g)	CHO (g)	SUGR (g)	DFIB (g)	A (RE)	C (mg)	B-2 (mg)	B-6 (mg)	FOL (mcg)	Na (mg)	Ca (mg)	Mg (mg)	Zn (mg)	Mn (mg)
	WT (g)	FAT (g)	SFA (g)	MUFA (g)	PUFA (g)	CHOL (mg)	A (IU)	B-1 (mg)	NIA (mg)	B-12 (mcg)	PANT (mg)	K (mg)	P (mg)	Fe (mg)	Cu (mg)	REF
jr, Heinz	121		0.4	28.8				15	.04	.06		4	17		.13	
1 jar	213	0.4					87	.04	0.3			222	19	.43	.128	I
str, Heinz	73		0.3	17.3				16	.03	.04		3	10		.08	
1 jar	128	0.3					52	.03	0.2			133	12	.26	.077	I
apples, diced, Gerber Graduates	57		0.2	13.7	8.8	1.2		40	.02	.04		8	13	8		.050
4.5 oz	128	0.1					10	.02	0.1			58	15	.20	.030	I
apples, inst dry, Heinz	50		0.0	13.0				16	.01	.03		4	8		.04	
4 T	14	0.0					28	.02	0.1			104	9	.20	.040	I
apples, peaches, & strawberries, Beech-	93		0.0	22.3				16	.04						.38	
Nut Stage 2—4.5 oz	128	0.0					255	.01	0.5							I
apples, pears, & bananas, Beech-Nut	97		0.0	23.6				16	.05							
Stage 2—4.5 oz	128	0.0						.03	0.3							I
applesauce																
Beech-Nut Stage 1	54		0.0	13.0				16	.02							
2.8 oz	79	0.0						.01								I
Beech-Nut Stage 2	68		0.0	16.3				16	.03							
4.5 oz	128	0.0						.01								I
Beech-Nut Stage 3	87		0.0	21.1				16	.05							
6 oz	170	0.0						.03								I
Gerber 1st Foods	40		0.2	9.4	8.0	1.3		16	.02	.03		1	3	3		.030
2.5 oz	71	0.1					28	.01	0.1			68	7	.10	.020	I
Gerber 2nd Foods	58		0.2	13.8	10.7	1.5		16	.04	.05		1	4	4	.03	.040
4 oz	113	0.2					29	.02	0.1			101	9	.10	.030	I
Gerber 3rd Foods	86		0.3	20.6	16.1	2.5		16	.05	.07		2	6	7		.060
6 oz	170	0.3					36	.03	0.1			155	14	.20	.050	I
jr	79	190.6	0.0	21.9		3.6	2	81	.06	.06	4	4	11	6	.09	
1 jar	213	0.0	0.0	0.0	0.0	0	19	.03	0.1	.00	.21	164	13	.47	.075	803
str	52	113.4	0.3	14.0		2.2	3	49	.04	.04	2	3	5	4	.03	
1 jar	128	0.3	0.0	0.0	0.1	0	22	.02	0.1	.00	.14	91	9	.28	.049	803
applesauce & apricots																
Beech-Nut Stage 2	73		0.0	17.3				16	.01							
4.5 oz	128	0.0					704	.03	0.2							I
Gerber 2nd Foods	60		0.4	14.2	9.7	2.0		16	.05	.05		2	7	6	.05	.050
4 oz	113	0.2					713	.02	0.2			142	12	.20	.050	I
jr	77	149.1	0.3	19.7		3.1	66	32	.05	.05	2	5	10	7	.07	
1 jar	170	0.3	0.0	0.1	0.1	0	658	.02	0.2	.00	.20	204	15	.42	.070	803
str	53	98.2	0.2	14.0		2.0	38	20	.03	.03	2	3	7	5	.03	
1 jar	113	0.2	0.0	0.0	0.1	0	383	.02	0.2	.00	.14	123	11	.29	.050	803
applesauce & bananas, Beech-Nut	73		0.0	17.4				16	.01			3				
Stage 2—4.5 oz	128	0.0	0.0	0.0	0.0			.01	0.2							I
applesauce & bananas, Beech-Nut	95		0.0	23.5				16	.03							
Stage 3—6 oz	170	0.0	0.0	0.0	0.0			.02								I
applesauce & cherries																
Beech-Nut Stage 2	72		0.0	17.7				16	.04				13			
4.5 oz	128	0.0					90	.03							.51	I
Beech-Nut Stage 3	100		0.0	24.5				16	.03							
6 oz	170	0.0					80	.02	0.2						.68	I
jr	95	145.5	0.0	24.0		1.9	7	73	.05	.07	1	2	2	7	.05	
1 jar	170	0.0	0.0	0.0	0.0	0	77	.02	0.2	.00	.22	224	14	.51	.078	803
str	58	96.8	0.0	15.9		1.2	5	48	.03	.04	0	1	1	5	.03	
1 jar	113	0.0	0.0	0.0	0.0	0	51	.01	0.2	.00	.15	149	9	.34	.051	803
applesauce & pineapple, jr	83	189.8	0.2	22.4		3.2	4	57	.06	.08	4	4	9	9	.06	
1 jar	213	0.2	0.0	0.0	0.1	0	45	.05	0.2	.00	.22	162	13	.21	.077	803
applesauce & pineapple, str	47	114.6	0.1	12.9		1.9	3	36	.03	.05	2	3	5	4	.02	
1 jar	128	0.1	0.0	0.0	0.0	0	26	.03	0.1	.00	.13	100	8	.13	.045	803
apricots w/ mixed fruit, Gerber	69		0.6	16.3	10.0	1.9		16	.02	.02		6	8	13	.10	.040
2nd Foods—4 oz	113	0.2					1009	.01	0.0			104	19	.30	.070	I
apricots w/ mixed fruit, Gerber 3rd Foods	104		0.9	24.5	15.4	2.9		16	.02	.07		9	12	19	.20	.170
6 oz	170	0.3					1514	.01	0.4			306	28	.40	.100	I

Food	KCAL / WT (g)	H₂O / FAT (g)	PRO / SFA (g)	CHO / MUFA (g)	SUGR / PUFA (g)	DFIB / CHOL (g)(mg)	A RE / A IU	C (mg) / B-1 (mg)	B-2 / NIA (mg)	B-6 / B-12	FOL / PANT	Na / K (mg)	Ca / P (mg)	Mg / Fe (mg)	Zn / Cu (mg)	Mn / REF
apricots w/ pears & apples, Beech-Nut Stage 3—6 oz	112		1.2	26.2				16	.05							
	170	0.0					1428	.03	0.8					.68		I
apricots w/ pears & applesce, Beech-Nut Stage 2—4.5 oz	87		0.8	20.4				16	.04					14		
	128	0.0	0.0	0.0	0.0		1190	.03	0.6					.51		I
apricots w/ tapioca, jr — 1 jar	107	139.6	0.5	29.4		2.5	122	30	.02	.05	3	10	14	7	.07	
	170	0.0	0.0	0.0	0.0	0	1229	.01	0.3	.00	.23	213	17	.46	.061	803
apricots w/ tapioca, str — 1 jar	68	93.9	0.3	18.4		1.7	81	24	.01	.03	2	9	10	5	.05	
	113	0.0	0.0	0.0	0.0	0	819	.01	0.2	.00	.15	137	11	.34	.038	803
banana & pineapple, Gerber 3rd Foods — 6 oz	124		1.4	29.1	23.6	2.1		16	.06	.21		19	7	43	.30	.600
	170	0.2					73	.03	0.4			418	31	.40	.200	I
banana & yogurt, Beech-Nut Stage 2 — 4.5 oz	123		1.9	25.3				16	.10			29	54			
	128	1.5						.01	0.2							I
banana strawberry, Gerber 3rd Foods — 6 oz	159		1.6	37.7	32.5	2.2		16	.05	.22		17	8	48	.30	.480
	170	0.2					62	.01	0.4			494	38	.40	.160	I
banana van w/ tapioca, Gerber — 4 oz	96		0.5	21.0	16.1	0.5		32	.05	.07		12	16	11	.10	.240
	113	0.9					9	.01	0.2			97	15	.10	.030	I
bananas																
Beech-Nut Stage 1 — 2.8 oz	65		0.7	15.3				16	.04						.24	
	79	0.0					63	.02	0.4							I
Beech-Nut Stage 2 — 4.5 oz	108		1.2	25.3				16	.05							
	128	0.0					115	.03	0.5					.38		I
Gerber 1st Foods — 2.5 oz	71		0.8	16.6	13.1	1.1		16	.06	.27		2	3	20	.10	.260
	71	0.2					28	.02	0.5			244	17	.20	.060	I
Gerber 2nd Foods — 4 oz	101		1.2	23.8	20.9	1.7		16	.07	.30		7	5	35	.20	.340
	113	0.1					73	.01	0.1			340	25	.30	.130	I
inst dry, Heinz — 3 T	50		1.0	13.0				16	.04	.24		4	4		.10	
	14	0.0	0.0	0.0	0.0		60	.01	0.2			236	16	.20	.050	I
bananas, apples, & pears, Gerber 2nd Foods—4 oz	95		1.0	22.4	16.7	1.5		16	.03	.32		11	5	30	.20	.290
	113	0.1					62	.01	0.6			260	22	.30	.090	I
bananas w/ apples & pears, Gerber 3rd Foods—6 oz	142		1.5	33.6	26.1	2.3		16	.02	.50		16	7	44	.20	.430
	170	0.2					94	.01	0.9			390	33	.40	.140	I
bananas w/ pears & apples, Beech-Nut Stage 3—6 oz	133		1.0	31.3				16	.03							
	170	0.0					160	.03	0.5					.51		I
bananas w/ pears & applesce, str, Beech-Nut Stage 2—4.5 oz	96		0.8	23.0				16	.06							
	128	0.0						.03	0.6					.38		I
bananas w/ pineapple & tapioca, jr — 1 jar	111	138.9	0.3	30.3		2.7	7	33	.03	.14	9	10	12	10	.07	
	170	0.0	0.0	0.0	0.0	0	70	.03	0.3	.00	.24	116	9	.39	.066	803
bananas w/ pineapple & tapioca, str — 1 jar	77	91.6	0.2	20.8		1.8	5	24	.02	.10	6	9	8	7	.04	
	113	0.1	0.0	0.0	0.0	0	45	.02	0.2	.00	.17	88	6	.15	.045	803
bananas w/ tapioca, jr — 1 jar	114	138.5	0.7	30.3		2.7	7	44	.03	.24	11	15	14	20	.12	
	170	0.3	0.1	0.0	0.1	0	75	.03	0.4	.00	.29	184	15	.51	.078	803
bananas w/ tapioca, str — 1 jar	64	94.9	0.5	17.3		1.8	5	19	.04	.13	6	10	6	11	.07	
	113	0.1	0.0	0.0	0.0	0	49	.01	0.2	.00	.17	99	8	.23	.045	803
fruit juice snacks, Gerber Graduates — 1 oz	96		0.0	24.1	16.9	0.4		8	.01	.01		27	2	2		.010
	28	0.0	0.0	0.0	0.0			.00	0.0			24	2		.030	I
fruit salad, Gerber 3rd Foods — 6 oz	105		0.6	25.1	19.7	2.9		16	.05	.10		5	9	15	.10	.550
	170	0.2					186	.03	0.4			196	20	.30	.080	I
guava & papaya w/ tapioca, str — 1 jar	81	105.6	0.3	21.8			23	104	.03	.02	3	5	9	6	.08	
	128	0.1					236	.01	0.3	.00		95	8	.26		803
guava w/ mixed fruit, Gerber — 4 fl oz	62		0.3	14.8	13.9	0.6		35	.04	.04		6	15	9	.10	.070
	127	0.1					42	.02	0.4			135	17	.20	.030	I
guava w/ tapioca, str — 1 jar	86	103.9	0.4	23.4		2.3	38	97	.09	.05	3	3	9	3	.10	
	128	0.0	0.0	0.0			383	.02	0.5	.00	.21	93	6	.26		803
mango w/ tapioca, Gerber — 4 oz	84		0.2	20.2	13.0	0.7		32	.02	.07		4	7	6	.04	.060
	113	0.2					734	.02	0.2			85	7	.10	.040	I
mango w/ tapioca, str — 1 jar	90	87.8	0.3	24.4		1.1	76	141	.03	.13	2	5	5	5	.07	
	113	0.2	0.1	0.1	0.0	0	751	.03	0.3	.00	.22	67	7	.11	.031	803
mixed fruit & yogurt, Beech-Nut Stage 2 — 4.5 oz	123		1.4	27.0				16	.06			20	42			
	128	1.0					77	.05	0.1							I
mixed fruit & yogurt, Beech-Nut Stage 3 — 6 oz	160		1.9	35.2				16	.09			31	56			
	170	1.2					94	.05	0.2							I

	KCAL / WT (g)	H₂O (g) / FAT (g)	PRO (g) / SFA (g)	CHO (g) / MUFA (g)	SUGR (g) / PUFA (g)	DFIB (g) / CHOL (mg)	A (RE) / A (IU)	C (mg) / B-1 (mg)	B-2 (mg) / NIA (mg)	B-6 (mg) / B-12 (mcg)	FOL (mcg) / PANT (mg)	Na (mg) / K (mg)	Ca (mg) / P (mg)	Mg (mg) / Fe (mg)	Zn (mg) / Cu (mg)	Mn (mg) / REF
mixed fruit, diced, Gerber Graduates	56		0.0	13.4	10.4	1.3		40	.01	.05		8	11	8		.040
4.5 oz	128	0.1					109	.01	0.3			70	16	.20	.030	I
mixed fruit, inst dry, Heinz	50		1.0	13.0				17	.02	.04		2	9		.08	
4 T	14	0.0					212	.01	0.5			167	9	.20	.060	I
papaya & applesce w/ tapioca, str	90	103.2	0.3	24.2		1.8	10	145	.04	.03	3	6	9	6	.04	
1 jar	128	0.1					97	.01	0.1	.00	.36	101	6	.56	.056	803
papaya w/ tapioca, Gerber	72		0.2	17.5	11.2	0.4		31	.01	.01		4	7	6		.040
4 oz	113	0.1					124	.01	0.1			73	5	.10	.020	I
peaches																
Beech-Nut Stage 1	47		0.8	10.7				16	.03							
2.8 oz	79	0.0					387	.01	0.8							I
Beech-Nut Stage 2	61		1.0	14.3				16	.04							
4.5 oz	128	0.0					614	.01	1.0							I
Beech-Nut Stage 3	82		1.4	19.0				16	.05							
6 oz	170	0.0					816	.02	1.4							I
diced, Gerber Graduates	63		0.7	14.6	11.5	1.1		40	.04	.05		10	10	10	.10	.060
4.5 oz	128	0.2					258	.02	0.6			105	22	.30	.060	I
Gerber 1st Foods	30		0.5	6.8	2.8	1.1		16	.03	.04		1	3	5	.10	.040
2.5 oz	71	0.2					169	.01	0.5			108	12	.10	.040	I
Gerber 2nd Foods	78		1.0	18.0	12.2	1.6		16	.04	.04		6	7	12	.10	.070
4 oz	113	0.2					279	.01	0.7			171	28	.20	.090	I
Gerber 3rd Foods	117		1.5	27.0	18.0	2.3		16	.06	.03		9	11	18	.20	.110
6 oz	170	0.3					417	.02	1.1			256	42	.20	.130	I
inst dry, Heinz	50		1.0	13.0				16	.01	.04		2	12		.14	
3 T	14	1.0					224	.01	0.5			202	20	.40	.070	I
jr	121	136.2	0.8	32.1		2.5	31	32	.05	.03	7	9	9	9	.10	
1 jar	170	0.3	0.0	0.1	0.2	0	303	.02	1.1	.00	.22	264	19	.46	.085	803
str	80	90.5	0.6	21.4		1.7	18	35	.04	.02	4	7	7	7	.10	
1 jar	113	0.2	0.0	0.1	0.1	0	182	.01	0.7	.00	.15	183	14	.27	.060	803
peaches & yogurt, Beech-Nut Stage 2	118		1.9	24.8				16	.09			28	54			
4.5 oz	128	1.2					294	.05	0.5							I
pears																
Beech-Nut Stage 1	48		0.0	11.4				16	.03							
2.8 oz	79	0.0						.01	0.2							I
Beech-Nut Stage 2	69		0.0	16.6				16	.03							
4.5 oz	128	0.0						.03	0.3							I
Beech-Nut Stage 3	92		0.0	22.1				16	.05				2			
6 oz	170	0.0						.03	0.5							I
diced, Gerber Graduates	64		0.3	15.3	9.0	1.7		40	.02	.04		7	12	9		.040
4.5 oz	128	0.2						.02	0.2			62	16	.20	.060	I
Gerber 1st Foods	40		0.3	9.6	4.6	2.1		16	.02	.01		1	7	5	.10	.040
2.5 oz	71	0.1					5	.01	0.1			83	9	.10	.060	I
Gerber 2nd Foods	81		0.5	19.5	12.2	3.1		16	.03	.02		3	12	12	.10	.070
4 oz	113	0.1					11	.02	0.3			158	19	.20	.080	I
Gerber 3rd Foods	122		0.8	29.3	26.8	4.6		16	.05	.03		4	18	18	.30	.100
6 oz	170	0.1					16	.03	0.4			237	28	.30	.120	I
jr	92	187.0	0.6	24.7		7.7	6	47	.06	.02	8	4	17	19	.17	
1 jar	213	0.2	0.0	0.0	0.0	0	72	.03	0.4	.00	.20	245	26	.53	.170	803
str	52	113.2	0.4	13.8		4.6	4	31	.04	.01	5	3	10	10	.10	
1 jar	128	0.3	0.0	0.1	0.1	0	42	.02	0.2	.00	.12	166	15	.31	.083	803
pears & applesce, Beech-Nut Stage 2	81		0.0	19.5				16	.04							
4.5 oz	128	0.0						.03	0.3							I
pears & pineapple																
Beech-Nut Stage 2	79		0.0	19.3				16	.05				13			
4.5 oz	128	0.0						.04	0.3							I
Gerber 2nd Foods	63		0.4	14.5	10.8	3.3		16	.03	.03		1	10	8	.10	.160
4 oz	113	0.2					15	.02	0.2			125	13	.20	.090	I
jr	94	187.0	0.6	24.3		5.5	6	36	.05	.03	6	2	21	15	.27	
1 jar	213	0.4	0.0	0.1	0.1	0	68	.05	0.4	.00	.20	251	21	.45	.224	803

	KCAL / WT (g)	H₂O (g) / FAT (g)	PRO (g) / SFA (g)	CHO (g) / MUFA (g)	SUGR (g) / PUFA (g)	DFIB (g) / CHOL (mg)	A (RE) / A (IU)	C (mg) / B-1 (mg)	B-2 (mg) / NIA (mg)	B-6 (mg) / B-12 (mcg)	FOL (mcg) / PANT (mg)	Na (mg) / K (mg)	Ca (mg) / P (mg)	Mg (mg) / Fe (mg)	Zn (mg) / Cu (mg)	Mn (mg) / REF
str	52	113.3	0.4	14.0		3.3	4	35	.04	.02	4	5	13	9	.08	
1 jar	128	0.1	0.0	0.0	0.0	0	37	.03	0.3	.00	.11	148	12	.32	.179	803
plums & apples, Gerber 2nd Foods	78		0.6	18.8	15.2	2.0		16				7	20	11	.20	.090
4 oz	113	0.1					95					164	18	.20	.210	I
plums & apples, Gerber 3rd Foods	117		0.9	28.2	22.8	3.0		0	.06	.06		10	16	16	.30	.140
6 oz	170	0.2					143	.02	0.4			247	25	.30	.330	I
plums w/ rice, Beech-Nut Stage 2	111		0.0	27.1				5	.03			9				
4.5 oz	128	0.0					166	.01	0.4							I
plums w/ tapioca, jr	126	134.6	0.2	34.7		2.0	15	1	.05	.05	2	14	10	7	.14	
1 jar	170	0.0	0.0	0.0	0.0	0	160	.01	0.4	.00	.19	141	10	.37	.065	803
plums w/ tapioca, str	96	108.0	0.1	26.6		1.6	14	1	.04	.03	1	8	8	5	.11	
1 jar	135	0.0	0.0	0.0	0.0	0	128	.01	0.3	.00	.15	115	8	.27	.050	803
prunes & apples, Gerber 2nd Foods	85		0.7	20.2	13.1	2.3			.09	.09		14	14	12	.02	.090
4 oz	113	0.2					193	.01	0.6			208	21	.30	.140	I
prunes, Gerber 1st Foods	72		0.7	17.1	12.4	1.8			.15	.08		4	15	13	.10	.080
2.5 oz	71	0.1					276	.01	0.6			216	21	.20	.070	I
prunes w/ pears, Beech-Nut Stage 2	138		1.3	32.9					.09				28			
4.5 oz	128	0.0					141	.03	0.8					.64		I
prunes w/ tapioca, jr	119	136.2	1.0	31.8		4.6	70	1	.14	.15	0	3	26	17	.17	
1 jar	170	0.2	0.0	0.1	0.0	0	692	.04	0.9	.00	.24	275	26	.56	.105	803
prunes w/ tapioca, str	79	90.7	0.7	20.9		3.1	51	1	.08	.09	0	6	17	11	.10	
1 jar	113	0.1	0.0	0.1	0.0	0	512	.02	0.6	.00	.16	200	17	.40	.069	803
strawberry fruit bar, Gerber Graduates	37		0.5	6.6	3.5	0.3			.02	.01		8	4	2		.040
.3 oz	9	0.9	0.2					.03	0.2			13	9	.20	.010	I
tropical fruit medley w/ tapioca, Gerber	73		0.1	17.3	10.7	0.2		32	.02	.04		4	6	5		.190
4 oz	113	0.1					140	.02	0.1			44	4	.10	.020	I

19.7 MEATS

beef

	KCAL / WT (g)	H₂O (g) / FAT (g)	PRO (g) / SFA (g)	CHO (g) / MUFA (g)	SUGR (g) / PUFA (g)	DFIB (g) / CHOL (mg)	A (RE) / A (IU)	C (mg) / B-1 (mg)	B-2 (mg) / NIA (mg)	B-6 (mg) / B-12 (mcg)	FOL (mcg) / PANT (mg)	Na (mg) / K (mg)	Ca (mg) / P (mg)	Mg (mg) / Fe (mg)	Zn (mg) / Cu (mg)	Mn (mg) / REF
& beef broth, Beech-Nut Stage 1	85		10.0	0.0	0.0				.11			37				
2.8 oz	79	5.0						.02	1.8					1.11		I
& gravy, Gerber 2nd Foods	76		8.5	3.5	0.1	0.5		0	.09	.09		31	8	10	2.10	
2.5 oz	71	3.2					4	.01	1.8			134	78	.90	.040	I
jr	105	79.1	14.4	0.0	0.0	0.0	31	2	.16	.12	6	65	8	9	1.98	
1 jar	99	4.9	2.6	1.8	0.2	27	58	.01	3.3	1.46	.35	188	71	1.63	.091	803
str	106	79.8	13.5	0.0	0.0	0.0	20	2	.14	.14	5	80	7	17	2.43	
1 jar	99	5.3	2.6	2.2	0.2	29	67	.01	2.8	1.41	.34	218	83	1.46	.043	803

chicken

	KCAL / WT (g)	H₂O (g) / FAT (g)	PRO (g) / SFA (g)	CHO (g) / MUFA (g)	SUGR (g) / PUFA (g)	DFIB (g) / CHOL (mg)	A (RE) / A (IU)	C (mg) / B-1 (mg)	B-2 (mg) / NIA (mg)	B-6 (mg) / B-12 (mcg)	FOL (mcg) / PANT (mg)	Na (mg) / K (mg)	Ca (mg) / P (mg)	Mg (mg) / Fe (mg)	Zn (mg) / Cu (mg)	Mn (mg) / REF
& chicken broth, Beech-Nut Stage 2	60		10.4	0.0	0.0				.13			43	23			
2.8 oz	79	2.2						.02	2.0					1.26		I
& gravy, Gerber 2nd Foods	81		7.8	2.3	0.1	0.2		0	.09	.09		32	67	10	.80	.010
2.5 oz	71	4.5						.01	2.6			111	104	.80	.040	I
jr	148	75.2	14.6	0.0	0.0	0.0	12	1	.16	.19	11	50	54	11	1.00	
1 jar	99	9.5	2.4	4.3	2.3	58	40	.01	3.4	.40	.72	121	89	.98	.045	803
str	129	76.7	13.6	0.1		0.0	16	2	.15	.20	10	47	63	13	1.20	
1 jar	99	7.8	2.0	3.5	1.9	61	52	.01	3.2	.40	.67	140	96	1.39	.045	803
chicken sticks, jr	133	48.5	10.4	1.0		0.1	2	1	.14	.07	8	340	52	10	.72	
1 jar	71	10.2	2.9	4.4	2.1	55	8	.01	1.4	.28	.52	75	86	1.11	.032	803
chicken sticks, toddler, Gerber	95		10.8	1.0	0.7	0.8		0	.09	.08		299	66	9	1.00	.010
2.5 oz	71	5.4						.02	1.8			77	98	.80	.040	I

ham

	KCAL / WT (g)	H₂O (g) / FAT (g)	PRO (g) / SFA (g)	CHO (g) / MUFA (g)	SUGR (g) / PUFA (g)	DFIB (g) / CHOL (mg)	A (RE) / A (IU)	C (mg) / B-1 (mg)	B-2 (mg) / NIA (mg)	B-6 (mg) / B-12 (mcg)	FOL (mcg) / PANT (mg)	Na (mg) / K (mg)	Ca (mg) / P (mg)	Mg (mg) / Fe (mg)	Zn (mg) / Cu (mg)	Mn (mg) / REF
Gerber 2nd Foods	69		7.9	2.8	0.1	0.4		0	.10	.14		27	6	10	1.30	
2.5 oz	71	2.9						.11	2.3			140	81	.50	.050	I
jr	124	77.7	14.9	0.0	0.0	0.0	10	2	.19	.20	2	66	5	11	1.68	
1 jar	99	6.6	2.2	3.1	0.9	29	32	.14	2.8	.10	.53	208	88	1.00	.067	803
str	110	78.6	13.8	0.0	0.0	0.0	11	2	.15	.25	2	41	6	13	2.22	
1 jar	99	5.7	1.9	2.7	0.8	24	38	.14	2.6	.10	.50	202	80	1.02	.064	803

	KCAL / WT (g)	H₂O (g) / FAT (g)	PRO (g) / SFA (g)	CHO (g) / MUFA (g)	SUGR (g) / PUFA (g)	DFIB (g) / CHOL (mg)	A (RE) / A (IU)	C (mg) / B-1 (mg)	B-2 (mg) / NIA (mg)	B-6 (mg) / B-12 (mcg)	FOL (mcg) / PANT (mg)	Na (mg) / K (mg)	Ca (mg) / P (mg)	Mg (mg) / Fe (mg)	Zn (mg) / Cu (mg)	Mn (mg) / REF
lamb																
& lamb broth, Beech-Nut Stage 2	60		10.4	0.0	0.0				.13			45	10			
2.8 oz	79	2.1						.02	2.5					1.03		I
Gerber 2nd Foods	66		8.3	3.6	0.1	0.3		0	.10	.70		30	8	10	1.80	.010
2.5 oz	71	2.1						.01	1.7			130	76	.80	.050	I
jr	111	78.8	15.0	0.0	0.0	0.0	8	2	.19	.18	2	72	7	10	2.57	
1 jar	99	5.1	2.5	2.0	0.2	38	27	.02	3.2	2.25	.42	209	90	1.64	.056	803
str	102	79.5	14.0	0.1		0.0	10	1	.20	.15	2	61	7	13	2.73	
1 jar	99	4.7	2.3	1.9	0.2	38	32	.02	2.9	2.17	.41	203	96	1.48	.054	803
meat sticks, Gerber Graduates	109		10.0	1.1	0.6	1.4		0	.08	.08		330	24	7	2.40	.010
2.5 oz	71	7.2					4	.03	1.2			85	74	1.00	.040	I
meat sticks, jr	131	49.3	9.5	0.8		0.1	15	2	.12	.06	6	388	24	8	1.35	
1 jar	71	10.4	4.1	4.6	1.1	50	49	.04	1.1	.21	.34	81	73	.98	.048	803
pork, str	123	77.6	13.9	0.0	0.0	0.0	12	2	.20	.20	2	42	5	10	2.25	
1 jar	99	7.0	2.4	3.5	0.8	48	38	.14	2.2	.98	.27	221	93	.99	.071	803
turkey																
& gravy, Gerber 2nd Foods	75		7.3	2.8	0.2	0.3		1	.11	.09		37	58	10	1.50	.030
2.5 oz	71	3.9					3	.01	1.5			112	92	.80	.050	I
& turkey broth, Beech-Nut Stage 2	82		9.5	0.0	0.0				.15			43	29			
2.8 oz	79	4.9						.02	2.2					.79		I
jr	128	76.7	15.2	0.0	0.0	0.0	10	2	.25	.16	12	71	28	12	1.78	
1 jar	99	7.0	2.3	2.6	1.7	53	33	.02	3.4	1.06	.60	178	94	1.34	.043	803
str	113	78.1	14.2	0.1		0.0	14	2	.21	.18	11	54	23	14	1.81	
1 jar	99	5.7	1.9	2.2	1.4	58	47	.02	3.6	.99	.56	229	125	1.19	.040	803
turkey sticks, Gerber Graduates	96		9.6	1.0	0.7	0.0		1	.11	.07		311	52	8	1.60	.010
2.5 oz	71	6.0					2	.01	1.4			82	88	.70	.040	I
turkey sticks, jr	129	49.6	9.7	1.0		0.4	4	1	.11	.05	8	343	51	11	1.30	
1 jar	71	10.1	2.9	3.3	2.6	46	13	.01	1.2	.71	.40	65	73	.88	.028	803
veal																
& gravy, Gerber 2nd Foods	66		8.3	2.5	0.1	0.2		1	.10	.11		36	5	9	1.50	.010
2.5 oz	71	2.5					1	.02	2.5			129	76	.50	.040	I
& veal broth, Beech-Nut Stage 2	51		10.6	0.0	0.0				.17			46				
2.8 oz	79	1.0						.02	3.2					.63		I
jr	109	79.0	15.1	0.0	0.0	0.0	15	2	.18	.12	7	68	6	11	2.49	
1 jar	99	5.0	2.4	2.1	0.2	27	50	.02	3.8	1.29	.45	234	97	1.24	.074	803
str	100	80.1	13.4	0.0	0.0	0.0	14	2	.16	.15	6	63	7	12	1.98	
1 jar	99	4.8	2.3	2.0	0.2	25	46	.02	3.5	1.29	.43	214	97	1.26	.040	803

19.8 VEGETABLES

	KCAL / WT (g)	H₂O (g) / FAT (g)	PRO (g) / SFA (g)	CHO (g) / MUFA (g)	SUGR (g) / PUFA (g)	DFIB (g) / CHOL (mg)	A (RE) / A (IU)	C (mg) / B-1 (mg)	B-2 (mg) / NIA (mg)	B-6 (mg) / B-12 (mcg)	FOL (mcg) / PANT (mg)	Na (mg) / K (mg)	Ca (mg) / P (mg)	Mg (mg) / Fe (mg)	Zn (mg) / Cu (mg)	Mn (mg) / REF
beets, str	44	115.3	1.7	9.9		2.4	4	3	.06	.03	39	106	18	18	.15	
1 jar	128	0.1	0.0	0.0	0.0	0	42	.01	0.2	.00	.13	233	18	.41	.090	803
broccoli w/ carrots & cheese, Gerber 3rd	75		2.7	12.2	2.0	1.6		13	.05	.09		76	49	15	.40	.250
Foods—6 oz	170	1.7					4329	.03	0.5			169	71	.30	.030	I
carrots																
Beech-Nut Stage 1	26		0.7	5.7					.03			17	21			
2.8 oz	79	0.0					9401	.02	0.4							I
Beech-Nut Stage 2	41		1.0	8.8					.04			82	35			
4.5 oz	128	0.0					13952	.03	0.6					.38		I
Beech-Nut Stage 3	60		1.4	12.9					.09			32	32			
6 oz	170	0.0					19210	.03	1.0							I
diced, Gerber Graduates	19		0.4	3.9	1.8	1.7		0	.02	.04		31	17	7	.10	.060
2.5 oz	71	0.2					10673	.01	0.2			86	15	.10	.040	I
Gerber 1st Foods	25		0.6	4.9	3.1			0	.03	.07		30	18	8	.10	.080
2.5 oz	71	0.2					11547	.02	0.3			161	21	.20	.030	I
Gerber 2nd Foods	34		0.9	7.1	4.4	2.2		1	.05	.10		35	27	12	.18	.120
4 oz	113	0.3					17411	.03	0.4			268	31	.30	.040	I

	KCAL / WT (g)	H₂O (g) / FAT (g)	PRO (g) / SFA (g)	CHO (g) / MUFA (g)	SUGR (g) / PUFA (g)	DFIB (g) / CHOL (mg)	A (RE) / A (IU)	C (mg) / B-1 (mg)	B-2 (mg) / NIA (mg)	B-6 (mg) / B-12 (mcg)	FOL (mcg) / PANT (mg)	Na (mg) / K (mg)	Ca (mg) / P (mg)	Mg (mg) / Fe (mg)	Zn (mg) / Cu (mg)	Mn (mg) / REF
Gerber 3rd Foods	65		1.4	14.3	9.8	3.2		0	.09	.16		50	36	25	.40	.480
6 oz	170	0.4					17131	.04	0.6			371	48	.40	.100	I
inst dry, Heinz	60		1.0	11.0				1	.05	.03		30	45		.22	
4 T	14	2.0					9056	.04	0.3			225	38	.60	.080	I
jr	68	193.8	1.7	15.3		3.6	2516	12	.09	.17	37	104	49	23	.37	
1 jar	213	0.4	0.1	0.0	0.2	0	25155	.05	1.1	.00	.59	430	43	.83	.100	803
str	35	118.1	1.0	7.7		2.2	1467	7	.05	.09	19	47	28	12	.19	
1 jar	128	0.1	0.0	0.0	0.1	0	14670	.03	0.6	.00	.31	251	26	.47	.052	803
corn, creamed																
Beech-Nut Stage 2	90		2.2	18.4					.10			22	26			
4.5 oz	128	0.8					179		0.6					.38		I
Gerber 2nd Foods	70		2.0	14.3	1.1	0.6		0	.04	.06		10	23	13	.30	.140
4 oz	113	0.5					8	.01	0.7			116	53	.20	.030	I
inst dry, Heinz	60		2.0	10.0				0	.01	.04		1	4		.24	
6 T	14	1.0					23	.02	0.3			91	30	.30	.020	I
jr	138	173.4	3.0	34.7		4.5	17	5	.10	.09	27	111	38	17	.49	
1 jar	213	0.9	0.2	0.2	0.4	2	164	.03	1.1	.04	.70	173	70	.58	.081	803
str	73	107.0	1.8	18.0		2.7	9	3	.06	.05	14	55	26	10	.24	
1 jar	128	0.5	0.1	0.1	0.2	1	96	.02	0.7	.03	.37	115	42	.36	.044	803
garden veg																
Beech-Nut Stage 2	54		2.9	10.6				5	.09			12	28			
4.5 oz	128	0.0					2522	.05	0.9					.90		I
Gerber 2nd Foods	44		2.5	7.4	3.3	2.6		3	.07	.09		17	36	24	.50	.240
4 oz	113	0.5					6014	.07	0.9			189	48	.80	.070	I
str	47	115.2	2.9	8.7		1.9	777	7	.09	.13	51	45	36	27	.33	
1 jar	128	0.3	0.0	0.0	0.1	0	7766	.08	1.0	.00	.33	215	36	1.06	.090	803
green beans																
Beech-Nut Stage 2	32		1.5	6.3					.10				51			
4.5 oz	128	0.0					461	.04	0.5					1.28		I
Beech-Nut Stage 3	44		2.0	8.5					.19				65			
6 oz	170	0.0					748	.07	0.6					2.21		I
creamed, jr	68	193.6	2.1	15.3		3.4	32	6	.12	.03	85	26	68	15	.34	
1 jar	213	0.9	0.2	0.1	0.5	2	320	.05	0.5	.11	.39	138	40	.55	.126	803
diced, Gerber Graduates	20		0.9	3.8	0.8	1.6		1	.03	.02		28	24	9	.10	.050
2.5 oz	71	0.1					289	.01	0.2			59	14	.30	.030	I
Gerber 1st Foods	22		0.9	4.3	1.8	1.4		1	.05	.04		2	27	15	.20	.270
2.5 oz	71	0.1					272	.02	0.2			127	22	.40	.030	I
Gerber 2nd Foods	33		1.5	6.3	1.8	2.4		3	.07	.07		3	41	23	.03	.360
4 oz	113	0.2					439	.03	0.4			202	35	.60	.060	I
jr	52	190.6	2.5	11.7		3.9	89	17	.21	.07	67	4	134	45	.40	
1 jar	206	0.2	0.0	0.0	0.1	0	892	.04	0.7	.00	.31	264	39	2.22	.101	803
str	32	117.8	1.7	7.6		2.4	58	7	.11	.05	44	3	50	31	.26	
1 jar	128	0.1	0.0	0.0	0.1	0	573	.03	0.4	.00	.20	202	26	.96	.065	803
w/ rice, Gerber 3rd Foods	69		2.0	15.2	2.4	2.3		2	.08	.07		163	37	26	.50	.340
6 oz	170	0.2					286	.03	0.8			154	42	.80	.070	I
mixed veg																
Beech-Nut Stage 2	52		1.4	10.6				2	.04			23	20			
4.5 oz	128	0.0					4826	.03	0.5					.51		I
diced, Gerber Graduates	36		1.4	6.8	1.3	2.0		1	.02	.03		37	18	10	.10	.100
2.5 oz	71	0.3					6533	.03	0.4			76	3	.30	.040	I
Gerber 2nd Foods	48		1.4	9.7	2.8	1.6		0	.03	.07		19	17	12	.20	.200
4 oz	113	0.4					5566	.03	0.5			157	34	.30	.040	I
Gerber 3rd Foods	76		2.1	16.0	3.4	2.5		1	.06	.18		201	24	22	.30	.100
6 oz	170	0.3					8105	.07	1.1			316	47	.60	.090	I
inst dry, Heinz	60		2.0	9.0				0	.04	.05		3	12		.25	
5 T	14	2.0					1556	.05	0.6			116	31	.30	.060	I
jr	87	190.4	3.0	17.5		3.2	895	5	.07	.17	9	77	23	23	.58	
1 jar	213	0.9	0.2	0.1	0.4	0	8935	.06	1.4	.00	.55	362	53	.87	.087	803

	KCAL / WT (g)	H₂O (g) / FAT (g)	PRO (g) / SFA (g)	CHO (g) / MUFA (g)	SUGR (g) / PUFA (g)	DFIB (g) / CHOL (mg)	A (RE) / A (IU)	C (mg) / B-1 (mg)	B-2 (mg) / NIA (mg)	B-6 (mg) / B-12 (mcg)	FOL (mcg) / PANT (mg)	Na (mg) / K (mg)	Ca (mg) / P (mg)	Mg (mg) / Fe (mg)	Zn (mg) / Cu (mg)	Mn (mg) / REF
str	52	114.9	1.5	10.2		1.9	511	2	.03	.07	5	17	17	13	.19	
1 jar	128	0.6	0.1	0.2	0.2	0	5108	.03	0.4	.00	.32	163	28	.41	.051	803
peas																
& carrots, Beech-Nut Stage 2	52		2.9	9.3				4	.08			28	27			
4.5 oz	128	0.0					7322	.04	1.0					.90		I
Beech-Nut Stage 1	40		2.1	7.4				3	.05				13			
2.8 oz	79	0.0					450	.06	0.9				22	.71		I
Beech-Nut Stage 2	65		2.9	12.5				4	.08				22			
4.5 oz	128	0.0					717	.09	1.5					1.15		I
creamed, inst dry, Heinz	60		3.0	8.0				0	.05	.06		2	12		.46	
5 T	14	2.0					142	.08	0.5			91	49	.60	.070	I
creamed, str	68	110.7	2.8	11.4		2.4	12	2	.07	.06	29	18	17	20	.50	
1 jar	128	2.4	0.5	0.6	1.2	5	110	.11	1.0	.10	.39	113	40	.72	.065	803
Gerber 1st Foods	34		2.1	5.5	1.8	2.1		0	.04	.04		4	15	13	.30	.170
2.5 oz	71	0.3					272	.05	0.6			67	41	.70	.050	I
Gerber 2nd Foods	54		3.4	9.0	4.1	3.2		4	.06	.07		6	23	21	.50	.240
4 oz	113	0.5					404	.09	1.2			114	65	1.10	.080	I
Gerber Graduates	45		2.7	7.2	1.5	3.0		5	.05	.03		32	17	15	.50	.280
2.5 oz	71	0.5					298	.07	0.7			59	47	.80	.080	I
str	51	112.0	4.5	10.4		2.7	72	9	.08	.09	33	5	26	19	.45	
1 jar	128	0.4	0.1	0.0	0.2	0	723	.10	1.3	.00	.36	143	55	1.23	.082	803
w/ rice, Gerber 3rd Foods	92		4.2	17.2	2.5	3.5		5	.11	.07		162	27	29	.70	.390
6 oz	170	0.8					339	.11	1.5			155	85	1.50	.100	I
potatoes, diced, Gerber Graduates	36		0.7	8.3	0.2	0.7		5	.01	.05		29	4	7	.10	.040
2.5 oz	71	0.0	0.0	0.0	0.0			.01	0.3			75	17	.02	.050	I
potatoes, Gerber 1st Foods	32		0.7	7.1	0.2	0.7		0	.01	.04		5	5	6	.10	.030
2.5 oz	71	0.1						.01	0.4			53	17	.20	.020	I
spinach, creamed, Gerber 2nd Foods	54		3.5	8.4	2.3	1.8		9	.14	.09		32	105	44	.70	.720
4 oz	113	0.7	0.2			1	4506	.04	0.3			237	75	.80	.060	I
spinach, creamed, str	47	114.7	3.2	7.3		2.3	534	11	.13	.10	78	63	114	70	.40	
1 jar	128	1.7	0.9	0.4	0.2	6	5338	.02	0.3	.08		244	69	.79	.077	803
squash																
Beech-Nut Stage 1	29		0.8	6.2				2	.02				13			
2.8 oz	79	0.0					2267	.03	0.5					.24		I
Beech-Nut Stage 2	47		1.5	10.4				2	.06				24			
4.5 oz	128	0.0					3699	.05	0.8					.38		I
Gerber 1st Foods	24		0.6	4.9	2.8	1.1		2	.03	.05		2	18	9	.10	.040
2.5 oz	71	0.2					692	.02	0.4			140	16	.10	.030	I
Gerber 2nd Foods	37		0.9	7.6	3.8	1.7		4	.05	.08		2	28	14	.10	.080
4 oz	113	0.2					1661	.01	0.5			197	23	.20	.030	I
Gerber 3rd Foods	66		1.1	14.5	10.4	2.8		6	.11	.14		83	40	20	.20	.050
6 oz	170	0.4					2218	.02	0.8			268	35	.40	.050	I
jr	51	197.7	1.7	11.9		4.5	428	17	.14	.15	33	2	51	26	.17	
1 jar	213	0.4	0.1	0.0	0.2	0	4290	.02	0.8	.00	.47	394	34	.75	.115	803
str	31	118.7	1.0	7.2		2.7	259	10	.07	.08	20	3	31	15	.18	
1 jar	128	0.3	0.1	0.0	0.1	0	2589	.01	0.5	.00	.28	229	19	.38	.069	803
sweet potatoes																
Beech-Nut Stage 1	51		0.9	11.9					.03			5	13			
2.8 oz	79	0.0					4819	.02	0.4					.32		I
Beech-Nut Stage 2	79		1.4	18.3				4	.04			6	19			
4.5 oz	128	0.0					7898	.04	0.5					.38		I
Beech-Nut Stage 3	102		1.9	23.5					.05			87	39			
6 oz	170	0.0					10234	.05	0.7							I
Gerber 1st Foods	47		0.8	10.5	6.0	1.0		0	.02	.07		9	10	10	.10	.190
2.5 oz	71	0.2					5851	.02	0.3			178	20	.20	.070	I
Gerber 2nd Foods	70		1.1	16.1	9.2	1.6		3	.06	.13		15	16	16	.20	.280
4 oz	113	0.2					7215	.03	0.5			282	30	.30	.090	I
Gerber 3rd Foods	104		1.8	23.5	13.2	2.5		3	.10	.20		20	23	24	.30	.380
6 oz	170	0.3					13407	.04	0.7			374	46	.50	.240	I

	KCAL	H₂O (g)	PRO (g)	CHO (g)	SUGR (g)	DFIB (g)	A (RE)	C (mg)	B-2 (mg)	B-6 (mg)	FOL (mcg)	Na (mg)	Ca (mg)	Mg (mg)	Zn (mg)	Mn (mg)
	WT (g)	FAT (g)	SFA (g)	MUFA (g)	PUFA (g)	CHOL (mg)	A (IU)	B-1 (mg)	NIA (mg)	B-12 (mcg)	PANT (mg)	K (mg)	P (mg)	Fe (mg)	Cu (mg)	RFF
inst dry, Heinz	50		1.0	11.0				1	.01	.05		15	21		.16	
4 T	14	0.0					6940	.03	0.2			246	24	.30	.100	I
jr	102	143.0	1.9	23.6		2.5	1129	16	.06	.19	18	37	27	20	.19	
1 jar	170	0.2	0.0	0.0	0.1	0	11281	.04	0.7	.00	.69	413	41	.66	.170	803
str	64	95.8	1.2	14.9		1.7	728	11	.04	.11	11	23	18	15	.23	
1 jar	113	0.1	0.0	0.0	0.0	0	7275	.03	0.4	.00	.44	297	27	.42	.092	803

20. MEAT ANALOGUE PRODUCTS

	KCAL	H₂O (g)	PRO (g)	CHO (g)	SUGR (g)	DFIB (g)	A (RE)	C (mg)	B-2 (mg)	B-6 (mg)	FOL (mcg)	Na (mg)	Ca (mg)	Mg (mg)	Zn (mg)	Mn (mg)
	WT (g)	FAT (g)	SFA (g)	MUFA (g)	PUFA (g)	CHOL (mg)	A (IU)	B-1 (mg)	NIA (mg)	B-12 (mcg)	PANT (mg)	K (mg)	P (mg)	Fe (mg)	Cu (mg)	RFF
bacon, simulated meat product	25	3.9	0.9	0.5		0.2	1	0	.04	.04	3	117	2	2	.03	.016
1 strip	8	2.4	0.4	0.6	1.2	0	7	.35	0.6	.00	.01	14	6	.19	.008	816
Bacos, General Mills	30		3.0	2.0	0.0	0.0	0	0	.00			90	0			
1.5 T	7	1.0	0.0			0	0	.00	0.0			100		.20		I
Better 'n Burger, Morningstar Farms	75	55.6	11.3	6.4	0.4	3.9	0	0	.06			351	79		.69	
1 patty	78	0.5				0	0	.00	0.0			398	166	2.66		I
Big Franks, cnd, Loma Linda	100	30.3	10.2	2.3	0.1	2.2	0	0	.46	.14		243	8		.89	
1 frank	51	6.7	1.1	1.8	3.8	2	0	.26	2.0	.14	1.36	51	74	.77		I
Breakfast Links, Morningstar Farms	63	26.8	8.4	1.9	0.4	1.9	0	0	.22	.33		338	15		.36	
2 links	45	2.4	0.5	0.7	1.3	1	0	6.95	5.2	3.41		59	52	2.14		I
Breakfast Patties, Morningstar Farms	68	20.4	8.3	2.5	0.3	2.0	0	0	.13	.19		264	15		.37	
1 patty	38	2.8	0.5	0.7	1.3	1	0	5.38	1.8	1.49		102	107	1.67		I
Chicken Nuggets, frzn, Loma Linda	245	39.7	12.1	13.3	0.8	4.5	0	0	.30	.45		709	40		.43	
5 pieces	85	15.9	2.5	4.0	8.8	2	0	.67	2.9	4.50	1.62	153	172	1.39		I
Chicken Supreme dry mix, Loma Linda	89	1.5	14.8	5.6	0.3	4.0	0	0	.42	.30		723	28		.48	
⅓ cup	26	0.8	0.3	0.3	0.2	1	0	.55	2.5	1.75	1.57	448	154	1.42		I
Chik Patties, Morningstar Farms	177	36.3	7.3	14.9	1.6	2.5	0	0	.16	.14		536	11		.31	
1 patty	71	9.8	1.3	2.6	5.9	2	0	2.15	1.5	.95		163	106	1.02		I
Chikstiks, Worthington	111	26.7	8.7	2.5	0.5	2.0	0	0	.03	.34		355	10		.31	
1 piece	47	7.3	1.2	2.4	3.6	1	0	.32	2.5	2.06		59	89	.84		I
Choplets, Worthington	94	66.0	16.7	3.1	0.4	2.4	0	0	.06	.06		500	6		.65	
2 slices	92	1.6	0.9	0.3	0.3	0	0	.05	0.0	.00		40	75	.37		I
Corn Dogs, frzn, Loma Linda	204	30.8	10.4	19.2	1.2	2.9	0	0	.61	.87		237	12		.43	
1 corn dog	71	9.6	1.6	2.9	5.0	2	0	.72	1.5	2.19	4.98	39	139	.85		I
Dinner Cuts, cnd, Loma Linda	78	48.1	12.4	3.5	0.4	3.1	0	0	.11	.03		352	7		.72	
2 cuts	66	1.6	0.4	0.5	0.7	0	0	.05	0.0	.00	.05	19	75	.72		I
Dinner Loaf, dry mix, Loma Linda	94	1.6	13.7	7.0	0.2	4.6	0	0	.05	.39		561	23		.38	
⅓ cup	26	1.3	0.3	0.0	0.6	1	0	.45	2.3	2.33	1.87	414	137	1.31		I
Frichik, Worthington	116	68.0	9.9	1.1	0.2	1.1	0	0	.14	.15		429	15		.38	
2 pieces	90	8.0	1.2	2.1	4.8	2	0	.08	0.6	2.16		145	98	.96		I
Fried Chick'n w/ gravy, cnd, Loma Linda	386	84.5	21.1	5.8	1.0	3.1	0	0	.69	.35		814	15		.62	
2 pieces	147	30.9	4.4	8.1	17.7	6	0	1.49	3.1	2.93	1.91	62	141	.89		I
Fripats, Worthington	132	36.4	14.5	4.2	0.3	3.5	0	0	.15	.65		323	63		.61	
1 piece	64	6.3	1.0	1.6	3.8	2	0	2.70	3.4	1.08		126	119	.95		I
Garden Vege Patties, Morningstar Farms	111	40.1	11.2	8.9	1.0	4.0		0	.10	.00		382	34		.59	
1 patty	67	2.6	0.5	0.6	1.4	1	201	6.47	0.0	.00		180	124	.72		I
Grillers, Morningstar Farms	140	35.4	14.3	5.0	0.6	3.2	0	0	.24	.37		256	43		.49	
1 patty	64	6.9	1.7	2.3	3.0	1	0	11.70	3.0	4.85		127	111	1.16		I
Ground Meatless, frzn, Morningstar Farms—½ cup	60	39.4	10.3	3.6	0.2	2.1	0	0				261	21		.68	
	55	0.5					0					105	108	1.76		I
Leanies, Worthington	106	21.6	7.3	1.7	0.6	1.4	0	0	.12	.18		425	25		.23	
1 link	40	7.8	1.3	2.9	3.5	1	0	.20	1.0	.84		43	94	.90		I
Lentil Rice Loaf, Natural Touch	166	57.2	7.7	14.5	0.8	3.9		0	.12			367	21		1.04	
1" slice	90	8.6	2.6	1.7	4.3	1	775	.05	0.0			161	202	1.16		I
Linketts, cnd, Loma Linda	72	21.0	6.9	1.1	0.2	0.9	0	0	.22	.29		160	4		.46	
1 link	35	4.5	0.7	1.2	2.5	1	0	.13	0.6	1.04	.58	29	41	.39		I
Little Links, cnd, Loma Linda	93	28.7	8.2	2.5	0.3	1.5	0	0	.43	.46		225	6		.56	
2 links	46	5.6	0.8	1.5	3.2	1	0	.34	1.3	1.71	1.00	16	56	.46		I
meat extender, simulated meat product	89	2.1	10.8	10.9		5.0	1	0	.25	.38	56	3	58	61	.63	.077
1 oz	28	0.8	0.1	0.2	0.5	0	9	.20	6.2	1.70	.42	539	181	3.40	.086	816

	KCAL / WT (g)	H₂O (g) / FAT (g)	PRO (g) / SFA (g)	CHO (g) / MUFA (g)	SUGR (g) / PUFA (g)	DFIB (g) / CHOL (mg)	A (RE) / A (IU)	C (mg) / B-1 (mg)	B-2 (mg) / NIA (mg)	B-6 (mg) / B-12 (mcg)	FOL (mcg) / PANT (mg)	Na (mg) / K (mg)	Ca (mg) / P (mg)	Mg (mg) / Fe (mg)	Zn (mg) / Cu (mg)	Mn (mg) / REF
Nine Bean Loaf, Natural Touch	147	55.2	7.7	13.2	0.9	5.6		1	.11			319	27		.88	
1" slice	85	7.0	1.2	2.4	3.4	2	1509	.06	0.0			187	180	.64		I
Nuteena, cnd, Loma Linda	163	32.1	5.5	5.8	0.5	1.5	0	0	.35	.45		119	9		.46	
⅜" slice	55	13.0	5.2	5.8	1.7	0	0	.10	1.0	2.09	1.69	166	95	.27		I
Ocean Platter, dry mix, Loma Linda	94	1.4	13.6	7.6	0.3	4.5	0	0	.44	.39		450	4		.47	
⅓ cup	26	1.1	0.3	0.3	0.5	1	0	1.76	0.9	1.61	1.44	448	149	1.33		I
Okara Pattie, Natural Touch	105	34.3	10.5	3.5	0.4	3.1	0	0	.15	.03		364	33		.50	
1 patty	64	5.5	1.0	1.2	3.2	1	0	.04	0.0	.00		175	92	.93		I
Patty Mix, dry, Loma Linda	90	1.5	13.9	6.5	0.4	4.9	0	0	.38	.31		477	22		.12	
⅓ cup	26	1.0	0.2	0.3	0.5	1	0	.43	2.5	1.55	1.65	405	160	1.38		I
Prime Patties, frzn, Morningstar Farms	115	50.2	19.5	4.7	1.0	3.3	0	2	.30	.50		301	56		.90	
1 patty	78	2.0	0.3	0.4	0.8	1	0	.62	1.1	4.42		173	153	2.61		I
Redi-Burger, cnd, Loma Linda	172	50.5	16.4	4.8	0.9	3.9	0	0	.30	.51		455	12		1.11	
⅝" slice	85	9.7	1.5	2.4	5.8	1	0	.14	1.9	1.51	1.58	121	140	1.06		I
Sandwich Spread, cnd, Loma Linda	85	37.9	3.9	7.2	0.5	3.1		0	.32	.46		255	20		.41	
¼ cup	55	4.5	0.9	2.1	1.4	0	104	.28	1.8	3.61	1.08	139	73	1.30		I
sausage, simulated meat product	64	12.6	4.6	2.5		0.7	16	0	.10	.21	7	222	16	9	.36	.181
1 link	25	4.5	0.7	1.1	2.3	0	160	.59	2.8	.00	.08	58	56	.93	.063	816
	97	19.2	7.0	3.7		1.1	24	0	.15	.31	10	337	24	14	.55	.275
1 patty	38	6.9	1.1	1.7	3.5	0	243	.89	4.3	.00	.12	88	86	1.41	.095	816
Spicy Black Bean Burger, Morningstar Farms—1 patty	113	47.1	11.1	15.2	1.4	4.8		0	.14	.21		499	56		.93	
	78	0.9	0.2	0.3	0.4	1	139	8.06	0.0	.07		269	150	1.84		I
Stakelets, Worthington	144	41.5	12.3	5.7	0.2	1.7	0	0	.12	.26		484	49		.50	
1 piece	71	8.0	1.4	2.7	3.9	2	0	1.51	3.1	1.58		95	148	.99		I
Stripples, Worthington	56	6.8	1.8	2.1	0.1	0.5	0	0	.04	.07		220	7		.05	
2 strips	16	4.4	0.7	1.1	2.6	0	0	.75	0.6	.39		15	48	.27		I
Strips, Morningstar Farms	56	6.8	1.8	2.1	0.1	0.5	0	0	.04	.07		220	7		.05	
2 strips	16	4.4	0.7	1.1	2.6	0	0	.75	0.6	.39		15	48	.27		I
Swiss Stake w/ gravy, cnd, Loma Linda	120	65.7	9.0	8.4	0.6	4.1	0	0	.65	1.00		433	24		.41	
1 piece	92	5.6	0.8	1.5	3.3	2	0	1.25	5.4	5.30	4.70	226	134	.31		I
Tender Bits, cnd, Loma Linda	111	58.7	10.8	6.8	0.4	3.1	0	0	.40	.12		436	10		.34	
6 pieces	85	4.5	0.7	1.1	2.6	0	0	.33	1.4	.11	1.55	55	89	.73		I
Tender Rounds w/ gravy, cnd, Loma Linda—6 rounds	118	53.9	13.8	4.6	0.7	3.1	0	0	.10	.14		326	15		.66	
	80	5.0	0.9	1.4	2.7	1	0	1.13	0.4	.80	.44	73	78	.58		I
Veg-Skallops, Worthington	86	62.6	15.2	3.2	0.2	2.5	0	0	.03	.01		412	5		.67	
½ cup	85	1.4	0.5	0.5	0.3	0	0	.03	0.0	.00		10	60	.56		I
Vegan Burger, Natural Touch	75	55.6	11.3	6.4	0.5	3.9						351	79		.69	
1 patty	78	0.5				0						398	166	2.70		I
Vege-Burger, cnd, Loma Linda	66	39.1	10.5	2.4	0.5	2.0	0	0	.25	.31		114	8		.58	
¼ cup	55	1.6	0.4	0.6	0.5	0	0	.20	0.8	.87	.95	30	58	.50		I
Vegetarian Burger, Worthington	61	39.2	8.7	2.2	0.2	1.1	0	0	.10	.24		269	4		.39	
¼ cup	55	1.9	0.3	0.5	1.1	0	0	.13	2.0	1.24		25	56	1.73		I
Veja-Links, Worthington	49	21.5	4.6	1.0	0.2	0.4	0	0	.11	.15		192	4		.10	
1 link	31	3.0	0.6	1.5	1.0	1	0	.12	1.5	.48		18	22	.73		I
Vita-Burger granules, dry, Loma Linda	75	1.2	9.9	6.3	1.4	3.7	0	0	.17	.12		353	27		4.79	
3 T	21	1.1	0.3	0.2	0.6	0	0	1.23	3.1	.36	.36	499	155	1.83		I

	KCAL	H₂O (g)	PRO (g)	CHO (g)	SUGR (g)	DFIB (g)	A (RE)	C (mg)	B-2 (mg)	B-6 (mg)	FOL (mcg)	Na (mg)	Ca (mg)	Mg (mg)	Zn (mg)	Mn (mg)
	WT (g)	FAT (g)	SFA (g)	MUFA (g)	PUFA (g)	CHOL (mg)	A (IU)	B-1 (mg)	NIA (mg)	B-12 (mcg)	PANT (mg)	K (mg)	P (mg)	Fe (mg)	Cu (mg)	REF

21. MEATS
21.1 BEEF

	KCAL	H₂O	PRO	CHO	SUGR	DFIB	A	C	B-2	B-6	FOL	Na	Ca	Mg	Zn	Mn
breakfast strips, ckd	153	8.9	10.6	0.5		0.0	0	0	.09	.11	3	766	3	9	2.17	.006
3 slices	34	11.7	4.9	5.7	0.5	40	0	.03	2.2	1.17	.12	140	80	1.07	.039	813
brisket, flat half																
sep lean & fat, braised, 0" fat trim	215	57.7	30.5	0.0	0.0	0.0	0	0	.21	.30	8	62	5	24	6.11	.016
3.5 oz	100	9.4	3.4	4.2	0.4	95	0	.07	3.7	2.58	.36	289	248	2.75	.120	813
sep lean & fat, braised, ¼" fat trim	364	46.4	25.1	0.0	0.0	0.0	0	0	.18	.26	6	56	8	19	4.82	.014
3.5 oz	100	28.5	11.0	12.4	1.1	95	0	.06	3.1	2.32	.30	243	201	2.29	.100	813
sep lean, braised, 0" fat trim	191	59.8	31.5	0.0	0.0	0.0	0	0	.22	.31	8	63	5	25	6.36	.017
3.5 oz	100	6.2	2.0	2.8	0.2	95	0	.07	3.9	2.63	.37	298	257	2.84	.124	813
sep lean, braised, ¼" fat trim	222	58.9	31.5	0.0	0.0	0.0	0	0	.22	.31	8	63	5	25	6.36	.017
3.5 oz	100	9.7	3.2	4.3	0.4	95	0	.07	3.9	2.63	.37	298	257	2.84	.124	813
brisket, point half																
sep lean & fat, braised, 0" fat trim	358	46.0	23.5	0.0	0.0	0.0	0	0	.19	.24	7	68	8	18	5.83	.014
3.5 oz	100	28.5	11.2	12.7	1.0	92	0	.06	3.0	2.33	.29	233	187	2.34	.097	813
sep lean & fat, braised, ¼" fat trim	404	43.4	22.1	0.0	0.0	0.0	0	0	.18	.23	6	65	9	17	5.35	.014
3.5 oz	100	34.3	13.6	15.2	1.2	92	0	.06	2.9	2.25	.28	221	175	2.20	.091	813
sep lean, braised, 0" fat trim	244	55.7	28.1	0.0	0.0	0.0	0	0	.23	.28	8	77	6	22	7.39	.017
3.5 oz	100	13.8	5.2	6.5	0.4	91	0	.07	3.6	2.58	.34	273	226	2.79	.115	813
sep lean, braised, ¼" fat trim	261	56.2	28.1	0.0	0.0	0.0	0	0	.23	.28	8	77	6	22	7.39	.017
3.5 oz	100	15.7	5.9	7.3	0.4	91	0	.07	3.6	2.58	.34	273	226	2.79	.115	813
brisket, whole																
sep lean & fat, braised, 0" fat trim	291	51.5	26.8	0.0	0.0	0.0	0	0	.20	.27	7	65	7	21	5.96	.015
3.5 oz	100	19.5	7.5	8.7	0.7	93	0	.07	3.4	2.45	.32	259	216	2.53	.108	813
sep lean & fat, braised, ¼" fat trim	385	44.8	23.5	0.0	0.0	0.0	0	0	.18	.24	6	61	8	18	5.10	.014
3.5 oz	100	31.6	12.4	13.9	1.1	94	0	.06	3.0	2.28	.29	231	187	2.24	.095	813
sep lean, braised, 0" fat trim	218	57.7	29.8	0.0	0.0	0.0	0	0	.22	.29	8	70	6	23	6.89	.017
3.5 oz	100	10.1	3.6	4.7	0.3	93	0	.07	3.7	2.60	.36	285	241	2.81	.119	813
sep lean, braised, ¼" fat trim	242	57.5	29.8	0.0	0.0	0.0	0	0	.22	.29	8	70	6	23	6.89	.017
3.5 oz	100	12.8	4.6	5.9	0.4	93	0	.07	3.7	2.60	.36	285	241	2.81	.119	813
chuck arm pot roast, sep lean																
braised, choice, 0" fat trim	219	57.6	33.0	0.0	0.0	0.0	0	0	.29	.33	11	66	9	24	8.66	.019
3.5 oz	100	8.7	3.2	3.6	0.3	101	0	.08	3.7	3.40	.38	289	268	3.79	.164	813
braised, choice, ¼" fat trim	225	57.3	33.0	0.0	0.0	0.0	0	0	.29	.33	11	66	9	24	8.66	.019
3.5 oz	100	9.3	3.4	3.9	0.4	101	0	.08	3.7	3.40	.38	289	268	3.79	.164	813
braised, select, 0" fat trim	198	59.5	33.0	0.0	0.0	0.0	0	0	.29	.33	11	66	9	24	8.66	.019
3.5 oz	100	6.3	2.3	2.6	0.3	101	0	.08	3.7	3.40	.38	289	268	3.79	.164	813
braised, select, ¼" fat trim	206	58.4	33.0	0.0	0.0	0.0	0	0	.29	.33	11	66	9	24	8.66	.019
3.5 oz	100	7.2	2.6	3.0	0.3	101	0	.08	3.7	3.40	.38	289	268	3.79	.164	813
chuck arm pot roast, sep lean & fat																
braised, choice, 0" fat trim	293	51.4	29.4	0.0	0.0	0.0	0	0	.26	.30	10	62	10	21	7.50	.017
3.5 oz	100	18.6	7.2	7.9	0.7	100	0	.07	3.4	3.12	.35	262	237	3.35	.145	813
braised, choice, ¼" fat trim	348	46.9	27.0	0.0	0.0	0.0	0	0	.24	.28	9	59	10	19	6.70	.016
3.5 oz	100	25.8	10.2	11.1	1.0	99	0	.07	3.1	2.92	.32	243	216	3.05	.132	813
braised, select, 0" fat trim	260	54.2	30.1	0.0	0.0	0.0	0	0	.26	.31	10	63	10	22	7.72	.017
3.5 oz	100	14.6	5.7	6.3	0.6	100	0	.07	3.4	3.17	.35	267	243	3.44	.149	813
braised, select, ¼" fat trim	315	49.2	27.9	0.0	0.0	0.0	0	0	.24	.29	9	60	10	20	6.99	.016
3.5 oz	100	21.7	8.6	9.3	0.8	100	0	.07	3.2	2.99	.33	250	224	3.16	.137	813

	KCAL	H₂O (g)	PRO (g)	CHO (g)	SUGR (g)	DFIB (g)	A (RE)	C (mg)	B-2 (mg)	B-6 (mg)	FOL (mcg)	Na (mg)	Ca (mg)	Mg (mg)	Zn (mg)	Mn (mg)
	WT (g)	FAT (g)	SFA (g)	MUFA (g)	PUFA (g)	CHOL (mg)	A (IU)	B-1 (mg)	NIA (mg)	B-12 (mcg)	PANT (mg)	K (mg)	P (mg)	Fe (mg)	Cu (mg)	REF
chuck blade roast, sep lean																
braised, choice, 0″ fat trim	265	54.0	31.1	0.0	0.0	0.0	0	0	.28	.29	6	71	13	23	10.27	.018
3.5 oz	100	14.7	5.7	6.3	0.5	106	0	.08	2.7	2.47	.35	263	235	3.68	.148	813
braised, choice, ¼″ fat trim	263	54.6	31.1	0.0	0.0	0.0	0	0	.28	.29	6	71	13	23	10.27	.018
3.5 oz	100	14.4	5.6	6.2	0.5	106	0	.08	2.7	2.47	.35	263	235	3.68	.148	813
braised, select, 0″ fat trim	238	55.7	31.1	0.0	0.0	0.0	0	0	.28	.29	6	71	13	23	10.27	.018
3.5 oz	100	11.7	4.5	5.0	0.4	106	0	.08	2.7	2.47	.35	263	235	3.68	.148	813
braised, select, ¼″ fat trim	237	56.3	31.1	0.0	0.0	0.0	0	0	.28	.29	6	71	13	23	10.27	.018
3.5 oz	100	11.6	4.5	5.0	0.4	106	0	.08	2.7	2.47	.35	263	235	3.68	.148	813
chuck blade roast, sep lean & fat																
braised, choice, 0″ fat trim	348	46.9	27.0	0.0	0.0	0.0	0	0	.25	.26	5	65	13	20	8.50	.016
3.5 oz	100	25.8	10.3	11.2	0.9	104	0	.07	2.4	2.30	.31	234	203	3.16	.127	813
braised, choice, ¼″ fat trim	363	46.0	26.2	0.0	0.0	0.0	0	0	.24	.25	5	64	13	19	8.14	.015
3.5 oz	100	27.8	11.1	12.0	1.0	103	0	.07	2.4	2.27	.30	228	197	3.05	.123	813
braised, select, 0″ fat trim	313	49.4	27.6	0.0	0.0	0.0	0	0	.25	.26	5	66	13	20	8.76	.016
3.5 oz	100	21.7	8.6	9.4	0.8	104	0	.07	2.5	2.33	.32	239	208	3.23	.130	813
braised, select, ¼″ fat trim	326	48.8	27.0	0.0	0.0	0.0	0	0	.25	.26	5	65	13	20	8.50	.016
3.5 oz	100	23.4	9.3	10.1	0.8	104	0	.07	2.4	2.30	.31	234	203	3.16	.127	813
corned beef, cnd, Libby's	120		15.0	0.0	0.0	0.0	0	0				490	0			
2 oz	56	7.0	3.0			50	0							1.40		I
corned beef, cured brisket, ckd	251	59.8	18.2	0.5		0.0	0	0	.17	.23	6	1134	8	12	4.58	.022
3.5 oz	100	19.0	6.3	9.2	0.7	98	0	.03	3.0	1.63	.42	145	125	1.86	.154	813
flank, choice																
sep lean & fat, braised, 0″ fat trim	263	55.0	27.0	0.0	0.0	0.0	0	0	.18	.35	9	70	6	23	5.77	.018
3.5 oz	100	16.4	6.9	6.9	0.5	72	0	.14	4.4	3.30	.37	337	256	3.33	.119	813
sep lean & fat, broiled, 0″ fat trim	226	59.6	26.4	0.0	0.0	0.0	0	0	.18	.34	8	81	7	23	4.66	.016
3.5 oz	100	12.5	5.3	5.1	0.5	68	0	.10	4.9	3.19	.35	402	230	2.51	.097	813
sep lean, braised, 0″ fat trim	237	57.3	28.0	0.0	0.0	0.0	0	0	.19	.36	9	72	6	24	6.05	.019
3.5 oz	100	13.0	5.5	5.4	0.4	71	0	.14	4.6	3.41	.38	351	267	3.47	.124	813
sep lean, broiled, 0″ fat trim	207	61.3	27.1	0.0	0.0	0.0	0	0	.19	.34	8	83	7	24	4.80	.016
3.5 oz	100	10.1	4.4	4.1	0.4	67	0	.11	5.0	3.25	.36	414	236	2.57	.099	813
ground, extra lean																
baked, med	250	58.6	24.5	0.0	0.0	0.0	0	0	.24	.22	9	49	7	17	5.34	.015
3.5 oz	100	16.1	6.3	7.1	0.6	82	0	.04	4.2	1.73	.27	224	124	2.28	.075	813
baked, well done	274	52.7	30.3	0.0	0.0	0.0	0	0	.31	.29	11	64	9	22	6.94	.020
3.5 oz	100	16.0	6.3	7.0	0.6	107	0	.05	5.4	1.86	.35	291	162	2.96	.097	813
broiled, med	256	57.3	25.4	0.0	0.0	0.0	0	0	.27	.27	9	70	7	21	5.45	.016
3.5 oz	100	16.3	6.4	7.2	0.6	84	0	.06	5.0	2.17	.35	313	161	2.35	.070	813
broiled, well done	265	53.9	28.6	0.0	0.0	0.0	0	0	.32	.32	11	82	9	25	6.43	.019
3.5 oz	100	15.8	6.2	6.9	0.6	99	0	.07	5.8	2.56	.42	369	190	2.77	.083	813
pan fried, med	255	57.6	25.0	0.0	0.0	0.0	0	0	.26	.27	9	70	7	21	5.42	.016
3.5 oz	100	16.4	6.5	7.2	0.6	81	0	.06	4.7	2.00	.25	312	160	2.36	.087	813
pan fried, well done	263	53.9	28.0	0.0	0.0	0.0	0	0	.30	.31	10	81	8	24	6.27	.018
3.5 oz	100	15.9	6.3	7.0	0.6	93	0	.07	5.4	2.32	.29	360	185	2.73	.101	813
ground, lean																
baked, med	268	56.9	23.9	0.0	0.0	0.0	0	0	.19	.20	9	56	9	17	5.10	.014
3.5 oz	100	18.3	7.2	8.0	0.7	78	0	.05	4.3	1.77	.27	224	128	2.09	.072	813
baked, well done	292	51.3	29.6	0.0	0.0	0.0	0	0	.24	.26	12	71	12	21	6.51	.018
3.5 oz	100	18.4	7.2	8.0	0.7	99	0	.07	5.5	2.26	.34	286	164	2.66	.092	813
broiled, med	272	55.7	24.7	0.0	0.0	0.0	0	0	.21	.26	9	77	11	21	5.36	.014
3.5 oz	100	18.5	7.3	8.1	0.7	87	0	.05	5.2	2.35	.38	301	158	2.11	.066	813
broiled, well done	280	52.9	28.2	0.0	0.0	0.0	0	0	.24	.30	11	89	12	24	6.20	.017
3.5 oz	100	17.6	6.9	7.7	0.7	101	0	.06	6.0	2.72	.44	349	182	2.45	.077	813
pan fried, med	275	55.6	24.2	0.0	0.0	0.0	0	0	.22	.28	9	77	10	20	5.20	.014
3.5 oz	100	19.1	7.5	8.3	0.7	84	0	.05	4.8	2.27	.32	299	159	2.18	.077	813
pan fried, well done	277	53.7	27.6	0.0	0.0	0.0	0	0	.24	.32	10	87	11	23	5.91	.016
3.5 oz	100	17.7	6.9	7.7	0.7	95	0	.06	5.5	2.58	.36	340	181	2.48	.088	813

	KCAL	H₂O (g)	PRO (g)	CHO (g)	SUGR (g)	DFIB (g)	A (RE)	C (mg)	B-2 (mg)	B-6 (mg)	FOL (mcg)	Na (mg)	Ca (mg)	Mg (mg)	Zn (mg)	Mn (mg)
	WT (g)	FAT (g)	SFA (g)	MUFA (g)	PUFA (g)	CHOL (mg)	A (IU)	B-1 (mg)	NIA (mg)	B-12 (mcg)	PANT (mg)	K (mg)	P (mg)	Fe (mg)	Cu (mg)	REF
ground, regular																
baked, med	287	55.1	23.0	0.0	0.0	0.0	0	0	.16	.23	9	60	10	15	4.89	.017
3.5 oz	100	20.9	8.2	9.2	0.8	87	0	.03	4.8	2.34	.22	221	137	2.41	.070	813
baked, well done	317	48.9	28.8	0.0	0.0	0.0	0	0	.20	.29	11	75	12	19	6.07	.021
3.5 oz	100	21.5	8.4	9.4	0.8	108	0	.04	5.9	2.90	.27	274	170	2.99	.086	813
broiled, med	289	54.2	24.1	0.0	0.0	0.0	0	0	.19	.27	9	83	11	20	5.18	.017
3.5 oz	100	20.7	8.1	9.1	0.8	90	0	.03	5.8	2.93	.33	292	170	2.44	.082	813
broiled, well done	292	52.0	27.2	0.0	0.0	0.0	0	0	.21	.30	10	93	12	22	5.81	.020
3.5 oz	100	19.5	7.7	8.5	0.7	101	0	.04	6.5	3.28	.37	327	191	2.74	.092	813
pan fried, med	306	52.3	23.9	0.0	0.0	0.0	0	0	.20	.24	9	84	11	20	5.07	.017
3.5 oz	100	22.6	8.9	9.9	0.8	89	0	.03	5.8	2.71	.34	300	171	2.45	.081	813
pan-fried, well done	286	52.7	27.0	0.0	0.0	0.0	0	0	.21	.27	10	93	13	22	5.62	.019
3.5 oz	100	18.9	7.4	8.3	0.7	98	0	.04	6.5	3.00	.38	332	189	2.71	.090	813
rib eye, small end (ribs 10-12), choice, broiled,	307	51.5	24.9	0.0	0.0	0.0	0	0	.19	.35	7	64	13	23	5.98	.014
sep lean & fat, 0" fat trim—*3.5 oz*	100	22.3	9.0	9.5	0.8	83	0	.09	4.2	3.01	.31	344	184	2.30	.090	813
rib eye, small end (ribs 10-12), choice,	225	58.7	28.0	0.0	0.0	0.0	0	0	.22	.40	8	69	13	27	6.99	.016
broiled, sep lean, 0" fat trim—*3.5 oz*	100	11.7	4.7	4.9	0.3	80	0	.10	4.8	3.32	.34	394	208	2.57	.100	813
rib, large end (ribs 6-9), sep lean																
choice, broiled, ¼" fat trim	240	57.5	25.2	0.0	0.0	0.0	0	0	.19	.26	7	72	9	23	6.28	.015
3.5 oz	100	14.7	6.0	5.9	0.6	76	0	.08	3.2	3.31	.41	372	217	2.57	.090	813
choice, roasted, 0" fat trim	253	56.8	27.5	0.0	0.0	0.0	0	0	.22	.26	9	73	8	25	7.46	.016
3.5 oz	100	15.0	6.0	6.3	0.4	81	0	.09	4.5	2.61	.45	357	209	2.82	.105	813
choice, roasted, ¼" fat trim	250	57.5	27.5	0.0	0.0	0.0	0	0	.22	.26	9	73	8	25	7.46	.016
3.5 oz	100	14.7	5.9	6.2	0.4	81	0	.09	4.5	2.61	.45	357	209	2.82	.105	813
prime, broiled, ¼" fat trim	294	53.4	24.6	0.0	0.0	0.0	0	0	.20	.32	7	70	8	24	6.25	.016
3.5 oz	100	20.9	8.9	9.3	0.6	82	0	.09	3.1	3.26	.41	369	199	2.48	.089	813
prime, roasted, ¼" fat trim	283	54.4	27.5	0.0	0.0	0.0	0	0	.22	.26	9	73	8	25	7.46	.016
3.5 oz	100	18.3	7.9	8.1	0.6	81	0	.09	4.5	2.61	.45	357	209	2.82	.105	813
select, broiled, ¼" fat trim	206	60.8	25.2	0.0	0.0	0.0	0	0	.19	.26	7	72	9	23	6.28	.015
3.5 oz	100	10.9	4.4	4.4	0.4	76	0	.08	3.2	3.31	.41	372	217	2.57	.090	813
select, roasted, ¼" fat trim	220	59.4	27.5	0.0	0.0	0.0	0	0	.22	.26	9	73	8	25	7.46	.016
3.5 oz	100	11.4	4.5	4.8	0.3	81	0	.09	4.5	2.61	.45	357	209	2.82	.105	813
rib, large end (ribs 6-9), sep lean & fat																
choice, broiled, ¼" fat trim	367	46.2	21.0	0.0	0.0	0.0	0	0	.16	.23	6	63	10	18	4.87	.013
3.5 oz	100	30.8	12.5	13.0	1.2	81	0	.07	2.7	2.82	.34	298	176	2.13	.077	813
choice, roasted, 0" fat trim	372	46.1	22.8	0.0	0.0	0.0	0	0	.19	.23	7	64	10	20	5.76	.013
3.5 oz	100	30.5	12.3	13.0	1.1	85	0	.07	3.6	2.33	.37	290	172	2.33	.088	813
choice, roasted, ¼" fat trim	383	45.4	22.3	0.0	0.0	0.0	0	0	.18	.22	7	63	10	19	5.58	.013
3.5 oz	100	31.9	12.9	13.7	1.1	85	0	.07	3.5	2.30	.36	283	168	2.27	.086	813
prime, broiled, ¼" fat trim	413	42.6	20.3	0.0	0.0	0.0	0	0	.17	.26	6	61	10	18	4.75	.013
3.5 oz	100	36.2	15.0	15.8	1.3	86	0	.07	2.6	2.75	.33	291	161	2.04	.075	813
prime, roasted, ¼" fat trim	402	43.7	22.5	0.0	0.0	0.0	0	0	.18	.22	7	63	10	19	5.64	.013
3.5 oz	100	33.9	14.1	14.8	1.2	85	0	.07	3.6	2.31	.36	286	169	2.29	.087	813
select, broiled, ¼" fat trim	324	50.2	21.5	0.0	0.0	0.0	0	0	.16	.23	6	64	10	19	5.06	.013
3.5 oz	100	25.8	10.5	10.9	1.0	80	0	.07	2.8	2.89	.35	308	182	2.19	.079	813
select, roasted, ¼" fat trim	340	48.8	23.1	0.0	0.0	0.0	0	0	.19	.23	7	65	10	20	5.88	.014
3.5 oz	100	26.7	10.8	11.4	0.9	85	0	.07	3.7	2.35	.37	295	174	2.36	.089	813
rib, shortribs, sep lean & fat, braised	471	35.7	21.6	0.0	0.0	0.0	0	0	.15	.22	5	50	12	15	4.88	.013
3.5 oz	100	42.0	17.8	18.9	1.5	94	0	.05	2.5	2.62	.25	224	162	2.31	.099	813
rib, shortribs, sep lean, braised	295	50.1	30.8	0.0	0.0	0.0	0	0	.20	.28	7	58	11	22	7.80	.018
3.5 oz	100	18.1	7.7	8.0	0.6	93	0	.07	3.2	3.46	.34	313	235	3.36	.107	813
rib, small end (ribs 10-12), sep lean																
choice, broiled, 0" fat trim	225	58.7	28.0	0.0	0.0	0.0	0	0	.22	.40	8	69	13	27	6.99	.016
3.5 oz	100	11.7	4.7	4.9	0.3	80	0	.10	4.8	3.32	.34	394	208	2.57	.100	813
choice, broiled, ¼" fat trim	233	57.3	28.0	0.0	0.0	0.0	0	0	.22	.40	8	69	13	27	6.99	.016
3.5 oz	100	12.6	5.1	5.3	0.4	80	0	.10	4.8	3.32	.34	394	208	2.57	.100	813
choice, roasted, ¼" fat trim	232	58.4	26.8	0.0	0.0	0.0	0	0	.19	.28	8	71	12	25	6.21	.016
3.5 oz	100	13.1	5.2	5.6	0.4	79	0	.07	3.7	3.33	.27	398	222	2.91	.089	813

	KCAL	H₂O (g)	PRO (g)	CHO (g)	SUGR (g)	DFIB (g)	A (RE)	C (mg)	B-2 (mg)	B-6 (mg)	FOL (mcg)	Na (mg)	Ca (mg)	Mg (mg)	Zn (mg)	Mn (mg)
	WT (g)	FAT (g)	SFA (g)	MUFA (g)	PUFA (g)	CHOL (mg)	A (IU)	B-1 (mg)	NIA (mg)	B-12 (mcg)	PANT (mg)	K (mg)	P (mg)	Fe (mg)	Cu (mg)	REF
prime, broiled, ¼″ fat trim	260	55.7	28.0	0.0	0.0	0.0	0	0	.22	.40	8	69	13	27	6.99	.016
3.5 oz	100	15.5	6.6	6.8	0.5	80	0	.10	4.8	3.32	.34	394	208	2.57	.100	813
prime, roasted, ¼″ fat trim	304	51.1	26.7	0.0	0.0	0.0	0	0	.19	.37	8	75	13	25	6.19	.016
3.5 oz	100	21.1	8.9	9.2	0.6	80	0	.08	3.6	3.37	.44	404	219	2.30	.089	813
select, broiled, 0″ fat trim	198	60.3	28.0	0.0	0.0	0.0	0	0	.22	.40	8	69	13	27	6.99	.016
3.5 oz	100	8.7	3.5	3.7	0.3	80	0	.10	4.8	3.32	.34	394	208	2.57	.100	813
select, broiled, ¼″ fat trim	207	58.7	28.0	0.0	0.0	0.0	0	0	.22	.40	8	69	13	27	6.99	.016
3.5 oz	100	9.7	3.9	4.1	0.3	80	0	.10	4.8	3.32	.34	394	208	2.57	.100	813
select, roasted, ¼″ fat trim	203	61.7	26.8	0.0	0.0	0.0	0	0	.19	.28	8	71	12	25	6.21	.016
3.5 oz	100	9.8	3.8	4.2	0.3	79	0	.07	3.7	3.33	.27	398	222	2.91	.089	813
rib, small end (ribs 10-12), sep lean & fat																
choice, broiled, 0″ fat trim	312	51.1	24.7	0.0	0.0	0.0	0	0	.19	.35	7	64	13	23	5.93	.014
3.5 oz	100	22.8	9.2	9.8	0.8	83	0	.09	4.2	3.00	.30	342	183	2.28	.090	813
choice, broiled, ¼″ fat trim	349	47.2	23.5	0.0	0.0	0.0	0	0	.18	.33	7	62	13	22	5.54	.014
3.5 oz	100	27.6	11.2	11.8	1.0	84	0	.09	4.0	2.88	.29	322	174	2.18	.086	813
choice, roasted, ¼″ fat trim	367	46.5	22.0	0.0	0.0	0.0	0	0	.16	.24	6	62	13	19	4.77	.013
3.5 oz	100	30.2	12.2	13.1	1.1	84	0	.06	3.1	2.82	.23	314	178	2.35	.076	813
prime, broiled, ¼″ fat trim	361	46.8	23.9	0.0	0.0	0.0	0	0	.19	.34	7	62	13	22	5.65	.014
3.5 oz	100	28.7	11.8	12.5	1.0	84	0	.09	4.0	2.91	.29	328	176	2.21	.087	813
prime, roasted, ¼″ fat trim	417	41.3	21.9	0.0	0.0	0.0	0	0	.16	.30	6	65	13	19	4.75	.013
3.5 oz	100	35.9	14.8	15.6	1.3	84	0	.06	3.0	2.84	.35	318	176	1.93	.076	813
select, broiled, 0″ fat trim	285	52.8	24.9	0.0	0.0	0.0	0	0	.19	.35	7	64	13	23	5.98	.014
3.5 oz	100	19.8	8.0	8.5	0.7	83	0	.09	4.2	3.01	.31	344	184	2.30	.090	813
select, broiled, ¼″ fat trim	321	49.1	23.9	0.0	0.0	0.0	0	0	.19	.34	7	62	13	22	5.65	.014
3.5 oz	100	24.3	9.8	10.4	0.8	84	0	.09	4.0	2.91	.29	328	176	2.21	.087	813
select, roasted, ¼″ fat trim	331	50.1	22.5	0.0	0.0	0.0	0	0	.16	.24	6	63	13	20	4.91	.013
3.5 oz	100	26.1	10.5	11.3	0.9	83	0	.06	3.1	2.87	.24	323	183	2.41	.077	813
rib, whole (ribs 6-12), sep lean																
choice, broiled, ¼″ fat trim	237	57.4	26.3	0.0	0.0	0.0	0	0	.20	.32	7	71	11	25	6.57	.016
3.5 oz	100	13.8	5.6	5.7	0.5	77	0	.09	3.8	3.32	.38	381	213	2.57	.094	813
choice, roasted, ¼″ fat trim	243	57.9	27.3	0.0	0.0	0.0	0	0	.21	.27	8	72	10	25	6.95	.016
3.5 oz	100	14.0	5.6	5.9	0.4	80	0	.08	4.2	2.91	.38	374	214	2.86	.099	813
prime, broiled, ¼″ fat trim	280	54.4	26.0	0.0	0.0	0.0	0	0	.21	.35	7	70	10	25	6.55	.016
3.5 oz	100	18.7	8.0	8.3	0.6	81	0	.09	3.8	3.28	.38	379	203	2.52	.093	813
prime, roasted, ¼″ fat trim	292	53.0	27.2	0.0	0.0	0.0	0	0	.21	.30	9	74	10	25	6.94	.016
3.5 oz	100	19.5	8.3	8.6	0.6	81	0	.08	4.1	2.92	.44	376	213	2.61	.098	813
select, broiled, ¼″ fat trim	206	59.9	26.3	0.0	0.0	0.0	0	0	.20	.32	7	71	11	25	6.57	.016
3.5 oz	100	10.4	4.2	4.3	0.4	77	0	.09	3.8	3.32	.38	381	213	2.57	.094	813
select, roasted, ¼″ fat trim	213	60.3	27.3	0.0	0.0	0.0	0	0	.21	.27	8	72	10	25	6.95	.016
3.5 oz	100	10.7	4.3	4.5	0.3	80	0	.08	4.2	2.90	.38	374	214	2.86	.099	813
rib, whole (ribs 6-12), sep lean & fat																
choice, broiled, ¼″ fat trim	360	46.6	22.0	0.0	0.0	0.0	0	0	.17	.27	6	62	12	19	5.13	.013
3.5 oz	100	29.5	12.0	12.6	1.1	82	0	.08	3.2	2.84	.32	308	175	2.15	.080	813
prime, broiled, ¼″ fat trim	392	44.3	21.7	0.0	0.0	0.0	0	0	.17	.29	6	62	11	20	5.11	.013
3.5 oz	100	33.1	13.7	14.5	1.1	85	0	.08	3.1	2.82	.32	306	167	2.11	.080	813
prime, roasted, ¼″ fat trim	409	42.6	22.2	0.0	0.0	0.0	0	0	.17	.26	7	64	11	19	5.27	.013
3.5 oz	100	34.8	14.4	15.2	1.2	85	0	.07	3.3	2.53	.36	299	172	2.14	.082	813
select, broiled, ¼″ fat trim	323	49.7	22.5	0.0	0.0	0.0	0	0	.17	.27	6	63	11	20	5.30	.013
3.5 oz	100	25.1	10.2	10.7	0.9	82	0	.08	3.3	2.90	.33	316	179	2.20	.082	813
select, roasted, ¼″ fat trim	336	49.3	22.9	0.0	0.0	0.0	0	0	.18	.23	7	64	11	20	5.48	.014
3.5 oz	100	26.5	10.7	11.4	0.9	84	0	.07	3.5	2.57	.32	306	178	2.38	.084	813
roast beef w/ gravy, cnd, Libby's	140		26.0	2.0	0.0	0.0	0	1				800	0			
⅔ cup	152	3.0	1.5			70	0							1.40		I
round, bottom, sep lean																
choice, braised, 0″ fat trim	213	57.2	31.6	0.0	0.0	0.0	0	0	.26	.36	11	51	5	25	5.48	.018
3.5 oz	100	8.7	2.9	3.8	0.3	96	0	.07	4.1	2.47	.42	308	272	3.46	.134	813
choice, braised, ¼″ fat trim	220	56.8	31.6	0.0	0.0	0.0	0	0	.26	.36	11	51	5	25	5.48	.018
3.5 oz	100	9.4	3.2	4.1	0.4	96	0	.07	4.1	2.47	.42	308	272	3.46	.134	813

	KCAL	H₂O (g)	PRO (g)	CHO (g)	SUGR (g)	DFIB (g)		A (RE)	C (mg)	B-2 (mg)	B-6 (mg)	FOL (mcg)		Na (mg)	Ca (mg)	Mg (mg)	Zn (mg)	Mn (mg)
	WT (g)	FAT (g)	SFA (g)	MUFA (g)	PUFA (g)	CHOL (mg)		A (IU)	B-1 (mg)	NIA (mg)	B-12 (mcg)	PANT (mg)		K (mg)	P (mg)	Fe (mg)	Cu (mg)	REF
choice, roasted, 0" fat trim	193	60.7	28.8	0.0	0.0	0.0		0	0	.24	.37	12		66	5	28	4.62	.016
3.5 oz	100	7.8	2.6	3.5	0.3	78		0	.08	4.1	2.70	.35		391	239	3.13	.109	813
choice, roasted, ¼" fat trim	198	60.1	28.8	0.0	0.0	0.0		0	0	.24	.37	12		66	5	28	4.62	.016
3.5 oz	100	8.3	2.8	3.8	0.3	78		0	.08	4.1	2.70	.35		391	239	3.13	.109	813
select, braised, 0" fat trim	192	58.9	31.6	0.0	0.0	0.0		0	0	.26	.36	11		51	5	25	5.48	.018
3.5 oz	100	6.3	2.1	2.8	0.2	96		0	.07	4.1	2.47	.42		308	272	3.46	.134	813
select, braised, ¼" fat trim	196	58.6	31.6	0.0	0.0	0.0		0	0	.26	.36	11		51	5	25	5.48	.018
3.5 oz	100	6.8	2.3	3.0	0.3	96		0	.07	4.1	2.47	.42		308	272	3.46	.134	813
select, roasted, 0" fat trim	171	63.0	28.8	0.0	0.0	0.0		0	0	.24	.37	12		66	5	28	4.62	.016
3.5 oz	100	5.4	1.8	2.5	0.2	78		0	.08	4.1	2.70	.35		391	239	3.13	.109	813
select, roasted, ¼" fat trim	179	62.2	28.8	0.0	0.0	0.0		0	0	.24	.37	12		66	5	28	4.62	.016
3.5 oz	100	6.2	2.1	2.8	0.2	78		0	.08	4.1	2.70	.35		391	239	3.13	.109	813
round, bottom, sep lean & fat																		
choice, braised, 0" fat trim	227	56.0	31.0	0.0	0.0	0.0		0	0	.25	.35	11		51	5	24	5.36	.018
3.5 oz	100	10.6	3.7	4.6	0.4	96		0	.07	4.0	2.44	.41		302	266	3.39	.131	813
choice, braised, ¼" fat trim	284	51.5	28.7	0.0	0.0	0.0		0	0	.24	.33	10		50	6	22	4.91	.016
3.5 oz	100	17.9	6.7	7.8	0.7	96		0	.07	3.7	2.35	.38		282	245	3.12	.122	813
choice, roasted, 0" fat trim	203	59.8	28.4	0.0	0.0	0.0		0	0	.24	.37	12		65	5	28	4.55	.015
3.5 oz	100	9.0	3.1	4.1	0.3	78		0	.08	4.0	2.68	.35		385	236	3.09	.108	813
choice, roasted, ¼" fat trim	260	54.7	26.4	0.0	0.0	0.0		0	0	.22	.34	11		63	6	25	4.20	.015
3.5 oz	100	16.4	6.2	7.2	0.6	80		0	.08	3.8	2.56	.32		355	218	2.86	.101	813
select, braised, 0" fat trim	201	58.1	31.2	0.0	0.0	0.0		0	0	.26	.36	11		51	5	25	5.40	.018
3.5 oz	100	7.6	2.6	3.3	0.3	96		0	.07	4.0	2.45	.42		304	268	3.41	.132	813
select, braised, ¼" fat trim	259	53.4	28.9	0.0	0.0	0.0		0	0	.24	.33	10		50	6	23	4.95	.017
3.5 oz	100	15.1	5.7	6.5	0.6	96		0	.07	3.8	2.36	.39		283	247	3.15	.122	813
select, roasted, 0" fat trim	177	62.6	28.6	0.0	0.0	0.0		0	0	.24	.37	12		66	5	28	4.59	.016
3.5 oz	100	6.0	2.0	2.7	0.2	78		0	.08	4.0	2.69	.35		388	238	3.11	.109	813
select, roasted, ¼" fat trim	234	57.4	26.8	0.0	0.0	0.0		0	0	.23	.35	11		63	6	26	4.26	.015
3.5 oz	100	13.2	5.0	5.8	0.5	80		0	.08	3.8	2.58	.33		361	221	2.90	.102	813
round, eye of, sep lean																		
roasted, choice, 0" fat trim	175	64.2	29.0	0.0	0.0	0.0		0	0	.17	.38	7		62	5	27	4.74	.016
3.5 oz	100	5.7	2.1	2.4	0.2	69		0	.09	3.8	2.17	.46		395	226	1.95	.100	813
roasted, choice, ¼" fat trim	175	64.9	29.0	0.0	0.0	0.0		0	0	.17	.38	7		62	5	27	4.74	.016
3.5 oz	100	5.7	2.1	2.4	0.2	69		0	.09	3.8	2.17	.46		395	226	1.95	.100	813
roasted, select, 0" fat trim	155	65.1	29.0	0.0	0.0	0.0		0	0	.17	.38	7		62	5	27	4.74	.016
3.5 oz	100	3.5	1.3	1.5	0.1	69		0	.09	3.8	2.17	.46		395	226	1.95	.100	813
roasted, select, ¼" fat trim	160	65.1	29.0	0.0	0.0	0.0		0	0	.17	.38	7		62	5	27	4.74	.016
3.5 oz	100	4.0	1.4	1.7	0.1	69		0	.09	3.8	2.17	.46		395	226	1.95	.100	813
round, eye of, sep lean & fat																		
roasted, choice, 0" fat trim	180	63.7	28.8	0.0	0.0	0.0		0	0	.17	.38	7		62	5	27	4.71	.016
3.5 oz	100	6.3	2.3	2.7	0.2	69		0	.09	3.7	2.16	.45		392	224	1.94	.099	813
roasted, choice, ¼" fat trim	241	58.9	26.6	0.0	0.0	0.0		0	0	.16	.35	6		59	6	24	4.31	.015
3.5 oz	100	14.1	5.5	6.1	0.5	72		0	.08	3.5	2.10	.42		359	206	1.83	.093	813
roasted, select, 0" fat trim	161	64.6	28.8	0.0	0.0	0.0		0	0	.17	.38	7		62	5	27	4.71	.016
3.5 oz	100	4.2	1.5	1.8	0.1	69		0	.09	3.7	2.16	.45		392	224	1.94	.099	813
roasted, select, ¼" fat trim	217	60.0	27.0	0.0	0.0	0.0		0	0	.16	.35	7		60	6	25	4.37	.015
3.5 oz	100	11.3	4.4	4.9	0.4	72		0	.08	3.5	2.11	.42		365	209	1.85	.094	813
round, full cut																		
sep lean & fat, choice, broiled, ¼" fat trim	240	56.3	27.4	0.0	0.0	0.0		0	0	.21	.38	9		61	6	25	4.32	.015
3.5 oz	100	13.6	5.2	5.8	0.5	80		0	.09	4.0	3.01	.38		392	238	2.53	.100	813
sep lean & fat, select, broiled, ¼" fat trim	223	58.1	27.4	0.0	0.0	0.0		0	0	.21	.38	9		62	6	26	4.33	.015
3.5 oz	100	11.7	4.1	4.6	0.4	55		0	.09	4.0	3.02	.39		392	238	2.54	.101	813
sep lean, choice, broiled, ¼" fat trim	191	60.5	29.2	0.0	0.0	0.0		0	0	.22	.40	10		64	5	28	4.64	.016
3.5 oz	100	7.3	2.6	3.1	0.3	78		0	.10	4.3	3.17	.41		422	256	2.70	.106	813
sep lean, select, broiled, ¼" fat trim	172	62.4	29.3	0.0	0.0	0.0		0	0	.22	.41	10		64	5	28	4.66	.016
3.5 oz	100	5.2	1.8	2.2	0.2	78		0	.10	4.3	3.17	.41		423	256	2.71	.107	813

	KCAL / WT (g)	H₂O (g) / FAT (g)	PRO (g) / SFA (g)	CHO (g) / MUFA (g)	SUGR (g) / PUFA (g)	DFIB (g) / CHOL (mg)	A (RE) / A (IU)	C (mg) / B-1 (mg)	B-2 (mg) / NIA (mg)	B-6 (mg) / B-12 (mcg)	FOL (mcg) / PANT (mg)	Na (mg) / K (mg)	Ca (mg) / P (mg)	Mg (mg) / Fe (mg)	Zn (mg) / Cu (mg)	Mn (mg) / REF
round, tip, sep lean																
roasted, choice, 0″ fat trim	180	65.1	28.7	0.0	0.0	0.0	0	0	.27	.40	8	65	5	27	7.07	.017
3.5 oz	100	6.4	2.2	2.5	0.3	81	0	.10	3.7	2.89	.47	386	242	2.94	.125	813
roasted, choice, ¼″ fat trim	188	64.6	28.7	0.0	0.0	0.0	0	0	.27	.40	8	65	5	27	7.07	.017
3.5 oz	100	7.3	2.5	2.9	0.3	81	0	.10	3.7	2.89	.47	386	242	2.94	.125	813
roasted, prime, ¼″ fat trim	213	61.1	28.7	0.0	0.0	0.0	0	0	.27	.40	8	65	5	27	7.07	.017
3.5 oz	100	10.1	3.7	4.1	0.4	81	0	.10	3.7	2.89	.47	386	242	2.94	.125	813
roasted, select, 0″ fat trim	170	65.5	28.7	0.0	0.0	0.0	0	0	.27	.40	8	65	5	27	7.07	.017
3.5 oz	100	5.3	1.9	2.1	0.2	81	0	.10	3.7	2.89	.47	386	242	2.94	.125	813
roasted, select, ¼″ fat trim	180	65.1	28.7	0.0	0.0	0.0	0	0	.27	.40	8	65	5	27	7.07	.017
3.5 oz	100	6.4	2.2	2.5	0.3	81	0	.10	3.7	2.89	.47	386	242	2.94	.125	813
round, tip, sep lean & fat																
roasted, choice, 0″ fat trim	200	63.2	28.0	0.0	0.0	0.0	0	0	.26	.39	8	64	5	26	6.84	.017
3.5 oz	100	9.0	3.3	3.7	0.3	82	0	.10	3.6	2.84	.46	375	235	2.86	.122	813
roasted, choice, ¼″ fat trim	247	59.1	26.5	0.0	0.0	0.0	0	0	.25	.37	7	62	6	24	6.39	.016
3.5 oz	100	14.9	5.7	6.2	0.6	83	0	.09	3.5	2.74	.43	354	222	2.71	.115	813
roasted, prime, ¼″ fat trim	274	55.6	26.4	0.0	0.0	0.0	0	0	.24	.37	7	62	6	24	6.33	.016
3.5 oz	100	17.9	6.9	7.6	0.7	83	0	.09	3.5	2.72	.43	351	220	2.70	.115	813
roasted, select, 0″ fat trim	186	64.1	28.2	0.0	0.0	0.0	0	0	.26	.39	8	64	5	26	6.90	.017
3.5 oz	100	7.3	2.6	3.0	0.3	81	0	.10	3.7	2.85	.46	378	237	2.88	.123	813
roasted, select, ¼″ fat trim	225	60.9	27.1	0.0	0.0	0.0	0	0	.25	.38	8	63	6	25	6.56	.016
3.5 oz	100	12.2	4.6	5.1	0.5	82	0	.09	3.5	2.78	.44	362	227	2.77	.118	813
round, top, sep lean																
choice, braised, 0″ fat trim	207	58.1	36.1	0.0	0.0	0.0	0	0	.25	.28	9	45	4	26	4.56	.018
3.5 oz	100	5.8	2.0	2.3	0.3	90	0	.07	3.8	2.70	.37	334	226	3.32	.124	813
choice, braised, ¼″ fat trim	213	56.9	36.1	0.0	0.0	0.0	0	0	.25	.28	9	45	4	26	4.56	.018
3.5 oz	100	6.5	2.2	2.5	0.3	90	0	.07	3.8	2.70	.37	334	226	3.32	.124	813
choice, broiled, ¼″ fat trim	189	61.2	31.7	0.0	0.0	0.0	0	0	.27	.56	12	61	6	31	5.57	.017
3.5 oz	100	5.9	2.0	2.3	0.3	84	0	.12	6.0	2.48	.49	442	246	2.88	.123	813
choice, pan fried, ¼″ fat trim	227	55.5	35.1	0.0	0.0	0.0	0	0	.28	.61	13	71	5	35	4.62	.020
3.5 oz	100	8.6	2.4	2.8	1.6	97	0	.11	5.5	3.43	.46	513	292	3.15	.131	813
prime, broiled, ¼″ fat trim	215	60.4	31.7	0.0	0.0	0.0	0	0	.27	.56	12	61	6	31	5.57	.017
3.5 oz	100	8.9	3.1	3.5	0.4	84	0	.12	6.0	2.48	.49	442	246	2.88	.123	813
select, braised, 0″ fat trim	190	59.3	36.1	0.0	0.0	0.0	0	0	.25	.28	9	45	4	26	4.56	.018
3.5 oz	100	4.0	1.4	1.6	0.2	90	0	.07	3.8	2.70	.37	334	226	3.32	.124	813
select, braised, ¼″ fat trim	196	58.0	36.1	0.0	0.0	0.0	0	0	.25	.28	9	45	4	26	4.56	.018
3.5 oz	100	4.6	1.6	1.8	0.2	90	0	.07	3.8	2.70	.37	334	226	3.32	.124	813
select, broiled, ¼″ fat trim	169	63.2	31.7	0.0	0.0	0.0	0	0	.27	.56	12	61	6	31	5.57	.017
3.5 oz	100	3.7	1.3	1.4	0.2	84	0	.12	6.0	2.48	.49	442	246	2.88	.123	813
round, top, sep lean & fat																
choice, braised, 0″ fat trim	216	57.3	35.6	0.0	0.0	0.0	0	0	.25	.28	9	45	4	25	4.50	.018
3.5 oz	100	7.1	2.5	2.8	0.3	90	0	.07	3.8	2.68	.37	330	223	3.27	.122	813
choice, braised, ¼″ fat trim	260	53.1	33.6	0.0	0.0	0.0	0	0	.24	.27	9	45	5	24	4.24	.017
3.5 oz	100	12.9	4.9	5.3	0.5	90	0	.07	3.6	2.59	.35	312	211	3.09	.116	813
choice, broiled, ¼″ fat trim	224	58.1	30.2	0.0	0.0	0.0	0	0	.26	.53	11	60	7	29	5.27	.016
3.5 oz	100	10.6	3.9	4.3	0.4	85	0	.11	5.7	2.42	.46	419	234	2.75	.117	813
choice, pan fried, ¼″ fat trim	277	51.4	32.4	0.0	0.0	0.0	0	0	.26	.56	12	68	6	32	4.27	.019
3.5 oz	100	15.4	5.9	5.9	1.8	97	0	.10	5.0	3.23	.42	470	268	2.92	.122	813
prime, broiled, ¼″ fat trim	229	59.1	31.1	0.0	0.0	0.0	0	0	.26	.55	12	60	6	30	5.44	.017
3.5 oz	100	10.7	3.9	4.3	0.5	84	0	.12	5.9	2.45	.48	432	241	2.83	.121	813
select, braised, 0″ fat trim	200	58.5	35.6	0.0	0.0	0.0	0	0	.25	.28	9	45	4	25	4.50	.018
3.5 oz	100	5.3	1.9	2.1	0.2	90	0	.07	3.8	2.68	.37	330	223	3.27	.122	813
select, braised, ¼″ fat trim	234	54.9	34.1	0.0	0.0	0.0	0	0	.24	.27	9	45	5	24	4.31	.017
3.5 oz	100	9.9	3.7	4.1	0.4	90	0	.07	3.6	2.61	.35	317	214	3.14	.118	813
select, broiled, ¼″ fat trim	206	60.0	30.2	0.0	0.0	0.0	0	0	.26	.53	11	60	7	29	5.27	.016
3.5 oz	100	8.5	3.2	3.5	0.3	85	0	.11	5.7	2.42	.46	419	234	2.75	.117	813
shank, crosscuts, choice, simmered, sep lean & fat, ¼″ fat trim—*3.5 oz*	263	53.1	30.7	0.0	0.0	0.0	0	0	.20	.34	9	61	30	27	9.31	.018
	100	14.7	5.7	6.5	0.5	80	0	.12	5.3	3.51	.37	404	239	3.50	.155	813

	KCAL	H₂O (g)	PRO (g)	CHO (g)	SUGR (g)	DFIB (g)	A (RE)	C (mg)	B-2 (mg)	B-6 (mg)	FOL (mcg)	Na (mg)	Ca (mg)	Mg (mg)	Zn (mg)	Mn (mg)
	WT (g)	FAT (g)	SFA (g)	MUFA (g)	PUFA (g)	CHOL (mg)	A (IU)	B-1 (mg)	NIA (mg)	B-12 (mcg)	PANT (mg)	K (mg)	P (mg)	Fe (mg)	Cu (mg)	REF
shank, crosscuts, choice, simmered, sep lean, ¼" fat trim—*3.5 oz*	201	58.2	33.7	0.0	0.0	0.0	0	0	.21	.37	10	64	32	30	10.49	.020
	100	6.4	2.3	2.9	0.2	78	0	.14	5.9	3.79	.41	447	263	3.86	.172	813
short loin porterhouse steak, ¼" fat trim, broiled, sep lean & fat—*3.5 oz*	327	50.1	22.4	0.0	0.0	0.0	0	0	.21	.34	7	62	8	22	4.36	.014
	100	25.6	9.9	11.3	0.9	75	0	.09	3.9	2.11	.30	307	179	2.62	.119	813
short loin porterhouse steak, ¼" fat trim, broiled, sep lean—*3.5 oz*	215	60.1	26.0	0.0	0.0	0.0	0	0	.25	.40	8	69	7	27	5.29	.016
	100	11.5	4.0	5.2	0.4	69	0	.11	4.6	2.27	.34	367	211	3.11	.143	813
short loin T-bone steak, ¼" fat trim, broiled, sep lean & fat—*3.5 oz*	309	52.0	23.2	0.0	0.0	0.0	0	0	.21	.33	7	64	8	23	4.45	.014
	100	23.3	9.1	10.2	0.8	67	0	.09	4.0	2.13	.29	321	184	2.71	.121	813
short loin T-bone steak, ¼" fat trim, broiled, sep lean—*3.5 oz*	205	61.5	26.8	0.0	0.0	0.0	0	0	.25	.39	8	71	6	28	5.31	.016
	100	10.1	3.6	4.5	0.3	59	0	.11	4.6	2.27	.33	378	215	3.17	.143	813
short loin, top loin, sep lean																
broiled, choice, 0" fat trim	209	59.5	28.6	0.0	0.0	0.0	0	0	.20	.42	8	68	8	27	5.22	.016
3.5 oz	100	9.6	3.7	3.9	0.3	76	0	.09	5.3	2.00	.37	396	218	2.47	.107	813
broiled, choice, ¼" fat trim	214	59.3	28.6	0.0	0.0	0.0	0	0	.20	.42	8	68	8	27	5.22	.016
3.5 oz	100	10.2	3.9	4.1	0.3	76	0	.09	5.3	2.00	.37	396	218	2.47	.107	813
broiled, prime, ¼" fat trim	245	57.1	28.6	0.0	0.0	0.0	0	0	.20	.42	8	68	8	27	5.22	.016
3.5 oz	100	13.6	5.5	5.7	0.5	76	0	.09	5.3	2.00	.37	396	218	2.47	.107	813
broiled, select, 0" fat trim	184	61.0	28.6	0.0	0.0	0.0	0	0	.20	.42	8	68	8	27	5.22	.016
3.5 oz	100	6.9	2.6	2.8	0.2	76	0	.09	5.3	2.00	.37	396	218	2.47	.107	813
broiled, select, ¼" fat trim	193	60.7	28.6	0.0	0.0	0.0	0	0	.20	.42	8	68	8	27	5.22	.016
3.5 oz	100	7.8	3.0	3.1	0.3	76	0	.09	5.3	2.00	.37	396	218	2.47	.107	813
short loin, top loin, sep lean & fat																
broiled, choice, 0" fat trim	228	57.9	27.9	0.0	0.0	0.0	0	0	.19	.41	8	67	8	26	5.07	.016
3.5 oz	100	12.0	4.7	4.9	0.4	77	0	.09	5.2	1.98	.36	385	212	2.41	.105	813
broiled, choice, ¼" fat trim	298	51.9	25.4	0.0	0.0	0.0	0	0	.18	.37	7	63	9	23	4.53	.014
3.5 oz	100	21.0	8.3	8.8	0.8	79	0	.08	4.7	1.93	.33	346	192	2.22	.096	813
broiled, prime, ¼" fat trim	323	50.2	25.4	0.0	0.0	0.0	0	0	.18	.37	7	63	9	23	4.53	.014
3.5 oz	100	23.8	9.6	10.1	0.9	79	0	.08	4.7	1.93	.33	346	192	2.22	.096	813
broiled, select, 0" fat trim	199	59.7	28.1	0.0	0.0	0.0	0	0	.19	.41	8	67	8	26	5.11	.016
3.5 oz	100	8.8	3.4	3.6	0.3	77	0	.09	5.2	1.99	.36	388	214	2.43	.105	813
broiled, select, ¼" fat trim	266	54.4	25.9	0.0	0.0	0.0	0	0	.18	.38	7	64	9	24	4.65	.015
3.5 oz	100	17.2	6.8	7.2	0.6	79	0	.08	4.8	1.94	.33	354	197	2.26	.098	813
tenderloin, sep lean																
choice, broiled, 0" fat trim	212	59.8	28.3	0.0	0.0	0.0	0	0	.30	.44	7	63	7	30	5.59	.017
3.5 oz	100	10.1	3.8	3.8	0.4	84	0	.13	3.9	2.57	.38	419	238	3.58	.179	813
choice, broiled, ¼" fat trim	222	59.2	28.3	0.0	0.0	0.0	0	0	.30	.44	7	63	7	30	5.59	.017
3.5 oz	100	11.2	4.2	4.2	0.4	84	0	.13	3.9	2.57	.38	419	238	3.58	.179	813
choice, roasted, ¼" fat trim	231	56.4	27.7	0.0	0.0	0.0	0	0	.33	.57	9	72	8	32	4.79	.019
3.5 oz	100	12.5	4.7	4.8	0.5	83	0	.18	4.5	3.87	.47	489	281	3.69	.145	813
prime, broiled, ¼" fat trim	232	58.6	28.3	0.0	0.0	0.0	0	0	.30	.44	7	63	7	30	5.59	.017
3.5 oz	100	12.4	4.8	4.8	0.5	84	0	.13	3.9	2.57	.38	419	238	3.58	.179	813
prime, roasted, ¼" fat trim	255	56.0	27.5	0.0	0.0	0.0	0	0	.32	.38	8	59	7	27	5.17	.016
3.5 oz	100	15.3	6.0	5.9	0.6	86	0	.10	3.4	2.77	.45	393	236	3.66	.167	813
select, broiled, 0" fat trim	200	60.4	28.3	0.0	0.0	0.0	0	0	.30	.44	7	63	7	30	5.59	.017
3.5 oz	100	8.8	3.3	3.3	0.3	84	0	.13	3.9	2.57	.38	419	238	3.58	.179	813
select, broiled, ¼" fat trim	199	61.0	28.3	0.0	0.0	0.0	0	0	.30	.44	7	63	7	30	5.59	.017
3.5 oz	100	8.7	3.3	3.3	0.3	84	0	.13	3.9	2.57	.38	419	238	3.58	.179	813
select, roasted, ¼" fat trim	211	57.5	27.7	0.0	0.0	0.0	0	0	.31	.29	9	61	7	27	4.79	.016
3.5 oz	100	10.3	3.9	4.0	0.5	83	0	.10	3.4	2.71	.28	391	239	3.69	.145	813
tenderloin, sep lean & fat																
choice, broiled, 0" fat trim	244	56.9	27.0	0.0	0.0	0.0	0	0	.28	.42	7	61	7	28	5.30	.016
3.5 oz	100	14.3	5.5	5.7	0.5	85	0	.12	3.8	2.50	.36	398	227	3.40	.170	813
choice, broiled, ¼" fat trim	304	51.9	25.1	0.0	0.0	0.0	0	0	.26	.39	6	59	8	26	4.84	.015
3.5 oz	100	21.8	8.6	8.9	0.8	86	0	.11	3.5	2.40	.34	365	209	3.13	.155	813
choice, roasted, ¼" fat trim	339	47.4	23.6	0.0	0.0	0.0	0	0	.27	.47	8	65	9	26	3.97	.016
3.5 oz	100	26.4	10.4	10.9	1.0	86	0	.15	3.8	3.33	.39	400	232	3.06	.121	813

	KCAL / WT (g)	H₂O (g) / FAT (g)	PRO (g) / SFA (g)	CHO (g) / MUFA (g)	SUGR (g) / PUFA (g)	DFIB (g) / CHOL (mg)	A (RE) / A (IU)	C (mg) / B-1 (mg)	B-2 (mg) / NIA (mg)	B-6 (mg) / B-12 (mcg)	FOL (mcg) / PANT (mg)	Na (mg) / K (mg)	Ca (mg) / P (mg)	Mg (mg) / Fe (mg)	Zn (mg) / Cu (mg)	Mn (mg) / REF
prime, broiled, ¼" fat trim	317	51.0	24.9	0.0	0.0	0.0	0	0	.26	.38	6	59	8	25	4.79	.015
3.5 oz	100	23.4	9.3	9.7	0.9	86	0	.11	3.5	2.39	.34	362	207	3.10	.154	813
prime, roasted, ¼" fat trim	353	47.5	23.7	0.0	0.0	0.0	0	0	.27	.33	7	55	9	22	4.31	.014
3.5 oz	100	27.9	11.1	11.6	1.1	88	0	.09	3.0	2.51	.38	330	199	3.06	.139	813
select, broiled, 0" fat trim	229	57.9	27.2	0.0	0.0	0.0	0	0	.29	.42	7	62	7	29	5.34	.016
3.5 oz	100	12.5	4.8	5.0	0.5	85	0	.12	3.8	2.51	.36	401	228	3.43	.171	813
select, broiled, ¼" fat trim	271	54.6	25.6	0.0	0.0	0.0	0	0	.27	.39	6	60	8	26	4.96	.015
3.5 oz	100	17.9	7.0	7.4	0.7	86	0	.12	3.6	2.43	.34	374	214	3.20	.159	813
select, roasted, ¼" fat trim	324	48.2	23.6	0.0	0.0	0.0	0	0	.26	.25	7	56	9	22	3.97	.014
3.5 oz	100	24.7	9.8	10.4	1.0	86	0	.08	3.0	2.45	.25	326	200	3.06	.121	813
top sirloin, sep lean																
choice, broiled, 0" fat trim	200	61.0	30.4	0.0	0.0	0.0	0	0	.29	.45	10	66	11	32	6.52	.017
3.5 oz	100	7.8	3.0	3.3	0.3	89	0	.13	4.3	2.85	.39	403	244	3.36	.146	813
choice, broiled, ¼" fat trim	202	61.6	30.4	0.0	0.0	0.0	0	0	.29	.45	10	66	11	32	6.52	.017
3.5 oz	100	8.0	3.1	3.4	0.3	89	0	.13	4.3	2.85	39	403	244	3.36	.116	813
choice, pan fried, ¼" fat trim	238	55.9	32.5	0.0	0.0	0.0	0	0	.33	.50	10	77	11	33	6.40	.019
3.5 oz	100	11.0	4.0	4.4	1.5	99	0	.14	4.3	3.69	.43	465	267	3.90	.149	813
select, broiled, 0" fat trim	180	62.4	30.4	0.0	0.0	0.0	0	0	.29	.45	10	66	11	32	6.52	.017
3.5 oz	100	5.6	2.2	2.4	0.2	89	0	.13	4.3	2.85	.39	403	244	3.36	.146	813
select, broiled, ¼" fat trim	186	62.9	30.4	0.0	0.0	0.0	0	0	.29	.45	10	66	11	32	6.52	.017
3.5 oz	100	6.2	2.4	2.6	0.2	89	0	.13	4.3	2.85	.39	403	244	3.36	.146	813
top sirloin, sep lean & fat																
choice, broiled, 0" fat trim	229	58.5	29.2	0.0	0.0	0.0	0	0	.28	.43	10	64	11	30	6.21	.016
3.5 oz	100	11.6	4.6	5.0	0.5	89	0	.12	4.1	2.78	.37	386	234	3.22	.140	813
choice, broiled, ¼" fat trim	269	55.6	27.6	0.0	0.0	0.0	0	0	.27	.41	9	62	11	28	5.80	.016
3.5 oz	100	16.7	6.7	7.2	0.6	90	0	.11	3.9	2.68	.35	363	220	3.04	.132	813
choice, pan fried, ¼" fat trim	326	48.4	28.1	0.0	0.0	0.0	0	0	.28	.43	9	70	12	28	5.40	.017
3.5 oz	100	22.8	8.9	9.6	1.7	98	0	.12	3.8	3.28	.38	396	229	3.33	.128	813
select, broiled, 0" fat trim	195	61.1	29.7	0.0	0.0	0.0	0	0	.29	.44	10	65	11	31	6.35	.017
3.5 oz	100	7.6	3.0	3.2	0.3	89	0	.12	4.2	2.81	.38	393	239	3.28	.143	813
select, broiled, ¼" fat trim	245	57.6	28.0	0.0	0.0	0.0	0	0	.27	.41	9	63	11	29	5.91	.016
3.5 oz	100	13.9	5.5	6.0	0.5	90	0	.11	4.0	2.70	.36	369	224	3.08	.134	813

21.2 GAME MEATS

	KCAL / WT (g)	H₂O (g) / FAT (g)	PRO (g) / SFA (g)	CHO (g) / MUFA (g)	SUGR (g) / PUFA (g)	DFIB (g) / CHOL (mg)	A (RE) / A (IU)	C (mg) / B-1 (mg)	B-2 (mg) / NIA (mg)	B-6 (mg) / B-12 (mcg)	FOL (mcg) / PANT (mg)	Na (mg) / K (mg)	Ca (mg) / P (mg)	Mg (mg) / Fe (mg)	Zn (mg) / Cu (mg)	Mn (mg) / REF
antelope, roasted	150	65.9	29.4	0.0	0.0	0.0	0	0	.73			54	4	28	1.68	.022
3.5 oz	100	2.7	1.0	0.6	0.6	126	0	.26				372	210	4.20	.213	817
bear, simmered	259	53.5	32.4	0.0	0.0	0.0	0	0	.82	.29	6	71	5	23	10.27	
3.5 oz	100	13.4	3.5	5.7	2.4	98	0	.10	3.4	2.47		263	170	10.73	.148	817
beaver, roasted	212	57.9	34.9	0.0	0.0	0.0	0	3	.31	.47	11	59	22	29	2.27	
3.5 oz	100	7.0	2.1	1.9	1.4	117	0	.05	2.2	8.30	.93	403	292	10.00	.189	817
beefalo, roasted	188	61.7	30.7	0.0	0.0	0.0	0	9	.11		18	82	24		6.40	
3.5 oz	100	6.3	2.7	2.7	0.2	58	0	.03	4.9	2.55	.58	459	250	3.05		817
bison, roasted	143	66.5	28.4	0.0	0.0	0.0	0	0	.27	.40	8	57	8	26	3.68	.008
3.5 oz	100	2.4	0.9	0.9	0.2	82	0	.10	3.7	2.86		361	209	3.42	.107	817
boar, wild, roasted	160	63.9	28.3	0.0	0.0	0.0	0	0	.14	.42	6	60	16	27	3.01	
3.5 oz	100	4.4	1.3	1.7	0.6	77	0	.31	4.2	.70		396	134	1.12	.056	817
buffalo, water, roasted	131	68.8	26.8	0.0	0.0	0.0	0	0	.25	.46	9	56	15	33	2.54	
3.5 oz	100	1.8	0.6	0.6	0.4	61	0	.03	6.3	1.75	.17	313	220	2.12	.178	817
caribou, roasted	167	62.4	29.8	0.0	0.0	0.0	0	3	.90	.32	5	60	22	27	5.26	.087
3.5 oz	100	4.4	1.7	1.3	0.6	109	0	.25	5.8	6.64	2.68	310	233	6.17	.263	817
deer, roasted	158	65.2	30.2	0.0	0.0	0.0	0	0	.60			54	7	24	2.75	.046
3.5 oz	100	3.2	1.3	0.9	0.6	112	0	.18	6.7			335	226	4.47	.300	817
eel, ckd by dry heat	201	50.4	20.1	0.0	0.0	0.0	966	2	.04	.07	15	55	22	22	1.77	.034
3 oz	85	12.7	2.6	7.8	1.0	137	3219	.16	3.8	2.45	.24	297	235	.54	.025	815
eel, raw	156	58.0	15.7	0.0	0.0	0.0	887	2	.03	.06	13	43	17	17	1.38	.030
3 oz	85	9.9	2.0	6.1	0.8	107	2954	.13	3.0	2.55	.20	231	184	.42	.020	815
elk, roasted	146	66.3	30.2	0.0	0.0	0.0	0	0				61	5	24	3.16	.013
3.5 oz	100	1.9	0.7	0.5	0.4	73	0					328	180	3.63	.142	817
goat, roasted	143	68.2	27.1	0.0	0.0	0.0	0	0	.61	.00	5	86	17	0	5.27	.042
3.5 oz	100	3.0	0.9	1.4	0.2	75	0	.09	4.0	1.19		405	201	3.73	.303	817

	KCAL / WT (g)	H₂O (g) / FAT (g)	PRO (g) / SFA (g)	CHO (g) / MUFA (g)	SUGR (g) / PUFA (g)	DFIB (g) / CHOL (mg)	A (RE) / A (IU)	C (mg) / B-1 (mg)	B-2 (mg) / NIA (mg)	B-6 (mg) / B-12 (mcg)	FOL (mcg) / PANT (mg)	Na (mg) / K (mg)	Ca (mg) / P (mg)	Mg (mg) / Fe (mg)	Zn (mg) / Cu (mg)	Mn (mg) / REF
horse, roasted	175	64.0	28.1	0.0	0.0	0.0	0	2	.12	.33		55	8	25	3.82	.022
3.5 oz	100	6.0	1.9	2.1	0.8	68	0	.10	4.8	3.16		379	247	5.03	.171	817
moose, roasted	134	67.8	29.3	0.0	0.0	0.0	0	5	.34	.37	4	69	6	24	3.68	.009
3.5 oz	100	1.0	0.3	0.2	0.3	78	0	.05	5.3	6.31		334	176	4.22	.079	817
muskrat, roasted	234	55.6	30.1	0.0	0.0	0.0	0	7	.71	.47	11	95	36	26	2.27	.032
3.5 oz	100	11.7				121	0	.08	7.2	8.30	.93	320	271	7.10	.189	817
opossum, roasted	221	58.3	30.2	0.0	0.0	0.0	0	0	.37	.47	10	58	17	34	2.28	
3.5 oz	100	10.2	1.2	3.8	3.0	129	0	.10	8.4	8.30		438	278	4.64	.189	817
rabbit, domesticated, roasted	197	60.6	29.1	0.0	0.0	0.0	0	0	.21	.47	11	47	19	21	2.27	.032
3.5 oz	100	8.1	2.4	2.2	1.6	82	0	.09	8.4	8.30	.93	383	263	2.27	.189	817
rabbit, domesticated, stewed	206	58.8	30.4	0.0	0.0	0.0	0	0	.17	.34	9	37	20	20	2.37	.032
3.5 oz	100	8.4	2.5	2.3	1.6	86	0	.06	7.2	6.51	.67	300	226	2.37	.176	817
rabbit, wild, stewed	173	61.4	33.0	0.0	0.0	0.0	0	0	.07	.34	8	45	18	31	2.38	
3.5 oz	100	3.5	1.1	0.9	0.7	123	0	.02	6.4	6.51		343	240	4.85	.176	817
raccoon, roasted	255	54.3	29.2	0.0	0.0	0.0	0	0	.52	.47	11	79	14	30	2.27	
3.5 oz	100	14.5	4.1	5.2	2.1	97	0	.59	4.7	8.30		398	261	7.10	.189	817
squirrel, roasted	173	62.1	30.8	0.0	0.0	0.0	0	0	.29	.37	9	119	3	28	1.78	.032
3.5 oz	100	4.7	0.8	1.3	1.5	121	0	.06	4.6	6.51	.93	352	211	6.81	.148	817
turtle, green, cnd	106	75.0	23.4	0.0												
3.5 oz	100	0.7														800
turtle, green, raw	89	78.5	19.8	0.0												
3.5 oz	100	0.5														800
whale meat, raw	156	70.9	20.6	0.0				6	.08			78	12			
3.5 oz	100	7.5	1.0				1860	.09				22	144			800

21.3 LAMB

	KCAL / WT (g)	H₂O (g) / FAT (g)	PRO (g) / SFA (g)	CHO (g) / MUFA (g)	SUGR (g) / PUFA (g)	DFIB (g) / CHOL (mg)	A (RE) / A (IU)	C (mg) / B-1 (mg)	B-2 (mg) / NIA (mg)	B-6 (mg) / B-12 (mcg)	FOL (mcg) / PANT (mg)	Na (mg) / K (mg)	Ca (mg) / P (mg)	Mg (mg) / Fe (mg)	Zn (mg) / Cu (mg)	Mn (mg) / REF
domestic, foreshank, choice, braised, sep lean & fat—3.5 oz	243	56.8	28.4	0.0	0.0	0.0	0	0	.19	.10	17	72	20	22	7.69	.025
	100	13.5	5.6	5.7	1.0	106	0	.05	5.5	2.28	.63	257	166	2.14	.123	817
domestic, foreshank, choice, braised, sep lean—3.5 oz	187	61.8	31.0	0.0	0.0	0.0	0	0	.19	.11	19	74	20	23	8.66	.028
	100	6.0	2.1	2.6	0.4	104	0	.04	5.1	2.26	.63	267	175	2.27	.129	817
domestic, ground, broiled	283	55.1	24.8	0.0	0.0	0.0	0	0	.25	.14	19	81	22	24	4.67	.024
3.5 oz	100	19.6	8.1	8.3	1.4	97	0	.10	6.7	2.61	.66	339	201	1.79	.128	817
domestic, leg																
shank half, choice, roasted, sep lean	180	64.9	28.2	0.0	0.0	0.0	0	0	.28	.17	24	66	8	26	5.02	.028
3.5 oz	100	6.7	2.4	2.9	0.4	87	0	.11	6.4	2.71	.71	342	208	2.06	.121	817
shank half, choice, roasted, sep lean & fat	225	60.7	26.4	0.0	0.0	0.0	0	0	.27	.16	22	65	10	25	4.66	.025
3.5 oz	100	12.4	5.1	5.3	0.9	90	0	.10	6.5	2.67	.70	326	198	1.98	.117	817
sirloin half, choice, roasted, sep lean	204	62.5	28.4	0.0	0.0	0.0	0	0	.31	.17	21	71	8	25	4.85	.028
3.5 oz	100	9.2	3.3	4.0	0.6	92	0	.12	6.3	2.58	.70	333	203	2.20	.119	817
sirloin half, choice, roasted, sep lean & fat	292	54.1	24.6	0.0	0.0	0.0	0	0	.28	.14	17	68	11	22	4.13	.022
3.5 oz	100	20.7	8.7	8.7	1.5	97	0	.11	6.6	2.53	.67	301	183	2.00	.112	817
whole (shank & sirloin), choice, roasted, sep lean—3.5 oz	191	63.9	28.3	0.0	0.0	0.0	0	0	.29	.17	23	68	8	26	4.94	.028
	100	7.7	2.8	3.4	0.5	89	0	.11	6.3	2.64	.71	338	206	2.12	.120	817
whole (shank & sirloin), choice, roasted, sep lean & fat—3.5 oz	258	57.5	25.6	0.0	0.0	0.0	0	0	.27	.15	20	66	11	24	4.40	.024
	100	16.5	6.9	7.0	1.2	93	0	.10	6.6	2.59	.68	313	191	1.98	.115	817
domestic, leg & shoulder, cubed for stew or kabob, sep lean,																
braised	223	56.2	33.7	0.0	0.0	0.0	0	0	.24	.12	21	70	15	28	6.58	.032
3.5 oz	100	8.8	3.1	3.5	0.8	108	0	.07	6.0	2.73	.59	260	205	2.80	.141	817
broiled	186	63.5	28.1	0.0	0.0	0.0	0	0	.30	.14	23	76	13	31	5.77	.029
3.5 oz	100	7.3	2.6	3.0	0.7	90	0	.11	6.6	3.03	.69	335	224	2.34	.151	817
domestic, loin																
sep lean & fat, choice, broiled	316	51.6	25.2	0.0	0.0	0.0	0	0	.25	.13	18	77	20	24	3.48	.022
3.5 oz	100	23.1	9.8	9.7	1.7	100	0	.10	7.1	2.47	.64	327	196	1.81	.130	817
sep lean & fat, choice, roasted	309	52.5	22.6	0.0	0.0	0.0	0	0	.24	.11	19	64	18	23	3.41	.020
3.5 oz	100	23.6	10.2	9.7	1.9	95	0	.10	7.1	2.21	.65	246	180	2.12	.119	817
sep lean, choice, broiled	216	61.0	30.0	0.0	0.0	0.0	0	0	.28	.16	24	84	19	28	4.13	.028
3.5 oz	100	9.7	3.5	4.3	0.6	95	0	.11	6.8	2.52	.66	376	226	2.00	.145	817

	KCAL	H₂O (g)	PRO (g)	CHO (g)	SUGR (g)	DFIB (g)	A (RE)	C (mg)	B-2 (mg)	B-6 (mg)	FOL (mcg)	Na (mg)	Ca (mg)	Mg (mg)	Zn (mg)	Mn (mg)
	WT (g)	FAT (g)	SFA (g)	MUFA (g)	PUFA (g)	CHOL (mg)	A (IU)	B-1 (mg)	NIA (mg)	B-12 (mcg)	PANT (mg)	K (mg)	P (mg)	Fe (mg)	Cu (mg)	REF
sep lean, choice, roasted	202	62.8	26.6	0.0	0.0	0.0	0	0	.27	.16	25	66	17	27	4.06	.026
3.5 oz	100	9.8	3.7	4.0	0.9	87	0	.10	6.8	2.16	.68	267	206	2.44	.132	817
domestic, rib																
sep lean & fat, choice, broiled	361	47.1	22.1	0.0	0.0	0.0	0	0	.22	.11	14	76	19	23	4.00	.020
3.5 oz	100	29.6	12.7	12.1	2.4	99	0	.09	7.0	2.54	.61	270	178	1.88	.121	817
sep lean & fat, choice, roasted	359	47.9	21.1	0.0	0.0	0.0	0	0	.21	.11	15	73	22	20	3.49	.019
3.5 oz	100	29.8	12.8	12.5	2.2	97	0	.09	6.8	2.23	.63	271	166	1.60	.115	817
sep lean, choice, broiled	235	58.8	27.7	0.0	0.0	0.0	0	0	.25	.15	21	85	16	29	5.27	.029
3.5 oz	100	12.9	4.7	5.2	1.2	91	0	.10	6.5	2.64	.63	313	213	2.21	.139	817
sep lean, choice, roasted	232	60.1	26.2	0.0	0.0	0.0	0	0	.23	.15	22	81	21	23	4.47	.028
3.5 oz	100	13.3	4.8	5.8	0.9	88	0	.09	6.2	2.16	.66	315	195	1.77	.129	817
domestic, shoulder, arm																
sep lean & fat, choice, braised	346	44.2	30.4	0.0	0.0	0.0	0	0	.25	.11	18	72	25	26	6.08	.023
3.5 oz	100	24.0	9.9	10.2	1.7	120	0	.07	6.7	2.58	.61	306	206	2.39	.139	817
sep lean & fat, choice, broiled	281	54.7	24.4	0.0	0.0	0.0	0	0	.27	.12	18	77	18	26	4.89	.023
3.5 oz	100	19.6	8.4	8.0	1.6	96	0	.10	7.0	2.86	.68	309	197	2.09	.133	817
sep lean & fat, choice, roasted	279	55.9	22.5	0.0	0.0	0.0	0	0	.25	.12	20	65	18	23	4.48	.021
3.5 oz	100	20.2	8.7	8.3	1.6	92	0	.09	6.7	2.55	.71	259	183	2.03	.113	817
sep lean, choice, braised	279	49.3	35.5	0.0	0.0	0.0	0	0	.27	.13	22	76	26	29	7.30	.028
3.5 oz	100	14.1	5.0	6.2	0.9	121	0	.07	6.3	2.65	.62	338	232	2.70	.154	817
sep lean, choice, broiled	200	62.3	27.7	0.0	0.0	0.0	0	0	.29	.14	23	82	17	30	5.73	.028
3.5 oz	100	9.0	3.4	3.6	0.8	92	0	.10	6.8	3.00	.71	340	219	2.31	.145	817
sep lean, choice, roasted	192	64.3	25.5	0.0	0.0	0.0	0	0	.27	.14	25	67	16	26	5.25	.026
3.5 oz	100	9.3	3.6	3.8	0.8	86	0	.10	6.3	2.61	.74	277	202	2.23	.120	817
domestic, shoulder, blade																
sep lean & fat, choice, braised	345	45.2	28.5	0.0	0.0	0.0	0	0	.21	.11	18	75	27	24	6.86	.027
3.5 oz	100	24.7	10.3	10.1	2.0	116	0	.06	6.0	2.83	.61	243	185	2.35	.121	817
sep lean & fat, choice, broiled	278	55.9	23.1	0.0	0.0	0.0	0	0	.25	.15	18	82	24	24	5.62	.024
3.5 oz	100	19.9	8.2	8.5	1.4	95	0	.09	6.4	2.73	.67	336	198	1.72	.122	817
sep lean & fat, choice, roasted	281	55.9	22.3	0.0	0.0	0.0	0	0	.23	.11	21	66	21	22	5.58	.022
3.5 oz	100	20.6	8.6	8.4	1.7	92	0	.09	5.9	2.67	.69	246	183	1.92	.106	817
sep lean, choice, braised	288	49.6	32.4	0.0	0.0	0.0	0	0	.22	.12	21	79	28	26	8.06	.032
3.5 oz	100	16.6	6.4	6.7	1.5	117	0	.06	5.6	2.94	.61	254	202	2.60	.128	817
sep lean, choice, broiled	211	62.5	25.5	0.0	0.0	0.0	0	0	.26	.17	21	88	24	26	6.48	.028
3.5 oz	100	11.3	4.0	5.0	0.7	91	0	.10	6.1	2.81	.69	368	216	1.81	.129	817
sep lean, choice, roasted	209	62.8	24.6	0.0	0.0	0.0	0	0	.25	.15	25	68	21	25	6.48	.026
3.5 oz	100	11.6	4.3	4.7	1.0	87	0	.09	5.5	2.74	.72	258	199	2.07	.110	817
domestic, shoulder, whole (arm & blade)																
sep lean & fat, choice, braised	344	45.2	28.7	0.0	0.0	0.0	0	0	.22	.10	17	75	25	24	6.37	.026
3.5 oz	100	24.6	10.3	10.0	2.0	116	0	.07	6.3	2.80	.61	248	186	2.40	.123	817
sep lean & fat, choice, broiled	278	55.0	24.4	0.0	0.0	0.0	0	0	.26	.12	19	78	21	26	5.72	.024
3.5 oz	100	19.3	8.0	7.9	1.6	97	0	.09	6.5	2.97	.67	301	198	2.03	.128	817
sep lean & fat, choice, roasted	276	56.3	22.5	0.0	0.0	0.0	0	0	.24	.13	21	66	20	23	5.23	.022
3.5 oz	100	20.0	8.4	8.2	1.6	92	0	.09	6.2	2.64	.70	251	184	1.97	.108	817
sep lean, choice, braised	283	50.0	32.8	0.0	0.0	0.0	0	0	.23	.12	21	79	26	27	7.52	.032
3.5 oz	100	15.9	6.2	6.5	1.4	117	0	.06	6.0	2.91	.62	261	204	2.67	.132	817
sep lean, choice, broiled	210	61.4	27.1	0.0	0.0	0.0	0	0	.28	.14	23	83	21	29	6.60	.028
3.5 oz	100	10.5	3.9	4.2	0.9	93	0	.10	6.2	3.11	.69	324	217	2.19	.137	817
sep lean, choice, roasted	204	63.3	24.9	0.0	0.0	0.0	0	0	.26	.15	25	68	19	25	6.04	.026
3.5 oz	100	10.8	4.1	4.4	0.9	87	0	.09	5.8	2.70	.73	265	200	2.13	.113	817
New Zealand, imported																
composite of trimmed retail cuts, sep lean & fat, ckd—3.5 oz	305	51.1	24.4	0.0	0.0	0.0	0	0	.41	.12	1	46	17	19	3.49	.023
	100	22.3	11.1	8.6	1.0	109	0	.12	7.8	2.81	.58	162	217	2.10	.100	817
composite of trimmed retail cuts, sep lean, ckd—3.5 oz	206	60.0	29.6	0.0	0.0	0.0	0	0	.50	.14	0	50	13	22	4.30	.029
	100	8.9	3.9	3.5	0.5	109	0	.13	7.7	2.95	.58	188	246	2.35	.114	817
foreshank, sep lean & fat, braised	258	56.8	27.0	0.0	0.0	0.0	0	0	.33	.08	1	47	14	15	4.80	.024
3.5 oz	100	15.8	7.8	6.1	0.7	102	0	.07	6.1	2.44	.41	118	175	2.07	.102	817

	KCAL / WT (g)	H₂O (g) / FAT (g)	PRO (g) / SFA (g)	CHO (g) / MUFA (g)	SUGR (g) / PUFA (g)	DFIB (g) / CHOL (mg)	A (RE) / A (IU)	C (mg) / B-1 (mg)	B-2 (mg) / NIA (mg)	B-6 (mg) / B-12 (mcg)	FOL (mcg) / PANT (mg)	Na (mg) / K (mg)	Ca (mg) / P (mg)	Mg (mg) / Fe (mg)	Zn (mg) / Cu (mg)	Mn (mg) / REF
foreshank, sep lean, braised	186	63.5	30.8	0.0	0.0	0.0	0	0	.36	.09	1	49	10	16	5.60	.028
3.5 oz	100	6.0	2.6	2.4	0.3	101	0	.07	5.6	2.45	.37	125	184	2.22	.112	817
leg, whole (shank & sirloin), sep lean & fat, roasted—3.5 oz	246	57.9	24.8	0.0	0.0	0.0	0	0	.45	.13	1	43	10	20	3.58	.023
	100	15.6	7.6	6.0	0.8	101	0	.12	7.6	2.60	.55	167	218	2.10	.103	817
leg, whole (shank & sirloin), sep lean, roasted—3.5 oz	181	63.9	27.7	0.0	0.0	0.0	0	0	.50	.14	0	45	7	21	4.04	.027
	100	7.0	3.0	2.8	0.4	100	0	.12	7.5	2.63	.54	183	234	2.24	.111	817
loin, sep lean & fat, broiled	315	50.4	23.4	0.0	0.0	0.0	0	0	.36	.11	1	49	23	19	2.65	.021
3.5 oz	100	23.9	12.0	9.2	1.1	112	0	.12	7.9	2.53	.50	159	208	2.05	.109	817
loin, sep lean, broiled	199	60.9	29.3	0.0	0.0	0.0	0	0	.43	.14	0	55	21	22	3.29	.028
3.5 oz	100	8.2	3.6	3.2	0.5	114	0	.13	7.9	2.58	.46	189	240	2.34	.130	817
rib, sep lean & fat, roasted	340	50.2	19.0	0.0	0.0	0.0	0	0	.27	.08	1	43	19	14	2.60	.017
3.5 oz	100	28.8	14.4	11.1	1.3	100	0	.09	6.8	2.33	.51	124	170	1.71	.071	817
rib, sep lean, roasted	196	64.3	24.4	0.0	0.0	0.0	0	0	.33	.11	0	48	14	16	3.43	.024
3.5 oz	100	10.2	4.4	4.0	0.6	94	0	.11	6.1	2.28	.45	146	191	1.89	.077	817
shoulder, whole (arm & blade), sep lean & fat, braised—3.5 oz	357	42.6	28.2	0.0	0.0	0.0	0	0	.32	.07	1	51	27	18	4.53	.025
	100	26.3	12.7	10.2	1.3	123	0	.08	6.4	3.40	.52	147	196	2.11	.103	817
shoulder, whole (arm & blade), sep lean, braised—3.5 oz	285	47.9	34.1	0.0	0.0	0.0	0	0	.36	.08	0	56	27	20	5.60	.032
	100	15.5	6.8	6.1	0.9	127	0	.08	5.8	3.71	.50	166	215	2.34	.116	817

21.4 PORK

	KCAL / WT (g)	H₂O (g) / FAT (g)	PRO (g) / SFA (g)	CHO (g) / MUFA (g)	SUGR (g) / PUFA (g)	DFIB (g) / CHOL (mg)	A (RE) / A (IU)	C (mg) / B-1 (mg)	B-2 (mg) / NIA (mg)	B-6 (mg) / B-12 (mcg)	FOL (mcg) / PANT (mg)	Na (mg) / K (mg)	Ca (mg) / P (mg)	Mg (mg) / Fe (mg)	Zn (mg) / Cu (mg)	Mn (mg) / REF
arm picnic																
cured, sep lean & fat, roasted	280	54.7	20.4	0.0	0.0	0.0	0	0	.19	.28	3	1072	10	14	2.51	.024
3.5 oz	100	21.4	7.7	10.1	2.3	58	0	.61	4.1	.93	.56	258	221	.95	.113	810
cured, sep lean, roasted	170	63.9	24.9	0.0	0.0	0.0	0	0	.23	.37	4	1231	11	16	2.94	.030
3.5 oz	100	7.0	2.4	3.2	0.8	48	0	.73	4.8	1.11	.65	292	243	1.08	.128	810
lean, braised	248	54.3	32.3	0.0	0.0	0.0	2	0	.36	.41	5	102	8	22	4.97	.017
3.5 oz	100	12.2	4.2	5.8	1.2	114	8	.60	5.9	.71	.67	405	226	1.95	.161	810
lean, roasted	228	60.3	26.7	0.0	0.0	0.0	2	0	.36	.41	5	80	9	20	4.07	.041
3.5 oz	100	12.6	4.3	6.0	1.2	95	7	.58	4.3	.78	.59	351	247	1.42	.128	810
sep lean & fat, braised	329	47.6	28.0	0.0	0.0	0.0	3	0	.31	.35	4	88	18	19	4.18	.014
3.5 oz	100	23.2	8.5	10.4	2.3	109	9	.54	5.2	.65	.59	369	212	1.61	.138	810
sep lean & fat, roasted	317	52.0	23.5	0.0	0.0	0.0	2	0	.30	.35	4	70	19	17	3.45	.033
3.5 oz	100	24.0	8.8	10.7	2.4	94	8	.52	3.9	.71	.53	325	228	1.18	.111	810
bacon bits, Oscar Mayer	24	2.0	2.8	0.2	0.2	0.0	0	0				221	2	4	.34	
.25 oz	7	1.4	0.5	0.7	0.2	6	0					39	43	.19	.030	I
bacon, canadian style, grilled	87	29.0	11.4	0.6		0.0	0	0	.09	.21	2	727	5	10	.80	.013
2 slices	47	4.0	1.3	1.9	0.4	27	0	.39	3.3	.37	.24	183	139	.39	.025	810
bacon, canadian style, unheated	89	38.2	11.8	1.0		0.0	0	0	.10	.22	2	803	5	10	.79	.013
2 slices	57	4.0	1.3	1.8	0.4	28	0	.43	3.6	.38	.30	196	139	.39	.026	810
bacon, cured																
broiled/pan fried	109	2.5	5.8	0.1		0.0	0	0	.05	.05	1	303	2	5	.62	.008
3 med slices	19	9.4	3.3	4.5	1.1	16	0	.13	1.4	.33	.20	92	64	.31	.032	810
broiled/pan fried	732	16.4	38.7	0.7		0.0	0	0	.36	.34	6	2027	15	30	4.14	.052
4.48 oz (yield from 1 lb raw)	127	62.5	22.1	30.1	7.4	108	0	.88	9.3	2.22	1.34	617	427	2.04	.216	810
center cut, ckd, Oscar Mayer	62	2.1	3.8	0.2	0.2	0.0	0	0				266	1	4	.43	
2 slices	12	5.1	1.9	2.6	0.6	13	0					63	51	.22	.030	I
ckd, Oscar Mayer	70	2.8	4.4	0.1	0.1	0.0	0	0				290	3	7	.48	
2 slices	14	5.8	2.0	2.9	0.7	15	0					74	62	.23	.050	I
lower sodium, ckd, Oscar Mayer	72	2.8	4.3	0.1	0.1	0.0	0	0				175	2	6	.43	
2 slices	14	6.1	2.4	2.9	0.6	12	0					164	52	.20	.050	I
raw	378	21.5	5.9	0.1		0.0	0	0	.07	.10	1	496	5	6	.78	.005
3 med slices	68	39.1	14.5	17.9	4.6	46	0	.25	1.9	.63	.24	104	97	.41	.044	810
thick sliced, ckd, Oscar Mayer	60	2.4	3.8	0.0	0.0	0.0	0	0				249	2	6	.42	
1 slices	12	5.0	1.7	2.5	0.6	12	0					63	53	.20	.040	I
blade roll, cured, sep lean & fat, roasted	287	56.2	17.3	0.4		0.0	0	3	.28	.21	3	973	7	13	2.45	.023
3.5 oz	100	23.5	8.4	11.0	2.5	67	0	.46	2.4	1.05	.77	194	156	.89	.076	810
boston blade (steaks/roasts)																
lean & fat, braised	319	48.4	28.7	0.0	0.0	0.0	3	0	.36	.27	2	70	32	18	5.02	.014
3.5 oz	100	21.7	7.9	9.6	2.0	113	10	.67	4.1	.91	.78	389	179	1.83	.151	810

	KCAL	H₂O (g)	PRO (g)	CHO (g)	SUGR (g)	DFIB (g)	A (RE)	C (mg)	B-2 (mg)	B-6 (mg)	FOL (mcg)	Na (mg)	Ca (mg)	Mg (mg)	Zn (mg)	Mn (mg)
	WT (g)	FAT (g)	SFA (g)	MUFA (g)	PUFA (g)	CHOL (mg)	A (IU)	B-1 (mg)	NIA (mg)	B-12 (mcg)	PANT (mg)	K (mg)	P (mg)	Fe (mg)	Cu (mg)	REF
lean & fat, broiled	259	57.3	25.6	0.0	0.0	0.0	3	0	.40	.28	4	69	36	21	4.51	.003
3.5 oz	100	16.6	6.0	7.4	1.5	95	9	.69	4.1	1.06	.73	326	210	1.40	.058	810
lean & fat, roasted	269	57.5	23.1	0.0	0.0	0.0	2	1	.35	.23	5	67	28	18	3.96	.012
3.5 oz	100	18.9	7.0	8.3	1.8	86	7	.64	4.1	.88	.67	332	197	1.45	.114	810
lean, braised	273	52.0	31.1	0.0	0.0	0.0	3	0	.40	.29	2	75	29	20	5.57	.016
3.5 oz	100	15.6	5.5	7.0	1.3	116	9	.72	4.3	.98	.85	412	182	2.05	.165	810
lean, broiled	227	60.1	26.7	0.0	0.0	0.0	2	0	.44	.31	5	74	33	24	5.02	.009
3.5 oz	100	12.5	4.5	5.6	1.1	94	8	.75	4.3	1.13	.82	343	220	1.56	.059	810
lean, roasted	232	60.9	24.2	0.0	0.0	0.0	3	1	.40	.44	8	88	27	26	4.23	.015
3.5 oz	100	14.3	5.2	6.3	1.3	85	9	1.12	5.0	1.16	1.08	427	235	1.56	.121	810
breakfast strips, ckd	156	9.2	9.8	0.4		0.0	0	0	.13	.12	1	714	5	9	1.25	.015
3 slices	34	12.5	4.3	5.6	1.9	36	0	.25	2.6	.60	.31	158	90	.67	.052	810
center loin (loin chops/roasts), sep lean																
braised	202	61.4	29.8	0.0	0.0	0.0	2	1	.23	.40	3	62	23	20	2.26	.016
3.5 oz	100	8.3	3.1	3.7	0.6	85	7	.82	4.9	.51	.75	367	181	1.13	.076	810
broiled	202	61.1	30.2	0.0	0.0	0.0	2	0	.31	.47	6	60	31	27	2.38	.011
3.5 oz	100	8.1	3.0	3.6	0.6	82	8	1.15	5.5	.74	.69	375	241	.85	.045	810
pan fried	232	56.8	32.2	0.0	0.0	0.0	2	1	.33	.51	6	86	23	32	2.44	.012
3.5 oz	100	10.5	3.6	4.5	1.3	92	8	1.24	6.0	.76	1.00	449	271	.98	.078	810
roasted	199	63.0	27.6	0.0	0.0	0.0	2	1	.27	.37	4	66	25	22	2.09	.016
3.5 oz	100	9.0	3.3	4.0	0.7	79	7	.91	5.5	.58	.69	362	219	1.04	.070	810
center loin (loin chops/roasts), sep lean & fat																
braised	247	57.4	27.9	0.0	0.0	0.0	2	1	.21	.37	3	59	26	19	2.16	.015
3.5 oz	100	14.2	5.3	6.2	1.2	86	8	.77	4.6	.50	.70	353	179	1.05	.073	810
broiled	240	57.6	28.7	0.0	0.0	0.0	3	0	.29	.43	6	58	33	25	2.26	.003
3.5 oz	100	13.1	4.8	5.9	1.0	82	9	1.07	5.2	.73	.64	358	232	.80	.046	810
pan fried	277	53.0	29.9	0.0	0.0	0.0	2	1	.30	.47	6	80	27	29	2.31	.011
3.5 oz	100	16.6	6.0	7.1	1.9	92	8	1.14	5.6	.73	.92	425	259	.91	.075	810
roasted	234	59.8	26.3	0.0	0.0	0.0	2	1	.25	.35	4	63	27	20	2.02	.015
3.5 oz	100	13.5	5.1	5.9	1.2	80	7	.86	5.2	.57	.66	352	215	.99	.068	810
center rib (rib chops/roasts), sep lean																
braised	211	62.3	27.9	0.0	0.0	0.0	2	0	.26	.33	4	41	5	19	2.16	.010
3.5 oz	100	10.1	4.0	4.8	0.7	71	6	.55	4.5	.44	.64	405	173	.99	.074	810
broiled	216	57.0	29.5	0.0	0.0	0.0	2	0	.32	.40	9	65	31	28	2.38	.020
3.5 oz	100	10.1	3.6	4.6	0.6	81	6	.89	5.2	.70	.75	420	245	.82	.070	810
pan fried	224	60.9	27.7	0.0	0.0	0.0	2	0	.34	.39	8	52	5	27	2.14	.007
3.5 oz	100	11.8	4.3	5.3	1.5	70	6	.76	5.1	.61	.78	454	237	.78	.069	810
roasted	214	60.6	28.8	0.0	0.0	0.0	2	0	.31	.40	9	50	6	24	2.83	.011
3.5 oz	100	10.1	3.5	4.5	0.8	83	8	.64	5.4	.55	.58	363	222	1.00	.012	810
center rib (rib chops/roasts), sep lean & fat																
braised	255	58.1	26.3	0.0	0.0	0.0	2	0	.24	.31	4	40	5	17	2.07	.009
3.5 oz	100	15.8	6.1	7.2	1.3	73	7	.53	4.3	.44	.60	387	172	.92	.071	810
broiled	260	53.4	27.6	0.0	0.0	0.0	2	0	.30	.37	8	62	28	26	2.26	.018
3.5 oz	100	15.8	5.8	7.0	1.2	82	7	.83	4.9	.67	.70	401	237	.77	.068	810
pan fried	224	60.9	27.7	0.0	0.0	0.0	2	0	.34	.39	8	52	5	27	2.14	.007
3.5 oz	100	11.8	4.3	5.3	1.5	70	6	.76	5.1	.61	.78	454	237	.78	.069	810
roasted	252	57.3	27.0	0.0	0.0	0.0	3	0	.29	.36	8	48	6	22	2.64	.010
3.5 oz	100	15.2	5.3	6.7	1.3	81	9	.60	5.0	.56	.53	346	214	.93	.016	810
ham, cured (fully cooked as purchased)																
lean (4-5% fat), roasted	145	67.7	20.9	1.5		0.0	0	0	.20	.40	3	1203	8	14	2.88	.054
3.5 oz	100	5.5	1.8	2.6	0.5	53	0	.75	4.0	.65	.40	287	196	1.48	.079	810
lean (4-5% fat), cnd	120	73.5	18.5	0.0	0.0	0.0	0	0	.23	.45	6	1255	6	17	1.93	.025
3.5 oz	100	4.6	1.5	2.2	0.4	38	0	.84	5.3	.82	.49	364	224	.94	.084	810
lean (4-5% fat), cnd, roasted	136	69.5	21.2	0.5		0.0	0	0	.25	.45	5	1135	6	21	2.23	.024
3.5 oz	100	4.9	1.6	2.5	0.4	30	0	1.03	4.9	.71	.57	348	209	.92	.050	810
patties, grilled	205	30.8	8.0	1.0		0.0	0	0	.11	.10	2	638	5	6	1.14	.013
1 patty	60	18.5	6.7	8.8	2.0	43	0	.21	1.9	.42	.16	146	61	.97	.060	810

	KCAL	H₂O (g)	PRO (g)	CHO (g)	SUGR (g)	DFIB (g)	A (RE)	C (mg)	B-2 (mg)	B-6 (mg)	FOL (mcg)	Na (mg)	Ca (mg)	Mg (mg)	Zn (mg)	Mn (mg)
	WT (g)	FAT (g)	SFA (g)	MUFA (g)	PUFA (g)	CHOL (mg)	A (IU)	B-1 (mg)	NIA (mg)	B-12 (mcg)	PANT (mg)	K (mg)	P (mg)	Fe (mg)	Cu (mg)	REF
patties, unheated	205	35.4	8.3	1.1		0.0	0	0	.10	.10	2	707	5	7	1.02	.015
1 patty	65	18.3	6.6	8.6	2.0	46	0	.30	2.0	.70	.20	155	97	.68	.046	810
reg (11-13% fat), roasted	178	64.5	22.6	0.0	0.0	0.0	0	0	.33	.31	3	1500	8	22	2.47	.041
3.5 oz	100	9.0	3.1	4.4	1.4	59	0	.73	6.2	.70	.72	409	281	1.34	.145	810
reg (11-13% fat), cnd	190	66.5	17.0	0.0		0.0	0	0	.23	.48	5	1240	6	14	1.66	.023
3.5 oz	100	13.0	4.3	6.2	1.5	39	0	.96	3.2	.78	.39	316	175	.83	.067	810
reg (11-13% fat), cnd, roasted	226	60.9	20.5	0.4		0.0	0	14	.26	.30	5	941	8	17	2.50	.029
3.5 oz	100	15.2	5.0	7.1	1.8	62	0	.82	5.3	1.06	.73	357	243	1.37	.130	810
reg (11-13% fat), center slice, sep lean & fat, unheated—3.5 oz	203	63.5	20.2	0.1		0.0	0	0	.20	.47	4	1386	7	16	1.88	.031
	100	12.9	4.6	6.1	1.4	54	0	.84	4.8	.80	.50	337	215	.75	.074	810
steak, extra lean, ckd	122	72.2	19.6	0.0	0.0	0.0	0	32	.20	.37	4	1269	4	19	2.02	.037
3.5 oz	100	4.3	1.4	2.0	0.5	45	0	.80	5.1	.79	.62	325	260	1.00	.080	810
whole, sep lean & fat, roasted	243	58.4	21.6	0.0	0.0	0.0	0	0	.22	.38	3	1187	7	19	2.32	.014
3.5 oz	100	16.8	6.0	7.9	1.8	62	0	.60	4.5	.64	.46	286	214	.87	.083	810
whole, sep lean & fat, unheated	246	59.7	18.5	0.1		0.0	0		.19	.41	4	1284	7	15	1.76	.028
3.5 oz	100	18.5	6.6	8.7	1.6	56	0	.78	4.5	.74	.47	310	201	.71	.071	810
whole, sep lean, roasted	157	65.8	25.1	0.0	0.0	0.0	0	0	.25	.47	4	1327	7	22	2.57	.016
3.5 oz	100	5.5	1.8	2.5	0.6	55	0	.68	5.0	.70	.50	316	227	.94	.087	810
whole, sep lean, unheated	147	68.3	22.3	0.1		0.0	0	0	.23	.53	4	1516	7	18	2.04	.035
3.5 oz	100	5.7	1.9	2.6	0.7	52	0	.93	5.3	.87	.54	371	232	.81	.079	810
leg, sep lean & fat, roasted	273	55.0	26.8	0.0	0.0	0.0	3	0	.31	.40	10	60	14	22	2.96	.032
3.5 oz	100	17.6	6.5	7.9	1.7	94	10	.64	4.6	.68	.62	352	263	1.01	.100	810
leg, sep lean, roasted	211	60.7	29.4	0.0	0.0	0.0	3	0	.35	.45	12	64	7	25	3.26	.037
3.5 oz	100	9.4	3.3	4.5	0.8	94	9	.69	4.9	.72	.67	373	281	1.12	.108	810
loin blade (chops & roasts), sep lean																
braised	225	61.0	25.0	0.0	0.0	0.0	2	1	.27	.35	3	62	24	18	3.91	.014
3.5 oz	100	13.1	4.7	5.7	1.0	83	7	.53	3.9	.71	.64	326	161	1.35	.096	810
broiled	234	59.9	25.4	0.0	0.0	0.0	2	1	.35	.45	4	80	23	26	3.97	.009
3.5 oz	100	13.9	5.1	6.0	1.1	84	7	.74	4.6	.94	.70	374	226	1.09	.092	810
pan fried	241	59.3	24.7	0.0	0.0	0.0	2	1	.36	.41	4	78	22	26	3.87	.009
3.5 oz	100	15.1	5.2	6.3	1.9	82	7	.73	4.4	.97	.78	365	221	1.07	.090	810
roasted	247	58.2	26.6	0.0	0.0	0.0	2	0	.34	.44	5	29	29	24	3.81	.013
3.5 oz	100	14.8	5.3	6.5	1.1	93	8	.57	4.7	.80	.53	349	221	1.29	.086	810
loin blade (chops & roasts), sep lean & fat																
braised	323	51.8	21.9	0.0	0.0	0.0	2	1	.23	.30	2	55	31	15	3.27	.011
3.5 oz	100	25.4	9.5	10.9	2.3	85	8	.48	3.6	.65	.56	304	162	1.11	.085	810
broiled	320	51.8	22.5	0.0	0.0	0.0	2	1	.30	.38	4	70	29	22	3.37	.008
3.5 oz	100	24.9	9.3	10.7	2.3	86	8	.65	4.1	.83	.61	344	212	.93	.083	810
pan fried	342	50.0	21.5	0.0	0.0	0.0	3	1	.29	.34	4	67	30	21	3.19	.008
3.5 oz	100	27.7	10.2	11.7	3.1	85	8	.62	3.9	.84	.66	332	206	.88	.080	810
roasted	323	51.2	23.7	0.0	0.0	0.0	3	0	.30	.38	4	30	34	20	3.30	.011
3.5 oz	100	24.6	9.2	10.6	2.2	93	9	.52	4.2	.73	.49	326	210	1.11	.079	810
loin, sep lean																
braised	204	61.4	28.6	0.0	0.0	0.0	2	1	.27	.39	4	50	18	20	2.48	.013
3.5 oz	100	9.1	3.4	4.2	0.7	79	7	.66	4.6	.55	.68	387	183	1.13	.079	810
broiled	210	60.7	28.6	0.0	0.0	0.0	2	1	.34	.49	6	64	17	29	2.48	.009
3.5 oz	100	9.8	3.6	4.5	0.8	79	7	.92	5.2	.72	.73	438	253	.91	.075	810
roasted	209	61.0	28.6	0.0	0.0	0.0	2	1	.33	.55	7	58	18	28	2.53	.016
3.5 oz	100	9.6	3.5	4.3	0.8	81	8	1.02	5.9	.73	.78	425	249	1.09	.059	810
loin, sep lean & fat																
braised	239	58.3	27.2	0.0	0.0	0.0	2	1	.25	.37	3	48	21	19	2.38	.012
3.5 oz	100	13.6	5.1	6.1	1.2	80	7	.63	4.4	.54	.65	374	181	1.07	.077	810
broiled	242	57.9	27.3	0.0	0.0	0.0	2	1	.32	.46	5	62	19	28	2.39	.009
3.5 oz	100	13.9	5.2	6.2	1.2	80	7	.88	5.0	.70	.70	423	246	.87	.073	810
roasted	248	57.5	27.1	0.0	0.0	0.0	3	1	.31	.52	6	59	19	26	2.32	.011
3.5 oz	100	14.7	5.4	6.5	1.2	82	9	.99	5.6	.71	.76	408	242	.99	.056	810
rump, sep lean & fat, roasted	252	56.8	28.9	0.0	0.0	0.0	3	0	.33	.32	3	62	12	27	2.82	.023
3.5 oz	100	14.3	5.3	6.4	1.4	96	9	.75	4.7	.72	.62	374	272	1.05	.103	810

	KCAL / WT (g)	H₂O (g) / FAT (g)	PRO (g) / SFA (g)	CHO (g) / MUFA (g)	SUGR (g) / PUFA (g)	DFIB (g) / CHOL (mg)	A (RE) / A (IU)	C (mg) / B-1 (mg)	B-2 (mg) / NIA (mg)	B-6 (mg) / B-12 (mcg)	FOL (mcg) / PANT (mg)	Na (mg) / K (mg)	Ca (mg) / P (mg)	Mg (mg) / Fe (mg)	Zn (mg) / Cu (mg)	Mn (mg) / REF
rump, sep lean, roasted	206	61.0	30.9	0.0	0.0	0.0	3	0	.36	.34	3	65	7	29	3.01	.026
3.5 oz	100	8.1	2.9	3.8	0.8	96	9	.80	4.9	.75	.66	391	285	1.14	.109	810
sausage																
fresh, ckd	48	5.8	2.6	0.1	0.3	0.0	0	0	.03	.04	0	168	4	2	.33	.009
1 link	13	4.1	1.4	1.8	0.5	11	0	.10	0.6	.22	.09	47	24	.16	.018	810
fresh, ckd	100	12.0	5.3	0.3		0.0	0	1	.07	.09	1	349	9	5	.68	.019
1 patty	27	8.4	2.9	3.8	1.0	22	0	.20	1.2	.47	.19	97	50	.34	.038	810
fresh, w/ beef, ckd	51	5.8	1.8	0.4		0.0	0	0	.02	.01	0	105	1	2	.24	.005
1 link	13	4.7	1.7	2.2	0.5	9	0	.05	0.4	.06	.06	25	14	.15	.005	807
Little Friers, ckd, Oscar Mayer	165	23.8	7.8	0.5	0.4	0.0	0	0				401	8	9	1.25	
2 links	48	14.6	5.1	7.1	1.8	37	0					114	76	.83	.150	I
shank, sep lean & fat, roasted	289	53.8	25.3	0.0	0.0	0.0	3	0	.30	.40	5	59	15	22	3.06	.028
3.5 oz	100	20.1	7.4	9.0	1.9	92	9	.58	4.5	.66	.62	338	257	.98	.098	810
shank, sep lean, roasted	215	60.4	28.2	0.0	0.0	0.0	2	0	.34	.46	6	64	7	25	3.45	.034
3.5 oz	100	10.5	3.6	5.0	0.9	92	8	.63	4.9	.71	.69	360	278	1.11	.108	810
shoulder, sep lean & fat, roasted	292	54.8	23.3	0.0	0.0	0.0	2	1	.33	.29	5	68	24	18	3.71	.022
3.5 oz	100	21.4	7.9	9.5	2.0	90	8	.58	4.0	.80	.60	329	212	1.32	.113	810
shoulder, sep lean, roasted	230	60.6	25.3	0.0	0.0	0.0	2	1	.37	.32	5	75	18	20	4.16	.026
3.5 oz	100	13.5	4.8	6.2	1.3	90	7	.63	4.3	.86	.65	346	221	1.50	.124	810
sirloin (chops & roasts), sep lean																
braised	175	64.9	27.0	0.0	0.0	0.0	2	1	.28	.44	3	46	13	22	2.37	.014
3.5 oz	100	6.6	2.3	2.9	0.6	81	7	.70	4.0	.57	.69	356	182	1.11	.089	810
broiled	193	61.4	31.1	0.0	0.0	0.0	2	0	.40	.54	6	56	18	27	2.66	.010
3.5 oz	100	6.7	2.2	2.9	0.5	92	8	1.03	4.8	.84	.91	377	246	1.24	.053	810
roasted	198	61.3	28.9	0.0	0.0	0.0	2	1	.38	.47	5	56	17	27	2.53	.016
3.5 oz	100	8.3	3.0	3.6	0.7	86	7	.89	5.1	.76	.74	405	254	1.19	.095	810
sirloin (chops & roasts), sep lean & fat																
braised	189	63.6	26.5	0.0	0.0	0.0	2	1	.28	.43	3	46	13	21	2.34	.014
3.5 oz	100	8.4	3.0	3.7	0.8	81	7	.69	3.9	.57	.68	352	181	1.09	.088	810
broiled	208	60.1	30.5	0.0	0.0	0.0	2	0	.39	.53	6	56	18	27	2.62	.003
3.5 oz	100	8.6	2.9	3.8	0.7	91	8	1.01	4.7	.83	.88	372	243	1.21	.053	810
roasted	207	60.5	28.5	0.0	0.0	0.0	2	1	.37	.47	5	56	16	26	2.51	.016
3.5 oz	100	9.4	3.4	4.1	0.8	86	7	.88	5.1	.75	.73	402	252	1.17	.094	810
spareribs, sep lean & fat, braised	296	53.8	23.9	0.0	0.0	0.0	2	1	.26	.33	3	59	29	17	3.56	.012
3.5 oz	100	21.5	8.0	9.3	1.9	87	8	.51	3.8	.69	.61	328	167	1.22	.093	810
tenderloin, sep lean & fat, roasted	173	65.4	27.8	0.0	0.0	0.0	2	0	.38	.41	6	55	6	27	2.60	.038
3.5 oz	100	6.0	2.1	2.5	0.5	79	7	.93	4.7	.55	.68	433	257	1.45	.048	810
tenderloin, sep lean, roasted	164	66.3	28.1	0.0	0.0	0.0	2	0	.39	.42	6	56	6	28	2.63	.039
3.5 oz	100	4.8	1.7	1.9	0.4	79	7	.94	4.7	.55	.69	437	259	1.47	.048	810
top loin (chops & roasts), sep lean																
braised	202	61.0	29.1	0.0	0.0	0.0	2	0	.27	.34	5	42	23	20	2.18	.011
3.5 oz	100	8.6	3.1	4.0	0.6	73	6	.57	4.7	.46	.66	421	186	1.01	.078	810
broiled	203	60.7	31.1	0.0	0.0	0.0	2	0	.32	.40	9	65	31	28	2.38	.020
3.5 oz	100	7.8	2.7	3.6	0.5	80	6	.89	5.2	.70	.75	420	245	.82	.070	810
pan fried	225	57.6	30.5	0.0	0.0	0.0	2	0	.38	.43	8	57	22	30	2.29	.008
3.5 oz	100	10.5	3.6	4.6	1.3	77	6	.84	5.6	.67	.86	500	271	.85	.077	810
roasted	194	62.2	30.2	0.0	0.0	0.0	2	0	.31	.40	9	45	5	25	2.31	.011
3.5 oz	100	7.2	2.6	3.4	0.5	78	8	.64	5.4	.55	.58	354	221	1.06	.016	810
top loin (chops & roasts), sep lean & fat																
braised	233	58.2	27.8	0.0	0.0	0.0	2	0	.26	.33	4	42	21	19	2.11	.010
3.5 oz	100	12.7	4.7	5.7	1.0	75	7	.55	4.5	.46	.64	407	185	.96	.076	810
broiled	229	58.4	30.0	0.0	0.0	0.0	2	0	.31	.38	8	63	29	27	2.29	.003
3.5 oz	100	11.2	4.0	5.2	0.7	81	6	.85	5.0	.69	.70	405	238	.79	.069	810
pan fried	257	54.8	29.0	0.0	0.0	0.0	2	0	.35	.40	8	55	21	28	2.20	.007
3.5 oz	100	14.8	5.3	6.5	1.7	78	7	.80	5.4	.65	.81	479	262	.81	.075	810
roasted	226	59.2	28.8	0.0	0.0	0.0	3	0	.30	.37	8	44	5	23	2.21	.003
3.5 oz	100	11.4	4.2	5.3	0.8	78	8	.61	5.1	.55	.55	342	215	.80	.019	810

	KCAL	H₂O (g)	PRO (g)	CHO (g)	SUGR (g)	DFIB (g)	A (RE)	C (mg)	B-2 (mg)	B-6 (mg)	FOL (mcg)	Na (mg)	Ca (mg)	Mg (mg)	Zn (mg)	Mn (mg)
	WT (g)	FAT (g)	SFA (g)	MUFA (g)	PUFA (g)	CHOL (mg)	A (IU)	B-1 (mg)	NIA (mg)	B-12 (mcg)	PANT (mg)	K (mg)	P (mg)	Fe (mg)	Cu (mg)	REF

21.5 VEAL

ground, broiled	172	66.8	24.4	0.0	0.0	0.0	0	0	.27	.39	11	83	17	24	3.87	.035
3.5 oz	100	7.6	3.0	2.8	0.6	103	0	.07	8.0	1.27	1.16	337	217	.99	.103	817
leg & shoulder, cubed for stew, sep lean, braised—3.5 oz	188	59.3	34.9	0.0	0.0	0.0	0	0	.40	.38	16	93	29	28	6.01	.040
	100	4.3	1.3	1.4	0.5	145	0	.07	8.3	1.67	1.19	342	239	1.44	.153	817
leg (top round), sep lean																
braised	203	56.2	36.7	0.0	0.0	0.0	0	0	.36	.37	18	67	9	30	4.03	.040
3.5 oz	100	5.1	1.9	1.8	0.4	135	0	.06	10.7	1.19	1.04	387	252	1.32	.142	817
pan fried, breaded	206	53.1	28.4	9.8		0.2	10	0	.36	.42	20	455	39	32	2.87	.137
3.5 oz	100	6.3	1.6	2.2	1.4	113	34	.16	10.8	1.28	1.11	383	258	1.64	.074	817
pan fried, not breaded	183	60.7	33.2	0.0	0.0	0.0	0	0	.37	.51	16	77	7	32	3.38	.032
3.5 oz	100	4.6	1.3	1.6	0.4	107	0	.07	12.6	1.51	1.22	442	290	.87	.063	817
roasted	150	67.0	28.1	0.0	0.0	0.0	0	0	.33	.31	16	68	6	28	3.08	.031
3.5 oz	100	3.4	1.2	1.2	0.3	103	0	.06	10.1	1.18	1.00	393	236	.90	.130	817
leg (top round), sep lean & fat																
braised	211	55.5	36.2	0.0	0.0	0.0	0	0	.35	.36	18	67	8	29	3.96	.039
3.5 oz	100	6.3	2.5	2.4	0.5	134	0	.06	10.6	1.17	1.02	383	249	1.32	.140	817
pan fried, breaded	228	51.3	27.3	9.8		0.3	10	0	.35	.40	19	454	39	31	2.75	.135
3.5 oz	100	9.2	3.1	3.4	1.5	112	34	.16	10.3	1.24	1.07	371	250	1.64	.073	817
pan fried, not breaded	211	58.3	31.8	0.0	0.0	0.0	0	0	.35	.49	15	76	6	31	3.23	.031
3.5 oz	100	8.3	3.2	3.2	0.6	105	0	.07	12.1	1.45	1.17	425	279	.88	.062	817
roasted	160	66.1	27.7	0.0	0.0	0.0	0	0	.32	.31	16	68	6	28	3.04	.030
3.5 oz	100	4.7	1.8	1.7	0.3	103	0	.06	9.9	1.17	.99	389	234	.91	.129	817
loin																
sep lean & fat, braised	284	52.0	30.2	0.0	0.0	0.0	0	0	.30	.26	14	80	28	24	3.63	.034
3.5 oz	100	17.2	6.7	6.7	1.2	118	0	.04	9.0	1.21	.79	280	220	1.09	.091	817
sep lean & fat, roasted	217	60.7	24.8	0.0	0.0	0.0	0	0	.28	.34	15	93	19	25	3.03	.029
3.5 oz	100	12.3	5.3	4.8	0.8	103	0	.05	8.9	1.24	1.20	325	212	.87	.110	817
sep lean, braised	226	57.0	33.6	0.0	0.0	0.0	0	0	.34	.28	15	84	32	27	4.09	.038
3.5 oz	100	9.2	2.5	3.3	0.8	125	0	.05	10.1	1.32	.85	297	237	1.10	.099	817
sep lean, roasted	175	64.6	26.3	0.0	0.0	0.0	0	0	.30	.37	16	96	21	26	3.24	.030
3.5 oz	100	6.9	2.6	2.5	0.6	106	0	.06	9.5	1.31	1.27	340	222	.85	.117	817
rib																
sep lean & fat, braised	251	53.3	32.4	0.0	0.0	0.0	0	0	.29	.32	16	95	22	25	5.57	.038
3.5 oz	100	12.5	5.0	4.7	0.9	139	0	.05	7.5	1.45	1.07	306	210	1.41	.132	817
sep lean & fat, roasted	228	59.9	24.0	0.0	0.0	0.0	0	0	.27	.25	13	92	11	22	4.09	.030
3.5 oz	100	14.0	5.4	5.4	0.9	110	0	.05	7.0	1.46	1.28	295	197	.97	.099	817
sep lean, braised	218	56.1	34.4	0.0	0.0	0.0	0	0	.31	.34	16	99	24	26	5.98	.040
3.5 oz	100	7.8	2.6	2.6	0.7	144	0	.06	7.9	1.53	1.13	318	218	1.45	.140	817
sep lean, roasted	177	64.6	25.8	0.0	0.0	0.0	0	0	.29	.27	14	97	12	24	4.49	.032
3.5 oz	100	7.4	2.1	2.7	0.7	115	0	.06	7.5	1.58	1.38	311	207	.96	.106	817
shoulder, arm																
sep lean & fat, braised	236	55.3	33.6	0.0	0.0	0.0	0	0	.31	.29	18	87	28	29	5.81	.036
3.5 oz	100	10.2	4.0	4.0	0.7	148	0	.06	10.1	1.72	1.31	333	263	1.38	.128	817
sep lean & fat, roasted	183	64.7	25.5	0.0	0.0	0.0	0	0	.32	.29	17	90	26	26	4.18	.030
3.5 oz	100	8.3	3.5	3.2	0.5	108	0	.06	8.0	1.53	1.16	348	221	1.15	.141	817
sep lean, braised	201	58.2	35.7	0.0	0.0	0.0	0	0	.33	.30	19	90	30	30	6.24	.038
3.5 oz	100	5.3	1.5	1.9	0.5	155	0	.06	10.7	1.82	1.39	347	276	1.41	.135	817
sep lean, roasted	164	66.5	26.1	0.0	0.0	0.0	0	0	.33	.30	17	91	27	27	4.32	.030
3.5 oz	100	5.8	2.3	2.2	0.4	109	0	.07	8.2	1.57	1.19	356	226	1.16	.146	817
shoulder, blade																
sep lean & fat, braised	225	57.0	31.3	0.0	0.0	0.0	0	0	.35	.24	15	98	38	26	7.00	.036
3.5 oz	100	10.1	3.6	3.9	0.7	153	0	.06	5.5	1.93	1.52	297	244	1.44	.164	817

	KCAL	H₂O (g)	PRO (g)	CHO (g)	SUGR (g)	DFIB (g)	A (RE)	C (mg)	B-2 (mg)	B-6 (mg)	FOL (mcg)	Na (mg)	Ca (mg)	Mg (mg)	Zn (mg)	Mn (mg)
	WT (g)	FAT (g)	SFA (g)	MUFA (g)	PUFA (g)	CHOL (mg)	A (IU)	B-1 (mg)	NIA (mg)	B-12 (mcg)	PANT (mg)	K (mg)	P (mg)	Fe (mg)	Cu (mg)	REF
sep lean & fat, roasted	186	65.5	25.1	0.0	0.0	0.0	0	0	.35	.24	11	100	28	24	5.58	.030
3.5 oz	100	8.7	3.5	3.2	0.6	117	0	.07	5.7	2.01	1.38	306	212	1.00	.138	817
sep lean, braised	198	59.2	32.7	0.0	0.0	0.0	0	0	.36	.25	15	101	40	28	7.39	.038
3.5 oz	100	6.5	1.8	2.3	0.6	158	0	.06	5.7	2.01	1.59	305	252	1.47	.171	817
sep lean, roasted	171	66.9	25.6	0.0	0.0	0.0	0	0	.36	.24	11	102	28	24	5.72	.030
3.5 oz	100	6.9	2.6	2.5	0.6	119	0	.07	5.8	2.06	1.41	310	215	1.00	.141	817
shoulder, whole (arm & blade)																
sep lean & fat, braised	228	56.4	32.1	0.0	0.0	0.0	0	0	.34	.25	15	95	35	27	6.59	.036
3.5 oz	100	10.1	3.8	3.9	0.7	126	0	.06	6.4	1.84	1.53	309	250	1.42	.151	817
sep lean & fat, roasted	184	65.3	25.3	0.0	0.0	0.0	0	0	.34	.26	12	96	27	25	5.12	.030
3.5 oz	100	8.4	3.4	3.2	0.6	113	0	.07	6.3	1.82	1.30	322	215	1.03	.139	817
sep lean, braised	199	58.9	33.7	0.0	0.0	0.0	0	0	.35	.26	16	97	37	28	7.00	.038
3.5 oz	100	6.1	1.7	2.2	0.6	130	0	.06	6.7	1.94	1.61	319	260	1.45	.159	817
sep lean, roasted	170	66.7	25.8	0.0	0.0	0.0	0	0	.34	.26	13	97	27	25	5.25	.030
3.5 oz	100	6.6	2.5	2.4	0.5	114	0	.07	6.4	1.86	1.32	327	218	1.03	.142	817
sirloin																
sep lean & fat, braised	252	54.5	31.3	0.0	0.0	0.0	0	0	.35	.35	15	79	17	27	4.32	.035
3.5 oz	100	13.1	5.2	5.2	0.9	108	0	.05	6.6	1.48	1.01	321	243	1.20	.128	817
sep lean & fat, roasted	202	62.7	25.1	0.0	0.0	0.0	0	0	.35	.32	15	83	13	26	3.35	.029
3.5 oz	100	10.4	4.5	4.1	0.7	102	0	.06	8.9	1.42	1.26	351	223	.92	.129	817
sep lean, braised	204	58.5	34.0	0.0	0.0	0.0	0	0	.38	.38	16	81	19	29	4.75	.038
3.5 oz	100	6.5	1.8	2.3	0.6	113	0	.06	7.0	1.59	1.08	339	259	1.23	.138	817
sep lean, roasted	168	65.7	26.3	0.0	0.0	0.0	0	0	.37	.34	16	85	14	27	3.54	.030
3.5 oz	100	6.2	2.4	2.3	0.5	104	0	.06	9.3	1.49	1.32	365	231	.91	.136	817

21.6 VARIETY CUTS & INTERNAL ORGANS

	KCAL	H₂O (g)	PRO (g)	CHO (g)	SUGR (g)	DFIB (g)	A (RE)	C (mg)	B-2 (mg)	B-6 (mg)	FOL (mcg)	Na (mg)	Ca (mg)	Mg (mg)	Zn (mg)	Mn (mg)
belly, pork, raw	147	10.4	2.6	0.0	0.0	0.0	1	0	.07	.04	0	9	1	1	.29	.002
1 oz	28	15.0	5.5	7.0	1.6	20	3	.11	1.3	.24	.07	52	31	.15	.015	810
brain																
beef, pan fried	196	70.8	12.6	0.0	0.0	0.0	0	3	.26	.39	6	158	9	15	1.35	.032
3.5 oz	100	15.8	3.7	4.0	2.3	1995	0	.13	3.8	15.20	.57	354	386	2.22	.220	813
beef, simmered	160	73.3	11.1	0.0	0.0	0.0	0	1	.17	.24	7	120	9	14	1.25	.035
3.5 oz	100	12.5	2.9	2.5	1.4	2054	0	.08	2.2	8.60	.57	240	352	2.21	.240	813
lamb, braised	145	75.7	12.6	0.0	0.0	0.0	0	12	.24	.11	5	134	12	14	1.36	.059
3.5 oz	100	10.2	2.6	1.8	1.0	2043	0	.11	2.5	9.25	.99	205	337	1.68	.210	817
lamb, pan fried	273	60.7	17.0	0.0	0.0	0.0	0	23	.37	.23	7	157	21	22	2.00	.067
3.5 oz	100	22.2	5.7	4.0	2.3	2504	0	.17	4.5	24.10	1.56	358	495	2.04	.480	817
pork, braised	138	75.9	12.1	0.0	0.0	0.0	0	14	.22	.14	4	91	9	12	1.48	.085
3.5 oz	100	9.5	2.1	1.7	1.5	2552	0	.08	3.3	1.42	1.82	195	220	1.82	.263	810
pork w/ milk gravy, cnd, Armour Star	150		16.0	10.0	0.0	0.0	0	6				550	0			
⅔ cup	156	5.0	2.5			3500	0							1.80		I
veal, braised	136	76.9	11.5	0.0	0.0	0.0	0	13	.20	.17	3	156	16	16	1.61	.038
3.5 oz	100	9.6	2.2	1.7	1.5	3100	0	.08	2.4	9.65	1.00	214	385	1.67	.260	817
veal, pan fried	213	68.6	14.5	0.0	0.0	0.0	0	15	.36	.33	6	176	10	18	1.82	.044
3.5 oz	100	16.8	4.0	4.2	2.4	2120	0	.15	5.6	21.30	1.13	472	434	1.07	.300	817
chitterlings, pork, simmered	303	62.4	10.3	0.0	0.0	0.0	0	0	.08	.01	3	39	27	10	5.06	.012
3.5 oz	100	28.8	10.1	9.7	7.2	143	0	.00	0.1	1.03	.22	8	47	3.70	.233	810
ears, pork, simmered	184	80.6	17.7	0.2		0.0	0	0	.08	.01	0	185	20	8	.22	.011
1 ear	111	12.0	4.3	5.5	1.3	100	0	.02	0.6	.04	.04	44	27	1.67	.007	810
feet, pork, cured, pickled	203	68.6	13.5	0.0		0.0	0	0	.04	.38	4	923	32	4	1.24	.017
3.5 oz	100	16.1	5.6	7.6	1.8	92	0	.01	0.4	.62	.31	235	34	.62	.050	810
feet, pork, simmered	194	66.0	19.2	0.0	0.0	0.0	0	0	.06	.09	1	30	45	5	1.08	.005
3.5 oz	100	12.4	4.3	5.8	1.4	100	0	.01	0.5	.18	.24	146	48	.47	.044	810
heart																
beef, simmered	175	64.1	28.8	0.4		0.0	0	2	1.54	.21	2	63	6	25	3.13	.059
3.5 oz	100	5.6	1.7	1.3	1.4	193	0	.14	4.1	14.30	.87	233	250	7.51	.740	813
lamb, braised	185	64.2	25.0	1.9		0.0	0	7	1.19	.30	2	63	14	24	3.68	.055
3.5 oz	100	7.9	3.1	2.2	0.8	249	0	.17	4.4	11.20	1.37	188	254	5.52	.610	817

| | KCAL | H_2O (g) | PRO (g) | CHO (g) | SUGR (g) | DFIB (g) | A (RE) | C (mg) | B-2 (mg) | B-6 (mg) | FOL (mcg) | Na (mg) | Ca (mg) | Mg (mg) | Zn (mg) | Mn (mg) |
	WT (g)	FAT (g)	SFA (g)	MUFA (g)	PUFA (g)	CHOL (mcg)	A (IU)	B-1 (mg)	NIA (mg)	B-12 (mcg)	PANT (mg)	K (mg)	P (mg)	Fe (mg)	Cu (mg)	REF
pork, braised	191	87.8	30.4	0.5		0.0	9	3	2.20	.50	5	45	9	31	3.99	.094
1 heart	129	6.5	1.7	1.5	1.7	285	28	.72	7.8	4.89	3.19	266	230	7.52	.655	810
veal, braised	186	62.2	29.1	0.1		0.0	0	10	.93	.21	2	58	8	18	2.24	.061
3.5 oz	100	6.8	1.8	1.4	1.8	176	0	.35	4.9	14.46	1.65	199	250	4.32	.432	817
jowl, pork, raw	655	22.2	6.4	0.0	0.0	0.0	3	0	.24	.09	1	25	4	3	.84	.005
3.5 oz	100	69.6	25.3	32.9	8.1	90	9	.39	4.5	.82	.25	148	86	.42	.040	810
kidneys																
beef, simmered	144	68.8	25.5	1.0		0.0	373	1	4.06	.52	98	134	17	18	4.22	.185
3.5 oz	100	3.4	1.1	0.7	0.7	387	1241	.19	6.0	51.30	1.69	179	306	7.31	.680	813
lamb, braised	137	70.5	23.6	1.0		0.0	137	12	2.07	.12	81	151	18	20	3.80	.144
3.5 oz	100	3.6	1.2	0.8	0.7	565	455	.35	6.0	78.90	2.04	178	290	12.40	.370	817
pork, braised	151	68.7	25.4	0.0	0.0	0.0	78	11	1.59	.46	41	80	13	18	4.15	.149
3.5 oz	100	4.7	1.5	1.6	0.4	480	260	.40	5.8	7.79	2.87	143	240	5.29	.683	810
veal, braised	163	67.7	26.3	0.0	0.0	0.0	201	8	1.99	.18	21	110	29	24	4.25	.127
3.5 oz	100	5.7	1.7	1.2	1.1	791	669	.19	4.6	36.90	.86	159	372	3.04	.360	817
liver																
beef, braised	161	65.9	24.4	3.4		0.0	10602	23	4.10	.91	217	70	7	20	6.07	.413
3.5 oz	100	4.9	1.9	0.7	1.1	389	35679	.20	10.7	71.00	4.57	235	404	6.77	4.512	813
beef, pan fried	217	55.7	26.7	7.8		0.0	10729	23	4.14	1.43	220	106	11	23	5.45	.423
3.5 oz	100	8.0	2.7	1.6	1.7	482	36105	.21	14.4	111.80	5.92	364	461	6.28	4.466	813
lamb, braised	220	56.7	30.6	2.5		0.0	7490	4	4.03	.49	73	56	8	22	7.89	.520
3.5 oz	100	8.8	3.4	1.8	1.3	501	24945	.23	12.2	76.50	3.96	221	420	8.28	7.074	817
lamb, pan fried	238	56.2	25.5	3.8		0.0	7806	13	4.59	.95	400	124	9	23	5.63	.594
3.5 oz	100	12.7	4.9	2.6	1.9	493	25998	.35	16.7	85.70	6.33	352	427	10.20	9.830	817
pork, braised	165	64.3	26.0	3.8		0.0	5399	24	2.20	.57	163	49	10	14	6.72	.300
3.5 oz	100	4.4	1.4	0.6	1.1	355	17997	.26	8.4	18.67	4.77	150	241	17.92	.634	810
veal, braised	165	67.3	21.6	2.7		0.0	8049	31	1.94	.49	759	53	7	19	9.52	.112
3.5 oz	100	6.9	2.6	1.5	1.1	561	26883	.13	8.5	36.50	2.28	205	319	2.62	7.951	817
veal, pan fried	245	53.1	29.8	3.9		0.0	5628	22	3.36	.86	320	132	12	26	7.87	.206
3.5 oz	100	11.4	4.2	2.5	1.8	330	18798	.25	16.9	63.95	4.85	438	439	5.23	9.882	817
lungs																
beef, braised	120	76.4	20.4	0.0	0.0	0.0	12	33	.14	.02	8	101	11	10	1.64	.015
3.5 oz	100	3.7	1.3	0.9	0.5	277	39	.04	2.5	2.59	.62	173	178	5.40	.221	813
lamb, braised	113	75.8	19.9	0.0	0.0	0.0	32	28	.14	.06	8	84	12	11	1.93	.016
3.5 oz	100	3.1	1.1	0.8	0.4	284	106	.03	2.4	2.52		127	188	4.57	.234	817
pork, braised	99	80.0	16.6	0.0	0.0	0.0	0	8	.32	.08	2	81	8	12	2.45	.015
3.5 oz	100	3.1	1.1	0.7	0.4	387	0	.08	1.4	2.03	.66	151	186	16.41	.080	810
veal, braised	104	77.6	18.7	0.0	0.0	0.0	0	34	.13	.06	8	56	7	8	1.20	.015
3.5 oz	100	2.6	0.9	0.7	0.4	263	0	.03	2.3	2.38		142	232	3.61	.221	817
pancreas																
beef, braised	271	55.6	27.1	0.0	0.0	0.0	0	20	.48	.18	3	60	16	21	4.60	.208
3.5 oz	100	17.2	5.9	5.9	3.2	262	0	.18	4.0	16.60	4.25	246	453	2.61	.089	813
lamb, braised	234	59.6	22.8	0.0	0.0	0.0	0	20	.21	.05	13	52	12	19	2.68	.043
3.5 oz	100	15.1	6.8	5.5	0.7	400	0	.02	2.6	5.54	.85	291	431	2.12	.083	817
pork, braised	219	60.3	28.5	0.0	0.0	0.0	0	6	.66	.44	5	42	16	23	4.29	.198
3.5 oz	100	10.8	3.7	3.8	2.0	315	0	.09	3.2	17.07	4.74	168	291	2.69	.110	810
veal, braised	256	55.7	29.1	0.0	0.0	0.0	0	6	.51	.19	3	68	18	24	5.20	.235
3.5 oz	100	14.6	5.0	5.0	2.7		0	.19	4.1	17.33		278	512	2.38	.101	817
spleen																
beef, braised	145	70.0	25.1	0.0	0.0	0.0	0	50	.30	.04	4	57	12	19	2.79	.075
3.5 oz	100	4.2	1.4	1.1	0.3	347	0	.05	5.6	5.02	.88	284	305	39.36	.924	813
lamb, braised	156	66.4	26.5	0.0	0.0	0.0	0	26	.32	.08	4	58	13	21	3.94	.062
3.5 oz	100	4.8	1.6	1.3	0.3	385	0	.05	5.9	5.29		248	341	38.67	.139	817
pork, braised	149	66.7	28.2	0.0	0.0	0.0	0	12	.26	.06	4	107	13	15	3.54	.045
3.5 oz	100	3.2	1.1	0.9	0.2	504	0	.14	5.9	2.76	.89	227	283	22.23	.133	810
veal, braised	129	71.3	24.1	0.0	0.0	0.0	0	40	.29	.07	4	58	7	14	1.91	.075
3.5 oz	100	2.9	1.0	0.8	0.2	447	0	.05	5.3	4.82		215	312	7.36	.925	817

	KCAL	H₂O (g)	PRO (g)	CHO (g)	SUGR (g)	DFIB (g)		A (RE)	C (mg)	B-2 (mg)	B-6 (mg)	FOL (mcg)		Na (mg)	Ca (mg)	Mg (mg)	Zn (mg)	Mn (mg)
	WT (g)	FAT (g)	SFA (g)	MUFA (g)	PUFA (g)	CHOL (mg)		A (IU)	B-1 (mg)	NIA (mg)	B-12 (mcg)	PANT (mg)		K (mg)	P (mg)	Fe (mg)	Cu (mg)	REF
stomach, pork, raw	157	73.6	16.5	0.0	0.0	0.0		0	0	.12	.04	2		52	10	9	2.01	.011
3.5 oz	100	9.6	3.4	4.3	1.0	193		0	.09	4.5	.99	.64		201	155	2.18	.365	810
stomach sausage, cnd, Banner	90		9.0	1.0	0.0	0.0		0	0					430	0			
2 oz	56	5.0	3.0			95		0								.72		I
tail, pork, simmered	396	46.7	17.0	0.0	0.0	0.0		0	0	.07	.27	4		25	14	7	1.64	.006
3.5 oz	100	35.8	12.4	16.9	3.9	129		0	.07	1.1	.55	.42		157	47	.79	.067	810
thymus, beef, braised	319	52.8	21.9	0.0	0.0	0.0		0	30	.23	.08	1		116	10	10	2.20	.099
3.5 oz	100	25.0	8.6	8.6	4.7	294		0	.08	1.8	1.51	1.97		433	364	1.49	.043	813
thymus, veal, braised	174	64.5	31.6	0.0	0.0	0.0		0	74	.16	.09	1		66	3	17	3.10	.000
3.5 oz	100	4.3	1.5	1.5	0.8	469		0	.06	2.0	2.18			342	685	2.01	.000	817
tongue																		
beef, simmered	283	56.0	22.1	0.3		0.0		0	1	.35	.16	5		60	7	17	4.80	.026
3.5 oz	100	20.7	8.9	9.5	0.8	107		0	.03	2.1	5.90	.52		180	142	3.39	.220	813
lamb, braised	275	57.9	21.6	0.0	0.0	0.0		0	7	.42	.17	3		67	10	16	2.99	.033
3.5 oz	100	20.3	7.8	10.0	1.3	189		0	.08	3.7	6.30	.34		158	134	2.63	.210	817
pork, braised	271	56.9	24.1	0.0	0.0	0.0		0	2	.51	.23	4		109	19	20	4.53	.010
3.5 oz	100	18.6	6.4	8.8	1.9	146		0	.32	5.3	2.39	.51		237	174	4.99	.110	810
veal, braised	202	64.1	25.9	0.0	0.0	0.0		0	6	.35	.15	9		64	9	18	4.51	.047
3.5 oz	100	10.1	4.3	4.6	0.4	238		0	.07	1.5	5.30	.74		162	166	2.09	.210	817
tripe																		
beef, cnd, Armour Star	90		18.0	0.0	0.0	0.0		0	0					100	0			
3 oz	84	1.5	1.0			125		0								.36		I
beef, raw	98	81.4	14.6	0.0	0.0	0.0		0	3	.17	.04	2		46	9	8	2.47	.010
3.5 oz	100	4.0	2.0	1.3	0.1	95		0	.01	0.1	1.54	.56		270	79	1.95	.090	813
sausage, cnd, Banner	90		9.0	2.0	0.0	0.0		0	0					430	0			
2 oz	56	5.0	3.0			85		0								.72		I

22. MEATS, LUNCHEON

	KCAL	H₂O (g)	PRO (g)	CHO (g)	SUGR (g)	DFIB (g)		A (RE)	C (mg)	B-2 (mg)	B-6 (mg)	FOL (mcg)		Na (mg)	Ca (mg)	Mg (mg)	Zn (mg)	Mn (mg)
beef, chopped, Armour Star	170		7.0	2.0	2.0	0.0		0	0					810	0			
2 oz	56	15.0	7.0			40		0								.72		I
beef, loaved lunch meat	86	14.7	4.0	0.8		0.0		0	0	.06	.05	1		372	3	4	.71	.013
1 oz slice	28	7.3	3.1	3.4	0.2	18		0	.03	1.0	1.09	.15		58	33	.65	.034	807
beef, roast, Oscar Mayer	58	37.7	10.5	0.8	0.2	0.0		0	0					526	3	11	1.76	
4 slices	52	1.5	0.7	0.9	0.1	25		0						170	144	1.00	.070	I
beef, thin sliced lunch meat	37	12.2	5.9	1.2		0.0		0	0	.04	.07	2		302	2	4	.84	.008
5 slices	21	0.8	0.3	0.4	0.0	9		0	.02	1.1	.54	.12		90	35	.57	.007	813
berliner, pork & beef	53	14.0	3.5	0.6		0.0		0	0	.05	.05	1		298	3	3	.57	.009
1 slice	23	4.0	1.4	1.8	0.4	11		0	.09	0.7	.61	.16		65	30	.26	.018	807
blood sausage (blood pudding)	95	11.8	3.7	0.3		0.0		0	0	.03	.01	1		170	2	2	.33	.003
1 slice	25	8.6	3.3	4.0	0.9	30		0	.02	0.3	.25	.15		10	6	1.60	.010	807
bockwurst (pork, veal, milk), raw	200	36.5	8.7	0.3		0.0		4	0	.11	.15	4		718	10	12	1.01	.010
1 link	65	17.9	6.6	8.5	1.9	38		15	.27	2.7	.53	.44		176	95	.42	.039	807
bologna, beef	72	12.7	2.8	0.2	0.5	0.0		0	0	.03	.03	1		226	3	3	.50	.006
1 slice	23	6.6	2.8	3.2	0.3	13		0	.01	0.6	.33	.06		36	20	.38	.007	807
Oscar Mayer	89	15.2	3.1	0.6	0.4	0.0								310	3	4	.57	
1 oz slice	28	8.2	3.6	4.3	0.3	20								47	31	.38	.030	I
Oscar Mayer Light	56	18.2	3.3	1.6	0.6	0.0		0	0					314	4	4	.53	
1 slice	28	4.0	1.6	2.0	0.1	13		0						44	50	.34	.060	I
bologna, beef & pork	73	12.5	2.7	0.6		0.0		0	0	.03	.04	1		234	3	3	.45	.009
1 slice	23	6.5	2.5	3.1	0.6	13		0	.04	0.6	.31	.06		41	21	.35	.018	807
bologna, chicken, pork, & beef, Oscar Mayer—1 oz slice	89	15.0	3.1	0.7	0.4	0.0		0	0					289	19	6	.40	
	28	8.2	2.9	4.0	1.1	29		0						43	56	.50	.060	I
bologna, garlic, Oscar Mayer	130	22.0	4.5	1.0	0.6	0.0		0	0					424	28	9	.58	
1 slice	41	12.1	4.3	5.9	1.9	42		0						63	82	.73	.080	I

	KCAL	H₂O (g)	PRO (g)	CHO (g)	SUGR (g)	DFIB (g)	A (RE)	C (mg)	B-2 (mg)	B-6 (mg)	FOL (mcg)	Na (mg)	Ca (mg)	Mg (mg)	Zn (mg)	Mn (mg)
	WT (g)	FAT (g)	SFA (g)	MUFA (g)	PUFA (g)	CHOL (mg)	A (IU)	B-1 (mg)	NIA (mg)	B-12 (mcg)	PANT (mg)	K (mg)	P (mg)	Fe (mg)	Cu (mg)	REF
bologna, pork	57	13.9	3.5	0.2		0.0	0	0	.04	.06	1	272	3	3	.47	.008
1 slice	23	4.6	1.6	2.2	0.5	14	0	.12	0.9	.21	.17	65	32	.18	.018	807
bologna, pork, chicken, & beef, Oscar Mayer Light—*1 slice*	55	18.2	3.2	1.6	0.7	0.0	0	0				310	14	5	.44	
	28	4.0	1.6	2.1	0.4	16	0					46	52	.38	.060	I
bologna, turkey	56	18.2	3.8	0.3		0.0	0	0	.05	.06	2	246	24	4	.49	.004
1 slice	28	4.3	1.4	1.3	1.2	28	0	.02	1.0	.08	.20	56	37	.43	.008	807
bologna, turkey, beef, & pork, fat-free, Oscar Mayer—*1 slice*	23	21.8	3.5	1.7	0.6	0.0	0	0				274	4	6	.32	
	28	0.2	0.1	0.1	0.0	7	0					44	43	.26	.060	I
bologna, turkey, Louis Rich	52	18.9	3.2	1.3	0.3	0.0	0	0				270	35	6	.52	
1 oz slice	28	3.8	1.1	1.5	1.0	19	0					43	55	.46	.050	I
bologna, Wisconsin Ring, Oscar Mayer	175	30.7	6.7	1.5	1.2	0.0	0	0				463	9	8	1.04	
2 oz	56	15.8	6.2	7.9	1.1	35	0					78	59	.65	.070	I
bratwurst, pork, ckd	256	47.7	12.0	1.8		0.0	0	1	.16	.18	2	473	37	13	1.95	.039
1 link	85	22.0	7.9	10.4	2.3	51	0	.43	2.7	.81	.27	180	127	1.10	.076	810
braunschweiger (pork liver sausage)	65	8.6	2.4	0.6		0.0	760	0	.27	.06	8	206	2	2	.51	.028
1 slice	18	5.8	2.0	2.7	0.7	28	2529	.04	1.5	3.62	.61	36	30	1.68	.043	807
in tube, Oscar Mayer	190	27.8	8.0	1.3	0.4	0.0		5				626	5	7	1.77	
2 oz	56	17.0	6.1	8.7	2.1	90	9335					103	109	5.45	.220	I
Oscar Mayer	94	14.1	3.9	0.6	0.3	0.0		3				324	3	4	.95	
1 oz slice	28	8.4	3.1	4.3	1.0	49	4404					57	56	2.75	.140	I
brotwurst (pork & beef w/ nfdm)	226	35.9	10.0	2.1		0.0	0	0	.16	.09	4	778	34	11	1.47	.027
1 link	70	19.5	7.0	9.3	2.0	44	0	.17	2.3	1.43	.04	197	94	.72	.056	807
canadian style, Oscar Mayer	46	34.4	8.2	0.1	0.1	0.0		0				618	4	12	.94	
2 slices	46	1.4	0.6	0.7	0.1	24		.00				149	142	.53	.080	I
chicken breast																
baked, Carving Board	44	32.7	8.8	1.7	0.3	0.0	0	0				514	4	14	.40	
2 slices	45	0.3	0.1	0.1	0.1	23	0					131	127	.58	.110	I
grilled, Carving Board	44	32.7	8.8	1.7	0.3	0.0	0	0				514	4	14	.40	
2 slices	45	0.3	0.1	0.1	0.1	23	0					131	127	.58	.110	I
hickory smoked, Tyson	33	30.2	6.9	1.1	0.0	0.0	0	0				452	1			
2 slices (1.5 oz)	42	0.1	0.1			15	0							.13		I
honey flavor, Tyson	36	29.2	7.1	1.7	1.1	0.0	0	0				450	3			
2 slices (1.5 oz)	42	0.2	0.1			15	0							.15		I
chicken breast, oven roasted																
deluxe, Louis Rich	28	20.7	5.1	0.6	0.4	0.0	0	0				333	2	7	.20	
1 oz slice	28	0.6	0.2	0.4	0.1	14	0					74	74	.32	.060	I
fat-free, Oscar Mayer	44	39.4	9.5	0.8	0.5	0.0	0	0				646	6	19	.31	
4 slices	52	0.3	0.1	0.1	0.0	23	0					165	133	.69	.120	I
mesquite flavor, Tyson	33	29.9	7.1	1.0	0.1	0.0	0	0				437	2			
2 slices (1.5 oz)	42	0.2	0.1			15	0							.13		I
Oscar Mayer	57	36.5	10.2	2.3	2.2	0.0	0	0				721	5	18	.36	
4 slices	52	0.8	0.3	0.5	0.1	28	0					171	150	.59	.090	I
peppered, Tyson	35	29.6	7.3	1.0	0.0	0.0	0	1				478	0			
2 slices (1.5 oz)	42	0.2	0.1			15	0							.11		I
Tyson	33	29.9	7.1	0.9	0.0	0.0	0	1				457	3			
2 slices (1.5 oz)	42	0.2	0.1			15	0							.13		I
chicken roll, light meat	91	39.1	11.1	1.4		0.0	14	0	.07	.12	1	333	25	11	.41	.007
2 slices	57	4.2	1.2	1.7	0.9	28	47	.04	3.0	.09	.22	130	89	.55	.023	807
chicken salad																
Libby's Spreadables	140		7.0	7.0	4.0	2.0	0	0				340	20			
⅓ cup	80	9.0	1.5			25	0							.40		I
lite, cnd, Libby's Spreadables	120		9.0	8.0	3.0	0.0	0	0				560	20			
1 can	85	5.0	1.0			30	0							.40		I
Lunch Kit, Swanson	300		16.0	16.0	4.0	1.0	0	0				550	0			
3.7 oz kit	104	19.0	3.0			45	0							1.08		I
chicken spread	54	18.8	4.4	1.5		0.0	7	0	.03	.04	1	109	35	3	.33	.003
1 oz	28	3.3	1.0	1.4	0.7	15	25	.00	0.8	.04	.12	30	25	.66	.011	807
chicken, white, oven roasted, Louis Rich	36	20.0	4.7	0.7	0.3	0.0	0	0				335	5	7	.32	
1 oz slice	28	1.6	0.5	0.9	0.4	16	0					85	69	.44	.060	I

	KCAL	H₂O (g)	PRO (g)	CHO (g)	SUGR (g)	DFIB (g)	A (RE)	C (mg)	B-2 (mg)	B-6 (mg)	FOL (mcg)	Na (mg)	Ca (mg)	Mg (mg)	Zn (mg)	Mn (mg)
	WT (g)	FAT (g)	SFA (g)	MUFA (g)	PUFA (g)	CHOL (mg)	A (IU)	B-1 (mg)	NIA (mg)	B-12 (mcg)	PANT (mg)	K (mg)	P (mg)	Fe (mg)	Cu (mg)	REF
chorizo (pork & beef)	273	19.1	14.5	1.1		0.0	0	0	.18	.32	1	741	5	11	2.05	.024
1 link	60	23.0	8.6	11.0	2.1	53	0	.38	3.1	1.20	.67	239	90	.95	.048	807
corned beef, cnd, Armour Star	120		15.0	1.0	1.0	0.0	0	0				490	0			
2 oz	56	7.0	3.0			50	0							1.44		I
corned beef, loaf, jellied	43	19.3	6.4	0.0	0.0	0.0	0	0	.03	.03	2	267	3	3	1.15	.009
1 oz slice	28	1.7	0.7	0.8	0.1	13	0	.00	0.5	.36	.05	28	20	.57	.017	807
frankfurter																
beef	180	31.2	6.8	1.0		0.0	0	0	.06	.07	2	585	11	2	1.24	.019
1 frank (8 per 1 lb pkg)	57	16.2	6.9	7.8	0.8	35	0	.03	1.4	.88	.17	95	50	.82	.034	807
beef	142	24.6	5.4	0.8		0.0	0	0	.05	.05	2	462	9	1	.98	.015
1 frank (10 per 1 lb pkg)	45	12.8	5.4	6.1	0.6	27	0	.02	1.1	.69	.13	75	39	.64	.027	807
beef, 95% fat-free, Louis Rich	54	43.7	6.3	3.2	1.5	0.0	0	0				549	12	10	1.21	
1 frank	57	1.8	1.0	0.6	0.2	19	0					295	79	.89	.130	I
beef & pork	182	30.7	6.4	1.5	1.1	0.0	0	0	.07	.07	2	638	6	6	1.05	.018
1 frank	57	16.6	6.1	7.8	1.6	28	0	.11	1.5	.74	.20	95	49	.66	.046	807
beef, bun-length, Oscar Mayer	183	30.7	6.4	1.6	1.1	0.0	0	0				576	7	8	1.28	
1 frank	57	16.7	7.1	8.3	0.6	33	0					90	60	.89		I
beef, fat-free, Oscar Mayer	39	38.9	6.7	2.6	1.9	0.0	0	0				464	10	9	1.21	
1 frank	50	0.3	0.2	0.1	0.0	15	0					234	64	.98	.080	I
beef, Oscar Mayer	143	24.4	5.0	1.1	0.7	0.0	0	0				458	5	6	.90	
1 frank	45	13.1	5.6	6.6	0.6	29	0					77	41	.54	.040	I
beef, Oscar Mayer Light	110	38.1	6.1	2.4	1.2	0.0	0	0				615	12	10	1.20	
1 frank	57	8.4	3.6	4.3	0.6	28	0					228	93	.89	.120	I
chicken	116	25.9	5.8	3.1		0.0	17	0	.05	.14	2	617	43	5	.47	.007
1 frank	45	8.8	2.5	3.8	1.8	45	59	.03	1.4	.11	.37	38	48	.90	.023	807
pork & turkey, bun-length, Oscar Mayer	184	30.4	6.2	1.7	1.0	0.0	0	0				550	34	10	.98	
1 frank	57	17.0	5.8	8.5	2.6	41	0					92	78	.66	.150	I
pork & turkey, little, Oscar Mayer	177	31.4	6.2	1.3	0.9	0.0	0	0				592	7	7	1.05	
6 franks	54	16.4	6.4	8.2	1.5	31	0					91	55	.58	.060	I
pork & turkey, Oscar Mayer	145	24.0	4.9	1.3	0.8	0.0	0	0				435	27	8	.77	
1 frank	45	13.4	4.6	6.7	2.1	32	0					73	62	.52	.120	I
pork, turkey, & beef, Oscar Mayer Light	110	38.0	6.9	1.7	0.9	0.0	0	0				591	22	10	1.01	
1 frank	57	8.5	3.3	4.3	1.3	35	0					226	96	.73	.110	I
pork, turkey, & beef w/ cheese, Oscar	142	23.9	5.4	1.3	0.8	0.0	0	0				515	74	11	.83	
Mayer—1 frank	45	12.9	4.9	6.4	1.9	33	0					59	97	.67	.800	I
turkey	102	28.3	6.4	0.7		0.0	0	0	.08	.10	4	642	48	6	1.40	.007
1 frank	45	8.0	2.7	2.5	2.3	48	0	.02	1.9	.13	.32	81	60	.83	.045	807
turkey & beef, fat-free, Oscar Mayer	37	39.3	6.2	2.3	1.0	0.0	0	0				487	8	11	.60	
1 frank	50	0.3	0.1	0.1	0.1	14	0					235	81	.46	.110	I
turkey & chicken, bun-length, Louis Rich	107	38.1	6.4	3.1	0.9	0.0	0	0				647	75	13	1.06	
1 frank	57	7.7	2.5	3.6	2.0	53	0					91	84	1.24	.130	I
turkey & chicken, Louis Rich	81	28.7	4.8	2.3	0.7	0.0	0	0				488	56	10	.80	
1 frank	45	5.8	1.9	2.7	1.5	40	0					69	63	.94	.090	I
turkey & chicken, w/ cheese, Louis Rich	90	28.8	5.7	2.3	0.8	0.0	0	0				482	109	10	.81	
1 frank	45	6.5	2.3	2.8	1.3	42	77					71	92	.95	.090	I
turkey, chicken, & beef, 95 % fat-free,	57	43.3	6.3	3.2	1.4	0.0	0	0				551	25	10	1.02	
Louis Rich—1 frank	57	2.1	0.9	1.1	0.5	24	0					340	79	.64	.130	I
ham & cheese loaf, Oscar Mayer	64	17.0	4.0	1.0	0.9	0.0	0	0				350	19	5	.51	
1 oz slice	28	4.9	2.3	2.1	0.6	19	0					74	75	.24	.040	I
ham & cheese loaf/roll	73	16.4	4.7	0.4		0.0	7	0	.05	.07	1	381	16	5	.57	.008
1 oz slice	28	5.7	2.1	2.6	0.6	16	21	.17	1.0	.23	.15	83	72	.26	.023	807
ham & cheese spread	69	16.8	4.6	0.6		0.0	26	0	.06	.04	1	339	62	5	.64	.010
1 oz	28	5.3	2.4	2.0	0.4	17	86	.09	0.6	.21	.17	46	140	.22	.026	807
ham, baked, Carving Board	47	33.0	8.0	1.0	1.0	0.0	0	0				551	3	11	.96	
2 slices	45	1.2	0.4	0.6	0.1	24	0					145	130	.53		I
ham, baked, fat-free, Oscar Mayer	36	36.7	6.9	1.2	1.2	0.0	0	0				540	6	14	.68	
3 slices	47	0.4	0.1	0.2	0.1	18	0					134	87	.49	.090	I
ham, chopped, cnd, Armour Star	130		8.0	1.0	1.0	0.0	0	0				880	0			
2 oz	56	11.0	4.0			35	0							.30		I

	KCAL / WT (g)	H₂O (g) / FAT (g)	PRO (g) / SFA (g)	CHO (g) / MUFA (g)	SUGR (g) / PUFA (g)	DFIB (g) / CHOL (mg)	A (RE) / A (IU)	C (mg) / B-1 (mg)	B-2 (mg) / NIA (mg)	B-6 (mg) / B-12 (mcg)	FOL (mcg) / PANT (mg)	Na (mg) / K (mg)	Ca (mg) / P (mg)	Mg (mg) / Fe (mg)	Zn (mg) / Cu (mg)	Mn (mg) / REF
ham, cured																
baked, Oscar Mayer	65	47.1	10.4	0.8		0.0	0	0				765	6	20	1.14	
3 slices	63	2.2	0.9			30	0					169	147	.82	.150	I
boiled, Oscar Mayer	66	46.9	10.5	0.7	0.2	0.0	0	0				849	6	19	1.17	
3 slices	63	2.3	0.9	1.2	0.3	30	0					178	151	.93	.150	I
chopped, cnd	50	12.8	3.4	0.1		0.0	0	0	.03	.07	0	287	1	3	.38	.005
1 slice	21	4.0	1.3	1.9	0.4	10	0	.11	0.7	.15	.06	60	29	.20	.011	807
chopped, Oscar Mayer	51	18.3	4.5	0.8	0.7	0.0	0	0				329	3	6	.63	
1 oz slice	28	3.3	1.2	1.8	0.0	14	0					74	60	.36	.060	I
chopped, packaged	48	13.4	3.6	0.0	0.0	0.0	0	0	.04	.07	0	288	1	3	.41	.009
1 slice	21	3.6	1.2	1.7	0.4	11	0	.13	0.8	.19	.06	67	33	.17	.013	807
lower sodium, Oscar Mayer	69	46.1	10.4	1.6	1.5	0.0	0	0				526	4	15	1.25	
3 slices	63	2.4	0.9			29	0					582	160	.92	.140	I
minced	55	12.0	3.4	0.4		0.0	0	0	.04	.05	0	261	2	3	.40	.007
1 slice	21	4.3	1.5	2.0	0.5	15	0	.15	0.9	.20	.04	65	33	.17	.017	807
sliced, lean (5% fat)	37	19.7	5.4	0.3		0.0	0	0	.06	.13	1	400	2	5	.54	.009
1 oz slice	28	1.4	0.5	0.7	0.1	13	0	.26	1.4	.21	.13	98	61	.21	.020	807
sliced, reg (11% fat)	51	18.1	4.9	0.9		0.0	0	0	.07	.10	1	369	2	5	.60	.009
1 oz slice	28	3.0	0.9	1.4	0.3	16	0	.24	1.5	.23	.13	93	69	.28	.028	807
smoked, Oscar Mayer	62	47.8	10.4	0.1		0.0	0	0				765	6	19	1.14	
3 slices	63	2.2	0.9	1.3	0.3	30	0					169	147	.82	.150	I
ham, deviled, Armour Star	210		13.0	0.0	0.0	0.0	0	0				700	0			
⅓ cup	85	18.0	6.0			60	0							.72		I
ham, honey																
fat-free, Louis Rich	38	36.3	6.9	1.8	1.5	0.0	0	0				574	5	13	.67	
2 slices	47	0.3	0.1	0.2	0.0	19	0					133	95	.47	.090	I
fat-free, Oscar Mayer	38	36.3	6.9	1.8	1.5	0.0	0	0				574	5	13	.67	
3 slices	47	0.3	0.1	0.2	0.0	19	0					133	95	.47	.090	I
glazed, Carving Board	49	32.4	7.8	1.8	1.8	0.0	0	0				569	4	14	.91	
2 slices	45	1.2	0.5	0.6	0.1	23	0					151	122	.54	.130	I
Oscar Mayer	69	46.0	10.5	1.8	1.8	0.0	0	0				786	6	19	1.31	
3 slices	63	2.2	0.8	1.2	0.2	29	0					177	163	.85	.140	I
ham salad, Libby's Spreadables	110		8.0	8.0	2.0	4.0	0	0				620	0			
⅓ cup	81	4.5	1.0			20	0							.70		I
ham salad spread	61	17.7	2.5	3.0		0.0	0	0	.03	.04	0	259	2	3	.31	.004
1 oz	28	4.4	1.4	2.0	0.8	10	0	.12	0.6	.22	.09	43	34	.17	.020	807
ham, smoked																
Carving Board	46	33.4	8.1	0.4	0.3	0.0	0	0				566	3	13	.89	
2 slices	45	1.3	0.5	0.7	0.1	22	0					144	126	.51	.100	I
fat-free, Louis Rich	33	37.3	6.8	0.8	0.5	0.0	0	0				509	5	13	.74	
2 slices	47	0.3	0.1	0.1	0.1	18	0					110	92	.43	.090	I
fat-free, Oscar Mayer	33	37.3	6.8	0.8	0.5	0.0	0	0				509	5	13	.74	
3 slices	47	0.3	0.1	0.1	0.1	18	0					110	92	.43	.090	I
headcheese (pork)	59	18.1	4.5	0.1		0.0	0	0	.05	.05	1	352	4	3	.36	.005
1 oz slice	28	4.4	1.4	2.3	0.5	23	0	.01	0.3	.29	.06	9	17	.33	.034	807
headcheese (pork), Oscar Mayer	52	18.9	4.4	0.0	0.0	0.0	0	0				300	6	3	.33	
1 oz slice	28	3.8	1.3	2.1	0.4	26	0					8	18	.46	.600	I
honey loaf (pork & beef)	36	19.7	4.4	1.5		0.0	0	0	.07	.09	2	370	5	5	.68	.008
1 slice	28	1.3	0.4	0.6	0.1	10	0	.13	0.9	.30	.18	96	40	.38	.017	807
honey loaf (pork & beef), Oscar Mayer	33	19.8	5.1	1.1	1.1	0.0	0	0				378	6	6	.74	
1 oz slice	28	1.0	0.4	0.6	0.1	15	0					101	50	.36	.050	I
honey roll sausage (beef)	42	14.9	4.3	0.5		0.0	0	0	.04	.06	1	304	2	4	.75	.009
1 slice	23	2.4	0.9	1.1	0.1	12	0	.02	1.0	.54	.11	67	32	.51	.023	807
italian sausage, pork, ckd	216	33.5	13.4	1.0		0.0	0	1	.16	.22	3	618	16	12	1.60	.055
1 link	67	17.2	6.1	8.0	2.2	52	0	.42	2.8	.87	.30	204	114	1.01	.054	810
kielbasa/kolbassy (pork & beef w/ nfdm)	81	14.0	3.4	0.6		0.0	0	0	.06	.05	1	280	11	4	.53	.010
1 slice	26	7.1	2.6	3.4	0.8	17	0	.06	0.7	.42	.21	70	38	.38	.026	807
knockwurst/knackwurst (pork & beef)	209	37.7	8.1	1.2		0.0	0	0	.10	.12	1	687	7	7	1.13	.014
1 slice	68	18.9	6.9	8.7	2.0	39	0	.23	1.9	.80	.22	135	67	.62	.041	807

	KCAL	H₂O (g)	PRO (g)	CHO (g)	SUGR (g)	DFIB (g)	A (RE)	C (mg)	B-2 (mg)	B-6 (mg)	FOL (mcg)	Na (mg)	Ca (mg)	Mg (mg)	Zn (mg)	Mn (mg)
	WT (g)	FAT (g)	SFA (g)	MUFA (g)	PUFA (g)	CHOL (mg)	A (IU)	B-1 (mg)	NIA (mg)	B-12 (mcg)	PANT (mg)	K (mg)	P (mg)	Fe (mg)	Cu (mg)	REF
lebanon bologna (beef)	49	14.0	4.4	0.6		0.0	0	0	.04	.06	1	308	3	4	.92	.013
1 slice	23	3.0	1.3	1.4	0.1	16	0	.01	1.0	.59	.12	69	35	.57	.021	807
liver cheese, pork fat wrapped, Oscar Mayer—*1 slice*	115	20.4	5.7	0.6	0.5	0.0		1				419	3	5	1.50	
	38	10.0	3.5	4.9	1.3	80	8590					82	88	4.52	.200	I
liver cheese (pork liver)	116	20.4	5.8	0.8		0.0	1996	1	.85	.18	40	466	3	5	1.41	.076
1 slice	38	9.7	3.4	4.7	1.3	66	6646	.08	4.5	9.33	1.34	86	79	4.12	.146	807
liver pate																
chicken, cnd	57	18.6	3.8	1.9		0.0	62	3	.40	.07	91	109	3	4	.61	.046
1 oz	28	3.7	1.1	1.5	0.7	111	205	.01	2.1	2.29	.74	27	50	2.61	.051	807
goose, smoked, cnd	131	10.5	3.2	1.3		0.0	284	0	.08	.02	17	198	20	4	.26	.034
1 oz	28	12.4	4.1	7.3	0.2	43	945	.02	0.7	2.66	.34	39	57	1.56	.113	807
unspecified, cnd	90	15.3	4.0	0.4		0.0	283	1	.17	.02	17	198	20	4	.81	.034
1 oz	28	7.9	2.7	3.5	0.9	72	936	.01	0.9	.91	.34	39	57	1.56	.113	807
liver sausage/liverwurst (pork)	59	9.4	2.5	0.4		0.0	1494	0	.19	.03	5	155	5	2	.41	.028
1 slice	18	5.1	1.9	2.4	0.5	28	4980	.05	0.8	2.42	.53	31	41	1.15	.043	807
luncheon loaf, Oscar Mayer	65	16.5	3.8	2.0	1.3	0.0	0	0				343	31	7	.55	
1 oz slice	28	4.7	1.6	2.3	0.8	19	0					76	54	.38	.650	I
luncheon sausage (pork & beef)	60	13.5	3.5	0.4		0.0	0	0	.04		1	272	3	3	.56	.010
1 slice	23	4.8	1.8	2.3	0.5	15	0	.05	0.8	.45	.09	56	28	.33	.018	807
luxury loaf (pork)	39	19.1	5.2	1.4		0.0	0	0	.08	.09	1	343	10	6	.85	.011
1 oz slice	28	1.3	0.4	0.7	0.1	10	0	.20	1.0	.38	.14	106	52	.29	.028	807
mortadella (beef & pork)	47	7.8	2.5	0.5		0.0	0	0	.02	.02	0	187	3	2	.32	.004
1 slice	15	3.8	1.4	1.7	0.5	8	0	.02	0.4	.22	.07	24	15	.21	.009	807
Mother's Loaf (pork)	59	11.5	2.5	1.6		0.0	0	0	.04	.04	2	237	9	3	.30	.014
1 slice	21	4.7	1.7	2.2	0.5	9	0	.12	0.7	.22	.10	47	27	.28	.019	807
New England Brand Sausage (pork & beef)—*1 slice*	37	15.4	4.0	1.1		0.0	0	0	.06	.08	2	281	2	4	.62	.008
	23	1.7	0.6	0.8	0.2	11	0	.15	0.8	.31	.16	74	31	.22	.023	807
New England Brand Sausage (pork & beef), Oscar Mayer—*2 slices*	55	33.4	7.8	0.8	0.7	0.0	0	0				588	3	8	1.29	
	46	2.3	1.0	1.3	0.2	28	0					138	121	.52	.100	I
Old Fashioned Loaf, Oscar Mayer	65	16.5	3.7	2.2	1.2	0.0	0	0				332	30	6	.52	
1 oz slice	28	4.6	1.6	2.2	0.8	17	0					81	56	.37	.040	I
old fashioned loaf (pork & beef), Dutch Brand—*1 oz slice*	67	16.6	3.8	1.6		0.0	0	0	.08	.06	1	350	24	6	.48	.009
	28	5.0	1.8	2.3	0.5	13	0	.08	0.7	.37	.17	105	45	.35	.020	807
olive loaf (chicken, pork, & turkey), Oscar Mayer—*1 oz slice*	74	16.1	2.8	2.0	1.0	0.0	0	0				358	29	7	.29	
	28	6.1	2.0	3.2	0.8	20	0					51	36	.46	.060	I
olive loaf (pork)	66	16.3	3.3	2.6		0.0	6	0	.07	.06	1	416	31	5	.39	.010
1 oz slice	28	4.6	1.6	2.2	0.5	11	56	.08	0.5	.35	.22	83	36	.15	.014	807
peppered loaf (pork & beef)	41	18.9	4.8	1.3		0.0	0	0	.08	.08	1	426	15	6	.90	.018
1 slice	28	1.8	0.6	0.8	0.1	13	0	.11	0.9	.55	.15	110	48	.30	.034	807
pepperoni, Oscar Mayer	143	9.4	5.5	0.2	0.0	0.0	0	0				548	5	6	.84	
15 slices	30	13.3	5.2	6.6	1.2	25	0					90	57	.63	.060	I
pepperoni (pork & beef)	30	1.6	1.3	0.2		0.0	0	0	.01	.01	0	122	1	1	.15	.002
1 slice	6	2.6	1.0	1.3	0.3	5	0	.02	0.3	.15	.11	21	7	.08	.004	807
pickle & pimento loaf (chicken, pork, & turkey), Oscar Mayer—*1 oz slice*	75	15.7	2.7	2.5	1.9	0.0	0	0				357	31	8	.33	
	28	6.1	2.0	2.9	0.8	22	0					49	42	.61	.080	I
pickle & pimento loaf (pork)	73	16.0	3.2	1.7		0.0	2	0	.07	.05	1	389	27	5	.39	.008
1 oz slice	28	5.9	2.2	2.7	0.7	10	20	.08	0.6	.33	.22	95	39	.29	.035	807
picnic loaf (pork & beef)	65	16.9	4.2	1.3		0.0	0	0	.07	.08	1	326	13	4	.61	.008
1 slice	28	4.7	1.7	2.2	0.5	11	0	.10	0.6	.42	.19	75	35	.29	.020	807
polish sausage (pork)	92	15.1	4.0	0.5		0.0	0	0	.04	.05	1	248	3	4	.55	.014
1 oz	28	8.1	2.9	3.8	0.9	20	0	.14	1.0	.28	.13	67	39	.41	.026	807
pork & beef lunch meat	99	13.8	3.5	0.7		0.0	0	0	.04	.06	2	362	3	4	.46	.008
1 slice	28	9.0	3.2	4.2	1.0	15	0	.09	0.8	.36	.18	57	24	.24	.011	807
pork lunch meat, cnd	70	10.8	2.6	0.4		0.0	0	0	.04	.04	1	271	1	2	.31	.005
1 slice	21	6.4	2.3	3.0	0.7	13	0	.08	0.7	.19	.10	45	17	.15	.008	807
potted meat, Armour Star	100		8.0	0.0	0.0	0.0	0					550	40			
¼ cup	62	7.0	3.0			55	0							.72		I
potted meat, cnd, Libby's	110		10.0	0.0	0.0	0.0	0					440	0			
¼ cup	58	7.0	2.0			30	0							.40		I
poultry (chicken/turkey) salad spread	57	18.8	3.3	2.1		0.0	12	0	.02	.03	1	107	3	3	.29	.003
1 oz	28	3.8	1.0	0.9	1.8	9	39	.01	0.5	.11	.08	52	9	.17	.009	807

	KCAL	H₂O (g)	PRO (g)	CHO (g)	SUGR (g)	DFIB (g)	A (RE)	C (mg)	B-2 (mg)	B-6 (mg)	FOL (mcg)	Na (mg)	Ca (mg)	Mg (mg)	Zn (mg)	Mn (mg)
	WT (g)	FAT (g)	SFA (g)	MUFA (g)	PUFA (g)	CHOL (mg)	A (IU)	B-1 (mg)	NIA (mg)	B-12 (mcg)	PANT (mg)	K (mg)	P (mg)	Fe (mg)	Cu (mg)	REF
salami, beef	60	13.4	3.5	0.6	0.0	0.0	0	0	.04	.04	0	270	2	3	.50	.011
1 slice	23	4.8	2.1	2.2	0.2	15	0	.02	0.7	.70	.22	52	26	.50	.028	813
salami, beef & pork	58	13.9	3.2	0.5		0.0	0	0	.09	.05	0	245	3	3	.49	.013
1 slice	23	4.6	1.9	2.1	0.5	15	0	.05	0.8	.84	.20	46	26	.61	.053	807
salami, beef, Machiaeh	118	27.6	5.8	0.9	0.7	0.0	0	0				524	3	6	.81	
2 slices	46	10.2	4.8	5.2	0.5	33	0					87	94	1.01	.090	I
salami, beerwurst, beef	76	12.2	2.9	0.4		0.0	0	0	.03	.04	1	236	2	3	.56	.006
1 slice	23	6.9	3.0	3.2	0.3	14	0	.02	0.8	.45	.08	40	22	.35	.009	807
salami, beerwurst, pork	55	14.1	3.3	0.5		0.0	0	0	.04	.08	1	285	2	3	.40	.007
1 slice	23	4.3	1.4	2.1	0.5	14	0	.13	0.7	.20	.11	58	24	.17	.012	807
salami, cotto																
beef, chicken, & pork, Oscar Mayer	113	27.9	6.1	1.0	0.7	0.0	0	0				504	35	14	.91	
2 slices	46	9.3	3.9	4.7	0.8	37	0					100	114	1.33	.190	I
beef, Oscar Mayer	93	29.8	6.5	0.9	0.5	0.0	0	0				608	3	8	.96	
2 slices	46	7.1	3.1	3.2	0.4	38	0					95	103	1.25	.110	I
turkey, Louis Rich	43	19.9	4.1	0.2	0.1	0.0	0	0				285	9	6	.66	
1 oz slice	28	2.8	0.8	1.1	0.6	22	0					62	76	.46	.100	I
salami, dry/hard																
pork	41	3.6	2.3	0.2		0.0	0	0	.03	.06	0	226	1	2	.42	.007
1 slice	10	3.4	1.2	1.6	0.4	8	0	.09	0.6	.28	.11	38	23	.13	.016	807
pork & beef	42	3.5	2.3	0.3		0.0	0	0	.03	.05	0	186	1	2	.32	.004
1 slice	10	3.4	1.2	1.7	0.3	8	0	.06	0.5	.19	.11	38	14	.15	.008	807
pork & beef, Oscar Mayer	108	8.9	7.6	0.9	0.0	0.0	0	0				508	3	6	.85	
3 slices	27	8.2	3.2	4.3	0.8	26	0					96	49	.49	.050	I
salami, genoa (pork & beef), Oscar Mayer—*3 slices*	105	10.6	5.6	0.3	0.1	0.0	0	0				493	5	6	.91	
	27	9.0	3.3	4.5	0.7	28	0					90	55	.50	.070	I
salami, pork for beer, Oscar Mayer	102	29.1	6.3	0.9	0.5	0.0	0	0				566	4	8	.94	
2 slices	46	8.2	3.3	4.6	1.0	32	0					98	106	.54	.110	I
salami, turkey, ckd	112	37.5	9.3	0.3		0.0	0	0	.10	.14	2	572	11	9	1.03	.007
2 slices	57	7.9	2.3	2.6	2.0	47	0	.04	2.0	.12	.29	139	60	.92	.028	807
salami, turkey, Louis Rich	42	20.1	4.3	0.1	0.1	0.0	0	0				281	11	6	.65	
1 oz slice	28	2.7	0.9	1.0	0.8	21	0					61	74	.35	.050	I
sandwich spread (pork & beef), Oscar Mayer—*2 oz*	133	33.2	3.6	8.6	4.4	0.2		0				459	15	7	.49	
	56	9.3	3.8	4.7	1.6	25	56					66	38	.45	.100	I
smoked link sausage, beef, Oscar Mayer—*1 link*	128	24.0	5.4	0.8	0.5	0.0	0	0				425	5	7	1.26	
	43	11.5	4.8	5.4	0.4	27	0					73	96	.76	.090	I
smoked link sausage, pork	265	26.7	15.1	1.4		0.0	0	1	.17	.24	3	1020	20	13	1.92	.011
1 link	68	21.6	7.7	10.0	2.6	46	0	.48	3.1	1.11	.53	228	110	.79	.049	807
smoked link sausage, pork & beef	228	35.5	9.1	1.0		0.0	0	0	.12	.12	1	643	7	8	1.43	.025
1 link	68	20.6	7.2	9.6	2.2	48	0	.18	2.2	1.03	.30	129	73	.99	.041	807
Oscar Mayer	128	24.1	5.3	0.7	0.6	0.0	0	0				430	4	8	.89	
1 link	43	11.5	4.0	5.6	1.2	27	0					77	102	.50	.110	I
w/ american cheese	141	22.6	6.0	0.6		0.0	16	0	.07	.06	1	465	25	6	.97	.014
1 link	43	12.4	4.5	5.9	1.3	29	68	.11	1.2	.74	.33	89	77	.46	.030	807
w/ cheese, Oscar Mayer	130	23.7	5.6	0.8	0.7	0.0	0	0				450	19	7	.84	
1 link	43	11.6	4.4	5.6	1.2	30	0					78	124	.46	.090	I
w/ flour & nfdm	182	39.0	9.5	2.7		0.0	0	2	.12	.09	1	741	12	9	1.36	.035
1 link	68	14.6	5.3	6.8	1.5	59	0	.16	1.8	.90	.41	105	75	1.05	.061	807
w/ nfdm	213	36.7	9.0	1.3		0.0	0	0	.15	.12	1	798	28	11	1.33	.026
1 link	68	18.8	6.6	8.6	2.1	44	0	.13	1.9	1.07	.41	194	93	1.00	.061	807
smoked link sausage, pork & turkey, Oscar Mayer—*9 small links*	168	32.0	7.0	1.1	0.5	0.0	0	0				576	21	12	1.11	
	57	15.1	5.8	7.4	1.9	36	0					100	124	.73	.130	I
smoked link sausage, pork & turkey w/ cheese, Oscar Mayer—*6 links*	179	30.4	7.7	1.0	0.2	0.0	0	0				591	38	12	1.16	
	57	16.0	6.4	7.5	1.6	38	0					87	141	.71	.170	I
thuringer (cervelat/summer sausage)																
beef & pork	77	11.7	3.6	0.1		0.0	0	0	.08	.06	0	286	3	3	.59	.011
1 slice	23	6.8	2.8	3.0	0.3	17	0	.03	1.0	1.27	.23	62	26	.58	.035	807
beef & pork, Oscar Mayer	141	24.3	6.7	0.9	0.5	0.0	0	0				655	4	7	1.08	
2 slices	46	12.4	5.4	5.9	0.5	37	0					107	56	1.15	.090	I

	KCAL	H₂O (g)	PRO (g)	CHO (g)	SUGR (g)	DFIB (g)	A (RE)	C (mg)	B-2 (mg)	B-6 (mg)	FOL (mcg)	Na (mg)	Ca (mg)	Mg (mg)	Zn (mg)	Mn (mg)
	WT (g)	FAT (g)	SFA (g)	MUFA (g)	PUFA (g)	CHOL (mg)	A (IU)	B-1 (mg)	NIA (mg)	B-12 (mcg)	PANT (mg)	K (mg)	P (mg)	Fe (mg)	Cu (mg)	REF
beef, Oscar Mayer	140	24.5	6.9	0.4	0.3		0	0				658	4	7	.98	
2 slices	46	12.3	5.3	6.0	1.1	39	0					105	60	1.03	.080	I
Treet Luncheon Loaf, 50% less fat, Armour Star—2 oz	110		6.0	4.0	2.0	0.0	0	0				750	40			
	56	8.0	3.0			45	0								.72	I
Treet Luncheon Loaf, Armour Star	130		6.0	3.0	3.0	0.0	0	0				740	60			
2 oz	56	11.0	4.0			50	0								.72	I
tuna salad, Libby's Spreadables	130		7.0	6.0	3.0	3.0	0	0				370	0			
1 can	85	8.0	1.0			15	0								.40	I
tuna salad, lite, cnd, Libby's Spreadables	100		10.0	8.0	2.0	1.0		0				390	0			
1 can	85	3.0	0.5			10	500								.70	I
turkey breast	23	15.1	4.7	0.0	0.0		0	0	.02	.08	1	301	1	4	.24	.003
1 slice	21	0.3	0.1	0.1	0.1	9	0	.01	1.7	.42	.12	58	48	.08	.011	807
honey roasted, Louis Rich	29	20.6	4.6	1.3	0.8	0.0	0	0				321	2	6	.28	
1 oz slice	28	0.6	0.3	0.4	0.2	11	0					62	76	.22	.040	I
honey roasted, Oscar Mayer	54	37.9	9.4	2.3	1.3	0.0	0	0				504	3	15	.47	
4 slices	52	0.8	0.3	0.4	0.3	22	0					145	139	.40	.090	I
oven roasted, Carving Board	44	33.1	9.2	0.7	0.2	0.0	0	0				539	7	14	.42	
2 slices	45	0.5	0.2	0.2	0.1	19	0					139	140	.59	.080	I
oven roasted, fat-free, Louis Rich	24	21.4	4.3	1.2	0.5	0.0	0	0				334	3	8	.24	
1 slice	28	0.2	0.1	0.1	0.1	9	0					57	65	.31	.070	I
oven roasted, fat-free, Oscar Mayer	43	39.9	7.7	2.2	0.6	0.0	0	0				669	6	16	.42	
4 slices	52	0.3	0.1	0.1	0.1	14	0					107	121	.70	.150	I
oven roasted, Louis Rich	27	20.9	4.7	1.0	0.2	0.0	0	0				312	2	6	.28	
1 oz slice	28	0.5	0.2	0.3	0.2	10	0					62	69	.27	.050	I
roasted, Oscar Mayer	50	38.8	8.3	2.0	0.6	0.0	0	0				619	6	16	.50	
4 slices	52	1.0	0.3	0.3	0.2	23	0					134	123	.70	.090	I
rotisserie flavor, fat-free, Louis Rich	52	41.7	10.5	1.3	1.3	0.0	0	0				669	6	18	.60	
2 oz	56	0.5	0.2	0.2	0.1	21	0					168	158	.83	.080	I
smoked, Carving Board	42	33.4	8.9	0.7	0.1	0.0	0	0				537	7	14	.45	
2 slices	45	0.4	0.2	0.2	0.1	20	0					138	142	.66	.080	I
smoked, fat-free, Louis Rich	22	21.7	4.2	1.0	0.3	0.0	0	0				307	3	8	.24	
1 slice	28	0.2	0.1	0.0	0.0	9	0					61	68	.22	.070	I
smoked, fat-free, Oscar Mayer	41	40.4	7.8	1.8	0.6	0.0	0	0				569	5	15	.44	
4 slices	52	0.3	0.1	0.1	0.1	16	0					113	126	.40	.140	I
smoked, Louis Rich	28	21.0	4.9	0.7	0.3	0.0	0	0				257	3	10	.27	
1 slice	28	0.6	0.2	0.2	0.1	12	0					73	73	.21	.060	I
turkey ham (cured thigh meat)	73	40.7	10.8	0.2		0.0	0	0	.14	.14	3	568	6	9	1.68	.009
2 slices	57	2.9	1.0	0.7	0.9	32	0	.03	2.0	.14	.48	185	109	1.57	.063	807
chopped, Louis Rich	33	20.1	5.0	0.9	0.6	0.0	0					352	2	7	.71	
1 oz slice	28	1.1	0.3	0.3	0.2	19	0					80	84	.43	.060	I
honey cured, Louis Rich	33	20.1	5.0	0.9	0.6	0.0						352	2	7	.71	
1 slice	28	0.9	0.3	0.3	0.2	19						80	84	.43	.060	I
Louis Rich	31	20.5	5.1	0.3	0.3	0.0	0	0				366	2	6	.72	
1 oz slice	28	1.1	0.3	0.3	0.2	18						82	81	.36	.070	I
water added, Louis Rich	67	40.9	9.8	0.0	0.0	0.0	0	0				610	3	11	1.50	
2 oz	56	2.9	0.9	1.1	0.8	36	0					147	163	.71	.130	I
turkey pastrami	80	40.3	10.5	0.9		0.0	0	0	.14	.15	3	596	5	8	1.23	.007
2 slices	57	3.5	1.0	1.2	0.9	31	0	.03	2.0	.14	.33	148	114	.95	.028	807
turkey pastrami, Louis Rich	31	20.5	5.1	0.2	0.1	0.0	0	0				380	2	6	.67	
1 oz slice	28	1.1	0.3	0.3	0.2	18	0					77	81	.36	.050	I
turkey roll, light & dark meat	85	40.0	10.3	1.2		0.0	0	0	.16	.15	3	334	18	10	1.14	.007
2 slices	57	4.0	1.2	1.3	1.0	31	0	.05	2.7	.13	.32	154	96	.77	.040	807
turkey roll, light meat	84	40.8	10.7	0.3		0.0	0	0	.13	.18	2	279	23	9	.89	.007
2 slices	57	4.1	1.2	1.4	1.0	25	0	.05	4.0	.14	.24	143	104	.73	.023	807
turkey salad, Libby's Spreadables	150		7.0	7.0	3.0	2.0	0	0				310	20			
⅓ cup	82	10.0	1.5			25	0								.40	I
turkey, white, smoked, Louis Rich	28	21.4	3.8	0.9	0.2	0.0	0	0				313	4	7	.39	
1 oz slice	28	1.0	0.3	0.4	0.3	10	0					60	61	.20	.050	I
vienna sausage																
25% less fat, cnd, Armour Star	130		6.0	1.0	0.0	0.0	0	0				420	40			
3 pieces	53	11.0	4.0			50	0								.72	I

	KCAL	H₂O (g)	PRO (g)	CHO (g)	SUGR (g)	DFIB (g)	A (RE)	C (mg)	B-2 (mg)	B-6 (mg)	FOL (mcg)	Na (mg)	Ca (mg)	Mg (mg)	Zn (mg)	Mn (mg)
	WT (g)	FAT (g)	SFA (g)	MUFA (g)	PUFA (g)	CHOL (mg)	A (IU)	B-1 (mg)	NIA (mg)	B-12 (mcg)	PANT (mg)	K (mg)	P (mg)	Fe (mg)	Cu (mg)	REF
beef & pork, cnd	45	9.6	1.6	0.3		0.0	0	0	.02	.02	1	152	2	1	.26	.005
1 sausage	16	4.0	1.5	2.0	0.3	8	0	.01	0.3	.16	.06	16	8	.14	.005	807
chicken, cnd, Libby's	100		6.0	0.0	0.0	0.0	0	0				450	20			
3 links	48	8.0	2.5			50	0							.70		I
chicken in beef stock, cnd, Armour Star	120		6.0	1.0	1.0	0.0	0	0				620	40			
3 pieces	53	10.0	3.5			65	0							.72		I
cnd, Libby's	130		5.0	0.0	0.0	0.0	0	0				300	20			
3 links	48	12.0	2.5			50	0							.70		I
hot 'n spicy, cnd , Armour Star	150		5.0	2.0	0.0	0.0	0	0				660	60			
3 pieces	61	13.0	5.0			50	0							.72		I
in bbq sce, cnd, Armour Star	150		5.0	3.0	3.0	0.0	0	0				580	40			
3 pieces	61	13.0	5.0			50	0							.72		I
in bbq sce, cnd, Libby's	140		5.0	2.0	1.0	0.0	0	0				310	20			
3 links w/ sce	60	12.0	2.5			50	0							.70		I
in beef stock, cnd, Armour Star	170		5.0	1.0	0.0	0.0	0	0				420	40			
3 pieces	53	16.0	6.0			50	0							.72		I
jalapeno, in beef stock, cnd, Armour Star	170		5.0	1.0	0.0	0.0	0	0				420	40			
3 pieces	53	16.0	6.0			50	0							.72		I
lite, 50% less fat, cnd, Armour Star	90		5.0	1.0	1.0	0.0	0	0				420	40			
3 pieces	53	7.0	2.5			40	0							1.08		I
smoked, in beef stock, cnd, Armour Star	150		5.0	0.0	0.0	0.0	0	0				430	40			
3 pieces	53	14.0	6.0			50	0							.72		I

23. MILK, MILK BEVERAGES, MILK MIXES & YOGURT
23.1 MILK, COW

	KCAL	H₂O (g)	PRO (g)	CHO (g)	SUGR (g)	DFIB (g)	A (RE)	C (mg)	B-2 (mg)	B-6 (mg)	FOL (mcg)	Na (mg)	Ca (mg)	Mg (mg)	Zn (mg)	Mn (mg)
	WT (g)	FAT (g)	SFA (g)	MUFA (g)	PUFA (g)	CHOL (mg)	A (IU)	B-1 (mg)	NIA (mg)	B-12 (mcg)	PANT (mg)	K (mg)	P (mg)	Fe (mg)	Cu (mg)	REF
buttermilk, cultured	99	220.8	8.1	11.7	11.8	0.0	20	2	.38	.08	12	257	285	27	1.03	.005
8 fl oz	245	2.2	1.3	0.6	0.1	9	81	.08	0.1	.54	.67	371	219	.12	.027	801
buttermilk, dry	27	0.2	2.4	3.4		0.0	4	0	.11	.02	3	36	83	8	.28	.002
1 T	7	0.4	0.3	0.1	0.0	5	15	.03	0.1	.27	.22	111	65	.02	.008	801
condensed, sweetened, cnd	122	10.3	3.0	20.7		0.0	31	1	.16	.02	4	48	108	10	.36	.002
1 fl oz	38	3.3	2.1	0.9	0.1	13	125	.03	0.1	.17	.29	141	96	.07	.006	801
condensed, sweetened, cnd, Carnation	130		3.0	22.0	22.0	0.0		0				45	100			
2 T	38	3.0	2.0			10	100							.00		I
evaporated																
cnd, Carnation	40		2.0	3.0	3.0	0.0	0	0	.10			30	80			
2 T[1]	32	2.0	1.5			10	0					90	60	.00		I
lowfat, cnd, Carnation	25		2.0	3.0	3.0	0.0		0				35	80			
2 T	32	0.5	0.0	0.0	0.0	5	100	.10				100	60	.00		I
nonfat, cnd	25	25.4	2.4	3.6		0.0	37	0	.10	.02	3	37	93	9	.29	.002
1 fl oz	32	0.1	0.0	0.0	0.0	1	125	.01	0.1	.08	.24	106	62	.09	.005	801
nonfat, cnd, Carnation	25		2.0	4.0	4.0	0.0		0	.10			40	80			
2 T	32	0.0	0.0	0.0	0.0	0	100					110		.00		I
whole, cnd	43	23.7	2.2	3.2		0.0	17	1	.10	.02	3	34	83	8	.25	.002
1 fl oz	32	2.4	1.5	0.7	0.1	9	78	.02	0.1	.05	.20	97	65	.06	.005	801
whole, cnd	169	93.3	8.6	12.7		0.0	68	2	.40	.06	10	133	329	30	.97	.008
4 fl oz	126	9.5	5.8	2.9	0.3	37	306	.06	0.2	.21	.80	382	255	.24	.020	801
lowfat																
1% fat	102	219.8	8.0	11.7		0.0	144	2	.41	.10	12	123	300	34	.95	.005
8 fl oz	244	2.6	1.6	0.7	0.1	10	500	.10	0.2	.90	.79	381	235	.12	.024	801
1% fat, pro fortified	119	218.3	9.7	13.6		0.0	145	3	.47	.12	15	143	349	39	1.11	.005
8 fl oz	246	2.9	1.8	0.8	0.1	10	499	.11	0.2	1.05	.92	444	273	.15	.025	801
1% fat w/ nfdm	104	220.0	8.5	12.2		0.0	145	2	.42	.11	13	128	313	35	.98	.005
8 fl oz	245	2.4	1.5	0.7	0.1	10	500	.10	0.2	.94	.82	397	245	.12	.025	801
2% fat	121	217.7	8.1	11.7		0.0	139	2	.40	.10	12	122	297	33	.95	.005
8 fl oz	244	4.7	2.9	1.4	0.2	18	500	.10	0.2	.89	.78	377	232	.12	.020	801
2% fat, pro fortified	137	215.8	9.7	13.5		0.0	140	3	.48	.13	15	145	352	40	1.11	.005
8 fl oz	246	4.9	3.0	1.4	0.2	19	499	.11	0.2	1.05	.92	447	276	.15	.020	801

	KCAL	H₂O (g)	PRO (g)	CHO (g)	SUGR (g)	DFIB (g)	A (RE)	C (mg)	B-2 (mg)	B-6 (mg)	FOL (mcg)	Na (mg)	Ca (mg)	Mg (mg)	Zn (mg)	Mn (mg)
	WT (g)	FAT (g)	SFA (g)	MUFA (g)	PUFA (g)	CHOL (mg)	A (IU)	B-1 (mg)	NIA (mg)	B-12 (mcg)	PANT (mg)	K (mg)	P (mg)	Fe (mg)	Cu (mg)	REF
2% fat w/ nfdm	125	217.7	8.5	12.2		0.0	140	2	.42	.11	13	128	313	35	.98	.005
8 fl oz	245	4.7	2.9	1.4	0.2	18	500	.10	0.2	.94	.82	397	245	.12	.020	801
nonfat	86	222.5	8.4	11.9	10.8	0.0	149	2	.34	.10	13	126	302	28	.98	.005
8 fl oz	245	0.4	0.3	0.1	0.0	4	500	.09	0.2	.93	.81	406	247	.10	.027	801
dry	109	0.9	10.8	15.6	15.1	0.0	2	2	.46	.11	15	161	377	33	1.22	.006
¼ cup	30	0.2	0.1	0.1	0.0	6	11	.12	0.3	1.21	1.07	538	290	.10	.012	801
dry, Ca reduced	100	1.4	10.1	14.7		0.0	1	2	.47	.08	14	646	79	17	1.14	.002
1 oz[1]	28	0.1	0.0	0.0	0.0	1	2	.05	0.2	1.13	.94	193	287	.09	.005	801
dry, inst	326	3.6	31.9	47.5		0.0	646	5	1.59	.31	45	499	1120	107	4.01	.018
1 ⅓ cups (3.2 oz pkt)[2]	91	0.7	0.4	0.2	0.0	17	2157	.38	0.8	3.63	2.94	1552	896	.28	.037	801
dry, inst, Carnation	80		8.0	12.0	12.0	0.0		1	.43	.08		125	300	24		
⅓ cup	23	0.0	0.0	0.0	0.0	3	500	.90	0.0	.90	.80	387	200	.00		I
dry, inst, Sanalac	85		8.0	13.1	12.2	0.0		2				117	302			
¼ cup	24	0.1	0.0			6								.13		I
pro fortified	100	219.8	9.7	13.7		0.0	150	3	.48	.12	15	144	352	40	1.11	.005
8 fl oz	246	0.6	0.4	0.2	0.0	5	499	.11	0.2	1.05	.92	446	275	.15	.027	801
w/ nfdm	90	221.4	8.7	12.3		0.0	149	2	.43	.11	13	130	316	36	1.00	.005
8 fl oz	245	0.6	0.4	0.2	0.0	5	500	.10	0.2	.95	.83	418	255	.12	.027	801
whole																
3.3% fat	150	214.7	8.0	11.4		0.0	76	2	.40	.10	12	120	291	33	.93	.010
8 fl oz	244	8.1	5.1	2.4	0.3	33	307	.09	0.2	.87	.77	370	228	.12	.024	801
3.7% fat	157	214.0	8.0	11.3		0.0	83	4	.39	.10	12	119	290	33	.93	.010
8 fl oz	244	8.9	5.6	2.6	0.3	35	337	.09	0.2	.87	.76	368	227	.12	.024	801
dry	159	0.8	8.4	12.3	11.5	0.0	90	3	.39	.10	12	119	292	27	1.07	.013
¼ cup	32	8.5	5.4	2.5	0.2	31	295	.09	0.2	1.04	.73	426	248	.15	.026	801
low sodium	149	215.2	7.6	10.9		0.0	78	2	.26	.08	12	6	246	12	.93	.010
8 fl oz	244	8.4	5.3	2.4	0.3	33	317	.05	0.1	.88	.74	617	209	.12	.024	801

23.2 MILK, COW, BEVERAGES

	KCAL	H₂O (g)	PRO (g)	CHO (g)	SUGR (g)	DFIB (g)	A (RE)	C (mg)	B-2 (mg)	B-6 (mg)	FOL (mcg)	Na (mg)	Ca (mg)	Mg (mg)	Zn (mg)	Mn (mg)
carob flavor mix in whole milk	9	10.1	0.4	1.1		0.0	4	0	.02	.01	1	6	14	2	.04	.000
3 t powder in 8 fl oz milk	12	0.4	0.2	0.1	0.0	2	14	.00	0.0	.04	.04	17	11	.03	.001	814
choc dairy drink w/ aspartame, from mix, prep w/	63	185.2	5.3	10.6		0.4	73	0	.41	.02	9	171	192	47	.82	.157
water—¾ oz pkt in 4 oz water w/ 3 ice cubes	204	0.6	0.4	0.1	0.0	2	245	.02	0.3	.51	.46	479	182	1.65	.182	814
choc flavor nonfat dry milk in water,	80		6.0	13.0				1	.29	.06		120	310			
Alba—8 fl oz	250	1.0					378	.07	0.2				169	.24		I
choc malted milk, whole milk	228	214.9	9.0	29.9	18.0	0.3	80	3	.44	.14	16	172	305	48	1.09	.005
3 hp t powder in 8 fl oz milk	265	9.0	5.5	2.6	0.4	34	326	.13	0.6	.93	.77	498	265	.61	.066	814
choc malted milk, whole milk w/ added	225	215.2	9.0	29.1		0.3	901	34	1.26	1.02	32	244	384	53	1.17	.135
nutrients—4-5 hp t powder in 8 fl oz milk	265	8.7	5.5	2.6	0.4	34	3058	.73	10.9	.87	.91	620	313	3.76	.156	814
choc milk																
1% fat milk	158	211.3	8.1	26.1		1.3	148	2	.42	.10	12	152	287	33	1.02	.193
8 fl oz	250	2.5	1.5	0.8	0.1	7	500	.10	0.3	.86	.76	426	257	.60	.163	801
2% fat milk	179	208.9	8.0	26.0		1.3	143	2	.41	.10	12	151	284	33	1.02	.188
8 fl oz	250	5.0	3.1	1.5	0.2	17	500	.09	0.3	.85	.75	422	254	.60	.158	801
lowfat w/ nutrasweet, Land O Lakes	110		8.0	14.0								200				
8 fl oz	244	3.0	2.0	1.0	0.0	5										I
whole milk	208	205.8	7.9	25.9		2.0	73	2	.41	.10	12	149	280	33	1.02	.193
8 fl oz	250	8.5	5.3	2.5	0.3	31	303	.09	0.3	.84	.74	417	251	.60	.163	801
whole milk w/ choc powder	226	215.2	8.8	30.9		1.3	77	2	.43	.10	12	165	301	53	1.28	.157
2-3 hp t powder in 8 fl oz milk	266	8.8	5.5	2.6	0.3	32	311	.10	0.3	.88	.77	497	255	.80	.176	814
whole milk w/ choc syrup	231	229.0	8.7	33.6		0.6	76	2	.41	.10	14	155	296	56	1.21	.149
2 T syrup in 8 fl oz milk	282	8.5	5.3	2.5	0.3	34	319	.10	0.3	.87	.77	454	276	.90	.217	814
cocoa (hot choc)																
prep w/ 2% milk	193	202.4	9.8	29.5		2.0	138	3	.43	.12	15	128	315	70	1.47	.285
8 fl oz	250	5.8	3.6	1.7	0.2	20	515	.10	0.4	.93	.82	500	293	1.15	.302	801
prep w/ water from mix	103	178.0	3.1	22.5		2.5	0	0	.16	.03	0	148	97	25	.45	.078
3-4 hp t powder in 6 fl oz water	206	1.2	0.7	0.4	0.0	2	4	.03	0.2	.37	.25	202	89	.35	.093	814

	KCAL	H₂O (g)	PRO (g)	CHO (g)	SUGR (g)	DFIB (g)	A (RE)	C (mg)	B-2 (mg)	B-6 (mg)	FOL (mcg)	Na (mg)	Ca (mg)	Mg (mg)	Zn (mg)	Mn (mg)
	WT (g)	FAT (g)	SFA (g)	MUFA (g)	PUFA (g)	CHOL (mg)	A (IU)	B-1 (mg)	NIA (mg)	B-12 (mcg)	PANT (mg)	K (mg)	P (mg)	Fe (mg)	Cu (mg)	REF
prep w/ water from mix, added nutrients	119	178.1	1.9	24.0		0.8	150	6	.17	.04	0	207	105	23	.27	.092
1 pkt in 6 fl oz water	209	2.9	1.8	1.0	0.1	0	502	.15	2.0	.42	.28	405	111	1.82	.111	814
prep w/ water from mix, aspartame sweet-	48	177.4	3.8	8.4		0.4	0	0	.21	.05	2	173	90	33	.56	.100
ened—*.53 oz pkt powder in 6 fl oz water*	192	0.4	0.3	0.1	0.0	2	4	.04	0.2	.29	.57	405	134	.75	.121	814
eggnog, nonalcoholic	342	188.9	9.7	34.4		0.0	203	4	.48	.13	2	138	330	47	1.17	.013
8 fl oz	254	19.0	11.3	5.7	0.9	149	894	.09	0.3	1.14	1.06	420	278	.51	.033	801
eggnog, nonalcoholic, mix in whole milk	261	214.6	8.2	38.9		0.8	76	2	.39	.10	12	163	291	33	.92	.005
2 hp t in 8 fl oz milk	272	8.4	5.1	2.5	0.3	33	307	.09	0.2	.87	.76	370	228	.38	.024	814
instant breakfast																
in whole milk, Resource	290		15.0	37.0		0.0		20	.71	.66	130	220	470	132	4.90	.010
1.23 oz mix in 8 fl oz milk[3]	279	9.0				40	1650	.50	6.6	2.00	3.30	660	420	5.90	.660	I
liquid pack, Resource	250		12.0	33.0				15	.42	.50	100	190	300	60	3.70	1.000
8 fl oz[4]	279	8.0				20	1250	.37	5.0	1.50	2.50	480	300	4.50	.500	I
rtd, cnd, Carnation	215		12.0	34.5	33.0	0.5		30	.43	.50	100	208	500	100	3.80	
10 fl oz can[5]	315	2.8	0.6			9	2250	.38	5.0	1.50	2.50	498	500	4.50	.500	I
malted milk, whole milk	236	215.2	10.3	27.3		0.0	95	3	.59	.19	22	223	355	53	1.14	.005
3 hp t powder in 8 fl oz milk	265	9.8	6.0	2.8	0.6	37	368	.20	1.3	1.03	.77	530	302	.27	.066	814
malted milk, whole milk w/ added nutrients	231	215.4	9.8	28.4		0.0	742	29	1.14	.87	22	204	371	48	1.09	.093
4-5 hp t powder in 8 fl oz milk	265	8.7	5.4	2.5	0.4	34	2531	.71	10.4	1.03	.77	572	307	3.60	.082	814
strawberry flavored mix in whole milk	234	215.2	8.0	32.7		0.0	74	2	.42	.10	12	128	293	32	.93	.005
2-3 hp t powder in 8 fl oz milk	266	8.2	5.1	2.4	0.3	32	309	.09	0.2	.88	.77	370	229	.21	.024	814

23.3 MILK MIXES

	KCAL	H₂O (g)	PRO (g)	CHO (g)	SUGR (g)	DFIB (g)	A (RE)	C (mg)	B-2 (mg)	B-6 (mg)	FOL (mcg)	Na (mg)	Ca (mg)	Mg (mg)	Zn (mg)	Mn (mg)
	WT (g)	FAT (g)	SFA (g)	MUFA (g)	PUFA (g)	CHOL (mg)	A (IU)	B-1 (mg)	NIA (mg)	B-12 (mcg)	PANT (mg)	K (mg)	P (mg)	Fe (mg)	Cu (mg)	REF
Alba, Fit 'n Frosty																
choc	70		6.0	11.0				1	.30			210	310			
21.26 g pkt	21	1.0					304	.07	0.4				176	.43		I
choc marshmallow	70		6.0	11.0				1	.29			250	310			
21.26 g pkt	21	1.0					305	.07	0.5				177	.39		I
double fudge	70		6.0	11.0				1	.28			170	310			
21.26 g pkt	21	1.0					305	.07	0.5				173	.42		I
strawberry	70		5.0	12.0				1	.36			150	310			
21.26 g pkt	21	0.0					265	.09	0.6				187	.10		I
van	70		5.0	12.0				1	.30			150	310			
21.26 g pkt	21	0.0					218	.08	1.9				182	.10		I
choc milk powder	77	0.2	0.7	19.9		1.3	0	0	.03	.00	1	46	8	22	.34	.156
2-3 hp t	22	0.7	0.4	0.2	0.0	0	4	.01	0.1	.00	.01	130	28	.69	.155	814
Gerber Graduates	79		0.2	19.2	14.4	0.3			.02	.00		4	26	6	1.60	.060
.7 oz	20	0.1						.00	0.0			45	18	2.00	.030	I
Hershey	111		0.5	22.3	20.9	0.6		9	.00	.20		47	24	24	.91	
3 T	24	0.3	0.1			0	750	.15	2.0	.60	.60	42	0	3.91	.130	I
malted	79	0.3	1.1	18.4		0.2	4	0	.04	.03	4	53	13	15	.17	.132
.75 oz (3 hp t)	21	0.8	0.5	0.2	0.1	1	19	.04	0.4	.04	.14	130	37	.48	.042	814
malted, Carnation	90	0.3	1.0	18.0	14.0	0.2		0	.04	.03	4	40	0	15	.17	
.75 oz (3 hp t)	21	1.0	0.5	0.2	0.1	0	11	.04	0.4	.04		115	37	.48	.040	I
malted w/ added nutrients	75	0.5	1.0	17.7		0.2	824	32	.86	.92	20	125	93	20	.22	.132
.75 oz (4-5 hp t)	21	0.7	0.4	0.2	0.1	1	2751	.64	10.7	.04	.14	251	84	3.65	.133	814
cocoa mix, powder	101	0.4	3.0	22.1		0.3	1	1	.16	.03	0	141	91	23	.41	.075
1 oz pkt (3-4 hp t)	28	1.1	0.7	0.4	0.0	1	4	.03	0.2	.37	.25	199	88	.33	.080	814
70-cal, Carnation	70	0.4	3.0	15.0	15.0	1.0		0	.11	.03	4	140	91	20	.30	.002
1 pkt	21	0.0	0.0	0.0	0.0	1	3	.03	0.1	.30	.30	210	82	.43	.010	I
Alba	62		5.4	10.2				1	.29			134	323			
.68 oz pkt	19	0.5				4	283	.06	0.2			425	238	.07		I
aspartame sweetened	48	0.5	3.8	8.5		0.4	1	0	.21	.05	2	168	86	31	.52	.100
.53 oz pkt	15	0.4	0.3	0.1	0.0	1	5	.04	0.2	.29	.57	405	134	.74	.110	814
choc flavors, Swiss Miss	145		1.9	27.5	24.3	1.3		0				198	41			
1.2 oz[6]	35	3.1	1.2			2								.70		I
diet, Swiss Miss	22		1.8	3.6	2.4	0.8		0				185	48			
.26 oz	7	0.3	0.2			0								.44		I
lite, Swiss Miss	76		1.6	17.5	14.5	1.7		0				177	36			
.75 oz	21	0.6	0.6	0.2		0								.47		I

	KCAL	H₂O (g)	PRO (g)	CHO (g)	SUGR (g)	DFIB (g)	A (RE)	C (mg)	B-2 (mg)	B-6 (mg)	FOL (mcg)	Na (mg)	Ca (mg)	Mg (mg)	Zn (mg)	Mn (mg)
	WT (g)	FAT (g)	SFA (g)	MUFA (g)	PUFA (g)	CHOL (mg)	A (IU)	B-1 (mg)	NIA (mg)	B-12 (mcg)	PANT (mg)	K (mg)	P (mg)	Fe (mg)	Cu (mg)	REF
marshmallow lovers, fat-free, Swiss Miss	65		3.3	12.6	9.9			0				155	39			
.6 oz	17	0.3	0.0			0								.57		I
milk choc, Carnation	110	0.5	2.0	24.0	20.0	1.0		0	.15	.04	2	95	76	20	.36	.001
1 oz pkt (4 hp t)	28	1.0	0.0	0.1	0.0	1	3	.04	0.1	.23	.38	237	90	.43	.151	I
milk choc, Swiss Miss	118		1.4	22.3	15.8	1.5		0				118	38			
1 oz	28	2.7	0.8			1								.42		I
milk choc w/ mini marshmallows, Swiss	118		1.4	22.3	17.4	1.3		0				123	40			
Miss—1 oz	28	2.6	0.8		0.0	0								.48		I
no sugar added, rich choc, Carnation	50	0.5	4.0	8.0	7.0	0.1	1		.20	.03	6	140	123	26	.40	
.5 oz pkt[7]	15	0.0	0.0	0.0	0.0	5	6	.05	0.1	.44	.49	270	124	.47	.015	I
no sugar added, w/ marshmallows,	56		2.5	9.7	5.5	0.8		0				146	62			
Swiss Miss—.53 oz	15	0.8	0.4			1										I
rich choc, Carnation	110	0.5	2.0	24.0	21.0	1.0		0	.15	.04	1	100	40	20	.30	.000
1 oz pkt (3-4 hp t)	28	1.0	0.0	0.6	0.0	5	3	.04	0.1	.17	.39	253	86	.45	.154	I
rich, no sugar added, Swiss Miss	54		2.3	9.6	5.7	1.0		0				165	72			
.53 oz	15	1.1	0.6			1								.50		I
rich, Swiss Miss	110		1.7	22.6	20.7	1.2		0				140	47			
1 oz	28	1.8	0.5			1								.31		I
w/ added nutrients	119	0.5	1.9	23.9		0.9	149	6	.17	.04	0	200	100	22	.22	.090
1.1 oz pkt	31	3.0	1.8	1.0	0.1	1	497	.15	2.0	.41	.28	401	110	1.79	.100	814
w/ marshmallows, Carnation	110	0.8	1.0	24.0	21.0	1.0		0	.14	.04	1	95	42			
1 oz pkt (3-4 hp t)	28	1.0	0.0	0.1	0.0	1	3	.03	0.1	.16	.37	239				I
eggnog mix, powder, nonalcoholic	109	0.1	0.1	27.3		0.9	3	0	.00	.00	1	43	1	0	.02	.000
2 hp T	28	0.3	0.1	0.1	0.0	7	10	.00	0.0	.02	1.72	1	3	.25	.006	814
Instant Breakfast																
cafe mocha, Carnation	130		4.5	28.0	23.0	0.4		27	.14	.40	100	100	350	80	3.00	
1.3 oz pkt	37	0.5	0.0			3	1750	.30	5.0	.60	2.00	340	250	4.50	.500	I
choc malt, Carnation	130		4.5	26.0	17.0	1.0		27	.07	.40	100	130	250	80	3.00	
1.25 oz pkt	36	1.5	0.5			3	1750	.30	5.0	.60	2.00	250	250	4.50	.500	I
choc malt, Pillsbury	126	1.1	5.7	25.1				23	.41			119	335			
1.2 oz pkt	35	0.5					1684	.47	5.8			263	125	5.60		I
choc, Pillsbury	130	0.9	5.7	25.7				23	.35			141	91			
1.2 oz pkt	35	0.5					1681	.46	5.8			256	89	5.64		I
creamy milk choc, Carnation	130		4.5	28.0	20.0	1.0		27	.14	.40	100	100	300	80	3.00	
1.30 oz pkt	37	1.0				2	1750	.30	5.0	.60	2.00	350	250	4.50	.500	I
french van, Carnation	130		4.5	27.0	17.0	0.0		27	.14	.40	100					
1.26 oz pkt	36	0.0	0.0	0.0	0.0	3	1750	.30	5.0	.60	2.00					I
strawberry, Carnation	130	1.2	4.5	28.0	18.0	0.0		27	.14	.40	100	160	350	80	3.00	
1.26 oz pkt	36	0.0	0.0	0.0			1750	.30	5.0	.60	2.00	250	250	4.50	.500	I
strawberry, Pillsbury	130	0.9	5.4	26.4				23	.32			130	91			
1.2 oz pkt	35	0.2					1681	.44	5.8			250	70	5.40		I
vanilla, Pillsbury	133	0.8	5.4	27.3				23	.23			198	79			
1.2 oz pkt	35	0.2					1686	.33	4.7			229	111	5.10		I
Instant Breakfast, no sugar added																
choc, Carnation	70		4.5	12.0	6.0	1.0		27	.10	.40	100	95	300	80	3.00	
.72 oz pkt	21	1.0	0.5			3	1750	.30	5.0	.60	2.00	350	250	4.50	.500	I
choc malt, Carnation	70		4.5	11.0	6.0	1.0		27	.10	.40	100	115	250	80	3.00	
.7 oz pkt	20	1.5	1.0			3	1750	.30	5.0	.60	2.00	290	250	4.50	.500	I
strawberry, Carnation	70		4.5	12.0	7.0	0.0		27	.14	.40	100					
.7 oz pkt	20	0.0	0.0	0.0	0.0	3	1750	.30	5.0	.60	2.00					I
van, Carnation	70	0.8	4.5	12.0	7.0	0.0		27	.14	.40	100	95	350	80	3.00	
.7 oz pkt	20	0.0	0.0	0.0	0.0	3	1750	.30	5.0	.60	2.00	250	250	4.50	.500	I
malted milk powder	87	0.4	2.4	15.9		0.1	18	1	.19	.09	10	104	63	20	.21	.089
.75 oz (3 hp t)	21	1.7	0.9	0.4	0.3	4	61	.11	1.1	.16	.14	159	75	.15	.042	814
Carnation	90	0.4	3.0	15.0	10.0	1.0		0	.14	.08	10	85	40	20	.21	
.75 oz (3 hp t)	21	2.0	1.0		0.0	5	40	.11	1.1	.16	.30	140	79	.16	.042	I
w/ added nutrients	80	0.7	1.8	17.1		0.1	668	27	.75	.76	10	85	79	14	.15	.089
¾ oz (4-5 hp t)	21	0.6	0.3	0.2	0.1	4	2222	.62	10.2	.16	.14	203	79	3.49	.059	814
strawberry flavor mix, powder	85	0.1	0.0	21.8	0.0		0	0	.02	.00	0	8	0	0	.00	.000
2-3 hp t	22	0.0	0.0	0.0	0.0	0	0	.00	0.0	.00	.00	1	0	.10	.004	814

	KCAL	H₂O (g)	PRO (g)	CHO (g)	SUGR (g)	DFIB (g)	Vitamins A (RE)	C (mg)	B-2 (mg)	B-6 (mg)	FOL (mcg)	Minerals Na (mg)	Ca (mg)	Mg (mg)	Zn (mg)	Mn (mg)
	WT (g)	FAT (g)	SFA (g)	MUFA (g)	PUFA (g)	CHOL (mg)	A (IU)	B-1 (mg)	NIA (mg)	B-12 (mcg)	PANT (mg)	K (mg)	P (mg)	Fe (mg)	Cu (mg)	REF
van milk mixer, Gerber Graduates	79		19.7	15.4					.00	.00		2	22	1	1.60	
.7 oz	20							.01	0.0			2	9	2.00	.010	I

23.4 MILK, OTHER

	KCAL	H₂O	PRO	CHO	SUGR	DFIB	A (RE)	C	B-2	B-6	FOL	Na	Ca	Mg	Zn	Mn
goat milk	168	212.4	8.7	10.9		0.0	137	3	.34	.11	1	122	326	34	.73	.044
8 fl oz	244	10.1	6.5	2.7	0.4	28	451	.12	0.7	.16	.76	499	270	.12	.112	801
human milk	22	27.1	0.3	2.1		0.0	20	2	.01	.00	2	5	10	1	.05	.008
1 fl oz	31	1.4	0.6	0.5	0.2	4	75	.00	0.1	.01	.07	16	4	.01	.016	801
indian buffalo milk	236	203.5	9.2	12.6		0.0	129	5	.33	.06	14	127	412	76	.54	.044
8 fl oz	244	16.8	11.2	4.4	0.4	46	434	.13	0.2	.89	.47	434	286	.29	.112	801
sheep milk	264	197.7	14.7	13.1		0.0	103	10	.87	.15	17	108	474	45	1.32	.044
8 fl oz	245	17.2	11.3	4.2	0.8	66	360	.16	1.0	1.74	1.00	334	387	.25	.113	801
soy milk	79	223.8	6.6	4.3		3.1	7	0	.17	.10	4	29	10	46	.55	.408
8 fl oz	240	4.6	0.5	0.8	2.0	0	77	.39	0.4	.00	.12	338	118	1.39	.288	816

23.5 YOGURT

	KCAL	H₂O	PRO	CHO	SUGR	DFIB	A (RE)	C	B-2	B-6	FOL	Na	Ca	Mg	Zn	Mn
cafe au lait, Yoplait	170		8.0	31.0	28.0	0.0	0	0	.34			90	200			
6 fl oz	170	2.0	1.0			10	0	.09				340	200	.00		I
coconut cream pie, Yoplait	200		7.0	35.0	31.0	0.0	0	0	.26			125	200			
6 fl oz	170	3.0	2.0			10	0	.06				340	150	.00		I
custard style																
fruit flavors, multipack, Yoplait	130		5.0	22.0	19.0	0.0	0	0	.17			70	150			
4 fl oz[8]	113	2.0	1.5			10	0	.03				210	100	.00		I
fruit flavors, Yoplait	190		8.0	32.0	30.0	0.0	0	0	.25			100	200			
6 fl oz[9]	170	3.0	2.0			15	0	.06				310	150	.00		I
light, Yoplait	90		6.0	15.0	9.0	0.0	0	0	.17			95	150			
6 fl oz[10]	170	0.0	0.0	0.0	0.0	5	0	.00				250	150	.00		I
van, Yoplait	190		8.0	32.0	29.0	0.0	0	0	.26			95	200			
6 fl oz	170	3.0	2.0			15	0	.06				320	150	.00		I
light																
apple crisp w/ cinn graham crunch, Yoplait—7 fl oz	140		7.0	24.0	14.0	0.0	0	0	.26			130	250			
	199	1.5	0.0			5	0	.09				310	150	.00		I
cherry cheesecake w/ graham crunch, Yoplait—7 fl oz	130		7.0	23.0	13.0	0.0	0	0	.26			115	250			
	199	1.5	0.0			5	0	.09				310	150	.00		I
fruit flavors, Yoplait	90		5.0	16.0	10.0	0.0	0	0	.26			75	200			
6 fl oz[11]	170	0.0	0.0	0.0	0.0	5	0	.03				230	100	.00		I
indulgent flavors, Yoplait	90		6.0	16.0	10.0	0.0	0	0	.26			95	200			
6 fl oz[12]	170	0.0	0.0	0.0	0.0	5	0	.03				240	150	.00		I
lemon creme crunch, Yoplait 7 fl oz	140		7.0	22.0	12.0	0.0	0	0	.26			135	250			
	199	2.0	0.0			5	0	.09				290	150	.00		I
strawberry w/ granola crunch, Yoplait 7 fl oz	140		8.0	25.0	13.0	2.0	0	0	.26			115	250			
	199	1.5	0.0			5	0	.09				310	150	.00		I
van w/ choc crunch, Yoplait 7 fl oz	140		8.0	22.0	13.0	0.0	0	0	.26			150	200			
	199	2.0	0.0			5	0	.09				330	150	.00		I
lowfat																
(1% milk fat), flavored, Breyers	251		8.1	48.5	46.5	0.3	0	1	.34			111	300			
8 fl oz[13]	227	2.5	1.5			15	0	.04		.90		411	250	.00		I
(1% milk fat), flavored, Light 'n Lively Kidpack—4.4 fl oz[14]	140		5.0	27.1	24.0	0.0	0	0	.17			65	150			
	125	1.0	0.6			10	0	.00		.48		235	150	.00		I
(1% milk fat), flavored, Light 'n Lively Multipack—4.4 fl oz[15]	140		5.0	26.6	23.7	0.0	0	2	.17			63	157			
	125	1.0	0.6			9	0	.02		.48		231	150	.00		I
(1.5% milk fat), flavored, Breyers	220		10.0	38.0	37.3	0.0		0	.43			137	350			
8 fl oz[16]	227	3.0	2.0			20	100	.06		.12		473	300	.00		I
(1.5% milk fat), plain, Breyers	130		11.0	15.0	15.0	0.0		0	.43			150	400			
8 fl oz	227	3.0	2.0			20	100	.06		1.20		520	300	.00		I
coffee/van flavor w/ nfdm	194	179.3	11.2	31.3		0.0	30	2	.46	.10	24	149	389	37	1.88	.009
8 fl oz	227	2.8	1.8	0.8	0.1	11	123	.10	0.2	1.20	1.25	498	306	.16	.030	801
fruit flavor w/ nfdm	225	170.9	9.0	42.3		0.0	27	1	.37	.08	19	121	314	30	1.52	.145
8 fl oz	227	2.6	1.7	0.7	0.1	10	111	.08	0.2	.97	1.01	402	247	.14	.179	801

							Vitamins					Minerals				
	KCAL	H₂O (g)	PRO (g)	CHO (g)	SUGR (g)	DFIB (g)	A (RE)	C (mg)	B-2 (mg)	B-6 (mg)	FOL (mcg)	Na (mg)	Ca (mg)	Mg (mg)	Zn (mg)	Mn (mg)
	WT (g)	FAT (g)	SFA (g)	MUFA (g)	PUFA (g)	CHOL (mg)	A (IU)	B-1 (mg)	NIA (mg)	B-12 (mcg)	PANT (mg)	K (mg)	P (mg)	Fe (mg)	Cu (mg)	REF
fruit flavors, multipack, Yoplait	120		4.0	22.0	20.0	0.0	0	0	.17			80	150			
4 fl oz	113	1.0	0.5			5	0	.03				220	100	.00		I
fruit flavors, Yoplait	180		7.0	33.0	30.0	0.0	0	0	.26			125	200			
6 fl oz	170	1.5	1.0			10	0	.06				330	150	.00		I
plain, Dannon	140		11.0	15.0				0	.51			125	400			
8 fl oz	227	4.0				15			0.0	.24			250			I
plain w/ nfdm	144	193.1	11.9	16.0		0.0	36	2	.49	.11	25	159	415	40	2.02	.009
8 fl oz	227	3.5	2.3	1.0	0.1	14	150	.10	0.3	1.28	1.34	531	326	.18	.030	801
Trix, multipack, Yoplait	110		4.0	19.0	16.0	0.0	0	0	.17			65	100			
4 fl oz[17]	113	1.5	1.0			5	0	.03				190	100	.00		I
Trix, Yoplait	160		7.0	28.0	24.0	0.0	0	0	.26			95	200			
6 fl oz[17]	170	2.0	1.0			5	0	.06				280	150	.00		I
nonfat																
caramel nut, Snackwell's	170		5.0	38.0	29.0	1.0						200				
¾ cup	170	0.0	0.0	0.0	0.0	5										I
choc almond, Snackwell's	170		5.0	38.0	29.0	1.0						200				
¾ cup	170	0.0	0.0	0.0	0.0	5										I
choc cherry, Snackwell's	190		6.0	41.0	30.0	2.0						200				
¾ cup	170	0.0	0.0	0.0	0.0	5										I
choc raspberry, Snackwell's	170		5.0	38.0	29.0	1.0						200				
¾ cup	170	0.0	0.0	0.0	0.0	5										I
double choc, Snackwell's	190		6.0	41.0	30.0	2.0						200				
¾ cup	170	0.0	0.0	0.0	0.0	5										I
flavored, Knudsen Free	165		8.0	32.3	29.3	0.0	0	0	.26			104	250			
6 fl oz[18]	170	0.0	0.0	0.0	0.0	5	0	.03		.90		365	200	.00		I
flavored, Light 'n Lively Free	174		8.0	35.1	31.8	0.0	0	0	.34			105	225			
6 fl oz[19]	170	0.0	0.0	0.0	0.0	5	0	.03		.90		354	200	.00		I
flavored, w/ aspartame, Knudsen Cal 70	70		7.0	11.2	8.3	0.0	0	0	.26			84	200			
6 fl oz[20]	170	0.0	0.0	0.0	0.0	5	0	.03		.60		277	150	.00		I
flavored, w/ aspartame, Light 'n Lively Free 50 Cal—4.4 fl oz[21]	50		5.0	8.2	6.0	0.0	0	0	.17			60	150			
	125	0.0	0.0	0.0	0.0	5	0	.00		.48		208	100	.00		I
flavored, w/ aspartame, Light 'n Lively Free 70 Cal—6 fl oz[22]	70		6.9	11.3	8.1	0.0	0	0	.26			87	200			
	170	0.0	0.0	0.0	0.0	5	0	.03		.60		275	150	.00		I
fruit on the bottom, Yoplait	160		7.0	34.0	30.0	0.0	0	0	.26			95	200			
6 fl oz[23]	170	0.0	0.0	0.0	0.0	5	0	.06				310	150	.00		I
milk choc, Snackwell's	170		5.0	38.0	29.0	1.0						200				
¾ cup	170	0.0	0.0	0.0	0.0	5										I
plain w/ nfdm	127	193.5	13.0	17.4		0.0	5	2	.53	.12	28	174	452	43	2.20	.011
8 fl oz	227	0.4	0.3	0.1	0.0	4	16	.11	0.3	1.39	1.46	579	355	.20	.034	801
plain, Yoplait	130		13.0	19.0	14.0	0.0	0	0	.60			170	450		.00	
8 fl oz	227	0.0	0.0	0.0	0.0	10	0	.12				550	350			I
van, Yoplait	200		10.0	40.0	32.0	0.0	0	0	.43			160	350			
8 fl oz	227	0.0	0.0	0.0	0.0	5	0	.09				430	300	.00		I
whole, plain	139	199.5	7.9	10.6		0.0	68	1	.32	.07	17	105	274	26	1.34	.009
8 fl oz	227	7.4	4.8	2.0	0.2	29	279	.07	0.2	.84	.88	351	215	.11	.020	801

1. Not fortified with vitamin A.
2. Reconstitutes to 1 quart of fluid nonfat milk.
3. Values are averages for chocolate, strawberry, and vanilla.
4. Includes chocolate, strawberry, and vanilla.
5. Values are averages for cafe mocha, chocolate, French vanilla, and strawberry creme.
6. Values are averages for chocolate almond mocha, chocolate english toffee, chocolate pralines & creme, chocolate raspberry truffle, chocolate sensation, cocoa & creme, marshmallow lovers, and swisse chocolate truffle.
7. The sugar in this product is lactose.
8. Includes peaches 'n cream, raspberry, strawberry, strawberry banana, and strawberry vanilla.
9. Includes banana, berry bust, blueberry, blueberries 'n cream, cherry, lemon, peaches 'n cream, raspberry, strawberry, strawberry banana, and strawberry vanilla.
10. Includes cherry vanilla, peach, strawberry, and vanilla.
11. Includes apricot mango, blueberry, cherry, peach, raspberry, raspberry peach melba, strawberry, strawberry banana, strawberry cheesecake and white chocolate strawberry.
12. Includes amaretto cheesecake, banana cream pie, boston cream pie, caramel apple, key lime pie, and lemon cream pie.
13. Values are averages for black cherry, blueberry, mixed berry, peach, pineapple, red raspberry, strawberry, and strawberry banana.
14. Values are averages for banana berry, berry blue, cherry, grape, outrageous orange, tropical punch, wild berry, and wild strawberry.

15. Values are averages for blueberry, peach, pineapple, red raspberry, strawberry, strawberry banana, and strawberry fruit cup.
16. Values are averages for coffee, creamy lemon, and vanilla.
17. Includes rainbow punch, raspberry rainbow, strawberry banana bash, and triple cherry.
18. Values are averages for lemon, mixed berry, peach, red raspberry, strawberry, and vanilla.
19. Values are averages for blueberry, lemon, mixed berry, peach, red raspberry, strawberry, strawberry fruit cup, and vanilla.
20. Values are averages for black cherry, blueberry, lemon, peach, pineapple, red raspberry, strawberry, strawberry banana, strawberry fruit basket, and van.
21. Values are averages for blueberry, peach, red raspberry, strawberry, strawberry banana, and strawberry fruit cup.
22. Values are averages for black cherry, blueberry, lemon, peach, red raspberry, strawberry, strawberry banana, and strawberry fruit cup.
23. Includes blueberry, cherry, peach, raspberry, strawberry, and strawberry banana.

	KCAL	H₂O (g)	PRO (g)	CHO (g)	SUGR (g)	DFIB (g)	A (RE)	C (mg)	B-2 (mg)	B-6 (mg)	FOL (mcg)	Na (mg)	Ca (mg)	Mg (mg)	Zn (mg)	Mn (mg)
	WT (g)	FAT (g)	SFA (g)	MUFA (g)	PUFA (g)	CHOL (mg)	A (IU)	B-1 (mg)	NIA (mg)	B-12 (mcg)	PANT (mg)	K (mg)	P (mg)	Fe (mg)	Cu (mg)	REF

24. NUTS, NUT PRODUCTS, & SEEDS

	KCAL/WT	H₂O/FAT	PRO/SFA	CHO/MUFA	SUGR/PUFA	DFIB/CHOL	A	C/B-1	B-2/NIA	B-6/B-12	FOL/PANT	Na/K	Ca/P	Mg/Fe	Zn/Cu	Mn/REF
acorn flour, full-fat	142	1.7	2.1	15.5			1	0	.04	.20	32	0	12	31	.18	.494
1 oz	28	8.6	1.1	5.4	1.6	0	14	.04	0.7	.00	.26	202	29	.34	.173	812
acorns, dried	144	1.4	2.3	15.2			0	0	.04	.20	32	0	15	23	.19	.386
1 oz	28	8.9	1.2	5.6	1.7	0	0	.04	0.7	.00	.27	201	29	.29	.232	812
acorns, raw	110	7.9	1.7	11.6			1	0	.03	.15	25	0	12	18	.14	.379
1 oz	28	6.8	0.9	4.3	1.3	0	11	.03	0.5	.00	.20	153	22	.22	.176	812
almond butter	101	0.2	2.4	3.4		0.6	0	0	.10	.01	10	2	43	48	.49	.377
1 T	16	9.5	0.9	6.1	2.0	0	0	.02	0.5	.00	.04	121	84	.59	.144	812
almond butter w/ honey & cinn	96	0.3	2.5	4.3			0	0	.10	.01	10	2	43	48	.48	.373
1 T	16	8.4	0.8	5.4	1.8	0	0	.02	0.5	.00	.04	120	83	.59	.155	812
almond flour, full-fat	168	0.9	5.6	6.3			0	0	.33	.03	17	2	62	87	.06	.403
1 oz	28	14.6	1.4	9.5	3.1	0	0	.06	0.7	.00	.13	201	172	.79	.196	812
almond flour, partially defatted	111	2.7	10.6	9.0			0	0	.18	.03	10	3	67	78	.86	.394
1 oz	28	4.5	0.4	2.9	1.0	0	0	.04	0.9	.00	.13	204	144	.99	.291	812
almond meal, partially defatted	116	2.0	11.2	8.2			0	0	.48	.03	16	2	120	82	.80	.626
1 oz	28	5.2	0.5	3.4	1.1	0	0	.09	1.8	.00	.13	397	259	2.41	.259	812
almond paste	130	4.0	2.6	13.6		1.4	0	0	.12	.01	21	3	49	37	.42	.570
1 oz	28	7.9	0.7	5.1	1.6	0	0	.02	0.4	.00	.12	89	73	.45	.129	812
almonds																
barbecue, Blue Diamond	166	0.4	6.1	4.8					.33			172	92			
1 oz	28	14.9						.03	1.0			116		1.07		I
blanched, Blue Diamond	174	1.4	6.0	5.2					.20	.03	10	1	73	86	.94	
1 oz	28	14.4	1.2		3.3	0		.04	0.9			173	150	1.09	.310	I
blanched, slivered, Blue Diamond	172	1.3	5.9	5.5		2.6			.19	.03	10	2	71	86	.98	
1 oz	28	14.4	1.0	9.3	3.1	0		.05	0.9			179	151	1.04	.330	I
cheese, Blue Diamond	156	0.4	6.1	7.4					.34			95	102			
1 oz	28	12.5						.03	0.8			126		1.04		I
chopped, Blue Diamond	175	1.3	6.0	5.0					.20	.03	10	0	77	85	.92	
1 oz	28	14.6	1.2		3.3	0		.06	0.9			174	151	1.15	.300	I
dried	165	1.2	5.6	5.7		3.1	0	0	.22	.03	16	3	74	83	.82	.636
1 oz (24 nuts)	28	14.6	1.4	9.5	3.1	0	0	.06	0.9	.00	.13	205	146	1.02	.264	812
dry roasted	166	0.9	4.6	6.9	1.7	3.9	0	0	.17	.02	18	3	80	86	1.39	.560
1 oz	28	14.6	1.4	9.5	3.1	0	0	.04	0.8	.00	.07	218	155	1.08	.347	812
dry roasted, hickory smoke, Blue Diamond—1 oz	166	0.7	5.9	4.9					.42			121	117			
	28	15.0						.08	1.4			109		1.31		I
dry roasted, lightly salted, Blue Diamond	172	0.4	6.2	5.3		3.0			.34			121	89	81	.90	
1 oz	28	15.3	1.1	8.9	3.7	0		.03	0.9			209	139	1.00		I
dry roasted, unsalted, Blue Diamond	169	0.6	6.0	5.4		3.1			.40			1	92	91	1.60	
1 oz	28	15.1	1.2	9.3	3.0	0		.01	0.6			200	145	1.35		I
honey roasted, Blue Diamond	169	0.5	5.2	7.9		2.6			.27			37	75	68	.74	
1 oz	28	14.1	1.0	7.8	3.6	0		.03	0.8			159	113	.80	.280	I
honey roasted, unblanched	168	0.5	5.2	7.9		3.9	0	0	.27	.02	9	37	75	68	.74	.568
1 oz (26 nuts)	28	14.1	1.3	9.2	3.0	0	0	.03	0.8	.00	.07	159	113	.80	.275	812
lightly roasted, salted, Blue Diamond	176	0.5	6.3	3.6		2.6			.31			128	87	73	.89	
1 oz	28	16.4	1.2	9.5	3.9	0		.03	1.0			168	142	1.07	.230	I

	KCAL / WT (g)	H₂O (g) / FAT (g)	PRO (g) / SFA (g)	CHO (g) / MUFA (g)	SUGR (g) / PUFA (g)	DFIB (g) / CHOL (mg)	A (RE) / A (IU)	C (mg) / B-1 (mg)	B-2 (mg) / NIA (mg)	B-6 (mg) / B-12 (mcg)	FOL (mcg) / PANT (mg)	Na (mg) / K (mg)	Ca (mg) / P (mg)	Mg (mg) / Fe (mg)	Zn (mg) / Cu (mg)	Mn (mg) / REF
oil roasted, blanched, salted, Blue Diamond—1 oz	174	0.7	5.9	4.0					.40			70	65			
	28	16.3						.02	1.2			165		1.40		I
oil roasted, salted, Blue Diamond 1 oz	174	0.4	6.3	3.4					.31			95	87			
	28	16.4						.03	1.0			132		1.07		I
oil roasted, unblanched 1 oz (22 nuts)	173	0.9	5.7	4.4		3.1	0	0	.28	.02	18	3	66	85	1.37	.553
	28	16.1	1.5	10.5	3.4	0	0	.04	1.0	.00	.07	191	153	1.07	.343	812
onion garlic, Blue Diamond 1 oz	160	0.5	6.1	6.3					.32			168	125			
	28	13.6						.02	0.9			112		1.12		I
Planters 1 oz	170		6.0	5.0	1.0	3.0						0				
	28	15.0	1.0	10.0	4.0	0						190				I
raw, Fisher 1 oz	170		6.0	6.0								0				
	28	15.0	1.0	11.0	3.0	0						0				I
sliced, natural, Blue Diamond 1 oz	171	1.3	5.9	5.3		2.9			.20	.03	10	0	77	85	.92	
	28	14.4	1.1	8.9	3.0	0		.06	0.9			174	151	1.15	.300	I
sliced, Planters ⅓ cup	200		7.0	6.0	1.0	4.0						0				
	33	18.0	1.5	12.0	4.0	0						230				I
slivered, Planters 2 oz pkg (⅓ cup)	340		12.0	11.0	2.0	6.0						0				
	57	31.0	2.5	20.0	7.0	0						390				I
Smokehouse, Blue Diamond 1 oz	172	0.5	6.0	4.5		2.8			.34			169	101	75	.76	
	28	15.7	1.2	10.0	2.7	0		.03	1.0			155	138	1.11	.400	I
toasted, unblanched 1 oz	167	0.7	5.8	6.5		3.2	0	0	.17	.02	18	3	80	86	1.39	.568
	28	14.4	1.4	9.3	3.0	0	0	.04	0.8	.00	.07	219	156	1.39	.349	812
whole, blanched, Blue Diamond 1 oz	174	1.4	6.0	5.2		2.6			.20			0	73	86	.90	
	28	14.3	1.0	9.3	3.1	0		.04	0.9			173	150	1.10	.300	I
whole, natural, Blue Diamond 1 oz	170	1.3	5.9	5.7		3.5		0	.25	.03	10	0	79	86	.92	.710
	28	14.2	1.0	10.7	3.3	0	0	.05	0.9	.00	.00	179	149	1.30	.300	I
beechnuts, dried 1 oz	163	1.9	1.8	9.5			0	4	.11	.19	32	11	0	0	.10	.380
	28	14.2	1.6	6.2	5.7	0	0	.09	0.2	.00	.26	288	0	.70	.190	812
brazilnuts, dried 1 oz (8 med nuts)	186	0.9	4.1	3.6	0.7	1.5	0	0	.03	.07	1	1	50	64	1.30	.219
	28	18.8	4.6	6.5	6.8	0	0	.28	0.5	.00	.07	170	170	.96	.502	812
breadfruit seeds																
boiled 1 oz	48	16.8	1.5	9.1			7	2	.05	.08	14	7	17	14	.24	.037
	28	0.7	0.2	0.1	0.3	0	67	.08	1.5	.00	.23	248	35	.17	.303	812
raw 1 oz	54	16.0	2.1	8.3			7	2	.09	.09	15	7	10	15	.26	.040
	28	1.6	0.4	0.2	0.8	0	73	.14	0.1	.00	.25	267	50	1.04	.325	812
roasted 1 oz	59	14.1	1.8	11.4			8	2	.07	.12	17	8	24	18	.29	.046
	28	0.8	0.2	0.1	0.4	0	83	.12	2.1	.00	.29	307	50	.26	.375	812
butternuts, dried 1 oz	174	0.9	7.1	3.4		1.3	3	1	.04	.16	19	0	15	67	.89	1.860
	28	16.2	0.4	3.0	12.1	0	35	.11	0.3	.00	.18	119	126	1.14	.128	812
cashew butter 1 oz	166	0.8	5.0	7.8		0.6	0	0	.05	.07	19	4	12	73	1.46	.231
	28	14.0	2.8	8.3	2.4	0	0	.09	0.5	.00	.34	155	130	1.43	.621	812
cashew halves w/ pieces, Planters 1 oz[1]	170		5.0	8.0	2.0						120					
	28	14.0	2.5	8.0	2.5	0										I
cashews																
dry roasted 1 oz	163	0.5	4.3	9.3		0.9	0	0	.06	.07	20	5	13	74	1.59	.234
	28	13.1	2.6	7.7	2.2	0	0	.06	0.4	.00	.35	160	139	1.70	.629	812
dry roasted, Fisher 1 oz	160		5.0	8.0								100				
	28	13.0	3.0	8.0	2.0	0										I
fancy, Planters 1 oz	170		5.0	8.0	1.0							120				
	28	14.0	3.0	8.0	2.5	0						150				I
honey roasted, Fisher 1 oz	150		4.0	7.0								90				
	28	13.0	3.0	7.0	3.0	0										I
honey roasted, Planters 1 oz	150		4.0	11.0	5.0	1.0						120				
	28	12.0	2.0	7.0	2.5	0						130				I
Lance 1.1 oz	192	1.2	5.6	7.9					.08			93	14			
	32	15.1	2.8	9.4	2.9	0		.07	0.9			101		1.68		I
oil roasted 1 oz (18 med nuts)	163	1.1	4.6	8.1		1.1	0	0	.05	.07	19	5	12	72	1.35	.229
	28	13.7	2.7	8.1	2.3	0	0	.12	0.5	.00	.34	150	121	1.16	.615	812
oil roasted, Fisher 1 oz	170		5.0	8.0								110				
	28	14.0	4.0	8.0	2.0	0										I

	KCAL / WT (g)	H₂O (g) / FAT (g)	PRO (g) / SFA (g)	CHO (g) / MUFA (g)	SUGR (g) / PUFA (g)	DFIB (g) / CHOL (mg)	A (RE) / A (IU)	C (mg) / B-1 (mg)	B-2 (mg) / NIA (mg)	B-6 (mg) / B-12 (mcg)	FOL (mcg) / PANT (mg)	Na (mg) / K (mg)	Ca (mg) / P (mg)	Mg (mg) / Fe (mg)	Zn (mg) / Cu (mg)	Mn (mg) / REF
cashews & almonds, Fisher	170		5.0	6.0								95				
1 oz	28	15.0	2.0	9.0	4.0	0										I
cashews w/ almonds & macadamias, Planters—1 oz	170		4.0	6.0	2.0							90				
	28	16.0	2.5	11.0	2.0	0						160				I
cashews w/ almonds & pecans, Planters	170		4.0	7.0	2.0							95				
1 oz	28	15.0	2.0	9.0	3.0	0						160				I
chestnuts, chinese																
boiled & steamed	43	17.5	0.8	9.5			4	7	.03	.08	13	1	3	16	.17	.311
1 oz	28	0.2	0.0	0.1	0.1	0	39	.03	0.2	.00	.11	87	19	.27	.071	812
dried	103	2.5	1.9	22.6			9	17	.08	.19	31	1	8	39	.40	.737
1 oz	28	0.5	0.1	0.3	0.1	0	93	.07	0.4	.00	.26	206	44	.65	.167	812
raw	64	12.5	1.2	13.9			6	10	.05	.12	19	1	5	24	.25	.454
1 oz	28	0.3	0.0	0.2	0.1	0	57	.05	0.2	.00	.16	127	27	.40	.103	812
roasted	68	11.4	1.3	14.8			0	11	.03	.12	20	1	5	26	.26	.484
1 oz	28	0.3	0.0	0.2	0.1	0	1	.04	0.4	.00	.17	135	29	.43	.110	812
chestnuts, european																
boiled & steamed	37	19.3	0.6	7.9			1	8	.03	.07	11	8	13	15	.07	.242
1 oz	28	0.4	0.1	0.1	0.2	0	5	.04	0.2	.00	.09	203	28	.49	.134	812
dried	106	2.7	1.8	21.9		3.3	0	4	.10	.19	31	10	19	21	.10	.369
1 oz	28	1.3	0.2	0.4	0.5	0	0	.08	0.2	.00	.25	280	50	.67	.184	812
raw	60	13.8	0.7	12.9	3.1	2.3	1	12	.05	.11	18	1	8	9	.15	.270
1 oz (2 ½ nuts)	28	0.6	0.1	0.2	0.3	0	8	.07	0.3	.00	.14	147	26	.29	.127	812
roasted	69	11.5	0.9	15.0		1.4	1	7	.05	.14	20	1	8	9	.16	.335
1 oz (3 ½ nuts)	28	0.6	0.1	0.2	0.2	0	7	.07	0.4	.00	.16	168	30	.26	.144	812
chestnuts, japanese																
boiled & steamed	16	24.4	0.2	3.6			0	3	.02	.03	5	1	3	5	.11	.163
1 oz	28	0.1	0.0	0.0	0.0	0	4	.04	0.2	.00	.02	34	7	.15	.058	812
dried	102	2.8	1.5	23.1			3	17	.11	.19	31	10	20	33	.73	1.052
1 oz	28	0.4	0.1	0.2	0.1	0	24	.23	1.0	.00	.14	218	48	.96	.372	812
raw	44	17.4	0.6	9.9			1	7	.05	.08	13	4	9	14	.31	.451
1 oz	28	0.2	0.0	0.1	0.0	0	10	.10	0.4	.00	.06	93	20	.41	.159	812
roasted	57	14.1	0.8	12.8			2	8		.12	17	5	10	18	.41	.585
1 oz	28	0.2	0.0	0.1	0.1	0	21	.13	0.2	.00	.13	121	26	.60	.207	812
coconut																
cnd, Angel Flake	70		1.0	7.0	5.0	1.0	0	0				0	0			
2 T	15	5.0	4.5			0	0					65		.00		I
dried	187	0.9	2.0	6.9		4.6	0	0	.03	.09	3	10	7	26	.57	.778
1 oz	28	18.3	16.2	0.8	0.2	0	0	.02	0.2	.00	.23	154	58	.94	.226	812
dried, sweetened, flaked, cnd	505	26.5	3.8	46.6		5.1	0	0	.02	.27	8	23	16	56	1.81	2.475
4 oz	114	36.1	32.0	1.5	0.4	0	0	.03	0.3	.00	.72	369	117	2.10	.351	812
dried, sweetened, flaked, packaged	351	11.6	2.4	35.2		3.2	0	0	.01	.19	6	189	10	36	1.29	1.767
1 cup	74	23.8	21.1	1.0	0.3	0	0	.02	0.2	.00	.52	234	74	1.33	.223	812
dried, sweetened, shredded	466	11.7	2.7	44.3	32.0	4.2	0	1	.02	.25	8	244	14	47	1.69	2.302
1 cup	93	33.0	29.3	1.4	0.4	0	0	.03	0.4	.00	.67	313	100	1.79	.291	812
dried, toasted	168	0.3	1.5	12.6			0	0	.03	.09	3	10	8	26	.58	.794
1 oz	28	13.3	11.8	0.6	0.1	0	0	.02	0.2	.00	.23	157	60	.96	.230	812
packaged, Angel Flake	70		1.0	7.0	5.0	1.0	0	0				45	0			
2 T	15	4.5	4.0			0	0					55		.00		I
raw	159	21.1	1.5	6.9	1.6	4.0	0	1	.01	.02	12	9	6	14	.50	.675
1 piece (2" x 2" x ½")	45	15.1	13.4	0.6	0.2	0	0	.03	0.2	.00	.14	160	51	1.09	.196	812
shredded, Bakers Premium	60		0.0	6.0	5.0	1.0	0	0				35	0			
2 T	15	4.0	4.0			0	0					50		.00		I
coconut cream, raw	792	129.4	8.7	16.0		5.3	0	7	.00	.11	55	10	26	67	2.30	3.130
1 cup²	240	83.2	73.8	3.5	0.9	0	0	.07	2.1	.00	.63	780	293	5.47	.907	812
coconut cream, sweetened, cnd	568	210.8	8.0	24.7		6.5	0	5	.12	.09	42	148	3	50	1.78	2.412
1 cup	296	52.5	46.5	2.2	0.6	0	0	.07	0.1	.00	.48	299	65	1.51	.699	812
coconut milk, cnd	445	164.7	4.6	6.4			0	2	.00	.06	31	29	41	104	1.27	1.736
1 cup³	226	48.2	42.7	2.0	0.5	0	0	.05	1.4	.00	.35	497	217	7.46	.504	812

						Vitamins					Minerals				
KCAL	H₂O (g)	PRO (g)	CHO (g)	SUGR (g)	DFIB (g)	A (RE)	C (mg)	B-2 (mg)	B-6 (mg)	FOL (mcg)	Na (mg)	Ca (mg)	Mg (mg)	Zn (mg)	Mn (mg)
WT (g)	FAT (g)	SFA (g)	MUFA (g)	PUFA (g)	CHOL (mg)	A (IU)	B-1 (mg)	NIA (mg)	B-12 (mcg)	PANT (mg)	K (mg)	P (mg)	Fe (mg)	Cu (mg)	REF
coconut milk, raw															
552	162.3	5.5	13.3		5.3	0	7	.00	.08	39	36	38	89	1.61	2.198
1 cup[3] 240	57.2	50.7	2.4	0.6	0	0	.06	1.8	.00	.44	631	240	3.94	.638	812
coconut water															
46	228.0	1.7	8.9		2.6	0	6	.14	.08	6	252	58	60	.24	.341
1 cup[4] 240	0.5	0.4	0.0	0.0	0	0	.07	0.2	.00	.10	600	48	.70	.096	812
cornuts															
124	0.4	2.4	20.8		2.0	0	0	.04	.06	0	156	3	32	.50	.129
1 oz 28	4.0	0.7	2.1	0.9	0	0	.01	0.5	.00	.10	79	78	.47	.033	819
barbeque															
124	0.5	2.6	20.3		2.4	10	0	.04	.05	0	277	5	31	.53	.138
1 oz 28	4.1	0.7	2.1	0.9	0	96	.10	0.4	.00	.11	81	80	.48	.039	819
nacho															
124	0.6	2.7	20.3		2.3	1	4	.02	.06	4	180	10	31	.51	.116
1 oz 28	4.0	0.7	2.1	0.9	1	11	.10	0.3	.00	.15	88	88	.48	.043	819
cottonseed flour, lowfat															
94	2.0	14.1	10.2			12	1	.11	.22	65	10	134	203	3.29	.604
1 oz 28	0.4	0.1	0.1	0.2	0	122	.59	1.1	.00	.13	499	450	3.57	.332	812
cottonseed flour, partially defatted															
18	0.3	2.0	2.0		0.2	2	0	.02	.04	11	2	24	36	.58	.107
1 T 5	0.3	0.1	0.1	0.1	0	22	.11	0.2	.00	.02	89	80	.63	.059	812
cottonseed kernels, roasted															
51	0.5	3.3	2.2		0.6	4	1	.03	.08	23	3	10	44	.60	.218
1 T 10	3.6	1.0	0.7	1.8	0	44	.08	0.3	.00	.05	135	80	.54	.120	812
cottonseed meal, partially defatted															
104	0.3	13.9	10.9			13	1	.12	.23	69	10	143	215	3.49	.641
1 oz 28	1.4	0.3	0.2	0.6	0	130	.63	1.2	.00	.13	530	477	3.78	.000	812
filberts (hazelnuts)															
chopped/sliced, Blue Diamond															
161	1.6	5.5	5.1				1	.07			0	38			
1 oz 28	14.4					0	.22	0.5			211		1.17		I
dried															
179	1.5	3.7	4.3		1.7	2	0	.03	.17	20	1	53	81	.68	.572
1 oz 28	17.8	1.3	13.9	1.7	0	19	.14	0.3	.00	.33	126	88	.93	.428	812
dry roasted															
188	0.5	2.8	5.1		2.0	2	0	.06	.18	21	1	55	84	.71	.593
1 oz 28	18.8	1.4	14.7	1.8	0	20	.06	0.8	.00	.34	131	92	.96	.444	812
oil roasted															
187	0.3	4.0	5.4		1.8	2	0	.06	.18	21	1	56	84	.71	.597
1 oz 28	18.0	1.3	14.1	1.7	0	20	.06	0.8	.00	.34	132	92	.97	.447	812
roasted, salted, Blue Diamond															
180	0.6	4.6	3.9				1	.06	.08	70	39	51	46	.65	
1 oz 28	17.7					0	.08	0.3	.00	.19	157	79	1.09	.350	I
whole, Blue Diamond															
166	1.7	4.9	5.0				0	.06			1	40			
1 oz 28	15.4	1.1		2.8	0	0	.17	0.3			167		1.18		I
ginkgo nuts															
cnd															
31	20.7	0.6	6.3		2.6	10	3	.02	.06	9	87	1	5	.06	.019
1 oz (14 med nuts) 28	0.5	0.1	0.2	0.2	0	96	.04	1.0	.00	.03	51	15	.08	.047	812
dried															
99	3.5	2.9	20.5			31	8	.05	.18	30	4	6	15	.19	.062
1 oz 28	0.6	0.1	0.2	0.2	0	309	.12	3.3	.00	.38	283	76	.45	.152	812
raw															
52	15.6	1.2	10.7			16	4	.03	.09	15	2	1	8	.10	.032
1 oz 28	0.5	0.1	0.2	0.2	0	158	.06	1.7	.00	.05	145	35	.28	.078	812
hickorynuts, dried															
186	0.8	3.6	5.2		1.8	4	1	.04	.05	11	0	17	49	1.22	1.307
1 oz 28	18.2	2.0	9.2	6.2	0	37	.25	0.3	.00	.49	124	95	.60	.209	812
lotus seeds, dried															
94	4.0	4.4	18.3			1	0	.04	.18	29	1	46	60	.30	.657
1 oz 28	0.6	0.1	0.1	0.3	0	14	.18	0.5	.00	.24	388	177	1.00	.099	812
lotus seeds, raw															
25	21.8	1.2	4.9			0	0	.01	.05	8	0	12	16	.08	.176
1 oz 28	0.2	0.0	0.0	0.1	0	4	.05	0.1	.00	.06	104	48	.27	.027	812
macadamia nuts															
dried															
199	0.8	2.4	3.9		2.6	0	0	.03	.06	4	1	20	33	.48	.167
1 oz 28	20.9	3.1	16.5	0.4	0	0	.10	0.6	.00	.12	104	39	.68	.084	812
dry roasted, Blue Diamond															
200	0.4	2.5	3.2		1.9		0	.03	.09	0	120	19	31	.40	
1 oz 28	21.1	2.5	16.3	0.6	0	79	.09	0.6	.00	.08	80	74	.70	.200	I
oil roasted															
204	0.5	2.1	3.7		2.6	0	0	.03	.06	5	2	13	33	.31	.169
1 oz (10-12 nuts) 28	21.7	3.2	17.1	0.4	0	3	.06	0.6	.00	.13	93	57	.51	.085	812
mixed nuts															
deluxe, Planters															
170		5.0	6.0	2.0							110				
1 oz 28	16.0	2.0	9.0	4.0	0						170				I
dry roasted															
168	0.5	4.9	7.2		2.6	0	0	.06	.08	14	3	20	64	1.08	.549
1 oz[5] 28	14.6	2.0	8.9	3.1	0	4	.06	1.3	.00	.34	169	123	1.05	.363	812
dry roasted, Fisher															
170		6.0	7.0								125				
1 oz 28	15.0	2.0	9.0	4.0	0										I

	KCAL / WT (g)	H₂O (g) / FAT (g)	PRO (g) / SFA (g)	CHO (g) / MUFA (g)	SUGR (g) / PUFA (g)	DFIB (g) / CHOL (mg)	A (RE) / A (IU)	C (mg) / B-1 (mg)	B-2 (mg) / NIA (mg)	B-6 (mg) / B-12 (mcg)	FOL (mcg) / PANT (mg)	Na (mg) / K (mg)	Ca (mg) / P (mg)	Mg (mg) / Fe (mg)	Zn (mg) / Cu (mg)	Mn (mg) / REF
dry-roasted, Planters	170		6.0	7.0	1.0	2.0						250				
1 oz[6]	28	14.0	2.0	9.0	3.0	0						180				I
oil roasted	175	0.6	4.8	6.1	1.1	2.8	1	0	.06	.07	24	3	31	67	1.44	.536
1 oz[7]	28	16.0	2.5	9.0	3.8	0	5	.14	1.4	.00	.35	165	132	.91	.471	812
oil roasted, Fisher	170		6.0	6.0								110				
1 oz	28	16.0	2.0	9.0	5.0	0										I
Planters	170		6.0	5.0	1.0	2.0						115				
1 oz[1]	28	15.0	2.5	8.0	4.0	0						180				I
w/o peanuts, oil roasted	174	0.9	4.4	6.3		1.6	1	0	.14	.05	16	3	30	71	1.32	.439
1 oz	28	15.9	2.6	9.4	3.2	0	6	.14	0.6	.00	.27	154	127	.73	.509	812
Nut Topping, Fisher	160		6.0	7.0								115				
1 oz	28	14.0	2.0	7.0	5.0	0										I
nuts, wheat-base formulated																
flavored	183	0.6	3.7	5.9		1.5	0	0	.09	.10	35	26	6	17	.84	1.970
1 oz[8]	28	17.7	2.7	7.3	6.9	0	0	.11	0.4	.00	.09	91	104	.74	.051	812
macadamia flavored	175	0.9	3.2	7.9		1.5	0	0	.06	.07	27	13	6	16	.83	1.461
1 oz[9]	28	16.0	2.4	6.7	6.2	0	0	.06	0.3	.00	.09	74	85	.57	.051	812
unflavored	176	0.7	3.9	6.7		1.5	0	0	.09	.11	40	143	7	16	.83	2.245
1 oz[10]	28	16.4	2.5	6.7	6.4	0	0	.09	0.4	.00	.09	90	105	.68	.051	812
peanut & cashew mix, honey roasted, Planters—1 oz	150		5.0	10.0	5.0	2.0						125				
	28	12.0	2.0	6.0	3.0	0										I
peanut butter																
chunk style/crunchy	188	0.4	7.7	6.9		2.1	0	0	.04	.14	29	156	13	51	.89	.597
2 T	32	16.0	3.1	7.5	4.5	0	0	.04	4.4	.00	.31	239	101	.61	.165	816
creamy/crunchy, Jif	190		8.0	7.0	3.5	2.0	0	0	.03			150				
2 T[11]	32	16.0	3.0	8.0	5.0	0	0		4.0			232	99			I
creamy/crunchy, red fat, Jif	190		8.0	15.0	4.0	2.0	0	0		.12	24	250	0	60	.90	
2 T[12]	36	12.0	2.5	3.0	6.0	0			5.0			180	113	.72	.200	I
creamy/crunchy, Simply Jif	190		8.0	6.0	2.0	2.0	0	0	.03			65	0			
2 T[13]	31	16.0	3.0	8.0	5.0	0			4.0			244	99	.72		I
creamy/smooth	190	0.4	8.1	6.2		1.9	0	0	.03	.15	24	149	12	51	.93	.143
2 T[14]	32	16.3	3.3	7.8	4.4	0	0	.03	4.3	.00	.26	214	118	.59	.044	816
no salt added, Peter Pan Creamy	197		8.0	5.6	1.0	1.9	0	0				10	18			
2 T	32	17.5	2.5			0	0							.70		I
Peter Pan Creamy	189		8.0	6.6	3.0	2.2	0	0				152	13			
2 T	32	16.0	3.3			0	0							.55		I
Peter Pan Crunchy	188		8.5	6.3	2.5	2.1	0	0				119	13			
2 T	32	15.9	3.2			0	0							.54		I
Skippy Creamy	190	0.5	9.4	4.6		0.6			.02			150	10	60	1.00	
2 T	32	16.5	3.3	8.2	4.9	0		.02	3.8		.40	210	120	.60		I
Skippy Super Chunk	190	0.4	9.3	4.4		0.6			.02			130	10	50	1.00	
2 T	32	16.9	3.3	8.5	5.0	0		.02	3.8		.40	200	120	.60		I
whipped, Peter Pan Creamy	142		6.0	4.9	2.3	1.6	0	0				114	10			
2 T	24	12.0	2.5			0	0							.42		I
whipped, Peter Pan Crunchy	141		6.4	4.7	1.9	1.6	0	0				89	10			
2 T	24	11.9	2.4			0	0							.41		I
peanut flour, defatted	93	2.2	14.8	9.8		4.5	0	0	.14	.14	70	51	40	105	1.45	1.389
1 oz	28	0.2	0.0	0.1	0.0	0	0	.20	7.7	.00	.78	366	215	.60	.510	816
peanut flour, low-fat	121	2.2	9.6	8.9		4.5	0	0	.05	.09	38	0	37	14	1.70	1.199
1 oz	28	6.2	0.9	3.1	2.0	0	0	.13	3.3	.00	.44	385	144	1.34	.578	816
peanuts																
boiled	102	13.4	4.3	6.8		2.8	0	0	.02	.05	24	240	18	33	.59	.327
½ cup	32	7.0	1.0	3.5	2.2	0	0	.08	1.7	.00	.26	58	63	.32	.160	816
cocktail, Planters	170		7.0	6.0	1.0	3.0						115				
1 oz[15]	28	14.0	2.0	7.0	4.0	0						200				I
dry roasted	166	0.4	6.7	6.1		2.3	0	0	.03	.07	41	230	15	50	.94	.591
1 oz	28	14.1	2.0	7.0	4.4	0	0	.12	3.8	.00	.40	187	101	.64	.190	816
dry roasted, Fisher	160		7.0	6.0								210				
1 oz	28	14.0	2.0	8.0	4.0	0										I

	KCAL / WT (g)	H₂O (g) / FAT (g)	PRO (g) / SFA (g)	CHO (g) / MUFA (g)	SUGR (g) / PUFA (g)	DFIB (g) / CHOL (mg)	**Vitamins** A (RE) / A (IU)	C (mg) / B-1 (mg)	B-2 (mg) / NIA (mg)	B-6 (mg) / B-12 (mcg)	FOL (mcg) / PANT (mg)	**Minerals** Na (mg) / K (mg)	Ca (mg) / P (mg)	Mg (mg) / Fe (mg)	Zn (mg) / Cu (mg)	Mn (mg) / REF
dry roasted, Planters	160		7.0	6.0	1.0	3.0						250				
1 oz[16]	29	13.0	2.0	7.0	4.0	0						180				I
grandstand, Planters	150		7.0	5.0	2.0							220				
1 oz	28	13.0	2.0	7.0	4.0	0										I
honey roasted, Fisher	150		6.0	5.0								115				
1 oz	28	13.0	2.0	7.0	4.0	0										I
honey roasted, Planters	150		6.0	10.0	7.0	2.0						115				
1 oz	28	11.0	1.5	6.0	3.0	0										I
honey roasted, red fat, Planters	130		6.0	12.0	9.0	2.0						150				
1 oz (⅓ cup)	28	7.0	1.0	4.0	2.0	0						160				I
hot spicy, Planters	160		7.0	5.0	1.0	2.0						190				
1 oz	28	14.0	2.0	7.0	4.0	0						200				I
oil roasted	165	0.6	7.5	5.4		2.6	0	0	.03	.07	36	123	25	52	1.88	.585
1 oz	28	14.0	1.9	6.9	4.4	0	0	.07	4.0	.00	.39	193	147	.52	.369	816
oil roasted, Fisher	160		7.0	6.0								130				
1 oz	28	14.0	2.0	7.0	5.0	0										I
roasted in shell, Fisher	160		7.0	5.0								165				
1 oz	28	14.0	2.0	8.0	4.0	0										I
salted, Lance	193	0.4	8.8	6.5					.05			93	27			
1.1 oz	32	15.1	2.8	7.9	4.4	0		.02	1.1					.63		I
sweet 'n crunchy, Planters	140		4.0	16.0	14.0	2.0						20				
1 oz	28	7.0	1.0	4.0	2.0	0						115				I
unroasted	161	1.8	7.3	4.6		2.4	0	0	.04	.10	68	5	26	48	.93	.548
1 oz	28	14.0	1.9	6.9	4.4	0	0	.18	3.4	.00	.50	200	107	1.30	.324	816
peanuts & cashews, honey roasted, Fisher	150		5.0	6.0								105				
1 oz	28	13.0	2.0	7.0	4.0	0										I
peanuts, spanish																
oil-roasted, w/ salt	165	0.5	8.0	5.0	—	2.5	0	0	.02	.07	36	123	28	48	.57	.671
1 oz	29	14.0	2.2	6.3	4.8	0	0	.09	4.3	.00	.40	221	110	.65	.188	816
Planters	150		7.0	6.0	1.0	3.0						105				
1 oz	28	13.0	3.0	6.0	4.0	0						180				I
raw, Fisher	160		7.0	5.0												
1 oz	28	14.0	2.0	8.0	4.0	0										I
unroasted	162	1.8	7.4	4.5		2.7	0	0	.04	.10	68	6	30	53	.60	.748
1 oz	28	14.1	2.2	6.3	4.9	0	0	.19	4.5	.00	.50	211	110	1.11	.255	816
peanuts, valencia, oil-roasted	167	0.6	7.7	4.6		2.5	0	0	.04	.07	36	219	15	45	.87	.488
1 oz	28	14.5	2.2	6.5	5.0	0	0	.03	4.1	.00	.39	174	90	.47	.238	816
peanuts, valencia, unroasted	162	1.2	7.1	5.9		2.5	0	0	.09	.10	70	0	18	52	.95	.561
1 oz	28	13.5	2.1	6.1	4.7	0	0	.18	3.7	.00	.51	94	95	.59	.332	816
peanuts, virginia																
oil-roasted	164	0.6	7.3	5.6		2.5	0	0	.03	.07	36	123	24	53	1.88	.569
1 oz	28	13.8	1.8	7.2	4.2	0	0	.08	4.2	.00	.39	185	143	.47	.361	816
Planters	170		7.0	5.0	2.0						140					
1 oz	28	15.0	2.0			0										I
unroasted	160	2.0	7.1	4.7		2.4	0	0	.04	.10	68	3	25	48	1.26	.481
1 oz	28	13.8	1.8	7.2	4.2	0	0	.19	3.5	.00	.50	196	108	.72	.315	816
pecan chips, Planters	390		5.0	9.0	1.0	7.0						0				
2 oz pkg	57	40.0	3.0	22.0	13.0	0						230				I
pecan flour	93	3.0	9.0	14.4			3	1	.03	.05	10	0	9	34	1.45	1.205
1 oz	28	0.4	0.0	0.2	0.1	0	34	.23	0.2	.00	.45	95	78	.56	.316	816
pecan halves/ pieces, Planters	190		3.0	4.0	2.0							0				
1 oz	28	20.0	1.5	11.0	6.0	0						115				I
pecans																
dried	189	1.4	2.2	5.2	1.2	2.2	4	1	.04	.05	11	0	10	36	1.55	1.277
1 oz (31 large nuts)	28	19.2	1.5	12.0	4.7	0	36	.24	0.3	.00	.48	111	82	.60	.335	812
dry roasted	187	0.3	2.3	6.3		2.6	4	1	.03	.06	12	0	10	38	1.61	1.334
1 oz	28	18.3	1.5	11.4	4.5	0	38	.09	0.3	.00	.50	105	86	.62	.350	812
oil roasted	194	1.2	2.0	4.6		1.9	4	1	.03	.05	11	0	10	37	1.56	1.292
1 oz (15 halves)	28	20.2	1.6	12.6	5.0	0	37	.09	0.3	.00	.49	102	83	.60	.339	812

	KCAL	H₂O (g)	PRO (g)	CHO (g)	SUGR (g)	DFIB (g)	Vitamins					Minerals				
							A (RE)	C (mg)	B-2 (mg)	B-6 (mg)	FOL (mcg)	Na (mg)	Ca (mg)	Mg (mg)	Zn (mg)	Mn (mg)
	WT (g)	FAT (g)	SFA (g)	MUFA (g)	PUFA (g)	CHOL (mg)	A (IU)	B-1 (mg)	NIA (mg)	B-12 (mcg)	PANT (mg)	K (mg)	P (mg)	Fe (mg)	Cu (mg)	REF
raw, Fisher	190		2.0	5.0								0				
1 oz	28	19.0	2.0	12.0	5.0	0										I
pilinuts, dried	204	0.8	3.1	1.1			1	0	.03	.03	17	1	41	86	.84	.656
1 oz (15 nuts)	28	22.6	8.8	10.6	2.2	0	12	.26	0.1	.00	.14	144	163	1.00	.272	812
pine nuts, pignolia, dried	160	1.9	6.8	4.0		1.3	1	1	.05	.03	16	1	7	66	1.20	1.218
1 oz	28	14.4	2.2	5.4	6.1	0	8	.23	1.0	.00	.06	170	144	2.61	.291	812
pine nuts, pinyon, dried	178	1.7	3.3	5.5		3.0	1	1	.06	.03	16	20	2	66	1.21	1.228
1 oz	28	17.3	2.7	6.5	7.3	0	8	.35	1.2	.00	.06	178	10	.87	.293	812
pistachios																
dried	164	1.1	5.8	7.0	1.9	3.1	7	2	.05	.07	16	2	38	45	.38	.093
1 oz (47 nuts)	28	13.7	1.7	9.3	2.1	0	66	.23	0.3	.00	.34	310	143	1.92	.337	812
dry roasted	172	0.6	4.2	7.8		3.1	7	2	.07	.07	17	2	20	37	.39	.094
1 oz	28	15.0	1.9	10.1	2.3	0	67	.12	0.4	.00	.34	275	135	.90	.343	812
dry roasted, Blue Diamond	162	0.8	5.8	6.0				1	.09	.04		173	41	33	.31	
1 oz	28	13.9	2.3		4.5	0	0	.16	0.3	.00	.06	230	51	1.20	.100	I
dry roasted, Planters	160		5.0	7.0	2.0	3.0						180				
1 oz	28	14.0	2.0	8.0	4.0	0										I
natural, Blue Diamond	162	0.5	5.8	5.5		3.1			.10	.10	41	192	34	32	.50	.300
1 oz	28	13.9	1.7	6.8	4.2	0		.17	0.3	.00	.06	252	137	1.20	.300	I
red, Blue Diamond	158	0.6	5.9	5.7		3.6		1	.07	.13		246	33	32	.60	.300
1 oz	28	13.2	1.6	6.4	4.2	0	50	.18	0.3			248	136	1.20	.400	I
red/natural, Fisher	170		5.0	7.0								85				
1 oz	28	14.0	2.0	8.0	4.0	0										I
pumpkin & squash seeds, dried	153	2.0	7.0	5.0		1.1	11	1	.09	.06	16	5	12	152	2.11	.856
1 oz (142 seeds)	28	13.0	2.5	4.0	5.9	0	108	.06	0.5	.00	.10	229	333	4.24	.393	812
pumpkin & squash seeds, roasted	148	2.0	9.3	3.8		1.1	11	1	.09	.03	16	5	12	151	2.11	.855
1 oz	28	11.9	2.3	3.7	5.4	0	108	.06	0.5	.00	.10	229	332	4.24	.392	812
pumpkin seeds, Planters	110		5.0	14.0	0.0	2.0						1000				
⅓ cup	32	5.0	1.0	1.5	2.0	0										I
safflower seed kernels, dried	147	1.6	4.6	9.7			1	0	.12	.33	45	1	22	100	1.43	.571
1 oz	28	10.9	1.0	1.4	8.0	0	14	.33	0.6	.00	1.14	195	183	1.39	.495	812
safflower seed meal, partially defatted	97	1.8	10.1	13.8			1	0	.12	.33	45	1	22	99	1.42	.566
1 oz	28	0.7	0.1	0.1	0.4	0	14	.33	0.6	.00	1.13	19	181	1.38	.491	812
sesame butter (tahini), from roasted & toasted kernels—1 T	89	0.5	2.5	3.2		1.4	1	0	.07	.02	15	17	64	14	.69	.218
	15	8.1	1.1	3.0	3.5	0	10	.18	0.8	.00	.10	62	110	1.34	.241	812
sesame butter (tahini), from unroasted kernels—1 T	85	0.4	2.5	2.5		1.3	1	0	.02	.02	14	0	20	49	1.46	.204
	14	7.9	1.1	3.0	3.5	0	9	.22	0.8	.00	.10	64	111	.89	.208	812
sesame flour																
high fat	149	0.3	8.7	7.5			2	0	.08	.04	9	12	45	102	3.02	.422
1 oz	28	10.5	1.5	4.0	4.6	0	20	.76	3.8	.00	.83	120	229	4.30	.431	812
lowfat	94	2.0	14.2	10.1			2	0	.08	.04	8	11	42	96	2.84	.396
1 oz	28	0.5	0.1	0.2	0.2	0	18	.71	3.6	.00	.78	113	215	4.03	.404	812
partially defatted	108	1.9	11.4	10.0			2	0	.08	.04	8	12	43	103	3.03	.398
1 oz	28	3.4	0.5	1.2	1.4	0	20	.72	3.6	.00	.78	120	230	4.05	.406	812
sesame meal, partially defatted	161	1.4	4.8	7.4			2	0	.08	.04	8	11	43	98	2.90	.405
1 oz	28	13.6	1.9	5.1	6.0	0	19	.73	3.6	.00	.80	115	219	4.12	.413	812
sesame nut mix, Planters	150		5.0	9.0	2.0							240				
¼ cup	28	12.0	2.0	7.0	3.0	0						130				I
sesame seeds																
kernels, dried	47	0.4	2.1	0.8	0.1	0.9	1	0	.01	.01	8	3	10	28	.82	.114
1 T	8	4.4	0.6	1.7	1.9	0	5	.06	0.4	.00	.05	33	62	.62	.117	812
kernels, toasted	161	1.4	4.8	7.4		4.8	2	0	.13	.04	27	11	37	98	2.90	.405
1 oz	28	13.6	1.9	5.1	6.0	0	19	.34	1.5	.00	.19	115	219	2.21	.413	812
whole, dried	52	0.4	1.6	2.1		1.1	0	0	.02	.07	9	1	88	32	.70	.221
1 T	9	4.5	0.6	1.7	2.0	0	1	.07	0.4	.00	.00	42	57	1.31	.367	812
whole, toasted & roasted	160	0.9	4.8	7.3		4.0	0	0	.07	.23	28	3	280	101	2.03	.708
1 oz	28	13.6	1.9	5.1	6.0	0	3	.23	1.3	.00	.01	135	181	4.18	.700	812
snack mix, caribbean crunch, Planters	170		4.0	14.0	8.0	2.0						115				
¼ cup[17]	32	11.0	3.0	4.0	4.0	0										I

	KCAL	H₂O (g)	PRO (g)	CHO (g)	SUGR (g)	DFIB (g)	A (RE)	C (mg)	B-2 (mg)	B-6 (mg)	FOL (mcg)	Na (mg)	Ca (mg)	Mg (mg)	Zn (mg)	Mn (mg)
	WT (g)	FAT (g)	SFA (g)	MUFA (g)	PUFA (g)	CHOL (mg)	A (IU)	B-1 (mg)	NIA (mg)	B-12 (mcg)	PANT (mg)	K (mg)	P (mg)	Fe (mg)	Cu (mg)	REF
snack mix, orchard crunch, Planters	140		4.0	14.0	8.0	2.0						190				
⅓ cup[17]	28	8.0	1.0	3.5	3.0	0						115				I
soybean nuts, dry roasted	387	0.7	34.0	28.1		7.0	2	4	.65	.19	176	2	232	196	4.10	1.878
½ cup	86	18.6	2.7	4.1	10.5	0	20	.37	0.9	.00	.41	1173	558	3.40	.928	816
soybean nuts, roasted	405	1.7	30.3	28.9		15.2	17	2	.12	.18	181	140	119	125	2.70	1.856
½ cup	86	21.8	3.2	4.8	12.3	0	172	.09	1.2	.00	.39	1264	312	3.35	.712	816
soybutter, roasted, Natural Touch	174	0.6	6.9	11.3	2.9	3.1	0	0	.04			148	27		.55	
2 T	32	11.3	2.0	2.9	6.5	0	0	.00	0.0			151	83	1.43		I
sunflower seed butter	93	0.2	3.1	4.4			1	0	.05	.13	38	0	20	59	.85	.338
1 T	16	7.6	0.8	1.5	5.0	0	8	.05	0.9	.00	1.13	12	118	.76	.293	812
sunflower seed flour, partially defatted	16	0.4	2.4	1.8		0.3	0	0	.01	.04	11	0	6	17	.25	.099
1 T	5	0.1	0.0	0.0	0.0	0	2	.16	0.4	.00	.33	3	34	.33	.086	812
sunflower seeds/kernels																
dried	160	1.5	6.2	5.0	3.3	2.8	1	0	.06	.22	43	1	34	100	1.42	.574
1 oz	28	14.0	1.7	3.6	8.7	0	3	.59	1.8	.00	1.90	196	200	1.40	.364	MUL
dry roasted	165	0.3	5.5	6.8		3.1	0	0	.07	.23	67	1	20	37	1.50	.598
1 oz	28	14.1	1.5	2.7	9.3	0	0	.03	2.0	.00	2.00	241	327	1.08	.519	812
dry roasted, Fisher	170		6.0	6.0								200				
1 oz	28	15.0	2.0	3.0	10.0	0										I
oil roasted	174	0.7	6.1	4.2		1.9	1	0	.08	.22	66	1	16	36	1.48	.590
1 oz	28	16.3	1.7	3.1	10.8	0	14	.09	1.2	.00	1.97	137	323	1.90	.511	812
oil roasted, Fisher	170		6.0	4.0								170				
1 oz	28	16.0	2.0	3.0	11.0	0										I
roasted & salted, Planters	160		6.0	5.0	0.0	2.0										
1 oz[18]	28	15.0	1.5	3.0	10.0	0										I
toasted	175	0.3	4.9	5.8		3.3	0	0	.08	.23	67	1	16	37	1.50	.599
1 oz	28	16.1	1.7	3.1	10.6	0	0	.09	1.2	.00	2.00	139	328	1.93	.520	812
trail mix, Sierra	150		4.0	20.0	17.0	3.0	0	4				65	40			
¼ cup	35	8.0	2.5			0	0							.72		I
walnuts																
black, dried	172	1.2	6.9	3.4		1.4	9	1	.03	.16	19	0	16	57	.97	1.211
1 oz	28	16.0	1.0	3.6	10.6	0	84	.06	0.2	.00	.18	149	132	.87	.289	812
english/persian, dried	182	1.0	4.1	5.2	0.6	1.4	3	1	.04	.16	19	3	27	48	.77	.822
1 oz (14 halves)	28	17.5	1.6	4.0	11.1	0	35	.11	0.3	.00	.18	142	90	.69	.393	812
english, raw, Fisher	180		4.0	5.0								0				
1 oz	28	18.0	2.0	5.0	11.0	0										I
halves/pieces, Planters	190		4.0	4.0	1.0	1.0						0				
1 oz	28	19.0	2.0	6.0	11.0	0										I
watermelon seeds, dried	158	1.4	8.0	4.3			0	0	.04	.03	16	28	15	146	2.90	.458
1 oz (95 large seeds)	28	13.4	2.8	2.1	8.0	0	0	.05	1.0	.00	.10	184	214	2.06	.194	812

1. The lightly salted product contains 55 mg sodium.
2. Liquid expressed from grated coconut.
3. Liquid expressed from grated coconut and coconut water.
4. Liquid from the coconut center.
5. Cashew, almonds, peanuts, filberts, and pecans.
6. The unsalted product contains 0 mg sodium.
7. Cashews, peanuts, brazilnuts, filberts, almonds, and pecans.
8. Hydrogenated soybean oil, wheat germ, sugar, sodium caseinate, soy protein, natural and artificial flavors, and artificial color.
9. Hydrogenated soybean oil, wheat germ, sugar, wheat starch, sodium caseinate, soy protein, natural and artificial flavor.
10. Hydrogenated soybean oil, wheat germ, fructose, wheat starch, sodium caseinate, soy protein, and salt.
11. Creamy Jif contains 150 mg sodium; crunchy Jif contains 120 mg sodium.
12. Creamy reduced fat Jif contains 250 mg sodium; crunchy reduced fat Jif contains 200 mg sodium.
13. Creamy Simply Jif contains 65 mg sodium; crunchy Simply Jif contains 50 mg sodium.
14. If no salt is added, sodium is 5 mg.
15. The lightly salted product contains 55 mg sodium; the unsalted product contains 0 mg sodium.
16. The lightly salted product contains 110 mg sodium; the unsalted product contains 0 mg sodium.
17. Contains nuts, fruit, and snack sticks.
18. 1 oz = ¾ cup with shell.

	KCAL	H₂O (g)	PRO (g)	CHO (g)	SUGR (g)	DFIB (g)	A (RE)	C (mg)	B-2 (mg)	B-6 (mg)	FOL (mcg)	Na (mg)	Ca (mg)	Mg (mg)	Zn (mg)	Mn (mg)
	WT (g)	FAT (g)	SFA (g)	MUFA (g)	PUFA (g)	CHOL (mg)	A (IU)	B-1 (mg)	NIA (mg)	B-12 (mcg)	PANT (mg)	K (mg)	P (mg)	Fe (mg)	Cu (mg)	REF

25. POULTRY
25.1 CHICKEN, BROILER/FRYER

dark meat w/o skin

fried	239	55.7	29.0	2.6		0.0	24	0	.25	.37	9	97	18	25	2.91	.033
3.5 oz	100	11.6	3.1	4.3	2.8	96	79	.09	7.1	.33	1.26	253	187	1.49	.089	805
roasted	205	63.1	27.4	0.0	0.0	0.0	22	0	.23	.36	8	93	15	23	2.80	.021
3.5 oz	100	9.7	2.7	3.6	2.3	93	72	.07	6.5	.32	1.21	240	179	1.33	.080	805
stewed	192	65.8	26.0	0.0	0.0	0.0	21	0	.20	.21	7	74	14	20	2.66	.020
3.5 oz	100	9.0	2.5	3.3	2.1	88	69	.06	4.7	.22	.89	181	143	1.36	.075	805
dark meat w/ skin, roasted	253	58.6	26.0	0.0	0.0	0.0	58	0	.21	.31	7	87	15	22	2.49	.021
3.5 oz	100	15.8	4.4	6.2	3.5	91	201	.07	6.4	.29	1.11	220	168	1.36	.077	805
dark meat w/ skin, stewed	233	63.0	23.5	0.0	0.0	0.0	54	0	.18	.17	6	70	14	18	2.26	.019
3.5 oz	100	14.7	4.1	5.8	3.2	82	186	.05	4.5	.20	.77	166	133	1.31	.068	805

light & dark meat w/o skin

flour coated & fried	219	57.5	30.6	1.7		0.1	18	0	.20	.48	7	91	17	27	2.24	.028
3.5 oz	100	9.1	2.5	3.4	2.1	94	59	.09	9.7	.34	1.17	257	205	1.35	.075	805
roasted	190	63.8	28.9	0.0	0.0	0.0	16	0	.18	.47	6	86	15	25	2.10	.019
3.5 oz	100	7.4	2.0	2.7	1.7	89	53	.07	9.2	.33	1.10	243	195	1.21	.067	805
stewed	177	66.8	27.3	0.0	0.0	0.0	15	0	.16	.26	6	70	14	21	1.99	.019
3.5 oz	100	6.7	1.8	2.4	1.5	83	50	.05	6.1	.22	.75	180	150	1.17	.061	805

light & dark meat w/ skin

batter dipped & fried	289	49.4	22.5	9.4		0.3	28	0	.19	.31	8	292	21	21	1.67	.057
3.5 oz	100	17.4	4.6	7.1	4.1	87	93	.12	7.0	.28	.89	185	155	1.37	.072	805
flour coated & fried	269	52.4	28.6	3.1		0.1	27	0	.19	.41	6	84	17	25	2.04	.034
3.5 oz	100	14.9	4.1	5.9	3.4	90	89	.09	9.0	.31	1.08	234	191	1.38	.075	805
roasted	239	59.5	27.3	0.0	0.0	0.0	47	0	.17	.40	5	82	15	23	1.94	.020
3.5 oz	100	13.6	3.8	5.3	3.0	88	161	.06	8.5	.30	1.03	223	182	1.26	.066	805
stewed	219	63.9	24.7	0.0	0.0	0.0	42	0	.15	.22	5	67	13	19	1.76	.019
3.5 oz	100	12.6	3.5	4.9	2.7	78	146	.05	5.6	.20	.67	166	139	1.16	.057	805

light meat w/o skin

fried	192	60.1	32.8	0.4		0.0	9	0	.13	.63	4	81	16	29	1.27	.020
3.5 oz	100	5.5	1.5	2.0	1.3	90	30	.07	13.4	.36	1.03	263	231	1.14	.054	805
roasted	173	64.8	30.9	0.0	0.0	0.0	9	0	.12	.60	4	77	15	27	1.23	.017
3.5 oz	100	4.5	1.3	1.5	1.0	85	29	.07	12.4	.34	.97	247	216	1.06	.050	805
stewed	159	68.0	28.9	0.0	0.0	0.0	8	0	.12	.33	3	65	13	22	1.19	.018
3.5 oz	100	4.0	1.1	1.4	0.9	77	27	.04	7.8	.23	.57	180	159	.93	.044	805

light meat w/ skin

flour coated & fried	246	54.7	30.4	1.8		0.1	20	0	.13	.54	4	77	16	27	1.26	.026
3.5 oz	100	12.1	3.3	4.8	2.7	87	68	.08	12.0	.33	.97	239	213	1.21	.058	805
roasted	222	60.5	29.0	0.0	0.0	0.0	32	0	.12	.52	3	75	15	25	1.23	.018
3.5 oz	100	10.8	3.0	4.3	2.3	84	110	.06	11.1	.32	.93	227	200	1.14	.053	805
stewed	201	65.1	26.1	0.0	0.0	0.0	28	0	.11	.27	3	63	13	20	1.14	.018
3.5 oz	100	10.0	2.8	3.9	2.1	74	96	.04	6.9	.20	.54	167	146	.98	.044	805

25.2 CHICKEN, BROILER/FRYER PARTS

back w/ skin, fried

	238	31.7	20.0	4.7			27	0	.17	.22	6	65	17	17	1.78	.036
½ back	72	14.9	4.0	5.9	3.5	64	89	.08	5.3	.20	.79	163	120	1.17	.066	805

breast w/o skin

flour coated & fried	161	51.8	28.8	0.4		0.0	6	0	.11	.55	3	68	14	27	.93	.018
½ breast	86	4.1	1.1	1.5	0.9	78	20	.07	12.7	.32	.89	237	212	.98	.046	805

	KCAL	H₂O (g)	PRO (g)	CHO (g)	SUGR (g)	DFIB (g)	A (RE)	C (mg)	B-2 (mg)	B-6 (mg)	FOL (mcg)	Na (mg)	Ca (mg)	Mg (mg)	Zn (mg)	Mn (mg)
	WT (g)	FAT (g)	SFA (g)	MUFA (g)	PUFA (g)	CHOL (mg)	A (IU)	B-1 (mg)	NIA (mg)	B-12 (mcg)	PANT (mg)	K (mg)	P (mg)	Fe (mg)	Cu (mg)	REF
roasted	142	56.1	26.7	0.0	0.0	0.0	5	0	.10	.52	3	64	13	25	.86	.015
½ breast	86	3.1	0.9	1.1	0.7	73	18	.06	11.8	.29	.83	220	196	.89	.042	805
stewed	143	64.9	27.5	0.0	0.0	0.0	6	0	.11	.31	3	60	12	23	.92	.017
½ breast	95	2.9	0.8	1.0	0.6	73	18	.04	8.0	.22	.54	178	157	.84	.041	805
breast w/ skin																
flour coated & fried	218	55.5	31.2	1.6		0.1	15	0	.13	.57	4	74	16	29	1.08	.025
½ breast	98	8.7	2.4	3.4	1.9	87	49	.08	13.5	.33	.98	254	228	1.17	.056	805
roasted	193	61.2	29.2	0.0	0.0	0.0	26	0	.12	.55	4	70	14	26	1.00	.018
½ breast	98	7.6	2.1	3.0	1.6	82	91	.06	12.5	.31	.92	240	210	1.05	.049	805
stewed	202	72.8	30.1	0.0	0.0	0.0	26	0	.13	.32	3	68	14	24	1.07	.020
½ breast	110	8.2	2.3	3.2	1.7	83	90	.05	8.6	.23	.60	196	172	1.01	.048	805
drumstick w/o skin, roasted	76	29.4	12.4	0.0	0.0	0.0	8	0	.10	.17	4	42	5	11	1.40	.009
1 drumstick	44	2.5	0.7	0.8	0.6	41	26	.03	2.7	.15	.57	108	81	.57	.035	805
drumstick w/ skin																
flour coated & fried	120	27.8	13.2	0.8		0.0	12	0	.11	.17	4	44	6	11	1.42	.014
1 drumstick	49	6.7	1.8	2.7	1.6	44	41	.04	3.0	.16	.60	112	86	.66	.039	805
roasted	112	32.6	14.1	0.0	0.0	0.0	16	0	.11	.18	4	47	6	12	1.49	.011
1 drumstick	52	5.8	1.6	2.2	1.3	47	52	.04	3.1	.17	.63	119	91	.69	.040	805
stewed	116	37.1	14.4	0.0	0.0	0.0	15	0	.11	.11	4	43	6	11	1.51	.011
1 drumstick	57	6.1	1.7	2.3	1.4	47	52	.03	2.4	.13	.49	105	80	.76	.040	805
leg w/o skin, stewed	187	67.1	26.5	0.0	0.0	0.0	18	0	.22	.21	8	79	11	21	2.81	.019
1 leg	101	8.1	2.2	3.0	1.9	90	61	.06	4.8	.23	.92	192	150	1.41	.078	805
leg w/ skin																
flour coated & fried	284	61.9	30.1	2.8		0.1	31	0	.26	.38	9	99	15	27	3.00	.036
1 leg	112	16.2	4.4	6.4	3.7	105	103	.10	7.3	.35	1.34	261	204	1.60	.095	805
roasted	264	69.4	29.6	0.0	0.0	0.0	44	0	.24	.38	8	99	14	26	2.96	.024
1 leg	114	15.3	4.2	6.0	3.4	105	154	.08	7.1	.34	1.32	257	198	1.52	.088	805
stewed	275	80.0	30.2	0.0	0.0	0.0	45	0	.24	.22	8	91	14	25	3.04	.024
1 leg	125	16.1	4.5	6.3	3.6	105	155	.07	5.7	.25	1.02	220	174	1.69	.089	805
neck w/o skin, simmered	32	12.1	4.4	0.0	0.0	0.0	6	0	.05	.03	1	12	8	3	.68	.009
1 neck	18	1.5	0.4	0.5	0.4	14	22	.01	0.7	.03	.12	25	23	.47	.023	805
neck w/ skin, flour coated & fried	120	17.1	8.6	1.5			21	0	.09	.09	2	30	11	7	1.11	.019
1 neck	36	8.5	2.3	3.5	2.0	34	68	.03	1.9	.09	.35	65	48	.87	.047	805
neck w/ skin, simmered	94	23.5	7.5	0.0	0.0	0.0	18	0	.09	.04	1	20	10	5	1.03	.017
1 neck	38	6.9	1.9	2.7	1.5	27	61	.02	1.3	.05	.20	41	46	.87	.037	805
thigh w/o skin, roasted	109	32.7	13.5	0.0	0.0	0.0	10	0	.12	.18	4	46	6	12	1.34	.011
1 thigh	52	5.7	1.6	2.2	1.3	49	34	.04	3.4	.16	.62	124	95	.68	.042	805
thigh w/ skin																
flour coated & fried	162	33.6	16.6	2.0		0.1	18	0	.15	.20	5	55	9	16	1.56	.022
1 thigh	62	9.3	2.5	3.6	2.1	60	61	.06	4.3	.19	.73	147	116	.92	.055	805
roasted	153	36.8	15.5	0.0	0.0	0.0	30	0	.13	.19	4	52	7	14	1.46	.013
1 thigh	62	9.6	2.7	3.8	2.1	58	102	.04	3.9	.18	.69	138	108	.83	.048	805
stewed	158	42.9	15.8	0.0	0.0	0.0	30	0	.13	.12	4	48	7	13	1.53	.013
1 thigh	68	10.0	2.8	4.0	2.2	57	103	.04	3.3	.13	.53	116	95	.93	.048	805
wing w/ skin																
flour coated & fried	103	15.6	8.4	0.8		0.0	12	0	.04	.13	1	25	5	6	.56	.009
1 wing	32	7.1	1.9	2.8	1.6	26	40	.02	2.1	.09	.28	57	48	.40	.020	805
roasted	99	18.7	9.1	0.0	0.0	0.0	16	0	.04	.14	1	28	5	6	.62	.006
1 wing	34	6.6	1.9	2.6	1.4	29	54	.01	2.3	.10	.30	63	51	.43	.019	805
stewed	100	24.9	9.1	0.0	0.0	0.0	16	0	.04	.09	1	27	5	6	.65	.007
1 wing	40	6.7	1.9	2.6	1.4	28	53	.02	1.8	.07	.20	56	48	.45	.018	805

	KCAL / WT (g)	H₂O (g) / FAT (g)	PRO (g) / SFA (g)	CHO (g) / MUFA (g)	SUGR (g) / PUFA (g)	DFIB (g) / CHOL (mg)	A (RE) / A (IU)	C (mg) / B-1 (mg)	B-2 (mg) / NIA (mg)	B-6 (mg) / B-12 (mcg)	FOL (mcg) / PANT (mg)	Na (mg) / K (mg)	Ca (mg) / P (mg)	Mg (mg) / Fe (mg)	Zn (mg) / Cu (mg)	Mn (mg) / REF

25.3 CHICKEN, CAPON, ROASTER, & STEWER

Food / Serving	KCAL/WT	H₂O/FAT	PRO/SFA	CHO/MUFA	SUGR/PUFA	DFIB/CHOL	A(RE)/A(IU)	C/B-1	B-2/NIA	B-6/B-12	FOL/PANT	Na/K	Ca/P	Mg/Fe	Zn/Cu	Mn/REF
capon, meat w/ skin, roasted	229	58.7	29.0	0.0	0.0	0.0	20	0	.17	.43	6	49	14	24	1.74	.021
3.5 oz	100	11.7	3.3	4.8	2.5	86	68	.07	8.9	.33	1.10	255	246	1.49	.069	805
roaster																
dark meat w/o skin, roasted	178	67.0	23.3	0.0	0.0	0.0	16	0	.19	.31	7	95	11	20	2.13	.019
3.5 oz	100	8.8	2.4	3.3	2.0	75	54	.06	5.7	.27	1.03	224	171	1.33	.070	805
light & dark meat w/o skin, roasted	167	67.4	25.0	0.0	0.0	0.0	12	0	.15	.41	5	75	12	21	1.52	.017
3.5 oz	100	6.6	1.8	2.5	1.5	75	41	.06	7.9	.29	.97	229	192	1.21	.057	805
light & dark meat w/ skin, roasted	223	62.1	24.0	0.0	0.0	0.0	25	0	.14	.35	5	73	12	20	1.45	.018
3.5 oz	100	13.4	3.7	5.4	2.9	76	83	.06	7.4	.27	.92	211	179	1.26	.058	805
light meat w/o skin, roasted	153	67.8	27.1	0.0	0.0	0.0	8	0	.09	.54	3	51	13	23	.78	.015
3.5 oz	100	4.1	1.1	1.5	0.9	75	25	.06	10.5	.31	.91	236	217	1.08	.042	805
stewer																
dark meat w/o skin, stewed	258	55.1	28.1	0.0	0.0	0.0	43	0	.35	.24	8	95	12	22	3.12	.023
3.5 oz	100	15.3	4.1	5.2	3.6	95	145	.13	4.6	.25	1.01	204	187	1.64	.144	805
light & dark meat w/o skin, stewed	237	56.4	30.4	0.0	0.0	0.0	33	0	.28	.31	6	78	13	22	2.06	.022
3.5 oz	100	11.9	3.1	4.0	2.8	83	112	.11	6.4	.26	.86	202	204	1.43	.116	805
light & dark meat w/ skin, stewed	285	53.1	26.9	0.0	0.0	0.0	39	0	.23	.25	5	73	13	20	1.77	.021
3.5 oz	100	18.9	5.1	7.2	4.2	79	131	.09	5.8	.23	.75	182	180	1.37	.100	805
light meat w/o skin, stewed	213	57.8	33.0	0.0	0.0	0.0	22	0	.20	.39	4	58	14	23	.83	.020
3.5 oz	100	8.0	2.0	2.7	1.9	70	73	.09	8.5	.27	.69	199	225	1.19	.085	805

25.4 CHICKEN, UNSPECIFIED

Food / Serving	KCAL/WT	H₂O/FAT	PRO/SFA	CHO/MUFA	SUGR/PUFA	DFIB/CHOL	A(RE)/A(IU)	C/B-1	B-2/NIA	B-6/B-12	FOL/PANT	Na/K	Ca/P	Mg/Fe	Zn/Cu	Mn/REF
breast, crispy baked, Butterball Requests	178		17.2	13.4	0.0	1.6		1				510	0			
1 piece (3.5 oz)[1]	99	6.2	2.2			42	0							.65		I
breast, fried, frzn, Banquet	410		23.0	18.0	2.0	4.0		5				600	60			
5.5 oz piece	156	26.0	13.0			85	0							.72		I
breast, half w/ ribs & back, roasted, frzn, Tyson—*5.18 oz*	252	95.1	33.7	0.5	1.3		0	0				674				
	145	12.9	3.8			108	0									I
breast, herb roasted, frzn, Swanson	260		21.2	30.9				2	.25			518	26			
7.8 oz entree	220	5.7	2.1		1.5	41		.14	8.4			369		1.30		I
breast patties, breaded, southern fried, frzn, Tyson—*2.6 oz patty*	182	40.5	11.4	8.0	0.4	0.3		0				358	8			
	73	11.6	2.4			32	0							.30		I
breast patties, fat-free, frzn, Banquet	100		9.0	15.0	0.0	1.0		0				350	0			
1 patty (2.63 oz)	75	0.0	0.0	0.0	0.0	20	0							.36		I
breast quarters, rotisserie ckd, frzn, Tyson—*6.2 oz*	245	116.0	43.4	0.7	0.3	1.0		0				1190	31			
	173	7.7	2.5	3.7	1.4	144	0							.67		I
breast tenders																
fat-free, frzn, Banquet	130		13.0	20.0	0.0	2.0	0	0				480	0			
3 pieces (3.5 oz)	99	0.0	0.0	0.0	0.0	30	0							.72		I
frzn, Banquet	240		12.0	15.0	1.0	0	1					480	0			
3 pieces (3.1 oz)	88	15.0	3.5			30	0							.72		I
premium, frzn, Tyson	222	46.6	13.7	8.4	0.3	1.3		0				292	6			
3 oz	85	14.9	3.1	6.7	2.3	34	0							.30		I
southern, frzn, Banquet	260		12.0	16.0	1.0	1.0	0	1				460	0			
3 pieces (3.1 oz)	89	16.0	4.0			15	0							.72		I
chunks																
frzn, Country Skillet	270		12.0	18.0	2.0	1.0	0	0				720	20			
5 chunks (3.3 oz)	94	16.0	3.0			20	0							1.44		I
in water, cnd, Swanson Premium	100		16.0	0.5	0.0	0.5	0	0				340	0			
3 oz	85	3.0	1.0			38	0							.00		I
southern, frzn, Banquet	270		12.0	16.0	4.0	2.0		1				570	20			
5 pieces (3 oz)	85	18.0	4.0			35	0							1.08		I
white in water, cnd, Swanson Premium	80		16.0	0.0	0.0	0.5	0	0				340	0			
3 oz	85	1.5				40	0							.00		I

	KCAL	H₂O (g)	PRO (g)	CHO (g)	SUGR (g)	DFIB (g)	A (RE)	C (mg)	B-2 (mg)	B-6 (mg)	FOL (mcg)	Na (mg)	Ca (mg)	Mg (mg)	Zn (mg)	Mn (mg)
	WT (g)	FAT (g)	SFA (g)	MUFA (g)	PUFA (g)	CHOL (mg)	A (IU)	B-1 (mg)	NIA (mg)	B-12 (mcg)	PANT (mg)	K (mg)	P (mg)	Fe (mg)	Cu (mg)	REF
w/ broth, cnd	234	97.5	30.9	0.0	0.0	0.0	48	3	.18	.50	6	714	20	17	2.00	.021
5 oz can	142	11.3	3.1	4.5	2.5	88	166	.02	9.0	.41	1.21	196	158	2.24	.065	805
w/ cheddar, frzn, Banquet	280		12.0	13.0	2.0	1.0		0				560	80			
4 pieces (3 oz)	85	19.0	6.0			25	0							.72		I
cutlets, plump & juicy, frzn, Swanson	198		12.4	10.5				0	.10			337	11			
3 oz	85	11.9					0	.08	4.4			141		.90		I
diced, boneless, skinless, frzn, ckd, Tyson—3 oz	134	55.1	25.8	0.0	0.1	0.0	0	0				40	6			
	84	3.4	0.9			78	0							.96		I
Drumlets, plump & juicy, frzn, Swanson	213		13.0	10.3				0	.11			363	13			
3 oz	85	13.3					0	.08	4.7			196		1.00		I
drumsticks, roasted, frzn, Tyson	329	101.2	40.1	0.8	1.3	0.0	0	0				869	13			
3 drumsticks (5.9 oz)	164	18.4	5.1			226	0							1.48		I
fried																
extra crispy, plump & juicy, frzn, Swanson—3 oz	249		12.2	14.2				0	.09			319	19			
	85	16.0					0	.10	4.5			224		1.80		I
frzn, Banquet	270		14.0	13.0	1.0	1.0		4				620	80			
3 oz	85	18.0	5.0			65	0							.72		I
frzn, Country Skillet	270		14.0	13.0	1.0	1.0		4				620	80			
3 oz	85	18.0	5.0			65	0							.72		I
frzn, Swanson Southern Style	267		14.3	16.3				0	.12			688	25			
3.2 oz	92	16.0					0	.11	3.9			167		1.40		I
half breast & back, plump & juicy, frzn, Swanson—4.5 oz	342		22.8	19.0				0	.18			782	34			
	127	19.4					0	.17	6.9			248		1.90		I
honey bbq, skinless, Banquet	210		18.0	7.0	1.0	2.0		6				480	20			
3 oz	85	13.0	3.0			55	0							.36		I
hot & spicy, frzn, Banquet	260		14.0	13.0	1.0	1.0		4				590	80			
3 oz	85	18.0	5.0			65	0							.72		I
lemon pepper, skinless, frzn, Banquet	210		18.0	7.0	1.0	2.0		6				560	20			
3 oz	85	13.0	3.0			55	0							.36		I
nibbles wing sections, frzn, Swanson	296		12.6	18.8				0	.13			681	24			
3.2 oz	92	19.0					0	.13	3.1			124		1.50		I
plump & juicy, frzn, Swanson	260		14.9	14.6				0	.17			603	31			
3.2 oz	92	15.7					4	.12	4.3			179	192	1.50		I
skinless, frzn, Banquet	210		18.0	7.0	1.0	2.0		6				480	20			
3 oz	85	13.0	3.0			55	0							.36		I
thighs, backs & drumsticks, frzn, Swanson—3.2 oz	274		15.2	15.2				0	.16			585	27			
	92	17.0					1	.10	3.1			177		1.50		I
half, ckd, frzn, Tyson	172	50.9	18.8	1.9	0.1	0.9	0					610	68			
3 oz	84	10.0	3.1	4.9	1.7	90	71							.79		I
nuggets																
breaded, frzn, Swanson	225		12.8	14.1				0	.10			356	13			
3.2 oz	90	13.0					0	.10	4.1			166		.90		I
breaded, frzn, Tyson	276	37.6	11.2	13.6	0.2	1.5		0				491	7			
3 oz	84	19.7	4.6			50	50							.64		I
frzn, Banquet	240		14.0	12.0	2.0	1.0		0				540	0			
6 pieces (3 oz)	85	15.0	3.0			35	0							1.08		I
frzn, Country Skillet	280		14.0	16.0	2.0	1.0		0				610	20			
10 pieces (3.3 oz)	94	17.0	4.0			25	0							1.44		I
southern fried w/ bbq sce, frzn, Banquet	340		16.0	22.0	0.0	2.0		2				840	20			
6 pieces (4.5 oz)	128	20.0	4.0			45	0							1.80		I
w/ sweet & sour sce, frzn, Banquet	320		16.0	25.0	0.0	2.0		1				670	20			
6 pieces (4.5 oz)	128	18.0	4.0			45	0							1.80		I
patty																
frzn, Banquet	180		15.0	10.0	2.0	1.0		0				360	0			
1 patty (2.25)	64	11.0	2.5			25	0							.72		I
frzn, Country Skillet	190		9.0	12.0	3.0	1.0		0				490	0			
1 patty (2.5 oz)	71	11.0	2.5			20	0							1.08		I
parmigiana, frzn, Banquet Family	160		10.0	8.0	1.0			0				620	0			
1 patty (4.7 oz)	132	10.0	4.5			35	0							1.08		I

	KCAL	H_2O (g)	PRO (g)	CHO (g)	SUGR (g)	DFIB (g)	A (RE)	C (mg)	B-2 (mg)	B-6 (mg)	FOL (mcg)	Na (mg)	Ca (mg)	Mg (mg)	Zn (mg)	Mn (mg)
	WT (g)	FAT (g)	SFA (g)	MUFA (g)	PUFA (g)	CHOL (mg)	A (IU)	B-1 (mg)	NIA (mg)	B-12 (mcg)	PANT (mg)	K (mg)	P (mg)	Fe (mg)	Cu (mg)	REF
southern, frzn, Banquet	170		10.0	10.0	1.0	1.0		1				430	0			
1 patty (2.25 oz)	64	10.0	2.0			20	0								.72	I
w/ cheese, breaded, frzn, Tyson	221	35.1	10.6	12.4	0.6	0.4	0	0				274	61			
2.6 oz patty	74	14.4	4.0			42	0								.43	I
roll, white meat, Tyson	63	25.5	6.6	0.2	0.1	0.0						296	4			
1.33 oz slice	37	3.9	1.1			17									.35	I
Rondelet, frzn, Tyson	174	41.7	10.3	10.2		1.0		0				406	20			
2.6 oz piece	74	10.3	2.3	4.1	2.0	4	0								.53	I
Take-Out, assorted pieces, frzn, Swanson	267		14.3	16.3				0	.12			688	25			
3.2 oz	92	16.0					0	.11	3.9			167		1.40		I
thigh w/ back, roasted, frzn, Tyson	267	58.4	22.1	1.0	0.8	0.0	0	0				489	0			
3.7 oz piece	103	19.5	5.6			138	0								.71	I
thighs & drums, fried, frzn, Banquet	260		15.0	10.0	1.0	2.0		5				540	20			
3 oz	85	18.0	5.0			65	0								.36	I
wings																
bbq, baked, frzn, Tyson	222	57.7	20.4	2.0	2.4	0.0	0	0				159	12			
4 wings (3.4 oz)	96	14.7	4.0			130	0								.28	I
hot 'n spicy, frzn, Tyson	218	57.7	20.5	0.8	0.4	0.0		3				558	12			
3.4 oz	96	14.8	3.7			109	318								.82	I
hot & spicy, frzn, Banquet	230		15.0	5.0	0.0	1.0	0	4				280	20			
4 pieces (4 oz)	113	16.0	5.0			85	0								.72	I

25.5 DUCK, GOOSE, & OTHER POULTRY

	KCAL	H_2O (g)	PRO (g)	CHO (g)	SUGR (g)	DFIB (g)	A (RE)	C (mg)	B-2 (mg)	B-6 (mg)	FOL (mcg)	Na (mg)	Ca (mg)	Mg (mg)	Zn (mg)	Mn (mg)
	WT (g)	FAT (g)	SFA (g)	MUFA (g)	PUFA (g)	CHOL (mg)	A (IU)	B-1 (mg)	NIA (mg)	B-12 (mcg)	PANT (mg)	K (mg)	P (mg)	Fe (mg)	Cu (mg)	REF
cornish game hen, w/o skin, roasted	147	79.1	25.6	0.0	0.0	0.0	22	1	.25	.39	2	69	14	21	1.68	.017
½ bird	110	4.3	1.1	1.4	1.0	117	72	.08	6.9	.33	.61	275	164	.85	.065	805
cornish game hen, w/ skin, roasted	296	66.9	25.4	0.0	0.0	0.0	36	1	.23	.35	2	73	15	21	1.70	.017
½ bird	114	20.8	5.8	9.1	4.1	149	121	.08	6.7	.32	.68	279	166	1.04	.070	805
duck w/o skin, roasted	201	64.2	23.5	0.0	0.0	0.0	23	0	.47	.25	10	65	12	20	2.60	.019
3.5 oz	100	11.2	4.2	3.7	1.4	89	77	.26	5.1	.40	1.50	252	203	2.70	.231	805
duck w/ skin, roasted	337	51.8	19.0	0.0	0.0	0.0	63	0	.27	.18	6	59	11	16	1.86	.019
3.5 oz	100	28.4	9.7	12.9	3.6	84	210	.17	4.8	.30	1.10	204	156	2.70	.227	805
goose w/o skin, roasted	238	57.2	29.0	0.0	0.0	0.0	12	0	.39	.47	12	76	14	25	3.17	.024
3.5 oz	100	12.7	4.6	4.3	1.5	96	40	.09	4.1	.49	1.83	388	309	2.87	.276	805
goose w/ skin, roasted	305	52.0	25.2	0.0	0.0	0.0	21	0	.32	.37	2	70	13	22	2.62	.023
3.5 oz	100	21.9	6.9	10.3	2.5	91	70	.08	4.2	.41	1.53	329	270	2.83	.264	805
guinea hen w/o skin, raw	110	74.4	20.6	0.0	0.0	0.0	12	2	.11	.47	6	69	11	24	1.20	.018
3.5 oz	100	2.5	0.6	0.7	0.6	63	41	.07	8.8	.37	.94	220	169	.77	.044	805
pheasant w/o skin, raw	133	72.8	23.6	0.0	0.0	0.0	49	6	.15	.74	6	37	13	20	.97	.016
3.5 oz	100	3.6	1.2	1.2	0.6	66	165	.08	6.8	.84	.96	262	230	1.15	.069	805
pheasant w/ skin, raw	181	67.8	22.7	0.0	0.0	0.0	53	5	.14	.66	6	40	12	20	.96	.017
3.5 oz	100	9.3	2.7	4.3	1.2	71	177	.07	6.4	.77	.93	243	214	1.15	.065	805
quail w/o skin, raw	134	70.0	21.8	0.0	0.0	0.0	17	7	.28	.53	7	51	13	25	2.70	.019
3.5 oz	100	4.5	1.3	1.3	1.2	70	57	.28	8.2	.47	.79	237	307	4.51	.594	805
squab (pigeon) w/o skin, raw	142	72.8	17.5	0.0	0.0	0.0	28	7	.28	.53	7	51	13	25	2.70	.019
3.5 oz	100	7.5	2.0	2.7	1.6	90	94	.28	6.9	.47	.79	237	307	4.51	.594	805

25.6 INTERNAL ORGANS

	KCAL	H_2O (g)	PRO (g)	CHO (g)	SUGR (g)	DFIB (g)	A (RE)	C (mg)	B-2 (mg)	B-6 (mg)	FOL (mcg)	Na (mg)	Ca (mg)	Mg (mg)	Zn (mg)	Mn (mg)
	WT (g)	FAT (g)	SFA (g)	MUFA (g)	PUFA (g)	CHOL (mg)	A (IU)	B-1 (mg)	NIA (mg)	B-12 (mcg)	PANT (mg)	K (mg)	P (mg)	Fe (mg)	Cu (mg)	REF
giblets																
chicken, fried	277	47.9	32.5	4.3		0.0	3579	9	1.52	.61	379	113	18	25	6.27	.222
3.5 oz	100	13.5	3.8	4.4	3.4	446	11929	.10	11.0	13.31	4.45	330	286	10.32	.422	805
chicken, simmered	157	67.6	25.9	0.9		0.0	2229	8	.95	.34	376	58	12	20	4.57	.170
3.5 oz	100	4.8	1.5	1.2	1.1	393	7431	.09	4.1	10.14	2.96	158	229	6.44	.255	805
turkey, simmered	167	65.3	26.6	2.1		0.0	1795	2	.90	.33	345	59	13	17	3.68	.175
3.5 oz	100	5.1	1.5	1.1	1.2	418	6036	.05	4.5	24.03	3.46	200	204	6.71	.391	805
gizzard																
chicken, simmered	153	67.3	27.1	1.1		0.0	56	2	.24	.12	53	67	10	20	4.38	.062
3.5 oz	100	3.7	1.0	0.9	1.1	194	188	.03	4.0	1.94	.71	179	155	4.15	.110	805
goose, raw	139	73.0	21.4	0.0	0.0											
3.5 oz	100	5.3														456

	KCAL / WT (g)	H₂O (g) / FAT (g)	PRO (g) / SFA (g)	CHO (g) / MUFA (g)	SUGR (g) / PUFA (g)	DFIB (g) / CHOL (mg)	A (RE) / A (IU)	C (mg) / B-1 (mg)	B-2 (mg) / NIA (mg)	B-6 (mg) / B-12 (mcg)	FOL (mcg) / PANT (mg)	Na (mg) / K (mg)	Ca (mg) / P (mg)	Mg (mg) / Fe (mg)	Zn (mg) / Cu (mg)	Mn (mg) / REF
turkey, simmered	163	65.4	29.4	0.6		0.0	55	2	.33	.12	52	54	15	19	4.16	.098
3.5 oz	100	3.9	1.1	0.8	1.1	232	185	.03	3.1	1.90	.85	211	128	5.44	.173	805
heart, chicken, simmered	185	64.8	26.4	0.1		0.0	9	2	.74	.32	80	48	19	20	7.30	.107
3.5 oz	100	7.9	2.3	2.0	2.3	242	28	.07	2.8	7.29	2.65	132	199	9.03	.502	805
heart, turkey, simmered	177	64.2	26.8	2.0		0.0	8	2	.88	.32	79	55	13	22	5.27	.092
3.5 oz	100	6.1	1.8	1.2	1.8	226	28	.07	3.3	7.15	2.72	183	205	6.89	.627	805
liver																
chicken, simmered	157	68.3	24.4	0.9		0.0	4913	16	1.75	.58	770	51	14	21	4.34	.297
3.5 oz	100	5.5	1.8	1.3	0.9	631	16375	.15	4.5	19.39	5.41	140	312	8.47	.370	805
duck, raw	136	71.8	18.7	3.5		0.0	11946	5	.89	.76	738	140	11	24	3.07	.258
3.5 oz	100	4.6	1.4	0.7	0.6	515	39907	.56	6.5	54.00	6.18	230	269	30.53	5.962	805
goose, raw	125	67.5	15.4	5.9		0.0	8728	4	.84	.71	694	132	40	23	2.89	.000
3.3 oz	94	4.0	1.5	0.8	0.2	484	29138	.53	6.1	50.76	5.81	216	245	28.70	7.071	805
turkey, simmered	169	65.5	24.0	3.4		0.0	3741	2	1.42	.52	666	64	11	15	3.09	.253
3.5 oz	100	6.0	1.9	1.5	1.1	626	12581	.05	5.9	47.50	5.96	194	272	7.80	.560	805

25.7 TURKEY

	KCAL / WT (g)	H₂O (g) / FAT (g)	PRO (g) / SFA (g)	CHO (g) / MUFA (g)	SUGR (g) / PUFA (g)	DFIB (g) / CHOL (mg)	A (RE) / A (IU)	C (mg) / B-1 (mg)	B-2 (mg) / NIA (mg)	B-6 (mg) / B-12 (mcg)	FOL (mcg) / PANT (mg)	Na (mg) / K (mg)	Ca (mg) / P (mg)	Mg (mg) / Fe (mg)	Zn (mg) / Cu (mg)	Mn (mg) / REF
bacon, Louis Rich	34	8.4	2.2	0.2	0.2	0.0	0	0				180	6	3	.36	
1 slice	14	2.7	0.8	1.1	0.7	13	0					29	27	.21	.030	I
breast																
hickory smoked, fat-free, Louis Rich	52	41.5	10.7	1.3	0.4	0.0	0	0				721	9	15	.49	
2 oz	56	0.4	0.2	0.2	0.1	23	0					161	169	.63	.110	I
honey roasted, fat-free, Louis Rich	57	40.3	10.8	2.6	2.2	0.0	0	0				661	8	16	.56	
2 oz	55	0.4	0.3	0.1	0.1	22	0					147	155	.62	.120	I
oven roasted, fat-free, Louis Rich	51	41.9	10.7	1.1	0.2	0.0	0	0				659	10	16	.54	
2 oz	56	0.4	0.2	0.1	0.1	22	0					150	160	.62	.110	I
w/ skin, prebasted, roasted	126	70.9	22.2	0.0	0.0	0.0	0	0	.13	.32	5	397	9	21	1.53	.015
3.5 oz	100	3.5	1.0	1.1	0.8	42	0	.05	9.1	.32	.49	248	214	.66	.041	805
chunk in water, cnd, Swanson Premium	100		15.0	2.0	0.0	0.0	0	0				230	0			
¼ cup	62	4.0	1.0			50	0							.72		I
chunk, white in water, cnd, Swanson	90		16.0	4.0	0.0	1.0	0	0				220	0			
Premium—¼ cup	62	2.0	0.5			35	0							.00		I
dark meat w/o skin, roasted	187	63.1	28.6	0.0	0.0	0.0	0	0	.25	.36	9	79	32	24	4.46	.023
3.5 oz	100	7.2	2.4	1.6	2.2	85	0	.06	3.6	.37	1.29	290	204	2.33	.160	805
dark meat w/ skin, roasted	221	60.2	27.5	0.0	0.0	0.0	0	0	.23	.32	9	76	33	23	4.16	.023
3.5 oz	100	11.5	3.5	3.6	3.1	89	0	.06	3.5	.36	1.16	274	196	2.27	.150	805
ground, ckd	193	48.7	22.4	0.0	0.0	0.0	0	0	.14	.32	6	88	21	20	2.35	.016
3 oz patty	82	10.8	2.8	4.0	2.6	84	0	.04	4.0	.27	.67	221	161	1.58	.074	805
ground, Louis Rich	176	80.1	20.6	0.0	0.0		0	0				143	29	30	3.33	
4 oz	112	10.4	3.4	4.1	3.1	96	0					272	184	1.70	.260	I
light & dark meat																
seasoned, diced	138	71.7	18.7	1.0		0.0	0	0	.11	.28	5	850	1	17	2.02	.013
3.5 oz	100	6.0	1.8	2.0	1.5	55	0	.04	4.8	.24	.59	310	240	1.80	.063	805
seasoned, frzn, roasted	155	67.8	21.3	3.1		0.0	0	0	.16	.27	5	680	5	22	2.54	.015
3.5 oz	100	5.8	1.9	1.2	1.7	53	0	.05	6.3	1.52	.81	298	244	1.63	.060	805
w/o skin, roasted	170	64.9	29.3	0.0	0.0	0.0	0	0	.18	.46	7	70	25	26	3.10	.021
3.5 oz	100	5.0	1.6	1.0	1.4	76	0	.06	5.4	.37	.94	298	213	1.78	.094	805
w/ skin, roasted	208	61.7	28.1	0.0	0.0	0.0	0	0	.18	.41	7	68	26	25	2.96	.021
3.5 oz	100	9.7	2.8	3.2	2.5	82	0	.06	5.1	.35	.86	280	203	1.79	.093	805
light meat w/o skin, roasted	157	66.3	29.9	0.0	0.0	0.0	0	0	.13	.54	6	64	19	28	2.04	.020
3.5 oz	100	3.2	1.0	0.6	0.9	69	0	.06	6.8	.37	.68	305	219	1.35	.042	805
light meat w/ skin, roasted	197	62.8	28.6	0.0	0.0	0.0	0	0	.13	.47	6	63	21	26	2.04	.020
3.5 oz	100	8.3	2.3	2.8	2.0	76	0	.06	6.3	.35	.63	285	208	1.41	.048	805
nuggets, breaded, Louis Rich	254	46.6	13.2	14.1	0.0	0.4	0	0				625	8	20	1.69	
4 nuggets	92	16.1	3.1	7.5	5.0	37	0					162	181	.80	.270	I

	KCAL	H₂O (g)	PRO (g)	CHO (g)	SUGR (g)	DFIB (g)	A (RE)	C (mg)	B-2 (mg)	B-6 (mg)	FOL (mcg)	Na (mg)	Ca (mg)	Mg (mg)	Zn (mg)	Mn (mg)
	WT (g)	FAT (g)	SFA (g)	MUFA (g)	PUFA (g)	CHOL (mg)	A (IU)	B-1 (mg)	NIA (mg)	B-12 (mcg)	PANT (mg)	K (mg)	P (mg)	Fe (mg)	Cu (mg)	REF
patty																
breaded & fried	266	46.7	13.2	14.8		0.5	10	0	.18	.19	8	752	13	14	1.35	.072
1 patty	94	16.9	4.4	7.0	4.4	58	35	.09	2.2	.21	.49	259	254	2.07	.066	805
breaded, Louis Rich	215	45.8	11.8	12.8	0.0	0.4	0	0				531	9	18	1.48	
1 patty	85	13.0	2.4	5.6	4.3	33	0					148	157	.71	.170	I
white, Louis Rich	166	84.2	18.8	0.0	0.0	0.0	0	0				441	8	24	1.82	
1 pattie	113	10.1	2.4	3.9	3.6	65	0					237	224	.96	.190	I
sausage																
Louis Rich	109	48.8	12.5	1.2	0.4	0.0	0	0				435	22	17	2.01	
2.5 oz	70	6.0				57	0					182	109	1.13	.180	I
polska kielbasa, Louis Rich	87	39.0	8.2	2.0	1.3	0.0	0	0				505	10	10	1.08	
2 oz	56	5.1	1.6	2.0	1.5	39	0					111	114	.68	.070	I
smoked, Louis Rich	90	38.7	8.1	2.2	1.6	0.0	0	0				515	14	12	1.20	
2 oz	56	5.4	1.5	2.0	1.5	36	0					113	114	.77	.100	I
sticks, breaded & fried	357	63.2	18.2	21.8			15	0	.23	.26	12	1073	18	19	1.87	.106
2 sticks	128	21.6	5.6	8.9	5.6	82	51	.13	2.7	.29	.68	333	300	2.82	.093	805
sticks, breaded, Louis Rich	235	43.1	12.2	13.1	0.0	0.4	0	0				577	8	18	1.56	
3 sticks	85	14.9	2.9	7.0	4.6	34	0					150	167	.74	.250	I
thigh w/ skin, prebasted, roasted	493	221.7	59.0	0.0	0.0	0.0	0	0	.80	.72	19	1372	25	53	12.94	.047
11.1 oz thigh	314	26.8	8.3	7.9	7.4	195	0	.26	7.6	.75	2.55	757	537	4.74	.436	805
white, oven roasted, Oscar Mayer	29	21.1	3.7	1.4	0.4	0.0	0	0				302	3	6	.31	
1 slice	28	1.0	0.3	0.4	0.2	10	0					55	67	.28	.050	I
white, smoked, Oscar Mayer	28	21.4	3.8	0.9	0.2	0.0	0	0				313	4	7	.39	
1 slice	28	1.0	0.3	0.4	0.3	10	0					60	61	.20	.050	I

1. Average of values for Italian style herb, lemon pepper, original parmesan, and southwestern.

26. SALAD DRESSINGS
26.1 LOW & REDUCED CALORIE

	KCAL	H₂O (g)	PRO (g)	CHO (g)	SUGR (g)	DFIB (g)	A (RE)	C (mg)	B-2 (mg)	B-6 (mg)	FOL (mcg)	Na (mg)	Ca (mg)	Mg (mg)	Zn (mg)	Mn (mg)
bacon & tomato, Kraft Red Cal	60		1.0	3.0	3.0	0.0	0	0				300	0			
2 T	31	5.0	1.0			5	0					40		.00		I
blue cheese																
Kraft Free	50		1.0	12.0	3.0	1.0	0	0				340	0			
2 T	35	0.0	0.0	0.0	0.0	0	0					40		.00		I
Marie's Lite	45		0.5	3.4				0	.01			186	16			
1 T	15	3.3	0.6		1.7	3	0	.01	0.0			11		.10		I
Walden Farms Red Cal	27		0.0	1.7								270				
1 T	15	1.9				1.0	5					15				I
Wish-Bone Lite Chunky	70		1.0	3.0	2.0	0.0		0	.00			420	20	0	.00	.000
1 fl oz	30 ml	6.0	1.0			0	0	.00	0.0			0		.00	.000	I
caesar, Kraft Red Cal	60		1.0	2.0	2.0	0.0	0	0				560	20			
2 T	31	5.0	1.0			5	0					10		.00		I
catalina, Kraft Free	45		0.0	11.0	7.0	1.0		0				360	0			
2 T	35	0.0	0.0	0.0	0.0	0	500					60		.00		I
french	21	11.1	0.0	3.5		0.0	21	0	.00	.00	0	126	2	0	.03	
1 T	16	0.9	0.1	0.2	0.5	0	208	.00	0.0	.00	.00	13	2	.06	.002	804
Catalina Red Cal	80		0.0	9.0	7.0	0.0		0				400	0			
2 T	34	4.0	0.5			0	500					75		.00		I
Kraft Red Cal	50		0.0	6.0	5.0	0.0		0				260	0			
2 T	32	3.0	0.5			0	500					15		.00		I

	KCAL / WT (g)	H₂O (g) / FAT (g)	PRO (g) / SFA (g)	CHO (g) / MUFA (g)	SUGR (g) / PUFA (g)	DFIB (g) / CHOL (mg)	A (RE) / A (IU)	C (mg) / B-1 (mg)	B-2 (mg) / NIA (mg)	B-6 (mg) / B-12 (mcg)	FOL (mcg) / PANT (mg)	Na (mg) / K (mg)	Ca (mg) / P (mg)	Mg (mg) / Fe (mg)	Zn (mg) / Cu (mg)	Mn (mg) / REF
Walden Farms Red Cal	33		0.0	2.6								132				
1 T	15	2.4			1.0	2						18				I
french style, Kraft Free	45		0.0	12.0	5.0	1.0		0				300	0			
2 T	35	0.0	0.0	0.0	0.0	0	500					40		.00		I
honey dijon, Kraft Free	50		1.0	11.0	5.0	1.0	0	0				330	0			
2 T	35	0.0	0.0	0.0	0.0	0	0					50				I
honey mustard, from mix, fat-free, Good Seasons—2 T[1]	20		0.0	5.0	4.0	0.0	0	0				280	0			
	30	0.0	0.0	0.0	0.0	0	0					30		.00		I
italian	16	12.3	0.0	0.7		0.0	0	0	.00	.00	0	118	0	0	.02	
1 T	15	1.5	0.2	0.3	0.9	1	0	.00	0.0	.00	.00	2	1	.03	.001	804
from mix, fat-free, Good Seasons	10		0.0	3.0	2.0	0.0	0	0				290	0			
2 T[1]	30	0.0	0.0	0.0	0.0	0	0					110		.00		I
from mix, red cal, Good Seasons	50		0.0	2.0	1.0	0.0	0	0				280	0			
2 T[2]	30	5.0	1.0			0	0					15		.00		I
garlic, Marie's Lite	43		0.4	3.4				0	.01			181	13			
1 T	15	3.1	0.6		1.7	3	0	.00	0.0			20		.10		I
Kraft Free	10		0.0	2.0	2.0	0.0	0	0				290	0			
2 T	31	0.0	0.0	0.0	0.0	0	0					40		.00		I
Kraft Oil-Free	5		0.0	2.0	1.0	0.0	0	0				450	0			
2 T	31	0.0	0.0	0.0	0.0	0	0					10		.00		I
Kraft Red Cal	70		0.0	3.0	2.0	0.0	0	0				240	0			
2 T	31	7.0	1.0			0	0					25		.00		I
no sugar added, Walden Farms Red Cal	6		0.0	1.5	0.0							180				
1 T	15	0.0	0.0		0.0	0						6				I
Seven Seas Free	10		0.0	2.0	2.0	0.0	0	0				480	0			
2 T	32	0.0	0.0	0.0	0.0	0	0					45		.00		I
Seven Seas Red Cal	45		0.0	2.0	2.0	0.0	0	0				390	0			
2 T	31	4.0	1.0			0	0					10		.00		I
soduium free, Walden Farms Red Cal	9		0.0	1.5								5				
1 T	15	0.0				0						75				I
Walden Farms Red Cal	9		0.0	1.5								300				
1 T	15	0.0	0.0		0.0	0						8				I
Wish-Bone Lite	15		0.0	2.0	1.0	0.0		0	.00			380	0			
1 fl oz	30 ml	0.5	0.0			0	0	.00	0.0					.00		I
w/ olive oil, Seven Seas Red Cal	50		0.0	2.0	2.0	0.0	0	0				450	0			
2 T	31	5.0	1.0			0	0					10		.00		I
zesty, from mix, fat-free, Good Seasons	10		0.0	2.0	2.0	0.0	0	0				260	0			
2 T[1]	34	0.0	0.0	0.0	0.0	0	0					70		.00		I
zesty, from mix, red cal, Good Seasons	50		0.0	2.0	1.0	0.0	0	0				260	0			
2 T[2]	30	5.0	1.0			0	0					30		.00		I
italian, creamy																
from mix, fat-free, Good Seasons	20		1.0	3.0	3.0	0.0	0	0				280	0			
2 T[3]	30	0.0	0.0	0.0	0.0	0	0					140		.00		I
Kraft Red Cal	60		0.0	2.0	2.0	0.0	0	0				450	0			
2 T	31	5.0	1.0			0	0					20		.00		I
Seven Seas Red Cal	60		0.0	2.0	2.0	0.0	0	0				490	0			
2 T	31	5.0	1.0			0	0					10		.00		I
w/ parmesan, Walden Farms Red Cal	35		0.0	3.0								210				
1 T	15	2.5			1.0	4						19				I
Miracle Whip Free, Kraft	15		0.0	3.0	2.0	0.0	0	0				120	0			
1 T	16	0.0	0.0	0.0	0.0	0	0					5		.00		I
Miracle Whip Light, Kraft	40		0.0	3.0	2.0	0.0	0	0				120	0			
1 T	15	3.0			0.0	0	0					0		.00		I
peppercorn ranch, Kraft Free	50		1.0	11.0	2.0	1.0	0	0				360	0			
2 T	35	0.0	0.0	0.0	0.0	0	0					60		.00		I
ranch																
from mix, red cal, Good Seasons	60		1.0	3.0	2.0	0.0	0	0				240	0			
2 T[4]	30	4.5	1.0			5	0					55		.00		I

	KCAL	H₂O (g)	PRO (g)	CHO (g)	SUGR (g)	DFIB (g)	A (RE)	C (mg)	B-2 (mg)	B-6 (mg)	FOL (mcg)	Na (mg)	Ca (mg)	Mg (mg)	Zn (mg)	Mn (mg)
	WT (g)	FAT (g)	SFA (g)	MUFA (g)	PUFA (g)	CHOL (mg)	A (IU)	B-1 (mg)	NIA (mg)	B-12 (mcg)	PANT (mg)	K (mg)	P (mg)	Fe (mg)	Cu (mg)	REF
Kraft Free	50		1.0	11.0	2.0	1.0	0	0				310	0			
2 T	35	0.0	0.0	0.0	0.0	0	0					50		.00		I
Kraft Red Cal	110		0.0	2.0	1.0	0.0	0	0				310	0		.00	
2 T	30	11.0	2.0			10	0					40				I
Marie's Lite	46		0.3	3.8				0	.00			212	14			
1 T	15	3.3	0.6		1.9	2	3	.01	0.0			14		.10		I
Seven Seas Free	50		1.0	12.0	3.0	1.0	0	0				330	20			
2 T	35	0.0	0.0	0.0	0.0	0	0					55		.00		I
Seven Seas Red Cal	100		0.0	5.0	1.0	0.0	0	0				320	0			
2 T	31	9.0	1.5			0	0					10		.00		I
Walden Farms Red Calorie	35		0.0	3.0								165				
1 T	15	2.0			1.0	8						27				I
Wish-Bone Lite	100		0.0	7.0	1.0	2.0		0	.00			340	0	0	.00	.000
1 fl oz	30 ml	8.0	1.0			5	0	.00	0.0			0	0	.00	.000	I
red wine vinegar & oil, Seven Seas Red Cal—2 T	60		0.0	2.0	2.0	0.0	0	0				310	0			
	31	5.0	1.0			0	0					10		.00		I
red wine vinegar, Kraft Free	15		0.0	3.0	3.0	0.0	0	0				400	0			
2 T	32	0.0	0.0	0.0	0.0	0	0					15		.00		I
red wine vinegar, Seven Seas Free	15		0.0	3.0	2.0	0.0	0	0				400	0			
2 T	32	0.0	0.0	0.0	0.0	0	0					15		.00		I
russian	23	10.4	0.1	4.4		0.0	3	1	.00	.00	1	139	3	0	.02	
1 T	16	0.6	0.1	0.1	0.4	1	9	.00	0.0	.02	.02	25	6	.10	.002	804
sour cream & dill, Marie's Lite	51		0.3	3.6				0	.02			169	12			
1 T	15	3.9	0.7		2.2	3	25	.00	0.0			17		.10		I
thousand island	24	10.4	0.1	2.4		0.2	14	0	.00	.00	1	150	2	0	.02	
1 T	15	1.6	0.2	0.4	0.9	2	48	.00	0.0	.03	.03	17	3	.09	.002	804
Kraft Free	45		0.0	11.0	6.0	1.0	0	0				300	0			
2 T	35	0.0	0.0	0.0	0.0	0	0					55		.00		I
Kraft Red Cal	70		0.0	8.0	5.0	0.0	0	0				320	0			
2 T	32	4.0	1.0			5	0					55		.00		I
Marie's Lite	44		0.2	4.2				0	.00			155	8			
1 T	15	3.0	0.5		1.7	3	48	.01	0.0			15		.10		I
Walden Farms Red Calorie	24		0.0	3.1								132				
1 T	15	1.7			1.0	8						10				I
Wish-Bone Lite	80		0.0	8.0	5.0	0.0		0	.00			280	0	0	.00	.000
1 fl oz	30 ml	5.0	1.0			10	0	.00	0.0			0	0	.00	.000	I

26.2 REGULAR

	KCAL	H₂O (g)	PRO (g)	CHO (g)	SUGR (g)	DFIB (g)	A (RE)	C (mg)	B-2 (mg)	B-6 (mg)	FOL (mcg)	Na (mg)	Ca (mg)	Mg (mg)	Zn (mg)	Mn (mg)
	WT (g)	FAT (g)	SFA (g)	MUFA (g)	PUFA (g)	CHOL (mg)	A (IU)	B-1 (mg)	NIA (mg)	B-12 (mcg)	PANT (mg)	K (mg)	P (mg)	Fe (mg)	Cu (mg)	REF
Avocado Goddess, Marie's	97		0.2					0	.01			93	4			
1 T	15	10.6	1.7		6.0	8	0	.00	0.0			6		.10		I
bacon & tomato, Kraft	140			2.0	2.0	0.0	0	0				260	0			
2 T	30	14.0	2.5			5	0					35		.00		I
blue (bleu) cheese	76	4.8	0.7	1.1		0.0	10	0	.01	.01	1	164	12	0	.04	
1 T	15	7.8	1.5	1.8	4.2	3	32	.00	0.0	.04	.06	6	11	.03	.002	804
chunky, Seven Seas	90		1.0	5.0	3.0	0.0	0	0				470	20			
2 T	33	7.0	4.0			10	0					50		.00		I
Marie's	94		0.6	0.8				0	.01			87	14			
1 T	15	9.8	1.8		5.5	9	0	.00	0.0			7		.10		I
Roka Brand	90		1.0	5.0	3.0	0.0	0	0				470	20			
2 T	33	7.0	4.0			10	0					50		.00		I
Wish-Bone Chunky	170		1.0	3.0	1.0	0.0		0	.00			290	0			
1 fl oz	30 ml	17.0	2.5			0	0	.00	0.0					.00		I
buttermilk																
farm style, from mix, Good Seasons	120		1.0	2.0	2.0	0.0	0	0				260	0			
2 T[4]	32	12.0	2.0			10	0					45		.00		I
ranch, Kraft	150		0.0	2.0	2.0	0.0	0	0				230	0			
2 T	29	16.0	3.0			5	0					20		.00		I
spice, Marie's	89		0.2	1.9				0	.01			123	6			
1 T	15	8.9	1.4		5.1	5	0	.00	0.0			5		.10		I

Each food item is listed across two rows. The first data row corresponds to the upper header labels (KCAL, H₂O, PRO, CHO, SUGR, DFIB, A (RE), C, B-2, B-6, FOL, Na, Ca, Mg, Zn, Mn); the second data row (beginning with the serving/WT) corresponds to the lower header labels (WT, FAT, SFA, MUFA, PUFA, CHOL, A (IU), B-1, NIA, B-12, PANT, K, P, Fe, Cu, REF).

	KCAL / WT (g)	H_2O (g) / FAT (g)	PRO (g) / SFA (g)	CHO (g) / MUFA (g)	SUGR (g) / PUFA (g)	DFIB (g) / CHOL (mg)	A (RE) / A (IU)	C (mg) / B-1 (mg)	B-2 (mg) / NIA (mg)	B-6 (mg) / B-12 (mcg)	FOL (mcg) / PANT (mg)	Na (mg) / K (mg)	Ca (mg) / P (mg)	Mg (mg) / Fe (mg)	Zn (mg) / Cu (mg)	Mn (mg) / REF
caesar																
creamy, Seven Seas	140		1.0	1.0	0.0	0.0	0	0				300	20			
2 T	29	15.0	2.5			10	0					10		.00		I
gourmet, from mix, Good Seasons	150		0.0	3.0	2.0	0.0	0	0				300	0			
2 T²	32	16.0	2.5			0	0					110		.00		I
Kraft	130		1.0	2.0	1.0	0.0	0	0				370	20			
2 T	30	13.0	2.5			5	0					10		.00		I
Seven Seas Viva	120		1.0	2.0	2.0	0.0	0	0				500	20			
2 T	31	12.0	2.0			0	0					30		.00		I
Wish-Bone	110		1.0	2.0	2.0	0.0		0	.00			300	6	0	.00	.000
1 fl oz	30 ml	10.0	2.0			15	3	.00	0.0			0	0	.00	.000	I
caesar ranch, Kraft	140		1.0	1.0	0.0	0.0	0	0				300	20			
2 T	29	15.0	2.5			10	0					10		.00		I
catalina w/ honey, Kraft	140		0.0	8.0	8.0	0.0		0				310	0			
2 T	32	12.0	2.0			0						40		.00		I
cheese garlic, from mix, Good Seasons	140		0.0	1.0	1.0	0.0	0	0				330	0			
2 T²	32	16.0	2.5			0	0					15		.00		I
ckd, homemade	25	11.1	0.7	2.4		0.0	20	0	.02	.00	1	117	13	1	.06	
1 T	16	1.5	0.5	0.6	0.3	9	66	.01	0.0	.06	.00	19	14	.08	.002	804
coleslaw, Kraft	150		0.0	8.0	8.0	0.0	0	0				420	0			
2 T	32	12.0	2.0			25	0					10		.00		I
creamy garlic, Kraft	110		0.0	2.0	2.0	0.0	0	0				350	0			
2 T	30	11.0	2.0			0	0					25		.00		I
cucumber ranch, Kraft	150		0.0	2.0	2.0	0.0	0	0				220	0			
2 T	30	15.0	2.5			0	0					20		.00		I
french	69	6.1	0.1	2.8		0.0	21	0	.00	.00	1	219	2	0	.01	
1 T	16	6.6	1.5	1.3	3.5	0	208	.00	0.0	.02	.03	13	2	.06	.002	804
Catalina	140		0.0	8.0	8.0	0.0		0				390	0			
2 T	32	11.0	2.0			0	500					40		.00		I
homemade	88	3.4	0.0	0.5		0.0	22	0	.00	.00	0	92	1	0	.00	
1 T	14	9.8	1.8	2.9	4.7	0	72	.00	0.0	.00	.00	3	0	.03		804
Kraft	120		0.0	4.0	4.0	0.0		0				260	0			
2 T	31	12.0	2.0			0	500					15		.00		I
sweet 'n spicy, Wish-Bone	130		0.0	6.0	5.0	0.0		1	.00			330	0			
1 fl oz	30 ml	12.0	2.0			0	0	.00	0.0					.00		I
Wish-Bone Deluxe	120		0.0	5.0	4.0	0.0		0	.00			170	0	0	.00	.000
1 fl oz	30 ml	11.0	1.5			0	100	.00	0.0			0	0	.00	.000	I
garlic & herbs, from mix, Good Seasons	140		0.0	1.0	1.0	0.0	0	0				340	0			
2 T²	32	15.0	2.0			0	0					10		.00		I
Green Goddess, Seven Seas	120		0.0	1.0	1.0	0.0	0	0				260	0			
2 T	29	13.0	2.0			0	0					15		.00		I
herbs & spices, Seven Seas	120		0.0	1.0	1.0	0.0	0	0				320	0			
2 T	30	12.0	2.0			0	0					10		.00		I
honey dijon, Kraft	150		0.0	4.0	3.0	0.0	0	0				200	0			
2 T	31	15.0	2.0			0	0					35		.00		I
honey mustard, from mix, Good Seasons	150		0.0	3.0	2.0	0.0	0	0				240	0			
2 T²	32	15.0	2.0			0	0					15		.00		I
italian	70	5.8	0.1	1.5		0.0	4	0	.00	.00	1	118	2	0	.02	
1 T	15	7.2	1.1	1.7	4.2	0	12	.00	0.0	.02	.03	2	1	.03	.002	804
Classic House, Wish-Bone	140		0.0	2.0	1.0	0.0		0	.00			360				
1 fl oz	30 ml	14.0	2.0			5		.00	0.0					.00		I
classic olive oil, Wish-Bone	70			4.0	3.0	0.0		0	.00			400	0			
1 fl oz	30 ml	6.0	1.0			0	0	.00	0.0					.00		I
from mix, Good Seasons	140		0.0	1.0	1.0	0.0	0	0				320	0			
2 T²	32	15.0	2.0			0	0					15		.00		I
garlic, Marie's	96		0.2	0.5				0	.01			139	7			
1 T	15	10.3	1.7		6.0	9	0	.00	0.0			9		.10		I
herb & romano, Marie's	95		0.3	0.8				0	.01			85	9			
1 T	15	10.1	1.7		5.9	8	0	.00	0.0			8		.10		I
house, Kraft	120		0.0	3.0	2.0	0.0	0	0				240	0			
2 T	30	12.0	2.0			5	0					25		.00		I

	KCAL	H_2O (g)	PRO (g)	CHO (g)	SUGR (g)	DFIB (g)	Vitamins A (RE)	C (mg)	B-2 (mg)	B-6 (mg)	FOL (mcg)	Minerals Na (mg)	Ca (mg)	Mg (mg)	Zn (mg)	Mn (mg)
	WT (g)	FAT (g)	SFA (g)	MUFA (g)	PUFA (g)	CHOL (mg)	A (IU)	B-1 (mg)	NIA (mg)	B-12 (mcg)	PANT (mg)	K (mg)	P (mg)	Fe (mg)	Cu (mg)	REF
mild, from mix, Good Seasons	150		0.0	2.0	2.0	0.0	0	0				370	0			
2 T[2]	34	15.0	2.5			0	0					10		.00		I
presto, Kraft	140		0.0	2.0	2.0	0.0	0	0				290	0			
2 T	30	15.0	2.5			0	0					15		.00		I
robusto, Wish-Bone	100		0.0	4.0	2.0	0.0		0	.00			620	1	0	.00	.000
1 fl oz	30 ml	10.0	2.0			0	0	.00	0.0			0	0	.00	.000	I
Seven Seas Viva	100		0.0	2.0	2.0	0.0	0	0				580	0			
2 T	30	11.0	1.5			0	0					10		.00		I
Wish-Bone	80		0.0	3.0	2.0	0.0		1	.00			490	1			
1 fl oz	30 ml	8.0	1.0			0	0	.00	0.0					.10		I
zesty, from mix, Good Seasons	140		0.0	1.0	1.0	0.0	0	0				220	0			
2 T[2]	32	15.0	2.0			0	0					15		.00		I
zesty, Kraft	110		0.0	2.0	2.0	0.0	0	0				530	0			
2 T	30	11.0	1.5			0	0					10		.00		I
italian, creamy																
Kraft	110		0.0	3.0	2.0	0.0	0	0				230	0			
2 T	30	11.0	4.0			0	0					20		.00		I
Seven Seas	110		0.0	2.0	2.0	0.0	0	0				510	0			
2 T	30	12.0	2.0			0	0					10		.00		I
Wish-Bone	110		1.0	5.0	2.0	0.0		0	.00			240	0	0	.00	.000
1 fl oz	30 ml	10.0	2.0			0	0	.00	0.0			0	0	.00	.000	I
mayonnaise type	58	6.0	0.1	3.6		0.0	13	0	.00	.00	1	107	2	0	.03	
1 T	15	5.0	0.7	1.3	2.7	4	33	.00	0.0	.03	.04	1	4	.03	.002	804
mexican spice, from mix, Good Seasons	140		0.0	2.0	1.0	0.0	0	0				310	0			
2 T[2]	32	15.0	2.5			0	0					65		.00		I
Miracle Whip, Kraft	70		0.0	2.0	1.0	0.0	0	0				85	0			
1 T	14	7.0	1.0			5	0					0		.00		I
oriental sesame, from mix, Good Seasons	150		0.0	3.0	2.0	0.0	0	0				360	0			
2 T[2]	32	16.0	2.5			0	0					15		.00		I
peppercorn ranch, Kraft	170		1.0	1.0	1.0	0.0	0	0				340	20			
2 T	29	18.0	3.0			10	0					20		.00		I
ranch																
from mix, Good Seasons	120		1.0	2.0	1.0	0.0	0	0				220	0			
2 T[4]	30	12.0	2.0			10	0					35		.00		I
Kraft	170		0.0	2.0	1.0	0.0	0	0				270	0			
2 T	29	18.0	3.0			5	0					10		.00		I
Marie's	96		0.2	0.8				0	.01			90	5			
1 T	15	10.2	1.6		6.0	8	32	.01	0.0			5		.10		I
Seven Seas	150		0.0	2.0	1.0	0.0	0	0				250	0			
2 T	29	16.0	2.5			5	0					10		.00		I
Wish-Bone	160		0.0	1.0	1.0	0.0		0	.00			200	0			
1 fl oz	30 ml	17.0	2.5			10		.00	0.0					.00		I
red wine vinegar & oil, Seven Seas	110		0.0	2.0	2.0	0.0	0	0				510	0			
2 T	31	11.0	2.0			0	0					15		.00		I
russian	74	5.2	0.2	1.6		0.0	31	1	.01	.00	2	130	3	0	.06	
1 T	15	7.6	1.1	1.8	4.4	3	104	.01	0.1	.04	.06	24	6	.09	.002	804
Kraft	130		0.0	10.0	9.0	0.0		0				280	0			
2 T	33	10.0	1.5			0	400					40		.00		I
Marie's	94		0.2	1.6				0	.00			105	3			
1 T	15	9.7	1.6		5.5	7	54	.01	0.1			12		.10		I
Seven Seas Viva	150		0.0	3.0	2.0	0.0	0	0				230	0			
2 T	30	16.0	2.5			0	0					20		.00		I
Wish-Bone	110		0.0	15.0	7.0	0.0		1	.00			350	2	0	.00	.000
1 fl oz	30 ml	6.0	1.0			0	100	.00	0.0			0	0	.00	.000	I
salsa ranch, Kraft	130		0.0	1.0	1.0	0.0	0	0				320	0			
2 T	29	13.0	2.0			10	0					20		.00		I
salsa, zesty garden, Kraft	70		0.0	3.0	3.0	1.0		0				280	0			
2 T	31	6.0	1.0			0	300					30		.00		I
sesame seed	66	5.9	0.5	1.3		0.1	31	0	.00	.00	0	150	3	0	.01	
1 T	15	6.8	0.9	1.8	3.8	0	104	.00	0.0	.00	.00	24	6	.09		804

	KCAL	H₂O (g)	PRO (g)	CHO (g)	SUGR (g)	DFIB (g)	Vitamins					Minerals				
							A (RE)	C (mg)	B-2 (mg)	B-6 (mg)	FOL (mcg)	Na (mg)	Ca (mg)	Mg (mg)	Zn (mg)	Mn (mg)
	WT (g)	FAT (g)	SFA (g)	MUFA (g)	PUFA (g)	CHOL (mg)	A (IU)	B-1 (mg)	NIA (mg)	B-12 (mcg)	PANT (mg)	K (mg)	P (mg)	Fe (mg)	Cu (mg)	REF
sour cream & dill, Marie's	96		0.3	0.9				0	.01			89	8			
1 T	15	10.2	1.7		5.9	7	36	.00	0.0			6		.10		I
sour cream & onion ranch, Kraft	170		0.0	1.0	1.0	0.0	0	0				240	0			
2 T	29	18.0	3.0			10	0					40		.00		I
thousand island	60	7.4	0.1	2.4		0.0	15	0	.00	.00	1	112	2	0	.02	
1 T	16	5.7	1.0	1.3	3.2	4	51	.00	0.0	.03	.04	18	3	.10	.002	804
Kraft	110		0.0	5.0	5.0	0.0	0	0				310	0			
2 T	31	10.0	1.5			10	0					35		.00		I
Marie's	81		0.1	2.7			0		.00			113	4			
1 T	15	7.8	1.3		4.5	7	86	.00	0.1			11		.10		I
Wish-Bone	130		0.0	7.0	6.0				.00			340	0		.00	.000
1 fl oz	30 ml	12.0	2.0			10		.00	0.0			0	0		.000	I
w/ bacon, Kraft	120		0.0	5.0	4.0	0.0	0	0				190	0			
2 T	29	12.0	2.0			0	0					30		.00		I
two cheese italian, Seven Seas	70		0.0	3.0	2.0	0.0	0	0				240	0			
2 T	31	7.0	1.0			0	0					25		.00		I
vinaigrette, olive oil, Wish-Bone	61		0.0	4.0	3.0	0.0		0	.00			250	0			
1 fl oz	30 ml	5.0	1.0			0	0	.00	0.0					.00		I
vinegar & oil, homemade	72	7.6	0.0	0.4		0.0	0	0	.00	.00	0	0	0	0	.00	
1 T	16	8.0	1.5	2.4	3.9	0	0	.00	0.0	.00	.00	1	0	.00	.000	804

1. Prepared with vinegar and water.
2. Prepared with vinegar, water, and oil.

3. Prepared with nonfat milk, vinegar, and water.
4. Prepared with whole milk and mayonnaise.

27. SAUCES, CONDIMENTS, & GRAVIES
27.1 GRAVIES

	KCAL	H₂O	PRO	CHO	SUGR	DFIB	A	C	B-2	B-6	FOL	Na	Ca	Mg	Zn	Mn
	WT	FAT	SFA	MUFA	PUFA	CHOL	A	B-1	NIA	B-12	PANT	K	P	Fe	Cu	REF
au jus																
cnd	24	140.8	1.8	3.7		0.0	0	1	.09	.01	3	75	6	3	1.49	.298
½ can	149	0.3	0.1	0.1	0.0	0	0	.03	1.3	.15	.03	121	45	.89	.149	806
cnd, Franco-American	9		0.6	1.5				0	.01			316	3			
2 oz	57	0.1					0	.00	0.6			39		.20		I
mix	31	0.3	0.9	4.7			0	0	.03	.02	8	1159	14	6	.07	.027
amt to make 1 cup	10	1.0	0.2	0.5	0.0	0	1	.05	0.4	.03	.02	28	15	.93	.012	806
beef, cnd	62	102.4	4.4	5.6		0.5	0	0	.04	.01	2	655	7	2	1.17	.234
½ can	117	2.8	1.3	1.1	0.1	4	0	.04	0.8	.12	.02	95	35	.82	.117	806
beef, cnd, Franco-American	25		1.1	2.8				0	.02			295	4			
2 oz	57	1.0					0	.02	0.5			33		.20		I
brown																
cnd, Heinz Homestyle	29		0.7	1.4				1	.02			130	0			
2 oz	57	2.3					0	.00	0.1			80		.05		I
from mix, Pillsbury	16		0.4	3.2				0	.00			328	4			
¼ cup	60	0.2					0	.01	0.0			5	3	.04		I
mix	81	1.1	2.4	13.1		0.4	1	0	.09	.02	3	1065	29	7	.24	.091
amt to make 1 cup	22	2.1	0.7	1.0	0.1	1	6	.04	0.8	.15	.02	58	45	.38	.042	806
w/ onions, cnd, Franco-American	25		0.4	3.7				0	.00			331	6			
2 oz	57	0.9					0	.01	0.1			26		.20		I
chicken																
cnd	94	101.6	2.3	6.4		0.5	132	0	.05	.01	2	687	24	2	.95	.238
½ can	119	6.8	1.7	3.0	1.8	2	439	.02	0.5	.12	.02	130	35	.56	.119	806

	KCAL / WT (g)	H₂O (g) / FAT (g)	PRO (g) / SFA (g)	CHO (g) / MUFA (g)	SUGR (g) / PUFA (g)	DFIB (g) / CHOL (mg)	A (RE) / A (IU)	C (mg) / B-1 (mg)	B-2 (mg) / NIA (mg)	B-6 (mg) / B-12 (mcg)	FOL (mcg) / PANT (mg)	Na (mg) / K (mg)	Ca (mg) / P (mg)	Mg (mg) / Fe (mg)	Zn (mg) / Cu (mg)	Mn (mg) / REF
cnd, Franco-American	42		0.8	2.6				0	.02			242	11			
2 oz	57	3.1					217	.01	0.2			26			.20	I
cnd, Heinz Homestyle	35		0.7	2.9				1	.02			110	0			
2 oz	57	2.3					0	.00	0.1			50			.04	I
country, cnd, Libby's	60		1.0	3.0	0.0	0.0	0	0				330	0			
¼ cup	61	4.0	0.5			5	0								.00	I
from mix, Pillsbury	25		1.0	4.0								230				
¼ cup	130	1.0										20				I
mix	88	0.9	2.6	14.3			9	0	.15	.05	25	955	34	9	.32	.050
amt to make 1 cup	23	2.2	0.7	1.1	0.4	4	71	.06	0.9	.11	.30	93	57	.31	.026	806
chicken giblet, cnd, Franco-American	29		1.1	2.7				0	.02			301	4			
2 oz	57	1.5					0	.00	0.2			15			.30	I
cream, cnd, Franco-American	34		0.6	4.2				0	.02			210	10			
2 oz	57	1.7					0	.02	0.1			20				I
homestyle, from mix, Pillsbury	16		0.5	3.1				0	.00			339	3			
¼ cup	60	0.1					0	.01	0.0			5	3	.03		I
mushroom																
cnd	75	132.6	1.9	8.2		0.6	0	0	.09	.03	18	849	10	3	1.04	.447
½ can	149	4.0	0.6	1.7	1.5	0	0	.05	1.0	.00	1.64	158	22	.98	.149	806
cnd, Franco-American	21		0.6	2.7				0	.03			287	3			
2 oz	57	0.8					0	.01	0.3			30			.20	I
cnd, Heinz Homestyle	21		0.4	2.7				1	.02			200	0			
2 oz	57	0.9					0	.00	0.1			70			.10	I
mix	69	0.7	2.1	13.6		1.0	0	1	.08	.02	3	1382	48	7	.32	.084
amt to make 1 cup	21	0.8	0.5	0.3	0.0	1	0	.04	0.8	.15	.02	55	43	.21	.112	806
onion, cnd, Heinz Homestyle	24		0.4	3.6				1	.02			150	0			
2 oz	57	0.8					0	.00	0.1			80			.11	I
onion mix	77	1.0	2.2	16.2		1.4	0	2	.10	.02	3	1005	67	8	.21	.096
amt to make 1 cup	24	0.7	0.4	0.2	0.0	0	0	.05	0.9	.17	.02	63	49	.24	.041	806
pork																
cnd, Franco-American	36		0.7	2.8				0	.01			333	4			
2 oz	57	2.5					39	.01	0.2			18			.20	I
cnd, Heinz Homestyle	31		1.8	2.1				1	.02			130	0			
2 oz	57	1.7					0	.00	0.1			80			.06	I
mix	77	0.9	1.8	13.3		0.5	6	0	.06	.02	3	1125	29	7	.22	.065
amt to make 1 cup	21	1.8	0.9	0.8	0.1	2	25	.03	0.5	.11	.07	49	39	.83	.032	806
sausage, country, cnd, Libby's	90		1.0	3.0	0.0	0.0	0	0				280	0			
¼ cup	64	7.0	1.5			5	0								.00	I
turkey																
cnd	76	132.0	3.9	7.6		0.6	0	0	.12	.01	3	860	6	3	1.19	.298
½ can	149	3.1	0.9	1.3	0.7	3	0	.03	1.9	.15	.03	162	43	1.04	.149	806
cnd, Franco-American	23		0.6	3.2				0	.03			292	3			
2 oz	57	0.9					66	.01	0.5			25			.90	I
cnd, Heinz Homestyle	29		0.8	2.1				1	.02			140	0			
2 oz	57	2.0					0	.00	0.0			90			.07	I
mix	92	1.2	2.6	16.3			2	0	.11	.05	17	1098	37	11	.32	.055
amt to make 1 cup	25	1.8	0.5	0.6	0.5	4	9	.05	0.7	.14	.25	107	64	.82	.033	806

27.2 SAUCES & CONDIMENTS

	KCAL / WT (g)	H₂O (g) / FAT (g)	PRO (g) / SFA (g)	CHO (g) / MUFA (g)	SUGR (g) / PUFA (g)	DFIB (g) / CHOL (mg)	A (RE) / A (IU)	C (mg) / B-1 (mg)	B-2 (mg) / NIA (mg)	B-6 (mg) / B-12 (mcg)	FOL (mcg) / PANT (mg)	Na (mg) / K (mg)	Ca (mg) / P (mg)	Mg (mg) / Fe (mg)	Zn (mg) / Cu (mg)	Mn (mg) / REF
A1 Steak Sauce	15		0.0	3.0	2.0							280				
1 T	17	0.0	0.0	0.0	0.0											I
A1 Steak Sauce, bold	20		0.0	5.0	4.0							250				
1 T	17	0.0	0.0	0.0	0.0											I
A1 Steak Sauce, Thick 'n Hearty	25		0.0	6.0	6.0							290				
1 T	18	0.0	0.0	0.0	0.0											I
barbeque sce	12	12.9	0.3	2.0		0.2	14	1	.00	.01	1	130	3	3	.03	.048
1 T	16	0.3	0.0	0.1	0.1	0	139	.00	0.1	.00	.05	28	3	.14	.032	806
Hunt	46		0.6	11.0	8.6	0.7	6	3				383	15			
2 T[1]	35	0.2	0.0			0									.25	I

	KCAL	H₂O (g)	PRO (g)	CHO (g)	SUGR (g)	DFIB (g)	A (RE)	C (mg)	B-2 (mg)	B-6 (mg)	FOL (mcg)	Na (mg)	Ca (mg)	Mg (mg)	Zn (mg)	Mn (mg)
	WT (g)	FAT (g)	SFA (g)	MUFA (g)	PUFA (g)	CHOL (mg)	A (IU)	B-1 (mg)	NIA (mg)	B-12 (mcg)	PANT (mg)	K (mg)	P (mg)	Fe (mg)	Cu (mg)	REF
Kraft	48		0.0	11.0	8.7	0.0	0					390	0			
2 T²	33	0.1	0.0			0	180					72		.18		I
bernaise sce mix	91	1.4	3.5	14.9			0	1	.05	.01	3	848	41	7	.17	.025
1 pkt	25	2.3	0.3	1.0	0.8	0	1	.03	0.1	.10	.10	73	37	.13	.025	806
catsup (ketchup)	16	10.0	0.2	4.1		0.2	15	2	.01	.03	2	178	3	3	.03	.020
1 T	15	0.1	0.0	0.0	0.0	0	152	.01	0.2	.00	.02	72	6	.10	.031	811
Healthy Choice	9		0.3	2.0	1.9	0.3	3	1				97	3			
1 T	16	0.1	0.0			0								.10		I
Hunt	16		0.2	3.5	3.8	0.0	7	1				198	3			
1 T³	17	0.1	0.0			0								.09		I
Chili Fixins sce, Hunt Homestyle	84		5.6	18.5	6.7	6.0	41	7				858	36			
½ cup	132	1.2	0.2			0								.01		I
chili hot dog sce																
Armour Star	120		4.0	5.0	2.0	0.0	0					310	0			
¼ cup	62	9.0	4.0			20	200							.72		I
Gebhardt	60		2.7	5.8	0.0	1.9	6	1				274	30			
¼ cup	64	2.8	1.3			1								.38		I
Just Rite	50		2.2	5.1	0.0	1.7		1				265	16			
¼ cup	62	2.9	1.3			35								.25		I
Open Range	61		2.9	6.4	1.0	2.4	15	1				255	16			
¼ cup	63	3.5	1.5			4								.11		I
chili sce, Hunt	35		0.7	8.0		0.7	7	1				393	5			
2 T	34	0.1	0.0			0								.11		I
cocktail sce, Sauceworks	60			13.0	11.0	1.0		6				800	0			
¼ cup	66	0.5	0.0			0	500					270		.36		I
curry sce mix	149	1.5	3.3	17.7			4	1	.07	.02	3	1428	62	14	.32	.035
1 pkt	35	8.1	1.2	3.5	3.0	0	36	.03	0.3	.14	.14	123	52	1.08	.035	807
enchilada sce, Gebhardt	35		0.7	3.6	0.0	0.5	10	1				218	8			
¼ cup	62	2.1	0.9			0								.09		I
enchilada sce, Rosarita	23		0.7	2.6	2.5	0.0	56	1				409	11			
¼ cup	61	1.1	0.2			0								.21		I
fettucini sce, Stouffers	141	37.1	3.1	2.6				0	.11			296	91			
2 oz	57	13.1				37	63	.02	0.0			63		.06		I
hollandaise sce																
mix w/ butterfat	188	0.7	3.7	10.9		0.4	173	0	.14	.41	17	1241	98	6	.54	.034
1 pkt	34	15.7	9.2	4.7	0.7	40	578	.03	0.0	.61	.68	99	100	.71	.102	806
mix w/ veg oil	94	1.3	3.4	15.6			1	0	.10	.03	4	650	64	7	.23	.025
1 pkt	25	2.3	0.5	1.0	0.7	0	2	.03	0.1	.20	.20	94	53	.07	.025	806
Stouffers	86	45.0	0.6	2.8				0	.03			217	9			
2 oz	57	8.0				46	29	.01	0.0			9		.11		I
horseradish, cream style/reg, Kraft	0		0.0	0.0	0.0	0.0	0	1				50	0			
1 t	5	0.0	0.0	0.0	0.0	0	0					10		.00		I
horseradish, prep	6	13.1	0.2	1.4								14	9			
1 T	15	0.0	0.0		0.0							44	5	.10		456
horseradish sce, Sauceworks	20		0.0	1.0	1.0	0.0	0	0				35	0			
1 t	5	1.5	0.0			5	0					0		.00		I
hot sce (cayenne pepper), Gebhardt	1		0.0	0.1	0.0	0.0	1	0				89	1			
1 t	5	0.0	0.0	0.0	0.0	0								.01		I
Manwich Sce																
bbq, Sloppy Joe, Hunt	57		0.9	14.0	9.7	1.0	8	11				887	11			
¼ cup	64	0.2	0.1			0								.85		I
bold, Hunt	62		0.5	13.1	11.1	0.8	31	5				802	28			
¼ cup	63	1.1	0.0			0								.23		I
Hunt	32		1.0	6.1	4.8	0.7	51	4				365	13			
¼ cup	64	0.4	0.0			0								.83		I
mexican, Hunt	27		1.2	5.0	5.0	0.8	32	4				552	18			
¼ cup	64	0.2	0.0			0								.41		I
thick & chunky, Hunt	44		1.4	8.5	6.6	0.8	53	4				737	19			
¼ cup	65	0.5	0.0			0								.09		I

	KCAL	H₂O (g)	PRO (g)	CHO (g)	SUGR (g)	DFIB (g)	A (RE)	C (mg)	B-2 (mg)	B-6 (mg)	FOL (mcg)	Na (mg)	Ca (mg)	Mg (mg)	Zn (mg)	Mn (mg)
	WT (g)	FAT (g)	SFA (g)	MUFA (g)	PUFA (g)	CHOL (mg)	A (IU)	B-1 (mg)	NIA (mg)	B-12 (mcg)	PANT (mg)	K (mg)	P (mg)	Fe (mg)	Cu (mg)	REF
marinara sce, Angela Mia	24		0.9	4.5	3.3	1.5	27	4				252	11			
¼ cup	63	0.8	0.2			0								1.23		I
marinara sce, Stouffers	38	49.0	0.8	4.0				29	.02			228	20			
2 oz	57	2.1					268	.02	0.4			148		.40		I
Meatloaf Fixins Sce, Hunt	23		1.5	3.9		0.7	20	3				600	11			
¼ cup	63	0.4	0.0			0								.43		I
mushroom sce mix	98	1.0	4.0	15.3			0	0	.14	.03	8	1744	3	5	.25	.028
1 pkt	28	2.7	0.4	1.1	1.0	0	0	.03	1.3	.00	.64	121	37	.28	.168	806
mustard																
Grey Poupon	5		1.0	1.0								81				
1 t[4]	5	0.0	0.0	0.0	0.0	0										I
honey, Grey Poupon	10		0.0	2.0	2.0							5				
1 t	6	0.0	0.0	0.0	0.0											I
Hunt	3		0.2	0.5	0.2	0.1	0	0				64	5			
1 t	5	0.1	0.0			0	0							.08		I
mild, Heinz	5	3.9	0.3	0.3								65	6			
1 t	5	0.3										7	7	.10		I
yellow	4	4.0	0.2	0.3								63	4			
1 t	5	0.2										7	4	.10		456
mustard/horseradish mustard, Kraft	0		0.0	0.0	0.0	0.0	0	0				58	0			
1 t	5	0.0	0.0	0.0	0.0	0	0					5		.00		I
Newburg Sce, Stouffers	90	43.9	1.5	3.0				0	.08			211	46			
2 oz	57	8.0				22	51	.02	0.0			68		.06		I
pasta sce																
Contadina Pasta Ready	60		1.0	10.0	6.0	1.8		14				534	60			
½ cup[5]	122	1.8	0.0			0	530							.65		I
Healthy Choice	46		2.2	9.8	7.0	2.4	22	9				335	37			
½ cup[6]	126	0.4	0.0			0	468							1.18		I
w/ three cheeses, Contadina Pasta Ready	70		2.0	10.0	7.0	2.0		15				490	80			
½ cup	122	2.0	0.5			4	500							.70		I
pepper/hot sce	1	4.5	0.0	0.1		0.1	2	4	.00	.01	0	132	0	0	.01	.002
1 t	5	0.0	0.0	0.0	0.0	0	15	.00	0.0	.00	.01	7	1	.02	.001	806
pepper sce, Tabasco	1	4.8	0.1	0.0		0.0	8	0	.00	.01	0	32	1	1	.01	.005
1 t	5	0.0	0.0	0.0	0.0	0	82	.00	0.0	.00	.01	6	1	.06	.004	806
pesto sce, Stouffers	157	33.1	7.4	2.2				3	.17			245	165			
2 oz	57	13.1				14	627	.03	0.3			131		.63		I
picante sce																
hot/med/mild, Del Monte	10		0.0	2.0	2.0	0.0		2				210	0			
2 T	32	0.0	0.0	0.0	0.0	0	100							.00		I
mild, Hunt Homestyle	11		0.5	2.1	1.3	0.5	12	2				256	5			
2 T	31	0.2	0.0			0								.07		I
Pace	10		0.0	2.0	1.0	0.0		0				220	0			
2 T	32	0.0	0.0	0.0	0.0	0	200							.00		I
zesty jalapeno, Rosarita	8		0.4	1.7	1.2	0.6	4	1				246	7			
2 T[7]	31	0.2	0.0			0								.14		I
pizza sce																
Angela Mia	25		1.7	4.9	2.7	2.1	25	11				221	18			
¼ cup[8]	64	0.5	0.0			0								.80	.	I
chunky, Contadina	27		0.8	4.3	3.0	1.0		0				250	7			
¼ cup[9]	63	0.2	0.0			0	100							.00		I
Contadina Original	25		1.0	4.0	3.0	1.0		6				300	20			
¼ cup	63	0.5	0.0			0	300							.70		I
Contadina Pizza Squeeze	38		1.0	6.0	1.0	1.0		5				385	20			
¼ cup[10]	63	1.5	0.0			0	400							.70		I
w/ italian cheeses, Contadina	30		0.8	4.0	0.8	0.9		4				380	20			
¼ cup	63	0.5	0.0			0	300							.40		I
w/ pepperoni, Contadina	30		1.0	4.0	3.0	1.0		5				360	0			
¼ cup	63	1.0	0.0			0	300							.40		I

							Vitamins					Minerals				
	KCAL	H₂O (g)	PRO (g)	CHO (g)	SUGR (g)	DFIB (g)	A (RE)	C (mg)	B-2 (mg)	B-6 (mg)	FOL (mcg)	Na (mg)	Ca (mg)	Mg (mg)	Zn (mg)	Mn (mg)
	WT (g)	FAT (g)	SFA (g)	MUFA (g)	PUFA (g)	CHOL (mg)	A (IU)	B-1 (mg)	NIA (mg)	B-12 (mcg)	PANT (mg)	K (mg)	P (mg)	Fe (mg)	Cu (mg)	REF
Ready Sauce, Hunt	22		1.0	3.9	3.3	1.0	18	6				306	22			
¼ cup[11]	63	0.5	0.0			0								.45		I
salsa																
alfresco, mild, Hunt Homestyle	10		0.5	2.0	1.9	0.4	6	0				161	15			
2 T	31	0.8	0.1			0								.13		I
Del Monte	10		0.0	2.0	2.0	0.0		2				210	0			
2 T[13]	32	0.0	0.0	0.0	0.0	0	100							.00		I
hot/med/mild, Pace Thick & Chunky	10		0.0	3.0	2.0	0.0	0	5				220	0			
2 T	32	0.0	0.0	0.0	0.0	0	0							.00		I
Hunt Homestyle	27		0.5	6.2	1.5	0.6	20	5				236	10			
2 T[14]	31	0.2	0.0			0								.06		I
Rosarita	8		0.4	1.6	1.3	0.5	3	2				223	9			
2 T[15]	31	0.2	0.0			0								.10		I
sandwich spread & burger sce, Kraft	50		0.0	3.0	3.0	0.0	0	0				100	0			
1 T	15	5.0	0.5			5	0					0		.00		I
sloppy joe sce																
Del Monte	70		1.0	17.0	14.0	0.0		1				690	0			
¼ cup[16]	68	0.0	0.0	0.0	0.0	0	1250							1.08		I
Libby's	45		1.0	10.0	4.0	1.0		6				430	20			
⅓ cup	78	0.0	0.0	0.0	0.0	0	300							.40		I
w/o meat, Armour Star	30		0.0	7.0	6.0	0.0		1				430	0			
¼ cup	62	0.0	0.0	0.0	0.0	0	100							.36		I
soy sce																
Kikkoman	38	39.7	5.1	4.5		0.0						3074				
¼ cup	58	0.0	0.0	0.0	0.0	0						232				I
Kikkoman Lite	43	41.6	4.9	5.8		0.0						1914				
¼ cup	58	0.0	0.0	0.0	0.0	0						174				I
LaChoy	11		1.5	1.0	1.0	0.0	0	0				1227	6			
1 T	18	0.0	0.0	0.0	0.0	0	0							.11		I
light, LaChoy	15		1.6	2.2	2.2	0.0	0	0				542	3			
1 T	15	0.0	0.0	0.0	0.0	0	0							.01		I
made w/ hydrolyzed veg protein	24	43.9	1.4	4.5		0.3	0	0	.06	.08	8	3300	3	3	.18	.207
¼ cup	58	0.0	0.0	0.0	0.0	0	0	.02	1.6	.00	.16	88	54	.86	.056	816
made w/ soy & wheat (shoyu)	31	41.2	3.0	4.9		0.5	0	0	.08	.10	9	3315	10	20	.21	.246
¼ cup	58	0.0	0.0	0.0	0.0	0	0	.03	1.9	.00	.19	104	64	1.17	.067	816
made w/ soy (tamari)	35	38.3	6.1	3.2		0.5	0	0	.09	.12	11	3240	12	23	.25	.289
¼ cup	58	0.1	0.0	0.0	0.0	0	0	.03	2.3	.00	.22	123	75	1.38	.078	816
spaghetti sce	142	216.4	3.5	20.5		4.0	95	20	.10	.28	25	1026	55	42	.42	.548
1 cup	249	5.1	0.7	2.2	1.8	0	934	.13	2.6	.00	.74	735	80	1.79	.279	811
cheese & garlic, Hunt	64		2.6	9.8	7.0	3.1	8	3				622	32			
½ cup	127	2.4	0.6			1								.65		I
chunky, Hunt	38		1.3	7.6	6.7	2.0	8	10				467	50			
½ cup	125	0.7	0.1			0								.51		I
chunky, Hunt	62		1.4	12.8	4.7	1.7	35	25				527	32			
½ cup[17]	124	1.0	0.1			0								1.17		I
D'Italia	50		2.0	8.8	6.8	1.0		2				445	80			
½ cup[18]	124	1.6	0.0			0	750							1.80		I
Del Monte	62		2.1	12.4	8.2	1.9		2				487	38			
½ cup[19]	125	1.2	0.0			0	667							1.16		I
garden combination, extra chunky, Prego	90		2.0	16.0	12.0	3.0		30				480	20			
½ cup	130	1.0	0.5			0	1250							.72		I
Hunt Classic	50		2.3	8.4	5.8	2.6	10	6				588	22			
½ cup[20]	125	1.5	0.2			0								1.37		I
Hunt Homestyle	49		2.3	9.0	6.6	2.6	10	10				598	19			
½ cup	125	1.3	0.2			0								.65		I
Hunt Traditional	67		2.2	11.4	9.1		7	13				477	17			
½ cup	126	2.0	0.2		1.1	0								.98		I

	KCAL / WT (g)	H_2O (g) / FAT (g)	PRO (g) / SFA (g)	CHO (g) / MUFA (g)	SUGR (g) / PUFA (g)	DFIB (g) / CHOL (mg)	A (RE) / A (IU)	C (mg) / B-1 (mg)	B-2 (mg) / NIA (mg)	B-6 (mg) / B-12 (mcg)	FOL (mcg) / PANT (mg)	Na (mg) / K (mg)	Ca (mg) / P (mg)	Mg (mg) / Fe (mg)	Zn (mg) / Cu (mg)	Mn (mg) / REF
light, Hunt	42		2.1	7.5	5.5	2.2	28	6				414	25			
½ cup	125	0.7	0.2			0								1.46		I
marinara, Prego	110		2.0	12.0	8.0	3.0		18				670	40			
½ cup	126	5.0	1.5			0	1000							.72		I
meat flavored, Prego	140		3.0	21.0	13.0	3.0		12				500	40			
½ cup	130	6.0	1.5			5	1250							1.80		I
mushroom & green pepper, extra chunky, Prego—½ cup	120		2.0	18.0	11.0	6.0		4				430	60			
	130	4.5	0.5			5	1000							1.08		I
mushroom & tomatoes, extra chunky, Prego—½ cup	110		2.0	19.0	8.0	3.0		9				510	20			
	130	3.0	1.0			0	1250							1.08		I
mushroom, Prego	150		2.0	23.0	14.0	3.0		15				670	40			
½ cup	130	5.0	1.5			0	1250							1.08		I
mushrooms supreme, extra chunky, Prego	130		3.0	21.0	13.0	3.0		6				490	40			
½ cup	130	4.5	0.5			5	1000							1.44		I
no salt added, Prego	110		2.0	11.0	7.0	3.0		4				25	40			
½ cup	126	6.0	1.5			0	1250							1.08		I
onion & garlic, Prego	110		2.0	19.0	12.0	3.0		21				420	40			
½ cup	130	3.0	0.5			0	1250							1.08		I
Prego	140		2.0	23.0	15.0	2.0		9				610	40			
½ cup	130	4.5	1.5			0	1000							1.44		I
sausage & green pepper, extra chunky, Prego—½ cup	180		4.0	22.0	12.0	3.0		21				570	60			
	130	9.0	2.5			10	1000							1.44		I
three cheese, Prego	100		3.0	18.0	14.0	3.0		15				460	60			
½ cup	130	2.0	1.0			5	750							.72		I
tomato, onion, & garlic, extra chunky, Prego—½ cup	110		2.0	19.0	13.0	3.0		15				480	40			
	130	3.5	1.0			0	750							.72		I
tomato supreme, extra chunky, Prego	120		2.0	20.0	14.0	3.0		9				580	60			
½ cup	130	3.0	0.5			0	1000							1.08		I
veg supreme, extra chunky, Prego	90		2.0	15.0	10.0			2				490	40			
½ cup	130	3.0	0.5			5	1250							.72		I
w/ bits, Angela Mia	49		1.5	10.6	5.9	2.5	33	2				607	16			
½ cup	125	0.5	0.0			0								1.15		I
w/ meat, Hunt	68		2.0	11.7	8.0	3.0	17	13				600	18			
½ cup	126	2.0	0.3			1								1.11		I
w/ meat, Hunt Homestyle	51		2.4	9.0	4.8	2.8	11	12				600	20			
½ cup	125	1.5	0.4			0								2.01		I
w/ mushrooms & onion, extra chunky, Prego—½ cup	110		2.0	18.0	11.0	3.0		9				500	40			
	130	3.0	1.0			0	750							.72		I
w/ mushrooms, Hunt	62		2.1	11.4	8.6	2.5	11	20				605	18			
½ cup	126	1.7	0.2			0								2.03		I
w/ mushrooms, Hunt Homestyle	48		2.3	8.5	5.7	2.7	14	7				530	17			
½ cup	125	1.4	0.2			0								1.27		I
steak sce, Hunt	10		0.3	2.3	1.7	0.3	3	1				256	6			
1 T	17	0.1	0.0			0								.00		I
stir-fry sce, Kikkoman	14	10.5	0.8	2.6		0.1						369				
1 T	15	0.0	0.0	0.0	0.0	1						36				I
stroganoff sce mix	161	2.1	5.6	26.5		0.5	67	0	.48	.05	4	1863	307	19	1.10	.184
1 pkt	46	4.4	2.8	1.2	0.1	12	222	.84	0.6	.28	.60	398	126	1.33	.070	806
sweet 'n sour sce																
Contadina	40		0.0	8.0	6.0	0.0	0	0				115	0			
2 T	33	1.0	0.0			0	0							.00		I
Kraft	80		0.0	19.0	16.0	0.0	0	0				180	0			
2 T	37	0.5	0.0			0	0					20		.00		I
Sauceworks	60		0.0	14.0	12.0	0.0	0	0				125	0			
2 T	35	0.0	0.0	0.0	0.0	0	0					20		.00		I
sweet & sour sce																
Kikkoman	17	10.7	0.3	4.3		0.1						97				
1 T	15	0.0	0.0	0.0	0.0	0						14				I
LaChoy	58		0.1	14.1	13.7	0.0	0	0				104	1			
2 T	34	0.2	0.0			0	0							.03		I

| | KCAL | H₂O (g) | PRO (g) | CHO (g) | SUGR (g) | DFIB (g) | Vitamins | | | | | Minerals | | | | |
| | | | | | | | A (RE) | C (mg) | B-2 (mg) | B-6 (mg) | FOL (mcg) | Na (mg) | Ca (mg) | Mg (mg) | Zn (mg) | Mn (mg) |
	WT (g)	FAT (g)	SFA (g)	MUFA (g)	PUFA (g)	CHOL (mg)	A (IU)	B-1 (mg)	NIA (mg)	B-12 (mcg)	PANT (mg)	K (mg)	P (mg)	Fe (mg)	Cu (mg)	REF
mix	222	0.3	0.6	54.8		1.1	0	0	.07	.28	2	587	31	7	.07	.000
1 pkt	57	0.1	0.0	0.0	0.0	0	0	.01	0.6	.00	.51	50	34	1.22	.021	806
sweet & sour stir fry sce, LaChoy	137		1.7	35.5	26.1	3.0	59	15				754	11			
½ cup	136	0.0	0.0			0								.14		I
tartar sce, nonfat, Kraft	25		0.0	5.0	3.0	1.0	0	0				210	0			
2 T	32	0.0	0.0	0.0	0.0	0	0					15		.00		I
tartar sce, Sauceworks	100		0.0	4.0	0.0	0.0	0	0				180	0			
2 T	30	10.0	4.0			10	0					10		.00		I
teriyaki sce																
bottled	15	12.2	1.1	2.9		0.0	0	0	.01	.02	4	690	5	11	.02	.000
1 T	18	0.0	0.0	0.0	0.0	0	0	.01	0.2	.00	.04	41	28	.31	.018	806
Kikkoman	15	10.2		3.2		0.0							626			
1 T	15	0.0	0.0	0.0	0.0	0						45				I
Kikkoman Baste & Glaze	24	8.8		5.2		0.1							310			
1 T	15	0.0	0.0	0.0	0.0	0						32				I
LaChoy	17		1.1	2.8	2.0	0.0	0	0				917	2			
1 T	18	0.1	0.0			0	0					90		.00		I
mix	130	0.5	4.1	27.6		0.9	0	0	.09	.14	28	4784	112	83	.14	.000
1 pkt	46	0.9	0.1		0.5	0	0	.04	1.3	.00	.28	215	213	2.79	.138	806
tomato cooking sce, Country Italian	70		1.3	12.7	8.0	2.0		17				630	40			
½ cup[21]	125	1.5	0.5			0	750							.97		I
tomato cooking sce, three cheese, Country Italian—*½ cup*	80		2.0	14.0	10.0	2.0		18				600	60			
	125	2.0	0.5			2	500							1.10		I
tomato sce	37	108.7	1.6	8.8		1.7	120	16	.07	.19	11	738	17	23	.30	.267
½ cup	122	0.2	0.0	0.0	0.1	0	1194	.08	1.4	.00	.38	453	39	.94	.239	811
chunky chili, Hunt	22		1.0	4.1	2.7	1.4	33	3				320	44			
¼ cup	63	0.4	0.0			0								.21		I
Contadina	15		0.5	3.0	1.0	0.6		0				280	0			
¼ cup	61	0.0	0.0	0.0	0.0	0	300							.40		I
Hunt	16		1.0	3.0		0.9	23	7				366	8			
¼ cup	62	0.2	0.0			0								.26		I
Hunt Special	21		0.8	3.8	3.2	0.6	18	5				144	8			
¼ cup	62	0.6	0.0			0								.05		I
italian, Hunt	33		1.1	5.1		1.3	23	8				264	17			
¼ cup	63	1.2	0.0			0								.67		I
italian style, Contadina	15		0.6	4.0	1.0	1.0		6				320	0			
¼ cup	61	0.0	0.0	0.0	0.0	0	300							.40		I
Libby's	20		0.1	4.0	1.0	0.5		0				280	0			
¼ cup	61	0.0	0.0	0.0	0.0	0	300							.40		I
no salt added, Hunt	16		1.0	3.0		0.9	23	7				12	18			
¼ cup	62	0.2	0.0			0								.51		I
spanish style	40	108.7	1.8	8.8		1.7	121	10	.08	.22	16	576	21	23	.41	.264
½ cup	122	0.3	0.0	0.0	0.1	0	1202	.09	1.6	.00	.34	450	59	4.25	.195	811
Thick & Zesty, Contadina	20		1.0	3.0	2.0	1.0		5				340	0			
¼ cup	62	0.0	0.0	0.0	0.0	0	400							.70		I
w/ herbs & cheese	72	101.8	2.6	12.5		2.7	121	12	.15	.02	10	662	45	23	.44	.229
½ cup	122	2.4	0.8	0.5	1.0	4	1204	.09	1.5		.34	434	66	1.06	.212	811
w/ herbs, Hunt	32		1.3	4.8		0.6	16	4				271	1			
¼ cup	62	1.0	0.0			0								.39		I
w/ mushrooms	43	107.3	1.8	10.3		1.8	116	15	.13	.16	11	551	16	23	.26	.229
½ cup	122	0.2	0.0	0.0	0.1	0	1165	.09	1.5	.00	.45	464	39	1.09	.243	811
w/ onions	51	105.0	1.9	12.1		2.2	104	15	.16	.33	27	672	21	23	.28	.367
½ cup	122	0.2	0.0	0.0	0.1	0	1037	.09	1.5	.00	.45	504	48	1.13	.221	811
w/ onions, green peppers, & celery	50	107.7	1.1	10.7		1.7	99	16	.15	.24	17	666	16	26	.34	.298
½ cup	122	0.9	0.2	0.1	0.4	0	988	.08	1.3	.00	.27	486	46	.93	.242	811
w/ tomato tidbits	39	108.7	1.6	8.6		1.7	98	26	.12	.19	11		12	24	.23	.268
½ cup	122	0.5	0.1	0.1	0.2	0	977	.09	1.4	.00	.27	455	51	.83	.017	811
Veloute Sce, Stouffers	100	42.2	1.6	3.0				0	.09			262	50			
2 oz	57	9.1				23	29	.02				68		.07		I

	KCAL	H₂O (g)	PRO (g)	CHO (g)	SUGR (g)	DFIB (g)	A (RE)	C (mg)	B-2 (mg)	B-6 (mg)	FOL (mcg)	Na (mg)	Ca (mg)	Mg (mg)	Zn (mg)	Mn (mg)
	WT (g)	FAT (g)	SFA (g)	MUFA (g)	PUFA (g)	CHOL (mg)	A (IU)	B-1 (mg)	NIA (mg)	B-12 (mcg)	PANT (mg)	K (mg)	P (mg)	Fe (mg)	Cu (mg)	REF
white sce																
med, homemade	184	93.6	4.8	11.5		0.3	69	1	.23	.05	6	443	148	18	.51	.054
½ cup²²	125	13.3	3.6	5.5	3.6	9	691	.09	0.5	.35	.41	195	123	.41	.020	806
thick, homemade	233	86.4	5.0	14.5		0.4	84	1	.24	.05	8	466	139	18	.50	.084
½ cup	125	17.3	4.3	7.3	4.9	8	841	.11	0.7	.33	.39	186	120	.63	.026	806
thin, homemade	131	100.8	4.7	9.3		0.1	50	1	.23	.05	6	410	158	19	.53	.030
½ cup	125	8.4	2.7	3.3	2.0	10	504	.07	0.3	.38	.42	204	126	.26	.016	806

1. Values are averages for bold hickory, bold original, hickory & brown sugar, honey hickory, honey mustard, hot & spicy, mesquite, mild, mild dijon, open range hickory, open range original, open range premium, original, and teriyaki.
2. Values are averages for 20 flavors.
3. Product with no salt contains 6 mg sodium.
4. Includes country dijon, dijon, horseradish, peppercorn, and spicy brown.
5. Values are averages for original, tomatoes primavera, tomatoes with mushrooms, tomatoes with olives, and tomatoes with spicy red pepper.
6. Values are averages for 12 types.
7. Values are averages for hot, medium, and mild.
8. Values are averages for regular, fully prepared, and premium choice.
9. Values are averages for original sauce, sauce with mushrooms, and sauce with three cheeses.
10. Values are averages for original and Italian cheese flavors.
11. Values are averages for chunky Italian, chunky Mexican, chunky salsa, chunky tomato, and garlic & herb.
12. Tomatoes, green chili peppers, and onions.
13. Includes hot, medium, and mild in 4 flavors: fire roasted, garlic, thick and chunky, and traditional.
14. Includes hot, medium, and mild.
15. Values are averages for dipping, medium chunky, medium tomatillo, mild roasted, and mild traditional.
16. Values are averages for original and hickory.
17. Values are averages for three flavored sauces.
18. Values are averages for classic marinara, four cheese, spicy red pepper, and tomato & basil.
19. Values are averages for chunky garden, chunky garlic & herb, chunky Italian herb, chunky tomato basil, traditional, with garlic & onion, with green peppers & mushrooms, with meat, and with mushrooms.
20. Values are averages for three flavors of sauce.
21. Values are averages for cacciatore, garden vegetable, and mushroom and roasted garlic.
22. Contains lowfat milk, margarine, flour, and salt.

28. SOUPS
28.1 CANNED, CONDENSED

bean w/ bacon, Campbell's	180		8.0	25.0	4.0	7.0		0				890	80			
½ cup	128	5.0	2.0			3	500							1.80		I
beef broth, double strength, Campbell's	15		3.0	1.0	0.0	0.0	0	0				900	20			
½ cup	124	0.0	0.0	0.0	0.0	3	0							.00		I
beef noodle, Campbell's	70		5.0	8.0	1.0	1.0		0				920	20			
½ cup	126	2.5	1.0			15	100							1.08		I
beef w/ veg & barley, Campbell's	80		5.0	11.0	1.0	2.0		1				920	40			
½ cup	126	2.0	1.0			8	1250							.36		I
beefy mushroom, Campbell's	70		5.0	6.0	1.0	1.0	0	0				1000	40			
½ cup	126	3.0	1.0			10	0							.00		I
black bean, Campbell's	120		6.0	19.0	4.0	5.0		0				1030	40			
½ cup	126	2.0	0.5			0	200							1.80		I
broccoli cheese																
Campbell's	110		3.0	9.0	2.0	2.0		1				860	40			
½ cup	124	7.0	3.0			10	1500							.36		I
crm of, 98% fat-free, Campbell's	80		3.0	11.0	2.0	1.0		0				850	60			
½ cup	126	3.0	1.5			10	1500							.00		I
crm of, Healthy Choice	87		3.3	14.9	0.5	2.0	20	3				561	90			
½ cup	124	1.9	1.0			6						424		.24		I
broccoli, crm of, 98% fat-free, Campbell's	80		2.0	12.0	3.0	1.0		6				730	40			
½ cup	126	3.0	1.0			3	200							.36		I
broccoli, crm of, Campbell's	100		2.0	9.0	2.0	1.0		2				770	20			
½ cup	124	6.0	2.5			3	300							.36		I
celery, crm of	220	259.1	4.0	21.4		1.8	73	1	.12	.03	6	2309	98	15	.37	.610
1 can	305	13.6	3.4	3.1	6.1	34	744	.07	0.8	.12	2.81	299	92	1.52	.345	806

	KCAL / WT (g)	H₂O (g) / FAT (g)	PRO (g) / SFA (g)	CHO (g) / MUFA (g)	SUGR (g) / PUFA (g)	DFIB (g) / CHOL (mg)	**Vitamins** A (RE) / A (IU)	C (mg) / B-1 (mg)	B-2 (mg) / NIA (mg)	B-6 (mg) / B-12 (mcg)	FOL (mcg) / PANT (mg)	**Minerals** Na (mg) / K (mg)	Ca (mg) / P (mg)	Mg (mg) / Fe (mg)	Zn (mg) / Cu (mg)	Mn (mg) / REF
98% fat-free, Campbell's	70	2.0		9.0	1.0	1.0	0					850	40			
½ cup	126	3.0	1.0			3	100							.36		I
Campbell's	110	2.0		9.0	1.0	1.0		0				900	20			
½ cup	124	7.0	2.5			3	300							.36		I
Healthy Choice	73	0.9		13.9	1.6	3.0	0	3				366	90			
½ cup	122	2.0	1.0			3	0							.24		I
cheese	311	198.3	10.8	21.0		2.1	218	0	.27	.05	8	1920	285	8	1.28	.514
1 can	257	20.9	13.3	5.9	0.6	59	2177	.03	0.8	.00	.18	308	272	1.49	.257	806
cheddar, Campbell's	90	4.0		10.0	2.0	1.0		0				950	100			
½ cup	124	4.0	3.0			15	1000							.00		I
nacho, Campbell's	140	5.0		11.0	2.0	2.0		1				810	100			
½ cup	124	8.0	4.0			15	1250							.36		I
chicken alphabet w/ veg, Campbell's	80	4.0		11.0	1.0	1.0		0				880	20			
½ cup	126	2.0	1.0			10	750							.72		I
chicken & broccoli, crm of, Campbell's	120	4.0		9.0	2.0			1				860	20			
½ cup	124	8.0	2.5			15	750							.36		I
chicken & stars, Campbell's	70	3.0		9.0	1.0	1.0		1				1010	20			
½ cup	126	2.0	0.5			1	750							.72		I
chicken broth, Campbell's	30	2.0		2.0	1.0	0.0	0	0				770	0			
½ cup	124	2.0	0.5			3	0							.00		I
chicken, crm of	284	249.3	8.3	22.5		0.6	137	0	.15	.04	4	2397	82	6	1.52	.915
1 can	305	17.9	5.1	8.0	3.6	24	1360	.07	2.0	.21	.52	214	92	1.46	.305	806
98% fat-free, Campbell's	80	3.0		10.0	0.0	0.0		0				830	20			
½ cup	126	3.0	1.5			10	400							.36		I
Campbell's	130	3.0		11.0	1.0	1.0		0				890	20			
½ cup	124	8.0	3.0			10	500							.36		I
Healthy Choice	80	1.9		12.6	0.9	3.0	11	0				349	11			
½ cup	123	2.9	1.0			4						318		.04		I
chicken dumplings, Campbell's	80	4.0		10.0	1.0	2.0		0				1050	20			
½ cup	126	3.0	1.0			25	400							.36		I
chicken gumbo, Campbell's	60	2.0		9.0	1.0	1.0		0				990	20			
½ cup	126	1.5	0.5			10	200							.34		I
chicken mushroom, Campbell's	130	3.0		9.0	1.0	1.0		0				1000	20			
½ cup	124	9.0	2.5			15	750							.36		I
chicken noodle																
Campbell's	70	3.0		9.0	1.0	1.0		0				980	20			
½ cup	126	2.0	1.0			15	300							.72		I
creamy, Campbell's	130	5.0		12.0	2.0	2.0		0				800	20			
½ cup	124	7.0	2.0			15	1250							.72		I
homestyle, Campbell's	70	4.0		9.0	1.0	1.0		1				970	20			
½ cup	126	2.5	1.5			20	750							.72		I
Chicken Noodle O's, Campbell's	80	4.0		10.0	1.0	1.0		1				980	20			
½ cup	126	3.0	1.0			15	1000							1.08		I
chicken rice, Campbell's	70	3.0		9.0	0.0	0.0		0				940	0			
½ cup	126	2.5	1.0			3	400							.36		I
chicken veg, Campbell's	80	3.0		12.0	4.0	2.0		0				940	20			
½ cup	126	2.0	0.5			10	2500							.72		I
chicken veg, southwestern style, Campbell's—½ cup	110	7.0		18.0	4.0	4.0		24				900	40			
	126	1.5	0.5			10	500							1.08		I
chicken w/ wild & white rice, Campbell's	70	3.0		9.0	1.0	1.0		15				900	20			
½ cup	126	2.0	0.5			10	400							.36		I
chili beef w/ beans, Campbell's	170	7.0		24.0	4.0	4.0		1				910	100			
½ cup	128	5.0	2.5			15	750							.72		I
clam chowder, manhattan style, Campbell's—½ cup	60	2.0		12.0	2.0	2.0		4				910	20			
	126	0.5	0.0			3	1500							.72		I
clam chowder, new england style, Campbell's—½ cup	100	4.0		15.0	1.0	1.0	0	1				980	20			
	126	2.5	1.0			3	0							1.08		I
consomme beef, Campbell's	25	4.0		2.0	2.0	0.0	0	0				820	20			
½ cup	124	0.0	0.0	0.0	0.0	5	0							.00		I
corn, golden, Campbell's	120	2.0		20.0	7.0	2.0		0				730	20			
½ cup	124	3.5	1.0			3	500							.36		I

	KCAL	H₂O (g)	PRO (g)	CHO (g)	SUGR (g)	DFIB (g)	A (RE)	C (mg)	B-2 (mg)	B-6 (mg)	FOL (mcg)	Na (mg)	Ca (mg)	Mg (mg)	Zn (mg)	Mn (mg)
	WT (g)	FAT (g)	SFA (g)	MUFA (g)	PUFA (g)	CHOL (mg)	A (IU)	B-1 (mg)	NIA (mg)	B-12 (mcg)	PANT (mg)	K (mg)	P (mg)	Fe (mg)	Cu (mg)	REF
Curly Chicken Noodle, Campbell's	80		3.0	12.0	1.0	1.0		0				840	20			
½ cup	126	2.5	1.0			15	750							1.08		I
double noodle in chicken broth, Campbell's—½ cup	100		4.0	15.0	1.0	2.0		0				810	20			
	126	2.5	1.0			15	1500							1.08		I
french onion, Campbell's	70		2.0	10.0	5.0	1.0	0	0				980	20			
½ cup	126	2.5	0.0			3	0							.36		I
garlic, crm of, Healthy Choice	57		0.5	12.7	0.0	3.0	0	0				489	8			
½ cup	124	0.8	0.5			2	0					67		.05		I
mexican pepper, crm of, Campbell's	110		2.0	10.0	1.0	2.0	0	1				860	20			
½ cup	124	7.0	2.0			3	0							.36		I
minestrone, Campbell's	100		5.0	16.0	3.0	4.0		1				960	40			
½ cup	126	2.0	0.5			0	1000							1.08		I
mushroom, crm of	314	247.7	4.9	22.6		0.9	0	3	.20	.03	9	2111	79	12	1.44	.610
1 can	305	23.1	6.3	4.4	10.8	3	0	.07	2.0	.30	.61	204	104	1.28	.305	806
98% fat-free, Campbell's	70		1.0	9.0	1.0	0.0	0	0				830	20			
½ cup	124	3.0	1.0			3	0							.00		I
Campbell's	110		2.0	9.0	1.0	1.0	0	0				870	20			
½ cup	124	7.0	2.5			3	0							.36		I
Healthy Choice	56		0.8	12.7	0.2	3.0	0	1				478	14			
½ cup	123	0.7	0.5			2	0					318		.17		I
mushroom, golden, Campbell's	80		2.0	10.0	1.0	1.0		0				930	20			
½ cup	124	3.0	1.0			5	730							.00		I
noodles & ground beef, Campbell's	100		5.0	11.0	1.0	2.0		0				900	20			
½ cup	126	4.0	2.0			25	1000							1.08		I
onion, crm of, Campbell's	110		2.0	13.0	4.0	1.0		0				910	20			
½ cup	124	6.0	1.5			20	300							.72		I
oyster stew, Campbell's	90		2.0	6.0	1.0	0.0	0	4				940	100			
½ cup	126	6.0	3.5			20	0							.36		I
pea, green, Campbell's	180		9.0	29.0	6.0	5.0		0				890	80			
½ cup	128	3.0	1.0			5	200							.36		I
pea, split w/ ham, Campbell's	180		10.0	28.0	4.0	5.0		0				860	20			
½ cup	128	3.5	2.0			3	500							1.80		I
pepperpot, Campbell's	100		4.0	9.0	1.0	1.0		1				1020	20			
½ cup	126	5.0	2.0			15	1000							.72		I
potato, crm of, Campbell's	90		2.0	14.0	2.0	1.0	0	0				890	20			
½ cup	124	3.0	1.5			10	0							.72		I
scotch broth, Campbell's	80		4.0	9.0	1.0	1.0		0				870	40			
½ cup	124	3.0	1.5			10	2000							.36		I
shrimp, crm of, Campbell's	100		2.0	8.0	1.0	1.0	0	0				890	20			
½ cup	124	7.0	2.0			20								.36		I
tomato	207	247.8	5.0	40.3		1.2	171	162	.12	.27	36	1690	34	18	.59	.610
1 can	305	4.7	0.9	1.0	2.3	0	1693	.21	3.4	.00	.37	641	82	4.27	.610	I
bisque, Campbell's	130		2.0	24.0	15.0	2.0		15				900	40			
½ cup	126	3.0	1.5			5	500							.72		I
Campbell's	100		2.0	18.0	10.0	2.0		18				730	20			
½ cup	124	2.0	0.0			0	500							.72		I
fiesta, Campbell's	70		1.0	16.0	8.0	1.0		6				860	100			
½ cup	126	0.0	0.0			0	400							.72		I
garden, Healthy Choice	80		1.9	17.8	11.0	3.4	9	3				298	92			
½ cup	127	1.1	0.2			0						847		.80		I
italian w/ basil & oregano, Campbell's	100		2.0	23.0	16.0	2.0		18				820	40			
½ cup	126	0.5	0.0			0	750							1.08		I
rice, Campbell's Old Fashioned	120		2.0	23.0	11.0	1.0		6				790	20			
½ cup	126	2.0	0.5			5	400							.36		I
turkey noodle, Campbell's	80		4.0	10.0	1.0	1.0		0				970	20			
½ cup	126	2.5	1.0			15	500							.72		I
turkey veg, Campbell's	80		3.0	11.0	2.0	2.0		0				840	20			
½ cup	126	2.5	1.0			10	2500							.72		I
veg																
beef, Campbell's	80		5.0	10.0	2.0	2.0		0				810	20			
½ cup	126	2.0	1.0			10	2000							.72		I

	KCAL / WT (g)	H₂O (g) / FAT (g)	PRO (g) / SFA (g)	CHO (g) / MUFA (g)	SUGR (g) / PUFA (g)	DFIB (g) / CHOL (mg)	A (RE) / A (IU)	C (mg) / B-1 (mg)	B-2 (mg) / NIA (mg)	B-6 (mg) / B-12 (mcg)	FOL (mcg) / PANT (mg)	Na (mg) / K (mg)	Ca (mg) / P (mg)	Mg (mg) / Fe (mg)	Zn (mg) / Cu (mg)	Mn (mg) / REF
calif style, Campbell's	60		3.0	10.0	2.0	2.0		30				850	20			
½ cup	126	1.0	0.0			0	1000								.36	I
Campbell's	80		3.0	14.0	7.0	2.0		1				920	20			
½ cup	126	1.5	0.5			3	1500								.72	I
Campbell's Old Fashioned	70		2.0	10.0	2.0	2.0		0				950	20			
½ cup	126	2.5	0.5			3	2500								.72	I
hearty w/ pasta, Campbell's	90		2.0	18.0	8.0	2.0		0				830	20			
½ cup	126	1.0	0.0			0	2250								.72	I
vegetarian, Campbell's	70		2.0	14.0	6.0	2.0		2				770	20			
½ cup	126	1.0	0.0			0	1750								.72	I
won ton, Campbell's	45		4.0	5.0	1.0	1.0		0				940	20			
½ cup	126	1.0	0.0			15	100								.36	I

28.2 CANNED, CONDENSED, PREPARED WITH MILK

	KCAL / WT (g)	H₂O (g) / FAT (g)	PRO (g) / SFA (g)	CHO (g) / MUFA (g)	SUGR (g) / PUFA (g)	DFIB (g) / CHOL (mg)	A (RE) / A (IU)	C (mg) / B-1 (mg)	B-2 (mg) / NIA (mg)	B-6 (mg) / B-12 (mcg)	FOL (mcg) / PANT (mg)	Na (mg) / K (mg)	Ca (mg) / P (mg)	Mg (mg) / Fe (mg)	Zn (mg) / Cu (mg)	Mn (mg) / REF
asparagus, crm of	161	213.3	6.3	16.4		0.7	84	4	.28	.06	30	1042	174	20	.93	.379
1 cup	248	8.2	3.3	2.1	2.2	22	600	.10	0.9	.50	.52	360	154	.87	.139	806
celery, crm of	164	214.4	5.7	14.5		0.7	67	1	.25	.06	8	1009	186	22	.20	.253
1 cup	248	9.7	3.9	2.5	2.7	32	461	.07	0.4	.50	1.51	310	151	.69	.154	806
cheese	231	206.9	9.5	16.2		1.0	148	1	.33	.08	10	1019	289	20	.69	.259
1 cup	251	14.6	9.1	4.1	0.5	48	1242	.06	0.5	.43	.48	341	251	.80	.141	806
chicken, crm of	191	210.4	7.5	15.0		0.2	94	1	.26	.07	8	1047	181	17	.67	.379
1 cup	248	11.5	4.6	4.5	1.6	27	714	.07	0.9	.55	.57	273	151	.67	.139	806
clam chowder, new england	164	211.4	9.5	16.6		1.5	40	3	.24	.13	10	992	186	22	.80	.253
1 cup	248	6.6	3.0	2.3	1.1	22	164	.07	1.0	10.24	.69	300	156	1.49	.139	806
mushroom, crm of	203	209.7	6.1	15.0		0.5	37	2	.28	.06	10	918	179	20	.64	.253
1 cup	248	13.6	5.1	3.0	4.6	20	154	.08	0.9	.50	.62	270	156	.60	.139	806
onion, crm of	186	209.6	6.8	18.4		0.7	69	2	.27	.07	22	1004	179	22	.62	.248
1 cup	248	9.4	4.0	3.3	1.6	32	451	.10	0.6	.50	.69	310	154	.69	.149	806
oyster stew	135	217.9	6.1	9.8		0.0	44	4	.23	.06	10	1041	167	20	10.34	.370
1 cup	245	7.9	5.0	2.1	0.3	32	225	.07	0.3	2.62	.49	235	162	1.05	1.605	806
pea, green	239	197.9	12.6	32.2		2.8	58	3	.27	.10	8	970	173	56	1.76	.660
1 cup	254	7.0	4.0	2.2	0.5	18	356	.15	1.3	.43	.56	376	239	2.01	.391	806
potato, crm of	149	214.9	5.8	17.2		0.5	67	1	.24	.09	9	1061	166	17	.67	.379
1 cup[1]	248	6.4	3.8	1.7	0.6	22	444	.08	0.6	.50	1.69	322	161	.55	.263	806
shrimp, crm of	164	214.3	6.8	13.9		0.2	55	1	.23	.45	10	1037	164	22	.80	.397
1 cup	248	9.3	5.8	2.7	0.3	35	312	.06	0.5	1.04	.55	248	146	.60	.136	806
tomato	161	209.8	6.1	22.3		2.7	109	68	.25	.16	21	744	159	22	.29	.253
1 cup	248	6.0	2.9	1.6	1.1	17	848	.13	1.5	.45	.55	449	149	1.81	.263	806
tomato bisque	198	204.6	6.3	29.4		0.5	110	7	.27	.14	21	1109	186	25	.63	.259
1 cup	251	6.6	3.1	1.9	1.2	23	878	.11	1.3	.43	.50	605	173	.88	.141	806

28.3 CANNED, CONDENSED, PREPARED WITH WATER

	KCAL / WT (g)	H₂O (g) / FAT (g)	PRO (g) / SFA (g)	CHO (g) / MUFA (g)	SUGR (g) / PUFA (g)	DFIB (g) / CHOL (mg)	A (RE) / A (IU)	C (mg) / B-1 (mg)	B-2 (mg) / NIA (mg)	B-6 (mg) / B-12 (mcg)	FOL (mcg) / PANT (mg)	Na (mg) / K (mg)	Ca (mg) / P (mg)	Mg (mg) / Fe (mg)	Zn (mg) / Cu (mg)	Mn (mg) / REF
asparagus, crm of	85	224.0	2.3	10.7		0.5	44	3	.08	.01	22	981	29	5	.88	.376
1 cup	244	4.1	1.0	1.0	1.9	5	444	.05	0.8	.05	.12	173	39	.81	.124	806
asparagus, crm of, Campbell's	90		3.0	11.0	3.0	1.0		2				860	40			
½ cup	124	3.5	1.0			5	100								.34	I
bean w/ bacon	172	212.9	7.9	22.8		8.6	89	2	.03	.04	32	951	81	46	1.03	.670
1 cup	253	5.9	1.5	2.2	1.8	3	888	.09	0.6	.05	.10	402	132	2.05	.402	806
bean w/ franks	188	207.6	10.0	22.0			88	1	.07	.13	30	1093	88	48	1.18	.787
1 cup	250	7.0	2.1	2.7	1.7	13	870	.11	1.0	.07	.10	478	165	2.35	.395	806
beef mushroom	73	225.9	5.8	6.3		0.2	0	5	.06	.05	10	942	5	10	1.46	.488
1 cup	244	3.0	1.5	1.2	0.1	7	0	.04	1.0	.20	.22	154	34	.88	.244	806
beef noodle	83	224.5	4.8	9.0		0.7	63	0	.06	.04	4	952	15	5	1.54	.273
1 cup	244	3.1	1.1	1.2	0.5	5	630	.07	1.1	.20	.20	100	46	1.10	.139	806
black bean	116	215.6	5.6	19.8		4.4	49	1	.05	.09	25	1198	44	42	1.41	.642
1 cup	247	1.5	0.4	0.5	0.5	0	506	.08	0.5	.02	.20	274	106	2.15	.385	806
celery, crm of	90	225.1	1.7	8.8		0.7	32	0	.05	.01	2	949	39	7	.15	.251
1 cup	244	5.6	1.4	1.3	2.5	15	307	.03	0.3	.24	1.12	122	37	.63	.142	806
cheese	156	217.7	5.4	10.5		1.0	109	0	.14	.02	5	958	141	5	.64	.257
1 cup	247	10.5	6.7	3.0	0.3	30	1087	.02	0.4	.00	.10	153	136	.74	.128	806

	KCAL	H₂O (g)	PRO (g)	CHO (g)	SUGR (g)	DFIB (g)	Vitamins A (RE)	C (mg)	B-2 (mg)	B-6 (mg)	FOL (mcg)	Minerals Na (mg)	Ca (mg)	Mg (mg)	Zn (mg)	Mn (mg)
	WT (g)	FAT (g)	SFA (g)	MUFA (g)	PUFA (g)	CHOL (mg)	A (IU)	B-1 (mg)	NIA (mg)	B-12 (mcg)	PANT (mg)	K (mg)	P (mg)	Fe (mg)	Cu (mg)	REF
chicken & dumplings	96	221.2	5.6	6.0		0.5	53	0	.07	.04	2	860	14	5	.37	.489
1 cup	241	5.5	1.3	2.5	1.3	34	518	.02	1.8	.17	.14	116	60	.63	.123	806
chicken broth	39	234.1	4.9	0.9		0.0	0	0	.07	.02	5	776	10	2	.25	.249
1 cup	244	1.4	0.4	0.6	0.3	0	0	.01	3.3	.24	.05	210	73	.51	.124	806
chicken, crm of	117	221.1	3.4	9.3		0.2	56	0	.06	.02	2	986	34	2	.63	.376
1 cup	244	7.4	2.1	3.3	1.5	10	561	.03	0.8	.10	.20	88	37	.61	.124	806
chicken gumbo	56	229.0	2.6	8.4		2.0	15	5	.05	.06	5	954	24	5	.38	.251
1 cup	244	1.4	0.3	0.7	0.3	5	137	.02	0.7	.02	.20	76	24	.90	.124	806
chicken mushroom	132	219.6	4.4	9.3		0.2	112	0	.11	.05	0	942	29	10	.98	.244
1 cup	244	9.2	2.4	4.0	2.3	10	1135	.02	1.6	.05	.24	154	27	.88	.244	806
chicken noodle	75	221.7	4.0	9.4		0.7	72	0	.06	.03	2	1106	17	5	.40	.289
1 cup[2]	241	2.5	0.7	1.1	0.6	7	711	.05	1.4	.14	.17	55	36	.77	.193	806
chicken rice	60	226.1	3.5	7.2		0.7	65	0	.02	.02	1	815	17	0	.26	.366
1 cup	241	1.9	0.5	0.9	0.4	7	660	.02	1.1	.14	.17	101	22	.75	.118	806
chicken veg	75	223.3	3.6	8.6		1.0	265	1	.06	.05	5	945	17	7	.37	.366
1 cup	241	2.8	0.8	1.3	0.6	10	2656	.04	1.2	.12	.17	154	41	.87	.123	806
chili beef	170	211.7	6.7	21.4		9.5	150	4	.07	.16	18	1035	43	30	1.40	1.050
1 cup	250	6.6	3.4	2.8	0.3	13	1510	.06	1.1	.33	.50	525	148	2.13	.395	806
clam chowder, manhattan style	78	224.2	2.2	12.2		1.5	98	4	.04	.10	10	578	27	12	.98	.378
1 cup	244	2.2	0.4	0.4	1.3	2	964	.03	0.8	4.05	.00	188	41	1.63	.132	806
clam chowder, new england style	95	220.9	4.8	12.4		1.5	0	2	.04	.08	4	915	44	7	.75	.251
1 cup	244	2.9	0.4	1.2	1.1	5	7	.02	1.0	8.00	.32	146	54	1.49	.124	806
consomme w/ gelatin	29	231.9	5.4	1.8		0.0	0	0	.03	.02	3	636	10	0	.37	.366
1 cup	241	0.0	0.0	0.0	0.0	0	0	.02	0.7	.00	.05	154	31	.53	.246	806
minestrone	82	220.1	4.3	11.2		1.0	234	1	.04	.10	16	911	34	7	.74	.366
1 cup	241	2.5	0.6	0.7	1.1	2	2338	.05	0.9	.00	.34	313	55	.92	.123	806
mushroom barley	73	225.5	1.9	11.7		0.7	20	0	.09	.17	5	891	12	10	.49	.122
1 cup	244	2.3	0.4	1.0	0.7	0	198	.02	0.9	.00	.12	93	61	.51	.244	806
mushroom, crm of	129	220.4	2.3	9.3		0.5	0	1	.09	.01	5	881	46	5	.59	.251
1 cup	244	9.0	2.4	1.7	4.2	2	0	.05	0.7	.05	.29	100	49	.51	.124	806
mushroom w/ beef stock	85	224.7	3.1	9.3		0.7	124	1	.10	.04	9	969	10	10	1.38	.376
1 cup	244	4.0	1.6	1.4	0.8	7	1254	.03	1.2	.00	.24	159	37	.83	.251	806
onion	58	224.3	3.8	8.2		1.0	0	1	.02	.05	15	1053	27	2	.61	.246
1 cup	241	1.7	0.3	0.7	0.7	0	0	.03	0.6	.00	.00	67	12	.67	.123	806
onion, crm of	107	220.8	2.8	12.7		1.0	29	1	.08	.02	7	927	34	5	.15	.244
1 cup	244	5.3	1.5	2.1	1.5	15	295	.05	0.5	.05	.29	120	37	.63	.146	806
oyster stew	58	228.6	2.1	4.1		7	3	.04	.01	2	981	22	5	10.29	.366	
1 cup	241	3.8	2.5	0.9	0.2	14	70	.02	0.2	2.19	.12	48	48	.99	1.593	806
pea, green	165	208.7	8.6	26.5		2.8	20	2	.07	.05	2	918	28	40	1.71	.657
1 cup	250	2.9	1.4	1.0	0.4	0	203	.11	1.2	.00	.13	190	125	1.95	.378	806
pea, split w/ ham	190	206.9	10.3	28.0		2.3	46	2	.08	.07	3	1007	23	48	1.32	.670
1 cup	253	4.4	1.8	1.8	0.6	8	445	.15	1.5	.25	.25	400	213	2.28	.369	806
pepperpot	104	217.3	6.4	9.4		0.5	87	1	.05	.06	10	971	24	5	1.22	.612
1 cup	241	4.6	2.0	2.0	0.4	10	865	.05	1.2	.17	.34	152	41	.89	.123	806
potato, crm of	73	225.7	1.8	11.5		0.5	29	0	.04	.04	3	1000	20	2	.63	.376
1 cup[1]	244	2.4	1.2	0.6	0.4	5	288	.03	0.5	.05	.83	137	46	.49	.251	806
scotch broth	80	221.1	5.0	9.5		1.2	217	1	.05	.07	10	1012	14	5	1.59	.366
1 cup	241	2.6	1.1	0.8	0.6	5	2179	.02	1.2	.27	.24	159	55	.84	.246	806
shrimp, crm of	90	225.0	2.8	8.2		0.2	15	0	.03	.05	4	976	17	10	.75	.366
1 cup	244	5.2	3.2	1.5	0.2	17	159	.02	0.4	.59	.15	59	32	.54	.122	806
stockpot	99	223.7	4.9	11.5			398	2	.05	.09	10	1047	22	5	1.16	.257
1 cup	247	3.9	0.9	1.0	1.8	5	3979	.04	1.2	.00	.35	237	54	.86	.128	806
tomato	85	220.5	2.0	16.6		0.5	68	66	.05	.11	15	695	12	7	.24	.251
1 cup	244	1.9	0.4	0.4	1.0	0	688	.09	1.4	.00	.15	264	34	1.76	.251	806
tomato beef w/ noodle	139	211.5	4.5	21.2		1.5	54	0	.09	.09	7	917	17	7	.75	.251
1 cup	244	4.3	1.6	1.7	0.7	5	534	.08	1.9	.20	.20	220	56	1.12	.124	806
tomato bisque	124	215.3	2.3	23.7		0.5	72	6	.07	.09	15	1047	40	10	.59	.257
1 cup	247	2.5	0.5	0.7	1.1	5	721	.07	1.1	.00	.12	417	59	.82	.128	806
tomato rice	119	217.6	2.1	21.9		1.5	77	15	.05	.08	14	815	22	5	.51	.385
1 cup	247	2.7	0.5	0.6	1.4	2	756	.06	1.1	.00	.12	331	35	.79	.128	806
turkey noodle	68	226.9	3.9	8.6		0.7	29	0	.06	.04	2	815	12	5	.58	.251
1 cup	244	2.0	0.6	0.8	0.5	5	293	.07	1.4	.15	.17	76	49	.95	.124	806

	KCAL / WT (g)	H₂O (g) / FAT (g)	PRO (g) / SFA (g)	CHO (g) / MUFA (g)	SUGR (g) / PUFA (g)	DFIB (g) / CHOL (mg)	Vitamins A (RE) / A (IU)	C (mg) / B-1 (mg)	B-2 (mg) / NIA (mg)	B-6 (mg) / B-12 (mcg)	FOL (mcg) / PANT (mg)	Minerals Na (mg) / K (mg)	Ca (mg) / P (mg)	Mg (mg) / Fe (mg)	Zn (mg) / Cu (mg)	Mn (mg) / REF
turkey veg	72	223.9	3.1	8.6		0.5	243	0	.04	.05	5	906	17	5	.61	.246
1 cup	241	3.0	0.9	1.3	0.7	2	2444	.03	1.0	.17	.48	176	41	.77	.123	806
veg beef	78	223.5	5.6	10.2		0.5	190	2	.05	.08	10	791	17	5	1.54	.315
1 cup[3]	244	1.9	0.9	0.8	0.1	5	1891	.04	1.0	.32	.34	173	41	1.12	.183	806
veg vegetarian	72	222.5	2.1	12.0		0.5	301	1	.05	.06	11	822	22	7	.46	.460
1 cup	241	1.9	0.3	0.8	0.7	0	3005	.05	0.9	.00	.34	210	34	1.08	.123	806
veg w/ beef broth	82	220.5	3.0	13.1		0.5	210	2	.05	.06	10	810	17	7	.80	.337
1 cup	241	1.9	0.4	0.6	0.8	2	2089	.05	1.0	.00	.34	193	39	.96	.154	806

28.4 CANNED OR HOMEMADE, READY-TO-SERVE[4]

	KCAL / WT (g)	H₂O (g) / FAT (g)	PRO (g) / SFA (g)	CHO (g) / MUFA (g)	SUGR (g) / PUFA (g)	DFIB (g) / CHOL (mg)	A (RE) / A (IU)	C (mg) / B-1 (mg)	B-2 (mg) / NIA (mg)	B-6 (mg) / B-12 (mcg)	FOL (mcg) / PANT (mg)	Na (mg) / K (mg)	Ca (mg) / P (mg)	Mg (mg) / Fe (mg)	Zn (mg) / Cu (mg)	Mn (mg) / REF
bean 'n ham, chunky, Campbell's	260		17.0	42.0	6.0	13.0		6				1130	100			
11 oz	312	3.0	1.0			10	2500							4.50		I
bean, salsa, Home Cookin'	160		7.0	31.0	12.0	7.0		6				730	80			
1 cup	245	1.0	0.0			0	500							1.80		I
bean w/ bacon, Campbell's Microwave	280		14.0	40.0	8.0	11.0		6				1300	40			
10.5 oz	298	6.0	2.0			15	1750							3.60		I
bean w/ ham																
chunky	231	191.1	12.6	27.1		11.2	396	4	.15	.12	29	972	78	46	1.07	.705
1 cup	243	8.5	3.3	3.8	0.9	22	3951	.15	1.7	.07	.10	425	143	3.23	.389	806
Healthy Choice	166		8.6	31.1	2.9	7.1	19	6				570	74			
1 cup	249	1.3	0.4			4						979		1.37		I
Home Cookin'	180		9.0	33.0	8.0	9.0		2				720	80			
1 cup	245	1.5	0.5			5	1500							2.70		I
beef & potatoes, Healthy Choice	116		11.2	15.8	2.8	0.3	5	5				452	21			
1 cup	243	1.1	0.5			5						919		.24		I
beef broth/bouillon	17	234.1	2.7	0.1		0.0	0	0	.05	.02	5	782	14	5	.00	.024
1 cup	240	0.5	0.3	0.2	0.0	0	0	.00	1.9	.17	.05	130	31	.41	.000	806
beef broth, College Inn	20		4.0	0.0	0.0							1240				
1 cup[5]	240 ml	0.0	0.0	0.0	0.0	0										I
beef broth, Swanson	20		2.0	1.0	1.0	0.0	0	0				820	0			
1 cup	235	1.0	0.5			0	0							.36		I
beef, chunky	170	200.0	11.7	19.6		1.4	262	7	.15	.13	13	866	31	5	2.64	.240
1 cup	240	5.1	2.5	2.1	0.2	14	2611	.06	2.7	.62	.43	336	120	2.33	.240	806
beef, chunky, Campbell's	180		13.0	20.0	4.0	4.0		4				1090	60			
10.75 oz	305	6.0	2.0			20	6000							1.80		I
beef pasta, chunky, Campbell's	190		16.0	23.0	6.0	3.0		1				1200	60			
10.75 oz	305	4.0	1.0			20	3500							2.70		I
beef w/ country veg, chunky, Campbell's	200		16.0	22.0	5.0	4.0		2				1130	40			
10.75 oz	305	5.0	1.5				9500							1.80		I
broccoli cheddar, Healthy Choice	116		4.1	21.9	1.1	2.2	57	1				304	55			
1 cup	238	1.8	1.1			4						130		.45		I
chicken alfredo w/ pasta, Healthy Choice	132		12.1	17.4	2.9	2.4	0	8				333	65			
1 cup	236	2.3	1.2			10	0					184		.59		I
chicken & pasta w/ mushrooms, chunky, Campbell's—10.75 oz	150		14.0	13.0	2.0	1.0		1				1150	40			
	305	4.5	1.5			30	750							.72		I
chicken broccoli cheese, chunky, Campbell's—10.75 oz	250		11.0	17.0	1.0	1.0		0				1400	40			
	305	15.0	6.0			30	1250							.72		I
chicken broth																
College Inn	25		1.0	1.0	1.0							1050				
1 cup[6]	240 ml	1.5	0.5	0.5	0.0											I
Healthy Request	20		3.0	1.0	1.0	0.0	0	9				450	0			
1 cup	245	0.0	0.0	0.0	0.0	0	0							.00		I
Swanson	30		2.0	1.0	0.0	0.0	0	0				1000	0			
1 cup	235	2.0	0.5			0	0							.00		I
chicken, chunky	178	211.1	12.7	17.3		1.5	131	1	.17	.05	5	889	25	8	1.00	.251
1 cup	251	6.6	2.0	3.0	1.4	30	1300	.09	4.4	.25	.40	176	113	1.73	.251	806
chicken corn chowder, chunky, Campbell's—10.75 oz	310		12.0	22.0	5.0	4.0		4				1080	40			
	305	19.0	9.0			30	4500							1.44		I

	KCAL / WT (g)	H₂O (g) / FAT (g)	PRO (g) / SFA (g)	CHO (g) / MUFA (g)	SUGR (g) / PUFA (g)	DFIB (g) / CHOL (mg)	A (RE) / A (IU)	C (mg) / B-1 (mg)	B-2 (mg) / NIA (mg)	B-6 (mg) / B-12 (mcg)	FOL (mcg) / PANT (mg)	Na (mg) / K (mg)	Ca (mg) / P (mg)	Mg (mg) / Fe (mg)	Zn (mg) / Cu (mg)	Mn (mg) / REF
chicken corn chowder, Healthy Choice	176		8.3	30.4	1.6	1.9	28	9				466	23			
1 cup	252	3.2	1.2			8						1101		.76		I
chicken, crm of, Home Cookin'	210		3.0	8.0	1.0	2.0	0	2				1170	20			
1 cup	245	18.0	6.0			15	0							.72		I
chicken, crm of, w/ veg, Healthy Choice	127		7.2	21.4	0.0	1.2	20	1				384	36			
1 cup	254	2.0	0.9			10						945		.50		I
chicken, hearty, Healthy Choice	136		8.9	19.8	1.1	2.9	66	5				482	45			
1 cup	249	2.9	0.9			21						1274		.47		I
chicken, Home Cookin'	130		3.0	24.0	4.0	4.0		2				750	60			
1 cup	245	2.5	0.5			0	4500							1.08		I
chicken mushroom chowder, chunky, Campbell's—*1 cup*	210		10.0	15.0	1.0	3.0	0	5				970	20			
	245	12.0	4.0			10	0							1.44		I
chicken noodle																
Campbell's Microwave	130		7.0	18.0	4.0	2.0		0				1320	40			
10.5 oz	298	4.0	1.0			25	2500							1.44		I
chunky	175	201.6	12.7	17.0		3.8	122	0	.17	.05	5	850	24	10	.96	.240
1 cup	240	6.0	1.4	2.7	1.5	19	1222	.07	4.3	.31	.36	108	72	1.44	.240	806
chunky, Campbell's	160		12.0	20.0		3.0		2				1310	40			
10.75 oz	305	3.5	1.0			25	3000							1.44		I
Healthy Request	160		9.0	25.0	3.0	2.0		0				480	40			
1 cup	245	3.0	1.0			20	2000							1.80		I
Lunch Bucket	80		2.0	13.0	0.0	0.0		0				830	20			
7.27 oz container	206	2.0	1.0			10	100							.72		I
chicken pasta, glass jar, Campbell's	90		6.0	14.0	2.0	1.0		1				850	40			
1 cup	245	1.0	0.0			5	2500							1.08		I
chicken rice																
Campbell's Microwave	120		5.0	20.0	4.0	2.0		0				1130	40			
10.5 oz	298	2.5	1.0			10	2500							.36		I
chunky	127	208.3	12.3	13.0		1.0	586	4	.10	.05	4	888	34	10	.96	.240
1 cup	240	3.2	1.0	1.4	0.7	12	5858	.02	4.1	.31	.36	108	72	1.87	.240	806
chunky, Campbell's	140		9.0	18.0	2.0	2.0		1				840	40			
1 cup	245	3.0	1.0			25	4000							.72		I
Healthy Request	100		6.0	15.0	2.0	1.0		0				480	20			
1 cup	245	2.0	0.5			40	1750							.36		I
Home Cookin'	140		8.0	21.0	5.0	2.0		4				1130	40			
10.75 oz	305	2.0	0.5			20	3000							1.08		I
chicken veg																
chunky	166	200.3	12.3	18.9			600	6	.17	.10	12	1068	26	10	2.16	.240
1 cup	240	4.8	1.4	2.2	1.0	17	5990	.04	3.3	.24	.34	367	106	1.46	.240	806
chunky, Campbell's	130		9.0	12.0	2.0	3.0		0				950	40			
1 cup	245	3.0	1.5			20	5000							1.08		I
Healthy Request	120		7.0	18.0	3.0	2.0		0				480	20			
1 cup	245	2.0	0.5			20	4500							.72		I
hearty, chunky, Campbell's	110		7.0	15.0	3.0	3.0		0				1000	20			
10.75 oz	305	2.5	0.5			15	2000							1.08		I
Home Cookin'	170		8.0	24.0	7.0	4.0		2				1020	60			
10.75 oz	305	4.0	1.0			10	4500							1.08		I
spicy, chunky, Campbell's	90		7.0	13.0	2.0	3.0		4				870	20			
1 cup	245	1.0	0.0			10	1750							1.80		I
chicken w/ noodles, Healthy Choice	137		9.2	19.1	0.0	0.9	53	6				402	37			
1 cup	250	3.0	1.1			9						1073		.87		I
chicken w/ noodles, Home Cookin'	120		9.0	14.0	5.0	2.0		0				1220	40			
10.75 oz	305	4.0	1.5			20	4000							1.08		I
chicken w/ pasta, Healthy Choice	119		6.8	17.5	0.0	1.4	38	3				493	37			
1 cup	246	3.0	1.2			6						758		.59		I
chicken w/ rice, Healthy Choice	119		8.7	19.0	3.4	2.6	66	5				324	18			
1 cup	246	2.0	0.8			6						672		.98		I
chili beef, Healthy Choice	189		15.0	31.7	4.9	4.7	41	1				441	88			
1 cup	258	2.3	0.7			12						1899		2.92		I

	KCAL	H₂O (g)	PRO (g)	CHO (g)	SUGR (g)	DFIB (g)	Vitamins A (RE)	C (mg)	B-2 (mg)	B-6 (mg)	FOL (mcg)	Minerals Na (mg)	Ca (mg)	Mg (mg)	Zn (mg)	Mn (mg)
	WT (g)	FAT (g)	SFA (g)	MUFA (g)	PUFA (g)	CHOL (mg)	A (IU)	B-1 (mg)	NIA (mg)	B-12 (mcg)	PANT (mg)	K (mg)	P (mg)	Fe (mg)	Cu (mg)	REF
chili beef w/ beans, chunky, Campbell's	300		21.0	38.0	4.0	9.0		9				1080	80			
11 oz	312	7.0	2.0			20	1500							4.50		I
clam chowder																
Healthy Choice	123		6.5	22.8	2.8	1.6	0	2				481	32			
1 cup	251	1.3	0.9			12	0					562		.20		I
manhattan style, chunky	134	206.5	7.2	18.8		2.9	329	12	.06	.26	9	1001	67	19	1.68	.240
1 cup	240	3.4	2.1	1.0	0.1	14	3293	.06	1.8	7.92	.24	384	84	2.64	.240	806
manhattan style, chunky, Campbell's	130		6.0	20.0	3.0	3.0		9				900	40			
1 cup	245	4.0	1.0			5	4000							1.80		I
new england style, Campbell's Healthy	120		5.0	17.0	2.0	1.0	0	0				480	100			
Request—*1 cup*	245	3.0	0.5			15	0							1.44		I
new england style, chunky, Campbell's	300		9.0	26.0	1.0	3.0	0	0				1210	60			
10.75 oz	305	18.0	7.0			15	0							1.80		I
new england style, chunky, Home	200		5.0	16.0	2.0	1.0	0	1				950	40			
Cookin'—*1 cup*	245	13.0	5.0			5	0							1.80		I
country veg, Healthy Choice	112		5.0	23.5	5.2	2.8	93	1				453	46			
1 cup	246	1.0	0.3			0						1444		1.30		I
crab	76	223.3	5.5	10.3		0.7	51	0	.07	.12	15	1235	66	15	1.46	.488
1 cup	244	1.5	0.4	0.7	0.4	10	505	.20	1.3	.20	.29	327	88	1.22	.488	806
escarole	27	240.3	1.5	1.8			218	4	.05	.22	35	3864	32	5	2.23	1.240
1 cup	248	1.8	0.5	0.8	0.4	2	2170	.07	2.3	.50	.17	265	79	.74	.372	806
garden veg, Healthy Choice	108		5.0	22.4	0.0	5.6	74	1				454	55			
1 cup	246	1.1	0.6			0						1210		.44		I
gazpacho	56	228.8	7.1	0.8		0.5	261	7	.02	.15	10	739	24	7	.24	.732
1 cup	244	0.2	0.0	0.0	0.1	0	2603	.05	0.9	.00	.17	224	37	.98	.146	806
lentil																
Healthy Choice	135		9.9	27.5	2.0	5.2	98	1				472	67			
1 cup	247	0.7	0.3			0						1455		2.69		I
savory, Home Cookin'	130		7.0	24.0	3.0	5.0		0				860	40			
1 cup	245	0.5	0.5			0	2000							3.60		I
w/ ham	139	212.7	9.3	20.2			35	4	.11	.22	50	1319	42	22	.74	.298
1 cup	248	2.8	1.1	1.3	0.3	7	360	.17	1.4	.30	.35	357	184	2.65	.174	806
minestrone																
chunky	127	208.1	5.1	20.7		5.8	434	5	.12	.24	31	864	60	14	1.44	.720
1 cup	240	2.8	1.5	0.9	0.3	5	4351	.06	1.2	.00	.72	612	110	1.78	.240	806
chunky, Campbell's	140		5.0	22.0	4.0	2.0		5				800	80			
1 cup	245	5.0	1.5			5	4500							1.80		I
glass jar, Campbell's	120		5.0	23.0	5.0	4.0		0				1150	60			
1 cup	245	1.0	0.5			0	3000							1.44		I
Healthy Choice	107		5.4	23.9	4.5	4.7	56	1				370	60			
1 cup	245	1.0	0.4			1						1073		1.27		I
Healthy Request	120		4.0	24.0	5.0	3.0		4				480	0			
1 cup	245	2.0	0.5			3	4500							1.08		I
Home Cookin'	120		4.0	19.0	5.0	3.0		1				990	60			
1 cup	245	2.0	1.0			5	3500							1.08		I
tuscany, Home Cookin'	160		5.0	21.0	4.0	5.0		2				880	80			
1 cup	245	7.0	1.5			5	3000							2.70		I
mushroom & rice, Home Cookin'	80		3.0	16.0	2.0	2.0		2				820	40			
1 cup	245	0.5	0.0			0	2500							.36		I
mushroom, crm of																
glass jar, Campbell's	260		0.0	10.0	0.0	1.0	0	1				1130	20			
1 cup	245	23.0	5.0			15	0							.36		I
Healthy Choice	77		4.3	13.8	0.0	0.5	0	1				450	112			
1 cup	250	0.7	0.4			0	0					360		.15		I
Home Cookin'	170		3.0	9.0	1.0	3.0	0	0				970	0			
1 cup	245	13.0	4.0			15	0							.00		I
pasta e fagioli, homemade	194	206.0	8.7	29.6		1.7		12	.11	.16	49	790	62	50	1.13	.556
1 cup[7]	253	4.9	0.9	3.0	0.6	3	1878	.19	1.6	.03	.27	522	122	2.72	.261	806

	KCAL / WT (g)	H₂O (g) / FAT (g)	PRO (g) / SFA (g)	CHO (g) / MUFA (g)	SUGR (g) / PUFA (g)	DFIB (g) / CHOL (mg)	A (RE) / A (IU)	C (mg) / B-1 (mg)	B-2 (mg) / NIA (mg)	B-6 (mg) / B-12 (mcg)	FOL (mcg) / PANT (mg)	Na (mg) / K (mg)	Ca (mg) / P (mg)	Mg (mg) / Fe (mg)	Zn (mg) / Cu (mg)	Mn (mg) / REF
penne pasta, zesty, Healthy Request	90		4.0	17.0	5.0	2.0		60				470	40			
1 cup	245	0.5	0.0			5	2250							.72		I
pepper steak, chunky, Campbell's	140		11.0	18.0	4.0	3.0		5				830	40			
1 cup	245	2.5	1.0			20	2500							1.80		I
potato ham chowder, chunky, Campbell's	270		7.0	20.0	1.0	3.0	0	0				1050	20			
10.75 oz	305	18.0	9.0			25	0							1.08		I
potato w/ roasted garlic, Home Cookin'	180		3.0	21.0	2.0	2.0	0	2				800	20			
1 cup	245	9.0	2.5			5	0							.72		I
ratatouille, homemade	266	173.2	2.4	11.8		1.3		41	.06	.25	34	329	56	32	.41	.323
1 cup[8]	214	24.7	3.3	17.9	2.2	0	815	.13	1.1	.00	.22	485	63	1.27	.190	806
sirloin burger w/ veg, chunky, Campbell's—10.75 oz	230		12.0	25.0	3.0	5.0		0				1160	40			
	305	11.0	4.5			25	6000							2.70		I
split pea w/ ham																
chunky	185	194.3	11.1	26.8		4.1	487	7	.09	.22	5	965	34	38	3.12	.600
1 cup	240	4.0	1.6	1.6	0.6	7	4872	.12	2.5	.24	.48	305	178	2.14	.240	806
chunky, Campbell's	240		18.0	33.0	6.0	4.0		6				1400	40			
10.75 oz	305	3.5	1.5			20	4000							2.70		I
Healthy Choice	164		11.3	26.3	6.3	4.8	56	13				468	50			
1 cup	250	1.8	0.7			7						1460		1.38		I
Healthy Request	170		9.0	28.0	6.0	4.0		1				480	20			
1 cup	245	2.0	0.5			15	2000							1.80		I
Home Cookin'	170		10.0	30.0	6.0	6.0		2				880	40			
1 cup	245	1.5	0.5			5	2000							1.80		I
steak 'n potato, chunky, Campbell's	200		15.0	24.0	1.0	4.0		4				1110	20			
10.75 oz	305	5.0	1.5			25	100							2.70		I
stroganoff beef, chunky, Campbell's	310		16.0	28.0	4.0	4.0		0				1180	80			
10.75 oz	305	16.0	6.0			45	2500							2.70		I
tomato, garden, Healthy Choice	101		4.4	19.3	8.1	5.4	103	1				468	70			
1 cup	244	1.2	0.7			1						961		1.24		I
tomato, garden, Home Cookin'	150		5.0	27.0	13.0	4.0		1				900	100			
10.75 oz	305	4.0	2.0			5	2500							1.44		I
tomato veg, glass jar, Campbell's	80		4.0	14.0	2.0	2.0		4				1000	40			
1 cup	245	0.5	0.5			5	2500							.72		I
tomato veg, Healthy Request	120		4.0	22.0	9.0	3.0		5				480	60			
1 cup	245	2.0	0.5			5	4500							1.08		I
tortellini w/ chicken & veg, chunky, Campbell's—1 cup	110		6.0	18.0	3.0	2.0		0				910	60			
	245	1.5	0.5			10	1750							1.08		I
turkey, chunky	135	203.8	10.2	14.1			715	6	.11	.31	11	923	50	24	2.12	.236
1 cup	236	4.4	1.2	1.8	1.1	9	7156	.04	3.6	2.12	.92	361	104	1.91	.236	806
turkey veg w/ wild rice, Healthy Request	120		7.0	17.0	3.0	2.0		2				480	40			
1 cup	245	2.5	1.0			15	6000							.72		I
turkey w/ rice, Healthy Choice	72		9.0	8.5	4.7	2.7	37					407	27			
1 cup	240	1.0	0.4			3	91					727		.40		I
veg & pasta, glass jar, Campbell's	110		4.0	21.0	7.0	2.0		2				720	60			
1 cup	245	0.5	0.5			5	3500							1.08		I
veg beef																
Campbell's Microwave	140		9.0	26.0	4.0	5.0		1				1240	80			
10.5 oz	298	0.5	0.0			10	2500							1.44		I
Healthy Choice	96		10.9	13.6	2.7	2.4	67	2				433	31			
1 cup	252	0.9	0.4			2						1434		1.10		I
Healthy Request	140		9.0	20.0	4.0	3.0		2				480	40			
1 cup	245	2.5	1.0			20	5000							1.08		I
Home Cookin'	150		8.0	22.0	7.0	4.0		0				1260	60			
10.75 oz	305	2.5	1.5			10	5000							1.44		I
veg broth, College Inn	20		0.0	5.0	4.0							820				
1 cup	240 ml	0.0	0.0	0.0	0.0											I
veg broth, Swanson	20		2.0	3.0	3.0	0.0		0				1000	0			
1 cup	235	1.0	0.0			0	200							.00		
veg, chunky	122	210.2	3.5	19.0		1.2	588	6	.06	.19	17	1010	55	7	3.12	.480
1 cup	240	3.7	0.6	1.6	1.4	0	5878	.07	1.2	.00	.34	396	72	1.63	.240	806

	KCAL / WT (g)	H₂O (g) / FAT (g)	PRO (g) / SFA (g)	CHO (g) / MUFA (g)	SUGR (g) / PUFA (g)	DFIB (g) / CHOL (mg)	A (RE) / A (IU)	C (mg) / B-1 (mg)	B-2 (mg) / NIA (mg)	B-6 (mg) / B-12 (mcg)	FOL (mcg) / PANT (mg)	Na (mg) / K (mg)	Ca (mg) / P (mg)	Mg (mg) / Fe (mg)	Zn (mg) / Cu (mg)	Mn (mg) / REF
veg, chunky, Campbell's	160		4.0	28.0	6.0	5.0		4				1090	60			
10.75 oz	305	4.0	1.0			0	5000							1.80		I
veg, country, Home Cookin'	130		4.0	26.0	8.0	2.0		1				940	80			
10.75 oz	305	2.0	0.0			5	6000							1.08		I
veg, country, Lunch Bucket	60		1.0	14.0	1.0	3.0		1				750	20			
7.27 oz container	206	0.5	0.0			0	500							.72		I
veg, harborside, Home Cookin'	80		3.0	13.0	4.0			5				770	40			
1 cup	245	1.5	1.0			5	2000							1.08		I
veg, hearty, Healthy Request	100		3.0	20.0	6.0	2.0		0				470	40			
1 cup	245	1.0	0.0			0	5000							1.08		I
veg, italian, Home Cookin'	100		3.0	14.0	6.0	2.0		2				860	60			
1 cup	245	4.0	1.5			5	6000							.72		I
veg, southwestern w/ black beans,	140		5.0	28.0	10.0	5.0		4				480	60			
Healthy Request—1 cup	245	1.0	0.5			0	500							1.44		I
veg w/ pasta, chunky, Campbell's Old	130		4.0	21.0	6.0	3.0	0	1				1080	80			
Fashioned—1 cup	245	3.0	0.5			0	0							1.80		I

28.5 DEHYDRATED

	KCAL / WT (g)	H₂O (g) / FAT (g)	PRO (g) / SFA (g)	CHO (g) / MUFA (g)	SUGR (g) / PUFA (g)	DFIB (g) / CHOL (mg)	A (RE) / A (IU)	C (mg) / B-1 (mg)	B-2 (mg) / NIA (mg)	B-6 (mg) / B-12 (mcg)	FOL (mcg) / PANT (mg)	Na (mg) / K (mg)	Ca (mg) / P (mg)	Mg (mg) / Fe (mg)	Zn (mg) / Cu (mg)	Mn (mg) / REF
asparagus, Knorr	60	1.1	2.5	8.7				5	.10			750	50			
amt for 8 fl oz	16	1.6					120	.05	0.3					.40		I
barley, Country, Knorr	120	1.9	4.6	22.5				10	.05			940	34			
amt for 10 fl oz	34	1.8					1405	.10	0.8					1.90		I
beef broth cube	14	0.2	1.0	1.4		0.0	0	0	.01	.01	2	1019	4	3	.00	.028
1 cube	6	0.5	0.3	0.2	0.0	1	3	.00	0.3	.06	.02	27	19	.06	.000	806
beef mushroom, Lipton	35		7.0	2.0			0	.00				640				
amt for 8 fl oz	11	0.0	0.0	0.0	0.0		0	.00	0.0							I
beefy onion, Lipton	25		0.0	5.0			0	.00				610				
amt for 8 fl oz	8	0.5	0.0			0	0	.00	0.0							I
broccoli & cheese, creamy, Lipton	70		2.0	9.0		1.0						540	20			
Cup-A-Soup—amt for 6 fl oz	16	3.0	1.5													I
cauliflower, Knorr	80	0.9	3.3	11.4				23	.12			730	50			
amt for 8 fl oz	20	1.9					70	.10	0.3					.50		I

chicken

	KCAL / WT (g)	H₂O (g) / FAT (g)	PRO (g) / SFA (g)	CHO (g) / MUFA (g)	SUGR (g) / PUFA (g)	DFIB (g) / CHOL (mg)	A (RE) / A (IU)	C (mg) / B-1 (mg)	B-2 (mg) / NIA (mg)	B-6 (mg) / B-12 (mcg)	FOL (mcg) / PANT (mg)	Na (mg) / K (mg)	Ca (mg) / P (mg)	Mg (mg) / Fe (mg)	Zn (mg) / Cu (mg)	Mn (mg) / REF
country, Soup Secrets Kettle Creations	100		4.0	18.0	1.0	1.0						740	20			
¼ cup	27	1.5	0.0			5	500							.72		I
creamy w/ veg, Lipton Cup-A-Soup	80		2.0	10.0	3.0							590				
amt for 6 fl oz	19	4.0	1.5			0										I
crm of, Lipton Cup-A-Soup	70		12.0	3.0		0						640				.000
amt for 6 fl oz	17	2.0	0.0				0								.000	I
hearty, Lipton Cup-A-Soup	60		3.0	10.0		0.0	0	.00				590			.00	.000
amt for 6 fl oz	16	1.0	0.0			15	0	.00	0.0					.36	.000	I
chicken 'n noodle, Soup Secrets Kettle	80		3.0	12.0	1.0	1.0						650				
Creations—3 T	20	2.0	0.5			15								.72		I
chicken 'n onion, Soup Secrets Kettle	120			24.0		1.0		1				730	20			
Creations—¼ cup	34	1.0	0.0			5								.72		I
chicken 'n pasta, Knorr	90	1.6	3.5	16.2				6	.02			850	23			
amt for 8 fl oz	26	1.6					1355	.05	1.1					.50		I
chicken broth cube	10	0.1	0.7	1.2		0.0	4	0	.02	.01	2	1200	10	3	.01	.019
1 cube	5	0.2	0.1	0.1	0.1	1	13	.01	0.2	.01	.03	19	10	.09	.000	806
chicken broth, fat-free, Lipton Cup-A-	20		1.0	3.0	0.0	0.0	0	.00				440	0	0	.00	.000
Soup—amt for 6 fl oz	6	0.0	0.0	0.0	0.0	0	0	.00	0.0				0	.00	.000	I

chicken noodle

	KCAL / WT (g)	H₂O (g) / FAT (g)	PRO (g) / SFA (g)	CHO (g) / MUFA (g)	SUGR (g) / PUFA (g)	DFIB (g) / CHOL (mg)	A (RE) / A (IU)	C (mg) / B-1 (mg)	B-2 (mg) / NIA (mg)	B-6 (mg) / B-12 (mcg)	FOL (mcg) / PANT (mg)	Na (mg) / K (mg)	Ca (mg) / P (mg)	Mg (mg) / Fe (mg)	Zn (mg) / Cu (mg)	Mn (mg) / REF
Campbell's	90		4.0	15.0	3.0	0.0	0	0				660	0			
3 T	24	1.5	0.5			10	0							.72		I
Knorr	100	1.9	4.0	17.9				0	.01			710	14			
amt for 8 fl oz	28	1.5					47	.02	0.6					.50		I
w/ chicken meat, Lipton Cup-A-Soup	50		2.0	8.0		0.0			.10			540				
amt for 6 fl oz	13	1.0				10		.10	1.0					.36		I

| | KCAL | H₂O (g) | PRO (g) | CHO (g) | SUGR (g) | DFIB (g) | A (RE) | C (mg) | B-2 (mg) | B-6 (mg) | FOL (mcg) | Na (mg) | Ca (mg) | Mg (mg) | Zn (mg) | Mn (mg) |
	WT (g)	FAT (g)	SFA (g)	MUFA (g)	PUFA (g)	CHOL (mg)	A (IU)	B-1 (mg)	NIA (mg)	B-12 (mcg)	PANT (mg)	K (mg)	P (mg)	Fe (mg)	Cu (mg)	RFF
chicken veg, Lipton Cup-A-Soup	50		1.0	10.0		0.0						520				
amt for 6 fl oz	14	1.0	0.0			10								.36		I
chicken w/ pasta, fat-free. Lipton Cup-A-Soup—*1 pkg*	45		2.0	8.0	0.0	0.0						450				
	13	0.0	0.0	0.0	0.0	0								.36		I
chicken w/ pasta, Soup Secrets Kettle Creations—*¼ cup*	110		5.0	19.0	1.0	3.0						700	20			
	30	1.5				5	500							1.08		I
clam chowder, manhattan style	66	0.8	2.1	10.9			102	4	.04	.11	10	1343	25	11	.99	.399
amt for 8 fl oz	19	1.6	0.3	0.7	0.5	0	1020	.03	0.9	4.37	.13	200	44	1.73	.133	806
clam chowder, new england style	96	0.8	2.8	13.1		1.2	1	2	.16	.07	3	755	78	7	.69	.230
amt for 8 fl oz	23	3.7	0.6	1.7	1.2	1	9	.02	0.9	8.97	.30	207	101	1.29	.115	806
double noodle chicken, Campbell's	170		7.0	32.0	4.0	1.0	0	0				740	20			
1 pkt	45	2.0	1.0			30	0							1.44		I
extra noodle, Soup Secrets	90		3.0	15.0	1.0							680				
3 T	23	1.5	0.5			25								.72		I
french onion, Knorr	50	0.6	1.4	9.1				2	.01			970	11			
amt for 8 fl oz	15	0.8					10	.01	0.1					.40		I
golden herb w/ lemon, Recipe Secrets	35		7.0									510				
1 ½ T	10	0.5	0.0			0										I
golden onion, Recipe Secrets	50		1.0	10.0	1.0							640				
1 ⅔ T	15	1.5				0										I
herb, Knorr	110	1.1	2.8	13.5				1	.16			970	38			
amt for 8 fl oz	25	4.6					145	.09	0.6					.70		I
herb w/ garlic, Recipe Secrets	30		1.0	6.0								480				
1 T	9	0.0	0.0	0.0	0.0	0										I
leek, Knorr	70	0.8	2.2	10.9				1	.04			770	20			
amt for 8 fl oz	18	2.0					3	.07	0.2					.60		I
lentil, Soup Secrets Kettle Creations	130		7.0	22.0	1.0	5.0						750				
¼ cup	36	1.0	0.0			0	500							1.80		I
minestrone, Hearty, Knorr	130	1.9	5.0	22.7				25	.06			940	50			
amt for 10 fl oz	35	2.0					835	.12	1.0					1.40		I
minestrone, Soup Secrets Kettle Creations—*¼ cup*	110		4.0	21.0	4.0	3.0		2				750	20			
	31	1.0	0.0			0	500							.90		I
mushroom, crm of, Lipton Cup-A-Soup	60		1.0	10.0	2.0	0.0		0				610				
amt for 6 fl oz	15	2.0					0	.00								I
mushroom, Knorr	80	0.8	2.8	9.9				2	.14			850	35			
amt for 8 fl oz	19	2.8					20	.07	0.9							I
noodle ring, Lipton Cup-A-Soup	50		2.0	9.0	0.0	0.0						560	0			
amt for 6 fl oz	14	1.0	0.0			10								.36		I
noodle w/ chicken broth, Campbell's	100		3.0	17.0	2.0	1.0	0	0				740	0			
3 T	25	1.5	0.5			0	0							.72		I
noodle w/ chicken broth, Lipton	60		2.0	9.0	1.0	0.0	0	0	.07		16	710	0			
amt for 8 fl oz	16	2.0				15	0	.22	1.2					.36		I
onion	21	0.3	0.8	3.7		0.7	0	0	.04	.01	1	627	10	4	.04	.044
amt for 6 fl oz	7	0.4	0.1	0.2	0.0	0	1	.02	0.4	.00	.00	47	23	.10	.011	806
Campbell's	20		0.0	5.0	3.0	0.0	0	0				530	0			
1 T	8	0.0	0.0	0.0	0.0	0	0							.00		I
Lipton	20		0.0	4.0	0.0	0.0		0	.00			610	0			
amt for 8 fl oz	7	0.0	0.0	0.0	0.0	0	0	.00	0.0					.00		I
onion mushroom, Lipton	30		6.0			0.0	0	.00				630	0	5	.00	.000
amt for 8 fl oz	10	1.0	0.0			0	0	.00	0.0			0	26	.00	.000	I
oriental, hot & sour, Knorr	50	0.9	1.4	8.8				1	.02			670	5			
amt for 8 fl oz	14	0.7					35	.01	0.1					.40		I
oxtail	64	0.8	2.6	8.1		0.2	3	0	.03	.03	5	1098	10	9	.00	.085
amt for 8 fl oz	17	2.3	1.2	1.0	0.1	3	9	.02	0.8	.17	.05	77	54	.17	.000	806
oxtail hearty beef, Knorr	70	0.7	2.2	10.2				14	.03			1120	10			
amt for 8 fl oz	19	2.3					264	.07	0.3					.70		I
pea, green, Lipton Cup-A-Soup	80		4.0	12.0	1.0	3.0		0				520	0	0	.00	.000
amt for 6 fl oz	21	1.0	0.0			0							0	.00	.000	I
pea, green/split	100	1.2	5.7	17.0		2.8	4	0	.11	.04	11	914	17	35	.44	.199
amt for 6 fl oz	28	1.2	0.4	0.7	0.3	0	36	.17	1.0	.28	.20	178	100	.75	.144	806

	KCAL / WT (g)	H₂O (g) / FAT (g)	PRO (g) / SFA (g)	CHO (g) / MUFA (g)	SUGR (g) / PUFA (g)	DFIB (g) / CHOL (mg)	A (RE) / A (IU)	C (mg) / B-1 (mg)	B-2 (mg) / NIA (mg)	B-6 (mg) / B-12 (mcg)	FOL (mcg) / PANT (mg)	Na (mg) / K (mg)	Ca (mg) / P (mg)	Mg (mg) / Fe (mg)	Zn (mg) / Cu (mg)	Mn (mg) / REF
ramen noodle																
baked, beef flavor, Campbell's	210		6.0	44.0	2.0	1.0	0	0				830	0			
1 pkg	59	1.0	0.0			0	0							1.44		I
baked, chicken flavor, Campbell's	140		4.0	30.0	2.0	1.0	0	0				720	0			
½ block	40	1.0	0.0			0	0							1.44		I
baked, chicken spicy flavor, Campbell's	140		4.0	30.0	2.0	1.0	0	0				780	0			
½ block	40	1.0	0.0			0	0							1.44		I
baked, oriental flavor, Campbell's	140		4.0	30.0	3.0	2.0		0				1300	40			
1 pkg	40	1.0	0.5			0	300							1.80		I
beef flavor, Campbell's	290		6.0	41.0	3.0	2.0		0				1220	20			
1 pkt	62	11.0	3.0			3	100							1.80		I
beef oriental flavor, Campbell's	170		3.0	26.0		1.0	0	0				750	0			
½ block	40	6.0	4.0			0	0							1.08		I
chicken flavor, Campbell's	290		6.0	41.0	3.0	2.0		0				1120	20			
1 pkg	62	11.0	3.0			0	100							1.80		I
chicken oriental flavor, Campbell's	170		3.0	26.0	2.0	1.0	0	0				730	0			
½ block	40	6.0	4.0			0	0							1.44		I
oriental flavor, Campbell's	170		3.0	26.0	2.0	1.0	0	0				780	0			
½ block	40	6.0	4.0			0	0							1.08		I
pork oriental flavor, Campbell's	170		4.0	26.0	2.0	1.0	0	0				850	0			
½ block	40	6.0	4.0			0	0							1.08		I
shrimp flavor, Campbell's	170		3.0	26.0	2.0	1.0	0	0				740	0			
½ block	40	6.0	4.0			0	0							1.08		I
Ring-O-Noodle w/ chicken broth, Lipton	70		2.0	10.0	1.0	0.0			.10			710				
amt for 8 fl oz	17	2.0	0.5			15		.23	1.2					.72		I
ruffled pasta, Soup Secrets	60		2.0	12.0	1.0							660				
2 T	18	1.0	0.0			0								.36		I
tomato	83	0.9	2.0	15.7		0.4	67	4	.04	.08	5	763	44	12	.17	.069
amt for 8 fl oz	23	1.9	0.9	0.7	0.2	1	673	.05	0.6	.07	.09	239	54	.34	.075	806
basil, Knorr	85	0.7	2.3	14.3				60	.07			940	35			
amt for 8 fl oz	23	2.6					1265	.08	1.0					.80		I
Lipton Cup-A-Soup	90		2.0	20.0	6.0		4					510	80			
amt for 6 fl oz	26	1.0				0	200									I
veg	127	1.5	4.6	23.4		1.2	43	14	.10	.12	23	2622	18	45	.38	.382
amt for 8 fl oz	39	2.0	0.9	0.7	0.2	1	434	.13	1.8	.00	.33	236	67	1.45	.074	806
veg																
Knorr	35	0.5	1.5	6.5				14	.02			840	30			
amt for 8 fl oz	12	0.4					1270	.03	0.4					.40		I
Lipton	30		7.0	0.0	0.0		2	.00			600					
amt for 8 fl oz	10	0.5	0.0			0	200	.00								I
spring, Lipton Cup-A-Soup	45		2.0	8.0	1.0				.10		500					
amt for 6 fl oz	13	1.0	0.0			10		.10	0.5					.36		I

28.6 DEHYDRATED, RECONSTITUTED

	KCAL / WT (g)	H₂O (g) / FAT (g)	PRO (g) / SFA (g)	CHO (g) / MUFA (g)	SUGR (g) / PUFA (g)	DFIB (g) / CHOL (mg)	A (RE) / A (IU)	C (mg) / B-1 (mg)	B-2 (mg) / NIA (mg)	B-6 (mg) / B-12 (mcg)	FOL (mcg) / PANT (mg)	Na (mg) / K (mg)	Ca (mg) / P (mg)	Mg (mg) / Fe (mg)	Zn (mg) / Cu (mg)	Mn (mg) / REF
asparagus, crm of	58	235.7	2.2	9.0			28	1	.05	.01	8	801	23	3	.68	.256
1 cup	251	1.7	0.1	0.8	0.7	0	271	.05	0.5	.03	.08	133	30	.50	.128	806
bean w/ bacon	106	237.8	5.5	16.4		9.0	5	1	.27	.03	8	928	56	29	.69	.530
1 cup	265	2.1	1.0	0.9	0.2	3	53	.05	0.4	.03	.05	326	90	1.32	.265	806
beef broth/ bouillon	20	237.0	1.3	1.9		0.0	0	0	.02	.00	0	1367	10	7	.07	.039
1 cup	245	0.7	0.3	0.3	0.0	0	5	.00	0.4	.00	.00	37	25	.02	.015	806
beef noodle	40	239.3	2.2	6.0		0.8	0	1	.06	.04	2	1042	5	10	.10	.100
1 cup[9]	251	0.8	0.3	0.4	0.2	3	8	.12	0.7	.00	.00	80	40	.33	.050	806
cauliflower	69	237.9	2.9	10.7			0	3	.08	.03	3	842	10	3	.26	.051
1 cup	256	1.7	0.3	0.7	0.6	5	5	.08	0.5	.18	.10	105	51	.51	.026	806
celery, crm of	64	237.4	2.6	9.8			28	0	.05	.00	2	838	36	5	.13	.229
1 cup	254	1.6	0.3	0.7	0.6	0	269	.03	0.3	.05	1.02	109	33	.51	.127	806
chicken broth/bouillon	22	236.2	1.3	1.4		0.0	12	0	.03	.00	2	1484	15	5	.01	.000
1 cup[10]	244	1.1	0.3	0.4	0.4	0	39	.01	0.2	.02	.05	24	12	.07	.000	806

	KCAL / WT (g)	H₂O (g) / FAT (g)	PRO (g) / SFA (g)	CHO (g) / MUFA (g)	SUGR (g) / PUFA (g)	DFIB (g) / CHOL (mg)	A (RE) / A (IU)	C (mg) / B-1 (mg)	B-2 (mg) / NIA (mg)	B-6 (mg) / B-12 (mcg)	FOL (mcg) / PANT (mg)	Na (mg) / K (mg)	Ca (mg) / P (mg)	Mg (mg) / Fe (mg)	Zn (mg) / Cu (mg)	Mn (mg) / REF
chicken, crm of	107	237.4	1.8	13.3		0.3	123	1	.20	.05	5	1185	76	5	1.57	.783
1 cup	261	5.3	3.4	1.2	0.4	3	407	.10	2.6	.26	.78	214	97	.26	.261	806
chicken noodle	53	237.3	2.9	7.4		0.8	5	0	.06	.01	2	1283	33	8	.20	.081
1 cup[11]	252	1.2	0.3	0.5	0.4	3	63	.07	0.9	.00	.01	30	33	.50	.035	806
chicken rice	61	237.4	2.5	9.3		0.8	0	0	.00	.03	1	982	8	0	.13	.202
1 cup	253	1.4	0.3	0.6	0.4	3	0	.00	0.4	.08	.08	10	10	.00	.051	806
chicken veg	50	237.5	2.7	7.8			3	1	.05	.09	3	808	15	23	.21	.251
1 cup	251	0.8	0.2	0.3	0.2	3	15	.07	0.7	.10	.25	68	33	.58	.025	806
consomme w/ gelatin	17	236.5	2.2	2.1		0.0	0	0	.02	.02	4	3299	7	7	.00	.050
1 cup	249	0.0	0.0	0.0	0.0	0	7	.00	0.6	.12	.05	57	40	.12	.000	806
leek	71	235.7	2.1	11.4		3.0	0	3	.03	.03	8	965	30	10	.24	.025
1 cup	254	2.1	1.0	0.9	0.1	3	5	.05	0.3	.03	.10	89	30	.51	.036	806
minestrone	79	232.8	4.4	11.9			30	1	.05	.10	18	1026	38	8	.76	.406
1 cup	254	1.7	0.8	0.7	0.1	3	295	.08	1.0	.00	.38	340	61	1.02	.127	806
mushroom	96	231.9	2.2	11.1		0.8	0	1	.11	.03	5	1020	66	5	.09	.253
1 cup	253	4.9	0.8	2.3	1.5	0	8	.28	0.5	.25	.24	200	76	.51	.030	806
onion	27	236.9	1.1	5.1		1.0	0	0	.06	.00	1	849	12	5	.06	.059
1 cup[12]	246	0.6	0.1	0.3	0.1	0	2	.03	0.5	.00	.00	64	30	.15	.015	806
oxtail	71	235.2	2.8	9.0		0.5	0	0	.03	.03	5	1209	10	10	.00	.101
1 cup	253	2.6	1.3	1.1	0.1	3	10	.03	0.8	.25	.05	83	61	.25	.000	806
pea, green/split	133	235.2	7.7	22.7		3.0	5	0	.15	.05	42	1220	22	46	.59	.268
1 cup[13]	271	1.6	0.4	0.7	0.3	3	49	.22	1.3	.27	.26	238	133	1.00	.192	806
tomato	103	237.7	2.5	19.4		0.5	82	5	.05	.10	7	943	53	13	.21	.080
1 cup[14]	265	2.4	1.1	0.9	0.2	0	832	.06	0.8	.08	.11	294	66	.42	.093	806
tomato veg	56	236.6	2.0	10.2		0.5	20	6	.05	.05	10	1146	8	20	.17	.177
1 cup[15]	253	0.9	0.4	0.3	0.1	0	190	.06	0.8	.00	.14	104	30	.63	.033	806
veg, crm of	107	237.1	1.9	12.3		0.5	3	4	.11	.03	8	1170	31	10	.26	.182
1 cup	260	5.7	1.4	2.5	1.5	0	36	1.22	0.5	.13	.16	96	55	.52	.104	806

1. Includes vichyssoise.
2. Includes chicken alphabet, chicken noodle-o's, chicken with stars, and curly noodle with chicken.
3. Includes beef, beef vegetable, and barley and vegetable beef.
4. Soups are canned unless specified as homemade.
5. The lower sodium product contains 620 mg sodium.
6. The lower sodium product contains 640 mg sodium.
7. Made with beef broth, white beans, pasta, tomatoes, potatoes, onions, carrots, celery, ham, olive oil, parsley, garlic, and pepper.
8. Made with zucchini, eggplant, tomatoes, green pepper, olive oil, onions, parsley, garlic, salt, and basil.
9. Includes beef and macaroni and beef flavored noodle.
10. Includes chicken consomme.
11. Includes chicken broth with noodles.
12. Includes french onion.
13. Includes pea with ham.
14. Includes cream of tomato.
15. Includes italian vegetable and spring vegetable.

29. SPECIAL DIETARY PRODUCTS

The four data lines for each product correspond to the four header rows below, in order.

Item	KCAL	H₂O (g)	PRO (g)	CHO (g)	SUGR (g)	DFIB (g)	A (RE)	C (mg)	B-2 (mg)	B-6 (mg)	FOL (mcg)	Na (mg)	Ca (mg)	Mg (mg)	Zn (mg)	Mn (mg)
(row 2)	WT (g)	FAT (g)	SFA (g)	MUFA (g)	PUFA (g)	CHOL (mg)	A (IU)	B-1 (mg)	NIA (mg)	B-12 (mcg)	PANT (mg)	K (mg)	P (mg)	Fe (mg)	Cu (mg)	
(row 3)	TRY (mg)	THR (mg)	ISO (mg)	LEU (mg)	LYS (mg)	MET (mg)	D (IU)	E (IU)	K (mcg)	BIO (mcg)	CHLN (mcg)	Cl (mg)	I (mcg)	Mo (mcg)	F (mcg)	
(row 4)	CYS (mg)	PHE (mg)	TYR (mg)	VAL (mg)	ARG (mg)	HIS (mg)	INOS (mg)	E (AT) (mg)								REF
Biosearch, Entrition 250 ml[1]	250	210.0	8.8	34.0				38	.43	.50	100	175	125	50	1.88	.500
	262	8.8					625	.38	5.0	1.50	2.50	300	125	2.25	.250	
																I
Biosearch, Entrition HN 250 ml[2]	250	210.0	11.0	28.5				29	.50	.58	115	230	193	77	2.90	.385
	260	10.3					961	.43	5.8	1.73	2.88	395	193	3.48	.385	
																I
McGaw, Hepatic-Aid II inst drink powder 3.1 oz pkt[3]	400		15.0	57.3												
	86	12.3														
																I
McGaw, Immun-Aid, inst drink powder 4.3 oz pkt	500		61.5	83.0				30	.43	.50	100	290	250	100	13.30	1.300
	123	11.0					1333	.38	5.0	1.50	2.50	530	250	4.50	1.000	
			7800	11700			100	25.0	20	75		444	38		0	
				9500	15400											I
Mead Johnson — Boost 8 fl oz	240	200.0	10.2	41.0			280	60	.43	.70	140	130	300	100	4.50	.700
	260	4.1	0.4	2.6	1.1	7	1250	.38	5.0	2.10	2.50	400	250	3.60	.400	
	140	430	540	980	780	250	100	30.0	30	75		340	38	20		
	88	450	450	640	330	260		20.0								I
Casec protein supplement, dry 3 ½ oz[4]	380	4.0	90.0									100	1400			
	100	2.0	1.1	0.6	0.1	10						10	800			
	1150	3700	5100	9000	7700	2600										
	260	4900	5100	6400	3600	2800										I
Choice dm RTH 1000 ml	1060	850.0	45.0	106.0		14.4	1230	250	1.80	2.10	420	850	1060	420	21.00	3.200
	1080	51.0	4.0	29.0	12.3	17	5300	1.60	21.0	6.40	10.60	1820	1060	19	2.100	
	570	1850	2500	4400	3700	1190	420	127.0	127	320	530	1270	159	106		
	260	2300	2300	3000	1630	1280	250	85.0								I
Choice dm RTH 8 fl oz	250	200.0	10.6	25.0		3.4	290	60	.43	.50	100	200	250	100	5.00	.750
	250	12.0	1.0	6.9	2.9	7	1250	.38	5.0	1.50	2.50	430	250	4.50	.500	
	145	450	560	1020	810	260	100	30.0	30	75	125	300	38	25		
	91	470	470	670	340	270	60	20.0								I
Comply 8 fl oz	355	182.0	14.2	43.0			340	43	.48	.80	142	280	280	114	5.70	.850
	260	14.5	1.0	7.5	3.1	2	1420	.43	5.7	4.30	2.80	440	280	5.10	.570	
	181	580	810	1420	1210	400	114	21.0	34	85	142	400	43	28		
	42	780	810	1020	570	450		14.1								I
Criticare HN 8 fl oz[5]	250	200.0	9.0	51.0			189	38	.54	.63	50	150	125	50	2.50	.630
	260	1.3	0.2	0.3	0.8	0	630	.48	6.3	1.88	3.10	310	125	2.30	.250	
	144	440	540	920	770	410	50	9.4	31	38	63	250	19			
	36	430	200	680	360	270		6.3								I
Deliver 2.0 8 fl oz	470	168.0	17.7	47.0			350	71	1.02	1.18	95	190	240	95	4.70	.710
	260	24.0	2.5	4.1	10.2	2	1180	.90	11.8	3.50	5.90	400	240	4.30	.470	
	230	730	1010	1770	1510	500	95	17.7	59	71	118	280		59		
	52	970	1010	1270	710	560		11.9								I
Infalyte 100 ml	13	98.0	0.0	3.2								115				
	102	0.0	0.0	0.0	0.0	0						98				
												160				
																I
Isocal 8 fl oz[6]	250	200.0	8.1	32.0			189	38	.54	.63	50	125	150	50	2.50	.380
	250	10.5	1.3	2.0	5.3	0	630	.48	6.3	1.88	3.10	310	125	2.20	.250	
	97	320	430	790	590	194	50	9.4	31	38	63	250		31		
	41	410	380	570	310	220		6.3								I

	KCAL / WT / TRY / CYS	H₂O (g) / FAT (g) / THR (mg) / PHE (mg)	PRO (g) / SFA (g) / ISO (mg) / TYR (mg)	CHO (g) / MUFA (g) / LEU (mg) / VAL (mg)	SUGR (g) / PUFA (g) / LYS (mg) / ARG (mg)	DFIB (g) / CHOL (mg) / MET (mg) / HIS (mg)	A (RE) / A (IU) / D (IU) / INOS (mg)	C (mg) / B-1 (mg) / E (IU) / E (AT) (mg)	B-2 (mg) / NIA (mg) / K (mcg)	B-6 (mg) / B-12 (mcg) / BIO (mcg)	FOL (mcg) / PANT (mg) / CHLN (mcg)	Na (mg) / K (mg) / Cl (mg)	Ca (mg) / P (mg) / I (mcg)	Mg (mg) / Fe (mg) / Mo (mcg)	Zn (mg) / Cu (mg) / F (mcg)	Mn (mg) / / / REF
Isolocal HN *8 fl oz²*	250 / 250 / 125 / 52	200.0 / 10.7 / 420 / 520	10.4 / 1.2 / 550 / 490	29.0 / 1.7 / 1010 / 730	/ 4.0 / 760 / 400	/ 1 / 250 / 280	300 / 1000 / 80 /	60 / .75 / 15.0 / 10.1	.85 / 10.0 / 25	1.00 / 3.00 / 60	80 / 5.00 / 100	220 / 380 / 340	200 / 200 / 30	80 / 3.60 / 20	4.00 / .400 /	.600 / / / I
Kindercal *8 fl oz*	250 / 250 / 104 / 29	200.0 / 10.5 / 330 / 440	8.1 / 0.7 / 460 / 450	32.0 / 5.0 / 810 / 570	/ 2.7 / 680 / 320	1.5 / 1 / 230 / 250	175 / 970 / 125 / 20	58 / .40 / 8.8 / 5.9	.50 / 4.9 / 8	.50 / 1.40 / 38	38 / 3.10 / 63	88 / 310 / 175	200 / 200 / 30	50 / 2.50 / 13	3.00 / .300 /	.400 / / / I
Lipisorb, 30KCal/fl oz *8 fl oz*	240 / 250 / 107 / 25	200.0 / 11.5 / 350 / 460	8.4 / 0.3 / 480 / 480	28.0 / 0.4 / 840 / 600	/ 1.0 / 720 / 340	/ 1 / 240 / 260	270 / 900 / 72 /	11 / .28 / 5.4 / 3.6	.31 / 3.6 / 14	.36 / 1.08 / 54	72 / 1.80 / 32	176 / 300 / 280	168 / 168 / 18	48 / 2.20 /	2.40 / .240 /	.360 / / / I
Lipisorb liquid *8 fl oz*	320 / 260 / 173 / 40	190.0 / 13.4 / 560 / 750	13.6 / 0.4 / 770 / 770	38.0 / 0.5 / 1360 / 970	/ 1.2 / 1160 / 550	/ 2 / 390 / 430	450 / 1500 / 120 /	18 / .46 / 9.0 / 6.0	.52 / 6.0 / 24	.60 / 1.80 / 90	120 / 3.00 / 50	320 / 400 / 520	200 / 200 / 30	80 / 3.60 / 20	4.00 / .400 /	.600 / / / I
Liposorb, 40KCal/fl oz *8 fl oz*	320 / 260 / 143 / 33	190.0 / 15.4 / 460 / 610	11.2 / 0.3 / 640 / 640	37.0 / 0.6 / 1120 / 800	/ 1.3 / 960 / 450	/ 1 / 320 / 350	360 / 1200 / 96 /	14 / .37 / 7.2 / 4.8	.42 / 4.8 / 19	.48 / 1.44 / 72	96 / 2.40 / 43	240 / 400 / 370	220 / 220 / 24	64 / 2.90 /	3.20 / .320 /	.480 / / / I
Magnacal Renal *8 fl oz*	470 / 260 / 230 / 52	168.0 / 24.0 / 730 / 970	17.7 / 1.7 / 1010 / 1010	47.0 / 12.4 / 1770 / 1270	/ 5.1 / 1510 / 710	/ 2 / 500 / 560	240 / 1180 / 24 /	24 / .90 / 10.6 / 7.1	1.02 / 11.8 / 28	2.37 / 3.50 / 71	189 / 5.90 / 118	190 / 300 / 280	240 / 189 / 35	47 / 4.30 / 24	4.70 / .470 /	.710 / / / I
MCT oil (medium chain tryglycerides) *1 T⁷*	115 / 14 / /	0.0 / 14.0 / /	0.0 / / /	0.0 / / /	0.0 / / /	/ 0 / /	/ / /	/ / /	/ /	/ /	/ /	/ /	/ /	/ /	/ /	/ / / I
Microlipid *1 T*	68 / 14 / /	6.7 / 7.5 / /	/ 0.7 / /	/ 0.9 / /	/ 5.9 / /	/ 0 / /	/ / /	/ / /	/ /	/ /	/ /	/ /	/ /	/ /	/ /	/ / / I
Moducal, dry *3 ½ oz⁸*	380 / 100 / /	5.0 / 0.0 / /	0.0 / 0.0 / /	95.0 / 0.0 / /	/ 0.0 / /	/ 0 / /	/ / /	/ / /	/ /	/ /	/ /	70 / / 150	/ /	/ /	/ /	/ / / I
Phenyl-Free, dry *3 ½ oz⁹*	400 / 100 / 240 / 300	3.0 / 6.6 / 790 / 0	19.8 / 2.1 / 930 / 2000	64.0 / 1.3 / 1470 / 1070	/ 2.9 / 1600 / 550	/ 0 / 530 / 400	360 / 1190 / 300 / 30	52 / .59 / 9.9 / 6.6	.99 / 7.9 / 99	.89 / 2.50 / 30	124 / 3.00 / 84	400 / 1340 / 910	790 / 790 / 45	149 / 11.90 / 36	11.90 / 1.190 /	.990 / / / I
Protain XL *8 fl oz*	267 / 260 / 172 / 40	200.0 / 7.1 / 560 / 740	13.5 / 0.5 / 770 / 770	31.0 / 3.7 / 1350 / 970	/ 1.5 / 1150 / 540	2.2 / 1 / 380 / 420	360 / 1660 / 95 /	57 / .57 / 18.2 / 12.2	.64 / 7.6 / 28	.76 / 3.50 / 85	114 / 2.80 / 118	220 / 420 / 320	189 / 189 / 35	76 / 4.30 / 35	7.10 / .570 /	1.420 / / / I
Respalor *8 fl oz*	360 / 260 / 230 / 53	183.0 / 16.8 / 740 / 990	18.0 / 0.8 / 1020 / 1020	35.0 / 7.2 / 1800 / 1290	/ 3.6 / 1540 / 720	/ 2 / 510 / 560	250 / 830 / 67 /	50 / .63 / 12.5 / 8.4	.72 / 8.3 / 13	.83 / 2.50 / 50	67 / 4.20 / 83	300 / 350 / 400	167 / 167 / 25	67 / 3 / 17	3.30 / .330 /	.500 / / / I
Sustacal *8 fl oz¹⁰*	240 / 260 / 160 / 58	200.0 / 5.5 / 570 / 740	14.5 / 0.9 / 770 / 710	33.0 / 2.4 / 1330 / 930	/ 2.2 / 1060 / 620	/ 1 / 350 / 390	330 / 1110 / 89 /	13 / .33 / 6.7 / 4.5	.40 / 4.7 / 56	.47 / 1.33 / 67	89 / 2.30 / 56	220 / 490 / 350	240 / 220 / 33	90 / 4 /	3.30 / .470 /	.670 / / / I

	KCAL / WT (g) / TRY (mg) / CYS (mg)	H_2O (g) / FAT (g) / THR (mg) / PHE (mg)	PRO (g) / SFA (g) / ISO (mg) / TYR (mg)	CHO (g) / MUFA (g) / LEU (mg) / VAL (mg)	SUGR (g) / PUFA (g) / LYS (mg) / ARG (mg)	DFIB (g) / CHOL (mg) / MET (mg) / HIS (mg)	A (RE) / A (IU) / D (IU) / INOS (mg)	C (mg) / B-1 (mg) / E (IU) / E (AT) (mg)	B-2 (mg) / NIA (mg) / K (mcg)	B-6 (mg) / B-12 (mcg) / BIO (mcg)	FOL (mcg) / PANT (mg) / CHLN (mcg)	Na (mg) / K (mg) / Cl (mg)	Ca (mg) / P (mg) / I (mcg)	Mg (mg) / Fe (mg) / Mo (mcg)	Zn (mg) / Cu (mg) / F (mcg)	Mn (mg) / REF
Sustacal Basic 8 fl oz	250 250 108 27	200.0 9.0 390 410	9.0 0.8 420 410	34.0 5.8 830 530	 2.4 650 320	 1 210 230	189 630 50 	38 .38 5.7 3.8	.43 5.0 10 	.50 1.50 75 	100 2.50 75 	200 370 310 	125 125 19 	50 2.30 19 	2.90 .250 	.620 I
Sustacal Plus 8 fl oz	360 260 184 42	185.0 13.6 590 790	14.4 1.8 820 820	45.0 3.4 1440 1030	 8.4 1230 580	 2 410 450	300 1000 80 	18 .45 6.0 4.0	.51 6.0 16 	.60 1.80 90 	120 3.00 50 	200 350 300 	200 200 30 	80 3.60 20 	4.00 .400 	.600 I
Sustacal Powder 1 pkt	200 54 260 62	 0.3 500 570	12.4 670 660	36.0 1230 750	 810 290	 280 270	390 1300 33 	20 .40 10.0 6.7	.20 6.8 	.55 1.00 93 	135 2.70 	189 560 220 	290 250 40 	105 6 	4.00 .700 	1.000 I
Sustacal Pudding 5 oz[11]	240 142 140 34	92.0 9.5 270 310	6.8 1.5 370 360	32.0 4.2 670 410	 3.8 450 160	 4 153 147	230 750 60 14	9 .23 4.5 3.0	.26 3.0 22 	.30 .90 45 	60 1.50 28 	120 320 200 	220 220 23 	60 2.70 	2.30 .300 	.670 I
Sustacal w/ Fiber 8 fl oz[1]	250 260 130 54	200.0 8.3 430 540	10.8 1.1 570 510	33.0 2.1 1050 760	 5.1 790 410	2.6 1 260 290	250 830 100 	30 .37 5.0 3.4	.43 5.0 23 	.50 1.50 75 	100 2.50 	170 330 330 	200 167 25 	67 3 	3.30 .330 	.420 I
TraumaCal 8 fl oz[12]	355 260 250 57	185.0 16.2 800 1070	19.5 1.7 1110 1110	34.0 2.8 2000 1400	 6.9 1660 780	 2 550 610	177 590 47 	35 .45 8.9 6.0	.51 5.9 30 	.59 1.77 35 	47 3.00 59 	280 330 380 	177 177 18 	47 2.10 	3.50 .350 	.590 I
Ultracal 8 fl oz	250 260 133 31	200.0 10.6 430 570	10.4 0.5 590 590	29.0 3.9 1040 740	 1.9 890 420	3.4 1 300 330	300 1000 80 	60 .75 15.0 10.1	.85 10.0 16 	1.00 3.00 60 	80 5.00 100 	220 380 340 	200 200 30 	80 3.60 20 	4.00 .400 	.600 I
Nestle Sweet Success bar, low-fat 1 bar[13]	114 32 	 3.3 	1.7 1.6 	23.1 	10.7 	2.1 2 	 750 60 	9 .23 4.5 	.26 3.0 	.30 .90 43 	60 1.50 	 	 	 	 	 I
Sweet Success, corn syrup-based, rtd, cnd 1 can[14]	200 366 	 0.5 	9.0 0.0 	41.0 	34.0 	5.0 25 	 2500 100 	60 .38 15.0 	.43 5.0 	.50 1.50 75 	100 2.50 	 	 	 	 	 I
Sweet Success, milk-based, rtd, cnd 1 can[15]	200 316 	 3.0 	11.0 1.0 	38.0 	30.0 	6.0 5 	 1750 140 	21 .53 10.5 	.60 7.0 	.70 2.10 105 	140 3.50 	226 506 	500 350 53 	140 6.30 	5.30 .700 	 I
Sweet Success powder 1 scoop[16]	90 32 	 0.8 	3.0 0.4 	23.8 	8.2 	6.0 2 	 1250 40 	21 .45 10.5 	.26 7.0 	.70 1.20 105 	140 3.00 	 	 	 	 	 I
NutraStart, choc, rtd 11 fl oz	220 350 	 3.0 	10.0 1.0 	42.0 	35.0 	5.0 5 	 1750 140 	21 .53 10.5 	.60 7.0 20 	.70 2.10 105 	120 3.50 	220 530 0 	400 350 53 	140 2.70 26 	2.25 .000 	.700 I
NutraStart, van, rtd 11 fl oz	220 350 	 3.0 	10.0 1.0 	38.0 	33.0 	5.0 5 	 1750 140 	21 .53 10.5 	.60 7.0 10 	.70 2.10 105 	120 3.50 	460 450 	400 350 53 	140 2.70 26 	2.25 	.700 I

	KCAL WT (g) TRY (mg) CYS (mg)	H₂O (g) FAT (g) THR (mg) PHE (mg)	PRO (g) SFA (g) ISO (mg) TYR (mg)	CHO (g) MUFA (g) LEU (mg) VAL (mg)	SUGR (g) PUFA (g) LYS (mg) ARG (mg)	DFIB (g) CHOL (mg) MET (mg) HIS (mg)	A (RE) A (IU) D (IU) INOS (mg)	C (mg) B-1 (mg) E (IU) E (AT) (mg)	B-2 (mg) NIA (mg) K (mcg)	B-6 (mg) B-12 (mcg) BIO (mcg)	FOL (mcg) PANT (mg) CHLN (mcg)	Na (mg) K (mg) Cl (mg)	Ca (mg) P (mg) I (mcg)	Mg (mg) Fe (mg) Mo (mcg)	Zn (mg) Cu (mg) F (mcg)	Mn (mg) REF
Pillsbury																
Figurine Diet Bar, choc *2 bars*	200 43	1.5 10.7	4.5	22.3			 1195	20 .48	.27 5.4	.50 .95	129	93 214	113 121	74 4.86	3.03 .525	 I
Figurine Diet Bar, choc caramel *2 bars*	202 43	1.5 11.2	4.4	21.2			 1195	20 .48	.27 5.3	.50 .95	129	113 180	120 113	74 4.62	3.03 .525	 I
Figurine Diet Bar, choc peanut butter, Pillsbury *2 bars*	200 43	1.5 11.4	5.8	20.0			 1195	20 .49	.27 6.2	.50 .95	129	93 209	116 122	74 4.73	3.03 .525	 I
Figurine Diet Bar, S'mores *2 bars*	203 43	1.3 10.8	4.2	22.6			 1195	20 .49	.27 5.3	.50 .95	129	92 170	113 102	74 4.61	3.03 .525	 I
Figurine Diet Bar, van *2 bars*	203 43	1.4 10.6	4.3	22.8			 1195	20 .37	.16 5.3	.50 .95	129	95 176	118 112	74 4.62	3.03 .525	 I
R&D Labs, Amin-Acid inst drink *5.2 oz pkt[17]*	665 147 250 	 15.7 500 1100	6.6 700 	124.3 1100 	 790 	 1100 250										 I
R&D Labs, Regain Nutrition bar *2 bars (3 oz)*	330 85 230 290	 7.0 750 690	15.0 2.0 850 560	53.0 3.5 1850 920	32.0 0.0 1450 540	4.0 380 390						95 65	90 100	15		 I
Ross Labs																
Alterna *8 fl oz*	87 239	221.6 3.7	2.4	11.2								96 260	85 120	12		 I
Enrich, van *8 fl oz[18]*	260 255 103 56	195.7 8.8 385 460	9.4 1.3 469 413	38.2 2.2 873 582	 4.8 694 385	3.4 5 225 244	 849	51 .39	.44 5.1	.51 1.60	102 2.55	200 399	170 170	68 3.05	3.83 .340	.850 I
Ensure *8 fl oz[19]*	250 253 97 44	200.0 8.8 343 413	8.8 1.3 430 360	34.2 2.2 799 536	 4.8 624 343	0.0 5 237 237	 624	37 .38	.43 5.0	.50 1.50	100 2.50	200 369	125 125	50 2.25	2.82 .250	.620 I
Ensure HN *8 fl oz[20]*	250 253 115 52	198.7 8.4 419 514	10.5 1.2 514 514	33.3 2.1 943 639	 4.6 765 398	 5 283 273	 891	54 .41	.46 5.4	.54 1.70	108 2.68	190 369	179 179	71 3.21	4.01 .360	.890 I
Ensure Plus *8 fl oz[21]*	354 259 143 65	181.7 12.6 506 610	13.0 1.8 636 532	47.2 3.2 1181 792	 6.9 921 506	 5 350 350	 833	50 .50	.57 6.7	.67 2.00	134 3.33	250 459	167 167	67 2.99	3.74 .340	.830 I
Ensure Plus HN *8 fl oz[22]*	354 260 162 74	181.7 11.8 591 724	14.8 1.7 724 724	47.2 3.0 1330 901	 6.5 1079 561	0.0 5 399 384	 1248	75 .75	.85 10.0	1.00 2.99	200 4.99	280 429	250 250	100 4.49	5.62 .500	1.250 I

	KCAL / WT (g) / TRY (mg) / CYS (mg)	H₂O (g) / FAT (g) / THR (mg) / PHE (mg)	PRO (g) / SFA (g) / ISO (mg) / TYR (mg)	CHO (g) / MUFA (g) / LEU (mg) / VAL (mg)	SUGR (g) / PUFA (g) / LYS (mg) / ARG (mg)	DFIB (g) / CHOL (mg) / MET (mg) / HIS (mg)	A (RE) / A (IU) / D (IU) / INOS (mg)	C (mg) / B-1 (mg) / E (IU) / E (AT) (mg)	B-2 (mg) / NIA (mg) / K (mcg)	B-6 (mg) / B-12 (mcg) / BIO (mcg)	FOL (mcg) / PANT (mg) / CHLN (mcg)	Na (mg) / K (mg) / Cl (mg)	Ca (mg) / P (mg) / I (mcg)	Mg (mg) / Fe (mg) / Mo (mcg)	Zn (mg) / Cu (mg) / F (mcg)	Mn (mg) / REF
Ensure Pudding	250	90.9	6.8	34.0				15	.29	.34	68	240	200	68	3.83	.850
5 fl oz[23]	142	9.7	2.4	6.2	0.8	10	849	.26	3.4	1.10	1.70	330	200	3.06	.340	
	102	299	340	673	530	184										
	54	319	306	435	224	163										I
Glucerna	237	206.6	9.9	22.2		3.4		50	.43	.50	100	220	167	67	3.74	.840
8 fl oz	239	13.2				5	833	.38	5.0	1.50	2.50	369	167	2.99	.340	
	109	395	504	909	741	296										
	40	474	544	632	356	277										I
Introlite	125	217.7	5.3	16.7				54	.46	.54	108	220	179	72	4.05	.900
8 fl oz	240	4.4				1	896	.40	5.4	1.61	2.70	371	179	3.24	.360	
	58	205	257	478	393	142										
	26	247	215	320	204	142										I
Jevity	250	196.7	10.5	35.8		3.4		54	.46	.54	108	220	214	71	4.01	.890
8 fl oz	246	8.7				5	891	.41	5.4	1.70	2.68	369	179	3.21	.360	
	115	419	535	964	786	314										
	42	503	504	671	377	293										I
Osmolite	250	198.7	8.8	34.2				37	.43	.50	100	150	125	50	2.82	.620
8 fl oz[24]	253	9.1	4.4	1.2	3.0	5	624	.38	5.0	1.50	2.50	240	125	2.25	.250	
	97	343	430	799	624	237										
	44	413	360	536	343	237										I
Osmolite HN	250	198.7	10.5	33.3				54	.46	.54	108	220	179	71	4.01	.890
8 fl oz[25]	253	8.7	4.2	1.2	2.8	5	891	.41	5.4	1.70	2.68	369	179	3.21	.360	
	115	409	514	954	744	283										
	52	493	430	639	409	283										I
Pediasure	237	199.7	7.1	26.0				24	.50	.62	88	90	230	47	2.80	.590
8 fl oz	245	11.8				5	609	.64	4.0	1.40	2.40	309	190	3.29	.240	
																I
Polycose liquid	200	70.0	0.0	50.0								70	20			
100 ml[26]	120	0.0	0.0		0.0	0						6	3			
	0	0	0	0	0	0										
	0	0	0	0	0	0										I
Polycose powder	380		6.0	94.0								110	30			
3.5 oz	100	0.0										10	5			
																I
Pro Mod	119	2.5	21.0	2.8								64	187			
1 oz[27]	28	2.5										276	140			
																I
Pulmocare	354	185.7	14.8	25.0				75	.85	1.00	200	309	250	100	5.62	1.250
8 fl oz[28]	250	21.8	3.2	5.4	12.0	5	1248	.75	10.0	2.99	4.99	409	250	4.49	.500	
	163	591	754	1359	1108	443										
	59	709	709	946	532	414										I
Replena	474	168.7	7.1	60.5				25	.68	2.04	250	186	303	100	5.62	1.250
8 fl oz	259	22.7					250	.60	8.0	2.40	3.99	265	173	4.49	.500	
																I
SLD (Surgical Liquid Diet)	166	194.0	8.9	32.3				18	.51	.59	118	198	198	79	4.50	.990
8 fl oz[29]	236	0.1	0.0		0.0	0	987	.46	5.9	1.77	2.96	213	198	3.55	.390	
	98	452	488	816	665	293										
	222	630	399	674	621	240										I

	KCAL / WT (g) / TRY (mg) / CYS (mg)	H₂O (g) / FAT (g) / THR (mg) / PHE (mg)	PRO (g) / SFA (g) / ISO (mg) / TYR (mg)	CHO (g) / MUFA (g) / LEU (mg) / VAL (mg)	SUGR (g) / PUFA (g) / LYS (mg) / ARG (mg)	DFIB (g) / CHOL (mg) / MET (mg) / HIS (mg)	A (RE) / A (IU) / D (IU) / INOS (mg)	C (mg) / B-1 (mg) / E (IU) / E (AT) (mg)	B-2 (mg) / NIA (mg) / K (mcg)	B-6 (mg) / B-12 (mcg) / BIO (mcg)	FOL (mcg) / PANT (mg) / CHLN (mcg)	Na (mg) / K (mg) / Cl (mg)	Ca (mg) / P (mg) / I (mcg)	Mg (mg) / Fe (mg) / Mo (mcg)	Zn (mg) / Cu (mg) / F (mcg)	Mn (mg) / / / REF
TwoCal HN	474	168.7	19.8	51.3				75	.68	.80	160	309	250	100	5.62	1.250
8 fl oz	262	21.5	6.0	4.9	9.6	7	1248	.60	8.0	2.40	3.99	579	250	4.49	.500	
	217	791	1008	1818	1482	593										
	79	949	949	1265	712	554										I
Vital High Nitrogen	237	205.0	9.9	43.7				47	.54	.63	126	134	158	63	3.55	.790
8 fl oz[30]	262	2.6	1.1	0.3	1.0	4	789	.47	6.3	1.89	3.15	331	158	2.84	.320	
	108	375	453	789	522	217										
	89	444	375	552	542	256										I
Sandoz Nutrition	170	1.0	10.5	31.1				60	.91	1.10	210	170	270	107	4.00	1.300
Citrotein, orange flavor	45	0.4				0	1330	.80	10.7	3.20	5.30	140	270	9.60	.530	
1.57 oz pkg[31]							107	8.0		160	9	200	40			
																I
Compleat DiabetiSource	250	212.0	12.5	22.5		1.1		50	.43	.50	100	250	167	67	3.83	.830
250 ml	262	12.2				21	1670	.38	5.0	1.50	2.50	350	217	3	.330	
							67	7.5	17	75	50	283	25	50		
																I
Compleat, mod formula	265	209.0	10.7	35.0				15	.43	.50	67	250	167	67	3.83	.670
250 ml can[32]	266	9.2				13	833	.38	5.0	1.50	1.67	350	217	3	.330	
							67	7.5	17	50	50	283	25	50		
																I
Compleat, reg formula	265	211.0	10.7	31.7				15	.43	.50	67	317	167	67	3.83	.670
250 ml can[33]	266	10.7				13	833	.38	5.0	1.50	1.67	350	300	3	.330	
							67	7.5	17	50	50	283	25	50		
																I
FiberSource	300	206.0	10.8	42.3		2.5		50	.57	.67	67	283	167	67	4.17	.830
250 ml can[34]	272	10.4				1	833	.50	6.7	2.00	3.33	450	167	3	.330	
							67	7.5	16	100	83	283	32	50		
																I
FiberSource HN	300	205.0	13.3	39.7		1.7		50	.57	.67	67	283	167	67	4.17	.830
250 ml can[35]	272	10.4				1	833	.50	6.7	2.00	3.33	450	167	3	.330	
							67	7.5	16	100	83	283	32	50		
																I
Impact	250	213.0	14.0	32.9				20	.43	.37	100	267	200	67	3.75	.500
250 ml[36]	273	6.9				14	1670	.50	5.0	2.00	1.67	350	200	3	.420	
							67	15.0	17	50	67	333	25	50		
																I
Impact 1.5	375	195.0	20.9	35.3				24	.51	.44	120	320	240	80	4.50	.600
250 ml	272	17.2				25	2000	.60	6.0	2.40	2.00	420	240	3.60	.500	
							80	18.0	20	60	80	400	30	60		
																I
Impact w/ fiber	250	217.0	14.0	33.8		2.5		20	.43	.37	100	267	200	67	3.75	.500
250 ml	273	6.9				14	1670	.50	5.0	2.00	1.67	350	200	3	.420	
							67	15.0	17	50	67	333	25	50		
																I
IsoSource 1.5	375	194.0	16.9	42.0		2.0		80	.91	1.07	161	322	268	107	8.04	1.340
250 ml	273	16.2				2	2680	.80	10.7	3.22	5.36	536	268	4.82	.540	
							107	16.1	27	121	134	402	40	67		
																I
IsoSource HN, van	300	205.0	13.3	39.2				5	.57	.67	67	267	167	67	4.17	.830
250 ml[2]	270	10.4				1	833	.50	6.7	2.00	3.33	417	167	3	.330	
							67	7.5	16	100	83	283	32	50		
																I

							Vitamins					Minerals				
	KCAL	H_2O (g)	PRO (g)	CHO (g)	SUGR (g)	DFIB (g)	A (RE)	C (mg)	B-2 (mg)	B-6 (mg)	FOL (mcg)	Na (mg)	Ca (mg)	Mg (mg)	Zn (mg)	Mn (mg)
	WT (g)	FAT (g)	SFA (g)	MUFA (g)	PUFA (g)	CHOL (mg)	A (IU)	B-1 (mg)	NIA (mg)	B-12 (mcg)	PANT (mg)	K (mg)	P (mg)	Fe (mg)	Cu (mg)	
	TRY (mg)	THR (mg)	ISO (mg)	LEU (mg)	LYS (mg)	MET (mg)	D (IU)	E (IU)	K (mcg)	BIO (mcg)	CHLN (mcg)	Cl (mg)	I (mcg)	Mo (mcg)	F (mcg)	
	CYS (mg)	PHE (mg)	TYR (mg)	VAL (mg)	ARG (mg)	HIS (mg)	INOS (mg)	E (AT) (mg)								REF
IsoSource Standard, van	300	205.0	10.8	41.7				50	.57	.67	67	300	167	67	4.17	.830
250 ml[1]	270	10.4				1	833	.50	6.7	2.00	3.33	417	167	3.00	.330	
							67	7.5	16	100	83	283	32	50		
																I
IsoSource VHN	250	212.0	15.6	32.0		2.5		60	.68	.80	120	320	200	80	6.00	1.000
250 ml	269	7.2				2	2000	.60	8.0	2.40	4.00	400	200	3.60	.400	
							80	12.0	20	90	100	340	30	50		
																I
Isotein HN	350	3.0	20.0	46.7				15	.43	.50	67	183	167	67	2.50	.670
2.9 oz powder[37]	82	10.0				45	833	.38	3.3	1.00	1.67	317	167	3	.330	
							67	5.0	17	50	17	283	25	50		
																I
Merimix custard, from mix	90		6.0	15.0				1	.27	.05		120	14	17	.18	
½ cup	113	0.0	0.0	0.0	0.0	10	23	.04	0.1	.44	.38	190	120	.12	.010	
								.0								
																I
Meritene, prep w/ whole milk	280	213.0	18.0	31.0				15	.68	.50	100	280	570	100	3.75	1.000
1.14 oz powder in 237 ml milk[38]	270	9.0				40	1250	.38	5.0	1.80	2.50	730	500	4.50	.500	
							100	7.5	20	80	75	570	38			
																I
Nutrisource custard, from mix	140		6.0	20.0				1	.20	.05		130	150	15	.49	
½ cup	113	4.0				20	180	.03	0.1	.45	.41	190	130	.11	.010	
							48	.0								
																I
Nutrisource custard, red cal, from mix	80		6.0	15.0				1	.20	.05		110	190	18	.46	
½ cup	113	0.0	0.0	0.0	0.0	5	485	.05	0.1	.65	.41	200	140	.77	.020	
							50	.0								
																I
Nutrisource custard, van, rte	140		7.0	18.0					.32	.07		125		22	.48	
½ cup	113	4.0				20	170	.07	0.2	.67	.57	275				
																I
Resource Diabetic, van	250	200.0	15.0	23.4		3.0		38	.43	.50	100	230	220	50	2.81	.630
237 ml	251	11.1				1250	.38	5.0	1.50	2.50	270	220	2.25	.250		
							50	5.6	12	75	38	215	25	19		
																I
Resource eggnog nonalcoholic mix in whole milk	290		15.0	37.0		0.0		11	.65	.16	0	220	470	59	1.14	.010
1.23 oz mix in 8 fl oz milk	257	9.0	5.7			35	1090	.29	4.2	1.90	1.30	600	370	3.70	.070	
							140	.0								
																I
Resource fortified pudding, from mix, prep w/whole milk	250		9.0	35.0				11	.37	.36	70	140	270	72	2.70	.010
½ cup[39]	164	8.0				20	900	.27	3.6	1.10	1.80	702	270	3.20	.360	
							72	5.4								
																I
Resource fortified pudding, frzn	250		9.0	35.0				12	.34	.04		160	200	80	3.00	
5 oz[40]	142	8.0					1000	.30	4.0	1.20		433	200	3.60	.440	
							80	6.0								
																I
Resource Fruit Beverage	180	207.0	8.8	36.0				38	.43	.50	50	135	50	3.75	.500	
237 ml	253						625	.38	5.0	1.50	1.25	160	2.25	.250		
							50	5.7	9	38	130	220	19			
																I

	KCAL	H$_2$O (g)	PRO (g)	CHO (g)	SUGR (g)	DFIB (g)		Vitamins					Minerals			
							A (RE)	C (mg)	B-2 (mg)	B-6 (mg)	FOL (mcg)	Na (mg)	Ca (mg)	Mg (mg)	Zn (mg)	Mn (mg)
	WT (g)	FAT (g)	SFA (g)	MUFA (g)	PUFA (g)	CHOL (mg)	A (IU)	B-1 (mg)	NIA (mg)	B-12 (mcg)	PANT (mg)	K (mg)	P (mg)	Fe (mg)	Cu (mg)	
	TRY (mg)	THR (mg)	ISO (mg)	LEU (mg)	LYS (mg)	MET (mg)	D (IU)	E (IU)	K (mcg)	BIO (mcg)	CHLN (mcg)	Cl (mg)	I (mcg)	Mo (mcg)	F (mcg)	
	CYS (mg)	PHE (mg)	TYR (mg)	VAL (mg)	ARG (mg)	HIS (mg)	INOS (mg)	E (AT) (mg)								REF
Resource Healthshake 4 fl oz	190		6.0	32.0				9	.26	.30		103	150	60	2.25	
	136					5	750	.23	3.0	.90	1.50	267	150	2.70	.300	
							60	4.5								
																I
Resource Healthshake, eggnog 6 fl oz	280		9.0	48.0				12	.34	.40		140	200	80	3.00	
	200	6.0				5	1000	.30	4.0	1.20	2.00	400	200	3.60	.400	
							80	6.0								
																I
Resource Healthshake, strawberry/van w/ aspartame 4 fl oz	190		8.0	23.0				9	.26	.30		160	150	60	2.25	
	136	6.0				5	750	.23	3.0	.90		250	150	2.70	.270	
							60	4.5								
																I
Resource high protein broth, beef/chicken, from mix 6 fl oz	120		7.0	22.0			0	0	.02	.01	2	370	10	3	.07	.030
	183	0.4				1	0	.05	0.1	.11	.02	125	110	.08	.020	
																I
Resource high protein gelatin, all flavors, from mix 4 fl oz	150		12.0	26.0					.26		0	120	10			
	140	0.0	0.0	0.0	0.0	0		.01	0.1	.06	.20	140	14	.16		
																I
Resource Just for Kids, van 237 ml	237	202.0	7.1	26.0				24	.50	.62	88	90	270	47	2.80	.590
	250	11.8				3	830	.64	4.0	1.40	2.40	310	190	3.30	.240	
							120	5.4	10	76	71	200	28	17		
																I
Resource Milk Shake, mix in whole milk 8 fl oz[41]	263		9.0	41.0				12	.34	.40		193	300	80	3.00	
	263	9.0				35	1000	.30	4.0	1.20		420	200	3.60	.390	
							120	6.0								
																I
Resource Milk Shake Plus, mix in whole milk 8 fl oz[41]	290		15.0	37.0				21	.76	.70		235	450	140	5.30	
	260	9.0				40	1750	.34	7.0	1.50		712	400	6.30	.700	
							140	11.0								
																I
Resource Nutritious Juice Drink, all flavors 6 fl oz	190		6.0	41.0				60	.34	.40		100	200	80	.30	
	186	0.0	0.0	0.0	0.0	0	1000	.30	4.0	1.20	2.00	50	200	3.60	.400	
							80	6.0								
																I
Resource Plus, van 237 ml[42]	355	181.0	13.0	47.3				38	.65	.75	75					
	256	12.6				890		.63	7.5	2.25	2.00					
							70	7.8	13	56	125					
																I
Resource Shake, lactose controlled 6 fl oz[41]	270		9.0	45.0				12	.34	.40		180	200	60	3.00	
	200	6.0				5	750	.30	4.0	1.20	2.00	333	200	3.60	.400	
							80	6.0								
																I
Resource Shake Plus 8 fl oz[41]	400		15.0	58.0				21	.60	.70	140	260	350	60	5.25	
	259	12.0				10	1750	.53	7.0	2.10	3.50	343	350	6.30	.700	
							140	10.5								
																I
Resource Shake, thickened, van 6 fl oz	270		9.0	45.0				12	.34	.40		190	200	60	3.00	
	200	6.0				5	750	.30	4.0	1.20	2.00	400	200	3.60	.400	
							80	6.0								
																I

	KCAL / WT (g) / TRY (mg) / CYS (mg)	H₂O (g) / FAT (g) / THR (mg) / PHE (mg)	PRO (g) / SFA (g) / ISO (mg) / TYR (mg)	CHO (g) / MUFA (g) / LEU (mg) / VAL (mg)	SUGR (g) / PUFA (g) / LYS (mg) / ARG (mg)	DFIB (g) / CHOL (mg) / MET (mg) / HIS (mg)	A (RE) / A (IU) / D (IU) / INOS (mg)	C (mg) / B-1 (mg) / E (IU) / E (AT)	B-2 (mg) / NIA (mg) / K (mcg)	B-6 (mg) / B-12 (mcg) / BIO (mcg)	FOL (mcg) / PANT (mg) / CHLN (mcg)	Na (mg) / K (mg) / Cl (mg)	Ca (mg) / P (mg) / I (mcg)	Mg (mg) / Fe (mg) / Mo (mcg)	Zn (mg) / Cu (mg) / F (mcg)	Mn (mg) / REF
Resource Standard, van 237 ml	250	199.0	8.8	34.3				38	.43	.50	50	210	125	50	3.75	.500
	253	8.8				625	.38	0.5	1.50	1.25	380	125	2.25	.250		
							50	5.7	9	38	130	238	19			
																I
Resource Thicken Up 1 T	15		0.0	4.0				4	.00	.13		10	10	5	1.00	
	4	0.0	0.0	0.0	0.0	0	333	.10	1.3	.04	.66	0	7	1.20	.130	
							27	2.0								
																I
SandoSource Peptide 250 ml	250	210.0	12.5	40.8				43	.49			300	143	57	3.29	.430
	270	4.4					1430	.43	5.7			400	143	2.57	.290	
							57	6.4	11		57	243	21	36		
																I
Tolerex 2.82 oz powder	300	4.8	6.2	68.0				10	.28	.33	67	141	167	67	2.50	.470
	80	0.4					833	.25	3.3	1.00	1.67	350	167	3	.330	
							67	5.0	11	50	12	283	25	25		
																I
Vivonex Pediatric 250 ml[43]	200	220.0	6.0	31.5				25	.45	.50	50	100	243	50	3.00	.500
	270	5.9					625	.38	5.0	.75	1.25	300	200	2.50	.300	
							125	7.5	10	25	50	250	30	19		
																I
Vivonex Plus 300 ml[44]	300	255.0	13.5	57.0				20	.57	.67	133	183	167	67	3.75	.500
	329	2.0					1250	.50	6.7	2.00	3.33	317	167	3	.330	
							100	7.5	13	100	67	283	27	42		
																I
Vivonex Ten 2.84 oz powder[45]	300	6.0	11.5	61.7				18	.51	.60	120	138	150	60	3.00	.280
	80	0.8					750	.45	6.0	1.80	3.00	235	150	2.70	.300	
							60	4.5	7	90	22	246	23	15		
																I
Slim Fast Foods Slim-Fast bar, dutch choc 1.2 oz	140		5.0	20.0	13.0	2.0		15	.43	.40	40	80	40	16	3.75	
	34	5.0	2.0			1250	.38	5.0	1.50	2.50	150	40	4.50	.500		
							80	7.5			75		38			
																I
Slim-Fast bar, peanut butter 1.2 oz	150		6.0	19.0	10.0	2.0		15	.43	.40	40	80	40	16	3.75	
	34	5.0	3.0			1250	.38	5.0	1.50	2.50	150	40	4.50	.500		
							80	7.5			75		38			
																I
Slim-Fast powder, choc 1 oz[46]	100		5.0	20.0	17.0	2.0		18	.26	.60	100	110	150	100	4.50	
	28	1.0	0.5			750	.45	7.0	1.20	2.50	270	100	6.30	.400		
							40	15.0			105		15			
																I
Slim-Fast powder, choc malt 1 oz[46]	100		5.0	20.0	17.0	2.0		18	.26	.60	100	120	150	100	4.50	
	28	1.0	0.5			750	.45	7.0	1.20	2.50	240	100	6.30	.400		
							40	15.0			105		15			
																I
Slim-Fast powder, strawberry 1 oz[46]	100		5.0	20.0	18.0	2.0		18	.26	.60	100	130	150	100	4.50	
	28	0.5	0.0			750	.45	7.0	1.20	2.50	210	100	6.30	.400		
							40	15.0			105		15			
																I
Slim-Fast powder, van 1 oz[46]	100		5.0	20.0	18.0	2.0		18	.26	.60	100	130	150	100	4.50	
	28	0.5	0.0			750	.45	7.0	1.20	2.50	210	100	6.30	.400		
							40	15.0			105		15			
																I

	KCAL	H₂O (g)	PRO (g)	CHO (g)	SUGR (g)	DFIB (g)	A (RE)	C (mg)	B-2 (mg)	B-6 (mg)	FOL (mcg)	Na (mg)	Ca (mg)	Mg (mg)	Zn (mg)	Mn (mg)
	WT (g)	FAT (g)	SFA (g)	MUFA (g)	PUFA (g)	CHOL (mg)	A (IU)	B-1 (mg)	NIA (mg)	B-12 (mcg)	PANT (mg)	K (mg)	P (mg)	Fe (mg)	Cu (mg)	
	TRY (mg)	THR (mg)	ISO (mg)	LEU (mg)	LYS (mg)	MET (mg)	D (IU)	E (IU)	K (mcg)	BIO (mcg)	CHLN (mcg)	Cl (mg)	I (mcg)	Mo (mcg)	F (mcg)	
	CYS (mg)	PHE (mg)	TYR (mg)	VAL (mg)	ARG (mg)	HIS (mg)	INOS (mg)	E (AT) (mg)								REF
Ultra Slim-Fast bar, chewy caramel crunch	120		1.0	22.0	18.0	2.0		4	.26	.30	60	45			.60	
1 oz	28	3.5	2.0			300		.09	3.0	.90	1.50			2.70		
							60	4.5			45		3			
																I
Ultra Slim-Fast bar, choc chip crunch	120		1.0	16.0	11.0	2.0		9	.26	.30	60	40	150		.60	
1 oz	28	4.0	2.0			0	750	.15	3.0	.90	1.50	110	150	2.70	.800	
							60	4.5			30		23			
																I
Ultra Slim-Fast bar, peanut butter crunch	120		2.0	19.0	13.0	2.0		9	.26	.30	60	45	150	16	.60	
1 oz	28	4.0	2.0			0	750	.23	3.0	.90	1.00	100	150	2.70		
							60	4.5			30		3			
																I
Ultra Slim-Fast bar, peanut caramel crunch	120		1.0	22.0	18.0	2.0		6	.26	.30	60	35	150		.60	
1 oz	28	4.0	2.0			500		.23	3.0	.90	1.00		150	2.70		
							60	4.5			30		3			
																I
Ultra Slim-Fast, Juice Base, rtd, apple cran raspberry	220		7.0	46.0	41.0	5.0		60	.43	.50	100	240	250	100	3.75	
11.5 fl oz	350	1.5	0.5			10	2500	.38	5.0	1.50	2.50	200	250	4.50		
							100	15.0			75		38			
																I
Ultra Slim-Fast, Juice Base, rtd, orange pineapple	220		7.0	48.0	43.0	5.0		60	.43	.50	100	260	250	100	3.75	
11.5 fl oz	350	1.5	0.5			10	2500	.38	5.0	1.50	2.50	190	250	4.50		
							100	15.0			75		38			
																I
Ultra Slim-Fast, Juice Base, rtd, orange strawberry banana	220		7.0	47.0	42.0	5.0		60	.43	.50	100	240	250	100	3.75	
11.5 fl oz	350	1.5	0.5			10	2500	.38	5.0	1.50	2.50	200	250	4.50		
							100	15.0			75		38			
																I
Ultra Slim-Fast powder, cafe mocha	120		5.0	24.0	18.0	5.0		27	.17	.60	100	110	150	100	4.50	.700
1.2 oz[46]	33	1.0	0.5			5	750	.45	10.0	2.10	4.00	210	100	6.30	.500	
							100	30.0	20		150	68	15	26		
																I
Ultra Slim-Fast powder, choc fudge	120		5.0	24.0	16.0	5.0		27	.17	.60	100	100	150	100	4.50	.700
1.2 oz[46]	33	2.0	1.0			5	750	.45	10.0	2.10	4.00	340	100	6.30	.500	
							100	30.0	20		150	68	15	26		
																I
Ultra Slim-Fast powder, choc malt	120		5.0	24.0	18.0	5.0		27	.17	.60	100	100	150	100	4.50	.700
1.2 oz[46]	33	1.0	0.5			5	750	.45	10.0	2.10	4.00	220	100	6.30	.500	
							100	30.0	20		150	68	15	26		
																I
Ultra Slim-Fast powder, choc royale	110		5.0	24.0	17.0	5.0		27	.17	.60	100	130	150	100	4.50	.700
1.2 oz[46]	33	1.0	0.5			5	750	.45	10.0	2.10	4.00	280	100	6.30	.500	
							100	30.0	20		150	68	15	26		
																I
Ultra Slim-Fast powder, fruit juice	120		5.0	24.0	18.0	5.0		27	.17	.60	100	110	150	100	4.50	.700
1.1 oz[46]	31	1.0	0.0			5	750	.45	10.0	2.10	4.00	210	200	6.30	.500	
							100	30.0	20		150	68	15	26		
																I
Ultra Slim-Fast powder, milk choc	120		5.0	24.0	15.0	6.0		27	.17	.60	100	120	150	100	4.50	.700
1.2 oz[46]	33	1.0	0.0				750	.45	10.0	2.10	4.00	340	100	6.30	.500	
							100	30.0	20		150	68	15	26		
																I

	KCAL / WT (g) / TRY (mg) / CYS (mg)	H₂O (g) / FAT (g) / THR (mg) / PHE (mg)	PRO (g) / SFA (g) / ISO (mg) / TYR (mg)	CHO (g) / MUFA (g) / LEU (mg) / VAL (mg)	SUGR (g) / PUFA (g) / LYS (mg) / ARG (mg)	DFIB (g) / CHOL (mg) / MET (mg) / HIS (mg)	Vitamins A (RE) / A (IU) / D (IU) / INOS (mg)	C (mg) / B-1 (mg) / E (IU) / E (AT) (mg)	B-2 (mg) / NIA (mg) / K (mcg)	B-6 (mg) / B-12 (mcg) / BIO (mcg)	FOL (mcg) / PANT (mg) / CHLN (mcg)	Minerals Na (mg) / K (mg) / Cl (mg)	Ca (mg) / P (mg) / I (mcg)	Mg (mg) / Fe (mg) / Mo (mcg)	Zn (mg) / Cu (mg) / F (mcg)	Mn (mg) / REF
Ultra Slim-Fast powder, strawberry 1.2 oz[46]	120		5.0	25.0	20.0	4.0		27	.17	.60	100	130	150	100	4.50	.700
	33	0.5	0.0			5	750	.45	10.0	2.10	4.00	170	100	6.30	.500	
							100	30.0	20		150	68	15	26		
																I
Ultra Slim-Fast powder, van 1.2 oz[46]	110		5.0	22.0	16.0	6.0		27	.17	.60	100	130	150	100	4.50	.700
	33	0.5	0.0			5	750	.45	10.0	2.10	4.00	140	100	6.30	.500	
							100	30.0	20		150	68	15	26		
																I
Ultra Slim-Fast, rtd, choc fudge 11 fl oz	220		10.0	42.0	34.0	5.0		21	.60	.70	120	300	400	140	2.25	.700
	350	3.0	1.0			5	1750	.53	7.0	2.10	3.50	530	350	2.70	.000	
							140	10.5	20		105	0	53	26		
																I
Ultra Slim-Fast, rtd, choc royale 11 fl oz	220		10.0	38.0	33.0	5.0		21	.60	.70	120	220	400	140	2.25	.700
	350	3.0	1.0			5	1750	.53	7.0	2.10	3.50	530	350	2.70	.000	
							140	10.5	20		105	0	53	26		
																I
Ultra Slim-Fast, rtd, coffee 11 fl oz	220		10.0	38.0	33.0	5.0		21	.60	.70	120	300	400	140	2.25	.700
	350	3.0	0.5			5	1750	.53	7.0	2.10	3.50	500	350	2.70	.000	
							140	10.5	20		105	0	53	26		
																I
Ultra Slim-Fast, rtd, milk choc 11 fl oz	220		10.0	42.0	35.0	5.0		21	.60	.70	120	220	400	140	2.25	.700
	350	3.0	1.0			5	1750	.53	7.0	2.10	3.50	530	350	2.70	.000	
							140	10.5	20		105	0	53	26		
																I
Ultra Slim-Fast, rtd, strawberry 11 fl oz	220		10.0	42.0	37.0	5.0		21	.60	.70	120	460	400	140	2.25	.700
	350	3.0	1.0			5	1750	.53	7.0	2.10	3.50	450	350	2.70	.000	
							140	10.5	20		105	0	53	26		
																I
Ultra Slim-Fast, rtd, van 11 fl oz	220		10.0	38.0	33.0	5.0		21	.60	.70	120	460	400	140	2.25	.700
	350	3.0	1.0			5	1750	.53	7.0	2.10	3.50	450	350	2.70	.000	
							140	10.5	20		105	0	53	26		
																I

1. Enteral formula.
2. High nitrogen enteral formula.
3. High branched chain, low aromatic amino acids for patients with chronic liver disease; for oral or tube feeding; available in chocolate, custard, and eggnog flavors; requires 280 g water to reconstitute.
4. Used to increase the protein content of the diets of children and adults.
5. Ready-to-use high nitrogen elemental diet.
6. Nutrionally complete formula to meet the dietary needs of most tube-fed patients.
7. Substitute or supplemental source of fat calories for patients with poor digestion, absorption, or utilization of conventional food fats. The lipid fraction (coconut oil) contains less than 6% fatty acids shorter than C8, 67% fatty acids with C8 (caprylic), and less than 4% fatty acids longer than C10.
8. Refined readily digestible carbohydrate which can be added to foods to increase caloric content for patients with increased caloric requirements; 100% maltodextrin from hydrolysis of corn starch.
9. Used in the management of phenylketonuria. Contains less than 2.5 mg phenylalaine.
10. Complete or supplemental oral formula for patients who have difficulty meeting nutritional requirements through normal diets.
11. Nutritionally complete dietary supplement.
12. Oral or tube nutritionally complete feeding for patients with multiple traumas or major burns having elevated caloric requirements, exceptional nitrogen needs, and volume restrictions.

13. Values are averages for apple cinnamon spice, caramel honey & nougat, chewy chocolate brownie, chewy chocolate chip, chewy chocolate peanut butter, oatmeal raisin & almond, and peanut butter & caramel.
14. Values are averages for berry, orange peach, orange pineapple, and strawberry banana.
15. Values are averages for chocolate mint, chocolate mocha supreme, chocolate raspberry, creamy milk chocolate, creamy vanilla delite, dark chocolate fudge, rich chocolate almond, and strawberries 'n cream.
16. Values are averages for chocolate mocha supreme, creamy milk chocolate, creamy vanilla delight, dark chocolate fudge, and rich chocolate almond.
17. Essential amino acids plus histidine for uremic patients; for oral or tube feeding; available in berry, lemon-lime, orange, and strawberry flavors; requires 250 g water to reconstitute.
18. Fiber-containing, nutritionally complete liquid formula suitable for patients who do not require a low-residue diet; may be fed orally or by tube.
19. Oral/tube, liquid, low-residue feeding; complete, balanced formula.
20. Nutrient-dense, high-nitrogen, low-residue liquid food for patients with energy requirements less than 2000 kcal/day (elderly, comatose) or those with elevated nitrogen requirements; may be fed orally or by tube.
21. Nutritionally complete, high-calorie liquid food providing 1.5 kcal/ml;

useful when extra energy and nutrients are needed with normal protein concentration in a limited volume; oral or tube feeding.

22. Nutritionally complete, high-calorie, high-nitrogen liquid food, designed to meet the needs of stressed patients with higher energy and protein needs or for those with limited volume tolerance.

23. Calorically dense supplement for patients in need of increased nutrient intake.

24. Isotonic, low-residue, liquid, complete, balanced formula for hospitalized patients who require tube feeding (nasogastric, nasoduodenal, jejunal); may also be used for oral feeding.

25. Nutrient-dense, high nitrogen, isotonic, low-residue liquid food for patients with energy requirements less than 2000 kcal/day or for patients with elevated nitrogen requirements who require tube feeding; may also be used for oral feeding.

26. Glucose polymers for energy support to be mixed with food or beverage; may be used as enteral carbohydrate supplement.

27. Protein supplement to be used enterally or orally.

28. High-fat, low-carbohydrate enteral formula designed to reduce carbon dioxide production, thereby minimizing carbon dioxide retention resulting from chronic obstructive pulmonary disease, or acute respiratory failure. Can be used for enteral tube feeding

29. Highly fortified, low-residue, low-fat formula for patients restricted to clear liquid diets.

30. Nutritionally complete elemental diet for patients with impaired gastrointestinal function.

31. Fruit flavored nutritional supplement for patients with elevated protein, calorie, and nutrient needs; appropriate for clear liquid diets.

32. Ready-to-use liquid tube feeding formulated from natural foods providing complete, balanced nutrition in a lactose-free, low sodium, isotonic fomula; for short and long term tube-fed patients with normal gastrointestinal tracts.

33. Ready-to-use liquid tube feeding formulated from natural foods for short and long term tube-fed patients with normal gastrointestinal tracts; complete, balanced nutrition.

34. Complete liquid formula with fiber for short and long term patients with maintenance protein needs.

35. High nitrogen, complete liquid formula with fiber for short and long term patients with elevated protein needs.

36. Ready-to-use enteral formula for nutritional support of the immune system under metabolic stress due to trauma, sepsis, cancer, burn, or surgery.

37. Nutritionally complete, lactose-free formula for oral or tube feeding.

38. Enteral formula available in chocolate, eggnog, milk chocolate, plain, and vanilla.

39. Values are averages for chocolate, lemon, and vanilla.

40. Values are averages for butterscotch, chocolate, and vanilla.

41. Values are averages for chocolate, strawberry, and vanilla.

42. Ready-to-use, high calorie nutritional formula; concentrated source of calories and essential nutrients in a lactose free formula; available in chocolate, strawberry, and vanilla.

43. Contains 1.7 oz powder in 220 ml water.

44. Contains 2.8 oz powder in 250 ml water.

45. Elemental chemically defined diet.

46. Contains aspartame.

	KCAL	H$_2$O (g)	PRO (g)	CHO (g)	SUGR (g)	DFIB (g)	A (RE)	C (mg)	B-2 (mg)	B-6 (mg)	FOL (mcg)	Na (mg)	Ca (mg)	Mg (mg)	Zn (mg)	Mn (mg)
	WT (g)	FAT (g)	SFA (g)	MUFA (g)	PUFA (g)	CHOL (mg)	A (IU)	B-1 (mg)	NIA (mg)	B-12 (mcg)	PANT (mg)	K (mg)	P (mg)	Fe (mg)	Cu (mg)	REF

30. SPICES, HERBS, & FLAVORINGS

	KCAL/WT	H₂O/FAT	PRO/SFA	CHO/MUFA	SUGR/PUFA	DFIB/CHOL	A(RE)/A(IU)	C/B-1	B-2/NIA	B-6/B-12	FOL/PANT	Na/K	Ca/P	Mg/Fe	Zn/Cu	Mn/REF
allspice, ground	5	0.2	0.1	1.4		0.4	1	1	.00	.01	1	2	13	3	.02	.059
1 t	2.0	0.2	0.1	0.0	0.0	0	11	.00	0.1	.00		21	2	.14	.011	802
anise seed	7	0.2	0.4	1.0		0.3	1	0	.01	.01	0	0	13	3	.11	.046
1 t	2.0	0.3	0.0	0.2	0.1	0	6	.01	0.1	.00	.02	29	9	.74	.018	802
basil, fresh	1	4.5	0.1	0.2		0.2	19	1	.00	.01	3	0	8	4	.04	.072
2 T	5	0.0	0.0	0.0	0.0	0	193	.00	0.0	.00	.01	23	3	.16	.014	802
basil, ground	3	0.1	0.1	0.6		0.4	9	1	.00	.01	3	0	21	4	.06	.032
1 t	1.0	0.0	0.0	0.0	0.0	0	94	.00	0.1	.00		34	5	.42	.014	802
bay leaf, crumbled	3	0.1	0.1	0.7		0.3	6	0	.00	.01	2	0	8	1	.04	.082
1 t	1.0	0.1	0.0	0.0	0.0	0	62	.00	0.0	.00		5	1	.43	.004	802
Butter Buds mix	5	0.0	0.0	1.5	0.0	0.0						75				
1 t [1]	2.0	0.0	0.0	0.0	0.0	0										I
capsicum, McCormick	2		0.1	0.3	0.0	0.2		0				0	1			
¼ t [2]	0.6	0.1	0.0			0	50					13		.00		I
caraway seed	7	0.2	0.4	1.0		0.8	1	0	.01	.01	0	0	14	5	.11	.026
1 t	2.0	0.3	0.0	0.1	0.1	0	7	.01	0.1	.00		27	11	.32	.018	802
cardamon, ground	6	0.2	0.2	1.4		0.6	0	0	.00			0	8	5	.15	.560
1 t	2.0	0.1	0.0	0.0	0.0	0	0	.00	0.0	.00		22	4	.28	.008	802
celery seed	8	0.1	0.4	0.8		0.2	0	0	.01	.01	0	3	35	9	.14	.151
1 t	2.0	0.5	0.0	0.3	0.1	0	1	.01	0.1	.00		28	11	.90	.027	802
chervil, dried	2	0.1	0.2	0.5		0.1	6	1	.01	.01	3	1	13	1	.09	.021
1 t	1.0	0.0	0.0	0.0	0.0	0	59	.00	0.1	.00		47	5	.32	.004	802
chili powder	9	0.2	0.4	1.6		1.0	105	2	.02	.06	3	30	8	5	.08	.065
1 t [3]	3	0.5	0.1	0.1	0.2	0	1048	.01	0.2	.00		57	9	.43	.013	802
chili powder, Gebhardt	1		0.0	0.2	0.1	0.1	12	0				0	1			
¼ t	0.3	0.0	0.0	0.0	0.0	0								.03		I

	KCAL / WT (g)	H₂O (g) / FAT (g)	PRO (g) / SFA (g)	CHO (g) / MUFA (g)	SUGR (g) / PUFA (g)	DFIB (g) / CHOL (mg)	A (RE) / A (IU)	C (mg) / B-1 (mg)	B-2 (mg) / NIA (mg)	B-6 (mg) / B-12 (mcg)	FOL (mcg) / PANT (mg)	Na (mg) / K (mg)	Ca (mg) / P (mg)	Mg (mg) / Fe (mg)	Zn (mg) / Cu (mg)	Mn (mg) / REF
Chili Quick seasoning mix, Gebhardt	1		0.0	0.1	0.1	0.1	78	0				985	29			
2 t	14	0.0	0.0	0.0	0.0	0								.44		I
chives																
dried, McCormick	0		0.0	0.0	0.0	0.0		0				0	1			
¼ t	0.1	0.0	0.0	0.0	0.0	0	14					2		.00		I
freeze-dried	2	0.0	0.2	0.5		0.2	55	5	.01	.02	1	1	7	5	.04	.011
¼ cup	0.8	0.0	0.0	0.0	0.0	0	546	.01	0.0	.00	.02	24	4	.16	.005	811
freeze dried, McCormick	0		0.0	0.0	0.0	0.0		0				0	1			
¼ t	0.1	0.0	0.0	0.0	0.0	0	20					2		.00		I
raw	1	2.7	0.1	0.1		0.1	13	2	.00	.00	3	0	3	1	.02	.011
1 T chopped	3	0.0	0.0	0.0	0.0	0	131	.00	0.0	.00	.01	9	2	.05	.005	811
cinnamon, ground	5	0.2	0.1	1.6		1.1	1	1	.00	.01	1	1	25	1	.04	.333
1 t	2.0	0.1	0.0	0.0	0.0	0	5	.00	0.0	.00		10	1	.76	.005	802
cloves, ground	6	0.1	0.1	1.2		0.7	1	2	.01	.03	2	5	13	5	.02	.601
1 t	2.0	0.4	0.1	0.0	0.1	0	11	.00	0.0	.00		22	2	.17	.007	802
coriander (cilantro)																
leaf, dried	3	0.1	0.2	0.5		0.1	6	6	.01	.01	3	2	12	7	.05	.064
1 t	1.0	0.0	0.0	0.0	0.0	0	59	.01	0.1	.00		45	5	.42	.018	802
leaf, fresh	1	3.7	0.1	0.1		0.1	11	0	.00	.00	0	1	4	1	.02	.004
¼ cup	4	0.0	0.0	0.0	0.0	0	111	.00	0.0	.00	.01	22	1	.08	.004	811
seed	6	0.2	0.2	1.1		0.8	0		.01		0	1	14	7	.09	.038
1 t	2.0	0.4	0.0	0.3	0.0	0	0	.00	0.0	.00		25	8	.33	.020	802
cumin, ground, McCormick	3		0.1	0.2		0.2		0				1	5			
¼ t	0.6	0.1	0.0			0	3					11		.20		I
cumin seed	7	0.2	0.4	0.9		0.2	3	0	.01	.01	0	3	19	7	.10	.067
1 t	2.0	0.4	0.0	0.3	0.1	0	25	.01	0.1	.00		36	10	1.33	.017	802
curry powder	7	0.2	0.3	1.2		0.7	2	0	.01	.01	3	1	10	5	.08	.086
1 t	2.0	0.3	0.0	0.1	0.1	0	20	.01	0.1	.00		31	7	.59	.016	802
dill seed	6	0.2	0.3	1.1		0.4	0	0	.01	.01	0	0	30	5	.10	.037
1 t	2.0	0.3	0.0	0.2	0.0	0	1	.01	0.1	.00		24	6	.33	.016	802
dill weed, dried	3	0.1	0.2	0.6		0.1	6	1	.00	.01		2	18	5	.03	.040
1 t	1.0	0.0	0.0			0	59	.00	0.0	.00		33	5	.49	.005	802
dill weed, fresh	4	7.7	0.3	0.6		0.2	69	8	.03	.02	14	5	19	5	.08	.114
1 cup sprigs	9	0.1	0.0	0.1	0.0	0	695	.01	0.1	.00	.04	66	6	.59	.013	802
fennel seed	7	0.2	0.3	1.0		0.8	0	0	.01			2	24	8	.07	.131
1 t	2.0	0.3	0.0	0.2	0.0	0	3	.01	0.1	.00		34	10	.37	.021	802
fenugreek seed	13	0.4	0.9	2.3		1.0	0	0	.01		2	3	7	8	.10	.049
1 t	4	0.3	0.1			0	2	.01	0.1	.00		31	12	1.34	.044	802
garlic powder	10	0.2	0.5	2.2		0.3	0	1	.00	.08	0	1	2	2	.08	.016
1 t	3	0.0	0.0	0.0	0.0	0	0	.01	0.0	.00		33	13	.08	.004	802
garlic salt, Morton	1		0.0	0.2								370	3			
¼ t	1.2	0.0	0.0	0.0	0.0							3				I
ginger, fresh	17	19.6	0.4	3.6		0.5	0	1	.01	.04	3	3	4	10	.08	.055
¼ cup slices	24	0.2	0.0	0.0	0.0	0	0	.01	0.2	.00	.05	100	6	.12	.054	811
ginger, ground	7	0.2	0.2	1.4		0.3	0	0	.00	.02	1	1	2	4	.09	.530
1 t	2.0	0.1	0.0	0.0	0.0	0	3	.00	0.1	.00		27	3	.23	.010	802
green onion, freeze dried, McCormick	1		0.0	0.2	0.0	0.1		0				1	2			
¼ t	0.3	0.0	0.0	0.0	0.0	0	20					4		.00		I
mace, ground	10	0.2	0.1	1.0		0.4	2	0	.01	.01	2	2	5	3	.05	.030
1 t	2.0	0.6	0.2	0.2	0.1	0	16	.01	0.0	.00		9	2	.28	.049	802
Imperial soft	100	2.3	0.0	0.1								105	2			
1 T	14	11.2	1.9		5.3	0	523					6	2			I
marjoram, dried	3	0.1	0.1	0.6		0.4	8	1	.00	.01	3	1	20	3	.04	.054
1 t	1.0	0.1	0.0	0.0	0.0	0	81	.00	0.0	.00		15	3	.83	.011	802
Menudo Spice Mix, Gebhardt	1		0.0	0.1	0.1	0.1	8	0				52	1			
¼ t	0.4	0.0	0.0	0.0	0.0	0								.01		I
Molly McButter Flavor Sprinkles																
butter	5		0.0	1.0	0.0	0.0	0	0				180	0			
1 t	2.0	0.0	0.0	0.0	0.0	0	0					0		.00		I

	KCAL / WT (g)	H₂O (g) / FAT (g)	PRO (g) / SFA (g)	CHO (g) / MUFA (g)	SUGR (g) / PUFA (g)	DFIB (g) / CHOL (mg)	A (RE) / A (IU)	C (mg) / B-1 (mg)	B-2 (mg) / NIA (mg)	B-6 (mg) / B-12 (mcg)	FOL (mcg) / PANT (mg)	Na (mg) / K (mg)	Ca (mg) / P (mg)	Mg (mg) / Fe (mg)	Zn (mg) / Cu (mg)	Mn (mg) / REF
cheese	5		0.0	1.0	0.0	0.0	0	0				125	0			
1 t	2.0	0.0	0.0	0.0	0.0	0	0					0		.00		I
light sodium butter	5		0.5	1.0	0.0	0.0	0	0				90	0			
1 t	2.0	0.0	0.0	0.0	0.0	0	0					0		.00		I
roasted garlic	5		0.0	1.0	0.0	0.0	0	0				125	0			
1 t	2.0	0.0	0.0	0.0	0.0	0	0					0		.00		I
mustard flour, ground, McCormick	3		0.2	0.1	0.0	0.0		0				0	1			
¼ t	0.6	0.2	0.0			0	0					4		.00		I
mustard seed, yellow	14	0.2	0.7	1.0		0.4	0	0	.01	.01	2	0	16	9	.17	.053
1 t	3	0.9	0.0	0.6	0.2	0	2	.02	0.2	.00		20	25	.30	.012	802
nutmeg, ground	10	0.1	0.1	1.0		0.4	0	0	.00	.01	2	0	4	4	.04	.058
1 t	2.0	0.7	0.5	0.1		0	2	.01	0.0	.00		7	4	.06	.021	802
onion powder	7	0.1	0.2	1.6		0.1	0	0	.00	.03	3	1	7	2	.05	.007
1 t	2.0	0.0	0.0	0.0	0.0	0	0	.01	0.0	.00		19	7	.05	.004	802
oregano, ground	6	0.1	0.2	1.3		0.9	14	1	.01	.02	5	0	32	5	.09	.093
1 t	2.0	0.2	0.1	0.0	0.1	0	138	.01	0.1	.00		33	4	.88	.019	802
paprika	6	0.2	0.3	1.1		0.4	121	1	.03	.04	2	1	4	4	.08	.017
1 t	2.0	0.3	0.0	0.0	0.2	0	1212	.01	0.3	.00	.04	47	7	.47	.012	802
parsley, dried	3	0.1	0.2	0.5		0.3	23	1	.01	.01	2	5	15	2	.05	.105
1 t	1.0	0.0	0.0	0.0	0.0	0	233	.00	0.1	.00		38	4	.98	.006	802
parsley, fresh	11	26.3	0.9	1.9	0.3	1.0	156	40	.03	.03	46	17	41	15	.32	.048
½ cup chopped	30	0.2	0.0	0.1	0.0	0	1560	.03	0.4	.00	.12	166	17	1.86	.045	811
pepper																
black	5	0.2	0.2	1.3		0.5	0	0	.00	.01	0	1	9	4	.03	.113
1 t	2.0	0.1	0.0	0.0	0.0	0	4	.00	0.0	.00		25	3	.58	.023	802
red/cayenne	6	0.2	0.2	1.1		0.5	83	2	.02	.04	2	1	3	3	.05	.040
1 t	2.0	0.3	0.1	0.1	0.2	0	832	.01	0.2	.00		40	6	.16	.007	802
white	6	0.2	0.2	1.4		0.5	0	0	.00	.01	0	0	5	2	.02	.086
1 t	2.0	0.0	0.0	0.0	0.0	0	0	.00	0.0	.00		1	4	.29	.018	802
poppy seed	16	0.2	0.5	0.7		0.3	0	0	.01	.01	2	1	43	10	.31	.205
1 t	3	1.3	0.1	0.2	0.9	0	0	.03	0.0	.00		21	25	.28	.049	802
poultry seasoning	6	0.2	0.2	1.3		0.2	5	0	.00	.02	3	1	20	4	.06	.137
1 t[4]	2.0	0.2	0.1	0.0	0.0	0	53	.01	0.1	.00		14	3	.71	.017	802
pumpkin pie spice	7	0.2	0.1	1.4		0.3	1	0	.00	.01	1	1	14	3	.05	.317
1 t[5]	2.0	0.3	0.1	0.0	0.0	0	5	.00	0.0	.00		13	2	.39	.010	802
rosemary, dried	7	0.2	0.1	1.3		0.9	6	1				1	26	4	.06	.037
1 t	2.0	0.3	0.2			0	63	.01		.00		19	1	.58	.011	802
saffron	3	0.1	0.1	0.7		0.0	1	1	.00	.01	1	1	1	3	.01	.284
1 t	1.0	0.1	0.0	0.0	0.0	0	5	.00	0.0	.00		17	3	.11	.003	802
sage, ground	3	0.1	0.1	0.6		0.4	6	0	.00	.01	3	0	17	4	.05	.031
1 t	1.0	0.1	0.1	0.0	0.0	0	59	.01	0.1	.00		11	1	.28	.008	802
salt	0	0.0	0.0	0.0	0.0	0.0	0	0	.00	.00	0	2325	1	0	.01	.006
1 t	6	0.0	0.0	0.0	0.0	0	0	.00	0.0	.00		0	0	.02	.002	802
iodized, Morton	0		0.0	0.0	0.0							590	1			
¼ t	1.5	0.0	0.0	0.0	0.0							0				I
kosher, Morton	0		0.0	0.0	0.0							480				
¼ t	1.2	0.0	0.0	0.0												I
non-iodized, Morton	0		0.0	0.0	0.0							590	1			
¼ t	1.5	0.0	0.0	0.0	0.0							0				I
seasoned, Morton	1		0.0	0.2								400	4			
¼ t	1.3	0.0	0.0	0.0	0.0							3				I
salt substitutes																
Morton Lite Salt	0		0.0	0.0	0.0							280	0	4		
¼ t	1.4	0.0	0.0	0.0	0.0	0						350				I
Morton Salt Substitute	0		0.0	0.0	0.0	0.0						0	7	0		
¼ t	1.2	0.0	0.0	0.0	0.0	0						600	5			I
Morton Seasoned Salt Substitute	1		0.0	0.1								0	8			
¼ t	1.1	0.0	0.0	0.0	0.0							480				I
savory, ground	3	0.1	0.1	0.7		0.5	5	1				0	21	4	.04	.061
1 t	1.0	0.1	0.0			0	51	.00	0.0	.00		11	1	.38	.008	802

	KCAL	H₂O (g)	PRO (g)	CHO (g)	SUGR (g)	DFIB (g)	A (RE)	C (mg)	B-2 (mg)	B-6 (mg)	FOL (mcg)	Na (mg)	Ca (mg)	Mg (mg)	Zn (mg)	Mn (mg)
	WT (g)	FAT (g)	SFA (g)	MUFA (g)	PUFA (g)	CHOL (mg)	A (IU)	B-1 (mg)	NIA (mg)	B-12 (mcg)	PANT (mg)	K (mg)	P (mg)	Fe (mg)	Cu (mg)	REF
seasoning blend																
Nature's Seasons, Morton	0		0.0	0.1	0.0							380	1			
¼ t	1.2	0.0	0.0	0.0	0.0							3				I
salt-free, extra spicy, Mrs. Dash	0		0.0	1.0		0.0	0	0				0	0			
½ t	1.3	0.0	0.0	0.0	0.0	0	0					20		.00		I
salt-free, lemon & pepper, Mrs. Dash	0		0.0	1.0	0.0	0.0	0	0				0	0			
½ t	1.5	0.0	0.0	0.0	0.0	0	0					15		.00		I
salt-free, low pepper-no garlic, Mrs. Dash	0		0.0	1.0	0.0	0.0	0	0				0	0			
½ t	1.4	0.0	0.0	0.0	0.0	0	0					20		.00		I
salt-free, original, Mrs. Dash	0		0.0	1.0	0.0	0.0	0	0				0	0			
½ t	1.4	0.0	0.0	0.0	0.0	0	0					20		.00		I
salt-free, table, Mrs. Dash	0		0.0	1.0	0.0	0.0	0	0				0	0			
½ t	1.3	0.0	0.0	0.0	0.0	0	0					20		.00		I
seasoning mix, Shake 'n Bake Perfect	25		1.0	3.5	1.0	0.0	0	0				375	20			
Potatoes—⅙ pkt[6]	7	1.0	0.8			3	0					33		.00		I
shallots, freeze dried, McCormick	1		0.0	0.1	0.0	0.0		0				0	0			
¼ t	0.1	0.0	0.0			0	0					2		.00		I
spearmint, McCormick	1		0.0	0.1	0.0	0.0						1	3			
¼ t	0.2	0.0	0.0	0.0	0.0	0	12					4		.40		I
tarragon, ground	6	0.2	0.5	1.0		0.1	8	1	.03	.02	5	1	23	7	.08	.159
1 t	2.0	0.1	0.0	0.0	0.1	0	84	.01	0.2	.00		60	6	.65	.014	802
thyme, fresh	1	0.7	0.1	0.2		0.1	5	2	.00	.00	0	0	4	2	.02	.017
1 t	1.0	0.0	0.0	0.0	0.0	0	48	.00	0.0	.00	.00	6	1	.17	.006	802
thyme, ground	3	0.1	0.1	0.6		0.4	4	1	.00	.01	3	1	19	2	.06	.079
1 t	1.0	0.1	0.0	0.0	0.0	0	38	.01	0.0	.00		8	2	1.24	.009	802
turmeric, ground	7	0.2	0.2	1.3		0.4	0	1	.00	.04	1	1	4	4	.09	.157
1 t	2.0	0.2	0.1	0.0		0	0	.00	0.1	.00		51	5	.83	.012	802
vanilla extract	6	1.1	0.0	0.3	0.0	0	0	0	.00	.00	0	0	0	0	.00	.005
1 t[7]	4	0.0	0.0	0.0	0.0	0	0	.00	0.0	.00	.00	3	0	.00	.001	802
imitation w/ alcohol	10	2.7	0.0	0.1		0.0	0	0	.00	.00	0	0	0	0	.00	.020
1 t[7]	4	0.0	0.0	0.0	0.0	0	0	.00	0.0	.00	.00	4	1	.01	.001	802
imitation w/o alcohol	2	3.6	0.0	0.6		0.0	0	0	.00	.00	0	0	0	0	.00	.000
1 t	4	0.0	0.0	0.0	0.0	0	0	.00	0.0	.00	.00	0	0	.00	.000	802

1. One teaspoon of mix is equivalent to 1 tablespoon of liquid. Sprinkles has the same nutrient values per 1 teaspoon (2 g) except that the sodium is 120 mg.
2. Contains chilies, chili pepper, and red pepper.
3. Contains red pepper, cumin, oregano, salt, and garlic powder.
4. Contains white pepper, sage, thyme, marjoram, savory, ginger, allspice, and nutmeg.
5. Contains cinnamon, ginger, nutmeg, allspice, and cloves.
6. Values are averages for crisp cheddar, and herb & garlic. Serving size coats ½ cup of raw potatoes.
7. Contains 1.4 g alcohol (ethanol) in 1 teaspoon.

31. SPREADS

	KCAL	H₂O	PRO	CHO	SUGR	DFIB	A (RE)	C	B-2	B-6	FOL	Na	Ca	Mg	Zn	Mn
butter	36	0.8	0.0	0.0		0.0	38	0	.00	.00	0	41	1	0	.00	.000
1 t	5	4.1	2.5	1.2	0.2	11	153	.00	0.0	.01	.01	1	1	.01	.001	801
	108	2.4	0.1	0.0		0.0	113	0	.01	.00	0	124	4	0	.01	.001
1 T	15	12.2	7.6	3.5	0.5	33	459	.00	0.0	.02	.02	4	3	.02	.002	801
sweet (unsalted)	36	0.8	0.0	0.0		0.0	38	0	.00	.00	0	0	1	0	.00	.000
1 t	5	4.1	2.5	1.2	0.2	11	153	.00	0.0	.01	.01	1	1	.01	.001	801
sweet (unsalted)	108	2.4	0.1	0.0		0.0	113	0	.01	.00	0	2	4	0	.01	.001
1 T	15	12.2	7.6	3.5	0.5	33	459	.00	0.0	.02	.02	4	3	.02	.002	801
whipped	29	0.6	0.0	0.0		0.0	30	0	.00	.00	0	33	1	0	.00	.000
1 t	4	3.2	2.0	0.9	0.1	9	122	.00	0.0	.01	.00	1	1	.01	.001	801
whipped	79	1.7	0.1	0.0		0.0	83	0	.00	.00	0	91	3	0	.01	.000
1 T	11	8.9	5.6	2.6	0.3	24	336	.00	0.0	.01	.01	3	3	.02	.002	801

KCAL	H₂O (g)	PRO (g)	CHO (g)	SUGR (g)	DFIB (g)	A (RE)	C (mg)	B-2 (mg)	B-6 (mg)	FOL (mcg)	Na (mg)	Ca (mg)	Mg (mg)	Zn (mg)	Mn (mg)
WT (g)	FAT (g)	SFA (g)	MUFA (g)	PUFA (g)	CHOL (mg)	A (IU)	B-1 (mg)	NIA (mg)	B-12 (mcg)	PANT (mg)	K (mg)	P (mg)	Fe (mg)	Cu (mg)	REF

margarine

KCAL/WT	H₂O/FAT	PRO/SFA	CHO/MUFA	SUGR/PUFA	DFIB/CHOL	A(RE)/A(IU)	C/B-1	B-2/NIA	B-6/B-12	FOL/PANT	Na/K	Ca/P	Mg/Fe	Zn/Cu	Mn/REF
Blue Bonnet, 31% oil, soft															
45		0.0	1.0	0.0	0.0						95				
15	5.0	1.0	1.5	1.0	0						5				I
Blue Bonnet, 40% oil, stick															
50		0.0	1.0		0.0						75				
14	6.0	1.0	1.5	1.0	0						5				I
Chiffon, 80% oil, soft															
100		0.0	0.0	0.0	0.0						115				
14	11.0	2.0	3.5	3.0	0										I
Chiffon, 80% oil, whipped															
70		0.0	0.0	0.0	0.0						70				
9	7.0	1.5	1.5	2.5	0										I
Chiffon Soft															
100		0.0	0.0	0.0	0.0		0				105	0			
14	11.0	2.0			0	500					10		.00		I
Chiffon, whipped															
70		0.0	0.0	0.0	0.0						70	0			
9	7.0	1.5			0	300					0		.00		I
Country Morning Blend, soft															
90		0.0	0.0	0.0							75				
13	9.0	3.0	3.0	3.0	15						0				I
Country Morning Blend, stick															
101		0.1	0.0	0.0			0	.00			108	2			
14	11.3	4.0	3.0	1.9	12	476	.00	0.0			3	2	.01		I
Country Morning Blend, whipped															
94		0.1	0.0	0.0			0	.00			99	2			
13	10.5	3.8	2.8	1.8	11	455	.00	0.0			3	2	.01		I
Fleischmann's, 31% oil, soft															
40		0.0	1.0		0.0						90				
14	4.5	0.0	2.5	1.0	0						5				I
Fleischmann's, 40% oil, stick															
50		0.0	1.0		0.0						75				
15	6.0	1.0	1.5	1.5	0						0				I
Fleischmann's, 80% oil, unsalted, stick															
100		0.0	0.0	0.0	0.0						0				
14	11.0	2.0	3.0	4.0	0						0				I
Fleischmann's, stick															
100		0.0	0.0	0.0	0.0						105				
14	11.0	2.0	3.0	4.0	0						5				I
Imperial Diet															
49	8.1	0.0	0.0	0.0							139	0			
14	5.6	0.9		2.6	0	523					4	0			I
Imperial Quarters, stick															
107	2.5	0.0	0.1								113	2			
15	12.0	2.2		3.2	0	560					6	2			I
Imperial soft															
14	100	2.3	0.0	0.1							105	2			
	11.2	1.9		5.3	0	523					6	2			I
Land O' Lakes Corn, stick															
101		0.0	0.0	0.0			0	.00			102	0			
14	11.2	1.8	5.8	3.6	0	511	.00	0.0			1	0	.00		I
Land O' Lakes Soy, stick															
105		0.0	0.0	0.0							105				
14	12.0	3.0	6.0	3.0	0						0				I
Mazola Red Cal															
50	8.1	0.0	0.0	0.0							130				
14	5.5	0.9	2.2	2.3	0	500									I
Mazola stick															
100	2.3	0.0	0.2								100				
14	11.2	1.9	5.2	3.9	0	500									I
Mrs. Filbert's Corn, soft															
100	2.3	0.0	0.1								105	2			
14	11.2	1.9		5.0	0	523					6	3			I
Mrs. Filbert's Gold, soft															
100	2.3	0.0	0.1								105	2			
14	11.2	1.9		5.3	0	523					6	2			I
Mrs. Filbert's Golden Quarters, stick															
107	2.5	0.0	0.1								113	2			
15	12.0	2.2		3.2	0	560					6	2			I
Nucoa Soft															
90	2.0	0.0	0.1								150				
13	10.5	2.0		4.2	0	520									I
Nucoa stick															
100	2.3	0.0	0.0	0.0							160				
14	11.3	2.4		3.3	0	500									I
Parkay Diet															
50		0.0	0.0	0.0	0.0		0				110	0			
14	6.0	1.0			0	500					0		.00		I
Parkay Soft															
100		0.0	0.0	0.0	0.0						110				
14	11.0	2.0	3.0	4.0	0										I
Parkay, whipped															
70		0.0	0.0	0.0	0.0						80				
10	8.0	1.5	2.0	3.0	0										I
Shedd's Soft															
99	2.5	0.0	0.0	0.0							110	0			
14	11.2	1.9		5.3	0	523					0	1			I
Shedd's, stick															
78	2.0	0.0	0.0	0.0							87	0			
11	8.8	1.6		3.0	0	411					0	1			I

	KCAL / WT (g)	H₂O / FAT (g)	PRO / SFA (g)	CHO / MUFA (g)	SUGR / PUFA (g)	DFIB / CHOL (mg)	A (RE) / A (IU)	C / B-1 (mg)	B-2 / NIA (mg)	B-6 / B-12 (mg/mcg)	FOL / PANT (mcg/mg)	Na / K (mg)	Ca / P (mg)	Mg / Fe (mg)	Zn / Cu (mg)	Mn / REF (mg)
Shedd's, whipped	78	1.9	0.0	0.0	0.0							87	0			
1 T	11	8.8	1.5		4.2	0	411					0	1			I
Willow Run Print, stick	107	2.5	0.0	0.0	0.0							152	0			
1 T	15	12.0	2.2		4.1	0	560					2	2			I
mayonnaise																
Best Foods/Hellmann's	100	2.5	0.2	0.1								80				
1 T	14	11.0	1.7	3.3	5.9	51										I
cholesterol-free, red cal, Best Foods/ Hellmann's—1 T	50	8.7	0.0	1.1								80				
1 T	15	4.9	0.7	1.7	2.4	0										I
imitation, soybean	35	9.4	0.0	2.4		0.0	0	0	.00	.00	0	75	0	0	.02	
1 T	15	2.9	0.5	0.7	1.6	4	0	.00	0.0	.00	.00	2	0	.00	.002	804
Kraft Free	10		0.0	2.0	1.0	0.0	0	0				105	0			
1 T	16	0.0	0.0	0.0	0.0	0	0					5		.00		I
Kraft Light	50		0.0	1.0	0.0	0.0	0	0				110	0			
1 T	15	5.0	1.0			0	0					10		.00		I
light, red cal, Best Foods/Hellmann's	50	8.5	0.1	1.0		0.0						115				
1 T	15	5.1	0.9	1.5	2.6	5										I
safflower & soybean	100	2.1	0.2	0.4		0.0	12	0	.00	.08	1	80	3	0	.02	
1 T	14	11.1	1.2	1.8	7.7	8	39	.00	0.0	.04	.04	5	4	.07		804
soybean	100	2.1	0.2	0.4		0.0	12	0	.00	.08	1	80	3	0	.02	
1 T	14	11.1	1.7	3.2	5.8	8	39	.00	0.0	.04	.03	5	4	.07	.001	804
sandwich spread	58	6.1	0.1	3.4		0.1	13	0	.00	.00	1	150	2	0	.12	
1 T	15	5.1	0.8	1.1	3.0	11	33	.00	0.0	.03	.00	5	4	.03	.002	804
Sandwich Spread, Best Foods/Hellmann's	55	6.8	0.1	2.4								170				
1 T	15	5.2	0.8	1.7	2.7	5										I
spread, fat-free																
buttery, Fleischmann's Squeeze	5		0.0	1.0		0.0						130				
1 T	15	0.0	0.0	0.0	0.0	0						25				I
cheddar, Fleischmann's Squeeze	10		0.0	1.0		0.0						135				
1 T	15	0.0	0.0	0.0	0.0	0						65				I
Fleischmann's	15		0.0	3.0		0.0						75				
1 T	15	0.0	0.0	0.0	0.0	0										I
spread, veg oil/animal fat																
Blue Bonnet, 45% oil, soft	60		0.0	0.0	0.0	0.0						110				
1 T	14	6.0	1.0	2.0	1.5	0						10				I
Blue Bonnet, 56% oil, stick	70		0.0	0.0	0.0	0.0						100				
1 T	14	8.0	1.5	2.0	1.5	0						5				I
Blue Bonnet, 68% oil	80		0.0	0.0	0.0	0.0						80				
1 T	14	10.0	1.5	3.0	2.0	0						5				I
Country Crock, 52% corn oil, soft	64	6.5	0.0	0.0		0.0						111	0			
1 T	14	7.3	1.2		3.2	0	523					3	1			I
Country Crock Churnstyle, 52% oil, soft	64	6.6	0.0	0.0		0.0						56	1			
1 T	14	7.3	1.2		3.4	0	523					4	1			I
Country Crock Classic, 64% oil, stick	85	5.0	0.0	0.1								121	1			
1 T	15	9.6	1.8		2.6	0	560					7	2			I
Country Crock Squeeze	79	4.6	0.0	0.1								113	1			
1 T	14	9.0	1.4		4.0	0	523					7	2			I
Country Crock whipped w/ honey, soft	69	0.8	0.0	1.8								70	0			
1 T	11	7.0	1.2		3.3	0	411					2	1			I
Dairybrook Quarters, stick	56	8.0	0.4	0.1								100	4			
1 T	15	6.0	3.1		0.2	16	567					9	4			I
Fleischmann's, 56% oil, stick	70		0.0	0.0	0.0	0.0						85				
1 T	14	8.0	1.5	2.0	2.5	0						10				I
Fleischmann's, 67% oil, soft	80		0.0	0.0	0.0	0.0						90				
1 T	14	9.0	1.5	2.5	4.0	0						10				I
Fleischmann's, 67% oil, soft, unsalted	80		0.0	0.0	0.0	0.0						0				
1 T	14	9.0	1.5	2.5	4.0	0						0				I
Imperial, 45% oil, soft	55	7.5	0.0	0.0		0.0						104	0			
1 T	14	6.3	1.1		3.0	0	523					3	1			I

	KCAL	H₂O (g)	PRO (g)	CHO (g)	SUGR (g)	DFIB (g)	A (RE)	C (mg)	B-2 (mg)	B-6 (mg)	FOL (mcg)	Na (mg)	Ca (mg)	Mg (mg)	Zn (mg)	Mn (mg)
	WT (g)	FAT (g)	SFA (g)	MUFA (g)	PUFA (g)	CHOL (mg)	A (IU)	B-1 (mg)	NIA (mg)	B-12 (mcg)	PANT (mg)	K (mg)	P (mg)	Fe (mg)	Cu (mg)	REF
Imperial Quarters, 60% oil, stick	79	5.7	0.0	0.1								120	1			
1 T	15	9.0	1.6		2.4	0	560					6	1			I
Imperial Savory Butter Squeeze	87	3.9	0.0	0.1								72	2			
1 T	14	9.8	1.5		4.4	0	523					6	2			I
Imperial Savory Squeeze	86	3.8	0.0	0.1								72	2			
1 T	14	9.8	1.5		4.4	0	523					6	2			I
Imperial, whipped	43	5.9	0.0	0.0	0.0							82	0			
1 T	11	5.0	0.8		2.3	0	411					2	0			I
Land O' Lakes, 64% soy oil, soft	75		0.0	0.0	0.0							75				
1 T	14	9.0	3.0	3.0	3.0	0						0				I
Land O' Lakes Sweet Cream Spread	76		0.0	0.0	0.0			0	.00			77	1			
1 T	14	8.4	1.5	3.2	3.5	1	504	.00	0.0			6	1	.00		I
Latta, soft	50	8.0	0.2	0.0	0.0							68	1			
1 T	14	5.6	1.0		1.3	0	523					6	1			I
Mazola light corn oil	50	8.2	0.0	0.0	0.0							100				
1 T	14	5.6	0.9	2.5	2.1	0	500									I
Move Over Butter, 72% oil, soft, whipped	60		0.0	0.0	0.0	0.0						75				
1 T	10	7.0	1.5	2.5	1.5	0						5				I
Move Over Butter, 72% oil, stick	90		0.0	0.0	0.0	0.0						100				
1 T	14	10.0	2.0	3.0	2.0	0						10				I
Mrs. Filbert's, 52% corn oil, soft	64	6.5	0.0	0.0	0.0							111	0			
1 T	14	7.3	1.2		3.2	0	523					3	1			I
Mrs. Filbert's, 52% oil, soft	64	6.5	0.0	0.0	0.0							111	0			
1 T	14	7.3	1.2		3.4	0	523					3	1			I
Parkay, 40% oil, soft	50		0.0	0.0	0.0	0.0						120				
1 T	15	6.0	1.0			0										I
Parkay, 48% oil, soft	60		0.0	0.0	0.0	0.0						120				
1 T	15	7.0	1.0	2.0	2.5	0										I
Parkay, 50% oil	60		0.0	0.0	0.0	0.0		0				110	0			
1 T	14	7.0	1.5			0	500					0		.00		I
Parkay, 53% oil	70		0.0	0.0	0.0			0				120	0			
1 T	14	7.0	1.5			0	500					0		.00		I
Parkay, 53% oil, stick	70		0.0	0.0	0.0							120				
1 T	15	8.0	1.5			0										I
Parkay, 70% oil	90		0.0	0.0	0.0			0				110	0			
1 T	14	10.0	2.0			0	500					5		.00		I
Parkay, 70% oil, stick	90		0.0	0.0	0.0	0.0						115				
1 T	14	10.0	1.5	3.0	2.0	0										I
Parkay Light, 40% oil	50		0.0	0.0	0.0			0				120	0			
1 T	14	6.0	1.0			0	500					0		.00		I
Parkay Squeeze, 64% oil	80		0.0	0.0	0.0	0.0						120				
1 T	14	9.0	1.5	2.0	4.5	0										I
Promise, 53% oil, soft	65	6.4	0.0	0.0	0.0							68	1			
1 T	14	7.4	1.1		3.6	0	523					4	1			I
Promise, 68% oil, soft	85	4.0	0.0	0.2								94	2			
1 T	14	9.5	1.4		4.6	0	523					9	3			I
Promise Extra Lite, 40% oil, soft	50	8.0	0.2	0.1								57	1			
1 T	14	5.6	0.9		2.5	0	523					7	2			I
Promise Quarters 40% oil, extra light, stick—1 T	55	8.3	0.4	0.1								61	2			
	15	6.0	1.0		2.5	0	560					8	2			I
Promise Quarters, 53% oil, stick	70	6.9	0.0	0.0	0.0							73	1			
1 T	15	8.0	1.2		3.2	0	560					5	1			I
Promise Quarters, 68% oil, stick	91	4.3	0.0	0.2								101	2			
1 T²	15	10.2	1.6		4.2	0	560					10	3			I
Shedd's Quarters, 52% oil, stick	69	6.9	0.0	0.0	0.0							119	0			
1 T	15	7.8	1.4		2.6	0	560					3	1			I
Shedd's Spread, 52% oil, soft	64	6.5	0.0	0.0	0.0							111	0			
1 T	14	7.3	1.2		3.4	0	523					3	1			I
Touch of Butter, 40% oil	60		0.0	0.0	0.0			0				110				
1 T	14	7.0	1.5			0	500					0		.00		I
Touch of Butter, 47% oil, soft	60		0.0	0.0	0.0	0.0						120				
1 T	15	7.0	1.5	2.0	2.0	0										I

	KCAL	H₂O (g)	PRO (g)	CHO (g)	SUGR (g)	DFIB (g)		A (RE)	C (mg)	B-2 (mg)	B-6 (mg)	FOL (mcg)		Na (mg)	Ca (mg)	Mg (mg)	Zn (mg)	Mn (mg)
	WT (g)	FAT (g)	SFA (g)	MUFA (g)	PUFA (g)	CHOL (mg)		A (IU)	B-1 (mg)	NIA (mg)	B-12 (mcg)	PANT (mg)		K (mg)	P (mg)	Fe (mg)	Cu (mg)	REF
Touch of Butter, 70% oil	90		0.0	0.0	0.0	0.0		0						110	0			
1 T	14	10.0	2.0			0		500						0		.00		I
Touch of Butter Squeeze, 64% oil	80		0.0	0.0	0.0	0.0								115	0			
1 T	14	9.0	1.5			0		500						0		.00		I

32. SUGARS, SYRUPS, & OTHER SWEETENERS

	KCAL	H₂O (g)	PRO (g)	CHO (g)	SUGR (g)	DFIB (g)		A (RE)/IU	C/B-1	B-2/NIA	B-6/B-12	FOL/PANT		Na/K	Ca/P	Mg/Fe	Zn/Cu	Mn/REF
apple butter	33	9.3	0.0	8.6		0.2		0	0	.00	.01	0		0	1	1	.01	.070
1 T	18	0.1	0.0	0.0	0.0	0		0	.00	0.0	.00	.01		16	1	.02	.014	819
fruit spread, grape/strawberry, red cal,	20		0.0	5.0	5.0	0.0		0	0					20	0			
Kraft—*1 T*	17	0.0	0.0	0.0	0.0	0		0						25		.00		I
honey, strained/extracted	64	3.6	0.1	17.3	17.2	0.0		0	0	.01	.01	0		1	1	0	.05	.017
1 T	21	0.0	0.0	0.0	0.0	0		0	.00	0.0	.00	.01		11	1	.09	.008	819
jam/jelly/marmalade/preserves, all flavors,	35		0.0	9.0		0.0								5				
Welch's Spreads—*2 t*	10	0.0				0								5				I
jam, Kraft	60		0.0	13.3	8.0	0.0		0	1					10	0			
1 T[1]	20	0.0	0.0	0.0	0.0	0		0						17		.00		I
jam/preserves	48	6.9	0.1	12.9		0.2		0	2	.00	.00	7		8	4	1	.01	.008
1 T	20	0.0	0.0	0.0	0.0	0		2	.00	0.0	.00	.00		15	2	.10	.020	819
jam, strawberry, Smuckers	38	4.6	0.0	9.4	6.6	0.3		0	1					1	1			
½ oz	14	0.1				0		50								.05		I
jelly	51	5.4	0.1	13.5		0.2		0	0	.00	.00	0		7	2	1	.01	.026
1 T	19	0.0	0.0	0.0	0.0	0		3	.00	0.0	.00	.04		12	1	.04	.003	819
concord grape, Smuckers	38	4.5	0.0	9.4	6.6	0.3		0						1				
½ oz	14	0.1				0		50						4				I
Kraft	53		0.0	13.4	7.6	0.0		0	0					10	0			
1 T[2]	20	0.0	0.0	0.0	0.0	0		0						16		.00		I
marmalade, orange	49	6.6	0.1	13.3		0.0		1	1	.00	.00	7		11	8	0	.01	.004
1 T	20	0.0	0.0	0.0	0.0	0		9	.00	0.0	.00	.00		7	1	.03	.018	819
molasses	53	5.2	0.0	13.8	10.9	0.0		0	0	.00	.13	0		7	41	48	.06	.306
1 T	20	0.0	0.0	0.0	0.0	0		0	.01	0.2	.00	.16		293	6	.94	.097	819
blackstrap	47	5.7	0.0	12.2		0.0		0	0	.01	.14	0		11	172	43	.20	.522
1 T	20	0.0	0.0	0.0	0.0	0		0	.01	0.2	.00	.18		498	8	3.50	.408	819
dark/light, Brer Rabbit	60		0.0	15.0	15.0									10				
1 T	21	0.0	0.0	0.0	0.0													I
preserves, Kraft	50		0.0	13.4	7.3	0.0		0	2					10	0			
1 T[3]	20	0.0	0.0	0.0	0.0	0		0						15		.00		I
sugar																		
brown	827	3.5	0.0	214.1	197.6	0.0		0	0	.02	.06	2		86	187	64	.40	.701
1 cup packed	220	0.0	0.0	0.0	0.0	0		0	.02	0.2	.00	.24		761	48	4.20	.656	819
white, granulated	15	0.0	0.0	4.0	3.9	0.0		0	0	.00	.00	0		0	0	0	.00	.000
1 t	4	0.0	0.0	0.0	0.0	0		0	.00	0.0	.00	.00		0	0	.00	.002	819
white, granulated	50	0.0	0.0	13.0	12.6	0.0		0	0	.00	.00	0		0	0	0	.00	.001
1 T	13	0.0	0.0	0.0	0.0	0		0	.00	0.0	.00	.00		0	0	.01	.006	819
white, granulated	774	0.0	0.0	199.8	193.6	0.0		0	0	.04	.00	0		2	2	0	.06	.014
1 cup	200	0.0	0.0	0.0	0.0	0		0	.00	0.0	.00	.00		4	4	.12	.086	819
white, powdered	31	0.0	0.0	8.0	7.4	0.0		0	0	.00	.00	0		0	0	0	.00	.001
1 T	8	0.0	0.0	0.0	0.0	0		0	.00	0.0	.00	.00		0	0	.00	.003	819
white, powdered	467	0.4	0.0	119.4	111.6	0.0		0	0	.00	.00	0		1	1	0	.04	.008
1 cup	120	0.1	0.0	0.0	0.1	0		0	.00	0.0	.00	.00		2	2	.07	.052	819
sugar substitute																		
NatraTaste	4	0.0	0.0	0.9	0.9	0.0												
1 pkt	1.0	0.0				0												I
Sprinkle Sweet, Pillsbury	2	0.2	0.0	0.5					0	.00				1	0			
1 t	0.7	0.0						0	.00	0.0				0	0	.00		I

	KCAL	H₂O (g)	PRO (g)	CHO (g)	SUGR (g)	DFIB (g)	A (RE)	C (mg)	B-2 (mg)	B-6 (mg)	FOL (mcg)	Na (mg)	Ca (mg)	Mg (mg)	Zn (mg)	Mn (mg)
	WT (g)	FAT (g)	SFA (g)	MUFA (g)	PUFA (g)	CHOL (mg)	A (IU)	B-1 (mg)	NIA (mg)	B-12 (mcg)	PANT (mg)	K (mg)	P (mg)	Fe (mg)	Cu (mg)	REF
Sugar Twin	0		0.0	1.0	1.0	0.0	0	0				0	0			
1 pkt (2 t)	0.8	0.0	0.0	0.0	0.0	0	0					0		.00		I
Sugar Twin, brown	0		0.0	0.0	0.0		0	0				0	0			
1 t	0.4	0.0	0.0	0.0	0.0	0	0					0		.00		I
Sweet 'n Low	4		0.0	0.9	0.9	0.0						0				
1 pkt	1.0	0.0	0.0	0.0	0.0	0						0				I
Sweet 10, Pillsbury	0	0.8	0.0	0.0	0.0			0	.00			2	0			
⅛ t	0.8	0.0					0	.00	0.0			0		.00		I
Sweet One	4	0.0	0.0	0.9	0.9	0.0						0				
1 pkt[4]	1.0	0.0	0.0	0.0	0.0	0						11				I
syrup, cane & 15% maple	56	4.8	0.0	15.0		0.0	0	0	.00	.00	0	21	3	1	.13	.114
1 T	20	0.0	0.0	0.0	0.0	0	0	.00	0.0	.00	.01	7	0	.16	.004	819
syrup, corn																
dark	56	4.6	0.0	15.3	7.4	0.0	0	0	.00	.00	0	31	4	2	.01	.020
1 T	20	0.0	0.0	0.0	0.0	0	0	.00	0.0	.00	.00	9	2	.07	.011	819
dark, Karo	60	5.4	0.0	15.0								40				
1 T[5]	21	0.0														I
high fructose	53	4.6	0.0	14.4	14.1	0.0	0	0	.00	.00	0	0	0	0	.00	.018
1 T	19	0.0	0.0	0.0	0.0	0	0	.00	0.0	.00	.00	0	0	.01	.006	819
light	56	4.6	0.0	15.3	12.7	0.0	0	0	.00	.00	0	24	1	0	.00	.018
1 T	20	0.0	0.0	0.0	0.0	0	0	.00	0.0	.00	.00	1	0	.01	.002	819
light, Karo	60	5.4	0.0	14.9								30				
1 T[6]	21	0.0														I
syrup, corn & sugar	64	3.1	0.0	16.8		0.0	0	0	.01	.00	1	14	5	2	.01	.018
1 T	20	0.0	0.0	0.0	0.0	0	0	.00	0.0	.00	.01	13	2	.15	.012	819
syrup, malt	76	5.1	1.5	17.1		0.0	0	0	.09	.12	3	8	15	17	.03	.024
1 T	24	0.0	0.0	0.0	0.0	0	0	.00	1.9	.00	.04	77	57	.23	.048	819
syrup, maple	52	6.4	0.0	13.4	12.0	0.0	0	0	.00	.00	0	2	13	3	.83	.660
1 T	20	0.0	0.0	0.0	0.0	0	0	.00	0.0	.00	.01	41	0	.24	.015	819
syrup, pancake & waffle	57	4.8	0.0	15.1	10.9	0.0	0	0	.00	.00	0	17	0	0	.01	.018
1 T	20	0.0	0.0	0.0	0.0	0	0	.00	0.0	.00	.00	0	2	.02	.043	819
70% Cal Reduced S&W	60			15.0	0.0		0					105	0			
¼ cup	60 ml	0.0	0.0	0.0	0.0	0	0					0		.00		I
Aunt Jemima	212	26.9	0.0	52.6	37.8	0.2	0	0	.00	.00	0	122	3	1	.17	
¼ cup	80	0.1	0.0	0.0	0.0	0	0	.00	0.0	.00	.00	8	12	.25	.050	I
butter flavor, Country Kitchen	200		0.0	53.0	40.0	0.0	0	0				200	0			
¼ cup	59 ml	0.0	0.0			0	0					0		.00		I
butter lite, Aunt Jemima	104	43.2	0.0	26.4	26.0	0.4	0	0	.00	.00	0	160	0	0	.00	
¼ cup	70	0.0	0.0	0.0	0.0	0	0	.00	0.0	.00	.00	0	10	.03	.000	I
butter rich, Aunt Jamima	209	27.4	0.1	51.9	28.9	0.2	0	0	.00	.00	0	172	0	0	.00	
¼ cup	80	0.2	0.0	0.0	0.0	0	0	.00	0.0	.00	.00	0	24	.21	.070	I
Country Kitchen	200		0.0	53.0	40.0	0.0	0	0				110	0			
¼ cup	59 ml	0.0	0.0	0.0	0.0	0	0					0		.00		I
Country Kitchen Lite	100		0.0	26.0	25.0	0.0	0	0				160	0			
¼ cup	60 ml	0.0	0.0			0	0					0		.00		I
Country Rich, Aunt Jemima	212	26.5	0.0	53.1	30.3	0.2	0	0	.00	.00	0	119	0	0	.00	
¼ cup	80	0.0	0.0	0.0	0.0	0	0	.00	0.0	.00	.00	0	12	.22	.070	I
Country Rich Lite, Aunt Jemima	103	43.1	0.0	26.4	21.6	0.6	0	0	.00	.00	0	229	6	0	.00	
¼ cup	70	0.0	0.0	0.0	0.0	0	0	.00	0.0	.00	.00	1	12	.03	.000	I
Golden Griddle	55	5.7	0.0	14.2								15				
1 T[7]	20	0.0														I
Karo	60	5.5	0.0	14.9								35				
1 T[8]	21	0.0														I
lite, Aunt Jemima	93	38.0	0.0	23.7	22.9	0.5	0	0	.00	.00	0	139	0	0	.00	
1 pkt	62	0.0	0.0	0.0	0.0	0	0	.00	0.0	.00	.00	0	9	.02	.000	I
lite, Mrs. Richardson's	103	43.6	0.0	25.9	25.2	0.2	0	0	.00	.00	0	161	0	0	.00	
¼ cup	70	0.0	0.0	0.0	0.0	0	0	.00	0.0	.00	.00	0	10	.02	.000	I
Log Cabin	200		0.0	52.0	31.0	0.0	0	0				60	0			
¼ cup	59 ml	0.0	0.0	0.0	0.0	0	0					0		.00		I
Log Cabin Lite	100		0.0	26.0	25.0	0.0	0	0				180	0			
¼ cup	60 ml	0.0	0.0	0.0	0.0	0	0					0		.00		I

	KCAL	H₂O (g)	PRO (g)	CHO (g)	SUGR (g)	DFIB (g)	A (RE)	C (mg)	B-2 (mg)	B-6 (mg)	FOL (mcg)	Na (mg)	Ca (mg)	Mg (mg)	Zn (mg)	Mn (mg)
	WT (g)	FAT (g)	SFA (g)	MUFA (g)	PUFA (g)	CHOL (mg)	A (IU)	B-1 (mg)	NIA (mg)	B-12 (mcg)	PANT (mg)	K (mg)	P (mg)	Fe (mg)	Cu (mg)	REF
Mrs. Butterworth	111		0.0	27.0		0.1						32	0			
1 fl oz	40	0.1				0						0				I
Mrs. Butterworth Lite	62		0.0	16.0		0.2						63	0			
1 fl oz	35	0.2				0						0				I
original recipe, Mrs. Richardson's	207	28.0	0.0	51.7	22.7	0.1	0	0	.00	.00	0	117	0	0	.00	
¼ cup	80	0.0	0.0	0.0		0	0	.00	0.0	.00	.00	3	19	.01	.000	I
red cal	25	8.2	0.0	6.6		0.0	0	0	.00	.00	0	30	0	0	.00	.013
1 T	15	0.0	0.0	0.0	0.0	0	0	.00	0.0	.00	.00	0	6	.00	.000	819
w/ 2% maple syrup	53	6.0	0.0	13.9		0.0	0	0	.00	.00	0	12	1	0	.05	.037
1 T	20	0.0	0.0	0.0	0.0	0	0	.00	0.0	.00	.00	1	2	.01	.009	819
w/ butter	59	4.8	0.0	14.8		0.0	3	0	.00	.00	0	20	0	0	.01	.017
1 T	20	0.3	0.2	0.1	0.0	1	12	.00	0.0	.00	.01	1	2	.02	.042	819
syrup, sorghum	61	4.3	0.0	15.7		0.0	0	0	.03	.14	0	2	32	21	.09	.321
1 T	21	0.0	0.0	0.0	0.0	0	0	.02	0.0	.00	.17	210	12	.80	.027	819

1. Values are averages for grape, red plum, and strawberry.
2. Values are averages for apple, apple strawberry, blackberry, grape, guava, red currant, and strawberry.
3. Values are averages for apricot, blackberry, orange marmalade, peach, pineapple, red raspberry, and strawberry.
4. The sugar in this product is dextrose.
5. Contains 0.3 g fructose, 3.1 g glucose, 0.6 g sucrose, 2.0 g maltose, 1.6 g trisaccharides, and 7.4 g other polysaccharides.
6. Contains 0.4 g fructose, 3.9 g glucose, 1.9 g maltose, 1.6 g trisaccharides, and 7.1 g other polysaccharides.
7. Contains 0.9 g fructose, 3.2 g glucose, 2.2 g disaccharides, 1.6 g trisaccharides, and 6.3 g other polysaccharides.
8. Contains 0.8 g fructose, 3.6 g glucose, 1.9 g maltose, 1.5 g trisaccharides, and 7.1 g other polysaccharides.

33. VEGETABLES, VEGETABLE PRODUCTS, & VEGETABLE SALADS

	KCAL	H₂O	PRO	CHO	SUGR	DFIB	A (RE)	C	B-2	B-6	FOL	Na	Ca	Mg	Zn	Mn
	WT	FAT	SFA	MUFA	PUFA	CHOL	A (IU)	B-1	NIA	B-12	PANT	K	P	Fe	Cu	REF
adzuki beans																
boiled	294	152.5	17.3	57.0			2	0	.15	.22	279	18	64	120	4.07	1.318
1 cup	230	0.2	0.1			0	14	.26	1.6	.00	.99	1224	386	4.60	.685	816
cnd, sweetened	702	120.1	11.2	162.8			3	0	.17	.25	316	645	65	92	4.62	1.492
1 cup	296	0.1	0.0			0	15	.30	1.9	.00	1.12	352	219	3.34	.784	816
w/ sugar (yokan)	112	15.2	1.4	26.1			0	0	.00	.00	4	36	12	8	.03	.060
3 ¼" slices	43	0.1	0.0			0	0	.00	0.0	.00	.04	19	17	.50	.012	816
alfalfa sprouts, raw	10	30.1	1.3	1.2		0.8	5	3	.04	.01	12	2	11	9	.30	.062
1 cup	33	0.2	0.0	0.0	0.1	0	51	.03	0.2	.00	.19	26	23	.32	.052	811
amaranth, boiled	14	60.4	1.4	2.7			183	27	.09	.12	37	14	138	36	.58	.568
½ cup	66	0.1	0.0	0.0	0.1	0	1828	.01	0.4	.00	.04	423	48	1.49	.104	811
american style veg, frzn, Pillsbury	67	89.1	2.2	14.0		2.8		18	.06			232	17			
½ cup	108	1.6					323	.03	1.0			181	53	.65		I
arrowhead, boiled	9	9.2	0.5	1.9			0	0	.01	.02	1	2	1	6	.03	.034
1 med corm	12	0.0				0	0	.02	0.1	.00	.05	106	24	.15	.016	811
artichoke, boiled	150	251.9	10.4	33.5	3.3	16.2	54	30	.20	.33	153	285	135	180	1.47	.777
1 med	300	0.5	0.1	0.0	0.2	0	531	.20	3.0	.00	1.03	1062	258	3.87	.699	811
artichoke, frzn, boiled	36	69.2	2.5	7.3		3.7	13	4	.13	.07	95	42	17	25	.29	.218
2.8 oz	80	0.4	0.1	0.0	0.2	0	131	.05	0.7	.00	.16	211	49	.45	.049	811
artichoke hearts, marinated in veg oil, cnd, S&W Fine Foods—½ heart	20		0.0	2.0	0.0	1.0		6				80	0			
	28	2.0	0.0			0	0					55		.00		I
arugula, raw	3	9.2	0.3	0.4		0.2	24	2	.01	.01	10	3	16	5	.05	.032
½ cup	10	0.1	0.0	0.0	0.0	0	237	.00	0.0	.00	.04	37	5	.15	.008	811
asparagus																
boiled	22	83.0	2.3	3.8	1.4	1.4	49	10	.11	.11	131	10	18	9	.38	.137
½ cup (6 spears)	90	0.3	0.1	0.0	0.1	0	485	.11	1.0	.00	.14	144	49	.66	.101	811
cnd	23	113.7	2.6	3.0		1.9	64	22	.12	.13	116	347	19	12	.48	.206
½ cup	121	0.8	0.2	0.0	0.3	0	643	.07	1.2	.00	.17	208	52	2.21	.116	811

	KCAL	H₂O (g)	PRO (g)	CHO (g)	SUGR (g)	DFIB (g)	A (RE)	C (mg)	B-2 (mg)	B-6 (mg)	FOL (mcg)	Na (mg)	Ca (mg)	Mg (mg)	Zn (mg)	Mn (mg)
	WT (g)	FAT (g)	SFA (g)	MUFA (g)	PUFA (g)	CHOL (mg)	A (IU)	B-1 (mg)	NIA (mg)	B-12 (mcg)	PANT (mg)	K (mg)	P (mg)	Fe (mg)	Cu (mg)	REF
cnd, 50% less salt, Green Giant	19	113.7	2.3	3.0		1.2		16	.10			215	16			
½ cup	121	0.2					340	.04	0.7			171	44	.48		I
cnd, Pillsbury	16	99.6	2.0	2.7		1.1		14	.10			376	14			
½ cup	106	0.2				0	298	.04	0.6			149	39	.42		I
frzn, boiled	17	54.7	1.8	2.9		1.0	49	15	.06	.01	81	2	14	8	.34	.111
4 spears	60	0.3	0.1	0.0	0.1	0	491	.04	0.6	.00	.09	131	33	.38	.103	811
asparagus pilaf, frzn, Garden Gourmet	250	217.4	4.8	31.2		2.7		13	.13			594	35			
Microwave—9.5 oz	269	12.6					375	.94	8.1			234	100	5.38		I
balsam pear, leafy tips, boiled	20	51.4	2.1	3.9		1.1	100	32	.16	.44	51	8	24	55	.17	.311
1 cup	58	0.1	0.0	0.0	0.0	0	1005	.09	0.6	.00	.03	349	45	.59	.117	811
balsam pear, pods, boiled	12	58.2	0.5	2.7		1.2	7	20	.03	.03	32	4	6	10	.48	.053
½ cup pieces	62	0.1	0.0	0.0	0.0	0	70	.03	0.2	.00	.12	198	22	.24	.020	811
bamboo shoots																
boiled	14	115.1	1.8	2.3		1.2	0	0	.06	.12	3	5	14	4	.56	.136
1 cup	120	0.3	0.1	0.0	0.1	0	0	.02	0.4	.00	.08	640	24	.29	.098	811
cnd	25	123.6	2.3	4.2		1.8	1	1	.03	.18	4	9	10	5	.85	.206
1 cup	131	0.5	0.1	0.0	0.2	0	10	.03	0.2	.00	.12	105	33	.42	.149	811
raw	21	69.2	2.0	4.0		1.7	2	3	.05	.18	5	3	10	2	.84	.199
½ cup	76	0.2	0.1	0.0	0.1	0	15	.11	0.5	.00	.12	405	45	.38	.144	811
bean salad																
3 bean, cnd, Joan of Arc	90	99.1	2.4	22.6		3.2		2	.08			738	46			
½ cup	127	0.3					194	.04	1.0			202	44	2.03		I
3 bean, cnd, Pillsbury	67	101.6	2.2	15.4		0.9		17	.10			411	36			
½ cup	121	0.2				0	363	.08	1.0			243	36	.97		I
4 bean, cnd, Joan of Arc	110	104.9	3.2	26.8		3.7		6	.08			752	61			
½ cup	138	0.6					258	.04	1.2			170	54	1.66		I
bean sprouts, cnd, LaChoy	11		1.3	1.2	0.0	1.1	0	20				17	36			
1 cup	83	0.1	0.0			0	0							1.09		I
Beans 'n Fixins, cnd, Big John	127		7.1	22.6	11.4	6.3	10	3				590	72			
½ cup	133	3.5	1.2			3								2.67		I
beans, baked, homemade	382	164.9	14.0	54.1		13.9	0	3	.12	.23	122	1068	154	109	1.85	.645
1 cup	253	13.0	4.9	5.4	1.9	13	0	.34	1.0	.00	.39	906	276	5.03	.402	816
beans, barbecue, cnd, Campbell's	170		7.0	29.0	10.0	6.0		0				460	80			
½ cup	130	2.5	0.5			5	200							1.80		I
beans, barbecue old fashioned, cnd,	170		7.0	29.0	10.0	6.0		0				460	100			
Campbell's—½ cup	130	2.5	0.5			5	200							1.44		I
beans, black, refried, low-fat, cnd,	107		7.6	22.5	0.4	7.4						569				
Rosarita—½ cup	128	0.6	0.0			0										I
beans, brown sugar & bacon, cnd,	170		5.0	29.0	13.0	7.0	0	0				490	80			
Campbell's—½ cup	130	3.0	1.0		0.7	5	0							1.80		I
beans, chili																
caliente style, cnd, Joan of Arc	76	87.0	5.7	16.7		5.9		0	.08			496	32			
½ cup	113	1.0					122	.06	0.8			292	87	1.92		I
cnd, Gebhardt	134		7.1	30.7	1.4	7.2	66	2				630	64			
½ cup	130	1.0	0.4			0								2.31		I
cnd, Hunt's	87		6.0	17.1	8.2	5.7	14	1				597	41			
½ cup	127	1.0	0.0			0								.51		I
in zesty sce, cnd, Campbell's	130		6.0	21.0	4.0	6.0		1				490	60			
½ cup	130	3.0	1.0			5	300							1.44		I
beans, cnd, Open Range	152		6.6	30.5	11.2	6.7	0	4				424	85			
½ cup	132	2.3	0.7			1								2.27		I
beans, fiesta, cnd, Rosarita	112		7.9	20.6	2.0	4.7	0	5				548	47			
½ cup[1]	132	1.3	0.0			1	0							1.80		I
beans, Mix & Serve, cnd, Hunt's	125		1.8	30.3	15.8	7.8	9	2				575	74			
½ cup	135	2.8	1.1			1								1.94		I
beans, new england style, cnd,	180		5.0	32.0	14.0	6.0	0	1				460	80			
Campbell's—½ cup	130	3.0	1.0			5	0							1.80		I
beans, old fashioned, cnd, Campbell's	180		5.0	32.0	14.0	6.0		1				460	100			
½ cup	130	3.0	1.0			5	0							1.44		I

	KCAL / WT (g)	H₂O (g) / FAT (g)	PRO (g) / SFA (g)	CHO (g) / MUFA (g)	SUGR (g) / PUFA (g)	DFIB (g) / CHOL (mg)	A (RE) / A (IU)	C (mg) / B-1 (mg)	B-2 (mg) / NIA (mg)	B-6 (mg) / B-12 (mcg)	FOL (mcg) / PANT (mg)	Na (mg) / K (mg)	Ca (mg) / P (mg)	Mg (mg) / Fe (mg)	Zn (mg) / Cu (mg)	Mn (mg) / REF
beans, ranch, cnd, Open Range	124		6.2	22.7	5.4	8.3	36	2				628	55			
½ cup	133	3.2	1.1			1										I
beans, refried																
cnd	238	192.2	13.9	39.3		13.4	0	15	.04	.36	28	756	89	83	2.96	.397
1 cup	253	3.2	1.2	1.4	0.4	20	0	.07	0.8	.00	.25	676	218	4.20	.423	816
cnd, Gebhardt	109		6.1	19.8	1.8	6.2	0	0				497	43			
½ cup	128	2.8	1.3			1	0							2.00		I
cnd, Rosarita	111		6.7	19.4	1.4	6.4	0	1				515	41			
½ cup[2]	128	2.5	1.2			1	0							1.82		I
jalapeno, cnd, Gebhardt	105		6.9	19.0	3.2	6.3	0	0				380	44			
½ cup	128	3.0	1.4			1	0							.89		I
no fat, cnd, Gebhardt	92		7.3	19.5	1.8	6.2	0	0				480	43			
½ cup	128	0.5	0.0			0	0							1.92		I
no fat, cnd, Rosarita	109		6.8	24.7	0.5	6.6		2				578	62			
½ cup[3]	128	0.2	0.7		0.3	0								1.79		I
spicy, cnd, Rosarita	118		7.2	21.7	1.5	6.1	0	0				574	46			
½ cup	128	2.7	1.1			0	0							1.95		I
vegetarian, cnd, Gebhardt	118		7.7	20.9	3.2	6.5	0	0				550	41			
½ cup	128	2.3	0.4			0	0							2.27		I
vegetarian, cnd, Rosarita	119		7.7	20.9	3.2	6.5	0	0				551	40			
½ cup	128	2.3	0.3		1.0	0	0							2.27		I
beans, Special Recipe, cnd, Hunt's Homestyle—*½ cup*	152		6.6	30.5	11.2	6.7	39	11				687	91			
	132	2.3	0.7			1								2.82		I
beans, vegetarian, cnd	236	184.5	12.2	52.1		12.7	43	8	.15	.34	61	1008	127	81	3.56	.879
1 cup	254	1.1	0.3	0.1	0.5	0	434	.39	1.1	.00	.24	752	264	.74	.523	816
beans w/ pork																
cnd, Hunt's	130		6.2	27.5	16.4	4.3	13	2				516	45			
½ cup	127	1.2	0.4			0								.84		I
cnd, Open Range	157		6.1	26.8	10.9	7.4	35	4				621	73			
½ cup	131	4.8	1.7			2								2.11		I
in sweet sce, cnd	281	178.9	13.4	53.1		13.2	28	8	.15	.22	95	850	154	86	3.79	.939
1 cup	253	3.7	1.4	1.6	0.5	18	288	.12	0.9	.00	.26	673	266	4.20	.253	816
in tomato sce, cnd	248	183.9	13.1	49.1		12.1	30	8	.12	.17	57	1113	142	89	14.83	1.240
1 cup	253	2.6	1.0	1.1	0.3	18	314	.13	1.3	.00	1.34	759	296	8.30	.643	816
in tomato sce, cnd, Campbell's	130		5.0	24.0	8.0	6.0		0				420	60			
½ cup	130	2.0	0.5			5	200							1.44		I
in tomato sce, cnd, Joan of Arc	104	99.8	5.6	24.3		6.9		1	.04			424	60			
½ cup	133	1.2					36	.05	0.8			215	81	1.60		I
beet greens, boiled	19	64.2	1.9	3.9		2.1	367	18	.21	.10	10	174	82	49	.36	.370
½ cup	72	0.1	0.0	0.0	0.1	0	3672	.08	0.4	.00	.24	654	30	1.37	.181	811
beets																
boiled	37	74.0	1.4	8.5		1.7	3	3	.03	.06	68	65	14	20	.30	.277
½ cup slices	85	0.2	0.0	0.0	0.1	0	30	.02	0.3	.00	.12	259	32	.67	.063	811
cnd	26	77.3	0.8	6.1		1.4	1	3	.03	.05	26	165	13	14	.18	.244
½ cup slices	85	0.1	0.0	0.0	0.0	0	9	.01	0.1	.00	.13	126	14	1.55	.050	811
cnd, harvard	90	98.6	1.0	22.4		3.1	1	3	.06	.07	36	199	14	23	.28	.296
½ cup slices	123	0.1	0.0	0.0	0.0	0	14	.01	0.1	.00	.18	202	21	.44	.119	811
cnd, pickled	74	93.3	0.9	18.6			1	3	.05	.06	30	301	13	17	.30	.251
½ cup slices	114	0.1	0.0	0.0	0.0	0	13	.01	0.3	.00	.16	169	19	.47	.132	811
black beans, boiled	227	113.1	15.2	40.8		15.0	2	0	.10	.12	256	2	46	120	1.93	.764
1 cup	172	0.9	0.2	0.1	0.4	0	10	.42	0.9	.00	.42	611	241	3.61	.359	816
black turtle beans, boiled	241	121.6	15.1	45.0		9.8	2	0	.10	.14	158	6	102	91	1.41	.605
1 cup	185	0.6	0.2	0.1	0.3	0	11	.42	1.0	.00	.48	801	281	5.27	.498	816
black turtle beans, cnd	218	181.5	14.5	39.7		16.6	0	6	.29	.13	146	922	84	84	1.30	.559
1 cup	240	0.7	0.2	0.1	0.3	0	10	.34	1.5	.00	.44	739	259	4.56	.461	816
borage, boiled	25	91.9	2.1	3.5			438	33	.17	.09	10	88	102	57	.22	.385
3.5 oz	100	0.8	0.2	0.2	0.1	0	4385	.06	0.9	.00	.04	491	55	3.64	.143	811

Food / Measure	KCAL / WT (g)	H₂O (g) / FAT (g)	PRO (g) / SFA (g)	CHO (g) / MUFA (g)	SUGR (g) / PUFA (g)	DFIB (g) / CHOL (mg)	A (RE) / A (IU)	C (mg) / B-1 (mg)	B-2 (mg) / NIA (mg)	B-6 (mg) / B-12 (mcg)	FOL (mcg) / PANT (mg)	Na (mg) / K (mg)	Ca (mg) / P (mg)	Mg (mg) / Fe (mg)	Zn (mg) / Cu (mg)	Mn (mg) / REF
broadbeans																
boiled	187	121.6	12.9	33.4	3.1	9.2	3	1	.15	.12	177	9	61	73	1.72	.716
1 cup	170	0.7	0.1	0.1	0.3	0	26	.16	1.2	.00	.27	456	213	2.55	.440	816
cnd	182	205.6	14.0	31.8		9.5	3	5	.13	.12	84	1160	67	82	1.59	.737
1 cup	256	0.6	0.1	0.1	0.2	0	26	.05	2.5	.00	.30	620	202	2.56	.279	816
falafel	170	17.7	6.8	16.2			1	1	.08	.06	40	150	28	42	.77	.352
3 patties (2 ¼" dia)⁴	51	9.1	1.2	5.2	2.1	0	7	.07	0.5	.00	.15	298	98	1.74	.132	816
broccoli																
boiled	22	70.7	2.3	3.9		2.3	108	58	.09	.11	39	20	36	19	.30	.170
½ cup	78	0.3	0.0	0.0	0.1	0	1083	.04	0.4	.00	.40	228	46	.66	.034	811
chopped, frzn, boiled	26	83.5	2.9	4.9		2.8	174	37	.07	.12	52	22	47	18	.28	.299
½ cup	92	0.1	0.0	0.0	0.1	0	1741	.05	0.4	.00	.25	166	51	.56	.040	811
cuts w/ cheese sce, frzn, Pillsbury	75	121.4	4.0	11.1		2.8		45	.24			665	91			
5 oz	142	2.7				2	1343	.06	0.7			328	246	.57		I
raw	12	39.9	1.3	2.3	0.7	1.3	68	41	.05	.07	31	12	21	11	.18	.101
½ cup chopped	44	0.2	0.0	0.0	0.1	0	678	.03	0.3	.00	.24	143	29	.39	.020	811
spears, frzn, boiled	26	83.5	2.9	4.9		2.8	174	37	.07	.12	28	22	47	18	.28	.299
½ cup	92	0.1	0.0	0.0	0.1	0	1741	.05	0.4	.00	.25	166	51	.56	.040	811
w/ butter sce, frzn, Pillsbury	40	94.3	2.1	5.9				31	.07			350	38			
½ cup	104	2.0			0.0	5	245	.02	0.4			250	47	.39		I
w/ butter sce, frzn, Pillsbury	46	114.3	2.9	7.2		2.7		55	.10			424	44			
4.5 oz	128	1.8			0.0	5	572	.04	0.6			197	59	.51		I
w/ cheddar cheese sce, frzn, Pillsbury	60	95.9	3.1	9.0				38	.10			530	70			
½ cup	113	2.0				2	308	.03	0.7			260	71	.33		I
w/ cheese sce, frzn, Birds Eye	116	117.4	4.8	11.6				43	.19	.13	68	488	109	20	.47	
½ cup	142	6.2	1.9		0.9	6	3490	.06	0.5	.30	.42	249	103	.76	.040	I
w/ creamy italian cheese sce, frzn, Birds Eye—½ cup	90	109.1	5.0	6.6				47	.15	.13	74	391	93	17	.43	
	128	5.6	3.0		0.4	14	1941	.06	0.5	.25	.32	225	86	.91	.036	I
broccoli & cauliflower, frzn, Medley, Valley Combinations—½ cup	49	98.3	2.3	10.2		3.1		22	.05			261	30			
	113	1.1				0	1475	.07	0.9			188	49	.45		I
broccoli & cauliflower w/ creamy italian cheese sce, frzn, Birds Eye—½ cup	89	109.6	4.6	6.7				45	.14	.12	60	388	79	15	.36	
	128	5.5	3.0		0.4	14	1084	.05	0.4	.25	.28	220	78	.77	.029	I
broccoli carrot fanfare, frzn, Valley Combinations—½ cup	20	68.4	1.4	5.3		2.1		24	.01			28	22			
	76	0.2				0	1699	.03	0.5			164	26	.38		I
broccoli, carrots, & pasta w/ lightly seasoned sce, Birds Eye—⅔ cup	87	76.6	2.2	10.6				22	.07	.12	35	269	35	13	.27	
	95	4.4	0.8		0.9	0	8850	.06	0.6	.00	.16	164	40	.76	.053	I
broccoli, carrots, & rotini w/ cheese sce, frzn, Pillsbury—5.5 oz	120		4.0	20.0								550				
	156	3.0				2						280				I
broccoli, carrots, & water chestnuts, frzn, Birds Eye—¾ cup	45	99.8	2.7	9.4		3.5		42	.11	.20	67	34	49	18	.37	
	113	0.3	0.0		0.1	0	6032	.06	0.7	.00	.30	278	54	.83	.087	I
broccoli, cauliflower, & carrots																
frzn, Birds Eye	33	102.8	2.4	6.8		2.7		45	.08	.17	60	33	42	15	.30	
¾ cup	113	0.3	0.0		0.1	0	7821	.06	0.6	.00	.22	234	48	.82	.048	I
frzn, Pillsbury	26	102.8	2.0	7.0		3.1		43	.08			43	35			
4 oz	113	0.2	0.0		0.0	0	2888	.03	0.8			224	40	.45		I
frzn, w/ cheese sce, Birds Eye	99	119.9	4.0	11.6				39	.15	.15	53	381	86	18	.40	
½ cup	142	4.7	1.5		0.7	4	6158	.06	0.6	.23	.35	257	84	.73	.042	I
w/ butter sce, frzn, Pillsbury	30	72.1	2.0	3.6				21	.05			240	24			
½ cup	85	1.2			0.0	5	1750	.02	0.6			120	26	.41		I
w/ cheese sce, frzn, Pillsbury	75	121.6	3.4	11.9		2.3		15	.21			616	81			
5 oz	142	2.4				5	1894	.04	0.4			304	207	.43		I
broccoli cauliflower supreme, frzn, Valley Combinations—½ cup	17	69.2	1.4	4.7		2.1		29	.05			29	24			
	76	0.2				0	1943	.02	0.6			150	27	.30		I
broccoli, corn, & red peppers, frzn, Birds Eye—⅔ cup	59	95.2	3.2	13.3		2.9		39	.09	.16	66	16	33	20	.40	
	113	0.5	0.1		0.2	0	1682	.07	1.2	.00	.23	225	66	.77	.047	I
broccoli fanfare, frzn, Valley Combinations—½ cup	67	93.8	3.0	13.0		2.8		27	.08			325	23			
	113	1.5				0	350	.06	0.7			160	57	.45		I
broccoli, green beans, pearl onions, & red peppers, frzn, Birds Eye—¾ cup	32	103.1	2.4	6.6		2.9		42	.09	.12	58	18	51	18	.29	
	113	0.2	0.0		0.1	0	1848	.06	0.6	.00	.19	199	44	.91	.052	I

	KCAL / WT (g)	H₂O (g) / FAT (g)	PRO (g) / SFA (g)	CHO (g) / MUFA (g)	SUGR (g) / PUFA (g)	DFIB (g) / CHOL (mg)	A (RE) / A (IU)	C (mg) / B-1 (mg)	B-2 (mg) / NIA (mg)	B-6 (mg) / B-12 (mcg)	FOL (mcg) / PANT (mg)	Na (mg) / K (mg)	Ca (mg) / P (mg)	Mg (mg) / Fe (mg)	Zn (mg) / Cu (mg)	Mn (mg) / REF
broccoli, peas & carrots, frzn, Pillsbury	48	65.4	2.9	8.4				34	.07			57	42			
2.7 oz	80	0.3					6032	.09	0.9			191	49	.90		I
broccoli, red peppers, bamboo shoots, &	29	103.6	2.8	5.6		3.0		51	.10	.12	66	21	43	14	.25	
straw mushrooms, frzn, Birds Eye—¾ *cup*	113	0.3	0.0		0.1	0	2233	.07	0.8	.00	.19	253	54	.81	.037	I
brussels sprouts																
boiled	30	68.1	2.0	6.8		2.0	56	48	.06	.14	47	16	28	16	.26	.177
½ cup	78	0.4	0.1	0.0	0.2	0	561	.08	0.5	.00	.20	247	44	.94	.065	811
frzn, boiled	33	67.7	2.8	6.5		3.2	46	36	.09	.23	79	18	19	19	.28	.250
½ cup	78	0.3	0.1	0.0	0.2	0	459	.08	0.4	.00	.27	254	42	.58	.055	811
w/ butter sce, frzn, Pillsbury	40	81.9	2.9	8.0				59	.08			280	28			
½ cup	94	1.0			0.0	5	785	.09	0.7			290	49	.45		I
w/ cheese sce, frzn, Birds Eye	113	103.0	5.0	12.5				56	.19	.13	90	417	77	21	.40	
½ cup	128	5.6	1.7		0.9	5	2622	.09	0.6	.26	.38	359	96	.84	.028	I
w/ cheese sce, frzn, Pillsbury	79	97.9	3.1	13.0				59	.18			493	67			
½ cup	118	1.5					610	.06	1.2			325	185	.52		I
brussels sprouts, cauliflower, & carrots,	40	100.6	3.0	8.2		3.7		58	.09	.21	87	26	31	18	.28	
frzn, Birds Eye—¾ *cup*	113	0.3	0.1		0.2	0	4047	.08	0.7	.00	.29	308	53	.81	.039	I
burdock root, boiled	110	94.5	2.6	26.4		2.3	0	3	.07	.35	24	5	61	49	.47	.338
1 cup	125	0.2	0.0		0.1	0	0	.05	0.4	.00	.44	450	116	.96	.111	811
butter beans, cnd, Joan of Arc	76	98.1	5.7	15.9		3.7		0	.04			405	34			
½ cup	122	0.4					27	.02	0.6			296	85	1.22		I
butterbur (fuki), boiled	8	96.7	0.2	2.2			3	19	.01	.05	4	4	59	8	.09	.156
3.5 oz	100	0.0				0	27	.01	0.1	.00	.02	354	7	.10	.059	811
cabbage, chinese																
pak-choi, boiled	10	81.2	1.3	1.5		1.4	218	22	.05	.14	35	29	79	9	.14	.122
½ cup shredded	85	0.1	0.0	0.0	0.1	0	2183	.03	0.4	.00	.07	315	25	.88	.016	811
pak-choi, raw	5	33.4	0.5	0.8		0.3	105	16	.02	.07	23	23	37	7	.07	.056
½ cup shredded	35	0.1	0.0	0.0	0.0	0	1050	.01	0.2	.00	.03	88	13	.28	.007	811
pe-tsai, boiled	17	113.3	1.8	2.9			115	19	.05	.21	64	11	38	12	.21	.182
1 cup shredded	119	0.2	0.0	0.0	0.1	0	1151	.05	0.6	.00	.10	268	46	.36	.035	811
pe-tsai, raw	6	35.9	0.5	1.2		1.2	46	10	.02	.09	30	3	29	5	.09	.072
½ cup shredded	38	0.1	0.0	0.0	0.0	0	456	.02	0.2	.00	.04	90	11	.12	.014	811
cabbage, green, boiled	17	70.2	0.8	3.3		1.7	10	15	.04	.08	15	6	23	6	.07	.088
½ cup shredded	75	0.3	0.0	0.0	0.1	0	99	.04	0.2	.00	.10	73	11	.13	.009	811
cabbage, green, raw	9	32.3	0.5	1.9	1.3	0.8	5	11	.01	.03	15	6	16	5	.06	.056
½ cup shredded	35	0.1	0.0	0.0	0.0	0	47	.02	0.1	.00	.05	86	8	.21	.008	811
cabbage, red, boiled	16	70.2	0.8	3.5	2.1	1.5	2	26	.01	.11	9	6	28	8	.11	.097
½ cup shredded	75	0.2	0.0	0.0	0.1	0	20	.03	0.2	.00	.17	105	22	.26	.052	811
cabbage, red, raw	9	32.0	0.5	2.1	1.9	0.7	1	20	.01	.07	7	4	18	5	.07	.063
½ cup shredded	35	0.1	0.0	0.0	0.0	0	14	.02	0.1	.00	.11	72	15	.17	.034	811
cabbage, savoy, boiled	18	67.2	1.3	3.9		2.0	65	12	.01	.11	34	18	22	18	.17	.111
½ cup shredded	73	0.1	0.0	0.0	0.0	0	649	.04	0.0	.00	12	134	24	.28	.038	811
cabbage, savoy, raw	9	31.8	0.7	2.1	1.0	1.1	35	11	.01	.07	28	10	12	10	.09	.063
½ cup shredded	35	0.0	0.0	0.0	0.0	0	350	.02	0.1	.00	.07	81	15	.14	.022	811
cardoon, boiled	22	93.5	0.8	5.3		1.7	12	2	.03	.04	22	176	72	43	.18	.133
3.5 oz	100	0.1	0.0	0.0	0.0	0	118	.02	0.3	.00	.10	392	23	.73	.029	811
carrots																
boiled	35	68.2	0.9	8.2	3.4	2.6	1915	2	.04	.19	11	51	24	10	.23	.587
½ cup slices	78	0.1	0.0	0.0	0.1	0	19152	.03	0.4	.00	.24	177	23	.48	.105	811
cnd	17	67.9	0.5	4.0	2.4	1.1	1005	2	.02	.08	7	177	18	6	.19	.329
½ cup slices	73	0.1	0.0	0.0	0.1	0	10055	.01	0.4	.00	.10	131	18	.47	.076	811
frzn, boiled	26	65.6	0.9	6.0		2.6	1292	2	.03	.09	8	43	20	7	.18	.296
½ cup slices	73	0.1	0.0	0.0	0.0	0	12922	.02	0.3	.00	.12	115	19	.34	.053	811
raw	31	63.2	0.7	7.3	4.8	2.2	2025	7	.04	.11	10	25	19	11	.14	.102
1 med	72	0.1	0.0	0.0	0.1	0	20253	.07	0.7	.00	.14	233	32	.36	.034	811
carrots, peas & pearl onions, frzn, Birds	48	81.8	2.1	10.1		2.0		9	.05	.16	22	61	29	14	.35	
Eye—½ *cup*	95	0.2	0.0		0.1	0	9344	.10	1.0	.00	.17	181	37	.86	.067	811
cassava, raw	120	68.5	3.1	26.9		1.6	1	48	.10	.30	22	8	91	66	.25	.411
3.5 oz	100	0.4	0.1	0.1	0.1	0	10	.23	1.4	.00	.33	764	70	3.60	.184	811

	KCAL / WT (g)	H₂O (g) / FAT (g)	PRO (g) / SFA (g)	CHO (g) / MUFA (g)	SUGR (g) / PUFA (g)	DFIB (g) / CHOL (mg)	A (RE) / A (IU)	C (mg) / B-1 (mg)	B-2 (mg) / NIA (mg)	B-6 (mg) / B-12 (mcg)	FOL (mcg) / PANT (mg)	Na (mg) / K (mg)	Ca (mg) / P (mg)	Mg (mg) / Fe (mg)	Zn (mg) / Cu (mg)	Mn (mg) / REF
cauliflower																
boiled	14	57.7	1.1	2.5		1.7	1	27	.03	.11	27	9	10	6	.11	.086
½ cup pieces	62	0.3	0.0	0.0	0.1	0	11	.03	0.3	.00	.31	88	20	.20	.017	811
frzn, boiled	17	84.6	1.4	3.4		2.4	2	28	.05	.08	37	16	15	8	.12	.135
½ cup pieces	90	0.2	0.0	0.0	0.1	0	20	.03	0.3	.00	.09	125	22	.37	.022	811
raw	13	46.0	1.0	2.6	1.2	1.3	1	23	.03	.11	29	15	11	8	.14	.078
½ cup pieces	50	0.1	0.0	0.0	0.0	0	10	.03	0.3	.00	.33	152	22	.22	.021	811
w/ butter sce, frzn, Pillsbury	30	80.1	1.1	3.5				24	.04			319	21			
½ cup	88	1.2					64	.02	0.4			123	24	.35		I
w/ cheese sce, frzn, Birds Eye	114	118.2	4.0	11.7				39	.16	.12	42	483	83	17	.35	
½ cup	142	6.1	1.9		0.9	6	2298	.06	0.4	.30	.33	240	88	.50	.026	I
w/ cheese sce, frzn, Pillsbury	76	133.5	3.1	14.0		3.3		44	.19			693	83			
5.5 oz	156	2.3				5	465	.05	0.9			298	218	.78		I
cauliflower & carrots, frzn, Pillsbury	60	97.7	2.2	7.0				27	.07			287	16			
½ cup	111	2.9					1485	.11	0.7			161	39	.67		I
cauliflower, carrots, & snow peas, frzn, Birds Eye—⅔ cup	38	101.9	2.0	8.1		2.9		33	.07	.18	33	33	33	15	.26	
	113	0.2	0.0		0.1	0	7670	.05	0.7	.00	.26	228	36	.88	.039	I
cauliflower, green, ckd	20	55.5	1.9	3.9		2.0	9	45	.06	.13	25	14	20	12	.39	.150
½ cup pieces	62	0.1	0.0	0.0	0.1	0	87	.04	0.4	.00	.42	172	35	.45	.025	811
cauliflower, green, raw	16	44.9	1.5	3.0		1.6	8	44	.05	.11	29	12	17	10	.32	.123
½ cup pieces	50	0.1	0.0	0.0	0.1	0	76	.04	0.4	.00	.35	150	31	.36	.021	811
celeriac, boiled	25	92.3	1.0	5.9		1.2	0	4	.04	.10	3	61	26	12	.20	.096
3.5 oz	100	0.2				0	0	.03	0.4	.00	.20	173	66	.43	.043	811
celeriac, raw	39	88.0	1.5	9.2		1.8	0	8	.06	.17	8	100	43	20	.33	.158
3.5 oz	100	0.3	0.1	0.1	0.1	0	0	.05	0.7	.00	.35	300	115	.70	.070	811
celery, boiled	14	70.6	0.6	3.0		1.2	10	5	.04	.06	17	68	32	9	.11	.080
½ cup diced	75	0.1	0.0	0.0	0.1	0	99	.03	0.2	.00	.15	213	19	.32	.027	811
celery, raw	6	37.9	0.3	1.5	0.4	0.7	5	3	.02	.03	11	35	16	4	.05	.041
1 stalk (7.5" long)	40	0.1	0.0	0.0	0.0	0	54	.02	0.1	.00	.07	115	10	.16	.014	811
celtuce, raw	22	94.5	0.8	3.6		1.7	350	20	.07	.05	46	11	39	28	.27	.688
12 leaves	100	0.3				0	3500	.06	0.6	.00	.18	330	39	.55	.040	811
chard, swiss, boiled	18	81.5	1.7	3.6		1.8	276	16	.08	.07	8	158	51	76	.29	.294
½ cup chopped	88	0.1	0.0	0.0	0.0	0	2762	.03	0.3	.00	.14	483	29	1.99	.143	811
chayote, boiled	19	74.7	0.5	4.1		2.2	4	6	.03	.09	14	1	10	10	.25	.135
½ cup pieces	80	0.4				0	38	.02	0.3	.00	.33	138	23	.18	.088	811
chickpeas (garbanzo beans)																
boiled	269	98.7	14.5	45.0	7.9	12.5	5	2	.10	.23	282	11	80	79	2.51	1.689
1 cup	164	4.2	0.4	1.0	1.9	0	44	.19	0.9	.00	.47	477	276	4.74	.577	816
cnd	286	167.3	11.9	54.3		10.6	5	9	.08	1.14	160	718	77	70	2.54	1.450
1 cup	240	2.7	0.3	0.6	1.2	0	58	.07	0.3	.00	.72	413	216	3.24	.418	816
hummus	421	159.7	12.1	49.6		12.5	5	19	.13	.98	146	600	123	71	2.71	1.400
1 cup[5]	246	20.8	3.1	8.7	7.8	0	62	.23	1.0	.00	.71	428	276	3.86	.561	816
chicory greens, raw	21	82.8	1.5	4.2		3.6	360	22	.09	.09	99	41	90	27	.38	.386
½ cup chopped	90	0.3	0.1	0.0	0.1	0	3600	.05	0.5	.00	1.04	378	42	.81	.266	811
chicory roots, raw	44	48.0	0.8	10.5			1	3	.02	.14	14	30	25	13	.20	.140
1 root	60	0.1	0.0	0.0	0.1	0	4	.02	0.2	.00	.19	174	37	.48	.046	811
chicory, witloof, raw	8	42.5	0.4	1.8		1.4	1	1	.01	.02	17	1	9	5	.07	.045
½ cup	45	0.0	0.0	0.0	0.0	0	13	.03	0.1	.00	.07	95	12	.11	.023	811
chiles, green, cnd, Rosarita	4		0.2	1.1	0.6	0.5	12	7				74	17			
¼ cup slices (1 whole)	35	0.1	0.0			0								.14		I
chiles, jalapeno, diced, cnd, Rosarita	5		0.4	0.8	0.3	0.6	14	1				85	10			
2 T	30	0.2	0.0			0								.19		I
chinese style veg, frzn, Birds Eye	68	80.3	2.2	7.7				16	.05	.08	32	299	32	24	.20	
½ cup[6]	95	3.9	0.7		0.7	0	1669	.04	0.4	.00	.15	148	32	.77	.038	I
chinese style veg, stir fry, frzn, Birds Eye	36	82.8	2.0	7.9		1.9		16	.11	.08	23	540	44	24	.27	
½ cup[7]	95	0.2	0.0		0.1	0	2153	.07	0.6	.00	.20	234	36	.98	.087	I
chop suey veg, cnd, LaChoy	10		0.8	2.3	0.0	1.0	17	4				241	37			
½ cup	63	0.1	0.0			0								.46		I
chow mein style veg, frzn, Birds Eye	89	75.5	1.6	12.4				6	.09	.09	20	368	25	16	.26	
½ cup[8]	95	4.2	0.8		0.8	0	2745	.06	0.6	.00	.20	202	36	.63	.097	I

						Vitamins					Minerals				
KCAL	H₂O (g)	PRO (g)	CHO (g)	SUGR (g)	DFIB (g)	A (RE)	C (mg)	B-2 (mg)	B-6 (mg)	FOL (mcg)	Na (mg)	Ca (mg)	Mg (mg)	Zn (mg)	Mn (mg)
WT (g)	FAT (g)	SFA (g)	MUFA (g)	PUFA (g)	CHOL (mg)	A (IU)	B-1 (mg)	NIA (mg)	B-12 (mcg)	PANT (mg)	K (mg)	P (mg)	Fe (mg)	Cu (mg)	REF
chrysanthemum, garland, boiled															
20	92.5	1.6	4.3		2.3	505	24	.16	.12	50	53	69	18	.20	.355
1 cup pieces															
100	0.1	0.0	0.0	0.0	0	5050	.02	0.7	.00	.04	569	43	3.74	.133	811
chrysanthemum, garland, raw															
4	23.1	0.4	1.1		0.7	367	9	.06	.03	19	13	14	4	.05	.093
1 cup pieces															
25	0.0				0	3669	.01	0.2	.00	.01	143	8	.78	.035	811
coleslaw, homemade															
41	48.9	0.8	7.4		0.9	49	20	.04	.08	16	14	27	6	.12	.058
½ cup[9]															
60	1.6	0.2	0.4	0.8	5	381	.04	0.2	.00	.08	109	19	.35	.014	811
collards, boiled															
35	117.6	1.7	7.8		3.6	349	15	.07	.07	8	20	29	9	.14	.289
1 cup chopped															
128	0.2	0.0	0.0	0.1	0	3491	.03	0.4	.00	.07	168	10	.20	.041	811
collards, frzn, boiled															
31	75.2	2.5	6.0		2.4	508	22	.10	.10	65	43	179	26	.23	.564
½ cup chopped															
85	0.3	0.1	0.0	0.2	0	5084	.04	0.5	.00	.10	213	23	.95	.047	811
corn broccoli bounty, frzn, Valley															
45	68.9	2.1	9.7		1.9		24	.02			14	17			
Combinations—*½ cup*															
82	0.6				0	284	.02	1.0			189	44	.49		I
corn, green beans, & pasta curls w/ light															
108	71.1	3.0	14.9				8	.07	.07	17	283	53	18	.37	
cream sce, frzn, Birds Eye—*½ cup*															
95	4.9	1.1		0.9	1	630	.07	0.9	.01	.10	141	68	.63	.040	I
corn pudding															
273	190.8	11.0	31.9			90	7	.32	.29	63	138	100	38	1.25	1.340
1 cup[10]															
250	13.3	6.3	4.3	1.7	250	615	1.03	2.5	.22	.61	403	143	1.40	.107	811
corn, white, cnd, vacuum pak, Pillsbury															
100	78.0	2.4	21.5		0.9		10	.07			287	5			
½ cup															
104	0.4				0	332	.06	1.6			219	67	.37		I
corn, white w/ butter sce, frzn, Pillsbury															
100	84.4	2.0	20.5				7	.06			280	7			
½ cup															
113	2.0			0.0	5	31	.03	1.0			230	63	.26		I
corn, yellow															
50% less salt, cnd, Green Giant															
45	69.7	1.2	10.7		1.2		2	.04			94	2			
½ cup															
82	0.2					37	.02	0.7			88	31	.06		I
boiled															
89	57.0	2.7	20.6	2.1	2.3	18	5	.06	.05	38	14	2	26	.39	.159
½ cup															
82	1.0	0.2	0.3	0.5	0	178	.18	1.3	.00	.72	204	84	.50	.043	811
cnd															
66	63.1	2.1	15.2	2.3	1.6	13	7	.06	.04	40	175	4	16	.32	.142
½ cup															
82	0.8	0.1	0.2	0.4	0	128	.03	1.0	.00	.55	160	53	.71	.048	811
cnd, vacuum pack															
83	80.4	2.5	20.4		2.1	25	9	.08	.06	52	286	5	24	.48	.070
½ cup															
105	0.5	0.1	0.2	0.2	0	253	.04	1.2	.00	.71	195	67	.44	.050	811
cnd w/ red & green peppers															
85	88.3	2.7	20.7			26	10	.09	.11	39	396	6	28	.42	.049
½ cup															
114	0.6	0.1	0.2	0.3	0	264	.03	1.1	.00	.51	174	71	.90	.068	811
cream style, frzn, Pillsbury															
110	97.5	2.9	25.6				5	.05			370	9			
½ cup															
126	0.6	0.0		0.0	0	166	.09	0.6			180	65	.26		I
creamstyle, cnd															
59	64.6	1.4	14.9		1.0	8	4	.04	.05	37	234	2	14	.43	.032
½ cup															
82	0.3	0.1	0.1	0.2	0	80	.02	0.8	.00	.15	110	42	.31	.043	811
frzn, boiled															
66	62.9	2.3	16.0	1.5	2.0	18	3	.06	.11	25	4	3	16	.33	.104
½ cup															
82	0.4	0.1	0.1	0.2	0	180	.07	1.1	.00	.15	121	47	.29	.030	811
on-the-cob, frzn, Birds Eye															
120	90.5	4.1	28.7				8	.11	.22	49	4	5	40	.87	
1 ear															
125	1.0	0.1		0.5	0	261	.15	2.1	.00	.37	378	113	.86	.063	I
on-the-cob, frzn, Ore-Ida															
183	103.8	5.1	38.7				13	.12			22				
5.3 oz ear															
150	0.9	0.2	0.3	0.6	0	515	.12	3.7			460		1.44		I
on-the-cob w/ butter sce, frzn, Pillsbury															
120	78.1	2.9	23.8		1.8		9	.14			125	3			
2 half ears															
107	1.6	0.0		0.0	10	216	.09	1.8			266	81	.43		I
w/ butter sce, frzn, Niblets															
110	99.6	2.9	21.8		2.2		9	.06			346	0			
4.5 oz															
128	2.2			0.0	5	129	.06	1.7			225	77	.92		I
w/ butter sce, frzn, Pillsbury															
100		3.0	19.0								310				
½ cup															
113	2.0	1.0			5						140				I
w/ peppers, cnd, Mexicorn															
79	77.8	2.0	19.4		3.1		4	.08			321	6			
½ cup															
101	0.6					86	.04	1.1			191	60	.40		I
cornsalad, raw															
6	26.0	0.6	1.0			199	11	.02	.08	4	1	11	4	.17	.101
½ cup[11]															
28	0.1				0	1986	.02	0.1	.00	.01	129	15	.61	.038	811
cowpeas (blackeye peas)															
boiled, immature															
160	124.5	5.2	33.5		8.3	130	4	.24	.11	210	7	211	86	1.70	.944
1 cup															
165	0.6	0.2	0.1	0.3	0	1305	.17	2.3	.00	.25	690	84	1.85	.219	811
cnd, Joan of Arc															
91	115.0	7.1	17.8		3.7			.06			298	55			
½ cup															
142	0.6				0	8	.06	0.4			229	129	1.28		I
cnd, mature															
185	191.1	11.4	32.7		7.9	2	6	.18	.11	123	718	48	67	1.68	.679
1 cup															
240	1.3	0.3	0.1	0.6	0	31	.18	0.8	.00	.46	413	168	2.33	.281	816
frzn, boiled															
112	56.2	7.2	20.2		5.4	7	2	.05	.08	120	4	20	43	1.21	.672
½ cup															
85	0.6	0.1	0.1	0.2	0	64	.22	0.6	.00	.18	319	104	1.80	.156	811

Each food item is given as two rows. The first row columns are: **KCAL | H₂O (g) | PRO (g) | CHO (g) | SUGR (g) | DFIB (g) | A (RE) | C (mg) | B-2 (mg) | B-6 (mg) | FOL (mcg) | Na (mg) | Ca (mg) | Mg (mg) | Zn (mg) | Mn (mg)**. The second (measure) row columns are: **WT (g) | FAT (g) | SFA (g) | MUFA (g) | PUFA (g) | CHOL (mg) | A (IU) | B-1 (mg) | NIA (mg) | B-12 (mcg) | PANT (mg) | K (mg) | P (mg) | Fe (mg) | Cu (mg) | REF**.

Item	KCAL / WT	H₂O / FAT	PRO / SFA	CHO / MUFA	SUGR / PUFA	DFIB / CHOL	A(RE) / A(IU)	C / B-1	B-2 / NIA	B-6 / B-12	FOL / PANT	Na / K	Ca / P	Mg / Fe	Zn / Cu	Mn / REF
young pods w/ seeds, boiled	16	42.1	1.2	3.3			66	8	.04	.06	12	1	26	19	.11	.103
½ cup	47	0.1	0.0	0.0	0.1	0	658	.04	0.4	.00	.30	92	23	.33	.033	811
cowpeas, catjang, boiled	200	119.2	13.9	34.7		6.2	2	1	.08	.16	242	32	44	164	3.20	.809
1 cup	171	1.2	0.3	0.1	0.5	0	17	.28	1.2	.00	.66	641	243	5.22	.463	816
cowpeas, leafy tips, boiled	12	48.4	2.5	1.5			31	10	.08	.07	32	3	37	33	.13	.218
1 cup chopped	53	0.1	0.0	0.0	0.0	0	305	.14	0.5	.00	.02	186	22	.58	.082	811
cranberry beans, boiled	241	114.4	16.5	43.3		17.7	0	0	.12	.14	366	2	89	89	2.02	.655
1 cup	177	0.8	0.2	0.1	0.4	0	0	.37	0.9	.00	.42	685	239	3.70	.409	816
cranberry beans, cnd	216	201.7	14.4	39.3		16.4	0	2	.10	.14	201	863	88	83	2.18	.520
1 cup	260	0.7	0.2	0.1	0.3	0	0	.10	1.3	.00	.37	676	224	4.03	.369	816
cucumber, raw	7	49.9	0.4	1.4	1.2	0.4	11	3	.01	.02	7	1	7	6	.10	.040
½ cup slices (⅙ cucumber)	52	0.1	0.0	0.0	0.0	0	112	.01	0.1	.00	.09	75	10	.14	.017	811
dandelion greens, boiled	17	46.7	1.0	3.3		1.5	608	9	.09	.08	7	23	73	12	.15	.120
½ cup	52	0.3	0.1	0.0	0.1	0	6084	.07	0.3	.00	.03	121	22	.94	.060	811
dandelion greens, raw	13	24.0	0.8	2.6		1.0	392	10	.07	.07	8	21	52	10	.11	.096
½ cup chopped	28	0.2	0.0	0.0	0.1	0	3920	.05	0.2	.00	.02	111	18	.87	.048	811
dock, boiled	20	93.6	1.8	2.9		2.6	347	26	.09	.10	8	3	38	89	.17	.303
3.5 oz	100	0.6				0	3474	.03	0.4	.00	.04	321	52	2.08	.114	811
dock, raw	15	62.3	1.3	2.1		1.9	268	32	.07	.08	9	3	29	69	.13	.234
½ cup chopped	67	0.5				0	2680	.03	0.3	.00	.03	261	42	1.61	.088	811
eggplant																
boiled	13	44.0	0.4	3.2		1.2	3	1	.01	.04	7	1	3	6	.07	.065
½ cup	48	0.1	0.0	0.0	0.0	0	31	.04	0.3	.00	.04	119	11	.17	.052	811
fried sticks, frzn, Mrs. Paul's	240		4.1	28.2				1	.08			582	22			
3.5 oz	99	12.3					0	.04	0.6			143		1.30		I
parmigiana, frzn, Mrs. Paul's	293		6.4	25.8				6	.23			715	138			
5.5 oz	156	18.2				7	745	.11	1.8			363		2.60		I
raw	11	37.7	0.4	2.5	1.4	1.0	3	1	.01	.03	8	1	3	6	.06	.053
½ cup	41	0.1	0.0	0.0	0.0	0	34	.02	0.2	.00	.10	89	9	.11	.023	811
endive, raw	4	23.4	0.3	0.8	0.3	0.8	51	2	.02	.01	36	6	13	4	.20	.105
½ cup chopped	25	0.1	0.0	0.0	0.0	0	513	.02	0.1	.00	.23	79	7	.21	.025	811
fennel bulb, raw	27	78.5	1.1	6.3		2.7	11	10	.03	.04	23	45	43	15	.17	.166
1 cup slices	87	0.2				0	117	.01	0.6	.00	.20	360	44	.63	.057	811
french beans, boiled	228	117.8	12.5	42.5		16.6	0	2	.11	.19	132	11	112	99	1.13	.676
1 cup	177	1.3	0.1	0.1	0.8	0	5	.23	1.0	.00	.39	655	181	1.91	.204	816
garden cress, boiled	16	62.9	1.3	2.6		0.5	524	16	.11	.11	25	5	41	18	.10	.253
½ cup	68	0.4	0.0	0.1	0.1	0	5236	.04	0.5	.00	.11	240	33	.54	.078	811
garden cress, raw	8	22.4	0.7	1.4		0.3	233	17	.07	.06	20	4	20	10	.06	.138
½ cup	25	0.2	0.0	0.1	0.1	0	2325	.02	0.3	.00	.06	152	19	.33	.043	811
garden medley, cnd, Pillsbury	45		1.0	9.0								360				
½ cup	117	0.0				0						130				I
garden salad, cnd, Joan of Arc	75	112.9	1.5	19.4		2.7		6	.10			556	39			
½ cup	136	0.3					1875	.04	1.0			212	34	.82		I
garlic, raw	13	5.3	0.6	3.0		0.2	0	3	.01	.11	0	2	16	2	.10	.150
3 cloves	9	0.0	0.0	0.0	0.0	0	0	.02	0.1	.00	.05	36	14	.15	.027	811
gourd, calabash (white-flowered), boiled	11	69.6	0.4	2.7			0	6	.02	.03	3	1	18	8	.51	.048
½ cup cubes	73	0.0	0.0	0.0	0.0	0	0	.02	0.3	.00	.11	124	9	.18	.019	811
gourd, dishcloth (towelgourd), boiled	50	75.0	0.6	12.8			23	5	.04	.09	11	19	8	18	.15	.198
½ cup slices	89	0.3	0.0	0.1	0.1	0	231	.04	0.2	.00	.45	403	28	.32	.076	811
great northern beans																
boiled	209	122.1	14.7	37.3		12.4	0	2	.10	.21	181	4	120	89	1.56	.917
1 cup	177	0.8	0.2	0.0	0.3	0	2	.28	1.2	.00	.47	692	292	3.77	.437	816
cnd	299	183.1	19.3	55.1		12.8	0	3	.16	.28	213	10	139	134	1.70	1.069
1 cup	262	1.0	0.3	0.0	0.4	0	3	.37	1.2	.00	.73	920	356	4.11	.419	816
cnd, Joan of Arc	78	98.8	5.8	17.9		5.6		0	.03			288	105			
½ cup	125	0.6				0	10	.04	0.5			151	90	2.13		I
green bean mushroom casserole, frzn, Stouffers—3 oz entree	121	63.8	2.3	9.4				1	.12			468	51			
	85	8.2				9	136	.03	0.3			136		.34		I
green bean salad, german style, cnd, Joan of Arc—½ cup	106	105.6	1.8	15.4		2.1		3	.08			537	44			
	132	4.0					305	.04	0.8			139	30	1.19		I

	KCAL / WT (g)	H₂O (g) / FAT (g)	PRO (g) / SFA (g)	CHO (g) / MUFA (g)	SUGR (g) / PUFA (g)	DFIB (g) / CHOL (mg)	A (RE) / A (IU)	C (mg) / B-1 (mg)	B-2 (mg) / NIA (mg)	B-6 (mg) / B-12 (mcg)	FOL (mcg) / PANT (mg)	Na (mg) / K (mg)	Ca (mg) / P (mg)	Mg (mg) / Fe (mg)	Zn (mg) / Cu (mg)	Mn (mg) / REF
green beans, bavarian style & spaetzle (noodles), frzn, Birds Eye—½ cup	98 / 95	74.8 / 5.3	2.4 / 1.0	11.5 /	/ 1.0	/ 14	/ 572	4 / .04	.06 / 0.3	.05 / .10	13 / .10	357 / 73	40 / 36	14 / .72	.25 / .046	/ I
green beans (snap beans)																
boiled — ½ cup[12]	22 / 62	55.3 / 0.2	1.2 / 0.0	4.9 / 0.0	1.4 / 0.1	2.0 / 0	42 / 413	6 / .05	.06 / 0.4	.03 / .00	21 / .05	2 / 185	29 / 24	16 / .79	.22 / .064	.182 / 811
cnd — ½ cup	14 / 68	63.4 / 0.1	0.8 / 0.0	3.1 / 0.0	1.1 / 0.0	1.3 / 0	24 / 237	3 / .01	.04 / 0.1	.03 / .00	22 / .09	178 / 74	18 / 13	9 / .61	.20 / .026	.136 / 811
cut, frzn, Birds Eye — ½ cup	25 / 85	77.4 / 0.1	1.4 / 0.0	5.8 / 0.0	/ 0.1	2.2 / 0	/ 455	9 / .05	.07 / 0.3	.05 / .00	11 / .06	3 / 131	35 / 23	17 / .73	.17 / .039	/ I
french style, frzn, Birds Eye — ½ cup	26 / 85	77.1 / 0.2	1.4 / 0.0	5.9 /	/ 0.1	2.2 / 0	/ 390	8 / .05	.07 / 0.3	.04 / .00	11 / .09	3 / 145	39 / 21	18 / .80	.22 / .044	/ I
french style w/ toasted almonds, frzn, Birds Eye—½ cup	52 / 85	71.2 / 1.6	2.5 / 0.2	8.4 /	/ 0.5	/ 0	/ 372	8 / .05	.06 / 0.4	.05 / .00	11 / .11	335 / 167	36 / 32	25 / .52	.28 / .070	/ I
frzn, boiled — ½ cup	19 / 68	62.2 / 0.1	1.0 / 0.0	4.4 / 0.0	/ 0.1	2.0 / 0	27 / 273	3 / .02	.06 / 0.3	.04 / .00	16 / .03	6 / 86	33 / 21	16 / .60	.33 / .041	.220 / 811
italian, frzn, Birds Eye — ½ cup	31 / 85	75.2 / 0.1	1.8 / 0.0	7.2 /	/ 0.1	2.7 / 0	/ 374	14 / .07	.10 / 0.5	.04 / .00	14 / .22	3 / 184	35 / 31	19 / .74	.25 / .050	/ I
whole, frzn, Birds Eye — 4 oz	30 / 113	103.9 / 0.2	1.7 / 0.1	6.7 /	/ 0.1	2.5 / 0	/ 776	12 / .07	.10 / 0.3	.05 / .00	13 / .18	2 / 200	44 / 28	23 / .87	.27 / .047	/ I
w/ butter sce, frzn Pillsbury — 5.5 oz	60 / 156	/ 2.0	2.0 / 1.0	10.0 /	/ 0.0	/ 5	/	/	/	/	/	360 / 230	/	/	/	/ I
hearts of palm, cnd — 1 heart	9 / 33	29.8 / 0.2	0.8 / 0.0	1.5 / 0.0	/ 0.1	0.8 / 0	0 / 0	3 / .00	.02 / 0.1	.01 / .00	13 / .04	141 / 58	19 / 21	13 / 1.03	.38 / .044	.460 / 811
hominy, cnd, white — 1 cup	115 / 160	132.0 / 1.4	2.4 / 0.2	22.8 / 0.4	/ 0.6	4.0 / 0	0 / 0	0 / .00	.01 / 0.1	.01 / .00	2 / .25	336 / 14	16 / 56	26 / .99	1.68 / .048	.112 / 820
horseradish tree, leafy tips, boiled — 1 cup chopped	25 / 42	34.3 / 0.4	2.2 / 0.1	4.7 / 0.2	/ 0.0	0.8 / 0	294 / 2945	13 / .09	.21 / 0.8	.39 / .00	9 / .04	4 / 144	63 / 28	63 / .97	.21 / .036	.365 / 811
horseradish tree, pods, boiled — 1 cup slices	42 / 118	104.3 / 0.2	2.5 / 0.0	9.7 / 0.1	/ 0.0	5.0 / 0	8 / 83	114 / .05	.08 / 0.7	.13 / .00	36 / .83	51 / 539	24 / 58	50 / .53	.50 / .092	.284 / 811
hyacinth beans, boiled — 1 cup	44 / 87	75.6 / 0.2	2.6 / 0.1	8.0 / 0.1	/ 0.0	/ 0	12 / 124	4 / .05	.08 / 0.4	.02 / .00	40 / .05	2 / 228	36 / 43	37 / .66	.33 / .042	.183 / 811
italian style veg																
frzn, Birds Eye — ½ cup[13]	102 / 95	74.7 / 5.5	2.1 / 1.0	11.1 /	/ 1.0	/ 0	/ 736	27 / .04	.08 / 0.4	.08 / .01	16 / .11	489 / 102	38 / 33	15 / .62	.17 / .057	/ I
frzn, Garden Gourmet Microwave — 9.5 oz pkg	229 / 269	215.2 / 9.7	7.3 /	33.1 /	/	5.4 /	/ 4217	12 / .27	.16 / 2.9	/	/	516 / 279	39 / 94	/ 1.83	/	/ I
frzn, Pillsbury — ½ cup	37 / 110	99.0 / 2.2	2.2 /	5.0 /	/	2.6 /	/ 426	42 / .04	.09 / 0.4	/	/	219 / 176	42 / 51	/ .77	/	/ I
japanese style veg																
frzn, Birds Eye — ½ cup[14]	89 / 95	76.6 / 5.0	2.0 / 0.9	10.0 /	/ 1.0	/ 0	/ 774	18 / .04	.06 / 0.2	.08 / .01	26 / .11	426 / 134	31 / 37	16 / .57	.23 / .048	/ I
frzn, Pillsbury — ½ cup	45 / 110	/ 0.9	2.0 /	7.2 /	/	/	/ 1235	23 / .03	.06 / 0.4	/	/	405 / 173	33 / 34	/ .77	/	/ I
stir fry, frzn, Birds Eye — ½ cup[15]	30 / 95	84.9 / 0.2	1.6 / 0.0	6.6 /	/ 0.1	/ 0	/ 917	24 / .05	.09 / 0.7	.09 / .00	29 / .28	516 / 157	28 / 35	12 / .70	.20 / .074	/ I
jerusalem artichoke, raw — ½ cup slices	57 / 75	58.5 / 0.0	1.5 / 0.0	13.1 / 0.0	/ 0.0	1.2 / 0	2 / 15	3 / .15	.04 / 1.0	.06 / .00	10 / .30	3 / 322	11 / 59	13 / 2.55	.09 / .105	.045 / 811
jute, potherb, boiled — ½ cup	16 / 43	37.5 / 0.1	1.6 / 0.0	3.1 / 0.0	/ 0.0	0.9 / 0	223 / 2230	14 / .04	.08 / 0.4	.25 / .00	45 / .03	5 / 237	91 / 31	27 / 1.35	.34 / .110	.053 / 811
kale, boiled — ½ cup chopped	21 / 65	59.3 / 0.3	1.2 / 0.0	3.7 / 0.0	/ 0.1	1.3 / 0	481 / 4810	27 / .03	.05 / 0.3	.09 / .00	9 / .03	15 / 148	47 / 18	12 / .59	.16 / .101	.270 / 811
kale, frzn, boiled — ½ cup chopped	20 / 65	58.8 / 0.3	1.8 / 0.0	3.4 / 0.0	/ 0.2	1.3 / 0	413 / 4130	16 / .03	.07 / 0.4	.06 / .00	9 / .03	10 / 209	90 / 18	12 / .61	.12 / .031	.293 / 811
kale, scotch, boiled — ½ cup chopped	18 / 65	59.3 / 0.3	1.2 / 0.0	3.7 / 0.0	/ 0.1	0.8 / 0	129 / 1296	34 / .03	.03 / 0.5	.09 / .00	9 / .03	29 / 178	86 / 25	37 / 1.25	.16 / .101	.271 / 811
kidney bean sprouts, boiled — 3.5 oz	33 / 100	89.3 / 0.6	4.8 / 0.1	4.7 / 0.0	/ 0.3	/ 0	0 / 2	36 / .36	.27 / 3.0	.09 / .00	47 / .38	7 / 194	19 / 38	23 / .89	.44 / .174	.199 / 811

						Vitamins					Minerals				
KCAL	H₂O (g)	PRO (g)	CHO (g)	SUGR (g)	DFIB (g)	A (RE)	C (mg)	B-2 (mg)	B-6 (mg)	FOL (mcg)	Na (mg)	Ca (mg)	Mg (mg)	Zn (mg)	Mn (mg)
WT (g)	FAT (g)	SFA (g)	MUFA (g)	PUFA (g)	CHOL (mg)	A (IU)	B-1 (mg)	NIA (mg)	B-12 (mcg)	PANT (mg)	K (mg)	P (mg)	Fe (mg)	Cu (mg)	REF
kidney beans, red															
boiled															
225	118.5	15.3	40.4		13.1	0	2	.10	.21	229	4	50	80	1.89	.844
1 cup															
177	0.9	0.1	0.1	0.5	0	0	.28	1.0	.00	.39	713	251	5.20	.428	816
calif, boiled															
150	136.9	9.3	27.6		11.3	0	2	.16	.04	90	604	42	50	.97	.428
1 cup															
177	0.6	0.1	0.0	0.3	0	0	.19	0.8	.00	.27	455	166	2.23	.266	816
cnd															
207	199.6	13.3	38.1		9.0	0	3	.18	.18	126	888	69	79	1.41	.556
1 cup															
256	0.8	0.1	0.1	0.4	0	0	.28	1.3	.00	.37	658	269	3.15	.384	816
cnd, Hunt's															
94		6.4	19.5	5.6	4.9	0	0				484	37			
½ cup															
127	0.5	0.0			0	0							.86		I
royal, boiled															
218	118.6	16.8	38.7		16.5	0	2	.12	.18	130	9	78	74	1.59	.451
1 cup															
177	0.3	0.0	0.0	0.2	0	5	.17	1.0	.00	.39	669	251	4.90	.464	816
kohlrabi, boiled															
24	74.0	1.5	5.5		0.9	3	44	.02	.13	10	17	21	16	.25	.116
½ cup slices															
82	0.1	0.0	0.0	0.0	0	29	.03	0.3	.00	.13	279	37	.33	.108	811
lambsquarters, boiled															
29	80.0	2.9	4.5		1.9	873	33	.23	.16	12	26	232	21	.27	.473
½ cup chopped															
90	0.6	0.0	0.1	0.3	0	8730	.09	0.8	.00	.06	259	41	.63	.177	811
le sueur style veg, frzn, Pillsbury															
64	92.7	4.5	12.4		5.4		33	.09			331	31			
½ cup															
113	2.3					398	.15	1.6			139	70	1.47		I
leeks															
boiled															
8	23.6	0.2	2.0		0.3	1	1	.01	.03	6	3	8	4	.02	.064
¼ cup chopped															
26	0.1	0.0	0.0	0.0	0	12	.01	0.1	.00	.02	23	4	.29	.016	811
freeze-dried															
3	0.0	0.1	0.6		0.1	0	1	.00	.01	3	0	3	1	.01	.021
¼ cup															
0.8	0.0	0.0	0.0	0.0	0	2	.01	0.0	.00	.01	19	3	.06	.005	811
raw															
16	21.6	0.4	3.7		0.5	3	3	.01	.06	17	5	15	7	.03	.125
¼ cup chopped															
26	0.1	0.0	0.0	0.0	0	25	.02	0.1	.00	.04	47	9	.55	.031	811
lentils, boiled															
230	137.9	17.9	39.9	3.6	15.6	2	3	.14	.35	358	4	38	71	2.51	.978
1 cup															
198	0.8	0.1	0.1	0.3	0	16	.33	2.1	.00	1.26	731	356	6.59	.497	816
lentils, sprouted, stir-fried															
101	68.7	8.8	21.3			4	13	.09	.16	67	10	14	35	1.60	.502
3.5 oz															
100	0.5	0.1	0.1	0.2	0	41	.22	1.2	.00	.57	284	153	3.10	.337	811
lettuce															
butterhead, raw															
2	14.3	0.2	0.3		0.1	15	1	.01	.01	11	1	5	2	.03	.020
2 leaves[16]															
15	0.0	0.0	0.0	0.0	0	146	.01	0.0	.00	.03	39	3	.04	.003	811
cos/romaine, raw															
4	26.6	0.5	0.7	0.6	0.5	73	7	.03	.01	38	2	10	2	.07	.178
½ cup shredded															
28	0.1	0.0	0.0	0.0	0	728	.03	0.1	.00	.05	81	13	.31	.010	811
iceberg, raw															
2	19.2	0.2	0.4	0.5	0.3	7	1	.01	.01	11	2	4	2	.04	.030
1 leaf[17]															
20	0.0	0.0	0.0	0.0	0	66	.01	0.0	.00	.01	32	4	.10	.006	811
looseleaf, raw															
5	26.3	0.4	1.0		0.5	53	5	.02	.02	14	3	19	3	.08	.210
½ cup shredded															
28	0.1	0.0	0.0	0.0	0	532	.01	0.1	.00	.06	74	7	.39	.012	811
lima beans															
baby, boiled, mature															
229	122.2	14.6	42.4		14.0	0	0	.10	.14	273	5	53	96	1.87	1.065
1 cup															
182	0.7	0.2	0.1	0.3	0	0	.29	1.2	.00	.86	730	231	4.37	.391	816
baby, frzn, boiled, immature															
95	65.1	6.0	17.5		5.4	15	5	.05	.10	14	26	25	50	.50	.732
½ cup															
90	0.3	0.1	0.0	0.1	0	150	.06	0.7	.00	.16	370	101	1.76	.177	811
boiled															
216	131.2	14.7	39.3	5.5	13.2	0	0	.10	.30	156	4	32	81	1.79	.970
1 cup															
188	0.7	0.2	0.1	0.3	0	0	.30	0.8	.00	.79	955	209	4.49	.442	816
cnd															
190	185.8	11.9	35.9		11.6	0	0	.08	.22	121	810	51	94	1.57	.875
1 cup															
241	0.4	0.1	0.0	0.2	0	0	.13	0.6	.00	.62	530	178	4.36	.434	816
fordhook, frzn, boiled															
85	62.5	5.2	16.0		4.9	16	11	.05	.10	18	45	19	29	.37	.264
½ cup															
85	0.3	0.1	0.0	0.1	0	162	.06	0.9	.00	.14	347	54	1.16	.047	811
w/ butter sce, frzn, Pillsbury															
100	73.7	6.0	17.0				14	.04			390	32			
½ cup															
113	3.0	1.0		0.0	5	222	.06	1.0			400	77	1.31		I
lotus root, boiled															
59	72.5	1.4	14.3		2.8	0	24	.01	.19	7	40	23	20	.29	.196
10 slices															
89	0.1	0.0	0.0	0.0	0	0	.11	0.3	.00	.27	323	69	.80	.193	811
lotus root, raw															
45	64.1	2.1	14.0		4.0	0	36	.18	.21	10	32	36	19	.32	.211
10 slices															
81	0.1	0.0	0.0	0.0	0	0	.13	0.3	.00	.31	450	81	.94	.208	811
lupins, boiled															
198	118.0	25.8	16.4		4.6	2	2	.09	.01	98	7	85	90	2.29	1.122
1 cup															
166	4.8	0.6	2.0	1.2	0	12	.22	0.8	.00	.31	407	212	1.99	.383	816
mandarin style veg, frzn, Birds Eye															
87	76.0	1.4	11.9				20	.07	.13	25	390	41	15	.21	
½ cup[18]															
95	4.1	0.8		0.8	0	4053	.04	0.6	.00	.20	223	32	.64	.052	I

	KCAL	H₂O (g)	PRO (g)	CHO (g)	SUGR (g)	DFIB (g)	A (RE)	C (mg)	B-2 (mg)	B-6 (mg)	FOL (mcg)	Na (mg)	Ca (mg)	Mg (mg)	Zn (mg)	Mn (mg)
	WT (g)	FAT (g)	SFA (g)	MUFA (g)	PUFA (g)	CHOL (mg)	A (IU)	B-1 (mg)	NIA (mg)	B-12 (mcg)	PANT (mg)	K (mg)	P (mg)	Fe (mg)	Cu (mg)	REF
mexican style veg, frzn, Pillsbury	141	105.0	4.9	23.5		4.2		24	.11			398	74			
½ cup	140	4.9					1812	.08	1.5			143	136	.50		I
mixed chinese veg, cnd, LaChoy	9		1.1	1.0	0.0	1.0	1	7				31	18			
⁷⁄₁₀ cup	84	0.1	0.0			0									.35	I
mixed veg																
cnd	39	71.3	2.1	7.6		2.5	955	4	.04	.06	19	122	22	13	.34	.466
½ cup[19]	82	0.2	0.0	0.0	0.1	0	9551	.04	0.5	.00	.12	239	34	.86	.060	811
frzn	54	75.7	2.6	11.9		4.0	389	3	.11	.07	17	32	23	20	.45	.345
½ cup[20]	91	0.1	0.0	0.0	0.1	0	3892	.06	0.8	.00	.14	154	46	.75	.076	811
frzn, Birds Eye	59	78.5	2.6	12.9		2.5		9	.07	.13	27	41	22	18	.40	
½ cup[21]	95	0.4	0.1		0.2	0	6507	.10	1.2	.00	.15	187	52	.81	.063	I
frzn, Pillsbury	40	54.3	2.1	9.6				5	.05			40	16			
½ cup	76	0.3				0	1627	.05	0.3			115	41	.54		I
w/ butter sce, frzn, Pillsbury	60	94.6	2.0	11.0				9	.07			300	23			
½ cup	113	1.7			0.0	0	2453	.06	0.9			150	56	.68		I
w/ onion sce, frzn, Birds Eye	97	55.6	2.2	11.6				5	.11	.10	15	340	43	15	.26	
⅓ cup[22]	76	5.2	1.1		1.0	1	4155	.06	0.6	.19	.24	182	59	.53	.041	I
mothbeans, boiled	207	122.5	13.8	37.1			2	2	.04	.16	254	18	5	184	1.04	.933
1 cup	177	1.0	0.2	0.1	0.5	0	18	.22	1.2	.00	.69	538	266	5.56	.290	816
mountain yam, hawaiian, steamed	59	55.5	1.2	14.4			0	0	.01	.15	9	9	6	7	.23	.204
½ cup cubes	72	0.1	0.0				0	.06	0.1	.00	.35	356	29	.31	.093	811
mung bean sprouts																
ckd	13	57.9	1.3	2.6		0.5	1	7	.06	.03	18	6	7	9	.29	.087
½ cup	62	0.1	0.0	0.0	0.0	0	9	.03	0.5	.00	.15	63	17	.40	.076	811
cnd	7	59.6	0.9	1.3		0.5	1	0	.04	.02	6	87	9	6	.17	.045
½ cup	62	0.0	0.0	0.0	0.0	0	14	.02	0.1	.00	.09	17	20	.27	.097	811
raw	16	47.0	1.6	3.1	1.1	0.9	1	7	.06	.05	32	3	7	11	.21	.098
½ cup	52	0.1	0.0	0.0	0.0	0	11	.04	0.4	.00	.20	77	28	.47	.085	811
stir-fried	31	52.3	2.7	6.6		1.2	2	10	.11	.08	43	6	8	20	.56	.181
½ cup	62	0.1	0.0	0.0	0.0	0	19	.09	0.7	.00	.35	136	49	1.18	.158	811
mung beans, boiled	212	146.8	14.2	38.7		15.4	4	2	.12	.14	321	4	55	97	1.70	.602
1 cup	202	0.8	0.2	0.1	0.3	0	48	.33	1.2	.00	.83	537	200	2.83	.315	816
mungo beans, boiled	212	146.5	15.2	37.0		12.9	6	2	.15	.12	191	14	107	127	1.68	.832
1 cup	202	1.1	0.1	0.1	0.7	0	63	.30	3.0	.00	.87	467	315	3.54	.281	816
mushrooms																
boiled	21	71.0	1.7	4.0		1.7	0	3	.23	.07	14	2	5	9	.68	.090
½ cup pieces	78	0.4	0.0	0.0	0.1	0	0	.06	3.5	.00	1.68	278	68	1.36	.393	811
breaded, frzn, Ore-Ida	137	49.8	3.6	14.0					.27			457	7			
2.67 oz	76	7.4	1.3	5.1	1.0	1		.07	2.0			188		1.37		I
cnd	19	71.0	1.5	3.9		1.9	0	0	.02	.05	10	332	9	12	.56	.067
½ cup pieces	78	0.2	0.0	0.0	0.1	0	0	.07	1.2	.00	.63	101	51	.62	.183	811
cnd, B&B	20	79.1	1.9	2.4		0.7		4	.14			448	6			
½ cup	85	0.3				0		.00	1.3			130	37	.51		I
enoki, raw	2	4.5	0.1	0.4		0.1	0	1	.01	.00	2	0	0	1	.03	.004
1 large	5	0.0	0.0	0.0	0.0	0	0	.00	0.2	.00	.05	19	6	.04	.003	811
oriental straw, cnd, Pillsbury	15	61.4	1.5	2.1		0.7		0	.07			286	4			
¼ cup	66	0.1				0	0	.00	0.6			59	29	.13		I
raw	9	32.1	0.7	1.6		0.4	0	1	.16	.03	7	1	2	4	.26	.039
½ cup pieces[23]	35	0.1	0.0	0.0	0.1	0	0	.04	1.4	.00	.77	130	36	.43	.172	811
shitake, ckd	40	60.1	1.1	10.3		1.5	0	0	.12	.11	15	3	2	10	.96	.147
4 mushrooms	72	0.2	0.0	0.0	0.0	0	0	.03	1.1	.00	2.59	84	21	.32	.645	811
shitake, dried	44	1.4	1.4	11.3		1.7	0	1	.19	.14	24	2	2	20	1.15	.176
4 mushrooms	15	0.1	0.0	0.0	0.0	0	0	.04	2.1	.00	3.28	230	44	.26	.775	811
w/ butter sce, cnd, Pillsbury	18	72.5	1.7	2.2		0.6		3	.12			411	6			
½ cup	78	0.3				0	0	.00	1.2			119	34	.47		I
mustard greens, boiled	11	66.1	1.6	1.5		1.4	212	18	.04	.07	51	11	52	11	.08	.192
½ cup chopped	70	0.2	0.0	0.1	0.0	0	2122	.03	0.3	.00	.08	141	29	.49	.059	811
mustard greens, frzn, boiled	14	70.3	1.7	2.3		2.1	335	10	.04	.08	52	19	76	10	.15	.220
½ cup chopped	75	0.0	0.0	0.1	0.0	0	3353	.03	0.2	.00	.01	104	18	.84	.044	811

	KCAL	H₂O (g)	PRO (g)	CHO (g)	SUGR (g)	DFIB (g)	A (RE)	C (mg)	B-2 (mg)	B-6 (mg)	FOL (mcg)	Na (mg)	Ca (mg)	Mg (mg)	Zn (mg)	Mn (mg)
	WT (g)	FAT (g)	SFA (g)	MUFA (g)	PUFA (g)	CHOL (mg)	A (IU)	B-1 (mg)	NIA (mg)	B-12 (mcg)	PANT (mg)	K (mg)	P (mg)	Fe (mg)	Cu (mg)	REF
mustard spinach (tendergreen), boiled	14	85.0	1.5	2.5		1.8	738	59	.06	.09	66	13	142	6	.10	.243
½ cup chopped	90	0.2				0	7380	.04	0.4	.00	.11	257	16	.72	.045	811
mustard spinach (tendergreen), raw	17	69.2	1.7	2.9		2.1	743	98	.07	.11	119	16	158	8	.13	.305
½ cup chopped	75	0.2				0	7425	.05	0.5	.00	.13	337	21	1.13	.056	811
navy bean sprouts, boiled	78	76.0	7.1	15.0			0	17	.23	.20	106	14	16	111	.97	.446
3.5 oz	100	0.8	0.1	0.1	0.5	0	4	.38	1.3	.00	.85	317	103	2.11	.389	811
navy beans, boiled	258	115.0	15.8	47.9		11.6	0	2	.11	.30	255	2	127	107	1.93	1.012
1 cup	182	1.0	0.3	0.1	0.4	0	4	.37	1.0	.00	.46	670	286	4.51	.537	816
navy beans, cnd	296	184.6	19.7	53.6		13.4	0	2	.14	.27	163	1174	123	123	2.02	.983
1 cup	262	1.1	0.3	0.1	0.5	0	3	.37	1.3	.00	.45	755	351	4.85	.545	816
new england style veg, frzn, Birds Eye	125	70.4	3.1	14.2				10	.08	.11	29	357	26	21	.24	
½ cup²⁴	95	6.2	1.2		1.6	0	885	.09	0.6	.01	.25	157	42	.61	.048	I
new zealand spinach, boiled	11	85.3	1.2	2.0			326	14	.10	.21	7	96	43	29	.28	.473
½ cup chopped	90	0.2	0.0	0.0	0.1	0	3260	.03	0.4	.00	.23	92	20	.59	.069	811
new zealand spinach, raw	4	26.3	0.4	0.7			123	8	.04	.09	4	36	16	11	.11	.179
½ cup chopped	28	0.1	0.0	0.0	0.0	0	1232	.01	0.1	.00	.09	36	8	.22	.026	811
nopales, ckd	22	140.5	2.0	4.9		3.0	69	8	.06	.10	4	30	244	70	.31	.608
1 cup	149	0.1	0.0	0.0	0.0	0	684	.02	0.4	.00	.22	291	24	.74	.073	811
nopales, raw	14	80.8	1.1	2.9		2.0	35	12	.04	.06	3	19	140	50	.25	.434
1 cup	86	0.1	0.0	0.0	0.0	0	357	.01	0.5	.00	.16	274	15	.58	.048	811
okra																
boiled	30	72.9	1.7	4.6		2.2	41	10	.10	.04	116	2	77	41	.50	.817
½ cup slices	80	0.2	0.1	0.0	0.1	0	411	.08	0.6	.00	.19	187	37	.54	.078	811
breaded, frzn, Ore-Ida	166	62.0	3.0	17.0				2	.12			666	56			
3.25 oz	92	9.6	1.7	6.6	1.3	4	701	.11	1.8			149		.99		I
raw	16	45.0	0.9	3.6	1.2	1.3	29	8	.03	.09	23	3	32	29	.28	.456
½ cup slices	50	0.1	0.0	0.0	0.0	0	288	.07	0.4	.00	.11	161	28	.23	.043	811
onion rings																
frzn, heated	285	19.9	3.7	26.7		0.9	16	1	.10	.05	9	263	22	13	.29	.294
7 rings²⁵	70	18.7	6.0	7.6	3.6	0	158	.20	2.5	.00	.16	90	57	1.18	.056	811
frzn, Mrs. Paul's	200		2.8	24.1				1	.05			367	20			
2.5 oz	71	10.2					24	.09	0.9			53		.90		I
frzn, Ore-Ida	142	29.5	1.8	17.7				3	.03			129	12			
2 oz	57	7.1	1.2	2.6	3.3		57	.05	0.7			104		.54		I
onions																
boiled	46	92.3	1.4	10.7		1.5	0	5	.02	.14	16	3	23	12	.22	.161
½ cup chopped	105	0.2	0.0	0.0	0.1	0	0	.04	0.2	.00	.12	174	37	.25	.070	811
boiled, frzn	28	92.2	0.8	6.6		1.8	3	3	.03	.07	13	12	16	6	.07	.071
3.5 oz	100	0.1	0.0	0.0	0.0	0	34	.02	0.1	.00	.10	108	19	.30	.019	811
chopped, frzn, Ore-Ida	20	51.9	0.6	4.2				2	.01			8	0			
2 oz	57	0.0	0.0	0.0	0.0	0		.03	0.5			91				I
cnd	21	105.4	1.0	4.5		1.3	0	5	.01	.15	11	416	50	7	.32	.114
½ cup chopped	112	0.1	0.0	0.0	0.0	0	0	.04	0.1	.00	.11	124	31	.15	.062	811
dehydrated flakes	45	0.6	1.3	11.7		1.3	0	11	.01	.22	23	3	36	13	.26	.194
¼ cup	14	0.0	0.0	0.0	0.0	0	0	.07	0.1	.00	.19	227	42	.22	.058	811
raw	30	71.7	0.9	6.9	5.0	1.4	0	5	.02	.09	15	2	16	8	.15	.110
½ cup chopped	80	0.1	0.0	0.0	0.0	0	0	.03	0.1	.00	.08	126	26	.18	.048	811
small, whole, frzn, Birds Eye	40	101.9	1.0	9.6				9	.03	.10	24	10	40	12	.13	
½ cup	113	0.1	0.0		0.0	0	19	.03	0.2	.00	.11	156	26	.52	.057	I
small w/ cream sce, frzn, Birds Eye	100	65.4	1.6	10.8				6	.10	.08	15	345	55	12	.12	
½ cup	85	5.9	1.2		1.1	1	251	.03	0.2	.22	.24	168	55	.36	.038	I
onions, spring, raw	16	44.9	0.9	3.7	1.6	1.3	20	9	.04	.03	32	8	36	10	.20	.080
½ cup chopped	50	0.1	0.0	0.0	0.0	0	193	.03	0.3	.00	.04	138	19	.74	.042	811
onions, welsh, raw	34	90.5	1.9	6.5			116	27	.09	.07	16	17	18	23	.52	.137
3.5 oz	100	0.4	0.1	0.1	0.2	0	1160	.05	0.4	.00	.17	212	49	1.22	.070	811
oriental style veg, frzn, Garden Gourmet	199	211.2	7.8	46.5		5.4		6	.22			702	43			
Microwave—9.5 oz pkg	269	0.4					108					331	145			I
parsley, freeze-dried	4	0.0	0.4	0.6		0.5	89	2	.03	.02	21	5	2	5	.09	.019
¼ cup	1.4	0.1				0	885	.01	0.1	.00	.04	88	8	.75	.006	811

	KCAL	H₂O (g)	PRO (g)	CHO (g)	SUGR (g)	DFIB (g)	A (RE)	C (mg)	B-2 (mg)	B-6 (mg)	FOL (mcg)	Na (mg)	Ca (mg)	Mg (mg)	Zn (mg)	Mn (mg)
	WT (g)	FAT (g)	SFA (g)	MUFA (g)	PUFA (g)	CHOL (mg)	A (IU)	B-1 (mg)	NIA (mg)	B-12 (mcg)	PANT (mg)	K (mg)	P (mg)	Fe (mg)	Cu (mg)	REF
parsnips, boiled	63	60.6	1.0	15.2		3.1	0	10	.04	.07	45	8	29	23	.20	.229
½ cup slices	78	0.2	0.0	0.1	0.0	0	0	.06	0.6	.00	.46	286	54	.45	.108	811
pasta primavera style veg, frzn, Birds Eye	122	69.0	5.0	14.3				17	.13	.10	29	338	95	20	.53	
½ cup26	95	5.2	1.4		0.9	3	4279	.14	1.1	.13	.23	172	97	.95	.067	I
peas & carrots, cnd	49	112.8	2.8	10.9		2.6	739	8	.07	.11	23	333	29	18	.74	.457
½ cup	128	0.3	0.1	0.0	0.2	0	7386	.09	0.7	.00	.15	128	59	.96	.132	811
peas & carrots, frzn	38	68.6	2.5	8.1		2.5	621	6	.05	.07	21	54	18	13	.36	.162
½ cup	80	0.3	0.1	0.0	0.2	0	6209	.18	0.9	.00	.13	126	39	.75	.061	811
peas & onions, cnd, drained	31	51.8	2.0	5.1		1.4	10	2	.04	.12	16	265	10	10	.35	.153
½ cup	60	0.2	0.0	0.0	0.1	0	97	.06	0.8	.00	.10	58	31	.52	.060	811
peas & onions, frzn, boiled	41	79.4	2.3	7.8		2.0	32	6	.06	.08	18	33	13	12	.26	.149
½ cup	90	0.2	0.0	0.0	0.1	0	312	.14	0.9	.00	.08	105	31	.85	.057	811
peas & pearl onions, frzn, Birds Eye	71	75.6	4.6	13.5		3.5		19	.08	.13	44	442	15	18	.48	
½ cup	95	0.2			0.1	0	636	.24	1.8	.00	.17	172	59	.85	.083	I
peas & pearl onions w/ cheese sce, frzn, Birds Eye—½ cup	137	111.6	5.7	18.1				15	.16	.13	43	446	76	25	.72	
	142	4.9	1.5		0.8	4	2145	.22	1.5	.23	.29	217	109	1.22	.094	I
peas & potatoes w/ cream sce, frzn, Birds Eye—½ cup	127	50.0	3.4	14.8				6	.13	.12	26	390	42	21	.48	
	76	6.2	1.3		1.1	1	520	.15	0.9	.23	.33	208	84	.74	.093	I
peas, green																
cnd	59	69.4	3.8	10.7	3.0	3.5	65	8	.07	.05	38	214	17	14	.60	.258
½ cup	85	0.3	0.1	0.0	0.1	0	653	.10	0.6	.00	.11	147	57	.81	.070	811
frzn, boiled	62	63.6	4.1	11.4	4.5	4.4	54	8	.08	.09	47	70	19	23	.75	.331
½ cup	80	0.2	0.0	0.0	0.1	0	534	.23	1.2	.00	.11	134	72	1.26	.111	811
w/ cream sce, frzn, Birds Eye	118	51.5	4.1	13.4		2.7		6	.13	.08	37	368	42	23	.63	
½ cup	76	5.6	1.1		1.0	1	637	.19	1.0	.20	.24	171	91	1.02	.089	I
w/ onions, red peppers, & garlic, cnd	57	98.6	3.5	10.5		2.3	49	13	.08	.11	33	290	17	17	.74	.306
½ cup	114	0.3	0.1	0.0	0.1	0	494	.11	0.8	.00	.10	139	62	1.37	.113	811
peas, green, early june																
cnd, Pillsbury	62	103.2	3.5	11.8		1.9		7	.07			322	22			
½ cup	120	0.2				0	325	.13	1.0			102	61	1.20		I
frzn, Le Sueur	60	60.8	4.7	9.1				11	.30			169	21			
½ cup	76	0.2					406	.18	1.4			116	74	1.14		I
w/ butter sce, frzn, Le Sueur	80		5.0	14.0								440				
½ cup	113	2.0			0.0	5						110				I
w/ butter sce, frzn, Pillsbury	81	102.1	5.0	16.8		5.6		11	.09			586	33			
4.5 oz	128	1.8			0.0	5	698	.20	1.4			147	89	1.41		I
peas, mature seeds, sprouted, boiled	118	74.4	7.0	21.9			11	7	.28	.13	36	3	26	41	.78	.325
3.5 oz	100	0.5	0.1	0.0	0.2	0	107	.22	1.1	.00	.68	268	24	1.67	.020	811
peas, split, boiled	231	136.2	16.3	41.4	5.7	16.3	2	1	.11	.09	127	4	27	71	1.96	.776
1 cup	196	0.8	0.1	0.2	0.3	0	14	.37	1.7	.00	1.17	710	194	2.53	.355	816
peas, sweet & cauliflower medley, frzn, Valley Combinations—3 oz	35	73.1	2.9	8.1		2.9		25	.06			70	22			
	85	0.3						.12	1.1			152	48	.77		I
peas, sweet & onions, cnd, Pillsbury	62	104.1	3.6	10.9		4.1		6	.05			508	23			
½ cup	121	0.4				0	313	.11	1.6			131	64	1.09		I
peas, sweet, carrots, & pearl onions, cnd, Pillsbury—½ cup	50		3.0	11.0								510				
	117	0.0				0						120				I
peas, sweet w/ butter sce, frzn, Pillsbury	80		5.0	14.0								410				
½ cup	113	2.0			0.0	5						135				I
pepeao, dried	36	1.3	0.6	9.7			0	0	.04	.11	19	8	14	18	.90	.138
½ cup	12	0.1				0	0	.10	0.4	.00	2.58	85	14	.74	.608	811
pepeao, raw	25	91.7	0.5	6.7			0	1	.20	.09	19	9	16	25	.65	.100
1 cup slices	99	0.0				0	0	.08	0.1	.00	1.97	43	14	.55	.441	811
peppers, chilpothe in spice sce, cnd, Del Monte—2 T	20		1.0	4.0	3.0	1.0		4				430	0			
	32	0.5	0.0			0	1000							.36		I
peppers, hot chili																
cnd	14	62.9	0.6	3.5		0.9	41	46	.03	.10	7	798	5	10	.12	.094
½ cup chopppped	68	0.1	0.0	0.0	0.0	0	415	.01	0.5	.00	.02	127	12	.34	.069	811
raw	18	39.5	0.9	4.3		0.7	35	109	.04	.13	11	3	8	11	.14	.107
1 pepper27	45	0.1	0.0	0.0	0.0	0	347	.04	0.4	.00	.03	153	21	.54	.078	811

	KCAL / WT (g)	H₂O (g) / FAT (g)	PRO (g) / SFA (g)	CHO (g) / MUFA (g)	SUGR (g) / PUFA (g)	DFIB (g) / CHOL (mg)	A (RE) / A (IU)	C (mg) / B-1 (mg)	B-2 (mg) / NIA (mg)	B-6 (mg) / B-12 (mcg)	FOL (mcg) / PANT (mg)	Na (mg) / K (mg)	Ca (mg) / P (mg)	Mg (mg) / Fe (mg)	Zn (mg) / Cu (µg)	Mn (mg) / REF
red, sun-dried	16	0.4	0.5	3.5		1.4	132	2	.06	.04	3	5	2	4	.05	.041
10 peppers	5	0.3	0.0	0.0	0.2	0	1324	.00	0.4	.00	.05	94	8	.30	.011	811
yellow, cnd, Del Monte	10		0.0	3.0	2.0	1.0	0	12				610	0			
4 peppers	28	0.0	0.0	0.0	0.0	0	0								.36	I
peppers, jalapeno																
cnd	16	61.1	0.5	3.3		1.3	116	9	.03	.14	9	995	18	8	.13	.126
½ cup chopped	68	0.4	0.0	0.0	0.2	0	1156	.02	0.3	.00	.73	92	12	1.90	.095	811
pickled, sliced, cnd, Del Monte	5		0.0	1.0	0.0		6					440	0			
2 T	28	0.0	0.0	0.0	0.0	0	100								.36	I
whole, cnd, Del Monte	3		0.0	0	4							230	0			
1 pepper	20	0.0	0.0	0.0	0.0	0	0								.00	I
peppers, sweet																
boiled	19	62.5	0.6	4.6		0.8	40	51	.02	.16	11	1	6	7	.08	.078
½ cup chopped[28]	68	0.1	0.0	0.0	0.1	0	403	.04	0.3	.00	.05	113	12	.31	.044	811
cnd	13	63.9	0.6	2.7		0.8	11	33	.02	.12	11	958	29	8	.13	.112
½ cup halves[29]	70	0.2	0.0	0.0	0.1	0	109	.02	0.4	.00	.03	102	14	.56	.091	811
freeze-dried	5	0.0	0.3	1.1		0.3	10	30	.02	.04	4	3	2	3	.04	.030
¼ cup[30]	1.6	0.0	0.0	0.0	0.0	0	100	.02	0.1	.00	.01	51	5	.17	.022	811
frzn, boiled	18	94.7	0.9	3.9		0.9	29	41	.03	.11	10	4	8	7	.05	.097
3.5 oz[31]	100	0.2	0.0	0.0	0.1	0	290	.05	1.1	.00	.02	72	13	.52	.044	811
raw	14	46.1	0.4	3.2	1.3	0.9	32	45	.01	.12	11	1	5	5	.06	.058
½ cup chopped[32]	50	0.1	0.0	0.0	0.1	0	316	.03	0.3	.00	.04	89	10	.23	.033	811
yellow, raw	50	171.2	1.9	11.8		1.7	45	341	.05	.31	48	4	20	22	.32	.218
1 large pepper	186	0.4				0	443	.05	1.7	.00	.31	394	45	.86	.199	811
pigeonpeas, boiled	203	115.2	11.4	39.1		11.3	0	0	.10	.08	186	8	72	77	1.51	.842
1 cup	168	0.6	0.1	0.0	0.3	0	5	.25	1.3	.00	.54	645	200	1.86	.452	816
pimientos, cnd	3	11.2	0.1	0.6		0.2	32	10	.01	.03	1	2	1	1	.02	.011
1 T	12	0.0	0.0	0.0	0.0	0	319	.00	0.1	.00	.00	19	2	.20	.006	811
pink beans, boiled	252	103.4	15.3	47.2		9.0	0	0	.11	.30	284	3	88	110	1.62	.926
1 cup	169	0.8	0.2	0.1	0.4	0	0	.43	1.0	.00	.51	859	279	3.89	.458	816
sprouts, boiled	22	93.4	1.9	4.1			0	6	.06	.05	29	51	15	18	.17	.123
3.5 oz	100	0.3	0.0	0.0	0.2	0	1	.07	0.7	.00	.23	98	30	.66	.107	811
pinto beans																
boiled	234	109.9	14.0	43.9		14.7	0	4	.16	.27	294	3	82	94	1.85	.951
1 cup	171	0.9	0.2	0.2	0.3	0	3	.32	0.7	.00	.49	800	274	4.46	.439	816
cnd	206	186.1	11.7	36.6		11.0	5	2	.15	.18	144	706	103	65	1.66	.550
1 cup	240	1.9	0.4	0.4	0.7	0	58	.24	0.7	.00	.33	583	221	3.50	.336	816
picante style, cnd, Joan of Arc	98	109.9	6.8	21.3		6.7			.06			578	50			
½ cup	142	1.3				0	342	.07	0.7			271	84	1.28		I
poi	134	86.0	0.5	32.7		0.5	2	5	.05	.33	26	14	19	29	.26	.444
½ cup	120	0.2	0.0	0.0	0.1	0	24	.16	1.3	.00	.35	220	47	1.06	.199	811
pokeberry shoots, boiled	16	76.2	1.9	2.5		1.2	713	67	.20	.09	7	15	43	11	.16	.276
½ cup	82	0.3	0.1	0.0	0.1	0	7134	.06	0.9	.00	.03	151	27	.98	.103	811
potato, baked																
microwaved w/o skin	156	114.7	3.3	36.3		2.5	0	24	.04	.50	19	11	8	39	.51	.265
1 potato	156	0.2	0.0	0.0	0.1	0	0	.20	2.5	.00	.93	641	170	.64	.370	811
microwaved w/ skin	212	145.5	4.9	48.7		4.6	0	31	.06	.69	24	16	22	55	.73	.590
1 potato	202	0.2	0.1	0.0	0.1	0	0	.24	3.5	.00	.92	903	212	2.50	.675	811
w/ butter flavor, frzn, Ore-Ida	211	97.8	4.5	28.2				0	.10			394	55			
5 oz potato	142	8.9	1.8	4.4	2.3	0	151	.09	3.0			746		1.09		I
w/ cheddar cheese, frzn, Ore-Ida	228	95.2	6.3	27.5				0	.16			565	80			
5 oz potato	142	10.8	7.2	3.3	0.3	6	75	.11	2.3			538		2.14		I
w/ cheese topping, frzn, Pillsbury	200	96.6	4.5	32.9		0.9		7	.07			521	42			
5 oz	142	5.5					339	.06	2.4			625	112	.85		I
w/o skin	145	117.7	3.1	33.6	2.7	2.3	0	20	.03	.47	14	8	8	39	.45	.251
1 potato	156	0.2	0.0	0.0	0.1	0	0	.16	2.2	.00	.87	610	78	.55	.335	811
w/ skin	220	143.8	4.6	51.0		4.8	0	26	.07	.70	22	16	20	55	.65	.463
1 potato	202	0.2	0.1	0.0	0.1	0	0	.22	3.3	.00	1.12	844	115	2.75	.616	811

	KCAL	H₂O (g)	PRO (g)	CHO (g)	SUGR (g)	DFIB (g)	A (RE)	C (mg)	B-2 (mg)	B-6 (mg)	FOL (mcg)	Na (mg)	Ca (mg)	Mg (mg)	Zn (mg)	Mn (mg)
	WT (g)	FAT (g)	SFA (g)	MUFA (g)	PUFA (g)	CHOL (mg)	A (IU)	B-1 (mg)	NIA (mg)	B-12 (mcg)	PANT (mg)	K (mg)	P (mg)	Fe (mg)	Cu (mg)	REF
w/ sour cream & chives, frzn, Pillsbury	231	93.7	4.7	30.7		1.1		5	.09			579	50			
5 oz	142	9.9					439	.07	2.4			575	111	.99		I
w/ sour cream, frzn, Ore-Ida	209		4.7	26.9				1	.10			445	39			
5 oz potato	142	8.9	1.8	4.4	2.3	0	77	.13	2.4			583		1.85		I
potato, boiled w/o skin	117	103.9	2.5	27.2		2.4	0	18	.03	.40	14	5	7	30	.41	.186
1 potato	135	0.1	0.0	0.0	0.1	0	0	.14	1.9	.00	.70	512	59	.42	.254	811
potato, boiled w/o skin, frzn	65	82.8	2.0	14.5		1.4	0	9	.03	.20	8	20	7	11	.25	.185
3.5 oz	100	0.1	0.0	0.0	0.1	0	0	.10	1.3	.00	.28	287	26	.84	.078	811
potato, cnd w/o skin	54	75.9	1.3	12.2		2.1	0	5	.01	.17	6	197	5	13	.25	.087
½ cup	90	0.2	0.0	0.0	0.1	0	0	.06	0.8	.00	.32	206	25	1.13	.051	811
potato garden casserole, frzn, Healthy Choice—9.25 oz	210		11.0	30.0	5.0	6.0		18				520	100			
	262	5.0	1.5			10	1250							.72		I
potato pancakes, homemade	101	17.5	2.3	10.6		0.7	5	8	.06	.14	9	188	9	12	.31	.152
1 med pancake[33]	37	5.6	1.1	1.7	2.4	36	53	.05	0.8	.07	.27	291	41	.58	.136	811
potato patties, golden, frzn, Ore-Ida	163	54.5	1.8	18.5				6				275				
3 oz	85	9.1	1.6	6.3	1.3	0		.07	1.6			338		.78		I
potato puffs, frzn, prep	138	32.8	2.1	18.9		2.0	1	4	.04	.14	10	463	19	12	.19	.168
½ cup	62	6.7	3.2	2.7	0.5	0	10	.12	1.3	.00	.41	236	30	.97	.037	811
potato, raw w/o skin	88	88.4	2.3	20.1		1.8	0	22	.04	.29	14	7	8	24	.44	.295
1 potato	112	0.1	0.0	0.0	0.0	0	0	.10	1.7	.00	.43	608	52	.85	.290	811
potato salad																
german style, cnd, Joan of Arc	126	98.8	2.0	24.2		1.7		2	.03			568	15			
½ cup	130	3.0					29	.05	0.9			248	39	.52		I
homemade	179	95.0	3.4	14.0		1.6	41	13	.07	.18	8	661	24	19	.39	.126
½ cup	125	10.3	1.8	3.1	4.7	85	261	.10	1.1	.00	.67	318	65	.81	.147	811
homestyle, cnd, Joan of Arc	179	85.2	1.9	17.0		1.6		2	.04			566	17			
½ cup	120	11.4					151	.04	1.7			212	49	.96		I
potato wedges, homestyle w/ peel, frzn, Ore-Ida—3 oz	109	60.4	2.0	18.9				10				16				
	85	2.8	0.5	2.0	0.3	0		.08	1.9			430		.71		I
potatoes & broccoli w/ cheese sce, frzn, Pillsbury—5.5 oz	130		4.0	19.0								720				
	156	5.0			2.0	5						390				I
potatoes au gratin																
from mix	127	108.2	3.2	17.6		1.2	42	4	.11	.05	9	601	114	21	.33	.178
⅙ of 5.5 oz pkg[34]	137	5.6	3.5	1.6	0.2	21	292	.03	1.3	.00	.33	300	130	.44	.063	811
frzn, Pillsbury	200		7.0	20.0								560				
5.5 oz	156	10.0	4.0		2.0	20						370				I
frzn, Stouffers	102	63.8	3.9	11.1				1	.11			383	102			
3 oz	85	4.7				13	26	.04	0.3			102		.17		I
homemade	161	90.3	6.2	13.7		2.2	46	12	.14	.21	10	528	145	24	.84	.196
½ cup[35]	122	9.3	5.8	2.6	0.3	28	322	.08	1.2	.00	.47	483	138	.78	.195	811
potatoes, fried																
cottage fries, frzn, heated	109	26.4	1.7	17.0		1.6	0	5	.02	.12	8	23	5	11	.20	.152
10 strips	50	4.1	1.9	1.7	0.3	0	0	.06	1.2	.00	.34	240	33	.74	.100	811
cottage fries, frzn, Ore-Ida	125	58.3	2.2	19.5				9				17				
3 oz	85	4.2	0.8	2.9	0.6	0		.09	2.0			382		.72		I
country style, frzn, Ore-Ida	111	60.4	2.1	18.9				11				10				
3 oz	85	3.0	0.5	2.0	0.4	0		.10	1.7			346		.57		I
Crinkle Cuts, frzn, Ore-Ida	155	53.8	2.1	22.1				5				18				
3 oz	85	6.5	1.1	4.5	0.9	0		.09	1.9			387		.82		I
Crinkle Cuts, frzn, Ore-Ida Microwave	182	63.3	2.5	26.0				6				21				
3.5 oz	100	7.6	1.3	5.3	1.0	0		.10	2.2			455		.96		I
Crinkle Cuts, Lite, frzn, Ore-Ida	89	64.5	1.7	16.3				10				22				
3 oz	85	1.8	0.3	1.2	0.3	0		.09	1.7			311		.70		I
Crispers, frzn, Ore-Ida	231	42.1	2.2	24.7				4				471				
3 oz	85	14.4	2.6	9.9	2.0	0		.08	2.0			353		.90		I
Crispy Crowns, frzn, Ore-Ida	172	52.1	1.8	20.4				2				412				
3 oz	85	9.4	1.6	6.5	1.3	0		.08	1.3			236		.81		I
fries, extruded, heated, frzn	167	17.7	1.8	19.8		1.6	0	3	.02	.11	11	307	6	12	.20	.142
10 pieces	50	9.4	3.0	5.7	0.7	0	0	.04	1.3	.00	.30	270	48	.83	.020	811

	KCAL	H₂O (g)	PRO (g)	CHO (g)	SUGR (g)	DFIB (g)	A (RE)	C (mg)	B-2 (mg)	B-6 (mg)	FOL (mcg)	Na (mg)	Ca (mg)	Mg (mg)	Zn (mg)	Mn (mg)
	WT (g)	FAT (g)	SFA (g)	MUFA (g)	PUFA (g)	CHOL (mg)	A (IU)	B-1 (mg)	NIA (mg)	B-12 (mcg)	PANT (mg)	K (mg)	P (mg)	Fe (mg)	Cu (mg)	REF
fries, frzn, heated	100	28.6	1.6	15.6		1.6	0	5	.01	.15	6	15	4	11	.20	.131
10 pieces	50	3.8	0.6	2.4	0.4	0	0	.06	1.0	.00	.17	209	41	.62	.059	811
fries, reg cut, frzn, Ore-Ida	156	53.3	2.0	22.5				7				15				
3 oz	85	6.4	1.1	4.4	0.9	0		.08	1.9			363		.77		I
Golden Crinkles, frzn, Ore-Ida	121	58.6	2.1	19.9				8				16				
3 oz	85	3.6	0.7	2.5	0.5	0		.08	1.8			402		.61		I
Golden Fries, frzn, Ore-Ida	123	59.1	2.0	20.1				7				17				
3 oz	85	3.9	0.7	2.6	0.5	0		.09	1.6			321		.88		I
Pixie Crinkles, frzn, Ore-Ida	142	56.1	1.9	21.0				9				30				
3 oz	85	5.4	0.9	3.7	0.8	0		.09	1.7			298		.82		I
shoestring, frzn, Ore-Ida	149	54.3	2.1	22.1				5				16				
3 oz	85	5.8	1.0	4.0	0.8	0		.09	1.7			333		.93		I
potatoes, hash brown																
frzn, Ore-Ida	68	67.5	1.7	15.0				8				27				
3 oz	85	0.1				0		.08	1.6			384		.64		I
frzn, Ore-Ida Microwave	117	35.4	1.3	12.8				2				133				
2 oz	57	6.7	1.2	4.7	0.9	0		.04	0.9			218		.54		I
frzn, prep	170	43.8	2.5	21.9		1.6	0	5	.02	.10	5	27	12	13	.25	.174
½ cup36	78	9.0	3.5	4.0	1.0	0	0	.09	1.9	.00	.35	340	56	1.18	.119	811
homemade	163	48.0	1.9	16.6	0.2	1.6	0	4	.02	.22	6	19	6	16	.23	.119
½ cup36	78	10.8	4.2	4.8	1.2	0	0	.06	1.6	.00	.39	250	33	.63	.141	811
southern style, frzn, Ore-Ida	70	66.8	1.5	16.0				5				20				
3 oz	85	0.1				0		.08	1.4			224		.59		I
toaster, frzn, Ore-Ida	99	30.9	1.0	12.2				1				173	0			
1.75 oz	50	5.9	2.7	2.2	0.2	3		.04	1.0			135				I
w/ butter sce, frzn, prep	178	63.7	2.5	24.1		3.8	16	4	.03	.27	13	101	33	15	.33	.244
3.5 oz	100	8.8	3.4	3.1	1.8	23	111	.05	1.4	.00	.37	327	38	.99	.102	811
w/ cheddar cheese, frzn, Ore-Ida	85	65.1	3.2	13.6				5	.03			365	29			
3 oz	85	2.1	1.4	0.6	0.1	3	36	.10	1.9			356		.71		I
potatoes, mashed																
from flakes	119	80.1	2.0	15.8		2.4	22	10	.05	.01	8	349	51	19	.19	.120
½ cup37	105	5.9	3.6	1.7	0.3	15	189	.12	0.7	.08	.13	245	59	.23	.017	811
from granules	83	85.5	2.1	13.8		1.9	14	3	.05	.21	7	246	33	17	.26	.107
½ cup38	105	2.3	0.7	0.7	0.7	2	95	.03	0.8	.00	.43	352	46	.63	.127	811
from mix, French's	130		2.0	16.0								340				
½ cup	105	6.0										270				I
from mix, Hungry Jack	140		3.0	17.0								380				
½ cup	105	7.0										320				I
homemade	111	80.1	2.0	17.5		2.1	21	6	.04	.24	8	310	27	19	.28	.120
½ cup39	105	4.4	1.1	1.9	1.3	2	177	.09	1.1	.00	.60	303	48	.27	.144	811
potatoes O'Brien																
frzn, Ore-Ida	62	69.1	1.3	13.9				13	.03			17	15			
3 oz	85	0.1				0	108	.08	1.3			189		.55		I
frzn, prep	204	62.0	2.2	21.9		1.7	19	10	.14	.38	12	43	20	34	.55	.226
3.5 oz	100	13.2	3.3	5.8	3.5	0	188	.05	1.4	.00	.73	473	93	.96	.241	811
homemade	157	154.4	4.6	30.0			111	32	.11	.41	16	421	70	35	.58	.235
1 cup40	194	2.5	1.5	0.7	0.1	8	933	.15	2.0	.00	.85	516	97	.91	.250	811
potatoes, scalloped																
from mix	127	108.5	2.9	17.5		1.5	29	5	.08	.06	13	467	49	19	.34	.248
⅙ of 5.5 oz pkg41	137	5.9	3.6	1.7	0.3	15	203	.03	1.4	.00	.45	278	77	.52	.067	811
frzn, Stouffers	89	65.5	3.1	11.9				1	.09			383	77			
3 oz	85	3.2				7	26	.04	0.3			128		.17		I
frzn, Swanson	313		19.3	29.2				14	.30			935	336			
9 oz entree	255	13.2					201	.36	2.8			288		1.30		I
homemade	105	98.7	3.5	13.2		2.3	23	13	.11	.22	11	409	70	23	.49	.203
½ cup42	122	4.5	2.8	1.3	0.2	15	165	.08	1.3	.00	.63	461	77	.70	.199	811

	KCAL	H2O (g)	PRO (g)	CHO (g)	SUGR (g)	DFIB (g)	Vitamins A (RE)	C (mg)	B-2 (mg)	B-6 (mg)	FOL (mcg)	Minerals Na (mg)	Ca (mg)	Mg (mg)	Zn (mg)	Mn (mg)
	WT (g)	FAT (g)	SFA (g)	MUFA (g)	PUFA (g)	CHOL (mg)	A (IU)	B-1 (mg)	NIA (mg)	B-12 (mcg)	PANT (mg)	K (mg)	P (mg)	Fe (mg)	Cu (mg)	REF
potatoes, Tater Tots																
bacon flavored, frzn, Ore-Ida	145	54.9	2.5	19.3				3	.03			530	14			
3 oz	85	6.5	1.1	4.4	0.9	0	5	.45	1.5			273		.82		I
frzn, Ore-Ida	146	55.3	1.8	19.8				4	.01			401				
3 oz	85	6.6	1.2	4.6	0.9	0		.06	1.4			258		.77		I
frzn, Ore-Ida Microwave	204	71.3	2.3	28.5				7				580				
4 oz	113	9.0	1.6	6.2	1.2	0		.09	2.2			352		.82		I
w/ onions, frzn, Ore-Ida	145	55.0	1.9	19.9				4				518				
3 oz	85	6.5	1.1	4.4	0.9	0		.07	1.5			254		.93		I
potatoes w/ cheddar & broccoli, frzn, Banquet—*10.5 oz entree*	310		13.0	53.0	8.0	8.0		27				550	200			
	298	5.0	2.0			15	300							1.80		I
pumpkin																
boiled	24	114.3	0.9	6.0		1.3	132	6	.10	.05	10	1	18	11	.28	.109
½ cup mashed	122	0.1	0.0	0.0	0.0	0	1320	.04	0.5	.00	.25	281	37	.70	.111	811
cnd	41	109.8	1.3	9.9		3.5	2691	5	.07	.07	15	6	32	28	.21	.182
½ cup	122	0.3	0.2	0.0	0.0	0	26908	.03	0.4	.00	.49	251	43	1.70	.131	811
cnd, Libby's Solid Pack	40		2.0	9.0	4.0	5.0						5	40			
½ cup	122	0.5	0.0			0	17500							1.80		I
pumpkin flowers, boiled	10	63.8	0.7	2.2		0.6	116	3	.02	.03	27	4	25	17	.07	
½ cup	67	0.1	0.0	0.0	0.0	0	1162	.01	0.2	.00		71	23	.59	.067	811
pumpkin flowers, raw	5	31.4	0.3	1.1			64	9	.02		19	2	13	8		
1 cup	33	0.0	0.0	0.0	0.0	0	643	.01	0.2	.00		57	16	.23		811
pumpkin leaves, boiled	15	65.7	1.9	2.4		1.9	175	1	.10	.14	18	6	31	27	.14	.252
1 cup	71	0.2	0.1	0.0	0.0	0	1757	.05	0.6	.00	.03	311	56	2.27	.094	811
pumpkin pie mix, cnd	140	96.5	1.5	35.6		11.2	1121	5	.16	.21	47	281	50	22	.36	.541
½ cup	135	0.2	0.1	0.0	0.0	0	11202	.02	0.5	.00	1.53	186	61	1.43	.092	811
pumpkin pie mix, cnd, Libby's	80		0.6	20.0	17.0	2.0		1	.26	.26		150	20			
⅓ cup	87	0.0	0.0	0.0	0.0	0	7500	.09	1.2	.30	2.07			.72		I
purslane, boiled	10	54.2	0.9	2.1			107	6	.05	.04	5	26	45	39	.10	.178
½ cup	58	0.1				0	1074	.02	0.3	.00	.02	283	21	.45	.066	811
radicchio, raw	5	18.6	0.3	0.9		0.2	1	2	.01	.01	12	4	4	3	.12	.028
½ cup shredded	20	0.1	0.0	0.0	0.0	0	5	.00	0.1	.00	.05	60	8	.11	.068	811
radish, oriental																
boiled	13	70.3	0.5	2.5		1.2	0	11	.02	.03	13	10	13	7	.10	.024
½ cup slices	74	0.2	0.1	0.0	0.1	0	0	.00	0.1	.00	.08	211	18	.11	.075	811
dried	157	11.4	4.6	36.8			0	0	.39	.36	171	161	365	99	1.24	.313
½ cup	58	0.4	0.1	0.1	0.2	0	0	.16	2.0	.00	1.08	2027	118	3.90	.946	811
raw	8	41.6	0.3	1.8		0.7	0	10	.01	.02	12	9	12	7	.07	.017
½ cup slices[43]	44	0.0	0.0	0.0	0.0	0	0	.01	0.1	.00	.06	100	10	.18	.051	811
radish, raw	8	42.7	0.3	1.6	1.2	0.7	0	10	.02	.03	12	11	9	4	.14	.032
10 radishes	45	0.2	0.0	0.0	0.0	0	4	.00	0.1	.00	.04	104	8	.13	.018	811
radish seeds, sprouted, raw	16	34.2	1.4	1.4			15	11	.04	.11	36	2	19	17	.21	.099
1 cup	38	1.0	0.3	0.2	0.4	0	149	.04	1.1	.00	.28	33	43	.33	.046	811
radishes, white icicle, raw	7	47.7	0.6	1.3		0.7	0	15	.01	.04	7	8	14	5	.07	.017
½ cup slices	50	0.1	0.0	0.0	0.0	0	0	.01	0.1	.00	.09	140	14	.40	.050	811
ratatouille, frzn, Stouffers	31	77.4	1.1	4.4			9		.03			400	25			
3 oz entree	85	1.0					281	.03	0.6			187		.43		I
red beans, cnd, Joan of Arc	83	97.9	5.6	19.1		5.6		0	.04			341	45			
½ cup	125	0.6				0	6	.06	0.4			224	75	1.38		I
red beans, small, cnd, Hunt's	89		6.2	18.9	3.8	5.5	0	0				713	32			
½ cup	127	0.5	0.0			0	0							.64		I
rhubarb, frzn, ckd, sweetened	139	81.3	0.5	37.4		2.4	8	4	.03	.02	6	1	174	14	.10	.088
½ cup	120	0.1	0.0	0.0	0.0	0	83	.02	0.2	.00	.06	115	10	.25	.032	809
rhubarb, frzn, raw	29	128.1	0.8	7.0		2.5	15	7	.04	.03	11	3	266	25	.14	.133
1 cup	137	0.2	0.0	0.0	0.1	0	147	.04	0.3	.00	.09	148	16	.40	.032	809
rutabaga, boiled	33	75.5	1.1	7.4		1.5	48	16	.03	.09	13	17	41	20	.30	.148
½ cup cubes	85	0.2	0.0	0.0	0.1	0	477	.07	0.6	.00	.13	277	48	.45	.035	811
salsify, boiled	46	55.1	1.9	10.5		2.1	0	3	.12	.15	10	11	32	12	.20	.143
½ cup slices	68	0.1	0.0	0.0	0.0	0		.04	0.3	.00	.19	192	38	.37	.048	811

	KCAL / WT (g)	H₂O (g) / FAT (g)	PRO (g) / SFA (g)	CHO (g) / MUFA (g)	SUGR (g) / PUFA (g)	DFIB (g) / CHOL (mg)	A (RE) / A (IU)	C (mg) / B-1 (mg)	B-2 (mg) / NIA (mg)	B-6 (mg) / B-12 (mcg)	FOL (mcg) / PANT (mg)	Na (mg) / K (ug)	Ca (mg) / P (mg)	Mg (mg) / Fe (mg)	Zn (mg) / Cu (mg)	Mn (mg) / REF
san francisco style veg, frzn, Birds Eye	90	77.0	2.2	10.4				10	.07	.07	25	334	21	15	.25	
½ cup44	95	4.5	0.9		0.9	0	489	.06	0.5	.00	.15	154	38	.53	.077	I
sauerkraut, bottled, Claussen	7	27.8	0.2	1.2	0.1	1.0	0	3				218	11	3	.05	
¼ cup	30	0.1	0.0	0.0	0.0	0	0					48	6	.18	.020	I
sauerkraut, cnd	22	109.2	1.1	5.1		2.9	2	17	.03	.15	28	780	35	15	.22	.178
½ cup	118	0.2	0.0	0.0	0.1	0	21	.02	0.2	.00	.11	201	24	1.73	.113	811
seaweed																
agar, dried	306	8.7	6.2	80.9		7.7	0	0	.22	.30	580	102	625	770	5.80	4.300
3.5 oz	100	0.3	0.1	0.0	0.1	0	0	.01	0.2	.00	3.02	1125	52	21.40	.610	811
agar, raw	26	91.3	0.5	6.8		0.5	0	0	.02	.03	85	9	54	67	.58	.373
3.5 oz	100	0.0	0.0	0.0	0.0	0	0	.01	0.1	.00	.30	226	5	1.86	.061	811
irishmoss, raw	49	81.3	1.5	12.3		1.3	12	3	.47	.07	182	67	72	144	1.95	.370
3.5 oz	100	0.2	0.0	0.0	0.1	0	118	.01	0.6	.00	.18	63	157	8.90	.149	811
kelp (kombu/tangle), raw	43	81.6	1.7	9.6		1.3	12	3	.15	.00	180	233	168	121	1.23	.200
3.5 oz	100	0.6	0.2	0.1	0.0	0	116	.05	0.5	.00	.64	89	42	2.85	.130	811
laver (nori), raw	35	85.0	5.8	5.1		0.3	520	39	.45	.16	146	48	70	2	1.05	.988
3.5 oz	100	0.3	0.1	0.0	0.1	0	5202	.10	1.5	.00	.52	356	58	1.80	.264	811
spirulina, dried	290	4.7	57.5	23.9		3.6	57	10	3.67	.36	94	1048	120	195	2.00	1.900
3.5 oz	100	7.7	2.6	0.7	2.1	0	570	2.38	12.8	.00	3.48	1363	118	28.50	6.100	811
spirulina, raw	26	90.7	5.9	2.4			6	1	.34	.03	9	98	12	19	.20	.186
3.5 oz	100	0.4	0.1	0.0	0.1	0	56	.22	1.2	.00	.33	127	11	2.79	.597	811
wakame, raw	45	80.0	3.0	9.1		0.5	36	3	.23	.00	196	872	150	107	.38	1.400
3.5 oz	100	0.6	0.1	0.1	0.2	0	360	.06	1.6	.00	.70	50	80	2.18	.284	811
shallots, freeze-dried	14	0.1	0.5	3.2			224	2	.00	.07	5	2	7	4	.08	.057
¼ cup	4	0.0	0.0	0.0	0.0	0	2244	.01	0.0	.00	.06	66	12	.24	.017	811
shallots, raw	7	8.0	0.3	1.7			125	1	.00	.03	3	1	4	2	.04	.029
1 T chopped	10	0.0	0.0	0.0	0.0	0	1248	.01	0.0	.00	.03	33	6	.12	.009	811
shellie beans, cnd	37	110.6	2.1	7.6		4.1	28	4	.07	.06	22	407	35	18	.33	.466
½ cup	122	0.2	0.0	0.0	0.1	0	278	.04	0.3	.00	.16	133	37	1.21	.098	811
snow peas, frzn, La Choy	35		2.0	4.0	2.0	2.0		15				0	20			
3 oz	85	1.5	0.0			0	200							.72		I
soybean product, miso	284	57.2	16.3	38.6		7.5	12	0	.34	.30	46	5033	91	58	4.58	1.185
½ cup	138	8.4	1.2	1.9	4.7	0	120	.13	1.2	.00	.36	226	211	3.78	.603	816
soybean product, natto	187	48.4	15.6	12.6		4.8	0	11	.17	.11	7	6	191	101	2.67	1.345
½ cup	88	9.7	1.4	2.1	5.5	0	0	.14	0.0	.00	.19	642	153	7.57	.587	816
soybean product, tempeh	165	45.6	15.7	14.1			57	0	.09	.25	43	5	77	58	1.50	1.187
½ cup	83	6.4	0.9	1.4	3.6	0	569	.11	3.8	.83	.29	305	171	1.88	.556	816
soybean product, tofu																
dried, frozen (koyadufu)	82	1.0	8.1	2.5		1.2	9	0	.05	.05	16	1	62	10	.83	.627
1 piece	17	5.2	0.7	1.1	2.9	0	88	.08	0.2	.00	.07	3	82	1.65	.200	816
fried	35	6.6	2.2	1.4		0.5	0	0	.01	.01	3	2	48	8	.26	.194
1 piece	13	2.6	0.4	0.6	1.5	0	0	.02	0.0	.00	.02	19	37	.63	.052	816
okara	47	49.8	2.0	7.6			0	0	.01	.07	16	5	49	16	.34	.246
½ cup	61	1.1	0.1	0.2	0.5	0	0	.01	0.1	.00	.05	130	37	.79	.122	816
raw	94	104.8	10.0	2.3		1.5	11	0	.06	.06	19	9	130	128	.99	.750
½ cup	124	5.9	0.9	1.3	3.3	0	105	.10	0.2	.00	.08	150	120	6.65	.239	816
raw, firm	183	88.0	19.9	5.4		2.9	21	0	.13	.12	37	18	258	118	1.98	1.488
½ cup	126	11.0	1.6	2.4	6.2	0	209	.20	0.5	.00	.17	299	239	13.19	.476	816
salted & fermented (fuyu)	13	7.7	0.9	0.6			2	0	.01	.01	3	316	5	6	.17	.129
1 block	11	0.9	0.1	0.2	0.5	0	18	.02	0.0	.00	.01	8	8	.22	.041	816
soybeans, green, boiled	127	61.7	11.1	9.9	2.7	3.8	14	15	.14	.05	100	13	131	54	.82	.452
½ cup	90	5.8	0.7	1.1	2.7	0	140	.23	1.1	.00	.12	485	142	2.25	.105	816
soybeans, mature																
boiled	298	107.6	28.6	17.1		10.3	2	3	.49	.40	93	2	175	148	1.98	1.417
1 cup	172	15.4	2.2	3.4	8.7	0	15	.27	0.7	.00	.31	886	421	8.84	.700	816
sprouted, steamed	38	37.3	4.0	3.1		0.4	0	4	.02	.05	38	5	28	28	.49	.334
½ cup	47	2.1	0.3	0.5	1.2	0	5	.10	0.5	.00	.35	167	63	.62	.155	811
sprouted, stir-fried	125	67.2	13.1	9.4		0.8	2	12	.19	.17	127	14	82	96	2.10	1.133
3.5 oz	100	7.1	1.0	1.6	4.0	0	17	.42	1.1	.00	1.19	567	216	.40	.527	811

	KCAL	H₂O (g)	PRO (g)	CHO (g)	SUGR (g)	DFIB (g)	A (RE)	C (mg)	B-2 (mg)	B-6 (mg)	FOL (mcg)	Na (mg)	Ca (mg)	Mg (mg)	Zn (mg)	Mn (mg)
	WT (g)	FAT (g)	SFA (g)	MUFA (g)	PUFA (g)	CHOL (mg)	A (IU)	B-1 (mg)	NIA (mg)	B-12 (mcg)	PANT (mg)	K (mg)	P (mg)	Fe (mg)	Cu (mg)	REF
spinach																
boiled	21	82.1	2.7	3.4		2.2	737	9	.21	.22	131	63	122	78	.68	.842
½ cup	90	0.2	0.0	0.0	0.1	0	7371	.09	0.4	.00	.13	419	50	3.21	.157	811
cnd	25	98.2	3.0	3.6		2.6	939	15	.15	.11	105	29	136	81	.49	.639
½ cup	107	0.5	0.1	0.0	0.2	0	9390	.02	0.4	.00	.05	370	47	2.46	.193	811
creamed, frzn, Birds Eye	59	72.7	2.1	5.1		1.5		11	.12	.06	16	312	72	27	.16	
⅓ cup	85	3.8	0.8		0.7	1	4231	.05	0.2	.13	.14	199	43	1.08	.042	I
creamed, frzn, Pillsbury	60	93.0	3.6	9.0				3	.22			510	130			
½ cup	113	2.0	1.0	0.0		2	1848	.67	0.1			440	84	.90		I
frzn, boiled	27	85.5	3.0	5.1		2.8	739	12	.16	.14	102	82	139	66	.66	.895
½ cup	95	0.2	0.0	0.0	0.1	0	7395	.06	0.4	.00	.08	283	46	1.44	.134	811
raw	6	25.6	0.8	1.0	0.1	0.8	188	8	.05	.05	54	22	28	22	.15	.251
½ cup chopped	28	0.1	0.0	0.0	0.0	0	1880	.02	0.2	.00	.02	156	14	.76	.036	811
w/ butter sce, frzn, Pillsbury	40	130.5	3.0	6.0				26	.26			380	207			
½ cup	142	2.0			0.0	5	2907	.06	1.1			670	36	2.25		I
squash, summer, all varieties, boiled	18	84.3	0.8	3.9		1.3	26	5	.04	.06	18	1	24	22	.35	.192
½ cup slices	90	0.3	0.1	0.0	0.1	0	258	.04	0.5	.00	.12	173	35	.32	.093	811
squash, summer, all varieties, raw	13	60.9	0.8	2.8	1.4	1.2	13	10	.02	.07	17	1	13	15	.17	.102
½ cup slices	65	0.1	0.0	0.0	0.1	0	127	.04	0.4	.00	.07	127	23	.30	.049	811
squash, summer, crookneck																
boiled	18	84.3	0.8	3.9		1.3	26	5	.04	.08	18	1	24	22	.35	.192
½ cup slices	90	0.3	0.1	0.0	0.1	0	258	.04	0.5	.00	.12	173	35	.32	.093	811
cnd	14	103.7	0.7	3.2		1.5	13	3	.03	.05	11	5	13	14	.31	.105
½ cup slices	108	0.1	0.0	0.0	0.0	0	131	.02	0.5	.00	.05	104	23	.77	.086	811
frzn, boiled	24	88.6	1.2	5.3		1.3	19	7	.05	.10	12	6	19	26	.33	.252
½ cup slices	96	0.2	0.0	0.0	0.1	0	187	.03	0.4	.00	.10	243	39	.50	.070	811
raw	12	61.2	0.6	2.6		1.2	22	5	.03	.07	15	1	14	14	.19	.102
½ cup slices	65	0.2	0.0	0.0	0.1	0	220	.03	0.3	.00	.07	138	21	.31	.066	811
squash, summer, scallop, boiled	14	85.5	0.9	3.0		1.7	8	10	.02	.08	19	1	14	17	.22	.115
½ cup slices	90	0.2	0.0	0.0	0.1	0	77	.05	0.4	.00	.07	126	25	.30	.075	811
squash, summer, scallop, raw	12	61.2	0.8	2.5			7	12	.02	.07	20	1	12	15	.19	.102
½ cup slices	65	0.1	0.0	0.0	0.1	0	72	.05	0.4	.00	.07	118	23	.26	.066	811
squash, summer, zucchini																
boiled	14	85.3	0.6	3.5		1.3	22	4	.04	.07	15	3	12	20	.16	.160
½ cup slices	90	0.0	0.0	0.0	0.0	0	216	.04	0.4	.00	.10	228	36	.32	.077	811
breaded, frzn, Ore-Ida	152	57.0	2.9	14.8				1	.11			348	16			
3 oz	85	9.0	1.6	6.2	1.2	2	190	.12	1.4			164		1.13		I
frzn, boiled	19	106.1	1.3	4.0		1.5	48	4	.04	.05	9	2	19	15	.22	.258
½ cup slices	112	0.1	0.0	0.0	0.1	0	484	.05	0.4	.00	.30	217	28	.54	.053	811
italian style, cnd, packed in tomato jce	33	103.3	1.2	7.8			62	3	.05	.17	34	426	19	16	.30	.274
½ cup slices	114	0.1	0.0	0.0	0.1	0	614	.05	0.6	.00	.31	312	33	.78	.112	811
raw	9	61.9	0.8	1.9		0.8	22	6	.02	.06	14	2	10	14	.13	.083
½ cup slices	65	0.1	0.0	0.0	0.0	0	221	.05	0.3	.00	.05	161	21	.27	.037	811
sticks, breaded, frzn, Mrs. Paul's	174		3.1	23.1				1	.09			389	26			
3 oz	85	7.7					51	.14	0.9			95		1.30		I
squash, winter																
acorn, baked	57	84.6	1.1	14.9		4.5	44	11	.01	.20	19	4	45	44	.17	.247
½ cup cubes	102	0.1	0.0	0.0	0.1	0	437	.17	0.9	.00	.51	446	46	.95	.088	811
acorn, boiled, mashed	41	109.4	0.8	10.7		3.2	32	8	.01	.14	14	4	32	32	.13	.178
½ cup	122	0.1	0.0	0.0	0.0	0	315	.12	0.6	.00	.37	321	33	.68	.063	811
all varieties, baked	40	90.8	0.9	8.9		2.9	363	10	.02	.07	29	1	14	8	.27	.215
½ cup cubes	102	0.6	0.1	0.0	0.3	0	3628	.09	0.7	.00	.36	446	20	.34	.097	811
all varieties, raw	21	51.5	0.8	5.1	2.2	0.9	235	7	.02	.05	13	2	18	12	.08	.097
½ cup cubes	58	0.1	0.0	0.0	0.1	0	2355	.06	0.5	.00	.23	203	19	.34	.038	811
butternut, baked	41	89.6	0.9	10.7			714	15	.02	.13	20	4	42	30	.13	.175
½ cup cubes	102	0.1	0.0	0.0	0.0	0	7141	.07	1.0	.00	.37	290	28	.61	.066	811
butternut, frzn, boiled	47	105.4	1.5	12.1			401	4	.05	.08	20	2	23	11	.14	.208
½ cup mashed	120	0.1	0.0	0.0	0.0	0	4007	.06	0.6	.00	.18	160	17	.70	.043	811

	KCAL	H₂O (g)	PRO (g)	CHO (g)	SUGR (g)	DFIB (g)	Vitamins A (RE)	C (mg)	B-2 (mg)	B-6 (mg)	FOL (mcg)	Minerals Na (mg)	Ca (mg)	Mg (mg)	Zn (mg)	Mn (mg)
	WT (g)	FAT (g)	SFA (g)	MUFA (g)	PUFA (g)	CHOL (mg)	A (IU)	B-1 (mg)	NIA (mg)	B-12 (mcg)	PANT (mg)	K (mg)	P (mg)	Fe (mg)	Cu (mg)	REF
hubbard, baked	51	86.8	2.5	11.0			616	10	.05	.18	17	8	17	22	.15	.173
½ cup cubes	102	0.6	0.1	0.0	0.3	0	6156	.08	0.6	.00	.46	365	23	.48	.046	811
hubbard, boiled, mashed	35	107.5	1.7	7.6		3.4	473	8	.03	.12	11	6	12	15	.12	.149
½ cup	118	0.4	0.1	0.0	0.2	0	4726	.05	0.4	.00	.35	253	17	.33	.055	811
spaghetti, boiled/baked	23	72.0	0.5	5.0		1.1	9	3	.02	.08	6	14	16	9	.16	.085
½ cup	78	0.2	0.0	0.0	0.1	0	86	.03	0.6	.00	.28	91	11	.27	.027	811
stew veg, frzn, Ore-Ida	51	71.9	1.5	10.6				7	.03			35	16			
3 oz	85	0.2				0	3732	.07	1.4			232		1.02		I
succotash																
boiled	110	65.6	4.9	23.4		4.3	28	8	.09	.11	31	16	16	51	.60	.738
½ cup	96	0.8	0.1	0.1	0.4	0	282	.16	1.3	.00	.54	394	112	1.46	.172	811
cnd	81	104.9	3.3	17.9		3.3	19	6	.07	.06	41	283	14	24	.64	.468
½ cup	128	0.6	0.1	0.1	0.3	0	187	.04	0.8	.00	.40	209	70	.68	.140	811
cnd w/ cream style corn	102	104.0	3.5	23.4		4.0	19	9	.09	.17	59	326	15	1	.57	.858
½ cup	133	0.7	0.1	0.1	0.3	0	188	.04	0.8	.00	.29	243	78	.73	.237	811
frzn, boiled	79	63.0	3.7	17.0		3.5	20	5	.06	.08	28	38	13	20	.38	.238
½ cup	85	0.8	0.1	0.1	0.4	0	196	.06	1.1	.00	.20	225	60	.76	.051	811
swamp cabbage, boiled	10	45.5	1.0	1.8		0.9	255	8	.04	.04	17	60	26	15	.08	.070
½ cup chopped	49	0.1	0.0	0.0	0.0	0	2548	.02	0.2	.00	.06	139	21	.65	.010	811
swamp cabbage, raw	11	51.8	1.5	1.8		1.2	353	31	.06	.05	32	63	43	40	.10	.090
1 cup chopped	56	0.1				0	3528	.02	0.5	.00	.08	175	22	.94	.013	811
sweet potato																
baked, frzn	88	64.9	1.5	20.6		1.6	1444	8	.05	.16	20	7	31	18	.26	.585
½ cup cubes	88	0.1	0.0	0.0	0.0	0	14441	.06	0.5	.00	.49	332	39	.48	.161	811
baked w/ skin	117	83.0	2.0	27.7		3.4	2487	28	.14	.27	26	11	32	23	.33	.638
1 sweet potato	114	0.1	0.0	0.0	0.1	0	24877	.08	0.7	.00	.74	397	63	.51	.237	811
boiled w/o skin	172	119.5	2.7	39.8		3.0	2796	28	.23	.40	18	21	34	16	.44	.553
½ cup mashed	164	0.5	0.1	0.0	0.2	0	27969	.09	1.0	.00	.87	302	44	.92	.264	811
candied	144	70.3	0.9	29.3		2.5	440	7	.04	.04	12	74	27	12	.16	.448
1 piece (2 ½" long & 2" dia)[45]	105	3.4	1.4	0.7	0.2	8	4398	.02	0.4	.00	.28	198	27	1.19	.107	811
candied, cnd, Joan of Arc	240		1.0	60.0								15				
½ cup	146	0.0				0						190				I
cnd	182	152.1	3.3	42.3		3.6	1596	53	.11	.38	33	106	44	44	.36	.910
1 cup pieces	200	0.4	0.1	0.0	0.2	0	15966	.07	1.5	.00	1.05	624	98	1.78	.278	811
cnd, mashed	258	188.4	5.0	59.2		4.3	3858	13	.23	.60	27	191	77	61	.54	2.519
1 cup	255	0.5	0.1	0.0	0.2	0	38571	.07	2.4	.00	1.31	536	133	3.39	.709	811
cnd, syrup pack	106	71.0	1.3	24.9		2.9	702	11	.04	.06	8	38	17	12	.16	.603
½ cup	98	0.3	0.1	0.0	0.1	0	7014	.02	0.3	.00	.39	189	25	.93	.164	811
frzn, Mrs. Paul's Family	194		1.0	46.8				2	.07			118	34			
4 oz	113	0.4				1	6308	.04	0.6			222		.80		I
heavy syrup, cnd, Joan of Arc	125	90.5	0.7	30.4		2.5		2	.02			16	9			
½ cup	124	0.0				0	6753	.01	0.5			118	15	.50		I
light syrup, cnd, Joan of Arc	118	81.4	1.1	28.2		2.3		3	.05			29	16			
½ cup	113	0.2				0	12769	.05	1.1			149	23	.33		I
mashed, cnd, Joan of Arc	92	87.0	1.0	24.9		3.1		6	.05			43	17			
½ cup	113	0.1				0	16272	.02	1.8			235	34	.90		I
whipped, frzn, Stouffer's	111	62.9	1.3	16.2				4	.04			272	20			
3 oz	85	4.4				13	6800	.03	0.2			145		.26		I
w/ pineapple orange sce, cnd, Joan of Arc—½ cup	220	85.2	0.7	54.4				5	.01			15	12			
	142	0.0				0	6380	.01	0.5			121	14	.43		I
sweet potatoes & apples, frzn, Stouffers	108	59.5	0.7	22.1				23	.03			68	19			
3 oz	85	1.9					5100	.03	0.2			119		.43		I
taro, ckd	94	42.1	0.3	22.8		3.4	0	3	.02	.22	13	10	12	20	.18	.296
½ cup slices	66	0.1	0.0	0.0	0.0	0	0	.07	0.3	.00	.22	319	50	.48	.133	811
taro leaves, steamed	18	68.2	2.0	3.0		1.5	314	26	.28	.05	36	1	64	15	.16	.275
½ cup	74	0.3	0.1	0.0	0.1	0	3136	.10	0.9	.00	.03	340	20	.87	.104	811
taro shoots, ckd	10	66.7	0.5	2.2			4	13	.04	.08	2	1	10	6	.38	.091
½ cup slices	70	0.1	0.0	0.0	0.0	0	36	.03	0.6	.00	.05	241	18	.29	.066	811
taro, tahitian, ckd	30	58.8	2.8	4.7			120	26	.13	.08	5	37	101	35	.07	.114
½ cup slices	68	0.5	0.1	0.0	0.2	0	1200	.03	0.3	.00	.09	424	46	1.06	.052	811

	KCAL	H₂O (g)	PRO (g)	CHO (g)	SUGR (g)	DFIB (g)	A (RE)	C (mg)	B-2 (mg)	B-6 (mg)	FOL (mcg)	Na (mg)	Ca (mg)	Mg (mg)	Zn (mg)	Mn (mg)
	WT (g)	FAT (g)	SFA (g)	MUFA (g)	PUFA (g)	CHOL (mg)	A (IU)	B-1 (mg)	NIA (mg)	B-12 (mcg)	PANT (mg)	K (mg)	P (mg)	Fe (mg)	Cu (mg)	REF
tomatillos, raw	11	31.2	0.3	2.0		0.6	4	4	.01	.02	2	0	2	7	.07	.052
1 med	34	0.3	0.0	0.1	0.1	0	39	.01	0.6	.00	.05	91	13	.21	.027	811
tomato, green, raw	30	114.4	1.5	6.3		1.4	79	29	.05	.10	11	16	16	12	.09	.123
1 tomato	123	0.2	0.0	0.0	0.1	0	790	.07	0.6	.00	.61	251	34	.63	.111	811
tomato paste, cnd	107	96.7	4.8	25.3	16.9	5.4	320	56	.25	.50	29	115	46	67	1.05	.681
½ cup	131	0.7	0.1	0.1	0.3	0	3203	.20	4.2	.00	.99	1227	103	2.54	.776	811
Contadina	30		2.0	6.0	3.0	1.0		6				20	0			
2 T	33	0.0	0.0	0.0	0.0	0	500							.70		I
garlic, Hunt	28		1.5	6.1	3.7	1.6	15	7				281	17			
2 T	33	0.3	0.0			0								.96		I
Hunt	30		1.0	5.7	3.7	2.0	24	7				88	13			
2 T	33	0.5	0.0			0								.60		I
italian, Hunt	27		1.2	5.8	3.7	2.0	23	8				264	17			
2 T	33	0.3	0.0			0								.67		I
Italian (pear), Contadina	35		1.0	7.0	4.0	1.0		6				290	0			
2 T	33	0.5	0.0			0	300							.70		I
no salt added, Hunt	30		1.0	5.7	3.7	2.0	24	7				7	10			
2 T	33	0.5	0.0			0								.23		I
tomato puree, cnd	100	218.6	4.2	23.9		5.0	320	26	.14	.38	28	85	43	60	.55	.640
1 cup	250	0.4	0.1	0.1	0.2	0	3188	.18	4.3	.00	1.10	1065	100	3.10	.408	811
Angela Mia	16		0.9	2.9	2.6	0.4	24	8				21	7			
¼ cup	62	0.3	0.0			0										I
Contadina	20		0.7	4.0	1.0	0.5		9				15	0			
¼ cup	63	0.0	0.0	0.0	0.0	0	500							.40		I
Hunt	24		1.0	5.0	3.4	1.5	31	14				98	24			
¼ cup	62	0.3	0.0			0								.56		I
tomato, red, boiled	32	110.6	1.3	7.0		1.2	89	27	.07	.11	16	13	7	17	.13	.158
½ cup	120	0.5	0.1	0.1	0.2	0	892	.08	0.9	.00	.35	335	37	.67	.112	811
tomato, red, crushed in tomato puree,	20		0.6	3.3	2.0	1.0		6				150	20			
cnd, Contadina—¼ cup[46]	61	0.0	0.0	0.0	0.0	0	267							.40		I
tomato, red, cut, cnd, Hunt Choice	23		1.1	4.8		1.3	29	14				325	30			
½ cup	121	0.2	0.0			0								.42		I
tomato, red, cut/diced, garlic/italian herb,	24		1.1	5.3		0.5	29	18				553	27			
cnd, Hunt—½ cup	121	0.0	0.0	0.0	0.0	0								.07		I
tomato, red, diced																
in jce, cnd, Angela Mia	20		1.1	4.0		0.5	49	18				477	0			
½ cup	121	0.1	0.0			0								.07		I
in puree, cnd, Hunt	23		1.3	4.7		0.6	53	19				304	0			
½ cup	122	0.2	0.0			0								.13		I
w/ green chilies, cnd, Hunt	1		0.1	0.3	0.2	0.1	3	0				24	4			
2 T	10	0.0	0.0	0.0	0.0	0								.04		I
tomato, red, dried																
bits, Hunt	11		0.8	2.1	1.4	1.0	2	3				7	4			
2 t	5	0.2	0.0			0								.25		I
halves, Hunt's	9		0.6	1.7	1.1	0.8	2	2				5	5			
2 pieces	4	0.2	0.0			0								.20		I
julienne, Hunt	11		0.8	2.1	1.4	1.0	2	3				7	6			
8 pieces	5	0.2	0.0			0								.25		I
marinated, halves, Hunt	43		0.2	2.5	0.9	1.0	3	2				6	4			
3 pieces	11	4.0	0.6			0								.16		I
tomato, red, italian (pear shaped), cnd,	25		1.0	4.0	3.0	1.0		12				220	20			
Contadina—½ cup	121	0.0	0.0	0.0	0.0	0	500							.70		I
tomato, red, italian (pear shaped),	29		0.9	7.2	6.4	1.5	53	11				286	19			
cnd, crushed, Hunt—½ cup	121	0.3	0.0			0								1.98		I
tomato, red, raw	26	115.3	1.0	5.7	3.4	1.4	76	23	.06	.10	18	11	6	14	.11	.129
1 tomato	123	0.4	0.1	0.1	0.2	0	766	.07	0.8	.00	.30	273	30	.55	.091	811
tomato, red, stewed	80	81.4	2.0	13.2		1.7	68	18	.08	.09	11	460	26	15	.18	.195
1 cup[47]	101	2.7	0.5	1.1	0.9	0	673	.11	1.1	.00	.26	249	38	1.07	.096	811
cnd	36	116.5	1.2	8.7		1.3	69	15	.04	.02	7	283	42	15	.22	.076
½ cup	128	0.2	0.0	0.0	0.1	0	692	.06	0.9	.00	.15	305	26	.93	.143	811

	KCAL / WT (g)	H₂O (g) / FAT (g)	PRO (g) / SFA (g)	CHO (g) / MUFA (g)	SUGR (g) / PUFA (g)	DFIB (g) / CHOL (mg)	A (RE) / A (IU)	C (mg) / B-1 (mg)	B-2 (mg) / NIA (mg)	B-6 (mg) / B-12 (mcg)	FOL (mcg) / PANT (mg)	Na (mg) / K (mg)	Ca (mg) / P (mg)	Mg (mg) / Fe (mg)	Zn (mg) / Cu (mg)	Mn (mg) / REF
cnd, Contadina	50		1.0	9.0	6.0	1.0	2					220	40			
½ cup	122	1.0	0.0			0	300							.70		I
cnd, Hunt	33		1.2	7.3	5.7	1.5	25	7				357	28			
½ cup	121	0.3	0.0			0								.91		I
cnd, no salt added, Hunt	33		1.2	7.3	5.7	1.5	25	7				31	36			
½ cup	121	0.3	0.0			0								1.02		I
italian style, cnd, Contadina	50		1.0	8.0	7.0	1.0	2					260	40			
½ cup	122	1.0	0.0			0	300							.70		I
mexican style, cnd, Contadina	50		1.0	10.0	6.0	1.0	1					290	40			
½ cup	122	1.0	0.0			0	200							.70		I
tomato, red, sun-dried	139	7.9	7.6	30.1		6.6	47	21	.26	.18	37	1131	59	105	1.07	.997
1 cup	54	1.6	0.2	0.3	0.6	0	472	.29	4.9	.00	1.13	1851	192	4.91	.768	811
tomato, red, sun-dried, cnd, packed in oil	234	59.2	5.6	25.7		6.4	142	112	.42	.35	25	293	52	89	.86	.513
1 cup	110	15.5	2.1	9.5	2.3	0	1415	.21	4.0	.00	.53	1722	153	2.94	.520	811
tomato, red, wedges in tomato jce, cnd	34	120.2	1.0	8.3			76	19	.04	.15	13	284	34	14	.21	.216
½ cup	131	0.2	0.0	0.0	0.1	0	757	.07	0.9	.00	.28	329	30	.60	.136	811
tomato, red, whole, peeled																
cnd	23	112.4	1.1	5.2		1.2	72	17	.04	.11	9	178	36	14	.19	.152
½ cup	120	0.2	0.0	0.0	0.1	0	714	.05	0.9	.00	.20	265	23	.66	.132	811
cnd, Contadina	25		1.0	4.0	3.0	1.0	12					220	20			
½ cup	121	0.0	0.0	0.0	0.0	0	500							.70		I
cnd, Hunt	24		1.7	4.7		0.7	36	20				433	37			
2 tomatoes	159	0.1	0.0			0								.07		I
no salt added, cnd, Hunt	21		1.5	4.1		0.6	31	17				9	32			
2 tomatoes	137	0.1	0.0			0								.07		I
tomato, red w/ green chili, cnd	18	113.1	0.8	4.3			47	7	.02	.12	11	481	24	13	.16	.158
½ cup	120	0.1	0.0	0.0	0.0	0	468	.04	0.8	.00	.18	128	17	.31	.108	811
tree fern, ckd	28	62.9	0.2	7.8		2.6	14	21	.21	.13	11	4	6	4	.22	.383
½ cup chopped	71	0.0	0.0	0.0	0.0	0	142	.00	2.5	.00	.04	4	3	.11	.143	811
turnip, boiled	14	73.0	0.6	3.8		1.6	0	9	.02	.05	7	39	17	6	.16	.078
½ cup cup	78	0.1	0.0	0.0	0.0	0	0	.02	0.2	.00	.11	105	15	.17	.050	811
turnip, frzn, boiled	23	93.6	1.5	4.3		2.0	2	4	.03	.07	8	36	32	14	.20	.100
3.5 oz	100	0.2	0.0	0.0	0.1	0	25	.04	0.6	.00	.14	182	26	.98	.063	811
turnip greens																
boiled	14	67.1	0.8	3.1		2.5	396	20	.05	.13	85	21	99	16	.10	.243
½ cup chopped	72	0.2	0.0	0.0	0.1	0	3959	.03	0.3	.00	.20	146	21	.58	.182	811
cnd	16	110.8	1.6	2.8		2.0	420	18	.07	.04	48	324	138	23	.27	.324
½ cup	117	0.4	0.1	0.0	0.1	0	4196	.01	0.4	.00	.05	165	25	1.77	.097	811
frzn, boiled	25	74.1	2.7	4.1		2.8	654	18	.06	.05	32	12	125	21	.34	.389
½ cup	82	0.3	0.1	0.0	0.1	0	6540	.04	0.4	.00	.06	184	28	1.59	.123	811
raw	8	25.5	0.4	1.6		0.9	213	17	.03	.07	54	11	53	9	.05	.130
½ cup chopped	28	0.1	0.0	0.0	0.0	0	2128	.02	0.2	.00	.11	83	12	.31	.098	811
turnip greens & turnips, frzn, boiled	17	94.2	2.1	2.9		1.8	516	9	.07	.06	22	15	91	12	.13	.177
3.5 oz	100	0.2	0.0	0.0	0.1	0	5161	.03	0.3	.00	.10	62	17	1.33	.041	811
veg & pasta mornay, frzn, Lean Cuisine	280		15.0	26.0			30		.34			1190	200			
9.3 oz entree	265	13.0	3.0		1.0	40	2000	.30	2.0			350		1.08		I
veg casserole primavera, Stouffers	93	94.9	3.1	7.9			3		.10			367	73			
4 oz entree	113	5.4				11	791	.05	0.5			203		.34		I
veg medley, breaded, frzn, Ore-Ida	162	54.2	3.3	17.0			20		.12			466	15			
3 oz	85	9.0	1.6	6.2	1.2	3	2276	.12	1.9			192		.88		I
veg pasta italiano, frzn, Banquet	240		9.0	48.0	8.0	6.0	2					480	60			
10 oz entree	284	1.5	0.5			5	500							2.70		I
vinespinach, raw	19	93.1	1.8	3.4			800	102	.15	.24	140	24	109	65	.43	.735
3.5 oz	100	0.3				0	8000	.05	0.5	.00	.05	510	52	1.20	.107	811
water chestnuts, chinese																
cnd	35	60.5	0.6	8.7		1.8	0	1	.02	.11	4	6	3	4	.27	.113
½ cup slices	70	0.0	0.0	0.0	0.0	0	3	.01	0.3	.00	.15	83	13	.61	.070	811
cnd, LaChoy	10		0.2	2.4	0.3	1.0	0	0				2	1			
2 T[48]	20	0.1	0.0			0	0							.05		I

	KCAL	H₂O (g)	PRO (g)	CHO (g)	SUGR (g)	DFIB (g)	Vitamins					Minerals				
							A (RE)	C (mg)	B-2 (mg)	B-6 (mg)	FOL (mcg)	Na (mg)	Ca (mg)	Mg (mg)	Zn (mg)	Mn (mg)
	WT (g)	FAT (g)	SFA (g)	MUFA (g)	PUFA (g)	CHOL (mg)	A (IU)	B-1 (mg)	NIA (mg)	B-12 (mcg)	PANT (mg)	K (mg)	P (mg)	Fe (mg)	Cu (mg)	REF
raw	66	45.5	0.9	14.8		1.9	0	2	.12	.20	10	9	7	14	.31	.205
½ cup slices	62	0.1	0.0	0.0	0.0	0	0	.09	0.6	.00	.30	362	39	.04	.202	811
watercress, raw	2	16.2	0.4	0.2		0.3	80	7	.02	.02	2	7	20	4	.02	.041
½ cup chopped	17	0.0	0.0	0.0	0.0	0	799	.02	0.0	.00	.05	56	10	.03	.013	811
wax beans, cut, cnd, Joan of Arc	25		1.3	4.5				6	.04			321	87			
½ cup	119	0.2					81	.04	0.3			261	17			I
waxgourd, boiled	11	83.6	0.3	2.6		0.9	0	9	.00	.03	3	93	16	9	.51	.049
½ cup cubes[49]	87	0.2	0.0	0.0	0.1	0	0	.03	0.3	.00	.11	4	15	.33	.019	811
white beans																
boiled	249	112.9	17.4	44.9		11.3	0	0	.08	.17	144	11	161	113	2.47	1.138
1 cup	179	0.6	0.2	0.1	0.3	0	0	.21	0.3	.00	.41	1004	202	6.62	.514	816
cnd	307	183.7	19.0	57.5		12.6	0	0	.10	.20	171	13	191	134	2.93	1.349
1 cup	262	0.8	0.2	0.1	0.3	0	0	.25	0.3	.00	.48	1189	238	7.83	.608	816
small, boiled	254	113.2	16.1	46.2		18.6	0	0	.11	.23	245	4	131	122	1.95	.913
1 cup	179	1.1	0.3	0.1	0.5	0	0	.42	0.5	.00	.45	829	303	5.08	.267	816
winged bean leaves, raw	74	76.8	5.8	14.1			809	45	.60	.23	16	9	224	8	1.28	1.367
3.5 oz	100	1.1	0.3	0.3	0.2	0	8090	.83	3.5	.00	.14	176	63	4.00	.456	811
winged beans, boiled	253	115.6	18.3	25.7			0	0	.22	.08	18	22	244	93	2.48	2.062
1 cup	172	10.0	1.4	3.7	2.7	0	0	.51	1.4	.00	.27	482	263	7.45	1.330	816
yam, boiled/baked	79	47.7	1.0	18.8		2.7	0	8	.02	.16	11	5	10	12	.14	.252
½ cup cubes	68	0.1	0.0	0.0	0.0	0	0	.06	0.4	.00	.21	456	33	.35	.103	811
yambean, boiled	38	90.1	0.7	8.8			2	14	.03	.04	8	4	11	11	.15	.057
3.5 oz	100	0.1				0	19	.02	0.2	.00	.12	135	16	.57	.046	811
yardlong bean, boiled	202	117.6	14.2	36.1		6.5	3	1	.11	.16	249	9	72	168	1.85	.833
1 cup	171	0.8	0.2	0.1	0.3	0	27	.36	0.9	.00	.68	539	310	4.51	.385	816
yellow beans, boiled	255	111.5	16.2	44.7		18.4	0	3	.18	.23	143	9	110	131	1.88	.805
1 cup	177	1.9	0.5	0.2	0.8	0	4	.33	1.3	.00	.41	575	324	4.39	.329	816

1. Values are averages for with bacon & jalapenos, with chiles & chicken, with chiles & chorizo, and with onions & peppers.
2. Values are averages for plain, with bacon, with green chiles, with nacho cheese, and with onions.
3. Includes with salsa and with chiles.
4. Made with broadbeans, soybean oil, onions, flour, salt, garlic, coriander, and cumin.
5. Made with chickpeas, lemon juice, tahini, olive oil, and garlic.
6. Bean sprouts, cabbage, pea pods, spinach, red peppers, and water chestnuts.
7. Snow peas, spinach, bean sprouts, celery, water chestnuts, and red peppers.
8. Bean sprouts, french green beans, water chestnuts, carrots, celery, straw mushrooms, and sce.
9. Made with cabbage, celery, table cream, sugar, green pepper, lemon juice, onion, pimento, vingegar, salt, dry mustard, and white pepper.
10. Made with yellow corn, whole milk, egg, sugar, butter, salt, and pepper.
11. European plant used as an herb and as salad greens.
12. Includes Italian, green, and yellow varieties.
13. Italian green beans, chickpeas, red peppers, onions, and ripe olives.
14. French green beans, broccoli, pearl onions, mushrooms, and red peppers.
15. Green beans, broccoli, green peppers, mushrooms, and red peppers.
16. Includes Boston and Bibb types.
17. Includes crisphead types.
18. Cabbage, carrots, bok choy, water chestnuts, snow pea pods, straw mushrooms, and sce.
19. Carrots, green peas, snap beans, and lima beans.
20. Corn, lima beans, snap beans, green peas, and carrots.
21. Corn, carrots, peas, and green beans.
22. Carrots, corn, green beans, peas, and pearl onions.
23. Agaricus bisporus.
24. French style green beans, corn, broccoli, and red peppers.
25. Breaded and parboiled in vegetable oil.
26. Peas, broccoli, carrots, red peppers, macaroni, and sce.
27. Vitamin A value for green varieties; red varieties contain 4838 IU.
28. Vitamin A value for green varieties; red varieties contain 2557 IU.
29. Vitamin A value for green varieties; red varieties contain 364 IU.
30. Vitamin A value for green varieties; red varieties contain 1236 IU.
31. Vitamin A value for green varieties; red varieties contain 3343 IU.
32. Vitamin A value for green varieties; red varieties contain 2850 IU. Vitamin C value for green varieties; red varieties contain 95 mg.
33. Contains potatoes, eggs, onion, margarine, flour, and salt.
34. Water, whole milk, and margarine added.
35. Potatoes, whole milk, cheddar cheese, butter, flour, and salt.
36. Pan fried in vegetable oil.
37. Whole milk and butter added.
38. Milk, water and margarine added.
39. Whole milk and margarine added.
40. Potatoes, whole milk, onions, green pepper, bread crumbs, salt, butter, and black pepper.
41. Water, whole milk, and butter added.
42. Potatoes, whole milk, butter, flour, and salt.
43. Includes daikon (Japanese) and Chinese radishes.
44. French style green beans, bean sprouts, celery, mushrooms, and red peppers.
45. Canned sweet potato and syrup, brown sugar, butter, and salt.
46. Values are averages for original tomatoes, tomatoes with Italian herbs, and tomatoes with roasted garlic.
47. Tomatoes, breadcrumbs, margarine, sugar, onions, salt, and pepper.
48. Values are averages for chopped, sliced, and whole.
49. Chinese preserving melon.

	KCAL / WT (g)	H₂O (g) / FAT (g)	PRO (g) / SFA (g)	CHO (g) / MUFA (g)	SUGR (g) / PUFA (g)	DFIB (g) / CHOL (mg)	A (RE) / A (IU)	C (mg) / B-1 (mg)	B-2 (mg) / NIA (mg)	B-6 (mg) / B-12 (mcg)	FOL (mcg) / PANT (mg)	Na (mg) / K (mg)	Ca (mg) / P (mg)	Mg (mg) / Fe (mg)	Zn (mg) / Cu (mg)	Mn (mg) / REF

34. MISCELLANEOUS

Food	KCAL	H₂O	PRO	CHO	SUGR	DFIB	A(RE)	C	B-2	B-6	FOL	Na	Ca	Mg	Zn	Mn
baking choc, unsweetened	146	0.4	2.9	7.9		4.3	3	0	.05	.03	2	4	21	87	1.12	.537
1 oz square	28	15.5	9.1	5.2	0.5	0	27	.02	0.3	.00	.06	233	117	1.77	.607	819
Bakers	140		3.0	9.0	0.0	4.0	0	0				0	20			
1 oz square	28	14.0	9.0			0	0					290		2.70		I
Hershey	89		2.0	4.1	0.1	2.2	0	0				3	12			
½ bar (.5 oz)	14	7.2	4.4			0	0							.82		I
liquid	132	0.3	3.4	9.5		3.7	1	0	.04	.02	2	3	15	74	1.03	.462
1 oz pkt	28	13.4	7.1	2.6	3.0	0	5	.01	0.6	.00	.05	326	95	1.16	.535	819
Nestle Chocobake	80		1.0	5.0	0.0	3.0	0	0				0	0			
.5 oz	14	8.0	5.0			0	0							.70		I
Nestle Toll House	80		2.0	5.0	0.0	3.0	0	0				0	0			
.5 oz	14	7.0	2.0			0	0							.70		I
baking powder																
Calumet	0		0.0	0.0	0.0	0.0	0	0				100	40			
¼ t	1.0	0.0	0.0	0.0	0.0	0	0							.00		I
double-acting, sodium aluminum sulfate	3	0.3	0.0	1.4		0.0	0	0	.00	.00	0	530	294	1	.00	.001
1 t	5	0.0	0.0	0.0	0.0	0	0	.00	0.0	.00	.00	1	110	.55	.001	818
double-acting, straight phosphate	3	0.2	0.0	1.2		0.0	0	0	.00	.00	0	395	368	2	.00	.001
1 t	5	0.0	0.0	0.0	0.0	0	0	.00	0.0	.00	.00	0	496	.56	.001	818
low sodium	5	0.3	0.0	2.3		0.1	0	0	.00	.00	0	5	217	1	.04	.021
1 t	5	0.0	0.0	0.0	0.0	0	0	.00	0.0	.00	.00	505	343	.41	.001	818
baking soda (sodium bicarbonate)	0	0.0	0.0	0.0	0.0	0.0	0	0	.00	.00	0	1368	0	0	.00	.000
1 t	5	0.0	0.0	0.0	0.0	0	0	.00	0.0	.00	.00	0	0	.00	.000	818
cocoa, unsweetened, dry powder	11	0.2	1.0	2.7		1.7	0	0	.01	.01	2	1	6	25	.34	.192
1 T	5	0.7	0.4	0.2	0.0	0	1	.00	0.1	.00	.01	76	37	.69	.189	819
baking, Nestle	15		1.0	3.0	0.0	2.0	0	0				0	0			
1 T	5	1.0	0.0			0	0							.36		I
european style, Hershey	21	0.1	1.2	2.6	0.0	1.4	0	0	.01	.01	2	3	8	28	.37	.289
1 T	5	0.5	0.3			0	0	.00	0.2	.00	.01	257	42	2.10	.197	MUL
Hershey	21		1.3	2.7	0.0	1.4	0	0				1	9			
1 T	5	0.5	0.3			0	0							.69		I
processed w/ alkali	11	0.1	0.9	2.7		1.5	0	0	.02	.01	2	1	6	24	.32	.187
1 t	5	0.7	0.4	0.2	0.0	0	1	.01	0.1	.00	.01	125	36	.78	.180	819
corn starch, Argo & Kingsford's	30	0.8	0.0	7.2		0.0						0				
1 T	8	0.0														I
corn starch, Cream	40		0.0	9.0	0.0	0.0	0	0				0	0			
1 T	10	0.0	0.0	0.0	0.0	0	0							.00		I
cream of tartar (potassium acid tartrate)	8	0.1	0.0	1.8		0.0	0	0	.00	.00	0	2	0	0	.01	.006
1 t	3	0.0	0.0	0.0	0.0	0	0	.00	0.0	.00	.00	495	0	.11	.006	818
fruit pectin	39	1.0	0.0	10.8		1.0	0	0	.01	.00	0	24	1	0	.06	.008
¼ pkt	12	0.0	0.0	0.0	0.0	0	0	.00	0.0	.00	.01	1	0	.33	.050	819
fruit pectin, Sure-Jell	5		0.0	1.0	1.0	0.0	0	0				1	0			
¼ t[1]	0.9	0.0	0.0	0.0	0.0	0	0					0	0	.00	.000	I
fruit protector, Ever-Fresh	5		0.0	1.0	1.0	0.0	0	60				0	0			
¼ t	1.0	0.0	0.0	0.0	0.0	0	0					0		.00		I
gelatin, dry, unsweetened	23	0.9	6.0	0.0	0.0	0.0	0	0	.02	.00	2	14	4	2	.01	.007
1 pkt	7	0.0	0.0	0.0	0.0	0	0	.00	0.0	.00	.01	1	3	.08	.151	819
gelatin, unflavored, Knox	35		6.0	3.0								15				
1 pkt	10	0.0	0.0	0.0	0.0											I
olives, pickled, ripe, manzanillo/mission	4	2.6	0.0	0.2		0.1	1	0	.00	.00	0	28	3	0	.01	.001
1 small	3.2	0.3	0.0	0.3	0.0	0	13	.00	0.0	.00	.00	0	0	.11	.008	809
	5	3.2	0.0	0.3		0.1	2	0	.00	.00	0	35	4	0	.01	.001
1 med	4	0.4	0.1	0.3	0.0	0	16	.00	0.0	.00	.00	0	0	.13	.010	809
	5	3.5	0.0	0.3		0.1	2	0	.00	.00	0	38	4	0	.01	.001
1 large	4.4	0.5	0.1	0.3	0.0	0	18	.00	0.0	.00	.00	0	0	.15	.011	809

Food	KCAL / WT (g)	H₂O (g) / FAT (g)	PRO (g) / SFA (g)	CHO (g) / MUFA (g)	SUGR (g) / PUFA (g)	DFIB (g) / CHOL (mg)	A (RE) / A (IU)	C (mg) / B-1 (mg)	B-2 (mg) / NIA (mg)	B-6 (mg) / B-12 (mcg)	FOL (mcg) / PANT (mg)	Na (mg) / K (mg)	Ca (mg) / P (mg)	Mg (mg) / Fe (mg)	Zn (mg) / Cu (mg)	Mn (mg) / REF
	7	4.8	0.1	0.4		0.2	2	0	.00	.00	0	52	5	0	.01	.001
1 extra large	6	0.6	0.1	0.5	0.1	0	24	.00	0.0	.00	.00	0	0	.20	.015	809
olives, pickled, ripe, sevillano/ascolano	7	7.0	0.1	0.5		0.2	3	0	.00	.00	0	75	8	0	.02	.002
1 jumbo	8	0.6	0.1	0.4	0.0	0	29	.00	0.0	.00	.00	1	0	.28	.019	809
	9	9.5	0.1	0.6		0.3	4	0	.00	.00	0	101	11	0	.02	.002
1 colossal	11	0.8	0.1	0.6	0.1	0	39	.00	0.0	.00	.00	1	0	.38	.026	809
	12	12.8	0.1	0.9		0.4	5	0	.00	.00	0	136	14	1	.03	.003
1 super colossal	15	1.0	0.1	0.8	0.1	0	53	.00	0.0	.00	.00	1	0	.50	.034	809
pickle relish																
hamburger	19	9.2	0.1	5.2		0.5	4	0	.01	.00	0	164	1	1	.02	.002
1 T	15	0.1	0.0	0.0	0.0	0	40	.00	0.1	.00	.00	11	3	.17	.012	811
hamburger, Del Monte	20		0.0	6.0	5.0		0				220	0				
1 T	17	0.0	0.0	0.0	0.0	0	200							.00		I
hot dog	14	10.7	0.2	3.5		0.2	3	0	.01	.00	0	164	1	3	.03	.002
1 T	15	0.1	0.0	0.0	0.0	0	25	.01	0.1	.00	.00	12	6	.19	.012	811
hot dog, Del Monte	15		0.0	4.0	3.0	0	0				140	0				
1 T	16	0.0	0.0	0.0	0.0	0	0							.00		I
sweet	20	9.3	0.1	5.3		0.2	2	0	.00	.00	0	122	0	1	.02	.002
1 T	15	0.1	0.0	0.0	0.0	0	23	.00	0.0	.00	.00	4	2	.13	.013	811
sweet, Del Monte	20		0.0	5.0	5.0	0.0	0	0				125	0			
1 T	16	0.0	0.0	0.0	0.0	0	0							.00		I
pickles, bread & butter	11	11.8	0.1	2.7			1	.00				101	5			
2 slices	15	0.0					20	.00	0.0				4	.30		456
Claussen	5	26.0	0.2	0.9	0.4	0.5	0	0				315	16	2	.04	
1 oz	28	0.1	0.0	0.0	0.0	0	0					45	9	.11	.030	I
Claussen	19	22.9	0.2	4.3	3.3	0.3	0	1				175	14	3	.08	
4 slices	28	0.1	0.0	0.0	0.0	0	0					32	13	.13	.040	I
Vlasic	30		0.0	7.0	7.0	0.0	0	0				180	0			
1 oz	28	0.0	0.0	0.0	0.0	0	0							.00		I
pickles, chow chow, sour	35	105.1	1.7	4.9								1605	38			
½ cup²	120	1.5											63	3.10		456
pickles, chow chow, sweet	142	84.1	1.8	33.1								645	28			
½ cup²	122	1.1											27	1.80		456
pickles, dill	1	5.5	0.0	0.2		0.1	2	0	.00	.00	0	77	1	1	.01	.001
1 slice	6	0.0	0.0	0.0	0.0	0	20	.00	0.0	.00	.00	7	1	.03	.005	811
	12	59.6	0.4	2.7		0.8	21	1	.02	.01	1	833	6	7	.09	.010
1 large (3 ¾" long, 1 ¼" dia)	65	0.1	0.0	0.0	0.1	0	214	.01	0.0	.00	.04	75	14	.34	.051	809
halves, Del Monte	5		0.0	0.0	0	0			370	40						
1 oz	28	0.0	0.0	0.0	0.0	0	0							.00		I
hamburger chips, Del Monte	5		0.0	0.0	0.0	0.0	0	0				300	20			
5 chips (1 oz)	28	0.0	0.0	0.0	0.0	0	0							.36		I
kosher halves, Claussen	4	32.1	0.3	0.7	0.3	0.3	0	1				326	18	4	.10	
1 spear	34	0.1	0.0	0.0	0.0	0	0					40	13	.22	.060	I
kosher halves, Claussen	4	26.4	0.1	0.5	0.2	0.3	0	1				325	19	2	.04	
½ pickle	28	0.1	0.0	0.0	0.0	0	0					30	16	.11	.020	I
kosher slices, Claussen	4	28.2	0.1	0.4	0.3	0.3	0	0				394	35	4	.07	
10 slices	30	0.2	0.1	0.0	0.1	0	0					29	5	.23	.060	I
kosher, tiny, Del Monte	5		0.0	1.0	0.0	0	0					240	20			
1 ½ pickles (1 oz)	28	0.0	0.0	0.0	0.0	0	0							.00		I
kosher, whole, Claussen	3	26.3	0.2	0.5	0.3	0.3	0	1				328	18	3	.05	
½ pickle	28	0.1	0.0	0.0	0.0	0	0					34	11	.12	.030	I
mini, Claussen	4	21.4	0.2	0.5	0.4	0.2	0	1				286	13	3	.05	
1 pickle	23	0.1	0.0	0.0	0.0	0	0					31	8	.15	.040	I
Vlasic	5		0.0	1.0	1.0	0.0	0	0				270	0			
1 oz³	28	0.0	0.0	0.0	0.0	0	0							.00		I
pickles, sour	4	32.9	0.1	0.8		0.4	5	0	.00	.00	0	423	0	1	.01	.004
1 med (3 ¾" long, 1 ½" dia)	35	0.1	0.0	0.0	0.0	0	51	.00	0.0	.00	.01	8	5	.14	.030	811
pickles, sour, half, New York Deli	4	26.4	0.3	0.5		0.3	0	1				266	18	4	.07	
Style, Claussen—*½ pickle*	28	0.1	0.0	0.0	0.0	0	0					36	6	.22	.070	I
pickles, sweet	41	22.8	0.1	11.1		0.4	5	0	.01	.01	0	329	1	1	.03	.005
1 large (3" long, ¾" dia)	35	0.1	0.0	0.0	0.0	0	44	.00	0.1	.00	.04	11	4	.21	.037	811

	KCAL / WT (g)	H_2O (g) / FAT (g)	PRO (g) / SFA (g)	CHO (g) / MUFA (g)	SUGR (g) / PUFA (g)	DFIB (g) / CHOL (mg)	A (RE) / A (IU)	C (mg) / B-1 (mg)	B-2 (mg) / NIA (mg)	B-6 (mg) / B-12 (mcg)	FOL (mcg) / PANT (mg)	Na (mg) / K (mg)	Ca (mg) / P (mg)	Mg (mg) / Fe (mg)	Zn (mg) / Cu (mg)	Mn (mg) / REF
Claussen	13	11.7	0.1	2.8	2.3	0.2	0	0				85	14	3	.03	
1 T	15	0.1	0.0	0.0	0.0	0	0					23	6	.08	.020	I
Del Monte	40		0.0	10.0	10.0	0	0					210	0			
1 oz[4]	28	0.0	0.0	0.0	0.0	0	0							.00		I
Vlasic	40		0.0	10.0	10.0	0	0	0				170	0			
1 oz	28	0.0	0.0	0.0	0.0	0	0							.00		I
rennin tablets, unsweetened	1	0.1	0.0	0.2		0.0	0	0	.00	.00	0	261	37	0	.06	.009
1 tablet	1.0	0.0	0.0	0.0	0.0	0	0	.00	0.0	.00	.00	3	3	.07	.002	819
soybean protein concentrate	94	1.6	16.5	8.8		1.6	0	0	.04	.04	96	1	103	89	1.25	1.188
1 oz	28	0.1	0.0	0.0	0.1	0	0	.09	0.2	.00	.02	624	238	3.06	.277	816
soybean protein isolate	96	1.4	22.9	2.1		1.6	0	0	.03	.03	50	285	50	11	1.14	.423
1 oz	28	1.0	0.1	0.2	0.5	0	0	.05	0.4	.00	.02	23	220	4.11	.453	816
tapioca, Minute	20		0.0	5.0	0.0	0.0	0	0				0	0			
1 ½ t	6	0.0	0.0	0.0	0.0	0	0							.00		I
tapioca, pearl, dry	183	5.6	0.1	45.2		0.5	0	0	.00	.00	2	1	10	1	.06	.056
⅓ cup	51	0.0	0.0	0.0	0.0	0	0	.00	0.0	.00	.07	6	4	.81	.010	820
tomato powder	302	3.1	12.9	74.7		16.5	1725	117	.76	.46	120	134	166	178	1.71	1.951
3.5 oz	100	0.4	0.1	0.1	0.2	0	17247	.91	9.1	.00	3.76	1927	295	4.56	1.241	811
vinegar																
cider	2	14.1	0.0	0.9								0	1			
1 T	15	0.0										15	1	.10		456
distilled	2	14.3	0.0	0.8								0				
1 T	15	0.0										2				456
Regina	0		0.0									0				
1 T[5]	15 ml	0.0	0.0	0.0	0.0											I
whey																
acid, dry	10	0.1	0.4	2.2		0.0	0	0	.06	.02	1	29	62	6	.19	.000
1 T	3	0.0	0.0	0.0	0.0	0	2	.02	0.0	.07	.17	69	40	.04	.002	801
acid, fluid	59	229.8	1.9	12.6		0.0	2	0	.34	.10	5	118	253	24	1.06	.005
1 cup	246	0.2	0.1	0.1	0.0	1	17	.10	0.2	.44	.94	352	191	.20	.007	801
sweet, dry	28	0.3	1.0	6.0		0.0	1	0	.18	.05	1	86	64	14	.16	.001
1 T	8	0.1	0.1	0.0	0.0	0	4	.04	0.1	.19	.45	166	75	.07	.006	801
sweet, fluid	66	229.1	2.1	12.6		0.0	10	0	.39	.08	2	132	115	20	.32	.002
1 cup	246	0.9	0.6	0.2	0.0	5	39	.09	0.2	.68	.94	396	112	.15	.010	801
yeast																
bakers, active dry	21	0.5	2.7	2.7		1.5	0	0	.38	.11	164	4	4	7	.45	.039
1 pkg (¼ oz)	7	0.3	0.0	0.2	0.0	0	0	.17	2.8	.00	.79	140	90	1.16	.035	818
bakers, compressed	18	11.7	1.4	3.1		1.4	0	0	.19	.07	133	5	3	7	1.69	.034
1 cake (.6 oz)	17	0.3	0.0	0.2	0.0	0	0	.32	2.1	.00	.83	102	57	.55	.025	818
brewers	80	1.4	11.0	10.9				0	1.21			34	60			
1 oz	28	0.3					0	4.43	10.7			537	497	4.90		456
yeast, torula																
	79	1.7	10.9	10.5				0	1.43			4	120			
1 oz	28	0.3					0	3.97	12.6			580	486	5.50		456

1. Values pertain to regular and lower sugar.
2. Pickled cucumber w/ cauliflower, onions, and mustard.
3. Values are averages for deli kosher dill spears, kosher baby dills, kosher dill sandwich stackers, Milwaukee plain dills, Polish dill spears, and zesty dill spears.
4. Values are averages for 3 midget sweet pickles, 5 sweet pickle chips, 2 sweet gherkin pickles, or 2 sweet whole pickles.
5. Includes red wine, red wine with garlic, white wine, white wine champagne, and white wine with tarragon.

Supplementary Tables

Alcohol (Ethanol) Content of Alcoholic Beverages

	WEIGHT (g)	VOLUME (%)
1. BEVERAGES		
1.1 Alcoholic & Malt Beverages		
ale, Elk Mountain Amber Ale—*12 fl oz (355 g)*	15.7	5.6
ale, Northstone Amber—*12 fl oz (360 g)*	13.7	4.9
beer—*12 fl oz (356 g)*	12.8	4.6
Big Sky—*12 fl oz (360 g)*	13.4	4.8
Black & Tan—*12 fl oz (355 g)*	13.4	4.8
Bud Dry—*12 fl oz (356 g)*	13.9	5.0
Bud Ice—*12 fl oz (355 g)*	15.3	5.5
Budweiser—*12 fl oz (357 g)*	13.9	5.0
Busch—*12 fl oz (355 g)*	13.8	4.9
Busch Ice—*12 fl oz (355 g)*	16.1	5.7
Elk Mountain Red—*12 fl oz (355 g)*	13.8	4.9
Faust—*12 fl oz (355 g)*	14.0	5.0
Genuine Draft—*12 fl oz (360 g)*	14.0	5.0
High Life—*12 fl oz (360 g)*	14.0	5.0
High Life Ice—*12 fl oz (360 g)*	16.5	5.9
Hurricane—*12 fl oz (355 g)*	16.6	5.9
Icehouse—*12 fl oz (360 g)*	14.0	5.0
Icehouse 5.5—*12 fl oz (360 g)*	15.4	5.5
King Cobra—*12 fl oz (355 g)*	16.5	5.9
Lowenbrau Special/Dark—*12 fl oz (360 g)*	13.7	4.9
Magnum—*12 fl oz (360 g)*	16.5	5.9
Meister Brau—*12 fl oz (360 g)*	12.6	4.5
Michelob—*12 fl oz (355 g)*	14.2	5.1
Michelob Amber Block—*12 fl oz (355 g)*	14.0	5.0
Michelob Classic Dark—*12 fl oz (355 g)*	14.2	5.1
Michelob Dry—*12 fl oz (355 g)*	13.9	4.9
Michelob Golden Draft—*12 fl oz (355 g)*	13.4	4.8
Michelob Malt—*12 fl oz (355 g)*	16.8	6.0
Miller—*12 fl oz (360 g)*	14.0	5.0
Milwaukee's Best—*12 fl oz (360 g)*	12.6	4.5
Milwaukee's Best Ice—*12 fl oz (360 g)*	16.5	5.9
Muenchener—*12 fl oz (355 g)*	13.7	4.9
Natural Ice—*12 fl oz (355 g)*	16.4	5.8
Natural Pilsner—*12 fl oz (355 g)*	14.0	5.0
Red Dog—*12 fl oz (360 g)*	14.0	5.0
Red Wolf—*12 fl oz (355 g)*	15.6	5.5
Ziegenbock—*12 fl oz (355 g)*	13.3	4.7
beer light—*12 fl oz (354 g)*	11.3	4.0
Big Sky Light—*12 fl oz (360 g)*	12.6	4.5
Bud Ice Light—*12 fl oz (355 g)*	11.6	4.1
Bud Light—*12 fl oz (356 g)*	11.7	4.2
Busch Light—*12 fl oz (355 g)*	11.7	4.2
Genuine Draft Light—*12 fl oz (360 g)*	12.6	4.5
High Life Light—*12 fl oz (360 g)*	12.6	4.5
Meister Brau Light—*12 fl oz (360 g)*	12.6	4.5
Michelob Golden Draft Light—*12 fl oz (355 g)*	11.7	4.2
Michelob Light—*12 fl oz (355 g)*	12.2	4.3
Miller Lite—*12 fl oz (360 g)*	12.6	4.5
Miller Lite Ice 5.0—*12 fl oz (360 g)*	14.0	5.0
Miller Lite Ice 5.5—*12 fl oz (360 g)*	15.4	5.5
Milwaukee's Best Light—*12 fl oz (360 g)*	12.6	4.5
Natural Light—*12 fl oz (355 g)*	11.7	4.2
Southpaw Light—*12 fl oz (360 g)*	14.0	5.0
bloody mary (tomato jce, vodka, & lemon jce)—*5 fl oz cocktail (148 g)*	13.9	9.3
bourbon & soda—*4 fl oz cocktail (116 g)*	15.1	12.6
daiquiri, cnd—*6.8 fl oz can (207 g)*	19.9	9.8
daiquiri (rum, lime jce, & sugar)—*2 fl oz cocktail (60 g)*	13.9	23.2
distilled spirits, all types, 80 proof—*1.5 fl oz jigger (42 g)*	14.0	31.1
gin, 90 proof—*1.5 fl oz jigger (42 g)*	15.9	35.3
gin & tonic (tonic water, gin, & lime jce)—*7.5 fl oz (225 g)*	16.0	7.1
liqueur		
coffee, 53 proof—*1.5 fl oz (52 g)*	11.3	25.1
coffee w/ cream, 34 proof—*1.5 fl oz (47 g)*	6.5	14.4
creme de menthe—*1.5 fl oz (50 g)*	14.9	33.1
malt beverage, nonalcoholic		
Bush NA—*12 fl oz (355 g)*	.7	.3
O'Doul's—*12 fl oz (361 g)*	1.1	.4
Sharp's—*12 fl oz (360 g)*	1.1	.4
manhattan (whiskey & vermouth)—*2 fl oz cocktail (57 g)*	17.4	29.0
martini (gin & vermouth)—*2.5 fl oz (70 g)*	22.4	29.9
pina colada, cnd—*6.8 fl oz can (222 g)*	20.0	9.8
pina colada (pineapple jce, rum, sugar, & coconut cream)—*4.5 fl oz cocktail (141 g)*	14.0	10.4
rum, 80 proof—*1.5 fl oz jigger (42 g)*	14.0	31.1
screwdriver (orange jce & vodka)—*7 fl oz cocktail (213 g)*	14.1	6.7
tequila sunrise, cnd—*6.8 fl oz can (211 g)*	19.8	9.6
la sunrise (orange jce, tequila, lime jce, & grenadine)—*5.5 fl oz cocktail (172 g)*	18.7	11.3
tom collins (club soda, gin, lemon jce, & sugar)—*7.5 fl oz cocktail (222 g)*	16.0	7.1
vodka, 80 proof—*1.5 fl oz jigger (42 g)*	14.0	31.1
whiskey, 86 proof—*1.5 fl oz (42 g)*	15.1	33.6
whiskey sour		
cnd—*6.8 fl oz can (209 g)*	19.9	14.7
lemon jce, whiskey, & sugar—*3 fl oz cocktail (90 g)*	15.1	16.8
prep from bottled mix—*2 fl oz mix & 1.5 fl oz whiskey (106 g)*	14.9	14.2
prep from powdered mix—*17 g pkt w/ 1.5 fl oz water & 1.5 fl oz whiskey (103 g)*	15.0	16.7
wine, dessert, dry—*2 fl oz (59 g)*	9.0	15.0
wine, dessert, sweet—*2 fl oz (59 g)*	9.0	15.0
wine, table, all types—*3.5 fl oz (103 g)*	9.6	9.1
red—*3.5 fl oz (103 g)*	9.6	9.1
rose—*3.5 fl oz (103 g)*	9.6	9.1
white—*3.5 fl oz (103 g)*	9.6	9.1
5. CHEESE & CHEESE PRODUCTS		
5.2 Cheese Products		
cheese fondue—*½ cup (108 g)*[1]	.3	0.3
30. SPICES, HERBS, & FLAVORINGS		
vanilla extract—*1 t (4 g)*	1.4	0.0
imitation w/ alcohol—*1 t (4 g)*	1.4	0.0

1. Contains table wine, swiss cheese, and all-purpose enriched flour.

Amino Acids (mg)

	TRY	THR	ISO	LEU	LYS	MET	CYS	PHE	TYR	VAL	ARG	HIS	REF
1. BEVERAGES													
1.1 Alcoholic & Malt Beverages													
beer—*12 fl oz (356 g)*	11	18	18	21	25	4	11	21	53	32	32	18	814
beer light—*12 fl oz (354 g)*	11	14	14	18	18	4	7	18	42	25	25	14	814
liqueur, coffee w/ cream, 34 proof—*1.5 fl oz (47 g)*	19	60	80	129	105	33	12	64	64	88	48	36	814
screwdriver (orange jce & vodka)—*7 fl oz cocktail (213 g)*	2	13	13	21	15	6	9	15	6	19	79	4	814
1.4 Cereal Grain Beverages													
powder—*1 t (2.3 g)*	2	4	5	9	5	2	3	6	4	6	6	3	814
prep from powder w/ water—*6 fl oz water & 1 t powder (180 g)*	2	4	5	9	5	2	2	5	4	7	7	2	814
prep from powder w/ whole milk—*6 fl oz milk & 1 t powder (185 g)*	85	278	368	598	481	154	57	296	294	409	224	165	814
1.5 Coffee													
brewed—*6 fl oz (177 g)*	0	2	4	9	2	0	4	5	4	5	2	4	814
inst powder—*1 rd t (1.8 g)*	1	3	3	9	2	0	4	5	3	5	1	3	814
cappuccino flavor, sugar sweetened—*2 rd t (14 g)*	1	5	6	15	3	1	7	8	5	9	2	5	814
decaffeinated—*1 rd t (1.8 g)*	1	2	3	8	2	0	3	5	3	5	1	3	814
french flavor, sugar sweetened—*2 rd t (12 g)*	1	6	7	19	4	1	8	10	6	11	2	6	814
mocha flavor, sugar sweetened—*2 rd t (12 g)*	5	14	14	24	17	3	6	18	14	21	18	7	814
w/ chicory—*1 rd t (1.8 g)*	0	2	2	6	1	0	3	3	2	4	1	2	814
prep from inst powder—*6 fl oz water & 1 rd t powder (179 g)*	0	2	4	9	2	0	4	5	4	5	2	4	814
cappuccino flavor, sugar sweetened—*6 fl oz water & 2 rd t powder (192 g)*	2	4	6	15	4	0	6	8	6	10	2	6	814
decaffeinated—*6 fl oz water & 1 rd t powder (179 g)*	0	2	4	9	2	0	4	5	4	5	2	4	814
french flavor, sugar sweetened—*6 fl oz water & 2 rd t powder (189 g)*	2	6	8	19	4	0	8	9	6	11	2	6	814
mocha flavor, sugar sweetened—*6 fl oz water & 2 rd t powder (188 g)*	6	13	13	24	17	4	6	17	13	21	19	8	814
w/ chicory—*6 fl oz water & 1 rd t powder (179 g)*	0	2	2	5	2	0	2	4	2	4	0	2	814
1.6 Juice Drinks & Fruit Flavored Beverages													
grape drink, cnd—*6 fl oz (188 g)*		0	0	0	0	0		0	0	0	2	0	814
orange breakfast drink, from frzn conc—*6 fl oz (188 g)*	0	2	2	4	4	2	2	4	2	4	13	2	814
orange gelatin drink, from powder—*1 pkt in 4 fl oz water (136 g)*	0	122	94	201	261	48		144	26	169	521	54	814
1.7 Tea, Hot/Iced													
iced, inst powder—*1 t (0.7 g)*	1	0	0	0	0	0	0	0	0	0	0	0	814
w/ lemon flavor—*1 rd t (1.4 g)*	1	0	0	0	0	0	1	0	0	0	1	0	814
w/ sodium saccharin & lemon flavor—*2 t (1.6 g)*	1	0	0	0	0	0	0	0	0	0	0	0	814
w/ sugar & lemon flavor—*3 rd t (23 g)*	1	1	1	1	1	0	1	0	1	1	1	0	814
2. CANDY & GUM													
butterscotch—*1 oz (5 pieces) (28 g)*	0	1	1	1	1	0	0	1	1	1	0	0	819
caramel, choc flavored roll—*2.25 oz bar (64 g)*	18	58	58	93	78	19	17	51	44	71	52	23	819
caramels—*2.5 oz (6 pieces) (71 g)*	43	136	183	296	240	76	28	146	146	202	110	82	819
choc chips, semi-sweet—*1 cup (6 oz pkg) (168 g)*	178	474	464	726	600	123	146	575	449	717	677	207	819

	TRY	THR	ISO	LEU	LYS	MET	CYS	PHE	TYR	VAL	ARG	HIS	REF
choc coated													
1 large patty (1.23 oz) (35 g)	10	27	27	42	34	7	8	33	26	41	39	12	819
fondant													
peanuts—*10 pieces (40 g)*	56	197	224	402	241	84	50	275	222	272	400	107	819
raisins—*10 pieces (10 g)*	4	16	17	30	20	10	4	19	16	23	17	9	819
choc, semi-sweet—*1 oz (28 g)*	30	80	78	122	101	21	25	97	76	121	114	35	819
choc, sweet, dark—*1.45 oz bar (41 g)*	24	63	62	97	80	16	20	77	60	96	91	27	819
confectioner's coating													
butterscotch—*1 oz (28 g)*	9	27	37	59	48	15	6	29	29	40	22	16	819
peanut butter—*1 oz (28 g)*	50	178	184	338	190	47	66	267	210	219	610	131	819
divinity—*.4 oz piece (11 g)*	2	6	8	11	9	5	3	8	5	8	7	3	819
fudge													
brown sugar w/ nuts—*.49 oz piece (14 g)*	5	13	17	28	16	8	7	16	13	20	39	9	819
choc—*.6 oz piece (17 g)*	4	12	14	23	19	5	3	13	12	18	12	6	819
choc marshmallow—*.7 oz piece (20 g)*	6	19	21	35	29	8	5	22	18	28	25	10	819
choc marshmallow w/ nuts—*.78 oz piece (22 g)*	9	25	29	48	35	11	9	30	24	38	52	15	819
choc w/ nuts—*.67 oz piece (19 g)*	8	21	26	44	27	11	10	27	21	33	57	14	819
peanut butter—*.56 oz piece (16 g)*	6	21	24	42	27	9	7	29	24	28	56	15	819
van—*.56 oz piece (16 g)*	2	7	10	16	13	4	1	8	8	11	6	4	819
van w/ nuts—*.53 oz piece (15 g)*	5	14	18	30	17	8	7	17	14	22	42	10	819
marshmallows—*1 regular (7 g)*	0	3	2	5	6	1	0	3	1	4	11	1	819
marshmallows, minature—*1 cup, not packed (46 g)*	0	16	13	30	35	7	1	19	5	23	68	8	819
milk choc—*1.55 oz bar (44 g)*	37	130	162	284	181	65	18	167	139	200	88	47	819
w/ almonds—*1.55 oz bar (44 g)*	51	154	190	334	196	70	35	207	161	231	206	70	819
w/ rice cereal—*1.45 oz bar (41 g)*	31	108	134	237	146	56	20	141	114	168	93	42	819
milk choc chips—*1 cup chips (168 g)*	139	497	620	1084	692	249	71	638	533	763	338	178	819
peanut bar—*1.6 oz bar (45 g)*	67	234	240	444	245	83	87	354	278	287	818	173	819
peanut brittle—*1 oz (28 g)*	21	73	75	138	77	26	27	110	87	90	253	54	819
praline—*1.38 oz piece (39 g)*	23	30	38	62	35	22	25	49	34	46	131	27	819
sesame crunch—*20 pieces (35 g)*	78	148	154	274	115	118	72	190	150	200	530	106	819
taffy—*.5 oz piece (15 g)*	0	0	0	0	0	0	0	0	0	0	0	0	819
toffee—*.42 oz piece (12 g)*	2	6	7	12	10	3	1	6	6	8	4	3	819
truffles—*.42 oz piece (12 g)*	8	29	37	63	42	15	4	37	31	45	20	11	819

3. CEREALS, COOKED

	TRY	THR	ISO	LEU	LYS	MET	CYS	PHE	TYR	VAL	ARG	HIS	REF
barley, pearled, ckd—*1 cup (157 g)*	60	121	130	242	132	68	79	199	102	174	177	80	820
buckwheat groats, roasted, ckd—*1 cup (198 g)*	97	255	251	420	341	87	115	263	123	343	495	156	820
bulgur, ckd—*1 cup (182 g)*	87	162	207	379	155	87	129	264	164	253	262	129	820
corn grits, inst, white, enr—*1 pkt prep (137 g)*	85	452	430	1474	338	252	216	590	489	608	599	367	808
corn grits, reg/quick, enr, ckd—*1 cup (242 g)*	24	131	123	423	97	73	63	169	140	174	172	106	808
corn grits, reg/quick, unenr, ckd—*1 cup (242 g)*	24	131	123	423	97	73	63	169	140	174	172	106	808
couscous, ckd—*1 cup (179 g)*	88	179	263	464	131	106	192	329	179	290	251	138	820
Cream of Rice, ckd—*¾ cup (183 g)*	24	81	27	134	68	48	27	68	90	104	132	48	808
Cream of Wheat													
inst, ckd—*¾ cup (181 g)*	45	105	145	252	85	62	74	179	105	161	143	76	808
inst, mix & eat—*1 pkt prep (142 g)*	38	87	121	209	72	51	62	149	88	135	122	62	808
inst, mix & eat, flavored—*1 pkt prep (150 g)*	35	78	106	186	65	47	56	132	78	119	110	57	808
quick, ckd—*¾ cup (179 g)*	38	86	120	206	70	50	61	147	86	132	118	63	808
reg, ckd—*¾ cup (188 g)*	39	90	126	216	73	53	64	154	90	137	124	66	808
farina													
ckd, enr—*¾ cup (175 g)*	31	67	98	172	49	39	72	123	67	107	93	51	808
ckd, unenr—*¾ cup (175 g)*	31	67	98	172	49	39	72	123	67	107	93	51	808
millet, ckd—*1 cup (240 g)*	91	271	355	1070	161	168	161	444	259	442	293	180	820
oatmeal, quick/reg/inst, ckd—*1 cup (234 g)*	84	206	248	459	250	112	145	321	206	335	426	145	808

	TRY	THR	ISO	LEU	LYS	MET	CYS	PHE	TYR	VAL	ARG	HIS	REF
4. CEREALS, READY-TO-EAT													
bran 100%—½ cup (1 oz) (28 g)	54	114	112	208	136	50	68	135	99	164	245	96	808
CW Post—¼ cup (1 oz) (28 g)	37	94	119	196	102	47	59	133	96	149	185	61	808
CW Post w/ raisins—¼ cup (1 oz) (28 g)	34	88	110	183	95	45	55	123	90	139	171	57	808
Frosted Rice Krinkles—⅞ cup (1 oz) (28 g)	20	68	72	113	57	41	23	58	76	88	111	41	808
granola, homemade—¼ cup (1 oz) (28 g)	41	126	151	246	150	59	71	165	109	186	307	86	808
puffed rice—1 cup (.5 oz) (14 g)	13	45	47	74	38	26	15	38	50	58	73	27	808
puffed wheat—1 cup (.5 oz) (14 g)	32	63	88	149	57	36	40	107	62	98	100	53	808
shredded wheat—1 oz (28 g)	59	103	122	213	95	54	59	149	90	152	160	72	808
—1 biscuit (.8 oz) (24 g)	50	88	104	182	81	46	50	127	77	130	137	61	808
Team Flakes, Nabisco—1 ¼ cups (2 oz) (57 g)	0	0	0	0	0	0	0	0	0	0	0	0	MUL
5. CHEESE & CHEESE PRODUCTS													
5.1 Cheese													
american processed—1 oz (28 g)	92	204	290	555	623	162	40	319	344	376	263	256	801
blue—1 oz (28 g)	88	223	319	544	525	166	30	308	367	441	202	215	801
brick—1 oz (28 g)	92	250	322	636	602	160	37	349	316	417	248	233	801
brie—1 oz (28 g)	91	213	288	547	525	168	32	328	340	380	208	203	801
camembert—1 oz (28 g)	87	203	274	522	501	160	31	313	325	363	199	194	801
caraway—1 oz (28 g)	92	254	443	684	594	187	36	376	345	477	270	251	801
cheddar—1 oz (28 g)	91	251	438	676	587	185	35	372	341	471	267	248	801
—3.5 oz (100 g)	320	886	1546	2385	2072	652	125	1311	1202	1663	941	874	801
—1 cup, not packed (113 g)	362	1001	1747	2695	2341	737	141	1481	1358	1879	1063	988	801
low-fat—1 oz (28 g)	81	226	394	608	529	167	31	334	306	424	240	223	801
low sodium—1 oz (28 g)	81	226	394	608	529	167	31	334	306	424	240	223	801
cheshire—1 oz (28 g)	85	236	411	634	551	174	33	349	320	442	250	233	801
colby—1 oz (28 g)	86	240	418	645	561	176	34	355	325	450	255	236	801
cottage cheese													
1% fat—1 cup (226 g)	312	1243	1645	2879	2265	843	260	1510	1492	1733	1277	931	801
2% fat—1 cup (226 g)	346	1376	1826	3193	2511	933	287	1675	1654	1923	1417	1033	801
creamed—1 rd T (28 g)	39	155	206	360	283	105	32	188	186	216	160	116	801
creamed—4 oz (113 g)	157	626	829	1451	1141	425	131	760	753	873	644	469	801
creamed—1 cup, not packed (210 g)	292	1163	1541	2696	2121	790	244	1413	1399	1623	1197	872	801
creamed w/ fruit—1 cup (226 g)	249	992	1315	2301	1810	673	208	1207	1193	1385	1022	744	801
dry curd—1 cup, not packed (145 g)	278	1111	1472	2575	2026	754	232	1350	1334	1550	1143	832	801
cream cheese—1 oz (2 T) (28 g)	19	91	113	207	192	51	19	119	102	126	81	77	801
edam—1 oz (28 g)	100	264	371	729	754	204	72	407	413	513	273	293	801
feta—1 oz (28 g)	57	181	228	395	346	104	24	191	189	302	133	113	801
fontina—1 oz (28 g)	102	265	392	755	660	200	74	424	432	546	237	272	801
gjetost—1 oz (28 g)	38	111	147	281	231	90	16	153	153	217	94	83	801
goat, hard—1 oz (28 g)	91	323	358	746	621	230	39	344	338	595	256	236	801
goat, semi-soft—1 oz (28 g)	64	228	253	528	439	163	28	244	239	421	181	167	801
goat, soft—1 oz (28 g)	55	196	217	453	377	140	24	209	205	361	156	143	801
gouda—1 oz (28 g)	100	264	370	727	752	204	72	406	412	512	273	293	801
gruyere—1 oz (28 g)	119	309	457	879	768	233	86	494	503	636	276	317	801
limburger—1 oz (28 g)	82	210	346	593	475	175	31	316	339	408	198	164	801
monterey—1 oz (28 g)	89	247	431	665	577	182	35	365	335	464	262	244	801
mozzarella													
low moisture—1 oz (28 g)	86	233	294	597	622	171	37	320	354	383	263	230	801
part skim—1 oz (28 g)	96	262	330	670	699	192	41	359	398	430	295	259	801
part skim, low moisture—1 oz (28 g)	109	297	374	759	791	217	46	407	450	487	335	293	801
whole milk—1 oz (28 g)	77	210	264	537	559	154	33	287	318	344	236	207	801
muenster—1 oz (28 g)	93	252	325	641	606	161	37	352	318	420	250	235	801
neufchatel—1 oz (28 g)	25	120	149	274	253	68	25	157	135	166	107	101	801
parmesan, grated—1 T (5 g)	28	77	110	201	192	56	14	112	116	143	77	80	801
parmesan, hard—1 oz (28 g)	137	373	537	979	937	272	67	545	566	696	373	392	801
pimento, processed—1 oz (28 g)	92	204	290	555	623	162	40	319	343	376	263	256	801
port du salut—1 oz (28 g)	97	248	410	704	563	208	38	375	403	484	234	194	801

	TRY	THR	ISO	LEU	LYS	MET	CYS	PHE	TYR	VAL	ARG	HIS	REF
provolone—*1 oz (28 g)*	98	278	309	651	750	194	33	365	431	465	290	316	801
queso anejo, mexican—*1 oz (28 g)*	61	207	299	572	412	153	24	317	337	379	198	192	801
queso asadero, mexican *1 oz (28 g)*	76	209	347	602	439	168	29	337	301	404	215	197	801
queso chihuahua, mexican—*1 oz (28 g)*	56	232	305	572	435	172	41	294	289	359	220	170	801
ricotta, part skim—*½ cup (124 g)*	157	649	739	1531	1678	352	124	697	739	868	792	575	801
ricotta, whole milk—*½ cup (124 g)*	155	641	730	1514	1659	348	123	689	730	858	784	569	801
romano—*1 oz (28 g)*	122	332	478	871	834	242	59	485	503	619	332	349	801
roquefort, sheep's milk—*1 oz (28 g)*	86	274	345	599	524	158	36	290	287	458	202	171	801
swiss—*1 oz (28 g)*	114	294	436	839	733	222	82	471	480	606	263	302	801
swiss, processed—*1 oz (28 g)*	102	227	324	620	696	181	45	356	384	420	293	286	801
tilsit, whole milk—*1 oz (28 g)*	100	255	421	722	578	214	39	385	413	497	241	200	801

5.2 Cheese Products

	TRY	THR	ISO	LEU	LYS	MET	CYS	PHE	TYR	VAL	ARG	HIS	REF
cheese fondue—*½ cup (108 g)*[1]	193	503	744	1434	1253	380	139	806	820	1038	449	515	801
cheese food													
american—*1 oz (28 g)*	81	181	257	491	552	144	36	282	304	333	233	227	801
american, cold pack—*1 oz (28 g)*	81	181	258	493	553	144	36	283	305	334	233	227	801
swiss—*1 oz (28 g)*	90	202	287	549	617	161	40	316	340	372	260	253	801
cheese product, mozzarella cheese substitute—*1 oz (28 g)*	43	113	162	262	225	80	14	149	162	193	110	81	801
cheese sauce, homemade—*2 T (30 g)*[2]	37	106	173	271	232	73	17	145	136	188	105	93	801
cheese spread, american—*1 T (16 g)*	38	100	133	285	241	86	17	149	142	219	87	81	801
1 oz (28 g)	68	178	236	505	427	153	30	264	252	387	155	144	801

6. CHIPS, PRETZELS, POPCORN, & OTHER SNACK FOODS

	TRY	THR	ISO	LEU	LYS	MET	CYS	PHE	TYR	VAL	ARG	HIS	REF
banana chips—*1 oz (28 g)*	8	22	21	45	30	7	11	24	15	29	29	51	819
beef & chicken stick, smoked—*.7 oz stick (20 g)*	37	166	164	295	304	91	58	160	119	190	304	106	819
cheese puffs/twists—*1 oz (28 g)*	27	111	104	222	129	43	39	85	73	115	80	51	819
corn-based cones—*1 oz (28 g)*	12	62	59	203	46	35	30	81	67	84	82	50	819
corn-based cones, nacho—*1 oz (28 g)*	16	71	75	215	74	40	30	90	78	99	86	56	819
corn-based snack, onion-flavor—*1 oz (28 g)*	17	82	81	257	68	44	38	107	88	109	114	66	819
corn cakes—*2 cakes (18 g)*	15	54	57	151	48	32	22	73	57	80	91	41	819
corn chips—*1 oz (28 g)*	13	70	67	228	52	39	34	91	75	94	92	57	819
barbecue—*1 oz (28 g)*	18	79	79	212	81	38	34	94	77	101	106	57	819
oriental mix, rice-based—*1 oz (28 g)*	54	181	191	352	193	70	72	276	211	226	596	134	819
popcorn cakes—*2 cakes (20 g)*	18	73	74	211	62	42	31	98	77	105	116	56	819
popcorn, caramel—*1 cup (1.24 oz) (35 g)*	16	53	55	99	98	26	14	54	38	62	82	38	819
w/ peanuts—*1 oz (28 g)*	15	65	64	182	56	32	29	91	74	86	139	52	819
popcorn, cheese—*2.6 cups (1 oz) (28 g)*	26	117	113	287	124	53	45	113	98	137	109	71	819
popcorn, plain													
air-popped—*3.5 cups (1 oz) (28 g)*	24	127	121	412	95	71	61	165	137	170	167	103	819
oil-popped—*2.6 cups (1 oz) (28 g)*	18	95	90	309	71	53	46	124	102	127	125	77	819
pork skins—*1 oz (28 g)*	33	517	392	942	789	136	150	550	342	686	1372	206	819
pork skins, barbecue—*1 oz (28 g)*	37	500	389	913	765	135	146	532	336	662	1289	204	819
potato chips, barbecue—*1 oz (28 g)*	31	91	98	143	142	36	31	95	78	121	108	50	I
potato chips, cheese—*1 oz (28 g)*	21	103	111	168	157	33	29	110	93	142	113	55	819
potato chips, cheese, from dried potatoes—*1 oz (28 g)*	19	82	93	144	135	31	23	91	80	117	91	48	819
potato chips, light—*1 oz (28 g)*	31	74	82	122	123	32	26	90	75	114	93	45	819
potato chips, light, from dried potatoes—*1 oz (28 g)*	12	69	70	105	100	18	21	73	63	93	77	35	819
potato chips, plain—*1 oz (28 g)*	31	72	80	119	120	31	25	88	73	111	91	43	819
from dried potatoes—*1 oz (28 g)*	13	73	74	110	105	20	22	77	66	98	81	37	819
potato chips, sour cream 'n onion—*1 oz (28 g)*	33	120	114	186	163	40	37	77	67	119	73	43	819
from dried potatoes—*1 oz (28 g)*	20	81	89	137	124	29	22	82	72	108	87	42	819
pretzels—*1 oz (28 g)*	31	73	98	180	63	46	56	128	75	111	99	57	819
choc coated—*2.6 minisize (1 oz) (28 g)*	27	70	80	149	71	37	41	100	66	93	86	46	819

	TRY	THR	ISO	LEU	LYS	MET	CYS	PHE	TYR	VAL	ARG	HIS	REF
whole wheat—*2 small (1 oz) (28 g)*	48	91	115	210	86	50	71	146	92	141	158	72	819
rice cakes, brown—*2 cakes (18 g)*	19	54	62	122	56	33	18	76	55	86	111	37	819
& buckwheat—*2 cakes (18 g)*	23	61	64	115	75	27	25	72	42	88	122	39	819
& corn—*2 cakes (18 g)*	17	55	61	141	53	33	21	76	57	84	102	40	819
& rye—*2 cakes (18 g)*	17	53	59	112	57	30	23	72	47	81	100	37	819
& sesame seed—*2 cakes (18 g)*	18	50	58	113	52	31	17	70	51	80	107	35	819
multigrain—*2 cakes (18 g)*	19	55	63	123	56	33	19	76	54	87	112	37	819
sesame sticks, wheat-based—*1 oz (28 g)*	41	94	119	217	102	54	57	155	100	133	184	73	819
taro chips—*12 chips (1 oz) (28 g)*	10	30	24	49	29	9	14	36	24	36	45	15	819
tortilla chips—*1 oz (28 g)*	14	75	72	246	56	42	36	99	82	101	100	61	819
nacho—*1 oz (28 g)*	19	80	84	250	82	46	35	106	90	114	110	67	819
nacho, light—*1 oz (28 g)*	20	89	94	280	90	51	39	118	100	126	122	74	819
ranch—*1 oz (28 g)*	16	81	79	247	70	44	37	101	84	108	109	63	819
taco flavor—*1 oz (28 g)*	19	83	89	252	85	46	36	109	90	117	114	68	819
trail mix—*1 oz (28 g)*	47	137	146	252	146	57	62	187	130	187	431	101	819
tropical—*1 oz (28 g)*	21	63	63	102	64	41	33	73	45	84	166	60	819
w/ choc chips—*1 oz (28 g)*	46	142	157	271	166	62	54	195	143	199	425	101	819

7. CREAMS & CREAM SUBSTITUTES

	TRY	THR	ISO	LEU	LYS	MET	CYS	PHE	TYR	VAL	ARG	HIS	REF
creamer, liquid/frzn w/ hydg veg oils—*½ fl oz (15 g)*[3]	2	6	8	13	10	2	3	8	6	8	12	4	801
creamer, liquid/frzn w/ lauric acid oils—*½ fl oz (15 g)*[4]	2	6	9	15	12	5	1	8	9	11	6	5	801
creamer, powdered—*1 t (2.0 g)*[4]	1	4	6	9	8	3	0	5	5	7	4	3	801
half & half (milk & cream)—*1 T (15 g)*	6	20	27	43	35	11	4	21	21	30	16	12	801
light (coffee/table) cream—*1 T (15 g)*	6	18	24	40	32	10	4	20	20	27	15	11	801
medium (25% fat) cream—*1 T (15 g)*	5	17	22	36	29	9	3	18	18	25	13	10	801
sour cream													
cultured—*1 T (12 g)*	5	17	23	37	30	10	3	18	18	25	14	10	801
half & half, cultured—*1 T (15 g)*	6	20	27	43	35	11	4	21	21	30	16	12	801
imitation—*1 oz (28 g)*	9	29	42	67	55	21	3	37	39	49	27	20	801
whipped topping													
from mix, prep w/ whole milk—*1 T (4 g)*	2	6	9	14	11	4	1	7	7	10	5	4	801
frzn—*1 T (4 g)*	1	2	3	5	4	2	0	3	3	4	2	1	801
pressurized—*1 T (4 g)*	1	2	2	4	3	1	0	2	2	3	2	1	801
whipping cream													
heavy, fluid—*1 T (15 g)*	4	14	19	30	24	8	3	15	15	21	11	8	801
light, fluid—*1 T (15 g)*	5	15	20	32	26	8	3	16	16	22	12	9	801
pressurized—*1 T (3 g)*	1	4	6	9	8	2	1	5	5	6	3	3	801

8. DESSERTS
8.1 Brownies & Bar Cookies

	TRY	THR	ISO	LEU	LYS	MET	CYS	PHE	TYR	VAL	ARG	HIS	REF
brownie—*1 large brownie (2¾″ x ⅞″) (56 g)*	36	106	125	202	146	63	59	135	93	148	143	57	818
from mix—*1 brownie (2″ sq) (33 g)*	19	49	56	93	63	23	25	65	46	72	77	27	818
homemade—*1 brownie (2¼″ x 1½″) (24 g)*	19	55	64	107	68	32	30	72	52	78	104	33	818

8.2 Cakes

	TRY	THR	ISO	LEU	LYS	MET	CYS	PHE	TYR	VAL	ARG	HIS	REF
angel food—*1/12 cake (1 oz) (28 g)*	21	70	88	136	103	52	42	95	62	100	86	37	818
from mix—*1/12 cake (50 g)*	39	130	162	249	190	96	77	172	113	184	158	67	818
homemade—*1/12 of 10″ cake (53 g)*	49	167	209	326	236	125	100	228	149	236	207	90	818
boston cream pie													
frzn—*1/6 of 19.5 oz cake (92 g)*	31	86	106	175	125	50	42	109	82	121	104	50	818
homemade—*1/12 of 9″ cake (93 g)*	54	158	193	335	210	95	78	212	158	222	191	99	818
carrot cake													
from mix—*1/12 of 9″ cake (70 g)*	43	132	158	265	165	81	73	177	122	178	172	80	818
w/ cream cheese icing, homemade—*1/12 of 9″ cake (111 g)*	59	178	214	373	226	111	101	244	172	248	321	120	818
cheesecake—*1/6 of 17 oz cake (80 g)*	51	178	225	371	298	109	57	206	178	251	201	106	818

	TRY	THR	ISO	LEU	LYS	MET	CYS	PHE	TYR	VAL	ARG	HIS	REF
from mix, no-bake type—⅛ of 9″ cake (99 g)	65	207	266	463	359	115	68	261	218	299	200	146	818
homemade—1/12 of 9″ cake (128 g)	86	357	435	769	664	212	114	458	374	485	369	265	818
w/ cherry topping, homemade—1/12 of 9″ cake (142 g)	70	285	346	612	527	168	92	365	297	388	294	212	818
cherry fudge w/ choc icing—⅛ of 20 oz cake (71 g)	21	74	77	128	105	33	28	70	53	88	79	33	818
choc cake													
from mix—1/12 of 9″ cake (65 g)	47	135	155	263	172	70	68	184	129	189	196	79	818
homemade—1/12 of 9″ cake (95 g)	65	192	228	387	255	110	93	252	187	269	240	114	818
w/ choc icing—⅛ of 18 oz cake (64 g)	36	106	123	198	151	54	47	130	99	151	133	56	818
choc pudding type, from mix—1/12 of 9″ cake (77 g)	48	142	166	270	203	79	69	177	131	199	182	77	818
coffee cake													
cheese (cream/neufchatel)—⅙ of 16 oz cake (76 g)	58	198	248	432	305	109	84	268	200	274	227	141	818
cinn w/ crumb topping—⅑ of 20 oz cake (63 g)	52	143	181	315	164	77	80	204	137	200	195	97	818
cinn w/ crumb topping, from mix—⅛ of cake (56 g)	37	106	137	236	128	67	62	152	104	154	125	69	818
cinn w/ crumb topping, homemade—1/12 of 8″ sq cake (60 g)	47	137	167	289	172	85	79	187	132	197	251	89	818
creme filled, w/ choc icing—⅙ of 19 oz cake (90 g)	52	145	183	326	151	83	92	218	139	206	186	101	818
fruit, from mix, Aunt Jemima—⅛ of 14 oz cake (50 g)	29	83	104	182	94	47	49	125	77	119	127	56	818
fruitcake—1 piece (1.5 oz) (43 g)	18	44	52	89	52	25	27	60	41	62	113	31	818
fruitcake, homemade—1/36 of 10″ cake (84 g)	38	92	100	178	105	66	60	127	86	123	182	71	818
german choc w/ coconut-nut icing, from mix—1/12 of 9″ cake (111 g)	56	148	172	282	203	85	80	192	138	209	250	84	818
gingerbread													
from mix—⅑ of 9″ sq cake (67 g)	36	96	117	200	135	52	56	132	89	131	137	60	818
homemade—⅑ of 8″ sq cake (74 g)	35	92	112	206	97	59	61	144	93	128	128	64	818
marble cake, from mix—1/12 of 9″ cake (73 g)	40	121	141	229	171	70	64	152	110	167	158	66	818
pineapple upside-down, homemade—⅑ of 8″ cake (115 g)	49	135	169	304	164	85	76	199	139	192	170	93	818
pound													
fat-free—1 oz (28 g)	20	61	78	123	90	42	35	82	56	88	73	34	818
made w/ butter—1/10 of 10.75 oz cake (30 g)	22	63	78	129	92	40	35	82	59	89	78	37	818
made w/ veg shortening—1/10 of 10.6 oz cake (30 g)	21	59	73	121	85	38	33	78	55	83	74	35	818
modified, made w/ butter, homemade—1/16 of loaf cake (54 g)[5]	40	119	145	252	153	76	65	164	117	164	151	75	818
modified, made w/ marg, homemade—1/16 of loaf cake (54 g)[5]	40	119	145	252	153	76	66	164	117	164	151	75	818
old-fashioned, made w/ butter, homemade—1/16 of loaf cake (53 g)[6]	41	130	155	264	169	84	73	174	122	175	170	78	818
old fashioned, made w/ marg, homemade—1/16 of loaf cake (53 g)[6]	41	130	155	264	170	84	73	174	122	175	170	78	818
shortcake, biscuit-type, homemade—1 shortcake (65 g)	49	120	155	292	128	75	75	196	132	177	156	91	818
sponge—1/12 of 16 oz cake (38 g)	27	81	95	159	113	48	45	100	71	107	100	45	818
sponge, homemade—1/12 of 10″ cake (63 g)	56	194	221	372	263	121	101	236	175	249	255	108	818
white													
from mix—1/12 of 9″ cake (62 g)	33	85	110	192	109	56	52	128	86	126	107	57	818
homemade—1/12 of 9″ cake (74 g)	50	141	180	310	178	95	82	208	141	204	174	92	818
pudding type, from mix—1/12 of 9″ cake (69 g)	34	89	117	193	127	59	54	128	86	132	108	55	818

	TRY	THR	ISO	LEU	LYS	MET	CYS	PHE	TYR	VAL	ARG	HIS	REF
w/ coconut icing, homemade—1/12 of 9" cake (112 g)	60	176	223	379	228	120	102	255	172	256	239	111	818
yellow													
from mix—1/12 of 9" cake (63 g)	39	110	139	231	161	68	59	145	105	157	134	66	818
homemade—1/12 of 8" cake (68 g)	45	130	160	282	167	82	70	181	130	182	162	84	818
light, 3% fat, from mix—1/12 of 9" cake (69 g)	39	101	130	216	144	63	62	148	96	147	139	63	456
light, 6% fat, from mix—1/12 of 9" cake (69 g)	47	135	165	274	195	81	75	179	125	185	184	79	818
light, from mix—1 oz (28 g)	18	40	52	92	54	21	26	63	40	59	59	28	818
pudding type, from mix—1/12 of 9" cake (69 g)	41	120	148	244	173	76	67	156	112	167	150	70	818
w/ choc icing—1/8 of 18 oz cake (64 g)	32	93	111	182	134	52	47	118	88	132	118	52	818
w/ van icing—1/8 of 18 oz cake (64 g)	29	91	113	186	138	56	43	111	87	127	104	52	818

8.3 Cakes, Snack

	TRY	THR	ISO	LEU	LYS	MET	CYS	PHE	TYR	VAL	ARG	HIS	REF
choc, creme filled w/ icing—1 snack cake (50 g)	24	56	68	117	73	29	33	79	53	82	71	34	818
cupcake, choc w/ icing, low-fat—1 cupcake (43 g)	26	71	89	143	100	45	41	98	66	104	89	40	818
sponge snack cake, creme filled—1 snack cake (43 g)	19	48	62	105	69	28	25	64	46	69	54	30	818

8.4 Cookies

	TRY	THR	ISO	LEU	LYS	MET	CYS	PHE	TYR	VAL	ARG	HIS	REF
animal crackers—11 pieces (1 oz) (28 g)	28	55	75	133	69	33	42	92	56	86	75	40	818
butter cookies—1 cookie (2" dia) (5 g)	4	11	14	24	15	7	6	15	11	16	13	7	818
choc chip													
(12-17% fat)—1 cookie (2¼" dia) (10 g)	8	17	23	42	22	10	11	28	18	27	22	12	818
(18-28% fat)—1 cookie (2¼" dia) (10 g)	7	17	22	40	22	10	10	26	17	26	19	10	818
from mix—2" cookie (16 g)	12	31	40	69	42	19	18	45	31	46	37	18	818
from refrig dough—1 cookie (2¼" dia) (12 g)	8	20	25	44	27	12	12	29	19	29	24	12	818
homemade w/ butter—1 cookie (2¼" dia) (16 g)	12	31	36	63	34	17	18	43	30	45	60	20	818
homemade w/ marg—1 cookie (2¼" dia) (16 g)	12	31	36	63	34	17	18	43	30	45	60	20	818
soft type—1 cookie (15 g)	8	18	23	40	23	10	10	27	18	27	21	11	818
choc coated graham crackers—2 crackers (1 oz) (28 g)	21	56	71	130	64	31	25	85	60	86	60	32	818
choc sandwich													
w/ creme filling—1 cookie (10 g)	7	15	18	32	19	7	9	22	15	23	20	9	818
w/ creme filling, choc coated—1 cookie (17 g)	10	25	26	44	31	9	11	30	22	35	31	12	818
w/ extra creme filling—1 cookie (13 g)	7	15	18	32	18	7	9	22	14	22	20	9	818
choc wafers—5 wafers (1 oz) (28 g)[7]	27	62	74	127	80	30	36	87	58	92	81	36	818
fig bar—1 bar (16 g)	7	18	21	36	22	8	12	23	20	25	19	11	818
fortune—1 cookie (8 g)	5	10	13	24	13	6	7	16	10	15	13	7	818
fudge, cake type—1 cookie (21 g)	12	31	37	64	47	15	14	43	28	47	56	18	818
gingersnaps—4 cookies (1 oz) (28 g)	23	44	60	108	55	27	34	75	45	70	60	32	818
graham crackers, plain/honey—4 crackers (1 oz) (28 g)[8]	26	54	69	135	46	34	43	98	59	81	83	44	818
ice cream cone													
cake/wafer—1 cone (4 g)	4	9	12	22	6	6	7	16	9	14	11	7	818
sugar—1 cone (10 g)	9	21	29	55	15	14	18	39	22	33	28	17	818
ladyfingers—1 ladyfinger (11 g)	15	51	57	95	75	29	25	56	45	64	67	27	818
macaroon, homemade—1 cookie (2" x 3/8") (24 g)	10	34	41	66	49	24	19	45	29	51	73	18	818
marshmallow, choc coated—1 sm cookie (1¾" x ¾") (13 g)	5	17	17	29	26	6	6	18	11	22	31	8	818
molasses—1 med cookie (3" x 3/8") (15 g)	12	23	31	57	29	14	18	39	24	37	32	17	818
oatmeal—1 cookie (18 g)	18	31	40	78	43	22	30	53	36	54	66	26	818
from mix—2" cookie (16 g)	20	38	49	92	55	24	34	61	43	63	73	27	818

	TRY	THR	ISO	LEU	LYS	MET	CYS	PHE	TYR	VAL	ARG	HIS	REF
from refrig dough—*1 cookie (12 g)*	12	24	30	55	34	16	20	37	26	39	45	17	818
homemade—*1 cookie (2⅝" dia) (15 g)*	13	35	42	77	41	21	23	53	35	52	59	24	818
soft type—*1 cookie (15 g)*	14	29	36	68	41	20	25	45	32	47	56	21	818
oatmeal raisin, fat-free—*2 cookies (1 oz) (28 g)*	23	50	62	113	60	31	37	79	49	78	85	38	818
homemade—*1 cookie (2⅝" dia) (15 g)*	12	33	38	70	38	20	21	48	32	48	57	23	818
peanut butter—*1 cookie (15 g)*	17	48	54	98	57	22	24	73	53	64	128	34	818
from refrig dough—*1 cookie (12 g)*	13	37	43	75	45	17	19	54	39	50	83	25	818
sandwich—*1 cookie (14 g)*	15	42	48	86	49	18	23	62	45	56	100	29	818
soft type—*1 cookie (15 g)*	9	26	30	54	30	10	13	40	29	35	69	19	818
peanut butter cookie mix, homemade—*1 cookie (3" dia) (20 g)*	20	60	68	125	64	30	30	92	66	79	147	43	818
raisin, soft type—*1 cookie (15 g)*	8	21	25	43	27	13	13	28	19	29	28	14	818
shortbread—*1 cookie (1⅝" sq) (8 g)*	7	16	20	36	20	10	11	24	15	23	21	10	818
homemade w/ butter—*1 cookie (1½" dia) (11 g)*	8	19	24	46	17	12	14	33	21	28	26	15	818
homemade w/ marg—*1 cookie (1½" dia) (11 g)*	8	19	24	47	17	12	14	33	21	28	27	15	818
pecan—*1 cookie (2" dia) (14 g)*	11	20	27	47	25	13	16	33	21	31	39	15	818
sugar—*1 cookie (15 g)*	11	27	35	59	38	17	16	38	26	39	33	17	818
from refrig dough—*1 cookie (12 g)*	8	18	24	41	25	12	13	28	18	27	25	12	818
homemade w/ butter—*1 cookie (3" dia) (14 g)*	10	26	32	60	27	16	17	42	27	37	35	19	818
homemade w/ marg—*1 cookie (3" dia) (14 g)*	10	26	32	60	27	17	17	42	27	37	35	19	818
sugar wafers, w/ creme filling—*8 wafers (1 oz) (28 g)*	17	33	44	80	41	20	25	55	33	51	44	24	818
vanilla sandwich w/ creme filling—*1 cookie (1¾" dia) (10 g)*	6	12	17	31	16	8	10	21	13	20	17	9	818
vanilla wafers													
(12-17% fat)—*7 wafers (1 oz) (28 g)*	19	48	60	103	65	30	31	69	45	69	63	30	818
(18-21% fat)—*5 wafers (1 oz) (28 g)*	18	37	48	86	47	21	26	57	35	55	46	25	818
8.5 Doughnuts													
cake—*1 doughnut (47 g)*	31	82	100	178	109	46	45	109	80	114	102	53	818
choc coated/frosted—*1 doughnut (43 g)*	29	80	93	160	111	37	37	101	76	109	110	48	818
choc, sugared/glazed—*1 doughnut (42 g)*	24	71	86	142	98	40	38	94	66	98	95	42	818
sugared/glazed—*1 doughnut (45 g)*	31	85	104	182	115	47	45	110	82	117	107	54	818
wheat, sugared/glazed—*1 doughnut (45 g)*	40	98	123	215	128	51	54	133	96	140	132	67	818
cruller, glazed—*1 cruller (3" dia) (41 g)*	18	43	54	95	60	23	25	60	41	61	56	28	818
yeast, glazed—*1 doughnut (60 g)*	46	128	160	281	139	68	78	186	120	177	163	86	818
w/ creme filling—*1 doughnut (85 g)*	66	182	230	407	205	100	108	264	173	256	230	125	818
w/ jelly filling—*1 doughnut (85 g)*	60	165	207	366	178	89	100	241	156	229	212	112	818
8.6 Frozen Desserts													
frozen yogurt													
soft serve—*½ cup (72 g)*	40	123	154	248	201	60	29	136	128	184	118	69	819
van, soft serve—*½ cup (72 g)*	38	122	164	265	215	68	25	130	130	181	98	73	819
ice cream													
french van, soft serve—*½ cup (86 g)*	41	145	185	304	255	78	31	151	146	207	148	85	819
van, reg (10% fat)—*½ cup (66 g)*	30	96	129	209	170	53	19	104	102	143	83	58	819
van, rich (16% fat)—*½ cup (74 g)*	30	102	135	221	184	56	20	110	105	152	100	61	819
ice milk, van—*½ cup (66 g)*	30	101	134	218	181	55	20	109	105	150	97	61	819
ice milk, van, soft serve—*½ cup (88 g)*	52	173	229	373	309	96	34	186	180	257	163	103	819
sherbet, orange—*½ cup (96 g)*	13	42	57	92	74	23	10	46	45	63	40	26	819
Simple Pleasures													
choc—*½ cup (89 g)*	85	394	474	808	721	299	123	448	289	562	343	304	I
choc chip—*½ cup (93 g)*	56	307	372	662	594	225	82	339	278	438	251	245	I
coffee—*½ cup (89 g)*	101	406	490	830	736	310	136	462	369	584	360	307	I

	TRY	THR	ISO	LEU	LYS	MET	CYS	PHE	TYR	VAL	ARG	HIS	REF
cookies'n cream—½ cup (90 g)	56	251	305	539	474	172	68	284	220	358	209	199	I
light, choc caramel sundae—½ cup (78 g)	64	265	274	487	445	124	70	231	191	297	148	148	I
light, chocolate—½ cup (74 g)	72	297	312	544	503	139	82	259	214	338	178	172	I
light, vanilla—½ cup (74 g)	62	257	277	486	477	119	68	226	183	294	144	152	I
light, vanilla fudge swirl—½ cup (77 g)	68	280	296	515	478	131	74	239	192	310	157	162	I
mint choc choc chip—½ cup (92 g)	64	272	325	574	516	189	73	302	232	386	232	213	I
peach—½ cup (89 g)	68	331	403	692	622	253	108	379	296	477	291	254	I
pecan praline—½ cup (91 g)	59	263	322	570	511	184	65	293	230	375	232	214	I
rum raisin—½ cup (89 g)	79	370	444	787	739	271	118	427	340	538	330	280	I
strawberry—½ cup (89 g)	62	324	387	670	605	262	102	363	291	458	280	244	I
toffee crunch—½ cup (89 g)	94	387	420	757	674	299	124	407	258	498	294	263	I
van—½ cup (89 g)	69	290	314	586	533	217	81	291	230	370	206	202	I

8.7 Fruit Cobblers & Turnovers

	TRY	THR	ISO	LEU	LYS	MET	CYS	PHE	TYR	VAL	ARG	HIS	REF
apple brown betty/crisp, homemade—½ cup (141 g)	28	75	99	176	75	44	51	120	72	111	96	54	819
strudel, apple—1 strudel (71 g)	28	84	104	182	109	48	41	107	82	116	96	54	818

8.8 Gelatin Desserts

	TRY	THR	ISO	LEU	LYS	MET	CYS	PHE	TYR	VAL	ARG	HIS	REF
dry mix													
all flavors—3 oz pkg (85 g)	0	128	100	213	301	53	0	151	26	181	575	58	819
aspartame-sweetened—.35 oz pkg (85 g)	0	906	711	1508	2126	373	0	1068	186	1279	4066	406	819
from mix													
all flavors—½ cup (140 g)	0	32	25	55	77	14	0	38	7	46	147	14	819
aspartame-sweetened—½ cup (140 g)	0	31	24	52	73	13	0	36	7	43	139	14	819
w/ fruit—½ cup (106 g)	3	27	20	42	50	14	5	29	11	35	93	27	819

8.9 Granola, Cereal, and Snack Bars

	TRY	THR	ISO	LEU	LYS	MET	CYS	PHE	TYR	VAL	ARG	HIS	REF
almond, hard—.83 oz bar (24 g)	34	53	69	140	75	32	55	94	68	97	143	43	819
chewy/soft—1 oz bar (28 g)	29	68	83	152	83	36	46	108	71	112	139	46	819
choc chip													
chewy/soft—1 oz bar (28 g)	26	65	77	142	79	35	43	99	68	106	134	44	819
chewy/soft w/ choc coating—1 oz bar (28 g)	20	63	76	133	81	32	18	81	68	97	67	29	819
hard—.83 oz bar (24 g)	32	51	66	132	75	32	53	88	66	95	124	39	819
choc, graham, & marshmallow, chewy/soft—1 oz bar (28 g)	24	59	70	130	70	33	40	90	60	96	128	42	819
crisped rice, choc chip—1 oz bar (28 g)	21	46	57	111	57	29	34	74	56	81	110	33	819
hard—1 oz bar (28 g)	50	75	100	205	113	50	86	136	100	144	191	61	819
nut & raisin, chewy/soft—1 oz bar (28 g)	28	74	85	154	85	39	46	110	73	113	180	53	819
peanut, hard—.83 oz bar (24 g)	41	79	96	192	106	44	67	135	102	132	233	63	819
peanut butter													
& choc chip, chewy/soft—1 oz bar (28 g)	29	94	99	182	101	37	39	141	110	123	297	67	819
chewy/soft—1 oz bar (28 g)	31	99	106	197	106	42	43	151	118	132	314	73	819
hard—.83 oz bar (24 g)	31	74	84	163	90	35	48	120	92	109	234	57	819
soft w/ choc coating—1.3 oz bar (37 g)	46	143	169	297	192	64	45	189	159	205	255	84	819
raisin, chewy/soft—1 oz bar (28 g)	31	73	86	160	85	40	49	112	72	117	166	52	819

8.10 Pastries

	TRY	THR	ISO	LEU	LYS	MET	CYS	PHE	TYR	VAL	ARG	HIS	REF
cream puff													
w/ custard filling, homemade—1 cream puff (130 g)	108	368	441	725	534	233	173	445	343	495	439	208	818
croissant—1 med croissant (57 g)	56	162	208	355	188	100	98	237	154	234	193	107	818
apple—1 med croissant (57 g)	49	146	185	317	181	86	80	205	139	210	176	95	818
cheese—1 med croissant (57 g)	62	173	232	394	211	107	100	259	172	258	207	121	818

	TRY	THR	ISO	LEU	LYS	MET	CYS	PHE	TYR	VAL	ARG	HIS	REF
danish pastry													
cheese (cream/neufchatel)—*1 pastry (4¼" dia) (71 g)*	63	208	263	457	305	124	97	285	208	293	230	146	818
cinn—*1 pastry (4¼" dia) (65 g)*	55	159	202	346	192	90	90	226	151	224	203	104	818
fruit—*1 pastry (4¼" dia) (71 g)*[9]	45	121	159	283	126	78	84	190	118	179	148	84	818
nut—*1 pastry (4¼" dia) (65 g)*[10]	57	155	198	344	176	90	90	219	153	226	280	108	818
eclair, w/ custard filling & choc glaze, homemade—*1 eclair (100 g)*	80	271	324	532	392	169	127	328	253	365	325	152	819
sweet roll/buns													
cheese (cream/neufchatel)—*1 roll (66 g)*	51	173	211	366	256	94	74	226	169	234	207	121	818
cinn raisin—*1 roll (2¾" sq) (60 g)*	44	127	155	275	146	70	72	180	120	175	170	87	818
cinn w/ icing, from refrig dough—*1 roll (30 g)*	20	48	59	115	42	29	35	80	50	67	65	36	818
raisin & nut—*1 roll (57 g)*	45	121	148	267	137	76	72	178	123	173	202	88	818
toaster pastry													
brown sugar cinn—*1 pastry (50 g)*	29	73	85	162	69	40	47	107	67	95	87	49	818
fruit—*1 pastry (52 g)*[11]	30	70	86	170	60	44	51	120	73	99	98	54	818
8.11 Pies													
apple													
frzn—*⅛ of 9" pie (125 g)*	33	68	91	161	88	40	50	110	68	105	93	48	818
homemade—*⅛ of 9" pie (155 g)*	45	102	129	254	87	65	78	183	112	150	149	82	818
apple pie filling, cnd—*⅛ can (74 g)*	1	2	2	4	4	1	1	1	1	3	1	1	819
banana cream													
from mix—*⅛ of 9" pie (92 g)*	42	126	155	262	186	61	46	148	121	167	144	77	818
homemade—*⅛ of 9" pie (148 g)*	81	244	300	530	343	136	101	305	249	339	275	172	818
blueberry													
frzn—*⅛ of 9" pie (125 g)*	31	64	86	156	78	39	49	107	64	100	90	46	818
homemade—*⅛ of 9" pie (147 g)*	43	107	132	263	84	68	75	187	106	159	166	82	818
butterscotch, homemade—*⅛ of 9" pie (127 g)*	76	231	286	499	334	130	90	282	237	321	255	147	818
cherry													
frzn—*⅛ of 9" pie (125 g)*	35	98	129	216	150	54	39	124	100	149	127	63	818
homemade—*⅛ of 9" pie (180 g)*	56	130	158	306	121	77	90	223	135	187	180	103	818
cherry pie filling, cnd—*⅛ can (74 g)*	1	7	7	10	12	1	1	6	4	9	5	4	819
choc cream													
frzn—*⅙ of 8" pie (113 g)*	38	99	107	186	128	40	47	128	81	141	155	54	818
homemade—*⅛ of 9" pie (142 g)*	88	260	315	548	365	139	102	322	266	365	298	162	818
choc mousse, from mix—*⅛ of 9" pie (95 g)*	46	132	157	264	191	59	48	158	126	181	159	78	818
coconut cream													
from mix—*⅛ of 9" pie (94 g)*	35	103	129	222	149	55	39	122	102	145	112	63	818
frzn—*⅙ of 7" pie (64 g)*	19	50	66	111	76	28	19	63	52	77	69	33	818
homemade—*⅛ of 9" pie (133 g)*	80	241	297	520	343	136	96	298	246	336	295	154	818
coconut custard—*⅙ of 8" pie (104 g)*	82	225	297	501	348	126	88	285	233	343	295	146	818
custard, egg—*⅙ of 8" pie (105 g)*	75	236	295	478	365	145	104	282	225	331	264	133	818
custard, egg, homemade—*⅛ of 9" pie (127 g)*	81	267	330	547	400	163	109	320	260	370	292	156	818
fruit, fried—*1 snack pie (5" x 3¾") (128 g)*[12]	54	114	154	270	155	67	76	177	115	177	143	79	818
lemon meringue													
frzn—*⅙ of 8" pie (113 g)*	21	68	75	131	95	34	33	75	61	84	92	38	818
homemade—*⅛ of 9" pie (127 g)*	58	182	215	371	230	117	105	246	171	244	243	110	818
mince, homemade—*⅛ of 9" pie (165 g)*	45	116	122	246	96	87	84	185	116	158	201	106	818
peach, frzn—*⅙ of 8" pie (117 g)*	26	67	78	143	75	41	41	95	61	101	77	43	818
pecan—*⅙ of 8" pie (113 g)*	73	167	205	338	227	110	106	229	159	235	324	107	818
homemade—*⅛ of 9" pie (122 g)*	84	231	272	454	303	153	135	305	217	311	397	142	818
pumpkin													
frzn—*⅙ of 8" pie (109 g)*	56	173	223	365	284	100	59	201	178	250	175	102	818

	TRY	THR	ISO	LEU	LYS	MET	CYS	PHE	TYR	VAL	ARG	HIS	REF
homemade—⅛ of 9″ pie (155 g)	91	279	350	583	428	163	104	339	290	392	308	169	818
van cream, homemade—⅛ of 9″ pie (126 g)	76	232	287	500	335	130	89	282	238	321	256	147	818

8.12 Puddings, Custards, & Pie Fillings

	TRY	THR	ISO	LEU	LYS	MET	CYS	PHE	TYR	VAL	ARG	HIS	REF
banana													
from inst mix w/ lowfat milk—½ cup (147 g)	54	175	234	379	307	97	35	187	187	259	140	104	819
from inst mix w/ whole milk—½ cup (147 g)	53	172	232	375	304	96	35	185	185	256	138	104	819
from reg mix w/ lowfat milk—½ cup (140 g)	55	176	237	382	309	98	36	188	188	260	141	106	819
from reg mix w/ whole milk—½ cup (140 g)	53	174	234	378	305	97	35	186	186	258	140	105	819
rte—5 oz can (142 g)	44	143	193	315	251	80	30	155	153	214	116	87	819
bread, homemade—½ cup (126 g)	79	268	328	537	402	168	108	312	257	372	302	165	819
choc													
from inst mix w/ lowfat milk—½ cup (147 g)	62	197	257	415	335	103	43	213	207	293	171	115	819
from inst mix w/ whole milk—½ cup (142 g)	60	187	246	396	321	98	41	203	199	280	163	111	819
from reg mix w/ lowfat milk—½ cup (142 g)	64	199	258	416	338	104	44	216	210	297	175	115	819
from reg mix w/ whole milk—½ cup (142 g)	62	195	254	409	331	101	43	212	206	291	170	114	819
homemade w/ lowfat milk—½ cup (157 g)	68	209	268	435	352	107	47	229	220	312	190	121	819
homemade w/ whole milk—½ cup (157 g)	66	207	267	430	349	105	46	228	218	309	188	119	819
rte—5 oz can (142 g)	51	163	210	341	273	84	37	179	172	243	148	94	819
choc mousse, homemade—½ cup (202 g)	111	398	463	764	644	198	105	390	386	525	424	216	819
coconut cream													
from inst mix w/ lowfat milk—½ cup (147 g)	56	182	243	395	318	101	40	197	194	272	169	110	819
from inst mix w/ whole milk—½ cup (147 g)	56	181	241	391	313	100	40	196	191	269	168	109	819
from reg mix w/ lowfat milk—½ cup (140 g)	57	183	244	396	318	101	39	197	193	273	172	111	819
from reg mix w/ whole milk—½ cup (140 g)	56	181	241	392	314	101	39	196	192	270	171	109	819
custard													
baked, homemade—½ cup (141 g)	92	323	403	643	529	193	107	351	313	447	326	178	819
from mix, made w/ lowfat milk—½ cup (133 g)	74	261	313	511	423	128	64	241	238	339	211	137	819
from mix, made w/ whole milk—½ cup (133 g)	74	258	310	507	420	128	63	238	237	336	210	136	819
flan/creme caramel													
from mix, made w/ lowfat milk—½ cup (133 g)	55	174	234	378	306	97	36	186	186	258	140	105	819
from mix, made w/ whole milk—½ cup (133 g)	53	172	231	374	303	96	35	184	184	255	138	104	819
homemade—½ cup (153 g)	89	318	389	620	511	193	115	346	300	433	335	171	819
lemon													
from inst mix w/ lowfat milk—½ cup (147 g)	54	175	234	379	307	97	35	187	187	259	140	104	819
from inst mix w/ whole milk—½ cup (147 g)	53	172	232	375	304	96	35	185	185	256	138	104	819
from reg mix w/ sugar, egg yolk, and water—½ cup (146 g)	12	54	51	91	80	25	19	44	45	57	73	26	819
rte—5 oz can (142 g)	0	3	4	13	3	1	3	6	4	6	6	3	819
rennin dessert													
choc, from mix w/ lowfat milk—½ cup (136 g)	58	188	246	398	324	101	39	201	199	279	160	110	819
choc, from mix w/ whole milk—½ cup (136 g)	58	185	245	394	321	99	39	200	196	276	159	110	819

	TRY	THR	ISO	LEU	LYS	MET	CYS	PHE	TYR	VAL	ARG	HIS	REF
van, from mix w/ lowfat milk—½ cup (133 g)	55	176	235	380	307	97	36	188	188	259	141	105	819
van, from mix w/ whole milk—½ cup (133 g)	53	173	233	376	305	96	36	185	185	257	140	104	819
van, homemade—½ cup (137 g)	53	173	232	375	304	96	36	185	185	256	138	104	819
rice													
from reg mix w/ lowfat milk—½ cup (144 g)	55	174	233	379	307	96	36	186	186	259	140	105	819
from reg mix w/ whole milk—½ cup (144 g)	53	173	232	374	302	95	35	184	184	256	138	104	819
homemade—½ cup (152 g)	68	223	286	480	354	134	65	255	230	339	263	143	819
rte—5 oz can (142 g)	37	119	159	264	202	68	27	133	129	180	114	72	819
tapioca													
from reg mix w/ lowfat milk—½ cup (141 g)	55	175	235	381	309	97	37	188	188	261	142	106	819
from reg mix w/ whole milk—½ cup (141 g)	54	173	233	378	305	96	37	186	186	258	141	104	819
homemade—½ cup (152 g)	91	324	404	644	530	195	109	353	313	448	328	179	819
rte—5 oz can (142 g)	38	121	162	263	212	68	27	131	129	180	104	74	819
van													
from inst mix w/ lowfat milk—½ cup (142 g)	53	169	226	366	297	94	34	180	180	250	135	101	819
from inst mix w/ whole milk—½ cup (142 g)	51	166	224	362	294	92	34	179	179	247	133	101	819
from reg mix w/ lowfat milk—½ cup (140 g)	55	178	238	389	309	98	36	190	190	263	143	108	819
from reg mix w/ whole milk—½ cup (140 g)	55	175	235	385	307	98	36	189	188	260	141	106	819
homemade—½ cup (123 g)	53	172	231	375	303	96	36	185	185	256	139	105	819
rte—½ cup (113 g)	34	112	149	244	195	62	23	120	119	165	90	68	819
8.13 Sauces, Syrups, & Toppings for Desserts													
choc fudge topping—1 T (21 g)	12	33	37	59	48	12	9	38	33	50	40	17	819
choc syrup—2 T (1 fl oz) (38 g)	10	24	24	38	31	6	8	30	24	36	35	11	819
icing/frosting, from mix													
choc creamy, made w/ butter—¹⁄₁₂ pkg prep (42 g)	7	19	19	31	25	5	6	23	18	29	26	9	819
choc creamy, made w/ marg—¹⁄₁₂ pkg prep (42 g)	7	19	19	31	25	5	6	23	18	29	26	9	819
van creamy, made w/ butter—¹⁄₁₂ pkg prep (43 g)	1	4	5	12	5	2	2	5	4	6	4	3	819
van creamy, made w/ marg—¹⁄₁₂ pkg prep (43 g)	1	4	5	12	5	2	2	5	4	6	4	3	819
white, fluffy, made w/ water—¹⁄₁₂ pkg prep (26 g)	4	17	21	31	26	12	9	22	14	24	24	8	819
icing/frosting, homemade													
choc creamy, made w/ butter—¹⁄₁₂ recipe (50 g)	10	26	28	45	37	9	8	31	26	40	33	13	819
choc creamy, made w/ marg—¹⁄₁₂ recipe (50 g)	10	26	28	45	37	9	8	31	26	40	33	13	819
glaze—¹⁄₁₂ recipe (27 g)	2	7	9	15	12	4	1	8	8	11	6	4	819
van creamy, made w/ butter—¹⁄₁₂ recipe (48 g)	4	12	17	27	22	7	2	13	13	19	10	8	819
van creamy, made w/ marg—¹⁄₁₂ recipe (48 g)	2	7	10	15	12	4	1	8	8	11	6	4	819
white, boiled (7 min)—¹⁄₁₂ recipe (32 g)	6	24	30	44	36	18	14	31	20	34	29	12	819
icing/frosting, rts													
choc creamy—¹⁄₁₂ tub (38 g)	6	16	16	25	21	4	5	20	16	25	23	7	819
coconut nut—¹⁄₁₂ tub (38 g)	12	18	22	36	21	12	13	27	19	28	78	15	819
cream cheese—¹⁄₁₂ tub (38 g)	0	1	1	2	1	0	0	1	1	1	1	0	819
sour cream—¹⁄₁₂ tub (38 g)	1	1	2	3	2	1	1	2	2	2	2	1	819
van creamy—¹⁄₁₂ tub (38 g)	1	2	3	5	3	1	1	2	2	3	2	2	819

	TRY	THR	ISO	LEU	LYS	MET	CYS	PHE	TYR	VAL	ARG	HIS	REF
marshmallow cream—*1 oz (28 g)*	0	10	8	18	21	4	1	12	3	14	41	5	819
walnut syrup topping—*2 T (41 g)*	24	57	72	127	50	36	44	80	56	92	269	46	819

9. EGGS, EGG DISHES, & EGG SUBSTITUTES

egg, chicken

	TRY	THR	ISO	LEU	LYS	MET	CYS	PHE	TYR	VAL	ARG	HIS	REF
boiled, hard/soft—*1 large (50 g)*	77	302	343	538	452	196	146	334	257	384	378	149	801
fried—*1 large (46 g)*	76	299	340	532	448	194	144	331	254	380	373	148	801
omelet, plain—*1 large egg (61 g)*	77	303	344	539	453	196	146	335	257	384	378	149	801
poached—*1 large (50 g)*	76	299	340	532	447	194	145	331	254	379	373	148	801
scrambled w/ milk—*1 large egg (61 g)*	83	322	371	582	488	207	149	356	279	414	393	161	801
white, fresh/frzn—*white of 1 large egg (33 g)*	43	158	196	293	236	119	90	203	135	221	189	78	I
whole, dried, stabilized (glucose reduced)—*1 T (5 g)*	39	118	151	212	163	78	57	136	100	173	154	58	801
whole, fresh/frzn—*1 large (50 g)*	76	300	341	534	449	195	145	332	255	381	375	148	I
yolk, fresh—*yolk of 1 large egg (17 g)*	33	151	144	250	226	71	51	122	127	159	203	74	I

egg, chicken dishes, souffle, spinach—*1 cup (136 g)*[13]

	TRY	THR	ISO	LEU	LYS	MET	CYS	PHE	TYR	VAL	ARG	HIS	REF
	166	458	650	994	782	298	143	574	487	719	533	313[13]	811

egg, other poultry

	TRY	THR	ISO	LEU	LYS	MET	CYS	PHE	TYR	VAL	ARG	HIS	REF
duck, whole—*1 egg (70 g)*	182	515	419	768	666	403	199	588	429	620	536	224	801
goose, whole—*1 egg (144 g)*	406	1148	932	1711	1483	899	445	1310	956	1380	1192	498	801
quail, whole—*1 egg (9 g)*	19	58	73	103	79	38	28	66	49	85	75	28	801
turkey, whole—*1 egg (79 g)*	173	531	675	949	730	349	258	611	450	778	692	261	801

egg substitutes

	TRY	THR	ISO	LEU	LYS	MET	CYS	PHE	TYR	VAL	ARG	HIS	REF
frzn—*¼ cup (60 g)*[14]	98	290	396	583	428	232	137	387	274	475	346	154	801
liquid—*1.5 fl oz (47 g)*[15]	90	260	352	509	370	200	137	360	233	417	368	139	801

10. ENTREES & MEALS
10.2 Canned & Shelf Stable Entrees

	TRY	THR	ISO	LEU	LYS	MET	CYS	PHE	TYR	VAL	ARG	HIS	REF
chili w/ beans—*1 cup (255 g)*	176	612	638	1163	1043	242	156	745	418	750	918	418	816
cowpeas w/ pork—*1 cup (240 g)*	82	250	269	504	446	94	72	384	214	314	456	204	816

10.5 Frozen Entrees

	TRY	THR	ISO	LEU	LYS	MET	CYS	PHE	TYR	VAL	ARG	HIS	REF
turkey, w/ gravy—*5 oz entree (142 g)*	95	372	435	666	787	241	87	331	329	443	582	260	805

11. FAST FOODS
11.1 Generic

biscuit

	TRY	THR	ISO	LEU	LYS	MET	CYS	PHE	TYR	VAL	ARG	HIS	REF
w/ egg—*1 biscuit (136 g)*	160	461	593	919	604	298	235	593	430	679	589	265	821
w/ egg & bacon—*1 biscuit (150 g)*	216	680	822	1313	1025	422	294	810	594	953	936	430	821
w/ egg & ham—*1 biscuit (192 g)*	273	876	1000	1657	1386	540	376	996	735	1083	1190	597	821
w/ egg & sausage—*1 biscuit (180 g)*	247	787	923	1505	1195	493	335	900	679	1053	1067	497	821
w/ egg & steak—*1 biscuit (148 g)*	229	747	872	1428	1183	460	296	829	641	980	1014	502	821
w/ egg, cheese, & bacon—*1 biscuit (144 g)*	213	619	772	1287	1109	405	242	783	635	917	841	462	821
w/ ham—*1 biscuit (113 g)*	166	544	580	1059	924	327	221	618	452	602	768	432	821
w/ sausage—*1 biscuit (124 g)*	140	428	485	898	649	260	186	534	394	549	599	322	821
w/ steak—*1 biscuit (141 g)*	157	495	560	1005	794	298	190	574	440	618	682	384	821

burritos

	TRY	THR	ISO	LEU	LYS	MET	CYS	PHE	TYR	VAL	ARG	HIS	REF
w/ beans—*2 burritos (217 g)*	171	529	586	1094	744	232	213	762	417	692	779	373	821
w/ beans & cheese—*2 burritos (186 g)*	177	506	711	1179	915	290	151	733	538	787	660	426	821
w/ beans & chili peppers—*2 burritos (204 g)*	192	557	620	1134	738	247	247	798	453	716	830	402	821
w/ beans & meat—*2 burritos (231 g)*	270	827	896	1679	1372	439	293	982	665	1028	1289	621	821
w/ beans, cheese, & beef—*2 burritos (203 g)*	175	530	658	1145	932	292	164	678	489	737	751	414	821
w/ beans, cheese, & chili peppers—*2 burritos (336 g)*	396	1109	1482	2574	1804	625	407	1663	1126	1673	1488	900	821
w/ beef—*2 burritos (220 g)*	323	988	1060	2000	1720	563	341	1087	807	1206	1566	763	821
w/ beef & chili peppers—*2 burritos (201 g)*	261	822	868	1628	1473	462	261	858	653	985	1307	629	821

	TRY	THR	ISO	LEU	LYS	MET	CYS	PHE	TYR	VAL	ARG	HIS	REF
w/ beef, cheese, & chili peppers—2 burritos (304 g)	492	1505	1745	3137	2797	879	447	1684	1325	1952	2298	1207	821
w/ fruit (apple/cherry)—1 large (155 g)	64	141	181	353	121	91	110	259	155	209	209	116	821
w/ fruit (apple/cherry)—1 small (74 g)	30	67	87	169	58	44	53	124	74	100	100	56	821
cheeseburger													
large—1 sandwich (185 g)	379	1127	1293	2396	2294	675	311	1278	1045	1530	1715	953	821
large w/ bacon—1 sandwich (195 g)	388	1203	1357	2478	2416	712	330	1332	1074	1611	1849	991	821
large w/ double meat, lettuce, & tomato—1 sandwich (258 g)	472	1465	1618	2990	2905	846	392	1551	1244	1886	2273	1182	821
large w/ ham, lettuce, & tomato—1 sandwich (254 g)	498	1516	1702	3129	3040	899	434	1681	1351	1963	2289	1267	821
large w/ lettuce & tomato—1 sandwich (219 g)	355	1051	1200	2210	2120	622	291	1187	964	1419	1588	878	821
large w/ triple meat—1 sandwich (304 g)	696	2225	2405	4466	4420	1274	568	2262	1827	2785	3490	1763	821
reg—1 sandwich (102 g)	186	534	630	1158	1018	316	167	648	493	754	803	447	821
reg w/ double meat—1 sandwich (155 g)	352	1048	1192	2213	2159	629	276	1169	972	1411	1593	888	821
reg w/ double meat & double-decker bun—1 sandwich (160 g)	278	813	942	1738	1613	485	235	946	749	1117	1230	682	821
reg w/ double meat, double-decker bun, lettuce, & tomato—1 sandwich (228 g)	374	1099	1272	2332	2164	652	317	1272	1003	1507	1660	917	821
reg w/ double meat, lettuce, & tomato—1 sandwich (166 g)	267	802	911	1682	1642	476	212	895	737	1076	1213	676	821
reg w/ lettuce & tomato—1 sandwich (154 g)	225	645	759	1388	1223	379	202	779	590	906	964	537	821
chicken, breaded & fried, boneless pieces—6 pieces (102 g)	203	682	855	1260	1268	447	247	710	567	832	972	496	821
w/ barbeque sce—6 pieces (130 g)	202	679	850	1253	1261	443	246	705	564	828	967	493	821
w/ honey sce—6 pieces (115 g)	201	676	848	1249	1257	443	245	704	562	826	964	491	821
w/ mustard sce—6 pieces (130 g)	202	679	850	1253	1261	443	246	705	564	828	967	493	821
w/ sweet & sour sce—6 pieces (130 g)	202	679	850	1253	1261	443	246	705	564	828	967	493	821
chicken, breaded & fried, dark meat—drumstick & thigh (148 g)	337	1212	1462	2170	2324	780	419	1184	962	1443	1843	861	821
chicken, breaded & fried, light meat—side breast & wing (163 g)	399	1439	1738	2577	2760	926	497	1405	1143	1715	2189	1024	821
chicken fillet sandwich—1 sandwich (182 g)	282	952	1212	1780	1744	608	333	1008	761	1199	1352	697	821
chicken fillet sandwich w/ cheese—1 sandwich (228 g)	347	1081	1370	2177	2107	702	383	1261	1005	1475	1585	857	821
chili con carne—1 cup (253 g)	293	992	1020	1860	1839	481	253	1012	716	1161	1543	719	821
chimichanga													
beef—1 chimichanga (174 g)	238	759	809	1514	1345	430	245	807	607	917	1197	578	821
beef & cheese—1 chimichanga (183 g)	242	727	880	1570	1321	437	232	867	670	985	1076	586	821
beef & red chili peppers—1 chimichanga (190 g)	224	692	737	1383	1210	386	230	752	555	836	1094	530	821
beef, cheese, & red chili peppers—1 chimichanga (180 g)	175	518	598	1089	900	299	180	616	457	673	788	410	821
clams, breaded & fried—¾ cup (115 g)	151	457	536	891	620	261	215	558	381	596	699	261	821
coleslaw—¾ cup (99 g)	18	52	68	81	71	20	19	50	32	64	87	30	821
cookies, animal crackers—1 box (67 g)	54	135	175	318	153	85	80	211	145	200	174	99	821
cookies, choc chip—1 box (55 g)	35	80	96	183	75	45	53	135	86	120	118	59	821
corn-on-the-cob w/ butter—1 ear (146 g)	32	180	180	483	191	93	37	209	171	258	181	124	821
corndog (frank w/ corn flour coating)—1 corndog (175 g)	151	635	751	1414	1150	364	236	660	555	802	1115	507	821
crab, baked—1 crab (3.8 oz meat) (109 g)	398	1151	1379	2256	2430	799	334	1215	950	1352	2448	580	821
crab cake—2.1 oz cake (60 g)	155	450	547	886	914	308	139	488	371	545	923	230	821

	TRY	THR	ISO	LEU	LYS	MET	CYS	PHE	TYR	VAL	ARG	HIS	REF
crab, soft shell, fried—*1 crab (4.4 oz meat) (125 g)*	143	393	491	816	699	255	145	485	321	519	758	224	821
croissant w/ egg													
& cheese—*1 croissant (127 g)*	184	476	634	1074	932	333	188	663	577	763	611	395	821
cheese & bacon—*1 croissant (129 g)*	224	606	787	1336	1186	415	231	815	702	948	800	498	821
cheese & ham—*1 croissant (152 g)*	255	768	903	1540	1374	494	307	921	731	1011	1041	587	821
cheese & sausage—*1 croissant (160 g)*	261	789	947	1602	1410	512	301	947	779	1106	1077	581	821
danish pastry													
cheese—*3.2 oz pastry (91 g)*	73	207	265	456	277	128	96	288	217	298	281	144	821
cinn—*3.1 oz pastry (88 g)*	63	167	214	365	197	106	97	244	167	245	220	112	821
fruit—*3.3 oz pastry (94 g)*	63	165	212	361	195	104	95	242	165	242	217	111	821
egg & cheese sandwich—*1 sandwich (146 g)*	218	588	781	1244	927	383	266	803	585	937	775	410	821
egg, scrambled—*2 eggs (94 g)*	199	618	786	1114	858	401	289	705	528	902	786	306	821
enchilada w/ cheese & beef—*1 enchilada (192 g)*	132	459	528	1081	785	261	132	516	434	612	670	372	821
enchilada w/ cheese & sour cream—*1 enchilada (163 g)*	99	324	461	879	570	205	83	440	390	526	380	287	821
enchirito w/ cheese, beef, & beans—*1 enchirito (193 g)*	197	674	786	1550	1183	376	181	774	627	905	977	540	821
english muffin, w/ butter—*1 muffin (63 g)*	60	153	187	344	161	88	95	242	157	215	209	112	821
w/ cheese & sausage—*1 sandwich (115 g)*	187	528	630	1179	1121	351	172	688	608	758	738	490	821
w/ egg, cheese, & canadian bacon—*1 sandwich (146 g)*	260	756	920	1564	1400	515	301	930	788	1073	1000	612	821
w/ egg, cheese, & sausage—*1 sandwich (165 g)*	281	807	983	1709	1563	533	295	1015	868	1165	1099	657	821
fish fillet, battered/breaded & fried—*3.2 oz fillet (91 g)*	153	570	615	1083	1135	379	159	548	450	692	775	387	821
fish sandwich w/ tartar sce—*1 sandwich (158 g)*	196	673	758	1322	1217	433	221	724	525	874	921	458	821
fish sandwich w/ tartar sce & cheese—*1 sandwich (183 g)*	245	796	924	1634	1554	525	245	900	701	1082	1082	593	821
french fries, fried in veg oil—*20-25 fries (76 g)*	41	138	131	182	161	34	19	129	76	154	144	51	821
french fries, fried in veg oil—*30-40 fries (115 g)*	62	208	198	276	244	52	29	196	115	233	217	77	821
french toast sticks—*5 sticks (141 g)*	103	288	341	606	324	155	158	410	279	385	376	196	821
french toast w/ butter—*2 slices (135 g)*	143	405	532	817	506	246	200	536	346	625	518	235	821
frijoles w/ cheese—*1 cup (167 g)*	130	431	513	873	760	185	102	563	351	586	600	316	821
ham & cheese sandwich—*1 sandwich (146 g)*	270	739	911	1667	1572	486	250	993	821	1073	1016	705	821
ham, egg, & cheese sandwich—*1 sandwich (143 g)*	265	752	935	1572	1404	493	290	958	764	1091	1014	599	821
hamburger													
large—*1 sandwich (137 g)*	274	875	948	1740	1580	485	255	908	660	1095	1375	660	821
large w/ double meat, lettuce & tomato—*1 sandwich (226 g)*	414	1354	1442	2649	2504	746	371	1354	1012	1648	2133	1017	821
large w/ lettuce & tomato—*1 sandwich (218 g)*	307	992	1070	1953	1775	541	292	1029	741	1234	1546	741	821
large w/ triple meat—*1 sandwich (259 g)*	614	2015	2129	3942	3838	1121	523	1958	1515	2427	3217	1523	821
reg—*1 sandwich (90 g)*	140	427	482	871	710	235	144	486	325	562	659	319	821
reg w/ double meat—*1 sandwich (176 g)*	315	1021	1096	2012	1869	563	285	1037	769	1257	1609	769	821
reg w/ lettuce & tomato—*1 sandwich (218 g)*	310	955	1079	1945	1583	523	323	1088	726	1256	1465	709	821
hash brown potatoes—*½ cup (72 g)*	26	89	84	117	103	22	12	83	49	99	92	32	821
hot dog—*1 hot dog (98 g)*	96	353	444	754	628	195	144	409	276	473	653	289	821
hot dog w/ chili—*1 hot dog (114 g)*	129	465	567	972	831	253	179	528	359	609	836	372	821
hush puppies—*5 pieces (78 g)*	52	201	227	520	226	119	90	245	201	283	257	135	821

	TRY	THR	ISO	LEU	LYS	MET	CYS	PHE	TYR	VAL	ARG	HIS	REF
ice milk, vanilla, soft serve w/ cone—*1 cone (103 g)*	52	160	213	350	268	90	40	181	171	237	137	100	821
nachos													
w/ cheese—*6-8 nachos (113 g)*	77	329	376	1019	375	197	129	442	376	485	420	279	821
w/ cheese & jalapeno peppers—*6-8 nachos (204 g)*	151	594	745	1795	812	369	208	812	702	918	728	522	821
w/ cheese, beans, ground beef, & peppers—*6-8 nachos (255 g)*	196	711	885	1912	1117	423	219	918	768	1056	913	599	821
w/ cinn & sugar—*6-8 nachos (109 g)*	51	270	257	882	203	150	130	353	293	365	359	220	821
onion rings—*8-9 rings (83 g)*	49	105	148	242	105	56	75	168	109	150	225	76	821
oysters, battered/breaded & fried—*6 oysters (139 g)*	149	470	528	880	681	267	206	531	388	573	739	256	821
pancakes w/ butter & syrup—*3 pancakes (232 g)*	102	304	385	712	420	174	128	401	318	452	350	206	821
pie, fruit (apple/cherry/lemon), fried—*1 pie (85 g)*	30	65	83	164	55	43	50	119	71	97	96	54	821
pizza													
cheese—*⅛ of 12" pizza (63 g)*	91	250	318	627	547	174	76	367	348	400	301	235	821
cheese, meat, & veg—*⅛ of 12" pizza (79 g)*	157	451	544	1062	962	297	130	598	553	672	589	403	821
pepperoni—*⅛ of 12" pizza (71 g)*	119	337	422	823	727	231	102	476	450	525	417	312	821
potato, baked													
w/ cheese sce—*1 potato (296 g)*	189	494	758	1157	1045	314	104	690	616	873	559	423	821
w/ cheese sce & bacon—*1 potato (299 g)*	233	646	939	1453	1346	404	141	855	750	1085	777	541	821
w/ cheese sce & broccoli—*1 potato (339 g)*	173	461	688	1034	946	281	98	620	546	797	542	380	821
w/ cheese sce & chili—*1 potato (395 g)*	292	810	1153	1821	1671	490	178	1063	912	1327	995	672	821
w/ sour cream & chives—*1 potato (302 g)*	100	257	305	468	435	121	79	299	263	390	290	154	821
potato salad—*⅓ cup (95 g)*	16	69	78	130	96	34	22	99	66	85	82	35	821
potatoes, mashed—*⅓ cup (80 g)*	28	70	83	127	119	34	22	83	73	108	80	42	821
roast beef sandwich—*1 sandwich (139 g)*	245	874	944	1655	1544	509	265	881	680	1049	1262	680	821
roast beef sandwich w/ cheese—*1 sandwich (176 g)*	373	1281	1417	2506	2392	762	378	1345	1084	1598	1827	1044	821
roast beef submarine sandwich—*1 sub (216 g)*	324	1147	1248	2177	1979	659	363	1179	888	1393	1639	881	821
salad, vegetable w/ dressing—*1½ cups (207 g)*	21	104	137	141	143	29	29	95	56	122	135	46	821
w/ cheese & egg—*1½ cups (217 g)*	102	341	499	690	599	200	102	414	330	527	401	226	821
w/ chicken—*1½ cups (218 g)*	198	735	924	1284	1445	460	222	689	576	863	1036	521	821
w/ pasta & seafood—*1½ cups (417 g)*	192	613	746	1197	1059	367	254	688	492	780	934	384	821
w/ shrimp—*1½ cup (236 g)*	198	604	734	1123	1149	392	198	637	486	741	1130	297	821
w/ turkey, ham, & cheese—*1½ cups (326 g)*	303	1073	1343	2090	2142	675	287	1134	988	1389	1487	808	821
scallops, breaded & fried—*6 scallops (144 g)*	186	609	674	1109	916	343	251	652	494	723	966	317	821
shake													
choc—*10 fl oz (283 g)*	136	436	583	945	764	241	88	464	464	645	348	263	814
strawberry—*10 fl oz (283 g)*	133	430	577	931	753	238	88	458	458	637	342	260	814
van—*10 fl oz (283 g)*	139	447	597	965	781	246	91	475	475	659	354	269	814
shrimp, breaded & fried—*6-8 shrimp (164 g)*	253	707	868	1433	1269	477	274	846	607	902	1348	392	821
steak sandwich w/ lettuce, tomato, & mayonnaise—*1 sandwich (204 g)*	369	1204	1287	2360	2217	663	335	1210	904	1475	1893	904	821
submarine sandwich—*1 sub (228 g)*[16]	249	743	903	1589	1288	438	287	987	750	1097	1015	620	821
sundae													
caramel—*1 sundae (155 g)*	98	313	422	680	550	174	64	336	336	467	251	191	821
hot fudge—*1 sundae (158 g)*	71	216	272	436	354	104	51	240	226	324	209	122	821
strawberry—*1 sundae (153 g)*	83	266	352	571	462	144	55	283	285	390	217	161	821
taco, large—*9.3 oz (263 g)*	352	1176	1486	2733	2249	707	279	1360	1168	1667	1625	981	821

	TRY	THR	ISO	LEU	LYS	MET	CYS	PHE	TYR	VAL	ARG	HIS	REF
taco salad—1½ cup (198 g)	149	503	616	1087	962	287	119	548	459	679	707	398	821
taco salad w/ chili con carne—1½ cups (261 g)	193	647	817	1449	1216	363	159	770	613	911	882	519	821
taco, small—6 oz (171 g)	229	764	966	1777	1462	460	181	884	759	1084	1057	638	821
tostada													
beans & cheese—1 tostada (144 g)	101	353	433	827	580	176	96	465	333	503	465	275	821
beans, beef, & cheese—1 tostada (225 g)	173	599	720	1370	1049	322	160	722	556	826	830	475	821
beef & cheese—1 tostada (163 g)	218	738	833	1581	1402	424	183	763	639	945	1105	588	821
w/ guacamole—2 tostadas (261 g)	123	415	556	1073	676	251	120	540	457	645	483	337	821
tuna salad submarine sandwich—9 oz sandwich (256 g)	343	1183	1334	2322	2156	755	384	1267	919	1526	1620	804	821

12. FATS, OILS, & SHORTENINGS
12.1 Animal Fats

	TRY	THR	ISO	LEU	LYS	MET	CYS	PHE	TYR	VAL	ARG	HIS	REF
beef separable fat, ckd—1 oz (28 g)	34	132	136	239	251	77	34	118	101	147	191	103	813
beef suet, raw—1 oz (28 g)	5	12	8	24	21	5	5	14	9	15	27	6	813
lamb fat, ckd—1 oz (28 g)	40	147	166	268	304	88	41	140	116	186	205	109	817
pork separable fat, ckd—1 oz (28 g)	11	107	90	221	269	48	28	122	60	153	308	45	810
salt pork, raw—1 oz (28 g)	5	47	38	100	119	21	12	54	23	69	148	16	810

13. FISH, SHELLFISH, & CRUSTACEA

	TRY	THR	ISO	LEU	LYS	MET	CYS	PHE	TYR	VAL	ARG	HIS	REF
abalone, fried—3 oz (85 g)[17]	191	713	726	1179	1219	375	222	608	533	731	1200	321	815
abalone, raw—3 oz (85 g)	163	626	633	1024	1087	328	191	521	465	635	1061	279	815
anchovy, cnd in olive oil—5 anchovies (20 g)	65	253	266	470	531	171	62	226	195	298	346	170	815
anchovy, raw—3 oz (85 g)	194	759	798	1407	1590	512	185	675	584	891	1035	509	815
bass, freshwater, ckd by dry heat—3 oz (85 g)	230	901	947	1670	1888	609	220	802	694	1059	1230	605	815
bass, freshwater, raw—3 oz (85 g)	179	703	739	1304	1473	475	172	626	542	826	959	472	815
bass, striped, ckd by dry heat—3 oz (85 g)	217	848	890	1572	1776	572	208	754	652	996	1157	569	815
bass, striped, raw—3 oz (85 g)	169	661	695	1226	1385	447	162	589	509	777	902	444	815
bluefish, ckd by dry heat—3 oz (85 g)	245	958	1007	1776	2007	646	234	853	737	1126	1307	643	815
bluefish, raw—3 oz (85 g)	191	747	785	1385	1565	504	183	665	575	878	1020	502	815
burbot, ckd by dry heat—3 oz (85 g)	236	923	970	1711	1934	623	225	822	711	1084	1260	620	815
burbot, raw—3 oz (85 g)	184	720	757	1335	1509	486	176	641	555	846	983	484	815
butterfish, ckd by dry heat—3 oz (85 g)	211	826	868	1532	1731	558	202	736	636	970	1128	555	815
butterfish, raw—3 oz (85 g)	165	645	677	1195	1350	435	157	574	496	757	879	433	815
carp, ckd by dry heat—3 oz (85 g)	218	852	896	1580	1786	576	208	759	657	1002	1163	572	815
carp, raw—3 oz (85 g)	170	665	699	1232	1393	449	162	592	512	782	907	447	815
catfish													
channel, breaded & fried—3 oz (85 g)[18]	170	672	711	1283	1358	448	174	617	529	802	916	451	815
farmed, cooked by dry heat—3 oz (85 g)	179	698	733	1294	1462	471	171	622	538	820	953	469	815
farmed, raw—3 oz (85 g)	148	580	610	1075	1215	391	142	516	447	681	792	390	815
wild, ckd by dry heat—3 oz (85 g)	176	689	724	1277	1443	465	168	613	531	810	941	463	815
wild, raw—3 oz (85 g)	156	611	642	1132	1279	412	150	543	470	718	833	410	815
caviar, black & red, granular—1 T (16 g)	52	202	166	341	293	103	72	171	155	202	254	104	815
cisco, raw—3 oz (85 g)	181	708	744	1312	1483	478	174	630	545	832	966	475	815
cisco, smoked—3 oz (85 g)	156	610	641	1131	1278	412	149	543	469	717	833	410	815
clam liquid, cnd—1 cup (240 g)		0	0	0	0			0	0	0	2	0	815
clams													
breaded & fried—3 oz (9 small) (85 g)[19]	143	512	541	871	844	276	174	467	395	553	838	238	815
ckd by moist heat—3 oz (19 small) (85 g)[20]	243	935	946	1529	1624	490	285	778	695	949	1585	417	815
cnd, drained—3 oz (85 g)	243	934	945	1528	1623	490	285	778	694	949	1584	417	815
raw—3 oz (4 large or 9 small) (85 g)	122	468	473	765	811	245	143	390	348	475	793	208	815
cod													
atlantic, ckd by dry heat—3 oz (85 g)	218	851	895	1579	1783	575	208	758	656	1000	1162	572	815
cnd—3 oz (85 g)	217	849	892	1573	1778	573	208	756	653	998	1158	570	815

	TRY	THR	ISO	LEU	LYS	MET	CYS	PHE	TYR	VAL	ARG	HIS	REF
dried & salted—*3 oz (85 g)*	599	2342	2462	4343	4907	1581	572	2085	1804	2752	3197	1573	815
raw—*3 oz (85 g)*	169	664	698	1231	1391	448	162	591	511	780	907	446	815
cod, pacific, ckd by dry heat—*3 oz (85 g)*	219	856	899	1586	1793	577	209	762	659	1005	1168	575	815
cod, pacific, raw—*3 oz (85 g)*	170	668	702	1237	1398	451	163	594	514	784	911	448	815
crab, alaska king													
ckd by moist heat—*3 oz (85 g)*	229	666	798	1306	1432	464	185	695	548	774	1437	334	815
imitation, made from surimi—*3 oz (85 g)*	62	494	478	810	934	347	110	401	412	519	679	236	815
raw—*3 oz (85 g)*	217	630	754	1235	1354	438	174	657	518	732	1359	316	815
crab, blue													
ckd by moist heat—*3 oz (85 g)*	239	696	833	1363	1495	484	192	725	572	808	1501	349	815
cnd—*3 oz (85 g)*	243	707	846	1385	1519	492	196	737	581	821	1525	355	815
raw—*3 oz (85 g)*	213	622	744	1219	1337	432	172	649	511	722	1341	312	815
crab cake—*1 cake (60 g)*[21]	169	497	598	970	1040	341	143	522	409	588	1038	248	815
crab, dungeness, ckd by moist heat—*3 oz (85 g)*	265	765	918	1504	1649	535	213	799	632	890	1655	386	815
crab, dungeness, raw—*3 oz (85 g)*	206	600	718	1175	1289	417	166	625	492	697	1294	301	815
crab, queen, ckd by moist heat—*3 oz (85 g)*	281	813	975	1597	1753	568	226	849	671	946	1759	410	815
crab, queen, raw—*3 oz (85 g)*	219	637	763	1249	1369	443	176	664	524	740	1374	320	815
crayfish													
farmed, ckd by moist heat—*3 oz (85 g)*	208	601	720	1180	1295	420	167	627	496	699	1300	303	815
farmed, raw—*3 oz (85 g)*	176	509	611	1000	1097	356	141	532	420	592	1101	257	815
wild, ckd by moist heat—*3 oz (85 g)*	199	575	690	1130	1239	401	160	600	475	668	1244	290	815
wild, raw—*3 oz (85 g)*	189	548	657	1076	1180	383	152	572	452	637	1185	276	815
croaker, atlantic, breaded & fried—*3 oz (85 g)*[19]	177	670	720	1259	1336	447	185	631	528	805	902	447	815
croaker, atlantic, raw—*3 oz (85 g)*	169	663	697	1229	1389	447	162	590	510	779	905	445	815
cusk, ckd by dry heat—*3 oz (85 g)*	232	907	954	1683	1902	613	222	808	699	1067	1239	610	815
cusk, raw—*3 oz (85 g)*	181	708	744	1313	1483	478	174	631	545	833	967	475	815
cuttlefish, ckd by moist heat—*3 oz (85 g)*	310	1189	1203	1945	2064	623	362	990	884	1207	2016	531	815
cuttlefish, raw—*3 oz (85 g)*	155	594	601	972	1032	311	181	495	442	603	1008	265	815
dolphinfish, ckd by dry heat—*3 oz (85 g)*	226	885	930	1640	1852	597	216	788	681	1039	1207	594	815
dolphinfish, raw—*3 oz (85 g)*	176	690	725	1279	1445	466	168	614	532	811	942	464	815
drum, freshwater, ckd by dry heat—*3 oz (85 g)*	214	839	881	1555	1756	566	205	747	646	986	1145	563	815
drum, freshwater, raw—*3 oz (85 g)*	167	654	687	1212	1370	441	160	583	503	769	892	439	815
fish pieces, frzn, reheated—*1 piece (4" x 2' x ½")* *(57 g)*[22]	111	368	425	722	640	242	129	398	307	476	483	239	815
fish sticks, frzn—*1 stick (4" x 2" x ½")* *(28 g)*[22]	55	183	211	359	318	120	64	198	153	237	240	119	815
flatfish (flounder/sole)													
ckd by dry heat—*3 oz (85 g)*	230	901	947	1670	1887	608	220	802	694	1059	1230	605	815
raw—*3 oz (85 g)*	179	703	738	1303	1472	475	172	626	541	826	959	472	815
gefiltefish w/ broth, sweet—*1 piece (42 g)*	36	205	204	340	354	107	47	207	160	230	250	110	815
grouper, ckd by dry heat—*3 oz (85 g)*	236	926	974	1717	1941	625	226	825	714	1089	1265	622	815
grouper, raw—*3 oz (85 g)*	185	722	759	1340	1513	488	177	643	556	849	986	485	815
haddock													
ckd by dry heat—*3 oz (85 g)*	231	904	950	1676	1894	611	221	805	696	1062	1234	607	815
raw—*3 oz (85 g)*	180	705	741	1307	1476	476	173	628	543	828	962	474	815
smoked—*3 oz (85 g)*	241	941	988	1744	1971	635	230	838	725	1106	1283	632	815
halibut, atlantic & pacific, ckd by dry heat—*3 oz (85 g)*	254	995	1046	1845	2085	672	243	886	766	1169	1358	668	815
halibut, atlantic & pacific, raw—*3 oz (85 g)*	198	776	816	1439	1625	524	190	691	598	912	1059	521	815
halibut, greenland, ckd by dry heat—*3 oz (85 g)*	175	687	722	1273	1439	464	168	612	529	807	937	461	815
halibut, greenland, raw—*3 oz (85 g)*	137	536	563	993	1123	361	131	477	412	629	731	360	815

	TRY	THR	ISO	LEU	LYS	MET	CYS	PHE	TYR	VAL	ARG	HIS	REF
herring, atlantic													
ckd by dry heat—3 oz (85 g)	219	859	902	1592	1799	580	210	765	662	1010	1172	577	815
kippered—1 piece (4⅜" x 1¾" x ¼") (40 g)	110	431	453	799	903	291	106	384	332	506	588	290	815
pickled—1 piece (1¾" x ⅞" x ½") (15 g)	24	93	98	173	195	63	23	83	72	110	127	63	815
raw—3 oz (85 g)	171	669	704	1242	1403	452	164	596	515	787	914	450	815
herring, pacific, ckd by dry heat—3 oz (85 g)	200	783	823	1453	1641	529	191	697	603	921	1069	526	815
herring, pacific, raw—3 oz (85 g)	156	612	642	1133	1281	412	150	544	470	719	834	411	815
ling, ckd by dry heat—3 oz (85 g)	232	907	954	1683	1902	613	222	808	699	1067	1239	610	815
ling, raw—3 oz (85 g)	181	708	744	1312	1483	478	174	630	545	832	966	475	815
lingcod, ckd by dry heat—3 oz (85 g)	216	845	887	1565	1768	570	207	752	650	992	1152	567	815
lingcod, raw—3 oz (85 g)	168	658	692	1220	1380	445	161	586	507	774	899	442	815
lobster, northern, ckd by moist heat—3 oz (85 g)	242	706	845	1384	1517	491	196	737	580	820	1523	355	815
lobster, northern, raw—3 oz (85 g)	223	647	775	1269	1391	450	179	675	532	752	1397	325	815
mackerel, atlantic, ckd by dry heat—3 oz (85 g)	227	889	935	1648	1863	600	218	792	685	1044	1214	597	815
mackerel, atlantic, raw—3 oz (85 g)	177	693	729	1286	1453	469	169	617	534	815	947	466	815
mackerel, jack, cnd—1 cup (190 g)	494	1932	2031	3582	4047	1303	473	1720	1488	2271	2637	1298	815
mackerel, king, ckd by dry heat—3 oz (85 g)	247	970	1019	1797	2031	655	237	863	747	1140	1323	651	815
mackerel, king, raw—3 oz (85 g)	193	756	795	1402	1584	510	185	674	583	889	1033	508	815
mackerel, pacific, and jack, ckd by dry heat—3 oz (85 g)	245	959	1008	1777	2009	648	235	854	739	1127	1309	644	815
mackerel, pacific, and jack, raw—3 oz (85 g)	191	748	787	1387	1567	505	183	666	577	879	1021	503	815
mackerel, spanish, ckd by dry heat—3 oz (85 g)	225	879	924	1630	1842	594	215	783	677	1033	1200	590	815
mackerel, spanish, raw—3 oz (85 g)	184	720	756	1334	1506	486	176	640	554	845	981	483	815
milkfish, ckd by dry heat—3 oz (85 g)	251	981	1032	1819	2056	663	240	874	756	1153	1340	659	815
milkfish, raw—3 oz (85 g)	196	765	805	1419	1604	517	187	682	589	900	1045	514	815
monkfish, ckd by dry heat—3 oz (85 g)	177	692	727	1283	1450	467	169	617	533	813	945	465	815
monkfish, raw—3 oz (85 g)	138	540	567	1001	1131	365	132	481	416	634	737	362	815
mullet, striped, ckd by dry heat—3 oz (85 g)	236	925	972	1715	1937	624	226	823	712	1087	1262	621	815
mullet, striped, raw—3 oz (85 g)	185	721	759	1338	1511	487	176	642	555	848	985	485	815
mussels, blue, ckd by moist heat—3 oz (85 g)	227	872	881	1425	1513	457	265	725	648	885	1477	389	815
mussels, blue, raw—3 oz (85 g)	113	435	441	713	756	228	133	362	324	442	738	194	815
ocean perch, atlantic, ckd by dry heat—3 oz (85 g)	227	890	936	1651	1865	601	218	793	686	1046	1215	598	815
ocean perch, atlantic, raw—3 oz (85 g)	178	695	730	1288	1455	469	170	618	535	816	948	466	815
octopus, ckd by moist heat—3 oz (85 g)	284	1091	1104	1785	1895	572	333	909	811	1108	1851	487	815
octopus, raw—3 oz (85 g)	142	546	552	892	947	286	167	454	406	554	925	243	815
orange roughy, ckd by dry heat—3 oz (85 g)	179	703	738	1303	1472	475	172	626	541	826	959	472	815
orange roughy, raw—3 oz (85 g)	140	548	576	1016	1148	370	134	488	422	644	748	368	815
oysters, eastern													
breaded & fried—3 oz (about 6 med) (85 g)[19]	89	310	337	543	495	169	111	299	247	348	498	149	815
cnd—3 oz (85 g)	67	259	261	423	449	135	79	215	192	262	438	116	815
farmed, ckd by dry heat—6 med (59 g)	46	178	180	291	309	93	54	148	132	181	301	79	815
farmed, raw—6 med (84 g)	50	189	191	309	328	99	58	157	140	192	320	84	815
wild, ckd by dry heat—6 med (59 g)	54	209	212	343	363	110	64	175	156	212	355	93	815
wild, ckd by moist heat—6 med (42 g)	66	255	258	417	442	134	78	212	189	259	432	114	815
wild, raw—6 med (84 g)	66	255	258	417	443	134	77	213	190	259	432	113	815
oysters, pacific, ckd by moist heat—3 oz (85 g)	180	691	700	1132	1201	362	211	576	515	703	1173	309	815
oysters, pacific, raw—3 oz (85 g)	90	346	350	566	600	181	105	288	257	351	586	154	815

	TRY	THR	ISO	LEU	LYS	MET	CYS	PHE	TYR	VAL	ARG	HIS	REF
perch													
ckd by dry heat—3 oz (85 g)	236	927	974	1718	1942	626	226	825	714	1089	1265	623	815
raw—3 oz (85 g)	185	723	759	1340	1515	488	177	644	557	850	987	486	815
pike, northern, ckd by dry heat—3 oz (85 g)	236	920	968	1707	1928	622	225	820	708	1082	1256	618	815
pike, northern, raw—3 oz (85 g)	184	718	754	1331	1504	485	175	640	553	844	980	482	815
pike, walleye, ckd by dry heat—3 oz (85 g)	234	915	962	1696	1917	617	224	815	704	1075	1249	614	815
pike, walleye, raw—3 oz (85 g)	182	714	750	1323	1495	481	174	635	549	839	974	479	815
pollock, atlantic, ckd by dry heat—3 oz (85 g)	237	930	976	1723	1947	628	227	828	715	1092	1268	624	815
pollock, atlantic, raw—3 oz (85 g)	185	725	762	1344	1519	490	177	646	558	852	990	486	815
pollock, walleye, ckd by dry heat—3 oz (85 g)	224	877	921	1625	1836	592	214	781	675	1030	1197	589	815
pollock, walleye, raw—3 oz (85 g)	163	640	674	1187	1342	433	156	571	493	753	874	430	815
pompano, florida, ckd by dry heat—3 oz (85 g)	225	883	929	1637	1850	596	216	787	680	1038	1205	593	815
pompano, florida, raw—3 oz (85 g)	176	689	724	1277	1443	465	168	613	531	810	941	463	815
pout, ocean, ckd by dry heat—3 oz (85 g)	203	795	836	1475	1666	537	195	708	612	935	1086	534	815
pout, ocean, raw—3 oz (85 g)	158	620	652	1150	1300	418	151	553	478	729	847	417	815
rockfish, pacific, ckd by dry heat—3 oz (85 g)	229	896	942	1662	1878	606	219	798	691	1053	1223	602	815
rockfish, pacific, raw—3 oz (85 g)	179	699	735	1296	1465	472	171	623	538	822	954	469	815
roe, mixed species, ckd by dry heat—1 oz (28 g)	106	370	415	711	618	201	141	397	408	475	465	221	815
roe, mixed species, raw—1 oz (28 g)	83	288	324	555	482	157	110	310	318	371	362	172	815
sablefish													
ckd by dry heat—3 oz (85 g)	164	641	674	1188	1343	433	156	571	493	754	875	430	815
raw—3 oz (85 g)	128	500	526	927	1048	338	122	446	385	588	683	336	815
smoked—3 oz (85 g)	168	658	692	1220	1380	445	161	586	507	774	899	442	815
salmon, atlantic													
farmed, ckd by dry heat—3 oz (85 g)	211	824	866	1527	1727	556	202	734	634	969	1124	554	815
farmed, raw—3 oz (85 g)	190	742	780	1375	1555	501	181	661	572	872	1013	498	815
wild, ckd by dry heat—3 oz (85 g)	242	948	997	1758	1987	640	232	845	731	1114	1294	637	815
wild, raw—3 oz (85 g)	189	740	777	1372	1550	499	181	659	570	869	1010	497	815
salmon, chinook													
ckd by dry heat—3 oz (85 g)	245	959	1008	1778	2009	647	235	854	738	1127	1309	644	815
raw—3 oz (85 g)	191	748	786	1386	1567	505	183	666	576	879	1021	502	815
smoked—3 oz (85 g)	174	681	716	1264	1428	460	167	607	525	801	930	458	815
salmon, chum													
ckd by dry heat—3 oz (85 g)	246	963	1012	1785	2017	650	236	857	742	1131	1314	646	815
cnd w/ bone—3 oz (85 g)	204	799	840	1482	1674	539	196	712	616	939	1090	537	815
raw—3 oz (85 g)	192	751	789	1392	1573	507	184	668	578	882	1025	504	815
salmon, coho													
farmed, ckd by dry heat—3 oz (85 g)	231	906	953	1680	1898	612	221	807	697	1065	1237	608	815
farmed, raw—3 oz (85 g)	202	793	833	1471	1661	535	194	706	611	932	1083	532	815
wild, ckd by dry heat—3 oz (85 g)	224	874	919	1621	1832	590	213	778	674	1027	1193	587	815
wild, ckd, moist heat—3 oz (85 g)	260	1021	1072	1892	2137	689	249	908	786	1199	1392	686	815
wild, raw—3 oz (85 g)	206	806	847	1493	1687	544	197	717	621	947	1100	541	815
salmon, pink													
ckd by dry heat—3 oz (85 g)	243	953	1002	1767	1997	644	233	849	734	1120	1301	640	815
cnd w/ bone—3 oz (85 g)	189	737	776	1368	1545	498	180	657	568	867	1007	495	815
raw—3 oz (85 g)	190	743	782	1379	1557	502	182	662	572	873	1015	499	815
salmon, sockeye													
ckd by dry heat—3 oz (85 g)	260	1018	1070	1887	2133	687	249	907	784	1197	1390	684	815
cnd w/ bone—3 oz (85 g)	195	763	802	1415	1599	515	186	680	588	897	1042	513	815
raw—3 oz (85 g)	203	794	835	1472	1664	536	194	708	612	933	1084	533	815
sardines, cnd, atlantic w/ soybean oil—2 sardines (24 g)	66	259	272	480	542	175	63	231	199	304	354	174	815

	TRY	THR	ISO	LEU	LYS	MET	CYS	PHE	TYR	VAL	ARG	HIS	REF
sardines, cnd, pacific w/ tomato sce—1 sardine (38 g)	60	302	302	516	532	181	53	301	238	352	399	258	815
scallops													
breaded & fried—2 large (31 g)[19]	65	238	248	401	397	126	78	213	182	254	392	110	815
imitation, made from surimi—3 oz (85 g)	66	525	508	860	993	368	117	426	438	551	721	250	815
mixed species, raw—3 oz (6 large) (85 g)	160	614	621	1004	1067	322	187	511	457	623	1041	274	815
scup, ckd by dry heat—3 oz (85 g)	230	902	948	1673	1891	609	220	804	695	1061	1232	606	815
scup, raw—3 oz (85 g)	179	703	740	1305	1474	475	172	627	542	827	960	473	815
sea bass, ckd by dry heat—3 oz (85 g)	225	881	926	1634	1846	594	215	785	679	1035	1203	592	815
sea bass, raw—3 oz (85 g)	175	687	722	1274	1440	464	168	612	529	808	938	462	815
seatrout, ckd by dry heat—3 oz (85 g)	204	800	841	1483	1676	540	196	713	617	941	1092	538	815
seatrout, raw—3 oz (85 g)	160	624	657	1158	1308	422	152	556	481	734	852	419	815
shad, american, ckd by dry heat—3 oz (85 g)	207	810	850	1500	1695	546	198	720	623	951	1105	543	815
shad, american, raw—3 oz (85 g)	162	631	663	1170	1323	426	155	562	486	742	862	424	815
shark, batter-dipped & fried—3 oz (85 g)	180	717	737	1289	1390	460	180	638	538	821	930	458	815
shark, raw—3 oz (85 g)	200	782	822	1450	1638	528	191	697	602	919	1067	526	815
sheepshead, ckd by dry heat—3 oz (85 g)	247	970	1020	1799	2033	655	237	864	747	1140	1324	651	815
sheepshead, raw—3 oz (85 g)	192	754	792	1397	1579	509	185	671	580	885	1029	506	815
shrimp													
breaded & fried—3 oz (11 large) (85 g)[19]	254	731	886	1444	1500	503	219	789	612	872	1517	372	815
ckd by moist heat—3 oz (15½ large) (85 g)	247	720	862	1411	1548	501	199	751	592	836	1553	361	815
cnd—3 oz (85 g)	273	794	952	1558	1709	553	220	829	653	924	1715	399	815
imitation, made from surimi—3 oz (85 g)	64	509	492	834	963	357	113	413	424	534	700	242	815
raw—3 oz (12 large) (85 g)	241	699	838	1371	1504	486	194	730	575	813	1510	351	815
smelt, rainbow, ckd by dry heat—3 oz (85 g)	215	843	885	1562	1766	569	206	750	649	990	1150	566	815
smelt, rainbow, raw—3 oz (85 g)	168	657	691	1219	1377	444	161	585	506	772	897	441	815
snapper, ckd by dry heat—3 oz (85 g)	250	981	1031	1818	2054	662	240	873	755	1152	1338	658	815
snapper, raw—3 oz (85 g)	196	765	804	1418	1601	516	187	681	589	898	1044	514	815
spiny lobster, ckd by dry heat—3 oz (85 g)	313	906	1085	1779	1952	633	252	945	748	1053	1959	457	815
spiny lobster, raw—3 oz (85 g)	244	709	849	1390	1524	493	196	740	583	824	1530	356	815
spot, ckd by dry heat—3 oz (85 g)	226	885	930	1641	1853	597	216	788	681	1040	1208	594	815
spot, raw—3 oz (85 g)	176	691	725	1280	1446	466	168	615	532	811	942	464	815
squid, fried—3 oz (85 g)[17]	172	649	663	1078	1114	343	206	558	490	668	1097	296	815
squid, raw—3 oz (85 g)	148	570	577	932	990	299	174	475	424	578	966	254	815
sturgeon													
ckd by dry heat—3 oz (85 g)	197	771	811	1431	1617	521	189	687	594	907	1053	518	815
raw—3 oz (85 g)	154	602	633	1116	1261	407	147	536	464	708	822	404	815
smoked—3 oz (85 g)	297	1163	1223	2157	2437	786	284	1036	896	1367	1588	782	815
sucker, white, ckd by dry heat—3 oz (85 g)	205	801	842	1485	1678	541	196	714	617	942	1094	538	815
sucker, white, raw—3 oz (85 g)	160	625	657	1158	1309	422	153	556	481	734	853	419	815
sunfish, pumpkinseed, ckd by dry heat—3 oz (85 g)	237	927	975	1720	1943	626	227	826	714	1089	1266	623	815
sunfish, pumpkinseed, raw—3 oz (85 g)	185	723	760	1341	1516	488	177	644	557	850	987	486	815
surimi—3 oz (85 g)[23]	78	624	603	1022	1180	438	139	506	521	655	857	298	815
swordfish, ckd by dry heat—3 oz (85 g)	242	947	995	1755	1983	639	231	843	729	1112	1292	635	815
swordfish, raw—3 oz (85 g)	189	738	776	1368	1546	498	180	657	568	868	1008	496	815
tilefish, ckd by dry heat—3 oz (85 g)	233	913	959	1692	1913	617	224	813	703	1073	1246	613	815
tilefish, raw—3 oz (85 g)	167	652	686	1209	1367	441	160	581	503	767	890	438	815
trout, mixed species, ckd by dry heat—3 oz (85 g)	253	993	1044	1840	2080	670	242	885	765	1167	1355	667	815
trout, mixed species, raw—3 oz (85 g)	198	775	814	1436	1622	523	190	690	596	910	1057	520	815

	TRY	THR	ISO	LEU	LYS	MET	CYS	PHE	TYR	VAL	ARG	HIS	REF
trout, rainbow													
farmed, ckd by dry heat—*3 oz (85 g)*	231	905	951	1677	1896	611	221	805	697	1063	1235	607	815
farmed, raw—*3 oz (85 g)*	199	778	818	1442	1630	526	191	693	599	914	1062	522	815
wild, ckd by dry heat—*3 oz (85 g)*	219	855	898	1584	1790	577	209	761	658	1004	1167	574	815
wild, raw—*3 oz (85 g)*	195	764	803	1415	1600	515	187	680	588	897	1042	513	815
tuna, bluefin, ckd by dry heat—*3 oz (85 g)*	285	1115	1172	2068	2336	753	273	993	859	1311	1522	748	815
tuna, bluefin, raw—*3 oz (85 g)*	222	870	914	1613	1822	587	213	775	669	1022	1187	584	815
tuna, cnd in oil, light, drained—*3 oz (85 g)*	277	1086	1141	2014	2275	733	265	967	836	1277	1482	730	815
tuna, cnd in oil, white, drained—*3 oz (85 g)*	253	989	1040	1834	2073	668	242	881	762	1163	1351	664	815
tuna, cnd in water, light, drained—*3 oz (85 g)*	243	951	999	1763	1993	642	232	847	732	1118	1299	639	815
tuna, cnd in water, white, drained—*3 oz (85 g)*	225	880	925	1633	1845	594	215	784	678	1035	1202	591	815
tuna salad—*½ cup (205 g)*[24]	369	1437	1515	2651	2987	963	353	1283	1105	1689	1982	957	815
tuna, skipjack, ckd by dry heat—*3 oz (85 g)*	269	1052	1106	1950	2203	710	257	936	810	1236	1436	706	815
tuna, skipjack, raw—*3 oz (85 g)*	209	820	862	1521	1718	554	201	731	632	964	1119	551	815
tuna, yellowfin, ckd by dry heat—*3 oz (85 g)*	286	1118	1175	2072	2341	754	273	995	861	1313	1526	750	815
tuna, yellowfin, raw—*3 oz (85 g)*	223	872	916	1616	1826	589	213	777	671	1024	1190	585	815
turbot, european, ckd by dry heat—*3 oz (85 g)*	196	767	806	1422	1607	518	188	683	591	902	1047	515	815
turbot, european, raw—*3 oz (85 g)*	153	599	629	1110	1254	404	146	533	461	703	816	402	815
whelk (sea snail), ckd by moist heat—*3 oz (85 g)*	526	1817	1408	3238	2492	1025	318	1402	1291	1765	4198	831	815
whelk (sea snail), raw—*3 oz (85 g)*	263	908	704	1619	1246	513	159	701	646	882	2099	415	815
whitefish													
ckd by dry heat—*3 oz (85 g)*	233	913	959	1692	1912	616	223	812	703	1072	1246	613	815
raw—*3 oz (85 g)*	182	712	748	1319	1491	481	174	634	548	836	971	478	815
smoked—*3 oz (85 g)*	223	873	917	1618	1828	589	213	777	672	1026	1191	586	815
whiting, ckd by dry heat—*3 oz (85 g)*	224	875	920	1623	1834	591	214	780	674	1029	1195	588	815
whiting, raw—*3 oz (85 g)*	174	683	718	1266	1431	461	167	608	526	802	932	458	815
wolffish, atlantic, ckd by dry heat—*3 oz (85 g)*	213	837	879	1551	1753	565	205	745	644	983	1142	562	815
wolffish, atlantic, raw—*3 oz (85 g)*	167	652	686	1209	1367	441	160	581	503	767	890	438	815
yellowtail, ckd by dry heat—*3 oz (85 g)*	282	1107	1163	2051	2318	747	270	985	852	1300	1510	742	815
yellowtail, raw—*3 oz (85 g)*	220	863	907	1600	1808	583	211	769	664	1014	1178	579	815
14. FRUIT & VEGETABLE JUICES													
clam & tomato jce, cnd—*5.5 fl oz (166 g)*	7	25	20	30	30	5	7	22	15	22	22	17	814
grape jce, cnd/bottled—*8 fl oz (253 g)*		40	18	30	25	3		30	8	25	119	18	809
grape jce, from frzn conc, sweetened—*8 fl oz (250 g)*		13	5	10	8			10	3	8	40	5	809
orange jce													
cnd—*8 fl oz (249 g)*	5	17	15	27	20	7	10	17	7	22	100	7	809
fresh—*8 fl oz (248 g)*	5	20	20	32	22	7	12	22	10	27	117	7	809
from frzn conc—*8 fl oz (249 g)*	5	20	17	32	22	7	12	20	10	27	112	7	809
tangerine jce													
cnd, sweetened—*8 fl oz (249 g)*	2	15	12	25	17	5	10	15	7	20	85	5	809
fresh—*8 fl oz (247 g)*	2	15	12	25	17	5	10	15	7	20	84	5	809
from frzn conc, sweetened—*8 fl oz (241 g)*	2	12	12	19	14	5	7	12	5	17	70	5	809
tomato jce—*6 fl oz (182 g)*	9	31	27	38	40	7	7	29	18	27	27	22	811
15. FRUITS													
apple													
boiled, w/o skin—*1 cup (171 g)*	3	15	17	27	27	5	7	12	9	21	14	7	809
cnd, sliced, sweetened—*½ cup (102 g)*	2	6	7	11	11	2	2	5	3	8	6	3	809
dried, sulfured—*10 rings (64 g)*	6	21	24	36	37	6	8	17	11	28	19	10	809

	TRY	THR	ISO	LEU	LYS	MET	CYS	PHE	TYR	VAL	ARG	HIS	REF
micro ckd w/o skin—*1 cup (170 g)*	5	17	19	29	31	5	7	14	9	22	15	7	809
raw, w/o skin—*1 med (128 g)*	1	6	8	12	12	3	3	5	4	9	6	3	809
raw, w/ skin—*1 med (138 g)*	3	10	11	17	17	3	4	7	6	12	8	4	809
applesauce, cnd													
sweetened—*½ cup (128 g)*	3	9	9	14	14	3	3	6	4	10	8	4	809
unsweetened—*½ cup (122 g)*	2	7	7	12	12	2	2	6	4	10	6	4	809
apricots													
cnd, heavy syrup—*4 halves (90 g)*	8	17	14	28	33	3	2	20	11	17	19	8	809
cnd, jce pack—*3 halves (84 g)*	9	19	16	31	37	3	2	22	13	19	20	8	809
cnd, light syrup—*3 halves (85 g)*	8	16	14	26	31	3	2	19	10	16	18	8	809
cnd, water pack—*4 halves (90 g)*	12	23	20	38	44	4	2	27	15	23	25	11	809
dried, sulfured—*10 halves (35 g)*	23	46	39	75	89	6	4	53	30	47	49	21	809
frzn, sweetened—*½ cup (121 g)*	10	29	24	47	59	4	2	31	18	29	27	16	809
raw—*3 med (106 g)*	16	50	43	82	103	6	3	55	31	50	48	29	809
avocado, raw, calif—*1 med (173 g)*	38	121	130	227	173	67	38	125	90	178	109	52	809
avocado, raw, florida—*1 med (304 g)*	52	161	173	301	228	88	52	164	119	237	143	70	809
banana, raw—*1 med (114 g)*	14	39	38	81	55	13	19	43	27	54	54	92	809
blueberries													
cnd, heavy syrup—*½ cup (128 g)*	4	23	26	50	15	13	9	29	10	35	42	13	809
frzn, sweetened—*1 cup (230 g)*	5	25	28	53	16	14	9	32	12	39	46	14	809
raw—*1 cup (145 g)*	4	26	30	58	17	16	10	35	12	41	49	15	809
breadfruit, raw—*¼ small (96 g)*		50	61	62	36	10	9	25	18	45			809
carambola, raw—*1 med (127 g)*	5	29	29	51	51	14		24	29	33	14	5	809
crabapples, raw—*1 cup slices (110 g)*	4	15	18	28	28	4	6	12	9	21	14	7	809
custard apple, raw—*3.5 oz (99 g)*	7				37	4							809
dates, dried—*10 dates (83 g)*	42	43	39	73	50	18	37	46	25	55	55	25	809
elderberries, raw—*1 cup (145 g)*	19	39	39	87	38	20	22	58	74	48	68	22	809
figs													
cnd, heavy syrup—*3 figs (85 g)*	3	10	10	14	13	3	5	8	14	12	8	4	809
dried—*10 figs (187 g)*	49	187	174	249	228	47	94	138	247	215	131	80	809
raw—*1 med (50 g)*	3	12	12	17	15	3	6	9	16	14	9	6	809
fruit snack													
fruit bar—*.81 oz bar (23 g)*	5	12	14	28	11	7	8	20	12	17	16	9	819
fruit bar w/ cream—*.85 oz bar (24 g)*	1	8	10	17	13	4	2	8	6	11	6	4	819
fruit pieces—*1 oz (28 g)*	3	9	9	17	10	3	4	11	9	10	12	6	819
fruit roll—*1 large roll (.74 oz) (21 g)*	2	6	5	11	10	1	2	6	6	7	8	4	819
grapefruit													
cnd, jce pack—*½ cup (124 g)*	2				22	2							809
cnd, light syrup—*½ cup (127 g)*	3				18	3							809
raw, pink & red—*½ med (123 g)*	2				20	2							809
raw, white—*½ med (118 g)*	2				21	2							809
grapes													
american (slip skin), raw—*1 cup (92 g)*	3	16	5	12	13	19	9	12	10	16	42	21	809
european (adherent skin), raw—*1 cup (160 g)*	5	29	8	22	24	35	18	22	19	29	78	38	809
thompson seedless, cnd, heavy syrup—*½ cup (128 g)*	3	17	5	13	14	20	10	13	10	17	45	23	809
guava, raw—*1 med (90 g)*	6	28	27	50	21	5		2	9	25	19	6	809
guava, strawberry, raw—*1 cup (244 g)*	12	54	51	95	39	10		2	17	49	37	12	809
lime, raw—*1 med (67 g)*	2				9	1							809
longans, dried—*3.5 oz (99 g)*		127	96	200	171	49		111	93	215	130	45	809
longans, raw—*31 fruits (100 g)*		34	26	54	46	13		30	25	58	35	12	809
loquats, raw—*6 med (100 g)*	5	15	15	26	23	4	6	14	13	21	14	7	809
lychees, dried—*3.5 oz (99 g)*	33				186	42							809
lychees, raw—*10 med (100 g)*	7				41	9							809
mammy apple, raw—*⅛ med (100 g)*	5				37	6							809
mandarin oranges, cnd, jce pack—*½ cup (124 g)*	7	12	21	19	38	16	7	25	12	32	53	14	809

	TRY	THR	ISO	LEU	LYS	MET	CYS	PHE	TYR	VAL	ARG	HIS	REF
mandarin oranges, cnd, light syrup—½ cup (126 g)	5	9	15	14	29	13	6	19	10	24	39	10	809
mango, raw—1 med (207 g)	17	39	37	64	85	10		35	21	54	39	25	809
orange, navel, raw—1 fruit (131 g)	13	22	37	34	68	29	14	45	22	58	94	25	809
orange, valencia, raw—1 med (121 g)	12	21	34	31	64	27	13	41	22	53	88	24	809
papaya, raw—1 med (304 g)	24	33	24	49	76	6		27	15	30	30	15	809
peach													
cnd, heavy syrup—1 cup (256 g)	3	46	33	67	38	28	10	36	31	64	31	20	809
cnd, heavy syrup, spiced—1 med (88 g)	1	14	11	20	11	9	3	11	10	20	9	7	809
cnd, jce pack—1 cup (248 g)	5	62	45	89	50	37	12	50	40	84	40	30	809
cnd, light syrup—1 cup (251 g)	3	45	33	63	35	28	10	35	30	63	28	20	809
cnd, water pack—1 cup (244 g)	2	41	32	61	34	27	10	34	27	59	27	20	809
dried, sulfured—10 halves (130 g)	13	183	135	265	151	113	38	148	122	256	120	87	809
frzn, sweetened—1 cup (250 g)	5	60	45	88	50	38	13	50	40	85	40	30	809
raw—1 med (87 g)	2	23	17	35	20	15	5	19	16	33	16	11	809
pear													
cnd, heavy pack—1 cup (255 g)		13	15	26	18	5	5	13	5	18	8	5	809
cnd, jce pack—1 cup (248 g)		22	25	42	30	10	7	22	7	30	15	10	809
cnd, light syrup—1 cup (251 g)		13	15	25	18	5	5	13	5	18	8	5	809
cnd, water pack—1 cup (244 g)		12	12	22	17	5	5	12	5	17	7	5	809
dried, sulfured—10 halves (175 g)		86	95	165	116	39	31	86	28	116	56	35	809
raw—1 med (166 g)		17	18	33	23	8	7	17	5	23	12	7	809
pear, asian, raw—1 pear (2½" high, 2½" dia) (122 g)	6	16	17	31	21	7	6	16	5	22	11	6	809
persimmon, japanese, dried—1 med (34 g)	8	24	20	34	27	4	10	21	13	24	20	9	809
persimmon, japanese, raw—1 med (168 g)	17	50	42	71	55	8	22	44	27	50	42	20	809
persimmon, raw—1 med (25 g)	4	10	9	15	11	2	5	9	6	11	9	4	809
pineapple													
cnd, heavy syrup—1 cup pieces (255 g)	13	23	23	33	41	23	3	23	20	28	31	20	809
cnd, jce pack—1 cup pieces (250 g)	13	25	25	40	48	28	3	25	25	33	35	23	809
raw—1 cup pieces (155 g)	8	19	20	29	39	17	3	19	19	25	28	14	809
plantain, ckd—1 cup slices (154 g)	14	32	34	55	57	15	18	42	31	43	102	60	809
plums													
cnd, heavy syrup—3 plums (133 g)		11	9	13	11	4	3	11	4	12	8	8	809
cnd, jce pack—3 plums (95 g)		10	10	13	10	4	3	10	4	11	9	8	809
raw—1 med (66 g)		11	11	14	11	4	3	11	4	13	9	9	809
sapodilla, raw—1 med (170 g)	9	20	26	41	66	5		22	24	27	29	27	809
sapote, raw—1 med (225 g)	52	131	104	189	216	36		119	124	173	124	95	809
soursop, raw—1 cup (225 g)	25				135	16							809
strawberries													
frzn, sweetened—1 cup (255 g)	15	41	31	66	54	3	10	38	43	38	56	26	809
frzn, unsweetened—1 cup (149 g)	7	19	15	33	25	1	6	18	21	18	27	12	809
raw—1 cup (149 g)	10	28	21	46	37	1	7	27	31	27	39	18	809
sugar apple, raw—1 med (155 g)	16				85	11							809
tamarind, raw—1 cup (120 g)	22				167	17							809
tangerine, raw—1 med (84 g)	5	8	14	13	27	11	6	18	9	23	37	10	809
watermelon, raw—1 cup (160 g)	11	43	30	29	99	10	3	24	19	26	94	10	809
16. GRAIN FRACTIONS													
amaranth—1 cup (195 g)	353	1088	1135	1714	1457	441	372	1057	642	1324	2067	759	820
arrowroot flour—1 cup (128 g)	5	15	13	24	17	8	8	15	12	18	15	5	820
buckwheat flour, whole groat—1 cup (120 g)	220	578	569	950	768	197	262	594	276	775	1122	353	820
carob (St. Johnsbread) flour—1 cup (103 g)	49	279	215	455	202	83	30	156	124	459	134	126	816
corn flour, masa harina, enr—1 cup (114 g)	75	400	381	1306	300	223	192	523	433	539	531	325	820
corn flour, whole grain—1 cup (117 g)	57	305	290	994	228	170	146	398	330	411	404	247	820

	TRY	THR	ISO	LEU	LYS	MET	CYS	PHE	TYR	VAL	ARG	HIS	REF
cornmeal, white													
bolted, enr, self-rising—1 cup (122 g)	71	379	361	1238	284	212	182	497	411	511	504	309	820
bolted, enr, self-rising, wheat flour added—1 cup (170 g)	111	519	510	1654	391	294	264	704	564	706	697	423	820
cornmeal, whole grain—1 cup (122 g)	70	372	355	1215	278	207	178	487	403	501	494	303	820
cracker meal—1 cup (115 g)	123	284	393	735	206	186	239	524	291	446	369	225	818
oat bran, ckd—½ cup (110 g)	63	95	125	259	143	63	109	171	125	182	241	77	820
raw—⅓ cup (31 g)	104	156	207	426	236	104	179	281	207	299	396	127	820
oats, reg/quick/inst, dry—⅓ cup (.95 oz) (27 g)	60	147	177	328	179	80	104	229	147	240	305	103	808
potato flour—½ cup (90 g)	120	292	311	443	431	112	73	329	234	372	390	173	811
quinoa—½ cup (85 g)		390	401	668	624	223		456	312	501	780	267	820
rice bran—1 oz (28 g)	31	157	161	290	184	87	90	180	117	250	300	101	820
rice flour, brown—1 cup (158 g)	145	419	483	945	436	258	139	589	428	670	866	291	820
rice flour, white—1 cup (163 g)	117	342	398	795	337	235	174	517	512	567	841	243	820
rye flour													
dark—1 cup (128 g)	204	622	692	1242	622	268	355	909	355	900	813	401	820
light—1 cup (102 g)	97	297	330	592	297	128	168	432	168	428	388	191	820
medium—1 cup (102 g)	108	332	369	662	332	143	189	485	189	479	434	213	820
semolina, enr—½ cup (84 g)	136	281	412	728	204	166	301	517	280	454	392	216	820
sorghum—½ cup (96 g)	119	332	416	1431	220	162	122	524	308	539	341	236	820
soy flour													
defatted—1 cup (85 g)	581	1736	1939	3254	2660	539	643	2085	1511	1994	3100	1078	816
full fat—1 cup (85 g)	427	1275	1424	2390	1953	396	473	1532	1110	1465	2277	791	816
full fat, roasted—1 cup (85 g)	430	1284	1435	2409	1969	399	477	1544	1119	1476	2295	797	816
low fat—1 cup (88 g)	595	1778	1986	3334	2725	552	660	2137	1549	2043	3177	1104	816
soy meal, defatted, raw—1 cup (122 g)	797	2381	2660	4465	3649	739	883	2862	2074	2736	4254	1479	820
triticale flour, whole grain—1 cup (130 g)	205	532	629	1196	480	268	361	837	503	800	881	408	820
wheat bran—½ cup (30 g)	85	150	146	278	180	70	111	178	131	218	326	129	820
wheat flour, white													
all purpose, enr—1 cup (125 g)	159	351	446	888	285	229	274	650	390	519	521	288	820
bread, enr—1 cup (137 g)	190	438	608	1134	316	288	369	810	449	688	570	348	820
cake, enr—1 cup (109 g)	129	247	339	608	311	150	194	423	255	392	342	182	820
self-rising, enr—1 cup (125 g)	151	336	428	850	274	219	263	623	373	496	499	275	820
tortilla mix—1 cup (111 g)25	132	292	371	737	236	190	228	539	323	431	433	239	820
wheat flour, whole wheat—1 cup (120 g)	254	474	610	1111	454	254	380	775	480	742	770	380	820
wheat germ													
crude—¼ cup (29 g)	92	281	246	456	426	132	133	269	204	347	541	186	
toasted—¼ cup (29 g)	115	353	309	573	536	166	167	339	257	437	681	235	820

17. GRAIN PRODUCTS
17.1 Bagels

	TRY	THR	ISO	LEU	LYS	MET	CYS	PHE	TYR	VAL	ARG	HIS	REF
cinn raisin—1 bagel (3½″) (71 g)	81	202	261	476	169	127	149	337	193	301	268	154	818
egg—1 bagel (3½″) (71 g)	89	217	292	531	185	135	164	371	219	327	280	164	818
oat bran—1 bagel (3½″) (71 g)	98	214	288	537	204	133	180	373	228	342	327	165	818
plain/nion/poppy seed/sesame seed—1 bagel (3½″) (71 g)	88	214	287	522	178	133	160	368	214	324	273	161	818

17.2 Biscuits

	TRY	THR	ISO	LEU	LYS	MET	CYS	PHE	TYR	VAL	ARG	HIS	REF
mixed grain, refrig dough—1 biscuit (3″ x 1″) (41 g)	36	81	102	202	68	51	63	146	87	120	123	66	818
plain/buttermilk—1 biscuit (2½″ x 1″) (35 g)	27	62	79	153	58	39	43	108	67	92	86	49	818
from mix—1 biscuit (3″ x 1½″) (57 g)	52	133	169	313	152	79	76	202	140	193	160	95	818
from refrig dough (12 -28% fat)—1 biscuit (2½″ x 1″) (27 g)	21	48	64	125	36	31	39	93	56	71	70	39	818
from refrig dough (2 -12% fat)—1 biscuit (2¼″ x 1″) (21 g)	20	44	56	113	36	29	35	82	49	66	66	36	818
homemade—1 biscuit (2½″ x 1½″) (60 g)	52	127	164	308	136	79	79	208	139	188	165	97	818

	TRY	THR	ISO	LEU	LYS	MET	CYS	PHE	TYR	VAL	ARG	HIS	REF
17.3 Breads, Quick													
banana													
homemade w/ marg—*1 slice (4⅜" x 2½" x ½") (60 g)*	32	90	109	196	108	56	54	131	89	125	119	68	818
homemade w/ veg shortening—*1 slice (4⅜" x 2½" x ½") (60 g)*	32	88	106	193	104	56	54	129	86	123	119	67	818
boston brown, cnd—*1 slice (3½" x 2") (45 g)*	33	73	84	158	70	41	52	105	67	105	115	58	818
cornbread, from mix—*1 slice (3¾" x 2 ½" x ¾") (60 g)*	47	160	186	388	190	98	82	215	161	223	200	109	818
cornbread, homemade w/ low fat milk—*1 slice (2½" x 1½") (65 g)*	44	168	189	441	192	99	76	215	174	232	203	118	818
cornbread, homemade w/ whole milk—*1 piece (2½" x 1½") (65 g)*	44	168	188	439	192	98	75	214	174	231	202	117	818
hush puppy, homemade—*1 hush puppy (2¼" x 1¼") (22 g)*	18	61	71	156	68	37	32	84	64	85	77	43	818
pumpkin, homemade—*1 slice (60 g)*	29	81	97	172	97	52	49	118	82	110	113	53	818
17.4 Breads, Yeast & Unleavened													
bread crumbs													
dry, grated—*1 cup (108 g)*	161	403	552	945	367	216	234	673	322	677	556	292	818
dry, grated, seasoned—*1 cup (120 g)*	205	509	703	1208	535	280	282	844	432	868	724	382	818
cracked wheat—*1 slice (25 g)*	28	65	85	152	61	37	48	105	63	97	87	48	818
egg—*1 slice (5" x 3" x ½") (40 g)*	45	122	158	277	124	76	83	190	117	177	154	84	818
french/vienna/sourdough—*1 med slice (4¾" x 4" x ½") (25 g)*	26	62	85	154	51	40	48	109	63	96	80	48	818
indian (navajo) fry—*5" dia (90 g)*	78	173	220	437	140	113	135	320	192	256	257	141	818
irish soda, homemade—*1 slice (60 g)*	43	121	140	262	131	83	73	180	121	170	174	95	818
italian—*1 slice (4½" x 3¼" x ¾") (30 g)*	31	74	100	184	59	47	58	130	74	113	95	56	818
mixed grain/whole grain/7-grain—*1 slice (26 g)*	34	80	101	182	82	43	56	126	74	120	115	58	818
oat bran—*1 slice (30 g)*	39	90	120	220	89	54	70	155	97	138	134	68	818
oatmeal—*1 slice (27 g)*	31	67	88	164	73	41	56	112	71	106	107	50	818
pita													
white—*1 pita (6½" dia) (60 g)*	63	154	209	380	131	96	118	268	154	236	197	117	818
whole wheat—*1 pita (6½" dia) (64 g)*	95	180	235	429	170	98	146	301	187	282	291	145	818
protein/gluten—*1 slice (19 g)*	28	70	89	163	71	38	47	113	69	98	104	51	818
pumpernickel—*1 slice (5" x 4" x ⅜") (32 g)*	31	85	107	193	79	50	61	135	76	127	115	63	818
raisin—*1 slice (26 g)*	22	58	75	134	52	33	40	94	53	86	94	43	818
rice bran—*1 slice (27 g)*	29	72	94	168	70	42	51	119	73	109	102	53	818
rye, american—*1 slice (5" x 4" x ½") (32 g)*	31	82	102	185	75	44	55	132	68	121	104	58	818
wheat bran—*1 slice (36 g)*	40	92	120	217	85	55	69	151	91	139	129	71	818
wheat germ—*1 slice (28 g)*	32	85	108	192	91	48	53	128	82	123	111	60	818
wheat/wheat berry—*1 slice (25 g)*	30	69	89	161	65	39	50	112	67	102	95	51	818
white—*1 slice (25 g)*	24	61	81	145	56	36	44	101	59	90	79	45	818
whole wheat—*1 slice (28 g)*	39	83	105	188	85	43	60	130	81	124	126	63	818
homemade—*1 slice (46 g)*	56	114	144	264	112	63	86	185	116	173	176	89	818
17.5 Breadsticks													
plain—*2 breadsticks (20 g)*	28	68	92	167	56	42	52	118	68	103	86	52	818
17.6 Crackers & Croutons													
cheese—*14 1" sq crackers (14 g)*	18	42	60	105	59	27	24	69	48	68	55	35	818
cheese w/ peanut butter filling—*1 sandwich (7 g)*	10	28	33	60	31	14	15	44	31	38	67	21	818
croutons—*1 cup (30 g)*	42	101	137	250	83	63	78	176	101	154	129	77	818
seasoned—*1 cup (40 g)*	50	130	171	310	138	78	87	210	132	195	161	98	818
matzo—*1 matzo (1 oz) (28 g)*	33	76	105	196	55	50	64	140	78	119	99	60	818
egg—*1 matzo (1 oz) (28 g)*	43	109	134	251	110	70	76	177	113	154	154	79	818
egg & onion—*1 matzo (1 oz) (28 g)*	35	84	105	199	80	54	60	142	89	121	123	63	818

	TRY	THR	ISO	LEU	LYS	MET	CYS	PHE	TYR	VAL	ARG	HIS	REF
whole wheat—*1 matzo (1 oz) (28 g)*	58	108	139	252	105	58	87	176	109	169	179	88	818
melba toast—*1 toast (5 g)*	7	17	23	42	14	11	13	30	17	26	22	13	818
rye/pumpernickel)—*1 toast (19 g)*	25	69	85	151	64	36	45	108	55	101	87	48	818
wheat—*1 toast (5 g)*	9	19	24	44	17	11	14	31	19	29	27	14	818
milk—*1 cracker (12 g)*	12	27	35	65	29	17	19	45	28	40	37	20	818
round—*1 cracker (3 g)*	3	6	8	15	5	4	5	11	7	9	9	5	818
rusk—*1 rusk (10 g)*	17	51	61	101	68	29	27	67	47	68	65	31	818
rye, crispbread—*1 cracker (10 g)*	9	29	32	56	30	12	16	40	17	40	37	18	818
rye w/ cheese filling—*1 sandwich (1.0 g)*	1	3	4	6	3	2	2	4	3	4	4	2	818
saltines—*1 saltine (3 g)*	4	8	10	19	8	5	6	14	8	12	11	6	818
fat-free, low-sodium—*3 crackers (15 g)*	21	43	57	107	43	27	34	77	46	66	62	34	818
sandwich w/ cheese filling—*1 sandwich (7 g)*	8	19	24	45	21	12	13	31	20	28	25	14	818
sandwich w/ peanut butter filling—*1 sandwich (7 g)*	5	10	14	26	10	7	8	19	11	16	15	8	818
wheat—*7 crackers (14 g)*	17	34	44	81	33	19	27	58	35	53	53	27	818
wheat w/ cheese filling—*1 sandwich (7 g)*	9	21	27	49	24	12	14	33	21	31	29	15	818
wheat w/ peanut butter filling—*1 sandwich (7 g)*	11	29	34	64	31	14	17	47	32	40	72	22	818
whole wheat—*1 sq cracker (4 g)*	5	10	13	24	10	5	8	17	10	16	17	8	818
17.7 English Muffins													
mixed grain/granola—*1 muffin (66 g)*	78	184	238	428	192	104	131	296	185	279	291	133	818
plain—*1 muffin (57 g)*	52	138	180	315	137	79	91	216	133	201	168	97	818
raisin cinn/apple cinn—*1 muffin (57 g)*	48	135	168	296	133	82	88	205	126	192	175	99	818
wheat—*1 muffin (57 g)*	64	152	194	340	154	83	103	235	145	223	205	110	818
whole wheat—*1 muffin (66 g)*	85	187	232	403	204	93	125	275	180	273	275	135	818
17.8 French Toast													
frzn—*1 slice (59 g)*	55	166	200	345	218	99	84	216	158	224	198	101	818
homemade w/ low-fat milk—*1 slice (65 g)*	61	198	244	404	268	122	101	253	183	272	237	116	818
homemade w/ whole milk—*1 slice (65 g)*	61	198	243	402	268	122	101	253	183	272	236	116	818
17.9 Muffins													
blueberry—*1 muffin (2½″ x 2¼″) (57 g)*	38	103	128	240	113	66	64	158	105	146	139	73	818
from mix—*1 muffin (50 g)*	35	85	108	185	114	53	57	125	81	124	113	54	818
homemade w/ 2% milk—*1 muffin (2¾″ x 2″) (57 g)*	46	125	157	284	150	78	71	185	129	179	158	86	818
homemade w/ whole milk—*1 muffin (2¾″ x 2″) (57 g)*	46	124	157	283	150	78	70	185	129	178	157	86	818
corn—*1 muffin (2½″ x 2¼″) (57 g)*	39	129	146	294	159	67	63	169	124	168	182	86	818
from mix—*1 muffin (2¼″ x 1½″) (50 g)*	41	137	159	330	162	83	70	184	138	190	171	92	818
homemade w/ 2% milk—*1 muffin (2¾″ x 2″) (57 g)*	44	149	173	373	173	89	72	199	154	207	182	104	818
homemade w/ whole milk—*1 muffin (2¾″ x 2″) (57 g)*	44	148	173	373	173	89	72	199	154	207	181	103	818
homemade w/ 2% milk—*1 muffin (2¾″ x 2″) (57 g)*	49	132	165	298	159	82	74	195	137	188	165	91	818
homemade w/ whole milk—*1 muffin (2¾″ x 2″) (57 g)*	48	131	165	298	158	82	74	194	136	188	165	91	818
oat bran—*1 muffin (2½″ x 2¼″) (57 g)*	60	120	149	288	158	70	104	197	133	207	269	89	818
toaster muffin													
blueberry—*1 muffin (31 g)*	20	60	68	116	86	22	25	75	53	72	100	38	818
corn—*1 muffin (31 g)*	20	61	70	145	65	39	37	90	61	84	83	43	818
wheat bran raisin—*1 muffin (34 g)*	25	67	74	134	85	32	36	89	61	85	111	46	818
wheat bran, from mix—*1 muffin (2¼″ x 1¾″) (50 g)*	49	116	133	230	155	67	75	150	105	164	183	78	818
wheat bran, homemade w/ 2% milk—*1 muffin (2¾″ x 2″) (57 g)*	59	141	164	294	182	80	81	184	137	202	212	102	I

	TRY	THR	ISO	LEU	LYS	MET	CYS	PHE	TYR	VAL	ARG	HIS	REF
wheat bran, homemade w/ whole milk—*1 muffin (2¾" x 2") (57 g)*	59	140	164	293	181	79	81	184	137	201	212	101	818
17.10 Pancakes													
blueberry, homemade—*4" pancake (38 g)*	29	86	107	185	115	53	42	115	86	121	102	55	818
buckwheat, from incomplete mix—*4" pancake (30 g)*[26]	32	92	111	188	130	50	42	111	83	130	119	57	818
buttermilk, homemade—*4" pancake (38 g)*	31	97	120	207	133	59	46	129	94	138	112	62	818
plain													
from complete mix—*4" pancake (38 g)*	22	71	82	169	80	40	36	97	69	98	84	48	818
from incomplete mix—*4" pancake (38 g)*[26]	36	113	143	250	154	68	54	146	111	163	130	71	818
frzn—*4" pancake (36 g)*	22	66	81	150	80	40	36	95	65	94	82	45	818
homemade—*4" pancake (38 g)*	30	90	113	195	122	56	44	121	91	127	106	58	818
whole wheat, from incomplete mix—*4" pancake (44 g)*[26]	52	139	174	297	193	80	73	184	137	206	190	90	818
17.11 Pasta													
corn, ckd—*1 cup (140 g)*	27	139	132	451	104	77	66	181	150	186	183	112	820
egg, homemade, ckd—*2 oz (57 g)*	38	94	126	217	94	57	81	149	88	140	126	63	820
egg, refrig, ckd—*2 oz (57 g)*	37	76	112	197	55	45	81	140	76	123	106	58	820
homemade w/o egg, ckd—*2 oz (57 g)*	32	66	96	170	48	39	70	120	65	105	91	50	820
lasagne, Mueller's—*2 oz dry (57 g)*	85	176	258	456	128	104	188	324	175	284	246	135	I
macaroni													
enr, ckd—*1 cup (140 g)*	85	176	258	456	127	104	188	323	175	284	246	136	820
protein-fortified, ckd—*1 cup (115 g)*	118	262	367	641	220	148	253	450	253	407	362	194	820
veg, ckd—*1 cup (134 g)*	78	163	235	414	125	94	168	292	161	260	225	123	820
whole wheat, ckd—*1 cup (140 g)*	97	200	290	510	165	120	155	371	195	323	263	175	820
noodles, chow mein—*1 cup (45 g)*	48	99	145	257	72	59	106	182	99	160	138	76	820
noodles, egg													
& spinach, ckd—*1 cup (160 g)*	107	251	349	582	242	149	213	402	238	390	344	170	820
enr, ckd—*1 cup (160 g)*	101	230	323	542	208	139	208	378	219	360	314	158	820
noodles, japanese, soba, ckd—*1 cup (176 g)*	127	312	343	581	377	127	165	382	185	438	558	209	820
noodles, japanese, somen, ckd—*1 cup (176 g)*	90	187	273	482	136	109	199	341	185	301	260	143	820
spaghetti													
enr, ckd—*1 cup (140 g)*	85	176	258	456	127	104	188	323	175	284	246	136	820
protein-fortified, ckd—*1 cup (140 g)*	144	319	447	780	267	181	308	547	308	496	441	237	820
spinach, ckd—*1 cup (140 g)*	81	172	248	437	132	99	176	308	171	274	238	130	820
whole wheat, ckd—*1 cup (140 g)*	97	200	290	510	165	120	155	371	195	323	263	175	820
spinach, refrig, ckd—*2 oz (57 g)*	38	90	124	207	86	53	76	143	84	139	122	61	820
17.12 Pastry Crust													
cream puff shell, homemade—*1 shell (66 g)*	73	242	284	474	328	157	131	308	221	320	312	138	818
phyllo dough—*1 sheet (16½" x 12") (19 g)*	17	37	47	93	30	24	29	68	41	54	55	30	818
pie crust, choc wafer, homemade—*⅛ of 9" crust (27 g)*	21	48	57	98	63	23	27	66	45	70	61	28	I
pie crust, graham, homemade—*⅛ of 9" crust (30 g)*	17	36	46	88	33	22	26	62	39	53	52	28	818
pie crust, plain													
from mix—*⅛ of 9" crust (20 g)*	15	36	49	92	26	23	30	66	36	56	46	28	818
frzn—*⅛ of 9" crust (16 g)*	10	20	27	48	25	12	15	33	20	31	27	14	818
homemade—*⅛ pf 9" crust (23 g)*	18	40	51	102	33	26	31	75	45	59	60	33	818
pie crust, van wafer, homemade,—*⅛ of 9" crust (22 g)*	11	29	36	62	40	17	17	40	27	41	36	18	818
puff pastry, frzn—*1 pastry (40 g)*	34	79	110	206	58	52	67	147	82	125	104	63	818
wonton wrappers—*1 wrapper (7" sq) (8 g)*	9	21	30	55	16	14	18	39	22	33	28	17	818

	TRY	THR	ISO	LEU	LYS	MET	CYS	PHE	TYR	VAL	ARG	HIS	REF
17.13 Rice & Rice Dishes													
brown rice													
long grain, ckd—*1 cup (195 g)*	64	185	213	417	193	113	60	259	189	294	382	129	820
med grain, ckd—*1 cup (195 g)*	59	166	191	372	172	101	55	232	170	265	341	115	820
white rice													
glutinous, ckd—*1 cup (241 g)*	55	174	210	402	176	113	99	260	161	296	405	113	820
long grain, enr, ckd—*1 cup (158 g)*	49	152	183	351	153	100	87	228	142	259	354	100	820
long grain, inst, ckd—*1 cup (165 g)*	40	122	147	281	122	79	69	182	114	208	284	79	820
long grain, parboiled, ckd—*1 cup (175 g)*	47	144	173	333	145	95	82	214	135	245	334	95	820
med grain, enr, ckd—*1 cup (186 g)*	52	158	192	366	160	104	91	236	149	270	368	104	820
short grain, enr, ckd—*1 cup (186 g)*	50	156	190	363	158	104	89	234	147	268	366	104	820
wild rice, ckd—*1 cup (164 g)*	80	208	274	453	279	195	77	320	277	380	505	171	820
17.14 Rolls													
dinner—*1 roll (28 g)*	28	71	96	171	67	43	50	118	71	107	88	52	818
egg—*1 roll (2½") (35 g)*	39	108	138	240	115	65	70	163	102	155	134	73	818
homemade w/ lowfat milk—*1 roll (2½") (35 g)*	37	99	124	224	116	61	57	149	103	141	127	69	818
homemade w/ whole milk—*1 roll (2½") (35 g)*	37	99	123	223	115	60	57	149	102	140	126	69	818
french—*1 roll (38 g)*	38	97	128	231	88	58	69	160	95	144	122	71	818
hamburger/hot dog—*1 roll (43 g)*	43	106	143	258	95	65	78	179	106	161	133	80	818
hamburger/hotdog, mixed-grain—*1 roll (43 g)*	52	121	154	282	109	69	92	197	114	183	174	91	818
hard/kaiser—*1 roll (3½" dia) (57 g)*	67	162	218	395	138	100	123	279	162	246	205	122	818
oat bran—*1 roll (33 g)*	40	90	121	222	89	54	71	157	98	140	135	68	818
popover													
from mix—*1 popover (2" x 2") (33 g)*	31	94	117	200	113	61	58	132	88	132	117	59	818
homemade w/ lowfat milk—*1 popover (2¾" x 4") (40 g)*	43	134	165	280	186	84	66	174	132	186	160	82	818
homemade w/ whole milk—*1 popover (2¾" x 4") (40 g)*	43	134	164	279	185	84	66	174	131	185	160	82	818
rye—*1 roll (28 g)*	34	89	112	202	80	49	61	145	74	133	114	64	818
wheat—*1 roll (28 g)*	33	68	91	168	58	41	56	119	70	107	100	55	818
whole wheat—*1 roll (28 g)*	38	74	94	170	75	39	56	117	74	114	115	58	818
17.15 Stuffing													
bread, from mix—*½ cup (100 g)*	41	97	120	228	96	57	64	161	101	137	136	74	818
bread, homemade—*½ cup (116 g)*	51	128	168	298	123	73	87	205	122	188	167	93	818
cornbread, from mix—*½ cup (100 g)*	31	95	108	256	85	55	57	145	101	132	128	73	818
17.16 Tortillas													
corn—*1 med (6-7" dia) (25 g)*	11	55	52	178	41	30	26	71	59	74	72	44	818
taco shell—*1 med (5" dia) (13 g)*	7	35	34	115	26	20	17	46	38	48	47	29	818
flour—*7-8" dia (35 g)*	37	86	107	210	75	54	63	152	93	125	125	68	818
17.17 Waffles													
buttermilk, homemade—*1 waffle (7" dia) (75 g)*	75	230	286	496	310	140	112	311	226	327	269	148	818
plain													
from complete mix—*1 waffle (7" dia) (75 g)*	53	176	203	394	214	103	89	230	166	239	211	111	818
frzn—*1 waffle (4" sq) (33 g)*	25	64	78	147	64	41	44	102	65	89	88	46	818
homemade—*1 waffle (7" dia) (75 g)*	74	217	272	473	288	134	109	296	220	307	259	140	818
19. INFANT, JUNIOR, & TODDLER FOODS													
19.1 Baked Products													
animal crackers, Gerber—*.3 oz (8 g)*	6	10	17	34	7	7	16	23	8	20	15	11	I
arrowroot cookie, Gerber Graduates—*.2 oz cookie (5 g)*	6	10	13	28	6	7	15	20	8	15	13	7	I

	TRY	THR	ISO	LEU	LYS	MET	CYS	PHE	TYR	VAL	ARG	HIS	REF
banana cookie, Gerber Graduates—.3 oz cookie (8 g)	7	12	19	38	12	11	20	24	9	23	19	12	I
biter biscuit, Gerber Graduates—.4 oz biscuit (11 g)	12	28	38	79	17	16	26	47	19	44	27	19	I
pretzels, Gerber Graduates—.2 oz (6 g)	11	22	28	56	13	12	24	39	14	32	26	15	I
teething biscuit—.4 oz biscuit (11 g)	21	62	93	161	39	30	17	58	73	97	66	44	803
veggie crackers, Gerber Graduates—.3 oz (8 g)	5	14	20	39	11	8	16	37	12	24	20	10	I
zwieback toast, Gerber Graduates—.2 oz piece (7 g)	9	22	30	56	14	14	24	41	17	34	25	15	I
19.2 Cereals													
barley, dry—1 T (2.4 g)	3	9	10	19	9	5	6	16	10	14	14	6	803
Gerber—.5 oz (15 g)	26	59	64	129	70	34	51	108	52	90	93	35	I
barley, prep w/ whole milk—1 oz (28 g)	17	53	67	114	79	29	19	68	57	80	54	33	803
cereal & egg yolks, jr—1 jar (213 g)	58	175	213	366	271	109	60	196	179	260	222	96	803
cereal & egg yolks, str—1 jar (128 g)	35	105	128	220	163	65	36	118	108	156	133	58	803
high protein, dry—1 T (2.4 g)	13	35	42	71	57	15	17	45	34	45	67	24	803
mixed, dry—1 T (2.4 g)	4	10	11	25	10	6	8	16	12	16	17	7	803
Gerber—.5 oz (15 g)	21	35	49	115	39	32	47	78	38	63	66	26	I
mixed, prep w/ whole milk—1 oz (28 g)	18	54	69	125	81	31	23	69	60	82	61	34	803
mixed w/ apples & bananas, Gerber 3rd Foods—6 oz (170 g)	36	61	77	175	85	43	75	117	66	105	133	48	I
mixed w/ applesce & bananas Gerber 2nd Foods—4 oz (113 g)	10	25	33	66	35	20	31	50	24	43	52	17	I
jr—1 jar (170 g)	22	58	73	146	60	41	44	105	73	99	111	46	803
str—1 jar (113 g)	15	40	50	99	41	28	31	71	50	67	76	32	803
mixed w/ bananas, dry—1 T (2.4 g)	3	9	10	23	11	5	5	13	11	14	12	8	803
mixed w/ bananas, dry, Gerber—.5 oz (15 g)	18	31	37	90	35	22	40	51	35	52	67	25	I
mixed w/ bananas, prep w/ whole milk—1 oz (28 g)	17	52	67	121	83	30	16	63	58	80	52	36	803
oatmeal, dry—1 T (2.4 g)	4	11	13	26	14	6	12	13	13	19	25	6	803
Gerber—.5 oz (15 g)	26	59	64	129	70	34	51	108	52	90	93	35	I
oatmeal, prep w/ whole milk—1 oz (28 g)	19	57	73	126	88	32	29	63	63	88	76	32	803
oatmeal w/ apples & cinn, Gerber 3rd Foods—6 oz (170 g)	27	54	68	150	77	36	71	100	54	92	121	39	I
oatmeal w/ apples & cinn, inst, Gerber Graduates—1 oz (28 g)	41	69	94	192	98	49	113	129	61	127	162	50	I
oatmeal w/ applesce & bananas Gerber 2nd Foods—4 oz (113 g)	10	25	33	66	35	20	31	50	24	43	52	17	I
jr—1 jar (170 g)	29	78	83	170	92	53	51	114	88	117	160	58	803
str—1 jar (113 g)	19	52	55	112	60	34	33	75	59	77	105	38	803
oatmeal w/ bananas, dry—1 T (2.4 g)	4	10	12	23	13	6	7	15	12	17	17	9	803
Gerber—.5 oz (15 g)	30	52	62	133	62	32	72	88	57	83	114	39	I
oatmeal w/ bananas, prep w/ whole milk—1 oz (28 g)	18	55	70	122	88	32	20	67	61	84	61	38	803
oatmeal w/ peaches & van, inst, Gerber Graduates—1 oz (28 g)	53	74	104	209	109	52	119	144	67	141	176	55	I
rice, dry—1 T (2.4 g)	2	8	7	13	7	4	4	9	8	11	16	5	803
Gerber—.5 oz (15 g)	17	35	51	100	46	36	35	70	41	70	93	26	I
rice, prep w/ whole milk—1 oz (28 g)	15	50	60	102	76	28	15	54	53	73	58	30	803
rice w/ apples, Gerber 2nd Foods—.5 oz (15 g)	14	21	30	66	34	25	24	40	29	43	61	16	I
rice w/ applesce & bananas, str—1 jar (113 g)	14	45	54	131	77	23	16	66	63	77	45	36	803
rice w/ applesce, Gerber 2nd Foods—4 oz (113 g)	12	21	25	59	38	22	22	37	23	35	55	14	I
rice w/ bananas, dry—1 T (2.4 g)	4	11	11	20	11	5	4	10	9	13	14	7	803
Gerber—.5 oz (15 g)	23	35	37	83	36	31	34	48	31	53	72	23	I

	TRY	THR	ISO	LEU	LYS	MET	CYS	PHE	TYR	VAL	ARG	HIS	REF
rice w/ bananas, prep w/ whole milk—*1 oz (28 g)*	18	56	69	115	83	30	16	56	55	77	56	34	803
rice w/ mixed fruit													
dry, Gerber—*.5 oz (15 g)*	17	30	39	86	36	36	35	50	38	57	81	20	I
Gerber 3rd Foods—*6 oz (170 g)*	27	44	56	124	77	39	29	68	48	73	71	32	I
19.3 Desserts													
banana pudding, str, Heinz—*1 jar (128 g)*								38					I
banana yogurt, Gerber 2nd Foods—*4 oz (113 g)*	13	34	40	90	67	29	17	58	27	54	29	34	I
blueberry buckle, Gerber 3rd Foods—*6 oz (170 g)*	3	5	7	14	7	7	11	10	5	9	11	3	I
cherry cobbler, Gerber 3rd Foods—*6 oz (170 g)*	3	6	10	21	11	7	12	14	6	12	12	6	I
fruit dessert													
Gerber 2nd Foods—*4 oz (113 g)*	2	7	7	14	11	6	5	12	6	10	15	8	I
Gerber 3rd Foods—*6 oz (170 g)*	3	9	9	20	15	8	9	10	7	14	16	9	I
hawaiian delight, Gerber—*4 oz (113 g)*	18	52	68	133	94	46	29	85	43	86	56	33	I
hawaiian delight, Gerber 2nd Foods—*6 oz (170 g)*	32	75	95	184	128	65	41	121	61	121	83	46	I
mixed fruit yogurt, Gerber 2nd Foods—*4 oz (113 g)*	13	29	37	81	63	29	18	38	26	47	34	22	I
orange pudding, str—*1 jar (113 g)*		51	64	128	102	17		47	51	79	96	35	803
peach cobbler													
Gerber 2nd Foods—*4 oz (113 g)*	9	9	8	18	10	11	6	24	6	11	10	6	I
Gerber 3rd Foods—*6 oz (170 g)*	3	15	17	39	26	12	19	24	12	22	20	12	I
raspberry cobbler, Gerber 3rd Foods—*6 oz (170 g)*	3	10	11	14	5	5	7	10	6	10	9	5	I
tutti frutti, jr, Heinz—*1 jar (213 g)*								34					I
tutti frutti, str, Heinz—*1 jar (128 g)*								8					I
van custard pudding													
Gerber 2nd Foods—*4 oz (113 g)*	39	87	114	220	177	71	42	111	78	134	96	50	I
Gerber 3rd Foods—*6 oz (170 g)*	46	116	138	267	185	82	43	131	90	168	109	63	I
jr—*1 jar (170 g)*		100	129	100	194	78		126	100	151	107	70	803
str—*1 jar (113 g)*		67	85	67	129	52		82	67	99	70	46	803
19.4 Dinners													
apples & ham, Gerber Simple Recipe—*4 oz (113 g)*	48	137	146	262	236	102	39	136	90	163	170	128	I
apples & turkey, Gerber Simple Recipe—*4 oz (113 g)*	38	131	151	255	225	134	44	141	86	157	178	102	I
au gratin potatoes & ham, Gerber Graduates—*6 oz (170 g)*	100	232	290	519	446	153	54	295	241	354	334	185	I
beef & egg noodles													
Gerber 2nd Foods—*4 oz (113 g)*	28	100	121	215	172	67	48	136	81	142	178	81	I
Gerber 3rd Foods—*6 oz (170 g)*	43	150	182	323	259	100	71	204	121	213	267	121	I
jr—*1 jar (213 g)*	58	211	294	443	394	113	62	249	198	281	334	158	803
str—*1 jar (128 g)*	32	114	159	238	212	60	33	134	106	151	180	84	803
beef & rice, toddler—*1 jar (177 g)*	81	354	434	694	666	218	96	349	285	487	598	227	803
beef lasagna, toddler—*1 jar (177 g)*	83	289	365	573	526	145	85	322	234	409	448	181	803
beef stew, toddler—*1 jar (177 g)*	94	372	435	687	697	251	94	356	281	481	625	227	803
broccoli & chicken, Gerber Simple Recipe—*4 oz (113 g)*	65	188	185	305	322	94	53	197	143	213	253	95	I
carrots & beef, Gerber Simple Recipe—*4 oz (113 g)*	48	155	156	279	266	100	46	148	103	178	238	135	I
carrots & white turkey, diced, Gerber Graduates—*2.1 oz (60 g)*	65	184	209	344	387	108	52	196	133	215	261	142	I
carrots, broccoli, & cheese w/ rice, Gerber Veggie Recipes—*4 oz (113 g)*	57	117	132	279	183	77	37	145	124	170	130	68	I
carrots, zucchini, & egg noodles, Gerber Veggie Recipes—*4 oz (113 g)*	39	67	108	200	155	54	58	119	83	132	138	45	I
cheese ravioli w/ tomato sce, Gerber Graduates—*6 oz (170 g)*	70	189	233	444	260	107	111	287	180	279	197	121	I

	TRY	THR	ISO	LEU	LYS	MET	CYS	PHE	TYR	VAL	ARG	HIS	REF
chicken & noodles													
Gerber 2nd Foods—*4 oz (113 g)*	32	110	126	231	179	75	68	137	88	142	204	76	I
Gerber 3rd Foods—*6 oz (170 g)*	53	138	150	282	208	100	245	187	114	177	253	82	I
jr—*1 jar (213 g)*	47	173	213	351	300	83	51	190	153	243	266	100	803
str—*1 jar (128 g)*	31	113	141	230	198	54	35	125	101	160	175	67	803
chicken stew, toddler—*1 jar (170 g)*	97	376	437	689	697	190	88	362	292	496	563	218	803
chicken stew w/ noodles, Gerber Graduates—*6 oz (170 g)*	73	274	298	524	478	163	167	306	196	333	425	255	I
chicken w/ broccoli in cheese sce, Gerber Graduates—*6 oz (170 g)*	117	236	291	526	500	167	71	272	230	335	276	218	I
corn & chicken, diced, Gerber Graduates—*2.5 oz (71 g)*	70	167	227	460	387	142	87	213	159	250	273	143	I
garden veg & pasta, Gerber Veggie Recipes—*4 oz (113 g)*	52	102	113	216	147	53	42	126	85	139	156	56	I
green beans & turkey, Gerber Simple Recipe—*4 oz (113 g)*	70	209	321	374	330	118	51	242	154	237	271	151	I
green beans & white turkey, diced, Gerber Graduates—*2.3 oz (65 g)*	75	192	218	357	404	122	60	206	138	228	268	149	I
harvest veg stew, Gerber Veggie Recipes—*4 oz (113 g)*	55	81	110	230	147	59	42	125	91	135	110	56	I
italian spaghetti in tomato sce w/ beef, Gerber 3rd Foods—*6 oz (170 g)*	65	129	146	311	177	87	87	194	116	174	192	104	I
lasagna w/ meat sce, Gerber 3rd Foods—*6 oz (170 g)*	40	111	127	234	185	70	60	133	87	148	155	81	I
macaroni & beef, in sce, Gerber Graduates—*6 oz (170 g)*	78	269	303	492	444	158	121	390	201	340	420	223	I
macaroni & cheese													
Gerber 2nd Foods—*4 oz (113 g)*	40	99	139	256	155	90	161	151	116	175	112	64	I
jr—*1 jar (213 g)*	68	166	277	498	315	192	68	281	262	313	217	132	803
str—*1 jar (128 g)*	41	100	166	300	189	115	41	169	157	188	131	79	803
macaroni, tomato, & beef													
Gerber 2nd Foods—*4 oz (113 g)*	26	96	109	202	139	64	45	119	81	126	142	68	I
jr—*1 jar (213 g)*	60	192	251	422	317	83	72	239	175	271	283	136	803
str—*1 jar (128 g)*	32	104	137	229	173	46	40	129	95	147	154	74	803
pasta shells & cheese, Gerber Graduates—*6 oz (170 g)*	77	198	254	493	320	135	93	324	217	315	211	120	I
pears & chicken, Gerber 2nd Foods—*4 oz (113 g)*	44	109	132	227	200	85	42	143	75	145	155	60	I
peas & chicken, diced, Gerber Graduates—*2.3 oz (65 g)*	97	233	261	447	498	139	74	241	169	278	385	154	I
spaghetti, tomato, & meat, toddler—*1 jar (177 g)*	115	349	474	731	554	184	117	427	326	506	503	250	803
spaghetti w/ mini meatballs & sce, Gerber Graduates—*6 oz (170 g)*	94	301	333	599	463	156	129	340	218	379	413	208	I
sweet potatoes & turkey, Gerber Simple Recipe—*4 oz (113 g)*	76	181	189	336	297	100	52	204	127	215	220	108	I
turkey & rice													
Gerber 2nd Foods—*4 oz (113 g)*	28	97	100	180	150	78	44	136	75	113	150	58	I
jr—*1 jar (213 g)*	40	158	192	307	309	104	40	162	138	217	281	92	803
str—*1 jar (128 g)*	26	100	122	195	196	67	26	102	87	137	178	58	803
turkey stew (white) w/ rice, Gerber Graduates—*6 oz (170 g)*	68	233	235	439	418	141	124	230	172	264	395	211	I
turkey w/ garden veg & rice, Gerber 3rd Foods—*6 oz (170 g)*	54	145	170	313	272	104	66	192	116	187	321	122	I
veg & bacon													
Gerber 2nd Foods—*4 oz (113 g)*	32	75	92	162	126	39	36	109	68	108	151	61	I
Gerber 3rd Foods—*6 oz (170 g)*	48	116	134	243	191	57	54	156	98	157	228	88	I
jr—*1 jar (213 g)*	36	130	175	273	232	79	55	164	121	207	258	85	803
str—*1 jar (128 g)*	19	69	84	133	109	41	29	79	70	109	142	44	803
veg & beef													
Gerber 2nd Foods—*4 oz (113 g)*	36	105	118	217	196	64	47	129	82	136	230	84	I
Gerber 3rd Foods—*6 oz (170 g)*	76	140	173	307	253	94	72	190	120	205	281	120	I

	TRY	THR	ISO	LEU	LYS	MET	CYS	PHE	TYR	VAL	ARG	HIS	REF
jr—1 jar (213 g)	49	181	213	345	358	81	49	175	130	256	302	113	803
str—1 jar (128 g)	26	91	106	173	179	41	24	87	65	128	151	56	803
veg & chicken													
Gerber 2nd Foods—4 oz (113 g)	34	102	111	211	198	58	42	119	81	126	200	61	I
Gerber 3rd Foods—6 oz (170 g)	51	129	122	236	185	83	60	126	94	143	197	63	I
str—1 jar (128 g)	27	88	116	174	155	46	35	100	76	133	151	49	803
veg & ham													
Gerber 2nd Foods—4 oz (113 g)	20	68	81	149	118	59	35	95	61	98	125	59	I
Gerber 3rd Foods—6 oz (170 g)	48	119	134	276	245	68	49	129	105	158	213	107	I
jr—1 jar (213 g)	55	194	232	381	354	109	55	194	158	271	343	141	803
str—1 jar (128 g)	23	84	100	165	152	47	23	84	68	118	148	60	803
veg & lamb													
jr—1 jar (213 g)	51	164	202	330	328	66	38	177	141	217	300	102	803
str—1 jar (128 g)	29	93	115	188	187	38	22	101	79	124	170	59	803
veg & turkey													
Gerber 2nd Foods—4 oz (113 g)	29	113	113	206	175	78	48	168	85	130	177	69	I
Gerber 3rd Foods—6 oz (170 g)	40	106	124	217	196	66	43	140	91	144	196	67	I
jr—1 jar (213 g)	38	145	175	281	266	81	38	136	124	204	228	77	803
str—1 jar (128 g)	23	84	102	165	156	47	23	79	73	120	134	45	803
toddler—1 jar (177 g)	106	329	441	689	586	156	92	354	308	492	522	202	803
veg pasta, Gerber 3rd Foods—6 oz (170 g)	58	129	156	291	180	82	71	170	116	192	160	77	I
veg stew w/ beef, Gerber Graduates—6 oz (170 g)	97	240	318	589	595	165	87	332	216	367	543	199	I
19.5 Fruit Juices													
apple w/ yogurt, Gerber 2nd Foods—4 fl oz (124 g)	42	72	118	225	183	70	29	116	86	144	86	55	I
apple apricot, str, Heinz—1 jar (130 g)								4					I
apple carrot, Gerber 3rd Foods—4 fl oz (125 g)	1	5	6	9	9	3	3	6	4	8	13	1	I
apple peach, Gerber 2nd Foods—4 oz (127 g)	1	2	3	3	4	1	3	3	1	3	3	1	I
apple pineapple, str, Heinz—1 jar (130 g)								7					I
apple sweet potato, Gerber 3rd Foods—4 fl oz (125 g)	4	11	11	17	16	6	6	14	8	16	12	5	I
banana medley w/ yogurt, Gerber 2nd Foods—4 fl oz (124 g)	43	83	125	245	193	79	36	124	89	156	122	76	I
mixed fruit, w/ yogurt, Gerber 2nd Foods—4 fl oz (124 g)	43	83	112	221	168	70	27	108	86	139	94	60	I
mixed tropical fruit, Gerber—4 fl oz (127 g)	4	11	12	24	22	17	11	16	11	17	47	14	I
orange banana pineapple, Gerber—4 fl oz (127 g)	3	27	14	32	26	13	9	16	10	24	66	23	I
pineapple carrot, Gerber 3rd Foods—4 fl oz (125 g)	4	14	15	23	26	13	11	14	14	21	24	8	I
white grape, Gerber 1st Foods—4 fl oz (127 g)	3	4	2	4	3	1	5	2	3	4	84	6	I
19.6 Fruits													
apple banana, Gerber 3rd Foods—6 oz (170 g)	6	15	21	50	35	12	14	23	12	36	28	35	I
apple blueberry, Gerber 2nd Foods—4 oz (113 g)	1	7	7	12	11	5	6	7	5	9	8	5	I
apple cinn fruit bar, Gerber Graduates—.3 oz (9 g)	7	12	19	36	12	11	17	22	8	23	21	8	I
apples & apricots, jr, Heinz—1 jar (213 g)								26					I
str, Heinz—1 jar (128 g)								15					I
apples & cranberries w/ tapioca, jr, Heinz—1 jar (213 g)								4					I

	TRY	THR	ISO	LEU	LYS	MET	CYS	PHE	TYR	VAL	ARG	HIS	REF
apples & cranberries w/ tapioca, str, Heinz—1 jar (128 g)								3					I
apples & pears, jr, Heinz—1 jar (213 g)								11					I
str, Heinz—1 jar (128 g)								6					I
apples, diced, Gerber Graduates—4.5 oz (128 g)	6	5	4	9	6	3	4	14	4	6	38	5	I
banana & pineapple, Gerber 3rd Foods—6 oz (170 g)	14	43	48	131	66	37	32	43	29	85	88	88	I
banana strawberry, Gerber 3rd Foods—6 oz (170 g)	8	42	37	127	100	19	26	36	22	79	71	111	I
banana van w/ tapioca, Gerber—4 oz (113 g)	7	14	16	41	34	14	12	17	10	25	18	19	I
bananas													
Gerber 1st Foods—2.5 oz (71 g)	4	19	23	66	31	14	15	37	11	44	37	57	I
Gerber 2nd Foods—4 oz (113 g)	3	32	26	101	48	20	23	36	16	63	56	82	I
bananas, apples, & pears, Gerber 2nd Foods—4 oz (113 g)	2	24	33	88	45	17	20	40	15	57	48	71	I
bananas w/ apples & pears, Gerber 3rd Foods—6 oz (170 g)	2	48	34	134	68	29	31	75	24	78	70	114	I
fruit salad, Gerber 3rd Foods—6 oz (170 g)	7	12	17	31	27	10	14	17	10	22	17	14	I
peaches, diced, Gerber Graduates—4.5 oz (128 g)	4	11	8	17	17	7	10	22	8	12	45	8	I
Gerber 1st Foods—2.5 oz (71 g)	6	11	9	16	16	6	7	13	6	11	10	6	I
Gerber 2nd Foods—4 oz (113 g)	15	27	22	42	41	15	18	69	15	29	26	15	I
Gerber 3rd Foods—6 oz (170 g)	22	41	32	63	61	22	27	104	22	44	39	22	I
pears													
diced, Gerber Graduates—4.5 oz (128 g)	11	9	8	15	11	4	5	14	6	11	51	6	I
Gerber 2nd Foods—4 oz (113 g)	6	9	14	24	20	5	5	14	8	16	14	6	I
Gerber 3rd Foods—6 oz (170 g)	10	17	17	32	26	14	10	37	10	22	19	10	I
plums & apples, Gerber 3rd Foods—6 oz (170 g)	15	16	15	29	25	7	11	36	10	19	17	10	I
prunes & apples, Gerber 2nd Foods—4 oz (113 g)	11	11	12	23	18	7	9	23	9	15	12	7	I
prunes, Gerber 1st Foods—2.5 oz (71 g)	6	11	13	23	16	6	6	28	9	18	20	10	I
strawberry fruit bar, Gerber Graduates—.3 oz (9 g)	7	12	20	37	13	12	18	23	8	23	20	9	I
19.7 Meats													
beef													
& gravy, Gerber 2nd Foods—2.5 oz (71 g)	121	375	366	665	707	228	116	358	257	402	579	315	I
jr—1 jar (99 g)	145	629	652	1150	1194	441	167	555	477	726	978	487	803
str—1 jar (99 g)	136	591	613	1080	1122	414	157	522	448	681	919	457	803
chicken													
& gravy, Gerber 2nd Foods—2.5 oz (71 g)	138	356	355	623	685	222	98	321	234	369	499	311	I
jr—1 jar (99 g)	165	653	686	1125	1216	390	191	593	466	733	1018	441	803
str—1 jar (99 g)	154	609	639	1047	1133	363	178	552	435	682	947	411	803
chicken sticks, jr—1 jar (71 g)	83	406	518	811	824	229	90	478	353	542	712	328	803
chicken sticks, toddler, Gerber—2.5 oz (71 g)	97	505	493	866	875	295	131	461	372	526	710	382	I
ham													
Gerber 2nd Foods—2.5 oz (71 g)	138	352	348	63	598	209	102	323	250	375	536	354	I
jr—1 jar (99 g)	148	649	711	1196	1270	382	184	570	501	771	1012	509	803
str—1 jar (99 g)	137	597	654	1100	1168	351	169	525	461	709	931	467	803
lamb													
Gerber 2nd Foods—2.5 oz (71 g)	136	415	361	668	692	230	119	324	271	395	585	240	I
jr—1 jar (99 g)	149	686	707	1188	1336	471	207	592	527	762	986	380	803
str—1 jar (99 g)	139	636	655	1101	1237	437	192	548	488	707	914	352	803
meat sticks, Gerber Graduates—2.5 oz (71 g)	96	450	445	793	778	255	116	432	357	484	606	301	I

	TRY	THR	ISO	LEU	LYS	MET	CYS	PHE	TYR	VAL	ARG	HIS	REF
meat sticks, jr—*1 jar (71 g)*	65	413	474	740	734	219	52	431	370	491	618	327	803
pork, str—*1 jar (99 g)*	135	611	673	1116	1146	394	152	564	505	695	939	443	803
turkey													
& gravy, Gerber 2nd Foods—*2.5 oz (71 g)*	117	317	326	569	605	209	101	301	223	337	499	220	I
jr—*1 jar (99 g)*	158	674	764	1213	1261	472	185	628	536	774	969	389	803
str—*1 jar (99 g)*	148	627	710	1127	1172	439	172	584	498	720	900	362	803
turkey sticks, Gerber Graduates—*2.5 oz (71 g)*	5	17	460	800	810	298	132	430	13	24	660	285	I
turkey sticks, jr—*1 jar (71 g)*	72	388	447	760	835	216	87	433	343	462	627	261	803
veal													
& gravy, Gerber 2nd Foods—*2.5 oz (71 g)*	128	330	318	581	618	211	108	301	224	358	524	258	I
jr—*1 jar (99 g)*	174	632	682	1168	1215	334	196	585	484	736	1004	464	803
str—*1 jar (99 g)*	154	558	604	1034	1074	295	173	518	428	650	888	411	803
19.8 Vegetables													
beets, str—*1 jar (128 g)*	15	41	49	59	44	13	9	23	45	58	38	27	803
broccoli w/ carrots & cheese, Gerber 3rd Foods—*6 oz (170 g)*	27	85	99	187	116	107	52	110	94	134	131	50	I
carrots													
diced, Gerber Graduates—*2.5 oz (71 g)*	5	17	18	31	23	9	7	27	13	24	26	8	I
Gerber 1st Foods—*2.5 oz (71 g)*	7	21	21	32	20	15	9	19	13	29	27	10	I
Gerber 2nd Foods—*4 oz (113 g)*	10	29	29	44	27	20	12	26	18	40	37	14	I
Gerber 3rd Foods—*6 oz (170 g)*	15	48	48	71	46	34	20	43	29	65	61	22	I
jr—*1 jar (213 g)*	23	49	51	70	45	19	13	53	43	66	111	28	803
str—*1 jar (128 g)*	14	28	31	41	26	12	8	31	24	38	64	15	803
corn, creamed													
Gerber 2nd Foods—*4 oz (113 g)*	23	62	79	196	79	52	35	111	71	100	83	51	I
jr—*1 jar (213 g)*	32	111	138	300	175	85	38	104	145	166	128	98	803
str—*1 jar (128 g)*	19	67	83	179	104	51	23	63	86	99	77	59	803
garden veg													
Gerber 2nd Foods—*4 oz (113 g)*	27	95	92	168	145	39	34	113	68	112	210	42	I
str—*1 jar (128 g)*	35	93	110	183	148	55	26	113	122	127	251	58	803
green beans													
creamed, jr—*1 jar (213 g)*	32	81	102	166	92	47	23	96	92	124	102	49	803
diced, Gerber Graduates—*2.5 oz (71 g)*	11	35	41	74	58	15	11	45	31	51	47	22	I
Gerber 1st Foods—*2.5 oz (71 g)*	17	38	35	70	47	43	17	47	29	48	43	24	I
Gerber 2nd Foods—*4 oz (113 g)*	32	65	59	108	69	28	25	70	46	77	65	33	I
jr—*1 jar (206 g)*	29	105	111	161	122	37	21	101	87	134	136	68	803
str—*1 jar (128 g)*	19	70	74	109	83	24	14	68	59	91	92	46	803
w/ rice, Gerber 3rd Foods—*6 oz (170 g)*	29	65	71	141	77	41	41	90	66	94	99	36	I
mixed veg													
diced, Gerber Graduates—*2.5 oz (71 g)*	13	50	47	107	59	21	19	54	35	58	73	24	I
Gerber 2nd Foods—*4 oz (113 g)*	15	39	48	84	46	37	32	65	39	64	82	24	I
Gerber 3rd Foods—*6 oz (170 g)*	31	78	73	121	105	34	31	102	63	107	129	37	I
jr—*1 jar (213 g)*	32	96	119	194	100	45	60	117	111	147	198	66	803
str—*1 jar (128 g)*	17	49	60	99	51	23	31	60	56	74	101	33	803
peas													
Gerber 1st Foods—*2.5 oz (71 g)*	20	89	84	144	131	29	28	83	52	101	241	40	I
Gerber 2nd Foods—*4 oz (113 g)*	34	140	128	220	211	43	43	139	82	153	346	61	I
Gerber Graduates—*2.5 oz (71 g)*	26	116	117	212	196	32	27	130	79	136	258	53	I
str—*1 jar (128 g)*	44	174	193	301	300	51	33	183	152	216	498	96	803
w/ rice, Gerber 3rd Foods—*6 oz (170 g)*	46	160	168	295	265	66	67	219	114	204	423	65	I
potatoes, diced, Gerber Graduates—*2.5 oz (71 g)*	9	28	27	49	41	16	13	39	25	39	38	12	I

	TRY	THR	ISO	LEU	LYS	MET	CYS	PHE	TYR	VAL	ARG	HIS	REF
potatoes, Gerber 1st Foods—*2.5 oz (71 g)*	13	15	23	37	35	11	9	28	23	36	37	13	I
spinach, creamed, Gerber 2nd Foods—*4 oz (113 g)*	45	134	159	299	189	85	56	173	133	180	172	71	I
spinach, creamed, str—*1 jar (128 g)*	46	129	143	283	189	70	40	123	147	193	195	82	803
squash													
Gerber 2nd Foods—*4 oz (113 g)*	17	28	34	54	39	22	23	52	24	37	51	16	I
Gerber 3rd Foods—*6 oz (170 g)*	15	31	37	63	43	16	18	36	26	43	45	16	I
jr—*1 jar (213 g)*	26	53	70	102	66	23	15	62	60	77	100	34	803
str—*1 jar (128 g)*	15	32	42	60	40	13	9	37	36	46	59	20	803
sweet potatoes													
Gerber 1st Foods—*2.5 oz (71 g)*	11	30	22	36	21	13	16	48	18	34	22	12	I
Gerber 2nd Foods—*4 oz (113 g)*	17	49	40	64	37	23	22	70	29	56	38	21	I
Gerber 3rd Foods—*6 oz (170 g)*	39	87	78	121	66	41	32	105	54	111	70	41	I
jr—*1 jar (170 g)*	36	90	85	129	73	39	26	104	68	121	90	43	803
str—*1 jar (113 g)*	25	61	58	88	50	27	17	70	46	82	61	29	803

20. MEAT ANALOGUE PRODUCTS

	TRY	THR	ISO	LEU	LYS	MET	CYS	PHE	TYR	VAL	ARG	HIS	REF
bacon, simulated meat product—*1 strip (8 g)*	13	36	45	73	58	12	14	49	32	47	70	24	816
meat extender, simulated meat product—*1 oz (28 g)*	163	458	566	925	736	147	178	619	405	600	885	303	816
sausage, simulated meat product,													
—*1 link (25 g)*	70	196	243	397	316	63	76	265	174	257	380	130	816
—*1 patty (38 g)*	106	298	369	603	480	96	116	403	264	391	577	197	816

21. MEATS
21.1 Beef

	TRY	THR	ISO	LEU	LYS	MET	CYS	PHE	TYR	VAL	ARG	HIS	REF
breakfast strips, ckd—*3 slices (34 g)*	97	402	460	782	816	247	136	383	347	468	657	339	813
brisket, flat half													
sep lean & fat, braised, 0" fat trim—*3.5 oz (100 g)*	341	1331	1370	2409	2536	780	341	1190	1024	1482	1926	1043	813
sep lean & fat, braised, ¼" fat trim—*3.5 oz (100 g)*	281	1094	1126	1980	2084	641	281	978	842	1218	1583	858	813
sep lean, braised, 0" fat trim—*3.5 oz (100 g)*	353	1377	1417	2491	2622	807	353	1230	1059	1533	1992	1079	813
sep lean, braised, ¼" fat trim—*3.5 oz (100 g)*	353	1377	1417	2491	2622	807	353	1230	1059	1533	1992	1079	813
brisket, point half													
sep lean & fat, braised, 0" fat trim—*3.5 oz (100 g)*	263	1028	1058	1859	1957	602	263	918	790	1144	1487	806	813
sep lean & fat, braised, ¼" fat trim—*3.5 oz (100 g)*	248	967	995	1749	1842	567	248	864	744	1077	1399	758	813
sep lean, braised, 0" fat trim—*3.5 oz (100 g)*	314	1225	1261	2217	2334	718	314	1095	942	1364	1773	960	813
sep lean, braised, ¼" fat trim—*3.5 oz (100 g)*	314	1225	1261	2217	2334	718	314	1095	942	1364	1773	960	813
brisket, whole													
sep lean & fat, braised, 0" fat trim—*3.5 oz (100 g)*	300	1170	1205	2118	2229	686	300	1046	900	1303	1693	917	813
sep lean & fat, braised, ¼" fat trim—*3.5 oz (100 g)*	263	1027	1057	1858	1956	602	263	918	790	1143	1485	805	813
sep lean, braised, 0" fat trim—*3.5 oz (100 g)*	333	1299	1338	2351	2475	762	333	1161	1000	1447	1880	1019	813
sep lean, braised, ¼" fat trim—*3.5 oz (100 g)*	333	1299	1338	2351	2475	762	333	1161	1000	1447	1880	1019	813
chuck arm pot roast, sep lean													
braised, choice, 0" fat trim—*3.5 oz (100 g)*	370	1442	1485	2610	2747	845	370	1289	1109	1606	2087	1131	813
braised, choice, ¼" fat trim—*3.5 oz (100 g)*	370	1442	1485	2610	2747	845	370	1289	1109	1606	2087	1131	813
braised, select, 0" fat trim—*3.5 oz (100 g)*	370	1442	1485	2610	2747	845	370	1289	1109	1606	2087	1131	813

	TRY	THR	ISO	LEU	LYS	MET	CYS	PHE	TYR	VAL	ARG	HIS	REF
braised, select, ¼" fat trim—3.5 oz (100 g)	370	1442	1485	2610	2747	845	370	1289	1109	1606	2087	1131	813
chuck arm pot roast, sep lean & fat													
braised, choice, 0" fat trim—3.5 oz (100 g)	330	1286	1324	2327	2449	754	330	1149	989	1432	1861	1008	813
braised, choice, ¼" fat trim—3.5 oz (100 g)	302	1178	1213	2132	2245	691	302	1053	906	1312	1705	924	813
braised, select, 0" fat trim—3.5 oz (100 g)	337	1315	1354	2380	2505	771	337	1176	1012	1465	1903	1031	813
braised, select, ¼" fat trim—3.5 oz (100 g)	312	1218	1253	2203	2319	714	312	1088	937	1356	1762	954	813
chuck blade roast, sep lean													
braised, choice, 0" fat trim—3.5 oz (100 g)	348	1357	1397	2455	2584	795	348	1213	1044	1511	1963	1064	813
braised, choice, ¼" fat trim—3.5 oz (100 g)	348	1357	1397	2455	2584	795	348	1213	1044	1511	1963	1064	813
braised, select, 0" fat trim—3.5 oz (100 g)	348	1357	1397	2455	2584	795	348	1213	1044	1511	1963	1064	813
braised, select, ¼" fat trim—3.5 oz (100 g)	348	1357	1397	2455	2584	795	348	1213	1044	1511	1963	1064	813
chuck blade roast, sep lean & fat, braised, choice, 0" fat trim—3.5 oz (100 g)	302	1178	1213	2132	2245	691	302	1053	907	1312	1705	924	813
braised, choice, ¼" fat trim—3.5 oz (100 g)	293	1143	1176	2068	2177	670	293	1021	879	1273	1654	896	813
braised, select, 0" fat trim—3.5 oz (100 g)	309	1205	1241	2181	2296	706	309	1077	927	1342	1744	945	813
braised, select, ¼" fat trim—3.5 oz (100 g)	302	1178	1213	2132	2245	691	302	1053	907	1312	1705	924	813
corned beef, cured brisket, ckd—3.5 oz (100 g)	166	686	785	1334	1392	421	232	654	593	799	1122	578	813
flank, choice													
sep lean & fat, braised, 0" fat trim—3.5 oz (100 g)	302	1178	1213	2132	2244	691	302	1053	906	1312	1705	924	813
sep lean & fat, broiled, 0" fat trim—3.5 oz (100 g)	296	1154	1188	2088	2198	676	296	1031	888	1285	1670	905	813
sep lean, braised, 0" fat trim—3.5 oz (100 g)	314	1224	1260	2215	2331	717	314	1094	941	1363	1771	959	813
sep lean, broiled, 0" fat trim—3.5 oz (100 g)	303	1183	1217	2140	2253	693	303	1057	910	1317	1711	927	813
ground, extra lean													
baked, med—3.5 oz (100 g)	274	1069	1100	1934	2036	626	274	955	822	1190	1546	838	813
baked, well done—3.5 oz (100 g)	339	1324	1362	2395	2521	776	339	1183	1018	1474	1915	1037	813
broiled, med—3.5 oz (100 g)	284	1109	1142	2008	2113	650	284	992	853	1235	1605	870	813
broiled, well done—3.5 oz (100 g)	320	1248	1285	2259	2378	732	320	1116	960	1390	1806	979	813
pan fried, med—3.5 oz (100 g)	280	1090	1122	1973	2077	639	280	975	839	1214	1578	855	813
pan fried, well done—3.5 oz (100 g)	313	1222	1258	2212	2329	716	313	1093	940	1361	1769	958	813
ground, lean													
baked, med—3.5 oz (100 g)	268	1045	1076	1892	1991	613	268	934	804	1164	1512	819	813
baked, well done—3.5 oz (100 g)	332	1293	1331	2340	2463	758	332	1156	995	1440	1871	1014	813
broiled, med—3.5 oz (100 g)	277	1080	1111	1954	2057	633	277	965	831	1202	1562	846	813
broiled, well done—3.5 oz (100 g)	316	1232	1268	2229	2346	722	316	1101	948	1372	1782	966	813
pan fried, med—3.5 oz (100 g)	271	1058	1089	1915	2016	620	271	946	814	1179	1531	830	813
pan fried, well done—3.5 oz (100 g)	309	1206	1241	2182	2296	707	309	1078	927	1342	1744	945	813
ground, regular													
baked, med—3.5 oz (100 g)	255	993	1022	1797	1892	582	255	888	764	1106	1437	779	813
baked, well done—3.5 oz (100 g)	323	1258	1295	2276	2396	737	323	1124	968	1401	1820	986	813
broiled, med—3.5 oz (100 g)	270	1051	1082	1902	2003	616	270	940	809	1171	1521	824	813
broiled, well done—3.5 oz (100 g)	305	1188	1223	2150	2263	696	305	1062	914	1323	1719	931	813
pan fried, med—3.5 oz (100 g)	268	1045	1075	1891	1990	612	268	934	804	1163	1512	819	813
pan-fried, well done—3.5 oz (100 g)	302	1179	1214	2134	2246	691	302	1054	907	1313	1706	924	813

	TRY	THR	ISO	LEU	LYS	MET	CYS	PHE	TYR	VAL	ARG	HIS	REF
rib eye, small end (ribs 10-12), choice, broiled, sep lean & fat, 0" fat trim—3.5 oz (100 g)	279	1088	1120	1969	2072	638	279	972	837	1212	1574	853	813
rib eye, small end (ribs 10-12), choice, broiled, sep lean, 0" fat trim—3.5 oz (100 g)	314	1225	1261	2216	2333	718	314	1095	942	1364	1772	960	813
rib, large end (ribs 6-9), sep lean													
choice, broiled, ¼" fat trim—3.5 oz (100 g)	282	1099	1132	1989	2094	644	282	983	846	1224	1591	862	813
choice, roasted, 0" fat trim—3.5 oz (100 g)	308	1203	1238	2176	2291	705	308	1075	925	1339	1740	943	813
choice, roasted, ¼" fat trim—3.5 oz (100 g)	308	1203	1238	2176	2291	705	308	1075	925	1339	1740	943	813
prime, broiled, ¼" fat trim—3.5 oz (100 g)	276	1076	1108	1948	2050	631	276	962	828	1198	1557	844	813
prime, roasted, ¼" fat trim—3.5 oz (100 g)	308	1203	1238	2176	2291	705	308	1075	925	1339	1740	943	813
select, broiled, ¼" fat trim—3.5 oz (100 g)	282	1099	1132	1989	2094	644	282	983	846	1224	1591	862	813
select, roasted, ¼" fat trim—3.5 oz (100 g)	308	1203	1238	2176	2291	705	308	1075	925	1339	1740	943	813
rib, large end (ribs 6-9), sep lean & fat,													
choice, broiled, ¼" fat trim—3.5 oz (100 g)	235	915	942	1657	1744	537	235	818	704	1019	1325	718	813
choice, roasted, 0" fat trim—3.5 oz (100 g)	255	996	1025	1802	1897	584	255	890	766	1109	1441	781	813
choice, roasted, ¼" fat trim—3.5 oz (100 g)	250	974	1003	1762	1855	571	250	871	749	1085	1409	763	813
prime, broiled, ¼" fat trim—3.5 oz (100 g)	227	887	913	1605	1689	520	227	793	682	988	1283	695	813
prime, roasted, ¼" fat trim—3.5 oz (100 g)	252	981	1010	1776	1869	575	252	877	755	1093	1420	769	813
select, broiled, ¼" fat trim—3.5 oz (100 g)	241	941	968	1702	1792	551	241	841	724	1048	1361	737	813
select, roasted, ¼" fat trim—3.5 oz (100 g)	259	1011	1040	1829	1925	592	259	903	778	1126	1463	792	813
rib, shortribs, sep lean & fat, braised—3.5 oz (100 g)	242	942	969	1704	1794	552	242	842	725	1049	1363	738	813
rib, shortribs, sep lean, braised—3.5 oz (100 g)	344	1343	1383	2431	2559	787	344	1201	1033	1496	1944	1053	813
rib, small end (ribs 10-12), sep lean,													
choice, broiled, 0" fat trim—3.5 oz (100 g)	314	1225	1261	2216	2333	718	314	1095	942	1364	1772	960	813
choice, broiled, ¼" fat trim—3.5 oz (100 g)	314	1225	1261	2216	2333	718	314	1095	942	1364	1772	960	813
choice, roasted, ¼" fat trim—3.5 oz (100 g)	301	1172	1207	2122	2233	687	301	1048	902	1306	1696	919	813
prime, broiled, ¼" fat trim—3.5 oz (100 g)	314	1225	1261	2216	2333	718	314	1095	942	1364	1772	960	813
prime, roasted, ¼" fat trim—3.5 oz (100 g)	299	1168	1202	2113	2225	684	299	1044	898	1301	1690	915	813
select, broiled, 0" fat trim—3.5 oz (100 g)	314	1225	1261	2216	2333	718	314	1095	942	1364	1772	960	813
select, broiled, ¼" fat trim—3.5 oz (100 g)	314	1225	1261	2216	2333	718	314	1095	942	1364	1772	960	813
select, roasted, ¼" fat trim—3.5 oz (100 g)	301	1172	1207	2122	2233	687	301	1048	902	1306	1696	919	813
rib, small end (ribs 10-12), sep lean & fat													
choice, broiled, 0" fat trim—3.5 oz (100 g)	277	1080	1112	1955	2058	633	277	966	831	1203	1563	847	813
choice, broiled, ¼" fat trim—3.5 oz (100 g)	263	1027	1057	1859	1957	602	263	918	790	1144	1486	805	813
choice, roasted, ¼" fat trim—3.5 oz (100 g)	246	960	988	1738	1829	563	246	858	739	1069	1389	753	813

	TRY	THR	ISO	LEU	LYS	MET	CYS	PHE	TYR	VAL	ARG	HIS	REF
prime, broiled, ¼" fat trim—3.5 oz (100 g)	267	1042	1073	1886	1986	611	267	932	802	1161	1508	817	813
prime, roasted, ¼" fat trim—3.5 oz (100 g)	245	957	985	1732	1823	561	245	855	736	1066	1385	750	813
select, broiled, 0" fat trim—3.5 oz (100 g)	279	1088	1120	1969	2072	638	279	972	837	1212	1574	853	813
select, broiled, ¼" fat trim—3.5 oz (100 g)	267	1042	1073	1886	1986	611	267	932	802	1161	1508	817	813
select, roasted, ¼" fat trim—3.5 oz (100 g)	252	981	1010	1776	1869	575	252	877	755	1093	1420	769	813
rib, whole (ribs 6-12), sep lean													
choice, broiled, ¼" fat trim—3.5 oz (100 g)	295	1151	1184	2082	2192	674	295	1028	885	1281	1665	902	813
choice, roasted, ¼" fat trim—3.5 oz (100 g)	305	1190	1225	2154	2267	698	305	1064	916	1325	1722	933	813
prime, broiled, ¼" fat trim—3.5 oz (100 g)	291	1137	1170	2057	2165	666	291	1016	874	1266	1645	891	813
prime, roasted, ¼" fat trim—3.5 oz (100 g)	305	1188	1223	2150	2264	697	305	1062	914	1323	1720	932	813
select, broiled, ¼" fat trim—3.5 oz (100 g)	295	1150	1184	2081	2191	674	295	1028	885	1281	1664	902	813
select, roasted, ¼" fat trim—3.5 oz (100 g)	305	1190	1225	2154	2267	698	305	1064	916	1325	1722	933	813
rib, whole (ribs 6-12), sep lean & fat													
choice, broiled, ¼" fat trim—3.5 oz (100 g)	246	960	988	1737	1828	563	246	858	738	1069	1389	752	813
prime, broiled, ¼" fat trim—3.5 oz (100 g)	243	949	977	1717	1807	556	243	848	730	1056	1373	744	813
prime, roasted, ¼" fat trim—3.5 oz (100 g)	249	970	998	1755	1848	568	249	867	746	1080	1403	760	813
select, broiled, ¼" fat trim—3.5 oz (100 g)	252	982	1011	1778	1871	576	252	878	756	1094	1421	770	813
select, roasted, ¼" fat trim—3.5 oz (100 g)	256	999	1028	1807	1902	585	256	893	768	1112	1445	783	813
round, bottom, sep lean													
choice, braised, 0" fat trim—3.5 oz (100 g)	354	1380	1420	2497	2628	809	354	1233	1061	1536	1996	1082	813
choice, braised, ¼" fat trim—3.5 oz (100 g)	354	1380	1420	2497	2628	809	354	1233	1061	1536	1996	1082	813
choice, roasted, 0" fat trim—3.5 oz (100 g)	322	1257	1294	2274	2394	737	322	1123	967	1400	1819	985	813
choice, roasted, ¼" fat trim—3.5 oz (100 g)	322	1257	1294	2274	2394	737	322	1123	967	1400	1819	985	813
select, braised, 0" fat trim—3.5 oz (100 g)	354	1380	1420	2497	2628	809	354	1233	1061	1536	1996	1082	813
select, braised, ¼" fat trim—3.5 oz (100 g)	354	1380	1420	2497	2628	809	354	1233	1061	1536	1996	1082	813
select, roasted, 0" fat trim—3.5 oz (100 g)	322	1257	1294	2274	2394	737	322	1123	967	1400	1819	985	813
select, roasted, ¼" fat trim—3.5 oz (100 g)	322	1257	1294	2274	2394	737	322	1123	967	1400	1819	985	813
round, bottom, sep lean & fat													
choice, braised, 0" fat trim—3.5 oz (100 g)	347	1352	1392	2447	2576	793	347	1209	1040	1506	1957	1060	813
choice, braised, ¼" fat trim—3.5 oz (100 g)	321	1252	1288	2265	2384	734	321	1119	963	1394	1811	981	813
choice, roasted, 0" fat trim—3.5 oz (100 g)	318	1241	1277	2246	2364	727	318	1109	955	1382	1796	973	813
choice, roasted, ¼" fat trim—3.5 oz (100 g)	296	1154	1188	2088	2198	676	296	1031	888	1285	1670	905	813
select, braised, 0" fat trim—3.5 oz (100 g)	349	1361	1401	2464	2593	798	349	1217	1047	1516	1970	1067	813
select, braised, ¼" fat trim—3.5 oz (100 g)	323	1261	1298	2282	2402	739	323	1127	970	1404	1824	988	813

	TRY	THR	ISO	LEU	LYS	MET	CYS	PHE	TYR	VAL	ARG	HIS	REF
select, roasted, 0" fat trim—*3.5 oz (100 g)*	320	1249	1286	2260	2379	732	320	1116	961	1391	1807	979	813
select, roasted, ¼" fat trim—*3.5 oz (100 g)*	300	1170	1204	2117	2228	686	300	1046	900	1303	1693	917	813
round, eye of, sep lean													
roasted, choice, 0" fat trim—*3.5 oz (100 g)*	325	1266	1303	2291	2412	742	325	1132	974	1410	1832	993	813
roasted, choice, ¼" fat trim—*3.5 oz (100 g)*	325	1266	1303	2291	2412	742	325	1132	974	1410	1832	993	813
roasted, select, 0" fat trim—*3.5 oz (100 g)*	325	1266	1303	2291	2412	742	325	1132	974	1410	1832	993	813
roasted, select, ¼" fat trim—*3.5 oz (100 g)*	325	1266	1303	2291	2412	742	325	1132	974	1410	1832	993	813
round, eye of, sep lean & fat													
roasted, choice, 0" fat trim—*3.5 oz (100 g)*	323	1258	1295	2277	2396	737	323	1125	968	1401	1820	986	813
roasted, choice, ¼" fat trim—*3.5 oz (100 g)*	298	1162	1196	2103	2213	681	298	1039	894	1294	1681	911	813
roasted, select, 0" fat trim—*3.5 oz (100 g)*	323	1258	1295	2277	2396	737	323	1125	968	1401	1820	986	813
roasted, select, ¼" fat trim—*3.5 oz (100 g)*	302	1178	1213	2132	2244	690	302	1053	906	1312	1705	923	813
round, full cut													
sep lean & fat, choice, broiled, ¼" fat trim—*3.5 oz (100 g)*	306	1195	1230	2162	2276	700	306	1068	919	1330	1729	937	813
sep lean & fat, select, broiled, ¼" fat trim—*3.5 oz (100 g)*	307	1197	1232	2165	2279	701	307	1069	920	1332	1731	938	813
sep lean, choice, broiled, ¼" fat trim—*3.5 oz (100 g)*	327	1276	1313	2309	2430	748	327	1140	981	1421	1846	1000	813
sep lean, select, broiled, ¼" fat trim—*3.5 oz (100 g)*	328	1278	1315	2312	2434	749	328	1142	983	1423	1849	1002	813
round, tip, sep lean													
roasted, choice, 0" fat trim—*3.5 oz (100 g)*	322	1254	1291	2269	2389	735	322	1121	965	1397	1815	983	813
roasted, choice, ¼" fat trim—*3.5 oz (100 g)*	322	1254	1291	2269	2389	735	322	1121	965	1397	1815	983	813
roasted, prime, ¼" fat trim—*3.5 oz (100 g)*	322	1254	1291	2269	2389	735	322	1121	965	1397	1815	983	813
roasted, select, 0" fat trim—*3.5 oz (100 g)*	322	1254	1291	2269	2389	735	322	1121	965	1397	1815	983	813
roasted, select, ¼" fat trim—*3.5 oz (100 g)*	322	1254	1291	2269	2389	735	322	1121	965	1397	1815	983	813
round, tip, sep lean & fat													
roasted, choice, 0" fat trim—*3.5 oz (100 g)*	313	1223	1258	2212	2329	717	313	1093	940	1361	1769	958	813
roasted, choice, ¼" fat trim—*3.5 oz (100 g)*	297	1159	1193	2098	2209	680	297	1036	892	1291	1678	909	813
roasted, prime, ¼" fat trim—*3.5 oz (100 g)*	295	1152	1185	2084	2194	675	295	1029	886	1282	1666	903	813
roasted, select, 0" fat trim—*3.5 oz (100 g)*	316	1230	1267	2227	2344	721	316	1100	947	1370	1780	965	813
roasted, select, ¼" fat trim—*3.5 oz (100 g)*	303	1183	1218	2141	2254	693	303	1057	910	1318	1712	927	813
round, top, sep lean													
choice, braised, 0" fat trim—*3.5 oz (100 g)*	405	1578	1624	2855	3006	925	405	1410	1214	1757	2283	1237	813
choice, braised, ¼" fat trim—*3.5 oz (100 g)*	405	1578	1624	2855	3006	925	405	1410	1214	1757	2283	1237	813
choice, broiled, ¼" fat trim—*3.5 oz (100 g)*	355	1384	1425	2505	2636	811	355	1237	1065	1541	2003	1085	813
choice, pan fried, ¼" fat trim—*3.5 oz (100 g)*	393	1532	1577	2772	2918	898	393	1369	1178	1706	2216	1201	813
prime, broiled, ¼" fat trim—*3.5 oz (100 g)*	355	1384	1425	2505	2636	811	355	1237	1065	1541	2003	1085	813

	TRY	THR	ISO	LEU	LYS	MET	CYS	PHE	TYR	VAL	ARG	HIS	REF

	TRY	THR	ISO	LEU	LYS	MET	CYS	PHE	TYR	VAL	ARG	HIS	REF
select, braised, 0" fat trim—3.5 oz (100 g)	405	1578	1624	2855	3006	925	405	1410	1214	1757	2283	1237	813
select, braised, ¼" fat trim—3.5 oz (100 g)	405	1578	1624	2855	3006	925	405	1410	1214	1757	2283	1237	813
select, broiled, ¼" fat trim—3.5 oz (100 g)	355	1384	1425	2505	2636	811	355	1237	1065	1541	2003	1085	813
round, top, sep lean & fat													
choice, braised, 0" fat trim—3.5 oz (100 g)	399	1556	1601	2815	2963	912	399	1390	1197	1732	2251	1219	813
choice, braised, ¼" fat trim—3.5 oz (100 g)	376	1467	1510	2654	2794	860	376	1311	1128	1633	2122	1150	813
choice, broiled, ¼" fat trim—3.5 oz (100 g)	338	1318	1356	2385	2510	772	338	1178	1014	1467	1907	1033	813
choice, pan fried, ¼" fat trim—3.5 oz (100 g)	363	1415	1456	2560	2694	829	363	1264	1088	1575	2047	1109	813
prime, broiled, ¼" fat trim—3.5 oz (100 g)	348	1357	1396	2455	2584	795	348	1212	1043	1511	1963	1063	813
select, braised, 0" fat trim—3.5 oz (100 g)	399	1556	1601	2815	2963	912	399	1390	1197	1732	2251	1219	813
select, braised, ¼" fat trim—3.5 oz (100 g)	382	1489	1533	2694	2836	873	382	1331	1145	1658	2154	1167	813
select, broiled, ¼" fat trim—3.5 oz (100 g)	338	1318	1356	2385	2510	772	338	1178	1014	1467	1907	1033	813
shank, crosscuts, choice, simmered, sep lean & fat, ¼" fat trim—3.5 oz (100 g)	344	1340	1380	2426	2553	786	344	1198	1031	1493	1939	1051	813
shank, crosscuts, choice, simmered, sep lean, ¼" fat trim—3.5 oz (100 g)	377	1471	1514	2662	2802	862	377	1315	1132	1638	2129	1153	813
short loin porterhouse steak, ¼" fat trim, broiled													
sep lean & fat—3.5 oz (100 g)	250	976	1005	1766	1859	572	250	873	751	1087	1412	765	813
sep lean—3.5 oz (100 g)	292	1138	1171	2058	2167	667	292	1017	875	1267	1646	892	813
short loin T-bone steak, ¼" fat trim, broiled, sep lean & fat—3.5 oz (100 g)	260	1015	1044	1836	1933	595	260	907	781	1130	1468	795	813
short loin T-bone steak, ¼" fat trim, broiled, sep lean—3.5 oz (100 g)	300	1170	1204	2117	2228	686	300	1045	900	1302	1692	917	813
short loin, top loin, sep lean													
broiled, choice, 0" fat trim—3.5 oz (100 g)	321	1250	1287	2262	2381	733	321	1117	962	1392	1809	980	813
broiled, choice, ¼" fat trim—3.5 oz (100 g)	321	1250	1287	2262	2381	733	321	1117	962	1392	1809	980	813
broiled, prime, ¼" fat trim—3.5 oz (100 g)	321	1250	1287	2262	2381	733	321	1117	962	1392	1809	980	813
broiled, select, 0" fat trim—3.5 oz (100 g)	321	1250	1287	2262	2381	733	321	1117	962	1392	1809	980	813
broiled, select, ¼" fat trim—3.5 oz (100 g)	321	1250	1287	2262	2381	733	321	1117	962	1392	1809	980	813
short loin, top loin, sep lean & fat													
broiled, choice, 0" fat trim—3.5 oz (100 g)	312	1219	1254	2205	2321	714	312	1089	937	1357	1763	955	813
broiled, choice, ¼" fat trim—3.5 oz (100 g)	284	1109	1141	2006	2112	650	284	991	853	1235	1604	869	813
broiled, prime, ¼" fat trim—3.5 oz (100 g)	284	1109	1141	2006	2112	650	284	991	853	1235	1604	869	813
broiled, select, 0" fat trim—3.5 oz (100 g)	314	1227	1262	2219	2336	719	314	1096	943	1366	1775	961	813
broiled, select, ¼" fat trim—3.5 oz (100 g)	290	1132	1166	2049	2157	664	290	1012	871	1261	1638	888	813
tenderloin, sep lean													
choice, broiled, 0" fat trim—3.5 oz (100 g)	316	1234	1270	2233	2350	723	316	1103	949	1374	1785	967	813
choice, broiled, ¼" fat trim—3.5 oz (100 g)	316	1234	1270	2233	2350	723	316	1103	949	1374	1785	967	813
choice, roasted, ¼" fat trim—3.5 oz (100 g)	310	1210	1246	2190	2305	709	310	1082	931	1348	1751	949	813

	TRY	THR	ISO	LEU	LYS	MET	CYS	PHE	TYR	VAL	ARG	HIS	REF
prime, broiled, ¼″ fat trim—3.5 oz (100 g)	316	1234	1270	2233	2350	723	316	1103	949	1374	1785	967	813
prime, roasted, ¼″ fat trim—3.5 oz (100 g)	308	1203	1238	2177	2291	705	308	1075	925	1339	1740	943	813
select, broiled, 0″ fat trim—3.5 oz (100 g)	316	1234	1270	2233	2350	723	316	1103	949	1374	1785	967	813
select, broiled, ¼″ fat trim—3.5 oz (100 g)	316	1234	1270	2233	2350	723	316	1103	949	1374	1785	967	813
select, roasted, ¼″ fat trim—3.5 oz (100 g)	310	1210	1246	2190	2305	709	310	1082	931	1348	1751	949	813
tenderloin, sep lean & fat													
choice, broiled, 0″ fat trim—3.5 oz (100 g)	303	1180	1215	2135	2248	692	303	1055	908	1314	1708	925	813
choice, broiled, ¼″ fat trim—3.5 oz (100 g)	281	1096	1128	1982	2087	642	281	979	843	1220	1585	859	813
choice, roasted, ¼″ fat trim—3.5 oz (100 g)	264	1031	1062	1866	1965	605	264	922	793	1149	1492	809	813
prime, broiled, ¼″ fat trim—3.5 oz (100 g)	279	1088	1120	1969	2072	638	279	972	837	1211	1574	853	813
prime, roasted, ¼″ fat trim—3.5 oz (100 g)	265	1034	1064	1871	1969	606	265	924	795	1151	1496	810	813
select, broiled, 0″ fat trim—3.5 oz (100 g)	305	1188	1223	2149	2263	696	305	1062	914	1323	1719	931	813
select, broiled, ¼″ fat trim—3.5 oz (100 g)	287	1119	1151	2024	2131	656	287	1000	860	1246	1619	877	813
select, roasted, ¼″ fat trim—3.5 oz (100 g)	264	1031	1062	1866	1965	605	264	922	793	1149	1492	809	813
top sirloin, sep lean													
choice, broiled, 0″ fat trim—3.5 oz (100 g)	340	1327	1365	2400	2527	777	340	1186	1020	1477	1919	1040	813
choice, broiled, ¼″ fat trim—3.5 oz (100 g)	340	1327	1365	2400	2527	777	340	1186	1020	1477	1919	1040	813
choice, pan fried, ¼″ fat trim—3.5 oz (100 g)	364	1419	1460	2567	2702	831	364	1268	1091	1580	2053	1112	813
select, broiled, 0″ fat trim—3.5 oz (100 g)	340	1327	1365	2400	2527	777	340	1186	1020	1477	1919	1040	813
select, broiled, ¼″ fat trim—3.5 oz (100 g)	340	1327	1365	2400	2527	777	340	1186	1020	1477	1919	1040	813
top sirloin, sep lean & fat													
choice, broiled, 0″ fat trim—3.5 oz (100 g)	327	1275	1312	2307	2428	747	327	1139	981	1420	1845	999	813
choice, broiled, ¼″ fat trim—3.5 oz (100 g)	309	1206	1241	2182	2297	707	309	1078	928	1343	1745	945	813
choice, pan fried, ¼″ fat trim—3.5 oz (100 g)	315	1228	1264	2222	2339	720	315	1098	945	1367	1777	963	813
select, broiled, 0″ fat trim—3.5 oz (100 g)	333	1297	1335	2348	2471	760	333	1160	998	1445	1877	1017	813
select, broiled, ¼″ fat trim—3.5 oz (100 g)	314	1223	1259	2213	2330	717	314	1093	941	1362	1770	959	813
21.2 Game Meats													
antelope, roasted—3.5 oz (100 g)		1362	1126	2489	2462	838	262	1166	1022	1310	1938	1401	817
beaver, roasted—3.5 oz (100 g)		1327	1489	2749	3240	792		1417	1087	1422	2141	1372	817
bison, roasted—3.5 oz (100 g)		1171	1198	2210	2219	674		1065	914	1287	1686	754	817
boar, wild, roasted—3.5 oz (100 g)	380	1331	1367	2300	2789	697	367	1132	1010	1517	1965	1435	817
buffalo, water, roasted—3.5 oz (100 g)	327	1284	1346	2309	2118	672	429	1075	1077	1427	1681	888	817
caribou, roasted—3.5 oz (100 g)	458	1273	1347	2457	2697	665	214	1324	976	1399	1771	1179	817
deer, roasted—3.5 oz (100 g)		1421	1194	2566	2639	745	338	1233	1069	1412	2175	1494	817
eel, ckd by dry heat—3 oz (85 g)	225	881	927	1634	1845	595	215	785	678	1035	1203	592	815
eel, raw—3 oz (85 g)	176	688	723	1274	1440	464	168	612	530	807	938	462	815
elk, roasted—3.5 oz (100 g)	545	1315	973	2546	2803	725		1198	1081	1066	2073	964	817
goat, roasted—3.5 oz (100 g)	403	1290	1371	2258	2016	726	323	941	833	1452	1989	565	817
horse, roasted—3.5 oz (100 g)	349	1262	1334	2232	2398	623	393	1157	882	1458	1843	1081	817
moose, roasted—3.5 oz (100 g)		1344	1405	2576	2655	749		1264	1077	1592	1892	983	817

	TRY	THR	ISO	LEU	LYS	MET	CYS	PHE	TYR	VAL	ARG	HIS	REF
muskrat, roasted—3.5 oz (100 g)		1237	1146	2373	2359	501		1242	823	1338	1444	895	817
rabbit, domesticated, roasted—3.5 oz (100 g)	384	1300	1379	2264	2544	727	365	1193	1035	1477	1795	815	817
rabbit, domesticated, stewed—3.5 oz (100 g)	401	1359	1441	2367	2660	760	382	1247	1082	1544	1877	852	817
rabbit, wild, stewed—3.5 oz (100 g)	436	1477	1567	2573	2891	826	415	1355	1176	1678	2040	926	817
squirrel, roasted—3.5 oz (100 g)		1172	1172	2211	2225	675		1191	921	1216	1605	803	817

21.3 Lamb

	TRY	THR	ISO	LEU	LYS	MET	CYS	PHE	TYR	VAL	ARG	HIS	REF
domestic, foreshank, choice, braised, sep lean & fat—3.5 oz (100 g)	332	1214	1369	2207	2505	728	339	1155	954	1531	1686	899	817
domestic, foreshank, choice, braised, sep lean—3.5 oz (100 g)	362	1327	1496	2412	2739	796	370	1262	1042	1673	1842	982	817
domestic, ground, broiled—3.5 oz (100 g)	289	1059	1194	1925	2186	635	295	1008	832	1335	1470	784	817
domestic, leg													
shank half, choice, roasted, sep lean—3.5 oz (100 g)	329	1206	1359	2191	2488	723	336	1147	947	1520	1674	892	817
shank half, choice, roasted, sep lean & fat—3.5 oz (100 g)	309	1130	1274	2054	2332	678	315	1075	888	1425	1569	837	817
sirloin half, choice, roasted, sep lean—3.5 oz (100 g)	331	1214	1368	2205	2504	728	338	1154	953	1530	1684	898	817
sirloin half, choice, roasted, sep lean & fat—3.5 oz (100 g)	288	1054	1188	1916	2175	632	294	1003	828	1329	1463	780	817
whole (shank & sirloin), choice, roasted, sep lean—3.5 oz (100 g)	331	1211	1365	2201	2499	726	338	1152	951	1527	1681	896	817
whole (shank & sirloin), choice, roasted, sep lean & fat—3.5 oz (100 g)	299	1094	1233	1987	2256	656	305	1040	859	1379	1518	809	817
domestic, leg & shoulder, cubed for stew or kabob, sep lean, braised—3.5 oz (100 g)	394	1442	1625	2620	2975	865	402	1372	1132	1818	2002	1067	817
domestic, leg & shoulder, cubed for stew or kabob, sep lean, broiled—3.5 oz (100 g)	328	1202	1355	2184	2479	720	335	1143	944	1515	1668	889	817
domestic, loin													
sep lean & fat, choice, broiled—3.5 oz (100 g)	294	1077	1214	1958	2223	646	300	1025	846	1358	1496	797	817
sep lean & fat, choice, roasted—3.5 oz (100 g)	264	965	1088	1754	1991	579	269	918	758	1217	1340	714	817
sep lean, choice, broiled—3.5 oz (100 g)	350	1283	1447	2332	2648	770	358	1221	1008	1618	1782	950	817
sep lean, choice, roasted—3.5 oz (100 g)	311	1138	1283	2068	2348	682	317	1083	894	1435	1580	842	817
domestic, rib													
sep lean & fat, choice, broiled—3.5 oz (100 g)	259	947	1068	1721	1954	568	264	901	744	1194	1315	701	817
sep lean & fat, choice, roasted—3.5 oz (100 g)	247	904	1019	1642	1865	542	252	860	710	1139	1254	669	817
sep lean, choice, broiled—3.5 oz (100 g)	324	1187	1338	2157	2449	712	331	1129	932	1497	1648	879	817
sep lean, choice, roasted—3.5 oz (100 g)	306	1119	1262	2034	2310	671	312	1065	879	1411	1554	829	817
domestic, shoulder, arm													
sep lean & fat, choice, braised—3.5 oz (100 g)	355	1301	1466	2364	2684	780	363	1237	1022	1640	1806	963	817
sep lean & fat, choice, broiled—3.5 oz (100 g)	286	1046	1179	1901	2158	627	292	995	821	1319	1452	774	817
sep lean & fat, choice, roasted—3.5 oz (100 g)	263	964	1087	1753	1990	578	269	917	757	1216	1339	714	817
sep lean, choice, braised—3.5 oz (100 g)	415	1521	1715	2764	3138	912	424	1447	1194	1918	2111	1126	817
sep lean, choice, broiled—3.5 oz (100 g)	324	1186	1337	2155	2447	711	331	1128	931	1495	1646	878	817

	TRY	THR	ISO	LEU	LYS	MET	CYS	PHE	TYR	VAL	ARG	HIS	REF
sep lean, choice, roasted—*3.5 oz (100 g)*	298	1090	1228	1980	2248	653	304	1036	856	1374	1513	807	817
domestic, shoulder, blade													
sep lean & fat, choice, braised—*3.5 oz (100 g)*	333	1220	1376	2218	2518	732	340	1161	958	1539	1694	903	817
sep lean & fat, choice, broiled—*3.5 oz (100 g)*	270	988	1113	1795	2038	592	275	940	776	1245	1371	731	817
sep lean & fat, choice, roasted—*3.5 oz (100 g)*	260	952	1073	1730	1964	571	266	906	748	1200	1322	705	817
sep lean, choice, braised—*3.5 oz (100 g)*	378	1385	1561	2516	2857	830	386	1317	1087	1746	1922	1025	817
sep lean, choice, broiled—*3.5 oz (100 g)*	298	1090	1229	1982	2250	654	304	1037	856	1375	1514	807	817
sep lean, choice, roasted—*3.5 oz (100 g)*	288	1053	1187	1914	2174	632	294	1002	827	1328	1462	780	817
domestic, shoulder, whole (arm & blade)													
sep lean & fat, choice, braised—*3.5 oz (100 g)*	335	1227	1384	2231	2532	736	342	1167	964	1547	1704	908	817
sep lean & fat, choice, broiled—*3.5 oz (100 g)*	285	1045	1178	1900	2157	627	292	994	821	1318	1451	774	817
sep lean & fat, choice, roasted—*3.5 oz (100 g)*	263	963	1086	1751	1988	578	269	916	756	1215	1337	713	817
sep lean, choice, braised—*3.5 oz (100 g)*	383	1404	1583	2552	2897	842	392	1336	1103	1770	1949	1039	817
sep lean, choice, broiled—*3.5 oz (100 g)*	317	1161	1308	2109	2395	696	324	1104	911	1463	1611	859	817
sep lean, choice, roasted—*3.5 oz (100 g)*	291	1067	1203	1940	2202	640	298	1015	838	1346	1482	790	817
New Zealand, imported													
composite of trimmed retail cuts, sep lean & fat, ckd—*3.5 oz (100 g)*	285	1045	1178	1900	2157	627	292	994	821	1318	1451	774	817
composite of trimmed retail cuts, sep lean, ckd—*3.5 oz (100 g)*	346	1267	1428	2302	2613	759	353	1205	995	1597	1758	937	817
foreshank, sep lean & fat, braised—*3.5 oz (100 g)*	315	1154	1301	2098	2382	692	322	1098	906	1455	1602	854	817
foreshank, sep lean, braised—*3.5 oz (100 g)*	359	1316	1484	2392	2716	789	367	1252	1034	1660	1827	974	817
leg, whole (shank & sirloin), sep lean & fat, roasted—*3.5 oz (100 g)*	290	1062	1197	1929	2190	637	296	1010	834	1338	1474	786	817
leg, whole (shank & sirloin), sep lean, roasted—*3.5 oz (100 g)*	323	1185	1335	2153	2444	710	330	1127	930	1494	1644	877	817
loin, sep lean & fat, broiled—*3.5 oz (100 g)*	274	1003	1130	1822	2069	601	280	954	787	1264	1392	742	817
loin, sep lean, broiled—*3.5 oz (100 g)*	343	1254	1414	2280	2588	752	350	1193	985	1581	1741	928	817
rib, sep lean & fat, roasted—*3.5 oz (100 g)*	222	812	916	1476	1676	487	227	773	638	1024	1127	601	817
rib, sep lean, roasted—*3.5 oz (100 g)*	285	1045	1178	1900	2157	627	292	994	821	1318	1451	774	817
shoulder, whole (arm & blade), sep lean & fat, braised—*3.5 oz (100 g)*	330	1207	1361	2194	2491	724	337	1148	948	1522	1676	894	817
shoulder, whole (arm & blade), sep lean, braised—*3.5 oz (100 g)*	398	1458	1643	2649	3007	874	406	1386	1145	1838	2023	1079	817
21.4 Pork													
arm picnic													
cured, sep lean & fat, roasted—*3.5 oz (100 g)*	227	885	861	1602	1728	516	294	871	637	894	1403	683	810
cured, sep lean, roasted—*3.5 oz (100 g)*	299	1109	1094	1980	2115	659	375	1078	818	1082	1620	894	810
lean, braised—*3.5 oz (100 g)*	410	1473	1511	2588	2901	854	411	1288	1124	1750	2005	1289	810
lean, roasted—*3.5 oz (100 g)*	339	1218	1249	2141	2399	706	340	1065	930	1447	1659	1066	810
sep lean & fat, braised—*3.5 oz (100 g)*	331	1240	1256	2203	2485	708	345	1105	929	1492	1809	1048	810
sep lean & fat, roasted—*3.5 oz (100 g)*	273	1032	1042	1838	2077	587	286	924	770	1246	1531	864	810
bacon, canadian style, grilled—*2 slices (47 g)*	113	457	430	802	897	310	142	370	345	454	621	414	810

	TRY	THR	ISO	LEU	LYS	MET	CYS	PHE	TYR	VAL	ARG	HIS	REF
bacon, canadian style, unheated—2 slices (57 g)	117	473	444	828	926	320	147	382	356	469	642	427	810
bacon, cured													
broiled/pan fried—3 med slices (19 g)	55	222	235	403	430	128	59	223	169	279	354	167	810
broiled/pan fried—4.48 oz (yield from 1 lb raw) (127 g)	371	1485	1571	2691	2871	853	396	1491	1126	1862	2363	1114	810
raw—3 med slices (68 g)	56	226	239	409	437	130	61	227	171	284	360	169	810
blade roll, cured, sep lean & fat, roasted—3.5 oz (100 g)	207	768	757	1371	1465	456	260	746	567	749	1122	619	810
boston blade (steaks/roasts)													
lean & fat, braised—3.5 oz (100 g)	350	1287	1310	2275	2560	740	358	1137	972	1540	1824	1103	810
lean & fat, broiled—3.5 oz (100 g)	325	1168	1198	2052	2300	677	326	1021	891	1388	1590	1022	810
lean & fat, roasted—3.5 oz (100 g)	283	1039	1059	1836	2064	598	289	917	785	1242	1467	893	810
lean, braised—3.5 oz (100 g)	395	1420	1456	2495	2796	823	397	1241	1083	1687	1933	1242	810
lean, broiled—3.5 oz (100 g)	340	1221	1252	2145	2405	708	341	1067	932	1451	1662	1068	810
lean, roasted—3.5 oz (100 g)	308	1106	1134	1943	2178	641	309	967	844	1314	1505	967	810
breakfast strips, ckd—3 slices (34 g)	95	378	400	685	731	217	101	379	287	474	601	284	810
center loin (loin chops/roasts), sep lean													
braised—3.5 oz (100 g)	378	1360	1395	2390	2678	789	380	1189	1038	1616	1851	1190	810
broiled—3.5 oz (100 g)	383	1379	1414	2422	2715	799	385	1205	1052	1638	1877	1206	810
pan fried—3.5 oz (100 g)	409	1470	1507	2582	2894	852	411	1285	1121	1746	2001	1286	810
roasted—3.5 oz (100 g)	350	1258	1290	2210	2477	729	351	1100	960	1495	1713	1101	810
center loin (loin chops/roasts), sep lean & fat													
braised—3.5 oz (100 g)	343	1257	1282	2220	2497	724	350	1109	951	1503	1771	1081	810
broiled—3.5 oz (100 g)	365	1311	1344	2304	2582	760	366	1146	1000	1558	1785	1147	810
pan fried—3.5 oz (100 g)	367	1345	1371	2377	2672	774	375	1187	1018	1608	1896	1157	810
roasted—3.5 oz (100 g)	325	1187	1211	2094	2354	684	331	1045	899	1417	1662	1024	810
center rib (rib chops/roasts), sep lean													
braised—3.5 oz (100 g)	355	1276	1309	2242	2513	740	356	1116	974	1516	1737	1116	810
broiled—3.5 oz (100 g)	374	1345	1379	2364	2649	780	376	1176	1026	1598	1831	1177	810
pan fried—3.5 oz (100 g)	352	1264	1296	2221	2489	733	353	1105	964	1502	1721	1106	810
roasted—3.5 oz (100 g)	366	1316	1349	2312	2591	763	367	1150	1004	1563	1791	1151	810
center rib (rib chops/roasts), sep lean & fat													
braised—3.5 oz (100 g)	322	1182	1205	2089	2349	680	329	1044	894	1414	1669	1016	810
broiled—3.5 oz (100 g)	339	1243	1267	2196	2469	715	346	1097	940	1486	1752	1069	810
pan fried—3.5 oz (100 g)	352	1264	1296	2221	2489	733	353	1105	964	1502	1721	1106	810
roasted—3.5 oz (100 g)	343	1232	1264	2166	2427	715	344	1077	940	1464	1678	1078	810
ham, cured (fully cooked as purchased), lean (4-5% fat), cnd—3.5 oz (100 g)	251	931	918	1661	1775	553	315	904	687	908	1360	750	810
lean (4-5% fat), cnd, roasted—3.5 oz (100 g)	210	826	796	1438	1589	482	219	713	607	829	1145	731	810
lean (4-5% fat), roasted—3.5 oz (100 g)	240	944	911	1645	1818	552	250	816	694	948	1310	836	810
patties, grilled—1 patty (60 g)	93	355	349	631	678	211	107	338	262	347	515	291	810
patties, unheated—1 patty (65 g)	97	370	363	657	706	219	112	352	272	361	536	303	810
reg (11-13% fat), cnd—3.5 oz (100 g)	238	882	870	1574	1682	524	298	857	651	860	1289	711	810
reg (11-13% fat), cnd, roasted—3.5 oz (100 g)	193	758	731	1320	1458	443	201	655	557	760	1051	671	810
reg (11-13% fat), center slice, sep lean & fat, unheated—3.5 oz (100 g)	233	916	883	1596	1764	535	243	791	673	920	1271	811	810
reg (11-13% fat), roasted—3.5 oz (100 g)	242	897	884	1601	1710	532	303	871	662	875	1310	723	810
steak, extra lean, ckd—3.5 oz (100 g)	235	870	858	1552	1658	516	295	845	641	848	1270	701	810
whole, sep lean & fat, roasted—3.5 oz (100 g)	245	941	918	1697	1825	551	315	922	682	941	1459	735	810
whole, sep lean & fat, unheated—3.5 oz (100 g)	210	806	787	1455	1565	473	270	791	584	807	1250	630	810
whole, sep lean, roasted—3.5 oz (100 g)	300	1114	1098	1988	2124	661	377	1082	822	1086	1627	898	810
whole, sep lean, unheated—3.5 oz (100 g)	268	992	978	1771	1892	589	336	964	732	967	1449	800	810

	TRY	THR	ISO	LEU	LYS	MET	CYS	PHE	TYR	VAL	ARG	HIS	REF
leg, sep lean & fat, roasted—*3.5 oz (100 g)*	324	1198	1218	2122	2390	687	333	1062	903	1437	1717	1022	810
leg, sep lean, roasted—*3.5 oz (100 g)*	374	1343	1377	2360	2645	779	375	1174	1025	1595	1828	1175	810
loin blade (chops & roasts), sep lean,													
braised—*3.5 oz (100 g)*	318	1143	1172	2008	2250	663	319	999	872	1358	1556	1000	810
broiled—*3.5 oz (100 g)*	322	1158	1187	2034	2280	671	323	1012	883	1376	1576	1013	810
pan fried—*3.5 oz (100 g)*	314	1130	1158	1985	2225	655	316	988	862	1342	1538	988	810
roasted—*3.5 oz (100 g)*	338	1215	1246	2135	2392	704	339	1062	927	1443	1654	1063	810
loin blade (chops & roasts), sep lean & fat													
braised—*3.5 oz (100 g)*	250	957	964	1709	1934	543	265	861	711	1159	1441	795	810
broiled—*3.5 oz (100 g)*	260	987	997	1759	1989	562	274	885	736	1192	1469	826	810
pan fried—*3.5 oz (100 g)*	243	935	940	1672	1894	529	259	843	693	1134	1421	773	810
roasted—*3.5 oz (100 g)*	278	1048	1060	1863	2104	597	291	936	784	1262	1540	882	810
loin, sep lean													
braised—*3.5 oz (100 g)*	363	1305	1338	2292	2569	756	364	1140	995	1550	1776	1141	810
broiled—*3.5 oz (100 g)*	363	1305	1338	2292	2569	756	364	1140	995	1550	1776	1141	810
roasted—*3.5 oz (100 g)*	364	1307	1340	2297	2574	758	365	1143	997	1553	1779	1143	810
loin, sep lean & fat													
braised—*3.5 oz (100 g)*	336	1229	1254	2168	2436	708	343	1082	931	1467	1719	1061	810
broiled—*3.5 oz (100 g)*	338	1234	1260	2177	2446	712	344	1086	936	1473	1723	1067	810
roasted—*3.5 oz (100 g)*	341	1232	1261	2168	2432	713	344	1080	938	1466	1693	1073	810
rump, sep lean & fat, roasted—*3.5 oz (100 g)*	354	1299	1324	2295	2581	748	362	1147	983	1553	1831	1117	810
rump, sep lean, roasted—*3.5 oz (100 g)*	393	1413	1449	2482	2782	819	395	1235	1078	1678	1923	1236	810
sausage													
fresh, ckd—*1 link (13 g)*	20	101	93	171	194	62	26	85	74	103	151	74	810
fresh, ckd—*1 patty (27 g)*	42	210	194	356	403	129	53	177	153	213	313	153	810
fresh, w/ beef, ckd—*1 link (13 g)*	17	72	69	127	141	43	18	62	53	77	111	54	807
shank, sep lean & fat, roasted—*3.5 oz (100 g)*	301	1125	1141	1997	2253	644	313	1001	845	1353	1634	954	810
shank, sep lean, roasted—*3.5 oz (100 g)*	358	1288	1321	2263	2537	747	360	1126	983	1530	1754	1127	810
shoulder, sep lean & fat, roasted—*3.5 oz (100 g)*	278	1036	1051	1837	2071	593	288	921	778	1244	1498	879	810
shoulder, sep lean, roasted—*3.5 oz (100 g)*	322	1157	1186	2032	2278	671	323	1011	883	1374	1575	1012	810
sirloin (chops & roasts), sep lean,													
braised—*3.5 oz (100 g)*	343	1233	1264	2166	2428	715	344	1078	941	1465	1678	1079	810
broiled—*3.5 oz (100 g)*	395	1422	1458	2498	2799	824	397	1243	1085	1689	1935	1244	810
roasted—*3.5 oz (100 g)*	366	1317	1351	2315	2594	764	368	1152	1005	1565	1793	1152	810
sirloin (chops & roasts), sep lean & fat,													
braised—*3.5 oz (100 g)*	334	1206	1235	2123	2382	698	337	1058	918	1436	1660	1050	810
broiled—*3.5 oz (100 g)*	388	1394	1429	2449	2745	808	389	1218	1063	1656	1897	1219	810
roasted—*3.5 oz (100 g)*	360	1298	1329	2282	2560	751	362	1136	988	1544	1778	1132	810
spareribs, sep lean & fat, braised—*3.5 oz (100 g)*	285	1062	1078	1883	2123	608	295	944	798	1275	1535	902	810
tenderloin, sep lean & fat, roasted—*3.5 oz (100 g)*	351	1266	1297	2227	2497	733	353	1109	964	1506	1735	1104	810
tenderloin, sep lean, roasted—*3.5 oz (100 g)*	357	1285	1318	2258	2531	745	359	1123	980	1527	1749	1124	810
top loin (chops & roasts), sep lean,													
braised—*3.5 oz (100 g)*	369	1327	1361	2332	2614	770	371	1160	1013	1577	1807	1161	810
broiled—*3.5 oz (100 g)*	396	1422	1458	2499	2800	825	397	1243	1085	1689	1936	1244	810
pan fried—*3.5 oz (100 g)*	387	1392	1427	2445	2741	807	389	1217	1062	1653	1895	1218	810
roasted—*3.5 oz (100 g)*	384	1381	1416	2426	2719	801	386	1207	1053	1640	1880	1208	810
top loin (chops & roasts), sep lean & fat,													
braised—*3.5 oz (100 g)*	345	1257	1284	2217	2491	725	351	1106	953	1500	1753	1087	810
broiled—*3.5 oz (100 g)*	381	1368	1403	2404	2694	793	382	1196	1044	1625	1862	1197	810
pan fried—*3.5 oz (100 g)*	359	1310	1337	2310	2596	755	365	1153	993	1563	1829	1132	810
roasted—*3.5 oz (100 g)*	366	1316	1349	2312	2591	763	367	1150	1004	1563	1791	1151	810

	TRY	THR	ISO	LEU	LYS	MET	CYS	PHE	TYR	VAL	ARG	HIS	REF
21.5 Veal													
ground, broiled—*3.5 oz (100 g)*	247	1065	1201	1940	2009	569	275	984	777	1347	1434	885	817
leg & shoulder, cubed for stew, sep lean, braised—*3.5 oz (100 g)*	354	1527	1721	2781	2879	815	394	1410	1114	1931	2055	1268	817
leg (top round), sep lean													
braised—*3.5 oz (100 g)*	372	1604	1808	2922	3025	857	414	1481	1170	2029	2159	1332	817
pan fried, breaded—*3.5 oz (100 g)*	295	1221	1394	2249	2235	657	340	1174	899	1573	1644	996	817
pan fried, not breaded—*3.5 oz (100 g)*	336	1449	1634	2640	2734	774	374	1339	1058	1834	1951	1204	817
roasted—*3.5 oz (100 g)*	284	1226	1382	2234	2313	655	317	1133	895	1552	1651	1019	817
leg (top round), sep lean & fat													
braised—*3.5 oz (100 g)*	366	1580	1781	2878	2980	844	408	1459	1153	1999	2127	1313	817
pan fried, breaded—*3.5 oz (100 g)*	284	1172	1339	2161	2144	631	328	1129	864	1512	1578	956	817
pan fried, not breaded—*3.5 oz (100 g)*	321	1387	1564	2527	2616	741	358	1281	1012	1755	1867	1152	817
roasted—*3.5 oz (100 g)*	280	1210	1364	2205	2282	646	313	1118	883	1531	1629	1005	817
loin													
sep lean & fat, braised—*3.5 oz (100 g)*	306	1319	1487	2403	2487	704	341	1218	962	1668	1775	1096	817
sep lean & fat, roasted—*3.5 oz (100 g)*	251	1083	1221	1974	2044	579	280	1001	791	1371	1459	900	817
sep lean, braised—*3.5 oz (100 g)*	340	1466	1653	2672	2766	783	379	1355	1070	1855	1974	1218	817
sep lean, roasted—*3.5 oz (100 g)*	266	1150	1296	2095	2169	614	297	1062	839	1455	1548	955	817
rib													
sep lean & fat, braised—*3.5 oz (100 g)*	328	1417	1597	2581	2673	757	366	1309	1034	1793	1908	1177	817
sep lean & fat, roasted—*3.5 oz (100 g)*	243	1047	1180	1907	1974	559	270	967	764	1324	1409	870	817
sep lean, braised—*3.5 oz (100 g)*	349	1504	1696	2741	2838	804	389	1390	1098	1903	2025	1250	817
sep lean, roasted—*3.5 oz (100 g)*	261	1125	1268	2050	2122	601	291	1040	821	1424	1515	935	817
shoulder, arm													
sep lean & fat, braised—*3.5 oz (100 g)*	340	1469	1656	2676	2771	785	380	1357	1072	1858	1978	1221	817
sep lean & fat, roasted—*3.5 oz (100 g)*	258	1112	1254	2027	2098	594	287	1028	812	1407	1498	924	817
sep lean, braised—*3.5 oz (100 g)*	362	1561	1760	2844	2944	834	403	1442	1139	1975	2101	1297	817
sep lean, roasted—*3.5 oz (100 g)*	265	1142	1287	2080	2153	610	295	1055	833	1444	1537	949	817
shoulder, blade													
sep lean & fat, braised—*3.5 oz (100 g)*	316	1366	1540	2488	2576	730	353	1262	997	1728	1839	1135	817
sep lean & fat, roasted—*3.5 oz (100 g)*	255	1099	1238	2002	2072	587	284	1015	802	1390	1479	913	817
sep lean, braised—*3.5 oz (100 g)*	331	1427	1608	2599	2691	762	369	1318	1041	1805	1921	1185	817
sep lean, roasted—*3.5 oz (100 g)*	259	1120	1262	2040	2112	598	289	1035	817	1417	1508	931	817
shoulder, whole (arm & blade)													
sep lean & fat, braised—*3.5 oz (100 g)*	325	1401	1579	2552	2642	748	362	1294	1022	1772	1886	1164	817
sep lean & fat, roasted—*3.5 oz (100 g)*	256	1106	1247	2015	2087	591	286	1022	807	1400	1489	919	817
sep lean, braised—*3.5 oz (100 g)*	341	1471	1658	2680	2775	786	380	1359	1074	1861	1981	1222	817
sep lean, roasted—*3.5 oz (100 g)*	261	1128	1271	2055	2127	602	291	1042	823	1427	1518	937	817
sirloin													
sep lean & fat, braised—*3.5 oz (100 g)*	316	1366	1539	2488	2576	729	353	1262	997	1728	1838	1135	817
sep lean & fat, roasted—*3.5 oz (100 g)*	254	1098	1238	2001	2072	587	284	1015	802	1390	1479	913	817
sep lean, braised—*3.5 oz (100 g)*	344	1483	1672	2703	2798	792	383	1371	1083	1877	1997	1233	817
sep lean, roasted—*3.5 oz (100 g)*	266	1150	1296	2095	2169	614	297	1062	839	1455	1548	956	817
21.6 Variety Cuts & Internal Organs													
belly, pork, raw—*1 oz (28 g)*	34	121	124	212	238	70	34	106	92	144	165	106	810
brain													
beef, pan fried—*3.5 oz (100 g)*	103	597	487	943	752	261	223	635	446	617	686	320	813
beef, simmered—*3.5 oz (100 g)*	90	526	429	831	662	230	197	560	393	544	604	282	813
lamb, braised—*3.5 oz (100 g)*	129	562	499	980	805	250	131	605	459	598	846	333	817
lamb, pan fried—*3.5 oz (100 g)*	175	760	675	1326	1088	338	177	818	621	808	1144	450	817
pork, braised—*3.5 oz (100 g)*	155	567	561	1058	954	241	214	618	509	691	635	326	810
veal, braised—*3.5 oz (100 g)*	115	568	467	886	711	252	120	604	445	546	629	287	817
veal, pan fried—*3.5 oz (100 g)*	145	716	589	1118	897	318	151	762	561	689	794	363	817
chitterlings, pork, simmered—*3.5 oz (100 g)*	61	451	420	809	656	194	90	410	379	502	840	215	810
ears, pork, simmered—*1 ear (111 g)*	34	529	405	971	813	142	158	566	354	708	1416	212	810
feet, pork, cured, pickled—*3.5 oz (100 g)*	27	365	230	595	582	149	119	392	216	338	1014	149	810

	TRY	THR	ISO	LEU	LYS	MET	CYS	PHE	TYR	VAL	ARG	HIS	REF
feet, pork, simmered—*3.5 oz (100 g)*	38	518	326	845	826	211	169	557	307	480	1440	211	810
heart													
beef, simmered—*3.5 oz (100 g)*	322	1359	1262	2547	2372	737	378	1303	1046	1502	1925	792	813
lamb, braised—*3.5 oz (100 g)*	271	1178	1082	2124	1881	547	209	1080	778	1243	1633	571	817
pork, braised—*1 heart (129 g)*	351	1335	1467	2748	2518	779	546	1344	1042	1613	2046	774	810
veal, braised—*3.5 oz (100 g)*	310	1288	1395	2287	2507	664	313	1263	955	1523	1808	783	817
jowl, pork, raw—*3.5 oz (100 g)*	21	210	168	446	528	95	56	239	104	305	659	72	810
kidneys													
beef, simmered—*3.5 oz (100 g)*	347	1231	1040	2043	1696	530	77	1223	958	1590	1496	665	813
lamb, braised—*3.5 oz (100 g)*	319	1113	941	1775	1533	480	270	1095	833	1387	1365	595	817
pork, braised—*3.5 oz (100 g)*	329	1053	1357	2280	1829	545	557	1199	914	1463	1561	610	810
veal, braised—*3.5 oz (100 g)*	338	1200	1119	2131	1751	552	292	1248	1009	1392	1622	636	817
liver													
beef, braised—*3.5 oz (100 g)*	351	1116	1116	2294	1693	616	374	1299	967	1506	1533	667	813
beef, pan fried—*3.5 oz (100 g)*	385	1223	1223	2514	1855	675	410	1424	1060	1650	1680	731	813
lamb, braised—*3.5 oz (100 g)*	355	1322	1316	2497	1653	664	320	1365	1090	1683	1714	718	817
lamb, pan fried—*3.5 oz (100 g)*	296	1104	1100	2086	1381	554	268	1140	910	1405	1432	600	817
pork, braised—*3.5 oz (100 g)*	366	1107	1320	2319	2007	645	491	1274	887	1607	1603	708	810
veal, braised—*3.5 oz (100 g)*	227	920	952	1761	975	342	239	1046	777	1210	1039	472	817
veal, pan fried—*3.5 oz (100 g)*	312	1267	1311	2424	1342	471	329	1440	1070	1665	1430	650	817
lungs													
beef, braised—*3.5 oz (100 g)*	186	761	973	1498	1446	408	313	829	460	1005	1234	620	813
lamb, braised—*3.5 oz (100 g)*	204	731	628	1591	1286	359	312	819	560	1095	1196	500	817
pork, braised—*3.5 oz (100 g)*	146	584	664	1288	1211	268	261	691	470	988	863	420	810
veal, braised—*3.5 oz (100 g)*	149	697	777	1071	1388	297	160	665	396	797			817
pancreas													
beef, braised—*3.5 oz (100 g)*	351	1257	1370	2116	1999	490	347	1127	1184	1453	1548	533	813
lamb, braised—*3.5 oz (100 g)*	292	840	804	1461	1972	329	292	767	548	986	1351	657	817
pork, braised—*3.5 oz (100 g)*	625	1281	1496	2130	1965	470	365	1222	1195	1537	1642	552	810
spleen													
beef, braised—*3.5 oz (100 g)*	261	988	968	2217	1815	462	727	1008	715	1510	1454	900	813
lamb, braised—*3.5 oz (100 g)*	292	1080	1677	2354	2049	504	339	1202	771	1727	1672	881	817
pork, braised—*3.5 oz (100 g)*	289	1128	1259	2306	2107	523	361	1205	790	1534	1539	672	810
veal, braised—*3.5 oz (100 g)*	236	975	1106	1529	1782	525	284	855	657	1118			817
stomach, pork, raw—*3.5 oz (100 g)*	98	510	560	990	874	288		525	412	692	924	246	810
tail, pork, simmered—*3.5 oz (100 g)*	102	595	391	952	1020	306	220	510	340	510	1173	306	810
thymus, beef, braised—*3.5 oz (100 g)*	168	790	745	1458	1818	304	280	626	454	947	1440	385	813
thymus, veal, braised—*3.5 oz (100 g)*	282	1485	1864	2393	2794	899		1241		1748			817
tongue													
beef, simmered—*3.5 oz (100 g)*	170	962	952	1652	1705	467	290	913	715	1058	1408	573	813
lamb, braised—*3.5 oz (100 g)*	218	975	843	1535	1527	457	236	805	639	1033	1421	477	817
pork, braised—*3.5 oz (100 g)*	278	1018	1099	1932	1970	540		999		1253	1488	605	810
veal, braised—*3.5 oz (100 g)*	279	1040	1108	1863	1901	533	257	1018	774	1186	1512	589	817
tripe, beef, raw—*3.5 oz (100 g)*	114	503	589	948	1044	315	168	471	396	613	995	363	813

22. MEATS, LUNCHEON

	TRY	THR	ISO	LEU	LYS	MET	CYS	PHE	TYR	VAL	ARG	HIS	REF
beef, loaved lunch meat—*1 oz slice (28 g)*	29	157	151	278	309	89	42	142	108	174	279	106	807
beef, thin sliced lunch meat—*5 slices (21 g)*	48	247	242	441	482	143	70	221	179	271	399	171	813
berliner, pork & beef—*1 slice (23 g)*	40	150	157	276	303	90	51	138	110	162	239	135	807
blood sausage (blood pudding)—*1 slice (25 g)*	47	146	82	357	269	53	47	211	88	263	175	181	807
bockwurst (pork, veal, milk), raw—*1 link (65 g)*	88	358	378	610	681	208	96	320	278	396	528	259	807
bologna, beef—*1 slice (23 g)*	25	105	120	204	213	64	36	100	91	123	172	89	807
bologna, beef & pork—*1 slice (23 g)*	24	118	117	207	203	64	31	106	83	143	161	73	807
bologna, pork—*1 slice (23 g)*	34	147	152	269	277	95	39	135	111	170	231	111	807
bologna, turkey—*1 slice (28 g)*	31	184	145	313	333	108	28	159	137	157	251	146	807
bratwurst, pork, ckd—*1 link (85 g)*	96	473	437	802	910	291	121	400	345	481	706	345	810

	TRY	THR	ISO	LEU	LYS	MET	CYS	PHE	TYR	VAL	ARG	HIS	REF
braunschweiger (pork liver sausage)—1 slice (18 g)	26	96	87	186	164	56	45	100	77	111	138	58	807
brotwurst (pork & beef w/ nfdm)—1 link (70 g)	92	419	424	756	797	258	114	379	310	473	662	305	807
chicken roll, light meat—2 slices (57 g)	127	465	569	821	923	301	146	437	366	545	686	335	807
chicken spread—1 oz (28 g)	51	184	229	327	369	120	56	173	146	216	266	134	807
chorizo (pork & beef)—1 link (60 g)	167	884	1324	1025	1448	282	166	689	449	548	1016	433	807
corned beef, loaf, jellied—1 oz slice (28 g)	46	250	241	444	493	142	67	227	172	278	444	168	807
frankfurter													
beef—1 frank (8 per 1 lb pkg) (57 g)	62	255	293	498	520	157	87	243	222	299	419	216	807
beef—1 frank (10 per 1 lb pkg) (45 g)	49	202	231	393	410	124	68	192	175	236	331	171	807
beef & pork—1 frank (57 g)	47	231	276	467	515	130	74	205	179	268	484	199	807
chicken—1 frank (45 g)	46	260	206	461	493	154	59	231	176	241	401	163	807
turkey—1 frank (45 g)	51	307	243	523	557	181	47	266	228	263	419	244	807
ham & cheese loaf/roll—1 oz slice (28 g)	59	204	214	384	428	124	67	196	159	227	317	192	807
ham & cheese spread—1 oz (28 g)	105	194	220	426	418	135	72	219	189	287	253	169	807
ham, cured													
chopped, cnd—1 slice (21 g)	38	151	145	262	290	88	40	131	111	151	209	134	807
chopped, packaged—1 slice (21 g)	44	160	162	289	322	95	54	145	112	168	252	146	807
minced—1 slice (21 g)	33	154	147	264	286	96	40	135	113	157	215	127	807
sliced, lean (5% fat)—1 oz slice (28 g)	65	241	237	430	459	143	81	234	178	235	352	194	807
sliced, reg (11% fat)—1 oz slice (28 g)	59	219	216	390	417	130	74	213	161	213	319	176	807
ham salad spread—1 oz (28 g)	25	116	114	206	219	65	14	100	79	127	168	99	807
headcheese (pork)—1 oz slice (28 g)	24	125	152	283	271	74	62	170	130	184	321	83	807
honey loaf (pork & beef)—1 slice (28 g)	51	221	204	384	415	134	43	187	162	217	301	171	807
honey roll sausage (beef)—1 slice (23 g)	35	179	175	319	349	103	51	160	129	196	289	124	807
italian sausage, pork, ckd—1 link (67 g)	108	531	490	900	1020	326	135	449	387	539	792	387	810
kielbasa/kolbassy (pork & beef w/ nfdm)—1 slice (26 g)	36	112	166	227	263	72	59	130	127	166	245	82	807
knockwurst/knackwurst (pork & beef)—1 slice (68 g)	73	326	317	558	634	195	100	277	245	350	482	245	807
lebanon bologna (beef)—1 slice (23 g)	36	186	182	332	363	107	53	167	135	204	300	129	807
liver cheese (pork liver)—1 slice (38 g)	78	247	240	506	448	130	125	272	177	306	315	149	807
liver pate, chicken, cnd—1 oz (28 g)	55	170	208	339	270	96	62	197	139	245	231	98	807
goose, smoked, cnd—1 oz (28 g)	46	144	172	292	245	77	43	161	114	204	198	86	807
unspecified, cnd—1 oz (28 g)	45	161	157	298	238	81	48	165	129	218	254	84	807
liver sausage/liverwurst (pork)—1 slice (18 g)	27	121	118	205	208	51	27	111	65	154	146	81	807
luncheon sausage (pork & beef)—1 slice (23 g)	37	153	181	294	333	81	65	143	141	200	260	114	807
luxury loaf (pork)—1 oz slice (28 g)	60	246	228	425	463	131	43	201	180	250	328	184	807
mortadella (beef & pork)—1 slice (15 g)	23	95	106	182	189	59	31	90	80	110	154	78	807
Mother's Loaf (pork)—1 slice (21 g)	36	127	134	236	247	75	43	120	94	140	191	112	807
New England Brand Sausage (pork & beef)—1 slice (23 g)	44	174	175	313	348	103	57	157	123	185	276	150	807
old fashioned loaf (pork & beef), Dutch Brand—1 oz slice (28 g)	41	173	156	301	301	90	30	143	125	173	224	115	807
olive loaf (pork)—1 oz slice (28 g)	29	132	118	244	227	84	40	117	107	142	163	82	807
peppered loaf (pork & beef)—1 slice (28 g)	56	213	219	389	423	125	68	195	155	231	328	182	807
pepperoni (pork & beef)—1 slice (6 g)	12	51	54	95	98	32	15	47	40	59	81	40	807
pickle & pimento loaf (pork)—1 oz slice (28 g)	32	146	137	265	251	71	33	123	109	156	186	96	807
picnic loaf (pork & beef)—1 slice (28 g)	40	184	163	321	334	106	45	150	128	180	249	122	807
polish sausage (pork)—1 oz (28 g)	39	168	173	305	315	107	45	153	126	192	262	126	807
pork & beef lunch meat—1 slice (28 g)	37	152	180	293	332	81	64	143	141	200	259	113	807
pork lunch meat, cnd—1 slice (21 g)	26	102	120	200	196	70	45	103	80	137	182	75	807
poultry (chicken/turkey) salad spread—1 oz (28 g)	37	141	166	249	286	91	40	129	117	167	221	98	807
salami, beef—1 slice (23 g)	32	131	150	254	265	80	44	124	113	152	214	110	813

	TRY	THR	ISO	LEU	LYS	MET	CYS	PHE	TYR	VAL	ARG	HIS	REF
salami, beef & pork—*1 slice (23 g)*	26	120	155	214	255	69	45	111	127	154	197	83	807
salami, beerwurst, beef—*1 slice (23 g)*	26	106	122	207	216	65	36	101	92	124	174	90	807
salami, beerwurst, pork—*1 slice (23 g)*	26	130	112	217	237	82	25	101	93	117	186	96	807
salami, dry/hard													
pork—*1 slice (10 g)*	25	101	108	163	188	47	29	94	69	112	137	61	807
pork & beef—*1 slice (10 g)*	21	96	97	173	182	59	26	87	71	108	152	70	807
salami, turkey, ckd—*2 slices (57 g)*	103	405	466	722	845	260	105	364	353	484	655	279	807
smoked link sausage, pork—*1 link (68 g)*	147	632	647	1151	1187	405	169	577	475	726	989	475	807
smoked link sausage, pork & beef, —*1 link (68 g)*	73	316	330	551	614	248	71	275	262	316	520	269	807
w/ american cheese—*1 link (43 g)*	64	233	266	472	498	154	65	243	222	298	360	203	807
w/ flour & nfdm—*1 link (68 g)*	95	389	422	732	734	244	110	367	312	460	591	295	807
w/ nfdm—*1 link (68 g)*	92	375	411	710	709	234	103	354	307	449	553	282	807
thuringer (cervelat/summer sausage), beef & pork—*1 slice (23 g)*	33	137	157	267	278	84	46	131	118	160	224	115	807
turkey breast—*1 slice (21 g)*	54	210	246	377	445	137	49	188	187	251	330	147	807
turkey ham (cured thigh meat)—*2 slices (57 g)*	123	480	561	860	1017	312	112	428	426	573	753	337	807
turkey pastrami—*2 slices (57 g)*	116	455	523	810	947	292	117	408	396	543	735	313	807
turkey roll, light & dark meat—*2 slices (57 g)*	114	451	518	803	940	291	114	405	392	538	729	311	807
turkey roll, light meat—*2 slices (57 g)*	117	465	534	827	968	299	117	417	404	555	752	320	807
vienna sausage, beef & pork, cnd—*1 sausage (16 g)*	17	57	89	128	127	42	28	68	55	92	113	44	807

23. MILK, MILK BEVERAGES, MILK MIXES & YOGURT
23.1 Milk, Cow

	TRY	THR	ISO	LEU	LYS	MET	CYS	PHE	TYR	VAL	ARG	HIS	REF
buttermilk, cultured—*8 fl oz (245 g)*	88	387	500	806	679	198	76	426	341	595	309	233	801
buttermilk, dry—*1 T (7 g)*	34	108	145	235	190	60	22	116	116	161	87	65	801
condensed, sweetened, cnd—*1 fl oz (38 g)*	43	136	182	295	238	75	28	145	145	201	109	81	801
evaporated													
nonfat, cnd—*1 fl oz (32 g)*	34	109	146	237	192	60	22	116	116	162	87	66	801
whole, cnd—*1 fl oz (32 g)*	31	98	132	213	173	55	20	105	105	146	79	59	801
whole, cnd—*4 fl oz (126 g)*	121	387	519	840	680	215	79	415	415	575	311	233	801
lowfat													
1% fat—*8 fl oz (244 g)*	112	364	486	786	637	203	73	388	388	537	290	217	801
1% fat w/ nfdm—*8 fl oz (245 g)*	120	385	517	835	676	213	78	412	412	571	309	230	801
2% fat—*8 fl oz (244 g)*	115	366	490	795	644	205	76	393	393	544	295	220	801
2% fat, pro fortified—*8 fl oz (246 g)*	138	438	588	952	770	244	91	470	470	649	352	263	801
2% fat w/ nfdm—*8 fl oz (245 g)*	120	385	517	835	676	213	78	412	412	571	309	230	801
lowfat, 1% fat, pro fortified—*8 fl oz (246 g)*	135	435	585	947	768	244	89	467	467	647	349	263	801
nonfat—*8 fl oz (245 g)*	118	377	505	818	662	211	78	404	404	559	301	225	801
dry—*¼ cup (30 g)*	153	490	656	1063	860	272	100	524	524	726	393	294	801
dry, Ca reduced—*1 oz (28 g)*	142	454	609	986	798	252	93	486	486	674	364	273	801
dry, inst—*1⅓ cups (3.2 oz pkt) (91 g)[27]*	450	1441	1933	3129	2533	801	296	1542	1542	2138	1157	866	801
pro fortified—*8 fl oz (246 g)*	138	440	590	954	772	244	91	470	470	652	352	263	801
w/ nfdm—*8 fl oz (245 g)*	123	394	529	858	693	221	81	421	421	586	316	238	801
whole													
3.3% fat—*8 fl oz (244 g)*	112	364	486	786	637	203	73	388	388	537	290	217	801
3.7% fat—*8 fl oz (244 g)*	112	361	483	783	634	200	73	386	386	537	290	217	801
dry—*¼ cup (32 g)*	119	380	509	825	668	211	78	407	407	564	305	228	801
low sodium—*8 fl oz (244 g)*	107	342	459	742	600	190	71	366	366	505	273	205	801

23.2 Milk, Cow, Beverages

	TRY	THR	ISO	LEU	LYS	MET	CYS	PHE	TYR	VAL	ARG	HIS	REF
carob flavor mix in whole milk—*3 t powder in 8 fl oz milk (12 g)*	5	17	23	37	30	9	3	18	18	25	14	10	814

	TRY	THR	ISO	LEU	LYS	MET	CYS	PHE	TYR	VAL	ARG	HIS	REF
choc dairy drink w/ aspartame, from mix, prep w/ water—¾ oz pkt in 4 oz water w/ 3 ice cubes (204 g)	78	235	298	479	390	114	53	259	247	349	218	133	814
choc malted milk, whole milk—3 hp t powder in 8 fl oz milk (265 g)	125	395	519	848	670	215	93	427	419	578	334	238	814
choc malted milk, whole milk w/ added nutrients—4-5 hp t powder in 8 fl oz milk (265 g)	111	363	485	784	636	201	74	387	387	538	292	217	814
choc milk													
1% fat milk—8 fl oz (250 g)	115	365	490	793	643	203	75	390	390	543	293	220	801
2% fat milk—8 fl oz (250 g)	113	363	485	785	638	203	75	388	388	538	290	217	801
whole milk—8 fl oz (250 g)	113	357	480	778	628	198	73	383	383	530	288	215	801
whole milk w/ choc powder—2-3 hp t powder in 8 fl oz milk (266 g)	122	388	511	825	668	207	80	418	412	575	325	229	814
whole milk w/ choc syrup—2 T syrup in 8 fl oz milk (282 g)	121	389	510	823	668	209	82	417	412	572	324	228	814
cocoa (hot choc)													
prep w/ 2% milk—8 fl oz (250 g)	133	415	538	865	703	215	90	453	438	620	370	240	801
prep w/ water from mix—3-4 hp t powder in 6 fl oz water (206 g)	43	130	163	262	212	62	29	142	134	192	119	72	814
prep w/ water from mix, added nutrients—1 pkt in 6 fl oz water (209 g)	27	79	100	161	132	38	19	88	84	117	73	46	814
eggnog, nonalcoholic—8 fl oz (254 g)	137	445	584	937	757	221	97	462	462	643	378	241	801
eggnog, nonalcoholic, mix in whole milk—2 hp t in 8 fl oz milk (272 g)	114	370	492	794	645	204	76	392	392	544	299	220	814
malted milk, whole milk—3 hp t powder in 8 fl oz milk (265 g)	138	427	559	925	702	236	122	469	456	620	382	265	814
strawberry flavored mix in whole milk—2-3 hp t powder in 8 fl oz milk (266 g)	112	364	487	787	638	202	74	388	388	537	290	218	814
23.3 Milk Mixes													
choc milk powder—2-3 hp t (22 g)	10	24	24	38	31	6	8	30	24	37	35	11	814
malted—.75 oz (3 hp t) (21 g)	12	30	34	61	34	13	20	39	32	41	43	21	814
cocoa mix, powder—1 oz pkt (3-4 hp t) (28 g)	42	127	160	258	210	62	29	140	133	188	118	72	814
w/ added nutrients—1.1 oz pkt (31 g)	26	79	99	160	130	38	18	86	82	117	73	45	814
eggnog mix, powder, nonalcoholic—2 hp T (28 g)	2	6	6	10	8	3	2	5	5	7	8	3	814
malted milk powder—.75 oz (3 hp t) (21 g)	26	63	73	140	67	34	49	82	68	83	90	49	814
23.4 Milk, Other													
goat milk—8 fl oz (244 g)	107	398	505	766	708	195	112	378	437	586	290	217	801
human milk—1 fl oz (31 g)	5	14	17	29	21	7	6	14	16	20	13	7	801
indian buffalo milk—8 fl oz (244 g)	129	444	495	893	683	237	117	395	447	534	278	190	801
sheep milk—8 fl oz (245 g)	206	657	828	1438	1257	380	86	696	688	1098	485	409	801
soy milk—8 fl oz (240 g)	103	271	346	578	430	96	113	362	269	338	514	170	816
23.5 Yogurt													
lowfat													
coffee/van flavor w/ nfdm—8 fl oz (227 g)	64	459	611	1128	1003	329	102	611	565	926	336	277	801
fruit flavor w/ nfdm—8 fl oz (227 g)	50	370	493	910	810	266	82	493	456	747	272	225	801
plain w/ nfdm—8 fl oz (227 g)	68	490	649	1201	1069	352	109	649	602	985	359	295	801
nonfat, plain w/ nfdm—8 fl oz (227 g)	73	533	711	1310	1167	384	118	711	656	1076	390	322	801
whole, plain—8 fl oz (227 g)	45	322	429	795	706	232	73	429	397	651	236	195	801
24. NUTS, NUT PRODUCTS, & SEEDS													
acorn flour, full-fat—1 oz (28 g)	26	82	99	169	133	36	38	93	64	119	164	59	812
acorns, dried—1 oz (28 g)	28	88	107	183	143	39	41	100	70	129	177	64	812
acorns, raw—1 oz (28 g)	21	67	81	139	109	29	31	76	53	98	134	48	812

	TRY	THR	ISO	LEU	LYS	MET	CYS	PHE	TYR	VAL	ARG	HIS	REF
almond butter—*1 T (16 g)*	43	89	105	188	81	28	43	135	85	124	302	68	812
almond butter w/ honey & cinn—*1 T (16 g)*	45	94	110	197	85	29	45	141	89	131	317	71	812
almond flour, full-fat—*1 oz (28 g)*	101	208	244	437	188	64	101	313	198	289	703	157	812
almond flour, partially defatted—*1 oz (28 g)*	191	394	461	826	355	121	191	593	375	547	1328	297	812
almond meal, partially defatted—*1 oz (28 g)*	201	415	486	871	374	128	201	625	395	577	1401	314	812
almonds													
blanched, Blue Diamond—*1 oz (28 g)*	48	184	223	416	192	45	133	320	164	266	708	144	I
blanched, slivered, Blue Diamond—*1 oz (28 g)*	49	204	238	448	230	34	133	374	193	284	822	164	I
chopped, Blue Diamond—*1 oz (28 g)*	48	187	227	419	192	39	138	326	167	266	722	144	I
dried—*1 oz (24 nuts) (28 g)*	100	207	242	435	186	64	100	312	197	288	699	156	812
dry roasted—*1 oz (28 g)*	83	172	201	360	155	53	83	258	164	239	579	130	812
honey roasted, unblanched—*1 oz (26 nuts) (28 g)*	80	163	192	343	147	51	80	247	156	228	552	123	812
oil roasted, unblanched—*1 oz (22 nuts) (28 g)*	102	212	248	444	191	65	102	319	202	294	714	160	812
sliced, natural, Blue Diamond—*1 oz (28 g)*	49	703	227	420	193	40	139	326	167	266	723	145	I
toasted, unblanched—*1 oz (28 g)*	104	214	251	450	193	66	104	322	204	298	723	162	812
whole, blanched, Blue Diamond—*1 oz (28 g)*	49	184	224	417	193	45	133	320	164	266	709	145	I
whole, natural, Blue Diamond—*1 oz (28 g)*	49	186	232	422	195	37	125	329	169	275	729	148	I
beechnuts, dried—*1 oz (28 g)*	20	63	69	104	104	41	56	74	49	98	126	49	812
brazilnuts, dried—*1 oz (8 med nuts) (28 g)*	74	130	170	337	153	287	99	211	130	258	678	114	812
breadfruit seeds													
boiled—*1 oz (28 g)*	25	78	90	114	116	20	24	162	111	109	100	42	812
raw—*1 oz (28 g)*	35	109	126	160	162	27	33	226	154	152	140	59	812
roasted—*1 oz (28 g)*	29	92	105	134	135	23	27	189	129	127	117	49	812
butternuts, dried—*1 oz (28 g)*	104	266	334	623	218	173	137	409	277	437	1378	229	812
cashew butter—*1 oz (28 g)*	77	192	238	418	266	89	92	257	160	338	566	130	812
cashews													
dry roasted—*1 oz (28 g)*	67	168	207	364	232	78	80	224	139	295	494	113	812
oil roasted—*1 oz (18 med nuts) (28 g)*	71	177	219	384	244	82	85	237	147	311	521	119	812
chestnuts, chinese													
boiled & steamed—*1 oz (28 g)*	10	33	31	50	44	20	21	37	24	43	84	24	812
dried—*1 oz (28 g)*	23	77	72	119	105	47	51	88	58	101	198	56	812
raw—*1 oz (28 g)*	14	47	45	73	65	29	31	54	35	62	122	34	812
roasted—*1 oz (28 g)*	15	50	47	78	69	31	33	58	38	67	130	37	812
chestnuts, european													
boiled & steamed—*1 oz (28 g)*	6	20	22	33	33	13	18	24	16	32	41	16	812
dried—*1 oz (28 g)*	20	65	71	107	107	43	57	77	50	101	130	50	812
raw—*1 oz (2½ nuts) (28 g)*	8	24	27	41	41	16	22	29	19	38	49	19	812
roasted—*1 oz (3½ nuts) (28 g)*	10	32	35	53	53	21	29	38	25	50	64	25	812
chestnuts, japanese													
boiled & steamed—*1 oz (28 g)*	3	9	11	14	15	6	7	9	7	14	15	6	812
dried—*1 oz (28 g)*	21	60	73	92	97	36	43	58	43	88	98	37	812
raw—*1 oz (28 g)*	9	26	31	39	42	15	18	25	18	38	42	16	812
roasted—*1 oz (28 g)*	12	34	41	52	55	20	24	33	24	50	55	21	812
coconut													
dried—*1 oz (28 g)*	23	71	77	145	86	37	39	99	60	118	320	45	812
dried, sweetened, flaked, cnd—*4 oz (114 g)*	44	139	150	284	169	72	75	194	119	231	628	88	812
dried, sweetened, flaked, packaged—*1 cup (74 g)*	28	88	95	180	107	45	48	123	75	147	398	56	812
dried, sweetened, shredded—*1 cup (93 g)*	32	98	105	199	118	50	53	136	83	163	440	61	812

	TRY	THR	ISO	LEU	LYS	MET	CYS	PHE	TYR	VAL	ARG	HIS	REF
dried, toasted—*1 oz (28 g)*	18	55	59	111	66	28	30	76	46	91	247	35	812
raw—*1 piece (2" x 2" x ½") (45 g)*	18	54	59	111	66	28	30	76	46	91	246	35	812
coconut cream, raw—*1 cup (240 g)*[28]	101	317	341	646	384	163	173	442	269	528	1428	199	812
coconut cream, sweetened, cnd—*1 cup (296 g)*	92	290	314	592	352	148	157	406	246	482	1308	184	812
coconut milk, cnd—*1 cup (226 g)*[29]	54	167	179	339	201	86	90	231	140	276	748	104	812
coconut milk, raw—*1 cup (240 g)*[29]	65	199	216	408	242	103	108	278	170	334	902	127	812
coconut water—*1 cup (240 g)*[30]	19	62	67	127	77	31	34	89	53	106	283	41	812
cottonseed flour, lowfat—*1 oz (28 g)*	213	522	509	965	717	229	371	880	509	725	1909	445	812
cottonseed flour, partially defatted—*1 T (5 g)*	31	76	74	140	104	33	54	128	74	105	277	65	812
cottonseed kernels, roasted—*1 T (10 g)*	49	121	117	223	165	53	86	203	117	167	440	103	812
cottonseed meal, partially defatted—*1 oz (28 g)*	210	515	502	951	706	226	365	867	502	714	1880	439	812
filberts (hazelnuts)													
dried—*1 oz (28 g)*	61	127	161	312	113	46	65	194	128	188	611	93	812
dry roasted—*1 oz (28 g)*	47	98	124	239	87	35	50	149	98	144	469	71	812
oil roasted—*1 oz (28 g)*	67	139	176	341	123	50	71	213	140	205	668	101	812
roasted, salted, Blue Diamond—*1 oz (28 g)*	36	164	184	345	121	90	85	176	130	263	710	124	I
whole, Blue Diamond—*1 oz (28 g)*	167	147	181	320	136	51	65	218	138	223	691	104	I
ginkgo nuts													
cnd—*1 oz (14 med nuts) (28 g)*	11	40	31	48	31	8	3	26	9	43	63	15	812
dried—*1 oz (28 g)*	48	181	142	214	140	38	16	116	41	192	285	69	812
raw—*1 oz (28 g)*	20	76	59	90	58	16	7	48	17	80	119	29	812
hickorynuts, dried—*1 oz (28 g)*	39	120	163	291	141	85	77	202	129	207	591	110	812
lotus seeds, dried—*1 oz (28 g)*	63	212	217	344	279	76	57	217	106	281	358	122	812
lotus seeds, raw—*1 oz (28 g)*	17	57	58	92	75	20	15	58	28	75	96	33	812
macadamia nuts													
dried—*1 oz (28 g)*	60	75	69	131	92	26	27	74	96	91	255	48	812
dry roasted, Blue Diamond—*1 oz (28 g)*	17	85	82	162	94	82	62	91	139	96	371	60	I
oil roasted—*1 oz (10-12 nuts) (28 g)*	53	65	61	115	81	23	24	64	84	80	223	42	812
mixed nuts													
dry roasted—*1 oz (28 g)*[31]	75	169	211	389	202	65	81	270	192	265	636	136	812
oil roasted—*1 oz (28 g)*[32]	70	161	205	381	187	96	83	261	186	265	574	134	812
w/o peanuts, oil roasted—*1 oz (28 g)*	71	161	199	359	193	98	86	232	145	270	564	118	812
nuts, wheat-base formulated													
flavored—*1 oz (28 g)*[33]	49	156	156	276	251	78	64	166	138	202	278	108	812
macadamia flavored—*1 oz (28 g)*[34]	39	135	138	242	217	68	52	145	121	176	231	92	812
unflavored—*1 oz (28 g)*[35]	46	164	157	281	258	79	71	171	137	207	302	111	812
peanut butter													
chunk style/crunchy—*2 T (32 g)*	75	263	270	499	276	94	99	399	313	323	920	195	816
creamy/smooth—*2 T (32 g)*	78	276	284	523	290	99	103	418	328	339	965	204	816
peanut flour, defatted—*1 oz (28 g)*	144	507	521	959	531	182	190	767	602	621	1770	374	816
peanut flour, low-fat—*1 oz (28 g)*	93	328	337	621	344	118	123	497	390	402	1146	242	816
peanuts													
boiled—*½ cup (32 g)*	42	148	152	280	155	53	55	224	176	181	517	109	816
dry roasted—*1 oz (28 g)*	65	230	236	435	241	82	86	348	273	282	803	170	816
oil roasted—*1 oz (28 g)*	73	256	263	484	268	92	96	387	304	313	893	189	816
unroasted—*1 oz (28 g)*	71	250	257	474	263	90	94	379	297	307	875	185	816
peanuts, spanish													
oil-roasted, w/ salt—*1 oz (29 g)*	78	273	281	518	286	98	102	414	325	335	954	202	816
unroasted—*1 oz (28 g)*	72	254	261	481	266	91	95	384	301	311	887	187	816
peanuts, valencia, oil-roasted—*1 oz (28 g)*	75	263	270	497	275	94	98	397	312	321	917	194	816
peanuts, valencia, unroasted—*1 oz (28 g)*	69	244	250	461	255	87	91	369	289	298	851	180	816

	TRY	THR	ISO	LEU	LYS	MET	CYS	PHE	TYR	VAL	ARG	HIS	REF
peanuts, virginia													
oil-roasted—*1 oz (28 g)*	71	251	258	475	263	90	94	380	298	308	877	185	816
unroasted—*1 oz (28 g)*	69	245	251	463	256	88	92	370	290	300	854	181	816
pecan flour—*1 oz (28 g)*	232	295	375	607	341	217	244	477	331	450	1289	264	816
pecans													
dried—*1 oz (31 large nuts) (28 g)*	56	72	91	147	83	53	59	116	81	109	313	64	812
dry roasted—*1 oz (28 g)*	58	74	94	152	85	54	61	119	83	113	322	66	812
oil roasted—*1 oz (15 halves) (28 g)*	50	64	82	132	74	47	53	104	72	98	281	58	812
pilinuts, dried—*1 oz (15 nuts) (28 g)*	54	115	137	252	105	112	54	141	108	199	430	72	812
pine nuts, pignolia, dried—*1 oz (28 g)*	86	216	265	490	255	122	123	261	249	352	1323	163	812
pine nuts, pinyon, dried—*1 oz (28 g)*	41	104	128	236	123	59	60	126	120	170	638	79	812
pistachios													
dried—*1 oz (47 nuts) (28 g)*	80	205	276	475	362	108	145	336	202	400	620	152	812
dry roasted—*1 oz (28 g)*	58	149	200	345	263	78	105	244	147	290	450	110	812
dry roasted, Blue Diamond—*1 oz (28 g)*	70	249	292	493	345	144	124	306	170	385	637	161	I
natural, Blue Diamond—*1 oz (28 g)*	70	250	290	490	350	140	120	310	170	390	160	160	I
pumpkin & squash seeds, dried—*1 oz (142 seeds) (28 g)*	122	256	358	589	520	156	85	346	289	559	1143	193	812
pumpkin & squash seeds, roasted—*1 oz (28 g)*	164	344	481	792	698	210	115	466	388	751	1536	259	812
safflower seed kernels, dried—*1 oz (28 g)*	52	166	203	327	151	81	88	229	151	291	496	128	812
safflower seed meal, partially defatted—*1 oz (28 g)*	114	366	448	720	333	177	194	503	331	640	1092	282	812
sesame butter (tahini), from roasted & toasted kernels—*1 T (15 g)*	56	106	110	195	82	84	51	135	107	143	378	75	812
sesame butter (tahini), from unroasted kernels—*1 T (14 g)*	55	104	108	193	81	83	51	133	105	140	373	74	812
sesame flour													
high fat—*1 oz (28 g)*	191	362	375	668	280	288	176	463	365	487	1294	257	812
lowfat—*1 oz (28 g)*	311	590	612	1089	456	469	287	754	595	794	2108	418	812
partially defatted—*1 oz (28 g)*	250	475	492	875	367	377	231	606	479	638	1695	337	812
sesame meal, partially defatted—*1 oz (28 g)*	105	200	207	368	154	159	97	255	201	268	713	141	812
sesame seeds													
kernels, dried—*1 T (8 g)*	38	94	103	172	66	72	42	122	90	118	266	54	812
kernels, toasted—*1 oz (28 g)*	105	200	207	368	154	159	97	255	201	268	713	141	812
whole, dried—*1 T (9 g)*	35	66	69	122	51	53	32	85	67	89	237	47	812
whole, toasted & roasted—*1 oz (28 g)*	105	200	207	368	154	159	97	255	201	268	713	141	812
soybean nuts, dry roasted—*½ cup (86 g)*	494	1478	1651	2772	2265	459	549	1777	1287	1699	2641	918	816
soybean nuts, roasted—*½ cup (86 g)*	440	1316	1470	2466	2016	409	488	1581	1146	1512	2350	817	816
sunflower seed butter—*1 T (16 g)*	48	128	157	229	129	68	62	161	92	182	332	87	812
sunflower seed flour, partially defatted—*1 T (5 g)*	37	98	120	175	99	52	48	123	70	139	253	67	812
sunflower seeds/kernels													
dried—*1 oz (28 g)*	0	0	0	0	0	0	0	0	0	0	1	0	MUL
dry roasted—*1 oz (28 g)*	84	223	274	399	225	119	109	281	160	316	578	152	812
oil roasted—*1 oz (28 g)*	92	247	303	441	249	131	120	311	177	350	639	168	812
toasted—*1 oz (28 g)*	75	199	244	356	201	106	97	250	143	282	515	135	812
walnuts													
black, dried—*1 oz (28 g)*	91	207	277	483	204	134	133	314	212	365	1038	193	812
english/persian, dried—*1 oz (14 halves) (28 g)*	54	127	160	281	110	79	98	178	124	205	596	102	812
watermelon seeds, dried—*1 oz (95 large seeds) (28 g)*	111	315	380	609	251	236	124	576	288	441	1388	220	812

25. POULTRY
25.1 Chicken, Broiler/Fryer

	TRY	THR	ISO	LEU	LYS	MET	CYS	PHE	TYR	VAL	ARG	HIS	REF
dark meat w/o skin													
fried—*3.5 oz (100 g)*	340	1221	1528	2176	2441	799	375	1156	978	1438	1742	897	805
roasted—*3.5 oz (100 g)*	320	1156	1445	2053	2325	757	350	1086	924	1357	1651	849	805

	TRY	THR	ISO	LEU	LYS	MET	CYS	PHE	TYR	VAL	ARG	HIS	REF
stewed—3.5 oz (100 g)	303	1097	1371	1949	2206	719	332	1030	877	1288	1566	806	805
dark meat w/ skin, roasted—3.5 oz (100 g)	289	1071	1288	1883	2105	688	348	1007	832	1258	1634	759	805
dark meat w/ skin, stewed—3.5 oz (100 g)	261	969	1167	1705	1906	623	314	911	754	1139	1477	687	805
light & dark meat w/o skin													
flour coated & fried—3.5 oz (100 g)	358	1289	1612	2294	2583	844	393	1217	1031	1516	1839	947	805
roasted—3.5 oz (100 g)	338	1222	1528	2171	2458	801	370	1148	977	1435	1745	898	805
stewed—3.5 oz (100 g)	319	1153	1441	2048	2318	755	349	1083	921	1353	1646	847	805
light & dark meat w/ skin													
batter dipped & fried—3.5 oz (100 g)	257	922	1125	1653	1765	591	311	899	732	1100	1378	655	805
flour coated & fried—3.5 oz (100 g)	323	1181	1439	2092	2320	762	382	1121	928	1392	1766	845	805
roasted—3.5 oz (100 g)	305	1128	1362	1986	2223	726	364	1061	879	1325	1711	802	805
stewed—3.5 oz (100 g)	276	1020	1233	1797	2011	657	329	959	796	1199	1545	726	805
light meat w/o skin													
fried—3.5 oz (100 g)	383	1386	1732	2463	2784	908	420	1303	1108	1628	1978	1018	805
roasted—3.5 oz (100 g)	361	1305	1632	2319	2626	855	396	1226	1043	1533	1864	959	805
stewed—3.5 oz (100 g)	337	1220	1525	2167	2454	799	370	1146	975	1433	1742	896	805
light meat w/ skin													
flour coated & fried—3.5 oz (100 g)	344	1262	1537	2231	2487	815	405	1192	991	1485	1888	904	805
roasted—3.5 oz (100 g)	326	1202	1458	2119	2374	776	385	1130	940	1412	1811	858	805
stewed—3.5 oz (100 g)	294	1084	1316	1910	2142	699	347	1019	848	1273	1629	774	805
25.2 Chicken, Broiler/Fryer Parts													
back w/ skin, fried—½ back (72 g)	226	822	1001	1463	1599	529	272	790	647	973	1235	587	805
breast w/o skin													
flour coated & fried—½ breast (86 g)	335	1214	1518	2158	2439	796	368	1142	970	1427	1733	892	805
roasted—½ breast (86 g)	311	1127	1409	2002	2266	739	341	1059	900	1324	1609	828	805
stewed—½ breast (95 g)	322	1163	1454	2066	2339	762	352	1092	929	1365	1661	855	805
breast w/ skin													
flour coated & fried—½ breast (98 g)	357	1300	1599	2306	2581	845	410	1228	1028	1531	1915	940	805
roasted—½ breast (98 g)	333	1219	1494	2154	2424	791	382	1146	960	1432	1800	879	805
stewed—½ breast (110 g)	343	1257	1541	2221	2499	815	395	1181	990	1476	1858	906	805
drumstick w/o skin, roasted—1 drumstick (44 g)	145	526	657	934	1057	345	159	494	420	617	751	386	805
drumstick w/ skin													
flour coated & fried—1 drumstick (49 g)	150	549	672	972	1085	355	174	518	432	646	815	395	805
roasted—1 drumstick (52 g)	158	583	708	1028	1152	376	186	548	456	684	876	417	805
stewed—1 drumstick (57 g)	163	599	730	1057	1187	388	191	563	470	704	897	429	805
leg w/o skin, stewed—1 leg (101 g)	310	1120	1401	1991	2253	734	339	1052	896	1316	1600	823	805
leg w/ skin													
flour coated & fried—1 leg (112 g)	340	1245	1520	2205	2452	804	400	1180	980	1467	1858	893	805
roasted—1 leg (114 g)	332	1225	1487	2160	2421	791	393	1153	959	1440	1847	876	805
stewed—1 leg (125 g)	339	1253	1520	2208	2474	808	401	1178	980	1471	1884	894	805
neck w/o skin, simmered—1 neck (18 g)	52	187	233	332	375	122	57	175	149	219	267	137	805
neck w/ skin, flour coated & fried—1 neck (36 g)	92	346	403	608	658	218	122	331	264	410	559	237	805
neck w/ skin, simmered—1 neck (38 g)	76	295	331	510	557	183	107	278	218	347	500	196	805
thigh w/o skin, roasted—1 thigh (52 g)	158	570	712	1012	1146	373	173	535	456	669	814	419	805
thigh w/ skin													
flour coated & fried—1 thigh (62 g)	187	685	835	1214	1345	442	222	652	539	808	1027	490	805
roasted—1 thigh (62 g)	174	643	779	1133	1269	415	206	605	502	755	971	458	805
stewed—1 thigh (68 g)	177	654	792	1153	1291	422	211	615	511	768	990	466	805
wing w/ skin													
flour coated & fried—1 wing (32 g)	90	338	396	592	650	214	116	321	258	398	538	233	805
roasted—1 wing (34 g)	98	370	432	645	714	234	126	348	281	435	592	255	805
stewed—1 wing (40 g)	98	370	434	646	716	235	125	348	282	435	588	256	805

	TRY	THR	ISO	LEU	LYS	MET	CYS	PHE	TYR	VAL	ARG	HIS	REF
25.3 Chicken, Capon, Roaster, & Stewer													
capon, meat w/ skin, roasted—*3.5 oz (100 g)*	325	1200	1455	2115	2370	774	384	1128	938	1409	1806	857	805
roaster													
dark meat w/o skin, roasted—*3.5 oz (100 g)*	272	982	1228	1745	1975	644	298	923	785	1153	1402	722	805
light & dark meat w/o skin, roasted—*3.5 oz (100 g)*	292	1056	1321	1877	2125	693	320	993	844	1240	1509	776	805
light & dark meat w/ skin, roasted—*3.5 oz (100 g)*	266	989	1191	1739	1945	636	320	929	769	1162	1506	701	805
light meat w/o skin, roasted—*3.5 oz (100 g)*	317	1146	1433	2036	2305	751	347	1077	916	1346	1637	842	805
stewer													
dark meat w/o skin, stewed—*3.5 oz (100 g)*	329	1189	1486	2112	2391	779	360	1117	950	1396	1698	874	805
light & dark meat w/o skin, stewed—*3.5 oz (100 g)*	356	1285	1606	2283	2585	842	389	1207	1027	1509	1835	944	805
light & dark meat w/ skin, stewed—*3.5 oz (100 g)*	301	1113	1348	1961	2197	717	357	1046	869	1307	1680	793	805
light meat w/o skin, stewed—*3.5 oz (100 g)*	386	1396	1744	2479	2807	914	423	1311	1115	1639	1993	1025	805
25.4 Chicken, Unspecified													
chunks, w/ broth, cnd—*5 oz can (142 g)*	345	1271	1541	2241	2505	815	422	1196	993	1494	1924	903	805
25.5 Duck, Goose, & Other Poultry													
cornish game hen w/o skin, roasted—*½ bird (110 g)*	299	1082	1353	1923	2178	710	328	1018	866	1272	1546	795	805
cornish game hen w/ skin, roasted—*½ bird (114 g)*	282	1044	1254	1835	2051	670	340	982	811	1225	1596	739	805
duck w/o skin, roasted—*3.5 oz (100 g)*	327	1003	1206	1983	2009	635	361	984	894	1228	1499	620	805
duck w/ skin, roasted—*3.5 oz (100 g)*	232	773	872	1465	1486	475	299	752	640	938	1284	462	805
goose w/o skin, roasted—*3.5 oz (100 g)*	403	1238	1488	2447	2480	783	445	1214	1103	1516	1849	765	805
goose w/ skin, roasted—*3.5 oz (100 g)*	332	1123	1183	2109	1988	608	390	1055	805	1232	1566	700	805
guinea hen w/o skin, raw—*3.5 oz (100 g)*	241	872	1090	1549	1754	571	264	819	697	1024	1245	641	805
pheasant w/o skin, raw—*3.5 oz (100 g)*	328	1180	1324	1995	2157	686	309	920	773	1305	1433	939	805
pheasant w/ skin, raw—*3.5 oz (100 g)*	304	1108	1228	1870	2015	643	305	876	724	1230	1412	864	805
quail w/o skin, raw—*3.5 oz (100 g)*	341	1090	1187	1866	1905	689	380	944	1010	1180	1379	825	805
squab (pigeon) w/o skin, raw—*3.5 oz (100 g)*	274	876	955	1501	1532	554	305	759	812	949	1109	664	805
25.6 Internal Organs													
giblets													
chicken, fried—*3.5 oz (100 g)*	373	1467	1630	2601	2348	810	437	1480	1067	1737	2159	759	805
chicken, simmered—*3.5 oz (100 g)*	295	1172	1297	2066	1886	646	343	1170	848	1379	1727	602	805
turkey, simmered—*3.5 oz (100 g)*	307	1204	1339	2140	1951	662	354	1207	877	1430	1768	625	805
gizzard													
chicken, simmered—*3.5 oz (100 g)*	243	1251	1281	1907	1877	712	356	1129	825	1216	1950	547	805
turkey, simmered—*3.5 oz (100 g)*	264	1356	1389	2067	2034	772	386	1224	895	1318	2114	593	805
heart, chicken, simmered—*3.5 oz (100 g)*	338	1196	1415	2303	2214	638	359	1183	946	1496	1694	693	805
heart, turkey, simmered—*3.5 oz (100 g)*	343	1212	1435	2333	2243	646	364	1199	959	1516	1717	702	805
liver													
chicken, simmered—*3.5 oz (100 g)*	343	1083	1294	2198	1843	577	327	1212	857	1535	1493	647	805
duck, raw—*3.5 oz (100 g)*	264	833	995	1691	1418	444	252	932	660	1181	1148	498	805
goose, raw—*3.3 oz (94 g)*	216	684	818	1388	1165	365	207	766	541	970	943	409	805
turkey, simmered—*3.5 oz (100 g)*	338	1066	1273	2163	1814	568	322	1193	844	1511	1469	637	805
25.7 Turkey													
breast, w/ skin, prebasted, roasted—*3.5 oz (100 g)*	246	967	1116	1725	2022	623	245	867	845	1155	1554	668	805
dark meat w/o skin, roasted—*3.5 oz (100 g)*	325	1271	1485	2276	2693	828	297	1134	1129	1518	1993	892	805

	TRY	THR	ISO	LEU	LYS	MET	CYS	PHE	TYR	VAL	ARG	HIS	REF
dark meat w/ skin, roasted—3.5 oz (100 g)	304	1200	1379	2138	2503	774	302	1076	1044	1432	1936	828	805
ground, ckd—3 oz patty (82 g)	251	987	1152	1766	2089	643	230	880	876	1178	1547	693	805
light & dark meat													
seasoned, diced—3.5 oz (100 g)	206	813	934	1447	1693	522	210	729	707	970	1313	559	805
seasoned, frzn, roasted—3.5 oz (100 g)	242	948	1109	1698	2009	617	222	846	843	1132	1487	665	805
w/o skin, roasted—3.5 oz (100 g)	333	1304	1525	2336	2763	849	305	1164	1159	1557	2045	915	805
w/ skin, roasted—3.5 oz (100 g)	311	1227	1409	2184	2557	790	308	1100	1066	1464	1979	845	805
light meat w/o skin, roasted—3.5 oz (100 g)	340	1330	1555	2383	2818	866	311	1187	1182	1588	2086	933	805
light meat w/ skin, roasted—3.5 oz (100 g)	315	1247	1432	2220	2599	803	314	1117	1084	1487	2013	859	805
patty, breaded & fried—1 patty (94 g)	157	562	673	1049	1091	359	164	556	509	696	858	391	805
sticks, breaded & fried—2 sticks (128 g)	218	776	929	1452	1495	495	228	773	703	961	1181	539	805
thigh w/ skin, prebasted, roasted—11.1 oz thigh (314 g)	659	2587	2996	4619	5423	1670	644	2314	2267	3090	4135	1793	805

26. SALAD DRESSINGS
26.1 Low & Reduced Calorie

	TRY	THR	ISO	LEU	LYS	MET	CYS	PHE	TYR	VAL	ARG	HIS	REF
russian—1 T (16 g)	1	4	5	7	5	2	1	4	4	5	6	2	804
thousand island—1 T (15 g)	2	6	7	10	8	3	2	5	5	7	8	3	804

26.2 Regular

	TRY	THR	ISO	LEU	LYS	MET	CYS	PHE	TYR	VAL	ARG	HIS	REF
blue (bleu) cheese—1 T (15 g)	11	26	38	65	62	20	4	37	43	52	24	26	804
french—1 T (16 g)	1	5	5	8	6	2	2	4	4	6	7	2	804
italian—1 T (15 g)	2	6	6	9	7	3	2	5	5	6	7	3	804
mayonnaise type—1 T (15 g)	2	7	8	12	9	3	2	6	6	8	9	3	804
russian—1 T (15 g)	4	13	14	20	16	6	4	11	11	15	17	6	804
sesame seed—1 T (15 g)	7	7	7	12	21	4	0	13	15	10	60	5	804
thousand island—1 T (16 g)	2	8	8	12	10	4	3	6	6	9	10	4	804

27. SAUCES, CONDIMENTS, & GRAVIES
27.2 Sauces & Condiments

	TRY	THR	ISO	LEU	LYS	MET	CYS	PHE	TYR	VAL	ARG	HIS	REF
catsup (ketchup)—1 T (15 g)	2	5	4	6	6	1	1	5	3	5	5	4	811
pepper/hot sce—1 t (5 g)	0	1	1	1	1	0	1	1	1	1	1	1	806
pepper sce, Tabasco—1 t (5 g)	1	2	2	3	3	1	1	2	1	3	3	1	806
soy sce													
made w/ soy & wheat (shoyu)—¼ cup (58 g)	43	121	142	240	171	43	53	158	109	148	207	78	816
made w/ soy (tamari)—¼ cup (58 g)	105	236	282	426	424	97	62	310	198	304	235	125	816
tomato sce—½ cup (122 g)	11	37	32	45	46	9	10	34	22	33	33	26	811
spanish style—½ cup (122 g)	12	40	34	49	50	9	11	37	23	35	35	28	811
w/ herbs & cheese—½ cup (122 g)	26	72	85	138	135	34	20	85	73	100	109	61	811
w/ mushrooms—½ cup (122 g)	21	52	45	67	90	17	9	48	28	50	51	34	811
w/ onions—½ cup (122 g)	20	45	51	60	72	12	22	44	35	41	139	31	811
w/ onions, green peppers, & celery—½ cup (122 g)	10	27	26	34	37	6	9	26	17	24	45	18	811
w/ tomato tidbits—½ cup (122 g)	11	37	32	45	46	9	10	34	22	33	33	26	811
white sce													
med, homemade—½ cup (125 g)[36]	54	173	233	375	304	96	35	185	185	256	139	104	806
thick, homemade—½ cup (125 g)	50	161	216	350	284	89	33	173	173	239	129	98	806
thin, homemade—½ cup (125 g)	58	184	248	400	324	103	38	196	196	274	148	111	806

28. SOUPS
28.1 Canned, Condensed

	TRY	THR	ISO	LEU	LYS	MET	CYS	PHE	TYR	VAL	ARG	HIS	REF
celery, crm of—1 can (305 g)	46	143	189	302	180	73	46	189	131	217	143	95	806
cheese—1 can (257 g)	144	380	645	1025	761	234	90	558	499	761	324	293	806
chicken, crm of—1 can (305 g)	104	317	415	640	522	195	122	372	287	421	406	223	806
mushroom, crm of—1 can (305 g)	70	189	235	384	265	95	61	226	183	262	204	113	806
tomato—1 can (305 g)	49	125	143	241	122	55	67	171	104	162	146	88	I

	TRY	THR	ISO	LEU	LYS	MET	CYS	PHE	TYR	VAL	ARG	HIS	REF
28.2 Canned, Condensed, Prepared with Milk													
asparagus, crm of—*1 cup (248 g)*	84	260	340	558	432	144	67	290	270	384	231	159	806
celery, crm of—*1 cup (248 g)*	74	241	322	518	394	131	55	273	248	360	206	149	806
cheese—*1 cup (251 g)*	128	371	567	906	700	218	83	474	444	650	309	256	806
chicken, crm of—*1 cup (248 g)*	99	312	414	657	533	181	87	347	312	444	312	201	806
clam chowder, new england—*1 cup (248 g)*	117	350	451	719	605	203	102	374	337	489	407	265	806
mushroom, crm of—*1 cup (248 g)*	84	260	340	553	429	141	62	288	270	377	231	156	806
pea, green—*1 cup (254 g)*	130	485	541	1016	831	206	117	572	447	711	853	279	806
potato, crm of—*1 cup (248 g)*[37]	82	243	320	513	402	131	64	278	255	362	221	149	806
tomato—*1 cup (248 g)*	77	233	303	494	370	124	64	265	238	335	206	146	806
tomato bisque—*1 cup (251 g)*	80	248	321	520	409	131	60	271	254	356	211	153	806
28.3 Canned, Condensed, Prepared with Water													
asparagus, crm of—*1 cup (244 g)*	29	78	98	163	112	41	29	95	76	115	85	49	806
bean w/ bacon—*1 cup (253 g)*	83	326	385	650	536	99	89	440	235	435	415	205	806
bean w/ franks—*1 cup (250 g)*	105	413	488	823	680	125	110	558	298	550	525	260	806
beef noodle—*1 cup (244 g)*	46	154	188	315	261	90	59	195	124	207	198	112	806
black bean—*1 cup (247 g)*	64	249	287	422	415	62	59	311	49	284	331	163	806
celery, crm of—*1 cup (244 g)*	20	59	78	124	73	29	20	78	54	90	59	39	806
cheese—*1 cup (247 g)*	72	190	321	511	380	116	44	279	249	380	163	146	806
chicken & dumplings—*1 cup (241 g)*	53	193	243	407	378	108	72	224	142	277	292	137	806
chicken, crm of—*1 cup (244 g)*	41	129	171	264	215	81	51	154	117	173	166	93	806
chicken gumbo—*1 cup (244 g)*	22	83	100	168	161	46	17	98	68	117	122	59	806
chicken noodle—*1 cup (241 g)*[38]	39	128	159	265	219	77	46	164	106	176	166	94	806
chicken rice—*1 cup (241 g)*	41	142	178	270	251	92	51	152	123	188	234	101	806
chicken veg—*1 cup (241 g)*	31	113	135	231	222	60	24	133	94	159	169	80	806
chili beef—*1 cup (250 g)*	70	275	328	553	455	85	73	373	200	368	350	175	806
clam chowder, new england style—*1 cup (244 g)*	54	149	183	288	251	90	56	159	127	195	229	137	806
minestrone—*1 cup (241 g)*	31	104	130	236	183	43	34	154	84	178	198	72	806
mushroom, crm of—*1 cup (244 g)*	34	90	112	181	127	44	27	107	88	122	95	54	806
pea, green—*1 cup (250 g)*	73	303	298	623	510	105	80	378	250	443	707	170	806
pea, split w/ ham—*1 cup (253 g)*	101	364	435	711	696	139	134	455	319	491	703	215	806
pepperpot—*1 cup (241 g)*	41	195	234	402	311	92	60	234	157	299	494	92	806
potato, crm of—*1 cup (244 g)*[37]	24	61	76	117	83	29	27	83	61	93	76	39	806
scotch broth—*1 cup (241 g)*	43	154	186	316	304	84	34	181	128	217	231	108	806
stockpot—*1 cup (247 g)*	42	151	183	311	299	82	35	178	126	215	227	109	806
tomato—*1 cup (244 g)*	20	51	59	100	51	22	27	71	41	66	61	37	806
tomato beef w/ noodle—*1 cup (244 g)*	41	144	171	290	242	83	54	181	115	193	183	102	806
tomato bisque—*1 cup (247 g)*	22	67	77	126	89	30	25	77	59	86	67	44	806
turkey noodle—*1 cup (244 g)*	37	124	151	254	212	73	46	156	102	168	159	90	806
turkey veg—*1 cup (241 g)*	27	96	116	198	190	53	22	113	82	135	145	67	806
veg beef—*1 cup (244 g)*[39]	49	173	210	359	344	95	39	205	146	246	261	122	806
veg vegetarian—*1 cup (241 g)*	14	75	99	147	99	24	24	99	48	99	99	48	806
veg w/ beef broth—*1 cup (241 g)*	22	72	92	164	125	31	24	106	58	125	137	51	806
28.4 Canned & Homemade, Ready-to-Serve													
beef, chunky—*1 cup (240 g)*	113	466	593	898	929	247	122	482	353	636	610	276	806
chicken, chunky—*1 cup (251 g)*	123	437	552	924	853	243	163	505	326	628	660	311	806
chicken noodle, chunky—*1 cup (240 g)*	122	437	552	924	854	245	163	504	326	629	662	312	806
split pea w/ ham, chunky—*1 cup (240 g)*	110	391	468	766	749	149	144	490	343	526	758	233	806
turkey, chunky—*1 cup (236 g)*	99	404	514	781	809	215	106	418	307	552	531	238	806
veg, chunky—*1 cup (240 g)*	26	108	161	271	190	26	26	161	82	190	190	82	806
30. SPICES, HERBS, & FLAVORINGS													
basil, fresh—*2 T (5 g)*	2	5	5	10	6	2	1	7	4	6	6	3	802

	TRY	THR	ISO	LEU	LYS	MET	CYS	PHE	TYR	VAL	ARG	HIS	REF
basil, ground—*1 t (1.0 g)*	2	6	6	11	6	2	2	7	4	7	7	3	802
caraway seed—*1 t (2.0 g)*	5	15	17	24	21	7	7	17	13	21	25	11	802
chives, freeze-dried—*¼ cup (0.8 g)*	2	7	7	10	8	2		5	5	7	12	3	811
raw—*1 T chopped (3 g)*	1	4	4	6	5	1		3	3	4	7	2	811
dill seed—*1 t (2.0 g)*		12	15	19	21	3		13		22	25	6	802
dill weed, fresh—*1 cup sprigs (9 g)*	1	6	18	14	22	1	2	6	9	14	13	6	802
fennel seed—*1 t (2.0 g)*	5	12	14	20	15	6	4	13	8	18	14	7	802
fenugreek seed—*1 t (4 g)*	16	36	50	70	67	14	15	44	31	44	99	27	802
garlic powder—*1 t (3 g)*	6	14	19	31	17	10	5	15	6	21	50	9	802
ginger, fresh—*¼ cup slices (24 g)*	3	9	12	18	14	3	2	11	5	18	10	7	811
ginger, ground—*1 t (2.0 g)*	1	4	5	8	6	1	1	5	2	8	5	3	802
mustard seed, yellow—*1 t (3 g)*	16	33	32	53	46	14	17	32	22	40	53	23	802
onion powder—*1 t (2.0 g)*	2	4	6	7	9	2	4	5	5	5	27	3	802
parsley, fresh—*½ cup chopped (30 g)*	13	37	35	61	54	13	4	43	25	52	37	18	811
poppy seed—*1 t (3 g)*	8	27	27	45	33	14	14	26	20	39	60	16	802
thyme, fresh—*1 t (1.0 g)*	1	2	3	3	1					3			802
thyme, ground—*1 t (1.0 g)*	2	3	5	4	2					5			802

31. SPREADS

	TRY	THR	ISO	LEU	LYS	MET	CYS	PHE	TYR	VAL	ARG	HIS	REF
butter													
—*1 t (5 g)*	1	2	3	4	3	1	0	2	2	3	2	1	801
—*1 T (15 g)*	2	6	8	12	10	3	1	6	6	9	5	3	801
sweet (unsalted)—*1 t (5 g)*	1	2	3	4	3	1	0	2	2	3	2	1	801
sweet (unsalted)—*1 T (15 g)*	2	6	8	12	10	3	1	6	6	9	5	3	801
whipped—*1 t (4 g)*	0	2	2	3	3	1	0	2	2	2	1	1	801
whipped—*1 T (11 g)*	1	4	6	9	7	2	1	5	5	6	3	3	801
mayonnaise													
safflower & soybean—*1 T (14 g)*	2	8	9	13	10	5	3	8	6	10	10	4	804
soybean—*1 T (14 g)*	2	8	9	13	10	5	3	8	6	10	10	4	804
sandwich spread—*1 T (15 g)*	2	7	8	12	9	3	2	6	6	8	9	3	804

32. SUGARS, SYRUPS, & OTHER SWEETENERS

	TRY	THR	ISO	LEU	LYS	MET	CYS	PHE	TYR	VAL	ARG	HIS	REF
honey, strained/extracted—*1 T (21 g)*	1	1	2	2	2	0	1	2	2	2	1	0	819
jam/preserves—*1 T (20 g)*	2	5	3	7	6	0	1	4	5	4	6	3	819
marmalade, orange—*1 T (20 g)*	1	1	2	1	3	1	1	2	1	3	4	1	819
syrup, malt—*1 T (24 g)*	18	50	50	91	64	26	16	62	41	73	68	32	819
syrup, pancake & waffle, w/ butter —*1 T (20 g)*	0	0	0	0	0	0	0	0	0	0	0	0	819

33. VEGETABLES, VEGETABLE PRODUCTS, & VEGETABLE SALADS

	TRY	THR	ISO	LEU	LYS	MET	CYS	PHE	TYR	VAL	ARG	HIS	REF
adzuki beans													
boiled—*1 cup (230 g)*	166	587	690	1454	1304	182	161	915	515	890	1118	455	816
cnd, sweetened—*1 cup (296 g)*	107	382	447	944	847	118	104	595	334	580	728	296	816
w/ sugar (yokan)—*three ¼" slices (43 g)*	14	48	56	119	107	15	13	75	42	73	92	37	816
alfalfa sprouts, raw—*1 cup (33 g)*		44	47	88	71			75		48			811
amaranth, boiled—*½ cup (66 g)*	18	56	67	110	72	20	17	75	45	78	69	29	811
asparagus													
boiled—*½ cup (6 spears) (90 g)*	23	65	86	102	111	23	28	55	37	90	109	36	811
cnd—*½ cup (121 g)*	25	73	96	113	122	25	30	62	41	99	121	40	811
frzn, boiled—*4 spears (60 g)*	17	49	65	77	84	17	21	42	28	68	83	28	811
bamboo shoots													
boiled—*1 cup (120 g)*	19	60	61	98	95	20	16	64		74	68	30	811
cnd—*1 cup (131 g)*	24	75	76	122	117	26	18	79		93	84	37	811
raw—*½ cup (76 g)*	21	65	67	106	102	23	17	68		81	74	32	811
beans, baked, homemade—*1 cup (253 g)*	170	577	612	1083	959	218	157	726	392	713	901	387	816
beans, refried, cnd—*1 cup (253 g)*	164	584	612	1108	954	210	152	751	392	726	860	387	816
beans, vegetarian, cnd—*1 cup (254 g)*	145	513	538	973	836	183	132	658	343	638	754	338	816

	TRY	THR	ISO	LEU	LYS	MET	CYS	PHE	TYR	VAL	ARG	HIS	REF
beans w/ pork													
in sweet sce, cnd—*1 cup (253 g)*	159	564	592	1073	921	205	147	726	377	703	832	374	816
in tomato sce, cnd—*1 cup (253 g)*	154	549	577	1042	896	197	142	706	367	683	807	364	816
beet greens, boiled—*½ cup (72 g)*	29	55	38	83	54	15	17	49	44	55	53	28	811
beets													
boiled—*½ cup slices (85 g)*	17	42	43	60	51	16	17	41	34	50	37	19	811
cnd—*½ cup slices (85 g)*	9	23	23	33	28	9	9	22	19	27	20	10	811
cnd, harvard—*½ cup slices (123 g)*	12	31	31	43	37	12	12	30	25	36	27	14	811
cnd, pickled—*½ cup slices (114 g)*	10	27	27	39	33	10	11	26	22	32	24	13	811
black beans, boiled—*1 cup (172 g)*	181	642	673	1218	1046	229	165	824	430	798	944	425	816
black turtle beans, boiled—*1 cup (185 g)*	179	636	668	1208	1040	228	165	818	426	792	938	422	816
black turtle beans, cnd—*1 cup (240 g)*	170	610	638	1154	994	218	158	782	408	756	895	403	816
broadbeans													
boiled—*1 cup (170 g)*	122	459	520	972	826	105	165	546	410	575	1193	328	816
cnd—*1 cup (256 g)*	133	497	566	1052	896	115	179	591	443	622	1293	356	816
falafel—*3 patties (2¼″ dia) (51 g)*[40]	68	251	289	481	437	95	93	361	173	287	653	186	816
broccoli													
boiled—*½ cup (78 g)*	24	76	90	108	117	28	16	70	52	106	121	41	811
chopped, frzn, boiled—*½ cup (92 g)*	29	93	111	133	144	34	20	86	64	131	148	51	811
raw—*½ cup chopped (44 g)*	13	40	48	58	62	15	9	37	28	56	64	22	811
spears, frzn, boiled—*½ cup (92 g)*	29	93	111	133	144	34	20	86	64	131	148	51	811
brussels sprouts													
boiled—*½ cup (78 g)*	22	71	78	89	90	19	12	58		91	119	44	811
frzn, boiled—*½ cup (78 g)*	31	101	112	128	129	27	18	83		130	170	64	811
burdock root, boiled—*1 cup (125 g)*	10	44	51	55	115	15	10	56	30	58	180	53	811
cabbage, chinese													
pak-choi, boiled—*½ cup shredded (85 g)*	13	43	76	77	79	8	14	39	26	59	74	23	811
pak-choi, raw—*½ cup shredded (35 g)*	5	17	30	31	31	3	6	15	10	23	29	9	811
pe-tsai, boiled—*1 cup shredded (119 g)*	18	58	101	105	106	11	20	52	35	79	100	31	811
pe-tsai, raw—*½ cup shredded (38 g)*	5	15	26	27	27	3	5	13	9	20	25	8	811
cabbage, green, boiled—*½ cup shredded (75 g)*	8	26	38	39	35	8	6	24	13	32	43	15	811
cabbage, green, raw—*½ cup shredded (35 g)*	5	17	25	26	23	5	4	16	8	21	28	10	811
cabbage, red, boiled—*½ cup shredded (75 g)*	8	27	40	41	38	8	7	26	13	34	45	16	811
cabbage, red, raw—*½ cup shredded (35 g)*	5	17	25	25	23	5	4	15	8	21	28	10	811
cabbage, savoy, boiled—*½ cup shredded (73 g)*	13	45	66	68	62	13	11	42	23	56	74	27	811
cabbage, savoy, raw—*½ cup shredded (35 g)*	7	24	35	36	33	7	6	22	12	30	40	14	811
carrots													
boiled—*½ cup slices (78 g)*	9	31	34	36	34	5	7	27	16	36	35	13	811
cnd—*½ cup slices (73 g)*	5	17	18	20	18	3	4	15	9	20	19	7	811
frzn, boiled—*½ cup slices (73 g)*	9	31	34	36	34	6	7	27	17	37	36	13	811
raw—*1 med (72 g)*	8	27	30	31	29	5	6	23	14	32	31	12	811
cassava, raw—*3.5 oz (100 g)*	43	65	61	90	100	26	65	60	40	79	314	45	811
cauliflower													
boiled—*½ cup pieces (62 g)*	15	42	43	66	61	16	13	41	25	57	55	23	811
frzn, boiled—*½ cup pieces (90 g)*	19	53	55	85	77	21	17	52	32	73	70	30	811
raw—*½ cup pieces (50 g)*	13	36	38	58	53	14	12	36	22	50	48	20	811
cauliflower, green, ckd—*½ cup pieces (62 g)*	25	68	72	110	101	27	22	67	41	95	91	38	811
cauliflower, green, raw—*½ cup pieces (50 g)*	20	54	56	86	79	21	17	53	32	74	71	30	811
celery, boiled—*½ cup diced (75 g)*	8	18	19	29	24	5	4	18	8	25	18	11	811
celery, raw—*1 stalk (7.5″ long) (40 g)*	4	9	9	14	12	2	2	9	4	12	9	5	811
celtuce, raw—*12 leaves (100 g)*	6	39	55	52	55	10	10	36	21	46	46	15	811
chard, swiss, boiled—*½ cup chopped (88 g)*	16	76	136	119	91	18		100		100	107	33	811

	TRY	THR	ISO	LEU	LYS	MET	CYS	PHE	TYR	VAL	ARG	HIS	REF
chayote, boiled—½ cup pieces (80 g)	6	25	26	46	24	1		29	19	38	21	9	811
chickpeas (garbanzo beans)													
boiled—1 cup (164 g)	139	540	623	1035	973	190	195	779	361	610	1369	400	816
cnd—1 cup (240 g)	115	442	509	845	794	156	161	636	295	499	1118	326	816
hummus—1 cup (246 g)[41]	116	426	487	905	768	101	155	509	381	536	1109	308	816
chicory greens, raw—½ cup chopped (90 g)	28	42	91	67	60	9		37		69	112	26	811
chicory, witloof, raw—½ cup (45 g)	7	11	24	18	16	2		10		18	30	7	811
coleslaw, homemade—½ cup (60 g)[42]	10	29	37	49	43	11	9	28	20	37	42	17	811
collards, boiled—1 cup chopped (128 g)	23	61	70	108	82	23	18	61	47	84	88	33	811
collards, frzn, boiled—½ cup chopped (85 g)	32	89	103	156	120	34	26	89	68	123	129	48	811
corn pudding—1 cup (250 g)[43]	133	495	588	1075	658	293	163	560	455	718	543	288	811
corn, yellow													
boiled—½ cup (82 g)	19	109	109	294	116	57	22	127	103	157	111	75	811
cnd—½ cup (82 g)	15	86	86	233	92	45	17	100	82	124	88	59	811
cnd, vacuum pack—½ cup (105 g)	18	102	102	273	107	53	21	118	97	145	103	69	811
cnd w/ red & green peppers—½ cup (114 g)	19	106	106	280	113	55	23	122	99	150	108	72	811
creamstyle, cnd—½ cup (82 g)	10	57	57	154	61	30	11	66	54	82	58	39	811
frzn, boiled—½ cup (82 g)	27	102	121	221	135	60	34	116	93	148	112	59	811
cornsalad, raw—½ cup (28 g)[44]	7	21	28	37	28	7	6	25	10	28	25	10	811
cowpeas (blackeye peas)													
boiled, immature—1 cup (165 g)	61	195	281	373	345	74	78	287	215	304	366	170	811
cnd, mature—1 cup (240 g)													
frzn, boiled—½ cup (85 g)	83	269	387	515	474	103	107	396	296	418	506	233	811
cowpeas, catjang, boiled—1 cup (171 g)	171	528	564	1065	941	198	154	812	450	662	963	431	816
cranberry beans, boiled—1 cup (177 g)	196	696	729	1320	1135	248	181	894	466	866	1023	460	816
cranberry beans, cnd—1 cup (260 g)	172	606	637	1152	991	216	156	780	406	754	892	400	816
cucumber, raw—½ cup sl (⅙ cucumber) (52 g)	3	10	11	15	15	3	2	10	6	11	23	5	811
dock, boiled—3.5 oz (100 g)		86	93	152	105	32		104	75	121	98	49	811
dock, raw—½ cup chopped (67 g)		63	68	112	77	23		76	56	89	72	36	811
eggplant													
boiled—½ cup (48 g)	4	14	17	25	19	4	2	17	11	21	22	9	811
raw—½ cup (41 g)	4	15	18	26	19	5	2	18	11	22	23	9	811
endive, raw—½ cup chopped (25 g)	1	13	18	25	16	4	3	13	10	16	16	6	811
french beans, boiled—1 cup (177 g)	147	526	550	997	857	188	136	674	352	653	773	347	816
garlic, raw—3 cloves (9 g)	6	14	20	28	25	7	6	16	7	26	57	10	811
gourd, calabash (white-flowered), boiled—½ cup cubes (73 g)	2	12	23	26	15	3		10		19	10	3	811
great northern beans													
boiled—1 cup (177 g)	175	621	651	1177	1012	221	161	798	416	772	913	411	816
cnd—1 cup (262 g)	228	812	852	1541	1326	291	210	1045	545	1011	1195	537	816
green beans (snap beans)[45]													
boiled—½ cup (62 g)	12	51	43	72	56	14	11	43	27	58	47	22	811
cnd—½ cup (68 g)	8	34	29	48	37	10	7	29	18	39	31	15	811
frzn, boiled—½ cup (68 g)	11	44	37	62	49	12	10	37	23	50	41	19	811
hearts of palm, cnd—1 heart (33 g)	8	32	33	56	30	14	6	32	16	38	59	18	811
hominy, cnd, white—1 cup (160 g)	13	80	93	323	53	50	53	122	90	123	109	72	820
horseradish tree, leafy tips, boiled—1 cup chopped (42 g)	34	97	106	186	126	29	33	115	82	144	125	46	811
hyacinth beans, boiled—1 cup (87 g)		108	175	267	177	23	17	57	46	190	175	108	811
jute, potherb, boiled—½ cup (43 g)	10	56	75	132	74	22	14	72	50	84	84	37	811
kale, boiled—½ cup chopped (65 g)	15	55	74	86	74	12	16	63	44	68	69	26	811
kale, frzn, boiled—½ cup chopped (65 g)	23	83	111	129	111	18	25	95	66	101	103	39	811
kale, scotch, boiled—½ cup chopped (65 g)	15	55	73	86	73	12	16	63	44	68	68	26	811
kidney bean sprouts, boiled—3.5 oz (100 g)	50	203	214	347	275	50	55	243	166	248	263	135	811

	TRY	THR	ISO	LEU	LYS	MET	CYS	PHE	TYR	VAL	ARG	HIS	REF
kidney beans, red													
boiled—*1 cup (177 g)*	182	646	678	1227	1053	230	166	830	432	804	950	428	816
calif, boiled—*1 cup (177 g)*	110	391	411	742	637	140	101	503	262	485	575	258	816
cnd—*1 cup (256 g)*	156	561	586	1062	911	200	146	719	374	696	824	371	816
royal, boiled—*1 cup (177 g)*	198	706	742	1340	1152	253	182	908	473	878	1039	467	816
kohlrabi, boiled—*½ cup slices (82 g)*	9	43	68	58	48	11	6	34		43	91	16	811
lambsquarters, boiled—*½ cup chopped (90 g)*	26	112	174	240	243	33	61	113	121	155	174	79	811
leeks													
boiled—*¼ cup chopped (26 g)*	2	9	7	14	11	3	4	8	6	8	11	4	811
freeze-dried—*¼ cup (0.8 g)*	1	5	4	8	6	1	2	4	3	5	6	2	811
raw—*¼ cup chopped (26 g)*	3	16	14	25	20	5	7	14	11	15	20	7	811
lentils, boiled—*1 cup (198 g)*	160	640	772	1295	1247	152	234	881	477	887	1380	503	816
lentils, sprouted, stir-fried—*3.5 oz (100 g)*		322	320	617	698	103	328	434	248	391	600	252	811
lettuce													
butterhead, raw—*2 leaves (15 g)*[46]	1	9	12	12	13	2	2	8	5	10	11	3	811
cos/romaine, raw—*½ cup shredded (28 g)*	3	21	29	27	29	6	5	19	11	24	25	8	811
iceberg, raw—*1 leaf (20 g)*[47]	2	11	15	14	15	3	3	10	6	12	13	4	811
looseleaf, raw—*½ cup shredded (28 g)*	3	17	24	22	24	4	4	15	9	20	20	6	811
lima beans													
baby, boiled, mature—*1 cup (182 g)*	173	632	770	1263	981	186	162	843	517	881	897	448	816
baby, frzn, boiled, immature—*½ cup (90 g)*	78	254	385	470	395	59	73	295	193	374	401	203	811
boiled—*1 cup (188 g)*	173	634	773	1265	983	186	162	844	519	882	899	447	816
cnd—*1 cup (241 g)*	140	513	624	1024	795	149	130	684	419	713	728	364	816
fordhook, frzn, boiled—*½ cup (85 g)*	68	218	332	405	341	51	63	254	166	322	345	175	811
lotus root, boiled—*10 slices (89 g)*	11	28	29	37	51	12	12	25	15	30	47	20	811
lotus root, raw—*10 slices (81 g)*	16	41	44	56	76	18	18	38	23	45	71	31	811
lupins, boiled—*1 cup (166 g)*	208	951	1154	1960	1381	183	319	1026	971	1079	2771	735	816
mixed veg													
cnd—*½ cup (82 g)*[48]	21	85	103	141	126	25	20	89	55	111	143	54	811
frzn—*½ cup (91 g)*[49]	26	105	126	173	155	31	24	109	67	136	176	66	811
mothbeans, boiled—*1 cup (177 g)*	89		687	929	752	133	71	620		443		466	816
mountain yam, hawaiian, steamed—*½ cup cubes (72 g)*	10	44	42	78	48	17	15	58	33	50	104	27	811
mung bean sprouts													
ckd—*½ cup (62 g)*	17	36	61	81	76	16	7	53	24	60	91	32	811
cnd—*½ cup (62 g)*	12	25	42	55	53	11	6	37	16	42	63	22	811
raw—*½ cup (52 g)*	19	41	69	91	86	18	9	61	27	68	102	36	811
stir-fried—*½ cup (62 g)*	36	76	128	171	162	33	16	113	50	126	192	68	811
mung beans, boiled—*1 cup (202 g)*	154	465	600	1099	990	170	125	859	424	735	994	414	816
mungo beans, boiled—*1 cup (202 g)*	158	529	778	1263	1010	222	141	889	473	854	992	426	816
mushrooms													
boiled—*½ cup pieces (78 g)*	40	79	69	107	177	34	5	69	37	80	87	47	811
cnd—*½ cup pieces (78 g)*	34	69	60	92	153	29	4	59	33	69	75	41	811
enoki, raw—*1 large (5 g)*	3	5	2	7	9	2		6	5	4	10	3	811
raw—*½ cup pieces (35 g)*[50]	16	33	29	45	74	14	2	28	16	34	36	20	811
shitake, ckd—*4 mushrooms (72 g)*	3	49	40	67	34	18	19	48	32	48	64	16	811
shitake, dried—*4 mushrooms (15 g)*	5	75	61	102	51	27	29	73	48	73	97	24	811
mustard greens, boiled—*½ cup chopped (70 g)*	18	42	57	48	72	15	24	42	83	62	116	28	811
mustard greens, frzn, boiled—*½ cup chopped (75 g)*	19	45	62	53	77	16	26	45	90	66	125	31	811
navy bean sprouts, boiled—*3.5 oz (100 g)*	74	297	314	508	403	74	80	357	243	363	385	198	811
navy beans, boiled—*1 cup (182 g)*	187	666	699	1265	1087	238	173	855	446	828	981	440	816
navy beans, cnd—*1 cup (262 g)*	233	831	870	1575	1355	296	215	1066	555	1032	1221	548	816
nopales, ckd—*1 cup (149 g)*	21	63	77	122	94	24	12	77	45	92	82	39	811

	TRY	THR	ISO	LEU	LYS	MET	CYS	PHE	TYR	VAL	ARG	HIS	REF
nopales, raw—1 cup (86 g)	12	34	42	66	51	13	7	42	25	51	45	22	811
okra													
boiled—½ cup slices (80 g)	14	54	58	87	67	18	16	54	73	76	70	26	811
raw—½ cup slices (50 g)	8	31	33	49	38	10	9	31	41	43	39	15	811
onion rings, frzn, heated—7 rings (70 g)[51]	49	105	150	245	106	57	76	170	110	151	228	76	811
onions													
boiled—½ cup chopped (105 g)	21	35	50	50	68	12	25	37	36	33	192	23	811
boiled, frzn—3.5 oz (100 g)	11	18	27	27	36	6	14	20	19	18	102	12	811
cnd—½ cup chopped (112 g)	13	22	32	31	44	8	17	24	22	21	122	15	811
dehydrated flakes—¼ cup (14 g)	18	30	44	44	60	10	22	32	31	29	168	20	811
raw—½ cup chopped (80 g)	14	22	33	33	44	8	17	24	23	22	125	15	811
onions, spring, raw—½ cup chopped (50 g)	10	36	39	55	46	10		30	27	41	66	16	811
onions, welsh, raw—3.5 oz (100 g)	21	74	81	113	95	21		61	55	84	137	33	811
parsley, freeze-dried—¼ cup (1.4 g)	7				44	3							811
peas & carrots, cnd—½ cup (128 g)	20	104	101	160	157	40	17	101	58	120	210	54	811
peas & carrots, frzn—½ cup (80 g)	18	93	90	143	140	35	15	90	51	107	187	48	811
peas & onions, cnd, drained—½ cup (60 g)	14	72	71	115	114	29	13	71	42	83	162	38	811
peas & onions, frzn, boiled—½ cup (90 g)	17	84	82	133	132	33	15	83	49	96	188	44	811
peas, green													
cnd—½ cup (85 g)	26	140	135	224	220	57	22	139	79	163	297	74	811
frzn, boiled—½ cup (80 g)	28	154	148	246	242	62	24	152	86	178	326	81	811
w/ onions, red peppers, & garlic, cnd—½ cup (114 g)	24	132	127	210	206	54	21	130	74	153	278	70	811
peas, mature seeds, sprouted, boiled—3.5 oz (100 g)		240	221	473	497	89	200	325	164	285	627	217	811
peas, split, boiled—1 cup (196 g)	182	580	674	1172	1180	167	249	753	474	772	1458	398	816
peppers, hot chili													
cnd—½ cup choppped (68 g)	8	22	20	32	27	7	12	19	13	26	29	12	811
raw—1 pepper (45 g)	12	33	29	47	40	11	17	28	19	38	43	18	811
red, sun-dried—10 peppers (5 g)	7	19	17	28	24	6	10	16	11	22	25	11	811
peppers, jalapeno, cnd—½ cup chopped (68 g)	7	20	18	29	24	7	10	17	12	23	26	11	811
peppers, sweet													
boiled—½ cup chopped (68 g)	8	23	20	33	28	7	12	20	13	27	30	13	811
cnd—½ cup halves (70 g)	7	20	18	29	25	7	10	18	12	24	27	11	811
freeze-dried—¼ cup (1.6 g)	4	11	9	15	13	3	6	9	6	12	14	6	811
frzn, boiled—3.5 oz (100 g)	12	35	31	49	42	11	18	29	20	40	45	19	811
raw—½ cup chopped (50 g)	6	17	15	23	20	6	9	14	9	19	22	9	811
yellow, raw—1 large pepper (186 g)	24	69	60	97	82	22	35	58	39	78	89	37	811
pigeonpeas, boiled—1 cup (168 g)	111	402	412	811	796	128	131	973	282	491	680	405	816
pimientos, cnd 1 T (12 g)	2	5	4	7	6	2	3	4	3	6	6	3	811
pink beans, boiled—1 cup (169 g)	181	644	676	1222	1051	230	167	828	431	801	948	426	816
pinto bean, sprouts, boiled—3.5 oz (100 g)	19	78	82	133	106	19	21	94	64	95	101	52	811
pinto beans, boiled—1 cup (171 g)	166	592	621	1122	964	212	152	759	395	735	870	392	816
cnd—1 cup (240 g)	139	492	514	931	802	178	127	631	326	612	725	324	816
potato, baked													
microwaved w/o skin—1 potato (156 g)	51	119	133	197	200	51	42	145	122	184	151	72	811
microwaved w/ skin—1 potato (202 g)	77	180	200	297	301	79	63	220	184	279	228	109	811
w/o skin—1 potato (156 g)	47	111	125	184	186	48	39	136	114	172	140	67	811
w/ skin—1 potato (202 g)	73	170	188	279	283	73	59	206	172	263	214	101	811
potato, boiled w/o skin—1 potato (135 g)	39	92	103	151	154	41	32	112	93	142	116	55	811
potato, boiled w/o skin, frzn—3.5 oz (100 g)	31	72	80	119	120	31	25	88	73	111	91	43	811
potato, cnd w/o skin—½ cup (90 g)	20	46	51	77	77	20	16	57	47	72	59	28	811

	TRY	THR	ISO	LEU	LYS	MET	CYS	PHE	TYR	VAL	ARG	HIS	REF
potato pancakes, homemade—1 med pancake (37 g)[52]	31	93	106	163	144	52	41	110	87	129	124	51	811
potato, raw w/o skin—1 potato (112 g)	36	84	94	139	141	37	29	103	86	131	106	50	811
potato salad, homemade—½ cup (125 g)	53	145	176	253	214	83	64	169	130	215	190	78	811
potatoes au gratin, homemade—½ cup (122 g)[53]	85	234	346	540	465	143	54	310	281	397	248	184	811
potatoes, fried													
cottage fries, frzn, heated—10 strips (50 g)	23	78	74	104	92	20	11	74	43	88	82	29	811
fries, extruded, heated, frzn—10 pieces (50 g)	24	81	77	107	94	20	12	76	45	90	84	30	811
fries, frzn, heated—10 pieces (50 g)	22	65	66	93	82	20	12	68	42	82	72	28	811
Golden Crinkles, frzn, Ore-Ida—3 oz (85 g)	24	68	60	97	83	22	36	57	39	79	89	38	I
potatoes, hash brown													
frzn, prep—½ cup (78 g)[54]	33	112	106	148	131	27	16	105	62	126	116	41	811
homemade—½ cup (78 g)[54]	26	86	81	114	100	21	12	80	48	96	90	32	811
potatoes, mashed													
from flakes—½ cup (105 g)[55]	20	89	102	158	140	34	23	95	86	125	88	48	811
from granules—½ cup (105 g)[56]	19	92	99	150	139	29	26	98	86	127	98	48	811
homemade—½ cup (105 g)[57]	30	77	91	139	130	37	24	90	80	118	86	46	811
potatoes O'Brien													
frzn, prep—3.5 oz (100 g)	34	80	89	131	132	34	30	95	79	120	111	48	811
homemade—1 cup (194 g)[58]	68	173	213	328	279	83	58	206	178	258	211	105	811
potatoes, scalloped, homemade—½ cup (122 g)[59]	51	140	176	275	234	71	41	165	148	212	144	85	811
pumpkin													
boiled—½ cup mashed (122 g)	11	26	28	41	48	10	2	28	37	31	48	13	811
cnd—½ cup (122 g)	16	39	41	62	73	15	4	43	56	46	72	21	811
pumpkin leaves, boiled—1 cup (71 g)	25	96	96	195	123	33	19	105	96	111	133	31	811
pumpkin pie mix, cnd—½ cup (135 g)	18	42	46	68	80	16	4	47	61	51	78	23	811
purslane, boiled—½ cup (58 g)	9	29	31	53	38	8	6	34	14	42	33	13	811
radicchio, raw—½ cup shredded (20 g)	5	8	17	12	11	2		7		13	21	5	811
radish, oriental													
boiled—½ cup slices (74 g)	3	21	21	26	24	4	4	16	10	23	29	10	811
dried—½ cup (58 g)	25	189	200	240	228	43	36	152	87	212	264	86	811
raw—½ cup slices (44 g)[60]	1	11	11	14	13	3	2	9	5	12	15	5	811
radish, raw—10 radishes (45 g)	2	13	14	17	16	3	2	10	6	14	18	6	811
radish, white icicle, raw—½ cup slices (50 g)	3	23	24	29	28	5	5	18	11	26	32	11	811
rutabaga, boiled—½ cup cubes (85 g)	12	43	45	35	36	9	10	29	21	43	135	27	811
seaweed													
kelp (kombu/tangle), raw—3.5 oz (100 g)	48	55	76	83	82	25	98	43	26	72	65	24	811
laver (nori), raw—3.5 oz (100 g)	43	232	259	501	222	145	100	273	254	402	285	140	811
spirulina, dried—3.5 oz (100 g)	929	2970	3209	4947	3025	1149	662	2777	2584	3512	4147	1085	811
spirulina, raw—3.5 oz (100 g)	96	306	331	509	312	118	68	286	266	362	427	112	811
wakame, raw—3.5 oz (100 g)	35	165	87	257	112	63	28	112	49	209	92	15	811
shallots, freeze-dried—¼ cup (4 g)	6	19	21	29	25	5		16	14	22	36	9	811
shallots, raw—1 T chopped (10 g)	3	10	11	15	13	3		8	7	11	18	4	811
soybean product, miso—½ cup (138 g)	197	882	1119	1558	911	206	131	822	500	1024	1031	454	816
soybean product, natto—½ cup (88 g)	196	715	819	1328	1008	183	194	828	489	896	800	451	816
soybean product, tempeh—½ cup (83 g)	234	639	832	1358	934	220	265	840	608	813	1093	413	816
soybean product, tofu													
dried, frozen (koyadufu)—1 piece (17 g)	127	333	404	619	537	104	113	397	273	411	542	237	816
fried—1 piece (13 g)	35	91	111	170	147	29	31	109	75	113	149	65	816
okara—½ cup (61 g)	31	80	97	149	129	25	27	96	66	99	131	57	816
raw—½ cup (124 g)	156	409	496	761	660	128	139	487	335	506	667	291	816

	TRY	THR	ISO	LEU	LYS	MET	CYS	PHE	TYR	VAL	ARG	HIS	REF
raw, firm—½ cup (126 g)	310	811	985	1511	1309	255	275	968	665	1003	1323	578	816
salted & fermented (fuyu)—1 block (11 g)	14	37	44	68	59	11	12	44	30	45	60	26	816
soybeans, green, boiled—½ cup (90 g)	135	443	489	795	665	135	102	503	399	494	895	299	816
soybeans, mature													
boiled—1 cup (172 g)	416	1244	1388	2331	1906	385	461	1495	1084	1429	2221	772	816
sprouted, steamed—½ cup (47 g)	48	153	176	285	228	42	48	195	145	188	275	106	811
sprouted, stir-fried—3.5 oz (100 g)	159	503	581	939	752	138	157	641	478	620	905	348	811
spinach													
boiled—½ cup (90 g)	36	114	137	208	164	50	32	121	102	151	151	59	811
cnd—½ cup (107 g)	41	128	154	234	184	56	36	136	113	169	170	66	811
frzn, boiled—½ cup (95 g)	40	127	152	232	182	55	36	135	113	168	169	66	811
raw—½ cup chopped (28 g)	11	34	41	62	49	15	10	36	30	45	45	18	811
squash, summer, all varieties, boiled—½ cup slices (90 g)	7	20	30	48	45	12	9	29	22	37	34	18	811
squash, summer, all varieties, raw—½ cup slices (65 g)	7	18	27	45	42	11	8	27	20	34	33	16	811
squash, summer, crookneck													
boiled—½ cup slices (90 g)	7	20	30	48	45	12	9	29	22	37	34	18	811
cnd—½ cup slices (108 g)	5	16	24	39	37	10	6	24	17	30	28	14	811
frzn, boiled—½ cup slices (96 g)	11	30	44	72	68	17	13	43	33	56	52	27	811
raw—½ cup slices (65 g)	5	15	22	36	34	9	7	21	16	27	26	13	811
squash, summer, scallop, boiled—½ cup slices (90 g)	8	23	33	55	51	14	10	32	25	42	40	20	811
squash, summer, scallop, raw—½ cup slices (65 g)	7	19	28	46	44	11	8	27	21	35	33	17	811
squash, summer, zucchini													
boiled—½ cup slices (90 g)	5	14	21	33	32	8	6	20	15	26	24	13	811
frzn, boiled—½ cup slices (112 g)	11	31	46	75	72	18	13	45	35	58	54	28	811
italian style, cnd, packed in tomato jce—½ cup slices (114 g)	10	29	42	68	65	17	13	41	31	52	49	25	811
raw—½ cup slices (65 g)	7	18	27	44	42	11	8	27	20	34	32	16	811
squash, winter													
acorn, baked—½ cup cubes (102 g)	16	34	45	65	42	14	10	45	39	49	63	21	811
acorn, boiled, mashed—½ cup (122 g)	12	24	32	46	31	10	7	32	28	35	45	16	811
all varieties, baked—½ cup cubes (102 g)	13	28	36	51	34	11	8	36	31	39	50	17	811
all varieties, raw—½ cup cubes (58 g)	12	25	33	48	31	10	8	33	28	36	47	16	811
butternut, baked—½ cup cubes (102 g)	13	28	36	52	34	11	8	36	31	40	51	17	811
butternut, frzn, boiled—½ cup mashed (120 g)	20	44	58	84	54	18	13	58	49	64	82	28	811
hubbard, baked—½ cup cubes (102 g)	21	45	59	86	56	18	13	59	51	65	84	29	811
hubbard, boiled, mashed—½ cup (118 g)	25	52	68	99	65	21	15	68	59	76	97	33	811
spaghetti, boiled/baked—½ cup (78 g)	7	14	19	27	17	5	4	19	16	20	26	9	811
succotash													
boiled—½ cup (96 g)	55	203	275	428	285	65	53	235	166	296	284	155	811
cnd—½ cup (128 g)	37	138	188	293	195	45	36	161	114	202	195	106	811
cnd w/ cream style corn—½ cup (133 g)	40	146	198	309	205	47	39	169	120	213	205	112	811
frzn, boiled—½ cup (85 g)	41	152	207	322	214	49	40	177	125	223	213	116	811
swamp cabbage, boiled—½ cup chopped (49 g)		55	41	57	43	17	11	50	31	53	58	18	811
swamp cabbage, raw—1 cup chopped (56 g)		78	58	82	61	25	16	71	45	76	83	26	811
sweet potato													
baked, frzn—½ cup cubes (88 g)	18	75	76	111	74	37	12	91	62	99	70	28	811
baked w/ skin—1 sweet potato (114 g)	24	98	98	144	97	48	16	117	81	128	91	36	811
boiled w/o skin—½ cup mashed (164 g)	33	134	134	198	133	67	21	162	112	177	126	51	811
candied—1 piece (2½" long & 2" dia) (105 g)[61]	12	45	46	68	46	22	7	55	38	60	42	18	811

	TRY	THR	ISO	LEU	LYS	MET	CYS	PHE	TYR	VAL	ARG	HIS	REF
cnd—1 cup pieces (200 g)	40	164	166	242	162	82	26	198	136	216	154	62	811
cnd, mashed—1 cup (255 g)	61	250	252	370	247	125	41	303	207	329	235	94	811
cnd, syrup pack—½ cup (98 g)	16	63	63	92	62	31	10	75	52	82	59	24	811
taro, ckd—½ cup slices (66 g)	5	16	13	25	15	5	7	18	13	18	24	8	811
taro leaves, steamed—½ cup (74 g)	19	67	105	158	99	32	26	79	72	104	89	46	811
tomato, green, raw—1 tomato (123 g)	11	37	36	54	54	12	20	38	26	38	36	22	811
tomato paste, cnd—½ cup (131 g)	33	109	93	134	138	24	28	102	66	98	97	76	811
tomato puree, cnd—1 cup (250 g)	28	95	80	118	123	23	25	88	55	85	83	65	811
tomato, red, boiled—½ cup (120 g)	10	32	31	47	47	11	17	34	22	32	31	19	811
tomato, red, raw—1 tomato (123 g)	7	26	25	38	38	9	14	27	18	27	26	16	811
tomato, red, stewed —1 cup (101 g)[62]	19	55	65	107	63	24	29	76	41	76	68	36	811
cnd—½ cup (128 g)	9	29	28	45	45	10	15	32	20	32	28	18	811
tomato, red, sun-dried—1 cup (54 g)	56	193	183	279	280	66	99	198	131	195	185	116	811
tomato, red, sun-dried, cnd, packed in oil—1 cup (110 g)	41	141	133	204	205	48	73	144	96	143	135	85	811
tomato, red, wedges in tomato jce, cnd—½ cup (131 g)	8	26	25	38	38	9	13	28	18	26	25	16	811
tomato, red, whole, peeled, cnd—½ cup (120 g)	8	29	26	41	41	10	14	29	19	29	28	17	811
turnip, boiled—½ cup cup (78 g)	5	16	23	20	22	7	3	11	9	18	15	9	811
turnip, frzn, boiled—3.5 oz (100 g)	15	42	62	57	61	19	9	30	23	51	41	24	811
turnip greens													
boiled—½ cup chopped (72 g)	14	45	42	76	53	19	9	50	32	56	52	20	811
cnd—½ cup (117 g)	27	87	82	145	103	36	18	97	62	108	99	39	811
frzn, boiled—½ cup (82 g)	48	151	142	252	179	62	31	169	107	187	172	66	811
raw—½ cup chopped (28 g)	7	23	22	38	27	10	5	26	16	29	26	10	811
turnip greens & turnips, frzn, boiled— 3.5 oz (100 g)	31	97	101	156	120	41	20	102	66	120	108	45	811
vinespinach, raw—3.5 oz (100 g)	28	55	53	101	86	19	27	85	48	65	70	39	811
watercress, raw—½ cup chopped (17 g)	5	23	16	28	23	3	1	19	11	23	26	7	811
waxgourd, boiled—½ cup cubes (87 g)[63]	2				8	3							811
white beans													
boiled—1 cup (179 g)	206	732	768	1389	1196	261	190	942	490	911	1078	485	816
cnd—1 cup (262 g)	225	799	838	1517	1305	286	207	1027	534	996	1176	529	816
small, boiled—1 cup (179 g)	190	675	709	1282	1103	242	175	868	453	840	993	448	816
winged bean leaves, raw—3.5 oz (100 g)	116	182	204	359	228	64	75	188	126	245	178	82	811
winged beans, boiled—1 cup (172 g)	401	619	771	1311	1121	187	286	750	765	803	991	415	816
yam, boiled/baked—½ cup cubes (68 g)	8	35	34	64	39	14	12	47	27	41	84	22	811
yambean, boiled—3.5 oz (100 g)		18	16	25	26	7	6	17	12	22	37	19	811
yardlong bean, boiled—1 cup (171 g)	174	540	576	1086	959	202	156	828	458	675	982	439	816
yellow beans, boiled—1 cup (177 g)	191	683	717	1296	1113	244	177	878	457	848	1004	451	816

34. MISCELLANEOUS

	TRY	THR	ISO	LEU	LYS	MET	CYS	PHE	TYR	VAL	ARG	HIS	REF
baking choc, unsweetened—1 oz square (28 g)	43	114	111	174	144	30	35	138	108	173	163	50	819
liquid—1 oz pkt (28 g)	51	135	132	206	171	35	41	164	128	204	193	59	819
cocoa, unsweetened, dry powder—1 T (5 g)	15	39	38	59	49	10	12	47	37	59	56	17	819
processed w/ alkali—1 T (5 g)	14	36	35	55	45	9	11	43	34	54	51	16	819
gelatin, dry, unsweetened—1 pkt (7 g)	0	103	81	172	242	42	0	122	21	146	463	46	819
olives, pickled, ripe, manzanillo/ mission													
—1 small (3.2 g)		1	1	2	1	0		1	1	1	2	1	809
—1 med (4.0 g)		1	1	2	1	0		1	1	2	3	1	809
—1 large (4.4 g)		1	1	2	1	1		1	1	2	3	1	809
—1 extra large (6.0 g)		2	2	3	2	1		2	1	2	4	1	809
olives, pickled, ripe, sevillano/ascolano													
—1 jumbo (8 g)		3	3	5	3	1		3	2	4	6	2	809
—1 colossal (11 g)		4	4	7	4	2		4	3	5	9	3	809
—1 super colossal (15 g)		5	5	9	6	2		5	4	7	12	4	809

	TRY	THR	ISO	LEU	LYS	MET	CYS	PHE	TYR	VAL	ARG	HIS	REF
pickle relish													
hamburger—*1 T (15 g)*	1	3	3	5	4	1	1	3	2	3	6	2	811
hot dog—*1 T (15 g)*	3	7	8	11	10	3	3	7	5	8	15	5	811
sweet—*1 T (15 g)*	1	2	2	3	2	1	0	2	1	2	3	1	811
pickles, dill—*1 slice (6 g)*	0	1	1	2	2	0	0	1	1	1	2	1	811
—*1 large (3¾" long x 1¼" dia) (65 g)*	3	11	12	17	17	3	3	11	7	13	26	6	809
pickles, sour—*1 med (3¾" long, 1½" dia) (35 g)*	1	3	4	5	5	1	1	3	2	4	7	2	811
pickles, sweet—*1 large (3" long, ¾" dia) (35 g)*	1	4	4	6	5	1	1	4	2	4	8	2	811
soybean protein concentrate—*1 oz (28 g)*	237	701	834	1394	1114	231	251	929	652	869	1316	447	816
soybean protein isolate—*1 oz (28 g)*	316	889	1206	1923	1510	320	297	1302	913	1162	1891	653	816
tapioca, pearl, dry—*⅓ cup (51 g)*	2	2	2	3	3	1	2	2	1	3	10	2	820
tomato powder—*3.5 oz (100 g)*	89	295	250	359	370	66	76	273	173	264	258	204	811
whey													
acid, dry—*1 T (3 g)*	7	18	17	33	30	7	6	12	9	17	10	7	801
acid, fluid—*1 cup (246 g)*	39	93	93	177	160	34	34	62	47	93	52	37	801
sweet, dry—*1 T (8 g)*	16	65	58	95	82	19	20	33	29	56	30	19	801
sweet, fluid—*1 cup (246 g)*	32	133	116	192	167	39	42	66	59	113	62	39	801
yeast													
bakers, active dry—*1 pkg (¼ oz) (7 g)*	34	139	152	214	221	53	36	130	111	164	148	70	818
bakers, compressed—*1 cake (.6 oz) (17 g)*	18	74	81	114	117	28	19	69	59	87	79	37	818

1. Contains table wine, swiss cheese, and all-purpose enriched flour.
2. Thin white sauce made with cheddar cheese and salt.
3. Contains hydrogenated vegetable oil and soy protein; vegetable oils are usually soybean, cottonseed, safflower, or blends thereof.
4. Contains lauric acid oils and sodium caseinate; lauric oils include modified coconut oil, hydrogenated coconut oil, and/or palm kernel oil.
5. Made with unequal weights of flour, sugar, fat, and eggs.
6. Made with equal weights of flour, sugar, fat, and eggs.
7. 28 wafers (168 g) = 1½ cups wafer crumbs.
8. Nine crackers (126 g) are equivalent to 1½ cups of cracker crumbs.
9. Includes apple, cinnamon, raisin, lemon, raspberry, and strawberry.
10. Includes almond, raisin nut, and cinnamon nut.
11. Includes apple, blueberry, cherry, and strawberry.
12. Includes apple, blueberry, cherry, lemon, peach, and strawberry.
13. Contains whole milk, spinach, egg white, cheddar cheese, egg yolk, butter, flour, salt, and pepper.
14. Contains egg whites, corn oil, and nonfat dry milk.
15. Contains egg white, hydrogenated soybean oil, and soy protein.
16. Contains cheese, salami, ham, lettuce, tomato, onion, and oil.
17. Dipped in flour and salt before frying.
18. Breading consists of cornmeal, egg, milk, and salt.
19. Breading consists of bread crumbs, egg, milk, and salt.
20. These values also apply to canned clams.
21. Prepared with crab meat, egg, onion, and margarine.
22. Prepared from walleye pollock, bread crumbs, egg, milk, and salt.
23. Prepared from walleye pollock.
24. Prepared with light tuna canned in oil, pickle relish, salad dressing, onion, and celery.
25. Contains enriched wheat flour, lard, salt, leavening agents, and calcium carbonate.
26. Lowfat milk, egg, and vegetable oil added to mix.
27. Reconstitutes to 1 quart of fluid nonfat milk.
28. Liquid expressed from grated coconut.
29. Liquid expressed from grated coconut and coconut water.
30. Liquid from the coconut center.
31. Cashew, almonds, peanuts, filberts, and pecans.
32. Cashews, peanuts, brazilnuts, filberts, almonds, and pecans.
33. Hydrogenated soybean oil, wheat germ, sugar, sodium caseinate, soy protein, natural and artificial flavors, and artificial color.
34. Hydrogenated soybean oil, wheat germ, sugar, wheat starch, sodium caseinate, soy protein, natural and artificial flavor.
35. Hydrogenated soybean oil, wheat germ, fructose, wheat starch, sodium caseinate, soy protein, and salt.
36. Contains lowfat milk, margarine, flour, and salt.
37. Includes vichyssoise.
38. Includes chicken alphabet, chicken noodle-o's, chicken with stars, and curly noodle with chicken.
39. Includes beef, beef vegetable, and barley and vegetable beef.
40. Made with broadbeans, soybean oil, onions, flour, salt, garlic, coriander, and cumin.
41. Made with chickpeas, lemon juice, tahini, olive oil, and garlic.
42. Made with cabbage, celery, table cream, sugar, green pepper, lemon juice, onion, pimento, vingegar, salt, dry mustard, and white pepper.
43. Made with yellow corn, whole milk, egg, sugar, butter, salt, and pepper.
44. European plant used as an herb and as salad greens.
45. Includes Italian, green, and yellow varieties.
46. Includes Boston and Bibb types.
47. Includes crisphead types.
48. Carrots, green peas, snap beans, and lima beans.
49. Corn, lima beans, snap beans, green peas, and carrots.
50. Agaricus bisporus.
51. Breaded and parboiled in vegetable oil.
52. Contains potatoes, eggs, onion, margarine, flour, and salt.
53. Potatoes, whole milk, cheddar cheese, butter, flour, and salt.
54. Pan fried in vegetable oil.
55. Whole milk and butter added.
56. Milk, water and margarine added.
57. Whole milk and margarine added.
58. Potatoes, whole milk, onions, green pepper, bread crumbs, salt, butter, and black pepper.
59. Potatoes, whole milk, butter, flour, and salt.
60. Includes daikon (Japanese) and Chinese radishes.
61. Canned sweet potato and syrup, brown sugar, butter, and salt.
62. Tomatoes, breadcrumbs, margarine, sugar, onions, salt, and pepper.
63. Chinese preserving melon.

Caffeine (mg)

1. BEVERAGES
1.2 Carbonated Beverages
Cherry Coca-Cola—*8 fl oz (240 g)*	31
Cherry RC—*12 fl oz (360 g)*	12
Coca-Cola Classic—*8 fl oz (240 g)*	31
Coke II—*8 fl oz (240 g)*	31
cola—*12 fl oz (370 g)*	37
Draft Cola, Royal Crown—*12 fl oz (360 g)*	43
Kick—*12 fl oz (360 g)*	58
Maxxvm Cola, Nehi—*12 fl oz (360 g)*	70
Mello Yello—*8 fl oz (240 g)*	35
Mountain Dew—*12 fl oz (360 g)*	55
Mr. Pibb—*8 fl oz (240 g)*	27
pepper type—*12 fl oz (368 g)*	37
Pepsi—*12 fl oz (360 g)*	37
Pepsi, wild cherry—*12 fl oz (360 g)*	38
RC Cola—*12 fl oz (360 g)*	43
Slice,	
cherry spice—*12 fl oz (360 g)*	35
cola—*12 fl oz (360 g)*	11
red—*12 fl oz (360 g)*	34

1.3 Carbonated Beverages, Low Calorie
diet cherry Coca-Cola—*8 fl oz (240 g)*	31
Diet Coke—*8 fl oz (248 g)*	31
diet cola, aspartame sweetened—*12 fl oz (355 g)*	50
diet cola, sodium saccharin sweetened—*12 fl oz (355 g)*	39
Diet Kick Citrus—*12 fl oz (360 g)*	58
Diet Mello Yello—*8 fl oz (240 g)*	35
Diet Mountain Dew—*12 fl oz (360 g)*	55
Diet Mr. Pibb—*8 fl oz (240 g)*	27
Diet Pepsi—*12 fl oz (360 g)*	36
Diet RC—*12 fl oz (360 g)*	48
Diet Rite Cola—*12 fl oz (360 g)*[1]	48
Tab—*8 fl oz (240 g)*	31

1.5 Coffee
brewed—*6 fl oz (177 g)*	103
ground, Folgers—*1 T (4 g)*[2]	59
inst powder—*1 rd t (1.8 g)*	57
cappuccino flavor, sugar sweetened—*2 rd t (14 g)*	73
decaffeinated—*1 rd t (1.8 g)*	2
french flavor, sugar sweetened—*2 rd t (12 g)*	51
mocha flavor, sugar sweetened—*2 rd t (12 g)*	33
w/ chicory—*1 rd t (1.8 g)*	37
prep from inst powder—*6 fl oz water & 1 rd t powder (179 g)*	57
cappuccino flavor, sugar sweetened—*6 fl oz water & 2 rd t powder (192 g)*	75
decaffeinated—*6 fl oz water & 1 rd t powder (179 g)*	2
french flavor, sugar sweetened—*6 fl oz water & 2 rd t powder (189 g)*	51
mocha flavor, sugar sweetened—*6 fl oz water & 2 rd t powder (188 g)*	34
w/ chicory—*6 fl oz water & 1 rd t powder (179 g)*	38

1.7 Tea, Hot/Iced
brewed, black, 3 min—*6 fl oz (178 g)*	36
iced, inst powder—*1 t (0.7 g)*	30
w/ lemon flavor—*1 rd t (1.4 g)*	25
w/ sodium saccharin & lemon flavor—*2 t (1.6 g)*	36
w/ sugar & lemon flavor—*3 rd t (23 g)*	29
prep from inst powder—*1 t powder in 8 fl oz water (237 g)*	31
w/ lemon flavor—*1 rd t powder in 8 fl oz water (238 g)*	26
w/ sodium saccharin & lemon flavor—*2 t powder in 8 fl oz water (238 g)*	36
w/ sugar & lemon flavor—*3 rd t powder in 8 fl oz water (259 g)*	28

2. CANDY & GUM
After Eight Mints—*2 mints (8 g)*	2
Baby Ruth—*2.1 oz bar (60 g)*	2
Butterfinger—*2.16 oz bar (61 g)*	2
choc chips, semi-sweet—*1 cup (6 oz pkg) (168 g)*	104
choc coated,	
peanuts—*10 pieces (40 g)*	9
peanuts, Goobers—*1.38 oz pkg (39 g)*	9
raisins—*10 pieces (10 g)*	3
raisins, Raisinets—*1.58 oz pkg (45 g)*	11
choc, semi-sweet—*1 oz (28 g)*	18
choc, sweet, dark—*1.45 oz bar (41 g)*	27
Special Dark, Hershey—*1.5 oz bar (41 g)*	31
Chunky—*1.4 oz bar (40 g)*	12
Crunch, Nestle—*1.4 oz bar (40 g)*	10
Golden Almond,	
Hershey—*3.2 oz bar (91 g)*	16
III, Hershey—*3.2 oz bar (91 g)*	15
Solitaires w/ almonds, Hershey—*3 oz pkg (85 g)*	14
Hundred Grand—*1.5 oz bar (43 g)*	11
Kit Kat Wafer, Hershey—*1.5 oz bar (42 g)*	5
Krackel choc bar, Hershey—*1.5 oz bar (41 g)*	7
milk choc—*1.55 oz bar (44 g)*	11
w/ almonds—*1.55 oz bar (44 g)*	10
w/ rice cereal—*1.45 oz bar (41 g)*	9
milk choc chips—*1 cup chips (168 g)*	43
Mr. Goodbar, Hershey—*1.75 oz bar (49 g)*	5
Peanut Butter Cups, Reese's—*2 pieces (1. 8 oz) (50 g)*	6
Rolo caramels w/ milk choc, Hershey—*9 pieces (1.9 oz) (53 g)*	4
Turtles, Demet's—*.6 oz piece (17 g)*	1
Twix, caramel—*2 oz pkg (2 pieces) (57 g)*	2

8. DESSERTS
8.6 Frozen Desserts
ice cream, choc—*½ cup (66 g)*	2

8.9 Granola, Cereal, and Snack Bars
peanut butter, soft w/ choc coating—*1.3 oz bar (37 g)*	2

8.12 Puddings, Custards, & Pie Fillings
choc, rte—*5 oz can (142 g)*	7

8.13 Sauces, Syrups, & Toppings for Desserts
choc fudge topping—*1 T (21 g)*	2
choc syrup—*2 T (1 fl oz) (38 g)*	5

23. MILK, MILK BEVERAGES, MILK MIXES & YOGURT
23.2 Milk, Cow, Beverages
choc dairy drink w/ aspartame, from mix, prep w/ water—*¾ oz pkt in 4 oz water w/ 3 ice cubes (204 g)*	22

choc malted milk, whole milk—*3 hp t powder in 8 fl oz milk (265 g)*	8
choc malted milk, whole milk wadded nutrients—*4-5 hp t powder in 8 fl oz milk (265 g)*	5
choc milk, whole milk wchoc powder—*2-3 hp t powder in 8 fl oz milk (266 g)*	8
whole milk wchoc syrup—*2 T syrup in 8 fl oz milk (282 g)*	6
cocoa (hot choc),	
prep w/ water from mix—*3-4 hp t powder in 6 fl oz water (206 g)*	4
prep w/ water from mix, added nutrients—*1 pkt in 6 fl oz water (209 g)*	6
prep w/ water from mix, aspartame sweetened—*.53 oz pkt powder in 6 fl oz water (192 g)*	15

23.3 Milk Mixes

choc milk powder—*2-3 hp t (22 g)*	8
malted—*.75 oz (3 hp t) (21 g)*	8
malted w/ added nutrients—*.75 oz (4-5 hp t) (21 g)*	6
cocoa mix, powder—*1 oz pkt (3-4 hp t) (28 g)*	5
aspartame sweetened—*.53 oz pkt (15 g)*	16
w/ added nutrients—*1.1 oz pkt (31 g)*	6

34. MISCELLANEOUS

baking choc, unsweetened—*1 oz square (28 g)*	57
cocoa, unsweetened, dry powder—*1 T (5 g)*	12
processed w/ alkali—*1 T (5 g)*	4

1. This product is available with caffeine (48 mg caffeine / 12 fl oz) and caffeine-free (0 mg caffeine / 12 fl oz).

2. The decaffeinated product contains 1 mg instead of 59 mg.

Calories & Carbohydrates in Chewing Gum, Mints, Candies, & Medications[1]

	KCAL	CHO (mg)		KCAL	CHO (mg)
Chewing Gum			Wrigleys—*1 piece*	10	2.3
1 stick (3.0 g)	10	2.9	**Mints/Candy**		
1 block (8.0 g)	27	7.7	Breath Savers, sugar free—*1 mint*	8	2.0
Beechies—*1 piece*	6	2.0	Certs, clear—*1 mint (2.2 g)*	8	2.1
Bubble Yum—*1 piece (8.0 g)*	25	6.0	Certs, pressed—*1 mint (1.7 g)*	6	1.5
Beech-Nut—*1 piece*	10	2.0	Certs, sugar free—*1 mint (1.7 g)*	7	1.6[2]
Bubblicious—*1 piece (7.9 g)*	25	6.2	Certs, sugar free mini-mints—*1 mint (0.4 g)*	1	0.4[2]
Bubblicious, sugar free—*1 piece (2.3 g)*	5	1.3[2]	Clorets, clear—*1 mint (2.2 g)*	8	2.1
Candilicious—*1 piece (8.5 g)*	30	7.6	Clorets, pressed—*1 mint (1.7 g)*	6	1.6
Carefree Sugarless—*1 piece*	8	2.0	Dynamints—*1 mint (0.4 g)*	2	0.4
Chewels—*1 piece (3.3 g)*	8	2.0[2]	Fiji-Fruits—*1 piece (1.3 g)*	5	1.3
Chiclets—*1 piece (1.6 g)*	6	1.5	Rascals—*1 piece (1.0 g)*	4	1.0
Clorets—*1 piece (1.6 g)*	6	1.5			
Clorets Stick—*1 piece (3.2 g)*	9	2.3	**Medications**		
Dentyne—*1 piece (1.9 g)*	6	1.5	Beech-Nut Cough Drops—*1 piece*	10	3.0
Dentyne, sugar free—*1 piece (1.9 g)*	5	1.1[?]	Halls Cough Tablets—*1 tablet (3.8 g)*	15	3.7
Freshen-Up—*1 piece (4.2 g)*	13	3.1	Listerine Throat Lozenges—*1 lozenge (2.2 g)*	9	2.0
Fruit Stripe—*1 stick (3.0 g)*	10	2.0	Pine Brothers Cough Drops, honey & wild cherry—*1 piece (2.2 g)*	10	2.4
Hubba Bubba Bubble Gum—*1 piece (8.0 g)*	23	5.8	Rolaids—*1 tablet (1.4 g)*	4	1.1
Sticklets—*1 piece (2.5 g)*	7	1.9	Rolaids Sodium Free, cherry[3]—*1 tablet (1.4 g)*	4	1.1
Trident Slab—*1 piece (1.9 g)*	5	1.3[2]			
Trident Soft Bubble Gum—*1 piece (3.3 g)*	9	2.2[2]			

1. These products contain negligible amounts of protein, fat, vitamins, and minerals.

2. Contains sorbitol and/or mannitol.
3. Contains 221 mg calcium per tablet.

SOURCES: Agriculture Handbook No. 8-19 and industry data.

Gluten[1]

GLUTEN-CONTAINING GRAINS	GLUTEN-FREE GRAINS & PRODUCTS
barley	corn flour
buckwheat	corn meal
oats	cornstarch
rye	gluten-free wheat starch
wheat	lima bean flour
	potato flour
	rice
	rice flour
	soy flour

1. Nontropical sprue and other malabsorption symptoms may be relieved or improved by a restriction of gluten-containing grains.

Iodine[1] (mcg/100 g)

1. BEVERAGES (AVG 1, RANGE 0–2 mcg/100 g)

beer	1
cherry drink, from powder	1
coffee, decaf, from inst	0
cola, carbonated	1
cola, carbonated, low cal	1
lemonade, frzn, reconstituted	1
lemon-lime, carbonated	1
orange drink, cnd	1
tea, brewed	2
water, tap	1
whiskey	0
wine, table	1

2. CANDY (AVG 39, RANGE 35–43 mcg/100 g)

caramels	35
milk choc	43

3. CEREALS, COOKED (AVG 14, RANGE 7–28 mcg/100 g)

corn grits, enr, ckd	28
farina, enr, ckd	8
oatmeal, ckd	7

4. CEREALS, READY-TO-EAT (AVG 58, RANGE 19–129 mcg/100 g)

corn flakes	93
crisped rice	66
fruit-flavored, sweetened	129
granola w/ raisins	26
oat ring	48
raisin bran	19
shredded wheat	28

5. CHEESE (AVG 39, RANGE 27–46 mcg/100 g)

american	46
cheddar, sharp/mild	43
cottage, 4% milk fat	27

6. CHIPS & POPCORN (AVG 21, RANGE 5–30 mcg/100 g)

corn chips	30
popcorn, popped in oil	27
potato chips	5

7. CREAMS & CREAM SUBSTITUTES (AVG 12, RANGE 7–17 mcg/100 g)

cream, half & half	17
cream substitute, powdered	7

8. DESSERTS (AVG 41, RANGE 12–76 mcg/100 g)

cake, choc w/ choc icing	23
cake, yellow w/ white icing	47
coffeecake, rte/frzn	29
cookies, choc chip	52
cookies, choc w/ creme filling	76
doughnut, cake type	25
gelatin dessert, strawberry, from inst mix	12
ice cream, choc	45
ice cream sandwich	59
ice milk, van	30
pastry, danish/sweet roll	45
pie, apple, frzn, heated	44
pie, pumpkin, frzn, heated	41
pudding, choc inst, made w/ whole milk	37
shake, choc, fast food	53

9. EGGS (AVG 47, RANGE 42–52 mcg/100 g)

fried	52
scrambled w/ milk	42
soft-boiled	48

10. ENTREES & MEALS (AVG 27, RANGE 9–95 mcg/100 g)

beef & veg stew, homemade	18
chicken, fried frzn dinner w/ mashed potatoes, cornbread, and/or veg, heated	24
chicken noodle casserole, homemade	25
chili con carne w/ beans, cnd	18
hamburger, ¼ lb w/ garnish, fast food	20
lasagna, homemade	33
macaroni & cheese, from box mix	34
pizza, cheese, frzn, heated	95
pork chow mein, homemade	9
pot pie, chicken, frzn, heated	39
spaghetti in tomato sce, cnd	23
spaghetti w/ meat sce, homemade	19

13. FISH & SHELLFISH (AVG 60, RANGE 20–116 mcg/100 g)

cod/haddock fillet, raw/frzn, baked	116
fish sticks, frzn, heated	63
shrimp, raw/ frzn, breaded, fried, homemade	41
tuna, cnd in oil	20

14. FRUIT & VEGETABLE JUICES (AVG 1, RANGE 1–3 mcg/100 g)

apple jce, cnd/bottled	3
grapefruit jce, frzn, reconstituted	1
grape jce, cnd/bottled	2
orange jce, frzn, reconstituted	1
pineapple jce, cnd/bottled	1
prune jce, bottled	1
tomato jce, cnd	1

15. FRUITS (4, RANGE 0–33 mcg/100 g)

apple, red w/ peel, raw	1
applesauce, sweetened, cnd	0
avocado, raw	1
banana, raw	2
cantaloupe, raw	2
cherries, sweet, raw	0
fruit cocktail, heavy syrup, cnd	33
grapefruit, raw	0
grapes, purple/green, raw	1
orange, navel/valencia, raw	1
peach, heavy syrup, cnd	1
peach, raw	1
pear, heavy syrup, cnd	1
pear, raw	1
pineapple, jce pack, cnd	1
plums, purple, raw	1
prunes	30
raisins	3
strawberries, raw	3
watermelon, raw	0

17. GRAIN PRODUCTS (AVG 63, RANGE 11–148 mcg/100 g)

biscuit, baking powder, enr, from refrig dough	35
bread, rye	49
bread, white	91
bread, whole wheat	63
cornbread, homemade	68
crackers, saltines	148
macaroni, enr, boiled	19
muffin, blueberry/plain	57
noodles, egg, enr, boiled	11
pancakes, from mix	56
rice, white, enr, ckd	63
roll, white, end	81
tortilla, flour	75

18/19. INFANT/JUNIOR FOODS & FORMULA (AVG 9, RANGE 0–28 mcg/100 g)

cereals	
mixed, prep w/ whole milk	17
oatmeal w/ applesce & bananas	1
formula	
milk-based, high iron, rts, cnd	9
milk-based, rts, cnd	9
fruits & juices, str/jr	
apple jce	3
applesce	1
bananas & pineapple	1
orange jce	2
peaches	1
pears	1
prunes/plums	0
desserts	
dutch apple/apple betty	1
fruit dessert	0
pudding/custard	9
dinners, str/jr	
beef & veg	18
chicken & noodles	8
chicken/turkey & veg	28
ham & veg	8
tomatoes, beef & macaroni	2
turkey & rice	6
veg w/ bacon/ham	2
veg w/ beef	1
veg w/ turkey/chicken	5
meats/poultry, str/jr	
beef	9
chicken/turkey	27
pork	7
vegetables, str/jr	
carrots	1
creamed corn	4
creamed spinach	10
green beans	1
mixed veg	1
peas	1
sweetpotatoes/yellow squash	1

21. MEATS (AVG 18, RANGE 6–42 mcg/100 g)

beef/calf liver, pan fried	42
beef	
chuck roast, baked	17
ground patty, pan fried	14
loin/sirloin steak, pan fried	15
round steak, stewed	18
lamb chop, pan fried	11
meatloaf, baked, homemade	38
pork	

bacon, pan fried	16
chop, pan fried	6
ham, cured, baked	12
roast loin, baked	11
sausage, pan fried	21
veal cutlet, breaded, pan fried	19

22. MEATS, LUNCHEON (AVG 20, RANGE 10–28 mcg/100 g)

bologna	21
frankfurter, boiled	10
salami	28

23. MILK & YOGURT (AVG 25, RANGE 20–38 mcg/100 g)

buttermilk	24
choc milk	24
evaporated milk	38
nonfat milk	21
2% fat milk	23
whole milk	20
yogurt, 2% fat, strawberry	20
yogurt, 2% fat, plain	33

24. NUTS & NUT PRODUCTS (AVG 6, RANGE 4–8 mcg/100 g)

peanut butter, creamy	4
peanuts, dry-roasted, salted	6
pecans, packaged, unsalted	8

25. POULTRY (AVG 24, RANGE 15–40 mcg/100 g)

chicken, baked	15
chicken, drumsticks & breasts, breaded, fried, homemade	17
turkey breast, baked	40

12/26/27/31. SAUCES, GRAVIES, SALAD DRESSINGS, OILS, & SPREADS (AVG 5, RANGE 1–19 mcg/100 g)

butter	3
corn oil	1
brown gravy, from mix	3
margarine, stick type	4
mayonnaise	4
salad dressing, italian	1
white sce, med, homemade	19

28. SOUPS (AVG 5, RANGE 3–11 mcg/100 g)

beef bouillon, cond, prep w/ water	2
chicken noodle, cond, prep w/ water	4
tomato, cond, prep w/ whole milk	11
veg beef, cond, prep w/ water	3

32. SUGARS, SYRUPS, & OTHER SWEETENERS (AVG 31, RANGE 5–85 mcg/100 g)

catsup	5
choc powder for milk	10
honey	38
jelly, grape	85
sugar, white, granulated	22
syrup, pancake	25

33. VEGETABLES, VEGETABLE PRODUCTS, AND VEGETABLE SALADS (AVG 9, RANGE 0–51 mcg/100 g)

asparagus, raw/frzn, boiled	0
beans w/ pork, cnd	5
beets, cnd	1
broccoli, raw/frzn, boiled	0
cabbage, boiled	0
carrot, raw	1
cauliflower, raw/frzn, boiled	1
celery, raw	1
coleslaw w/ dressing, homemade	4
collards, raw/frzn, boiled	1
corn, cnd	8
corn, creamed style, cnd	11
corn, raw/frzn, boiled	8
cowpeas, boiled	26
cucumber, raw	4
lettuce, crisphead	0
lima beans, immature, frzn, boiled	31
lima beans, mature, boiled	9
mixed veg, cnd	2
mushrooms, cnd	3
navy beans, boiled	39
onion, raw	1
onion rings, breaded, fried, frzn, heated	30
peas, green, cnd	4
peas, green, frzn, boiled	4
pepper, green, sweet, raw	1
pinto beans, boiled	15
potato	
baked w/ peel	31
boiled w/o peel	9
french fries, frzn, heated	29
mashed, from inst	51
scalloped, homemade	31
radishes, raw	1
red beans, boiled	21
sauerkraut, cnd	1
snap beans, green, cnd	2
snap beans, green, raw/frzn, boiled	1
spinach, cnd	5
spinach, raw/frzn, boiled	2
summer squash, raw/frzn, boiled	1
sweet potato, baked w/ peel	2
sweet potato, candied, homemade	15
tomato, cnd	1
tomato, raw	2
tomato sce, cnd	1
winter squash, hubbard/acorn, raw/frzn, boiled	1

34 MISCELLANEOUS

pickle, dill	2

1. These products and some of the other foods with higher iodine levels may contain erythrosine (a red food dye that is high in iodine) or iodine-containing dough conditioners. Another source of iodine is from iodophors that are commonly used in the dairy industry.

SOURCE: Pennington JAT, SA Schoen, GD Salmon, B Yound, RD Johnson, RW Marts. Composition of core foods of the US food supply, 1982-1991. III. Copper, manganese, selenium, and iodine. *J Food Comp Anal* 8:171-217, 1995.

Pectin (g)

1. BEVERAGES
1.1. Alcoholic Beverages
1.1.1. Ales, Beers & Malt Liquors
beer—*12 fl oz (356 g)* .71

1.1.2. Cocktails & Cocktail Mixes
whiskey sour, prep from bottled mix—*2 fl oz mix & 1.5 fl oz whiskey (106 g)* .11
whiskey sour mix, bottled[1]—*2 fl oz cocktail (65 g)* .13

1.5 Coffee
inst powder—*1 rd t (1.8 g)* .04
  mocha flavor, sugar sweetened—*2 rd t (11.5 g)* .10
prep from inst powder, mocha flavor, sugar sweetened—*6 fl oz water & 2 rd t powder (188 g)* .19

1.6 Fruit Juice Drinks & Fruit Flavored Beverages
lemonade, from frzn conc—*8 fl oz (240 g)* .25
orange breakfast drink, from frzn conc—*6 fl oz (188 g)* .19

1.8 Tea, Hot/Iced
tea, inst powder—*1 t (0.7 g)* .03

15. Fruits
apple
  raw, w/skin—*1 med (138 g)* 1.48
  raw, w/o skin—*1 med (128 g)* .49
  boiled, w/o skin—*1 cup (171 g)* .46
  cnd, sliced, sweetened—*½ cup (102 g)* .44
  cnd, sweetened, heated—*½ cup (102 g)* .50
  frzn, unsweetened—*½ cup (86 g)* .40
  frzn, unsweetened, heated—*½ cup (103 g)* .40
  micro ckd w/o skin—*1 cup (170 g)* .75

applesauce, cnd, sweetened—*½ cup (128 g)* .38
kiwifruit, raw—*1 med (76 g)* .32

24. Nuts, Nut Products & Seeds
almonds, dried—*1 oz (24 nuts) (28 g)* .38
chestnuts
  european, raw—*1 oz (2½ nuts) (28 g)* .34
  roasted—*1 oz (3½ nuts) (28 g)* .34

34. Vegetables, Vegetable Products & Vegetable Salads
broccoli
  frzn, chopped, boiled—*½ cup (92 g)* .92
  frzn, spears, boiled—*½ cup (92 g)* .92
brussels sprouts, frzn, boiled—*½ cup (78 g)* 1.09
carrots, raw—*1 med (72 g)* .72
corn, sweet, yellow/white, frzn, boiled—*½ cup (82 g)* .33
green beans (snap beans), frzn, boiled[2]—*½ cup (68 g)* .61
peas, green
  frzn—*½ cup (72 g)* .50
  frzn, boiled—*½ cup (80 g)* .48
spinach
  raw—*½ cup chopped (28 g)* .22
  boiled—*½ cup (90 g)* .72
  frzn, boiled—*½ cup (95 g)* 1.05
squash, summer
  all varieties, raw—*½ cup slices (65 g)* .39
  all varieties, boiled—*½ cup slices (90 g)* .45
  crookneck, raw—*½ cup slices (65 g)* .39
  crookneck, boiled—*½ cup slices (90 g)* .45
sweet potato
  baked w/skin—*1 sweet potato (114 g)* .91
  frzn, baked—*½ cup cubes (88g)* .70

1. Contains no alcohol.

2. Includes italian, green, and yellow varieties.

SOURCES: Agriculture Handbooks No. 8-9, 8-11, 8-12, 8-14, and 1989 Supplement.

Phytosterol (mg)

2. CANDY & GUM
fudge,
  brown sugar w/ nuts—*.49 oz piece (14 g)* 2
  choc marshmallow w/ nuts—*.78 oz piece (22 g)* 2
  choc w/ nuts—*.67 oz piece (19 g)* 3
  peanut butter—*.56 oz piece (16 g)* 2
  van w/ nuts—*.53 oz piece (15 g)* 2
peanut brittle—*1 oz (28 g)* 18
praline—*1.38 oz piece (39 g)* 15
truffles—*.42 oz piece (12 g)* 0

5. CHEESE & CHEESE PRODUCTS
5.2 Cheese Products
cheese sauce, homemade—*2 T (30 g)*[1] 3

6. CHIPS, PRETZELS, POPCORN, & OTHER SNACK FOODS
oriental mix, rice-based—*1 oz (28 g)* 7
trail mix, tropical—*1 oz (28 g)* 23

7. CREAMS & CREAM SUBSTITUTES
creamer, liquid/frzn w/ hydg veg oils—*½ fl oz (15 g)*[2] 2
creamer, liquid/frzn w/ lauric acid oils—*½ fl oz (15 g)*[3] 1

creamer, powdered—*1 t (2.0 g)*	1
sour cream, imitation—*1 oz (28 g)*	5
whipped topping	
frzn—*1 T (4 g)*	1
pressurized—*1 T (4 g)*	1

8. DESSERTS
8.7 Fruit Cobblers & Turnovers

apple brown betty/crisp, homemade—*½ cup (141 g)*	13

8.8 Gelatin Desserts

from mix, w/ fruit—*½ cup (106 g)*	3

8.12 Puddings, Custards, & Pie Fillings

bread, homemade—*½ cup (126 g)*	8
choc	
homemade w/ lowfat milk—*½ cup (157 g)*	3
homemade w/ whole milk—*½ cup (157 g)*	3

8.13 Sauces, Syrups, & Toppings for Desserts

icing/frosting, from mix	
choc creamy, made w/ marg—*1/12 pkg prep (42 g)*	12
van creamy, made w/ marg—*1/12 pkg prep (43 g)*	12
icing/frosting, homemade	
choc creamy, made w/ marg—*1/12 recipe (50 g)*	17
glaze—*1/12 recipe (27 g)*	6
van creamy, made w/ marg—*1/12 recipe (48 g)*	16

9. EGGS, EGG DISHES, & EGG SUBSTITUTES

egg, chicken	
fried—*1 large (46 g)*	6
omelet, plain—*1 large egg (61 g)*	6
scrambled w/ milk—*1 large egg (61 g)*	6
egg substitutes	
frzn—*¼ cup (60 g)*[4]	57
liquid—*1.5 fl oz (47 g)*[5]	2

12. FATS, OILS, & SHORTENINGS
12.3 Shortenings

beef tallow & cottonseed (for frying)—*1 T (13 g)*	4
hydg coconut & palm kernel (for confectionery)—*1 T (13 g)*	11
hydg palm (for confectionery)—*1 T (14 g)*	7
hydg soybean, 1% linoleic acid (for heavy duty frying)—*1 T (13 g)*	24
hydg soybean, 30% linoleic acid (for heavy duty frying)—*1 T (13 g)*	17
hydg soybean & cottonseed—*1 T (13 g)*	26
hydg soybean & cottonseed (for bread)—*1 T (13 g)*	26
hydg soybean & cottonseed (for frying)—*1 T (13 g)*	26
hydg soybean & palm (household)—*1 T (13 g)*	19
lard & veg oil—*1 T (13 g)*	2

12.4 Vegetable Oils & Sprays

almond oil—*1 T (14 g)*	37
apricot kernel oil—*1 T (14 g)*	37
babassu oil—*1 T (14 g)*	13
cocoa (cacao) oil—*1 T (14 g)*	28
coconut oil—*1 T (14 g)*	12
corn oil—*1 T (14 g)*	136
cottonseed oil—*1 T (14 g)*	45
hazelnut oil—*1 T (14 g)*	17
olive oil—*1 T (14 g)*	31
palm kernel oil—*1 T (14 g)*	13

peanut oil—*1 T (14 g)*	29
poppyseed oil—*1 T (14 g)*	39
rice bran oil—*1 T (14 g)*	167
safflower oil, commercial, 70% & over linoleic acid—*1 T (14 g)*	62
sesame oil—*1 T (14 g)*	121
sheanut oil—*1 T (14 g)*	50
soybean (hydg) & cottonseed oil—*1 T (14 g)*	21
soybean oil—*1 T (14 g)*	35
soybean oil, hydg—*1 T (14 g)*	18
sunflower oil, 60% & over linoleic acid—*1 T (14 g)*	14
sunflower oil, hydrg—*1 T (14 g)*	1
sunflower oil, southern crops (—*1 T (14 g)*	14
walnut oil—*1 T (14 g)*	25
wheat germ oil—*1 T (14 g)*	77

15. FRUITS

apple, raw, w/ skin—*1 med (138 g)*	17
apricots, raw—*3 med (106 g)*	19
banana, raw—*1 med (114 g)*	18
cantaloupe, raw—*1 cup pieces (160 g)*	16
cherries, sweet, raw—*10 cherries (68 g)*	8
figs, raw—*1 med (50 g)*	16
grapefruit, raw, white—*½ med (118 g)*	20
grapes, european (adherent skin), raw—*1 cup (160 g)*	6
lemon peel—*1 T (6 g)*	2
loquats, raw—*6 med (100 g)*	2
orange, navel, raw—*1 fruit (131 g)*	31
orange peel—*1 T (6 g)*	2
peach, raw—*1 med (87 g)*	9
pear, raw—*1 med (166 g)*	13
persimmon, japanese, raw—*1 med (168 g)*	7
pineapple, raw—*1 cup pieces (155 g)*	9
plums, raw—*1 med (66 g)*	5
pomegranate, raw—*1 med (154 g)*	26
strawberries, raw—*1 cup (149 g)*	18
watermelon, raw—*1 cup (160 g)*	3

16. GRAIN FRACTIONS

amaranth—*1 cup (195 g)*	47

17. GRAIN PRODUCTS
17.2 Biscuits

plain/buttermilk, homemade—*1 biscuit (2½" x 1½") (60 g)*	18

17.3 Breads, Quick

banana	
homemade w/ marg—*1 slice (4⅜" x 2½" x ½") (60 g)*	20
homemade w/ veg shortening—*1 slice (4⅜" x 2½" x ½") (60 g)*	14
cornbread, homemade w/ low fat milk—*1 slice (2½" x 1½") (65 g)*	8
pumpkin, homemade—*1 slice (60 g)*	17

17.4 Breads, Yeast & Unleavened

egg—*1 slice (5" x 3" x ½") (40 g)*	3
indian (navajo) fry—*5" diam (90 g)*	14
irish soda, homemade—*1 slice (60 g)*	8

17.9 Muffins

corn, homemade w/ whole milk—*1 muffin (2¾" x 2") (57 g)*	14

17.11 Pasta

egg, homemade, ckd—*2 oz (57 g)*	1
homemade w/o egg, ckd—*2 oz (57 g)*	1

19. INFANT, JUNIOR, & TODDLER FOODS
19.1 Baked Products

zwieback toast—*.2 oz piece (7 g)*	2

21. MEATS
21.4 Pork

center loin (loin chops/roasts), sep lean, pan fried—*3.5 oz (100 g)*	3
center loin (loin chops/roasts), sep lean & fat, pan fried—*3.5 oz (100 g)*	2
center rib (rib chops/roasts), sep lean, pan fried—*3.5 oz (100 g)*	3
center rib (rib chops/roasts), sep lean & fat, pan fried—*3.5 oz (100 g)*	3
loin blade (chops & roasts), sep lean, pan fried—*3.5 oz (100 g)*	4
loin blade (chops & roasts), sep lean & fat, pan fried—*3.5 oz (100 g)*	3
top loin (chops & roasts), sep lean, pan fried—*3.5 oz (100 g)*	3
top loin (chops & roasts), sep lean & fat, pan fried—*3.5 oz (100 g)*	2

21.5 Veal

leg (top round), sep lean, pan fried, breaded—*3.5 oz (100 g)*	3
leg (top round), sep lean & fat, pan fried, breaded—*3.5 oz (100 g)*	3

24. NUTS, NUT PRODUCTS, & SEEDS

almonds, dried—*1 oz (24 nuts) (28 g)*	40
cashews, dry roasted—*1 oz (28 g)*	45
chestnuts, european, raw—*1 oz (2½ nuts) (28 g)*	6
coconut, raw—*1 piece (2" x 2" x ½") (45 g)*	21
coconut milk, raw—*1 cup (240 g)*[6]	2
peanut butter	
chunk style/crunchy—*2 T (32 g)*	33
creamy/smooth—*2 T (32 g)*	33
peanuts, unroasted—*1 oz (28 g)*	62
pecans, dried—*1 oz (31 large nuts) (28 g)*	31
pine nuts, pignolia, dried—*1 oz (28 g)*	40
pistachios, dried—*1 oz (47 nuts) (28 g)*	31
sesame seeds, whole, dried—*1 T (9 g)*	64
sunflower seeds/kernels, dried—*1 oz (28 g)*	150
walnuts, english/persian, dried—*1 oz (14 halves) (28 g)*	31

26. SALAD DRESSINGS
26.1 Low & Reduced Calorie

french—*1 T (16 g)*	2
italian—*1 T (15 g)*	4
russian—*1 T (16 g)*	2
thousand island—*1 T (15 g)*	4

26.2 Regular

blue (bleu) cheese—*1 T (15 g)*	20
ckd, homemade—*1 T (16 g)*	4
french—*1 T (16 g)*	16
homemade—*1 T (14 g)*	25
italian—*1 T (15 g)*	18
mayonnaise type—*1 T (15 g)*	15
russian—*1 T (15 g)*	19
sesame seed—*1 T (15 g)*	17
thousand island—*1 T (16 g)*	16
vinegar & oil, homemade—*1 T (16 g)*	11

27. SAUCES, CONDIMENTS, & GRAVIES
27.2 Sauces & Condiments

catsup (ketchup)—*1 T (15 g)*	1
white sce	
med, homemade—*½ cup (125 g)*[7]	36
thick, homemade—*½ cup (125 g)*	50
thin, homemade—*½ cup (125 g)*	20

30. SPICES, HERBS, & FLAVORINGS

allspice, ground—*1 t (2.0 g)*	1
basil, ground—*1 t (1.0 g)*	1
caraway seed—*1 t (2.0 g)*	2
cardamon, ground—*1 t (2.0 g)*	1
celery seed—*1 t (2.0 g)*	1
chili powder—*1 t (3 g)*[8]	2
chives, raw—*1 T chopped (3 g)*	0
cinnamon, ground—*1 t (2.0 g)*	1
cloves, ground—*1 t (2.0 g)*	5
coriander (cilantro), seed—*1 t (2.0 g)*	1
cumin seed—*1 t (2.0 g)*	1
curry powder—*1 t (2.0 g)*	1
dill seed—*1 t (2.0 g)*	2
fennel seed—*1 t (2.0 g)*	1
fenugreek seed—*1 t (4 g)*	6
garlic powder—*1 t (3 g)*	0
ginger, fresh—*¼ cup slices (24 g)*	4
ginger, ground—*1 t (2.0 g)*	2
mace, ground—*1 t (2.0 g)*	1
marjoram, dried—*1 t (1.0 g)*	1
mustard seed, yellow—*1 t (3 g)*	4
nutmeg, ground—*1 t (2.0 g)*	1
onion powder—*1 t (2.0 g)*	2
oregano, ground—*1 t (2.0 g)*	4
paprika—*1 t (2.0 g)*	4
parsley, fresh—*½ cup chopped (30 g)*	2
pepper	
black—*1 t (2.0 g)*	2
red/cayenne—*1 t (2.0 g)*	2
white—*1 t (2.0 g)*	1
poppy seed—*1 t (3 g)*	3
poultry seasoning—*1 t (2.0 g)*[9]	2
pumpkin pie spice—*1 t (2.0 g)*[10]	1
rosemary, dried—*1 t (2.0 g)*	1
sage, ground—*1 t (1.0 g)*	2
savory, ground—*1 t (1.0 g)*	0
tarragon, ground—*1 t (2.0 g)*	2
thyme, ground—*1 t (1.0 g)*	2
turmeric, ground—*1 t (2.0 g)*	2

31. SPREADS

mayonnaise	
imitation, soybean—*1 T (15 g)*	9
safflower & soybean—*1 T (14 g)*	49
soybean—*1 T (14 g)*	31
sandwich spread—*1 T (15 g)*	11

33. VEGETABLES, VEGETABLE PRODUCTS, & VEGETABLE SALADS

asparagus, boiled—*½ cup (6 spears) (90 g)*	22
bamboo shoots, raw—*½ cup (76 g)*	14
cabbage, green, raw—*½ cup shredded (35 g)*	4
carrots, raw—*1 med (72 g)*	9
cauliflower, raw—*½ cup pieces (50 g)*	9

celery, boiled—½ cup diced (75 g)	5		potato pancakes, homemade—1 med pancake (37 g)[12]	10
celery, raw—1 stalk (7.5" long) (40 g)	2		potato, raw w/o skin—1 potato (112 g)	6
celtuce, raw—12 leaves (100 g)	11		radish, raw—10 radishes (45 g)	3
cucumber, raw—½ cup sl (⅙ cucumber) (52 g)	7		shallots, raw—1 T chopped (10 g)	1
eggplant, raw—½ cup (41 g)	3		soybeans, green, boiled—½ cup (90 g)	45
lettuce			spinach, raw—½ cup chopped (28 g)	3
iceberg, raw—1 leaf (20 g)[11]	2		tomato, red, boiled—½ cup (120 g)	11
looseleaf, raw—½ cup shredded (28 g)	11		tomato, red, raw—1 tomato (123 g)	9
mung bean sprouts, raw—½ cup (52 g)	8		tomato, red, stewed—1 cup (101 g)[13]	14
onions			turnip greens, raw—½ cup chopped (28 g)	3
boiled—½ cup chopped (105 g)	19			
raw—½ cup chopped (80 g)	12			

34. MISCELLANEOUS

peppers, sweet			pickles, dill—1 slice (6 g)	1
boiled—½ cup chopped (68 g)	6		—1 large (3¾" long x 1¼" dia) (65 g)	9
raw—½ cup chopped (50 g)	5		pickles, sour—1 med (3¾" long, 1½" dia) (35 g)	5
pimientos, cnd—1 T (12 g)	1		pickles, sweet—1 large (3" long, ¾" dia) (35 g)	5

1. Thin white sauce made with cheddar cheese and salt.
2. Contains hydrogenated vegetable oil and soy protein; vegetable oils are usually soybean, cottonseed, safflower, or blends thereof.
3. Contains lauric acid oils and sodium caseinate; lauric oils include modified coconut oil, hydrogenated coconut oil, and/or palm kernel oil.
4. Contains egg whites, corn oil, and nonfat dry milk.
5. Contains egg white, hydrogenated soybean oil, and soy protein.
6. Liquid expressed from grated coconut and coconut water.
7. Contains lowfat milk, margarine, flour, and salt.
8. Contains red pepper, cumin, oregano, salt, and garlic powder.
9. Contains white pepper, sage, thyme, marjoram, savory, ginger, allspice, and nutmeg.
10. Contains cinnamon, ginger, nutmeg, allspice, and cloves.
11. Includes crisphead types.
12. Contains potatoes, eggs, onion, margarine, flour, and salt.
13. Tomatoes, breadcrumbs, margarine, sugar, onions, salt, and pepper.

Purines[1]

FOODS HIGHEST IN PURINES (150–825 mg/100 g)

anchovies (363 mg/100 g)
brains
kidney (beef—200 mg/100 g)
game meats
gravies
herring
liver (calf/beef—233 mg/100 g)
mackerel
meat extracts (160–400 mg/100 g)
sardines (295 mg/100 g)
scallops
sweetbreads (825 mg/100 g)

FOODS HIGH IN PURINES (50–150 MG/100 G)

asparagus
breads & cereals, whole grain
cauliflower
eel
fish, fresh & saltwater
legumes, beans/lentils/peas
meat—beef/lamb/pork/veal
meat soups & broths
mushrooms
oatmeal
peas, green
poultry—chicken/duck/turkey
shellfish—crab/lobster/oysters
spinach
wheat germ & bran

FOODS LOWEST IN PURINES (0–50 mg/100 g)

beverages—coffee/tea/sodas
breads & cereals except whole grain
cheese
eggs
fats
fish roe
fruits & fruit juices
gelatin
milk
nuts
sugars, syrups, sweets
vegetables (except those listed above)
vegetable & cream soups

1. Purines are normally formed in the body during the metabolic breakdown of nucleoproteins. In certain genetic disorders, including gout, the relatively insoluble purine *uric acid* tends to accumulate and deposit in the toes and in other joints. Drug treatment is generally prescribed for patients with gout; however, dietary restriction of purine-yielding foods may also be advised.

Salicylates (mg/100 g)[1]

<.10 mg/100 g
FRUITS
apple (yellow), banana, paw paw, pear w/o skin, plum (green), pomegranate

VEGETABLES
Bamboo shoots, bean sprouts, blackeyed peas, brown beans, brussels sprouts, cabbage (green/red), celery, chives, garbanzo beans, leeks, lentils, lettuce, lima beans, mung beans, peas (green/split), potato w/o peel, shallots, soy beans, summer squash (chayote), swede

GRAINS & GRAIN PRODUCTS
arrowroot, barley, buckwheat, maize, millet, oats, rice (brown/white), rye, soy grits, wheat

NUTS & SEEDS
cashews, poppyseeds

ANIMAL PRODUCTS
beef, cheese, chicken, egg, kidney, lamb, liver, milk, oysters, pork, salmon, scallops, shrimp, tripe, tuna, yogurt

OTHER
carob powder, cocoa powder, coffee powder (decaffeinated), gin, maple syrup, Ovaltine powder, parsley leaves, saffron, soy sauce, sugar, tanodri powder, tea bag (camomile), vinegar (malt), vodka, whiskey

.10–.49 mg/100 g
FRUITS
apple (red), apple juice, apricot nectar, cherries (sour), custard apple, figs (fresh/cnd), grapes (light, seedless), grape juice (light), grapefruit juice, kiwi fruit, lemon, loquat, lychee, mango, nectarine, orange juice, passion fruit, peach nectar, pear w/skin, persimmon, pineapple juice, plum (red), tamarillo, watermelon

VEGETABLES
asparagus, beet, carrot, cauliflower, corn (reg/creamed), eggplant w/o peel, green french beans, horseradish, mushrooms (fresh), onion, parsnip, pimentos, potato w/ peel, pumpkin, rhubarb, spinach (frzn), squash (marrow), sweetpotato (yellow), tomato (fresh), tomato juice, turnip

NUTS & SEEDS
brazil nuts, coconut (dried), hazelnuts, peanut butter, pecans, sesame seeds, sunflower seeds, walnuts

OTHER
beer, brandy, caramels, cereal coffee powder, cider (hard), cola soda, coriander leaves, garlic, molasses, olives (black), sherry (dry), syrup (corn), tabasco sauce, tea bag (decaffeinated/fruit herbal/rose hip), wine (claret/rose/white), vermouth

.50–.99 mg/100 g
FRUITS
apple (cnd), apple (granny smith), avocado, cherries (sweet), figs (dried), grapes (red), grape juice (dark), grapefruit, mandarin orange, mulberries, peach, tangelo

VEGETABLES
alfalfa, broad beans, broccoli, chili peppers (green/yellow-green), cucumber w/o peel, eggplant w/peel, mushrooms (cnd), okra, spinach (fresh), squash, sweetpotato (white), tomato (canned), watercress

NUTS
macadamia nuts, pine nuts, pistachios

OTHER
coffee powder[2] fennel powder, sherry (sweet), wine (cabernet/claret riesling/sauvignon)

1.00–4.99 mg/100 g
FRUITS
apricot, blackberries, blueberries, boysenberries, cantaloupe, cherries (cnd), cranberries, cranberry sauce, currants (black/red), dates (fresh/dried), guava, grapes (sultana), loganberries, orange, pineapple, plum (dark red), raspberries (frzn), strawberries, youngberries

VEGETABLES
chicory, chili peppers (red), endive, mushrooms (cnd), peppers (sweet green), radishes, tomato paste, tomato sauce, zucchini

NUTS
almonds, peanuts, waterchestnuts

OTHER
bay leaves, basil, caraway, champagne, chili flakes, chili powder, ginger root, mints, nutmeg, olives (green), pepper (white), peppermints,[2] pimento powder, port, rum, tea bags/leaves (regular/herbal/peppermint),[2] vanilla flavoring, vinegar (white)

5.00–10.00 mg/100 g
FRUITS
raisins, prunes (cnd), raspberries (fresh)

OTHER
allspice, cardamom, cloves, dill (fresh), licorice, liqueurs,[2] mint (fresh), paprika (sweet), pepper (black), pickles

>10.00 mg/100 g
OTHER
aniseed, canella powder, cayenne, celery powder, cinnamon, cumin, curry, dill powder, fenugreek powder, garam masala, honey,[2] mace, mustard powder, oregano, paprika (hot), rosemary, sage, tarragon, tumeric, thyme, worcestershire sauce

---

1. Adapted from Swain AR, SP Dutton, AS Truswell. Salicylates in foods. *J Am Diet Assoc* 85:950–960, 1985. For information on the salicylate content of medications, see: Perry CA, J Dwyer, JA Gelf and, RR Couri's, WW McClockey. Health effects of salicylates in foods and drugs. *Nutr Rev* S4:225–240, 1996.

2. Salicylate ranges for these items (mg/100 g) are: coffee powder, 0–.96; honey, 2.5–11.24; liqueurs, .66–9.04; peppermints, .77–7.50; tea bags/leaves, 1.9–7.34.

Selenium (mcg/100 g)

1. BEVERAGES (AVG 0 mcg/100 g as consumed)

beer	0 (a)
cherry drink, from powder	0 (a)
cola, carbonated, low cal	0 (a)
coffee, brewed	0 (b)
coffee, decaf, from inst powder	0 (a)
coffee, from inst powder	0 (a)
coffee, inst powder	13 (b)
fruit punch, cnd	0 (b)
lemonade, from frzn conc	0 (a)
lemon-lime, carbonated	0 (a)
orange drink, cnd	0 (a)
orange drink, from powder	0 (b)
tea, brewed	0 (a)
tea, inst powder	5 (b)
Thirst Quencher drink, cnd	0 (b)
water, tap	0 (a)
whiskey, 80 proof	0 (a)
wine, white	0 (a)

2. CANDY (AVG 3, RANGE 0–5 mcg/100 gl)

caramels	0 (a)
Kit Kat Wafer	5 (b)
milk choc	1 (a)
Snickers	5 (b)

3. CEREALS, COOKED (AVG 6, RANGE 1–13 mcg/100 g)

bulgur, dry	2 (b)
corn grits, reg/quick/inst, ckd	1 (a)
Cream of Wheat, inst, ckd	11 (b)
Cream of Wheat, quick, ckd	13 (b)
farina, ckd	5 (a)
oatmeal, reg/quick/inst, ckd	6 (a)

4. CEREALS, READY-TO-EAT (AVG 15, RANGE 2–55 mcg/100 g)

All-Bran	9 (b)
Bran Buds	29 (b)
bran flakes, Kellogg's	11 (b)
Cheerios	38 (b)
Corn Chex	4 (b)
corn flakes	2 (a)
corn flakes, Kellogg's	5 (b)
Corn Pops	7 (b)
crisped rice	12 (a)
Froot Loops	7 (b)
Frosted Flakes, Kellogg's	4 (b)
Frosted Mini-Wheats	4 (b)
fruit-flavored, sweetened	6 (a)
Golden Crisp	49 (b)
granola w/raisins	19 (a)
Grape-Nuts	10 (b)
Honey Nut Cheerios	24 (b)
Life	24 (b)
Lucky Charms	20 (b)
Multi-Bran Chex	9 (b)
oat ring	33 (a)
100% Bran, Nabisco	8 (b)
100% Natural Cereal	17 (b)
Product 19	12 (b)
raisin bran	5 (a)
Rice Chex	4 (b)
Rice Krispies	15 (b)
rice, puffed	11 (b)
Special K	55 (b)
wheat, shredded	4 (a)
Wheaties	5 (b)

5. CHEESE & CHEESE PRODUCTS (AVG 14, RANGE 2–26 mcg/100 g)

cheese	
american processed	15 (a)
cheddar	14 (a)
cottage, creamed	7 (a)
cream	2 (b)
feta	15 (b)
mozzarella, low-moisture, part-skim	16 (b)
parmesan, grated	26 (b)
swiss	13 (b)
cheese food	16 (b)
cheese sauce, dry powder	14 (b)
cheese spread	11 (b)

6. CHIPS, PRETZELS, POPCORN, & OTHER SNACK FOODS (AVG 5, RANGE 3–7 mcg/100 g)

corn puffs/twists, cheese	3 (b)
corn-tortilla chips	3 (a)
popcorn, oil-popped	7 (a)
potato chips	4 (a)
pretzels, hard	6 (b)

7. CREAM & CREAM SUBSTITUTES (AVG 1, RANGE 0–2 mcg/100 g)

cream coffee/table	1 (b)
cream, half and half	0 (a)
cream, sour, cultured	2 (b)
cream substitute, powder	0 (a)

8. DESSERTS (AVG 5, RANGE 0–20 mcg/100 g)

cake	
choc w/ choc icing	0 (a)
coffeecake	17 (a)
yellow, from mix w/ white icing	0 (a)
yellow, pudding type, from mix w/ white icing	3 (b)
yellow w/ choc icing	3 (b)
cookies	
animal crackers	7 (b)
choc chip	1 (a)
choc w/ cream filling	1 (a)
fig bar	3 (b)
graham crackers	10 (b)
ice cream cone	5 (b)
oatmeal	10 (b)
peanut butter	6 (b)
peanut butter, from refrig dough, baked	5 (b)
peanut butter sandwich	8 (b)
peanut butter, soft	4 (b)

sugar	2 (b)
van wafers	11 (b)
doughnut, cake type	9 (a)
doughnut, yeast	20 (b)
frozen desserts	
ice cream, choc	0 (a)
ice cream sandwich	1 (a)
ice milk, van	0 (a)
gelatin dessert, from mix	0 (a)
pastry, danish/sweet roll	17 (a)
pastry, toaster, fruit	4 (b)
pie, apple	0 (a)
pie, pumpkin	0 (a)
pudding, choc, from mix	0 (a)
pudding, egg custard, from mix	14 (b)

9. EGGS (AVG 27, RANGE 22–31 mcg/100 g for whole eggs)

fried	28 (b)
raw, white	18 (b)
raw, whole	31 (b)
raw, yolk	45 (b)
scrambled	22 (a)
soft-boiled	27 (a)

10. ENTREES & MEALS (AVG 11, RANGE 0–22 mcg/100 g)

beef & veg stew, homemade	5 (a)
chicken noodle casserole, homemade	13 (a)
chili con carne w/ beans, cnd	0 (a)
frzn dinner, fried chicken, mashed potatoes, cornbread, &/or veg	11 (a)
lasagna, homemade	14 (a)
macaroni & cheese, from mix	16 (a)
meatloaf, homemade	15 (a)
pizza, cheese, frzn, heated	22 (a)
pork chow mein, homemade	7 (a)
pot pie, chicken, frzn, heated	8 (a)
spaghetti in tomato sce, cnd	10 (a)
spaghetti w/ meat sce, homemade	11 (a)

11. FAST FOODS (AVG 15, RANGE 0–21 mcg/100 g)

chicken nuggets	16 (b)
hamburger sandwich	
large	20 (b)
large w/ lettuce & tomato	15 (a)
regular	20 (b)
pizza, cheese/sausage	21 (b)
shake, choc	0 (a)

12. FATS, OILS, & SPREADS (AVG 4, RANGE 0–16 mcg/100 g)

butter	1 (a)
corn oil	0 (a)
lard	0 (b)
margarine, stick type	0 (a)
mayonnaise	0 (a)
pork fat, ckd	16 (b)
pork fat, raw	8 (b)

13. FISH & SHELLFISH (AVG 45, RANGE 13–80 mcg/100 g)

catfish, channel, raw	13 (b)
clams, cnd, drained	49 (b)
cod/haddock, baked	39 (a)
crab, blue, ckd w/ moist heat	40 (b)
crab, blue, cnd	32 (b)
fish sticks, frzn, heated	17 (a)
flounder	58 (b)
haddock	41 (b)
mackerel, atlantic, ckd	52 (b)
mackerel, atlantic, cnd	53 (b)
ocean perch, raw	43 (b)
oysters, ckd	72 (b)
oysters, raw	64 (b)
pollock, walleye, raw	22 (b)
salmon, pink, cnd	33 (b)
salmon, sockeye, ckd	38 (b)
salmon, sockeye, cnd	39 (b)
scallops, mixed species, raw	22 (b)
shrimp, breaded & fried	40 (a)
shrimp, cnd/frzn/ckd	40 (b)
snapper, raw	38 (b)
swordfish, raw	48 (b)
tuna, cnd in oil	79 (a)
tuna, light, cnd in water	80 (b)
tuna, white, cnd in water	66 (b)

14. FRUIT & VEGETABLE JUICES (AVG 0 mcg/100 g)

apple jce, cnd	0 (a)
grapefruit jce, from frzn, conc	0 (a)
grape juice, cnd	0 (a)
orange jce, from frzn conc	0 (a)
pineapple jce, cnd	0 (a)
prune jce, bottled	0 (a)
tomato/veg juice, cocktail	0 (a)

15. FRUITS (AVG 0, RANGE 0–1 mcg/100 g)

apple, raw	0 (a)
applesauce, cnd	0 (a)
avocado	0 (a)
banana, raw	1 (a)
cantaloupe, raw	0 (a)
cherries, sweet, raw	0 (a)
fruit cocktail, heavy syrup, cnd	0 (a)
grapefruit, raw	0 (a)
grapes, raw	0 (a)
orange, raw	0 (a)
peach, raw	0 (a)
peach, heavy syrup, cnd	0 (a)
pear, raw	0 (a)
pear, heavy syrup, cnd	0 (a)
pineapple, cnd	0 (a)
pineapple, raw	1 (b)
plums, purple, raw	0 (a)
prunes	0 (a)
raisins	0 (a)
strawberries, raw	0 (a)

strawberries, sweetened, frzn	1 (b)		rice, wild, dry	3 (b)
watermelon, raw	0 (a)		rolls	

16. GRAIN FRACTIONS (AVG 35, RANGE 3–79 mcg/100 g)

			dinner	28 (a)
corn flour, masa	15 (b)		hamburger/frankfurter	27 (b)
cornmeal, degermed	8 (b)		hard	39 (b)
cornstarch	3 (b)		stuffing, bread, dry mix	48 (b)
oat bran	45 (b)		tortilla, corn	6 (b)
rice bran	16 (b)		tortilla, flour	22 (b)
rye flour	36 (b)		waffle, frzn, toasted	16 (b)
wheat bran	78 (b)			
wheat germ	79 (b)			
wheat germ, toasted	65 (b)			
wheat flour, white				

18/19. INFANT FOODS & FORMULA (MEATS AVG 11, RANGE 3–15 mcg/100 g; DINNERS AVG 2, RANGE 0–7 mcg/100 g; OTHER FOODS AVG 0, RANGE 0–3 mcg/100 g)

all-purpose	34 (b)		cereals	
bread	40 (b)		mixed, prep w/ whole milk	3 (a)
cake	5 (b)		oatmeal w/ applesce & bananas	0 (a)
			desserts	

17. GRAIN PRODUCTS (AVG 21, RANGE 3–48 mcg/100 g)

			dutch apple/apple betty	0 (a)
bagel	32 (b)		fruit dessert	0 (a)
biscuit, refrig dough, baked	18 (a)		pudding/custard	0 (a)
bread			dinners	
cornbread, from mix	10 (b)		beef & veg	1 (a)
cornbread, homemade	10 (a)		chicken & noodles	1 (a)
cracked wheat	25 (h)		chicken/turkey & veg	6 (a)
french/vienna	32 (b)		ham & veg	7 (a)
italian	27 (b)		tomatoes, beef, & macaroni	1 (a)
pita, white	27 (b)		turkey & rice	0 (a)
pita, whole wheat	44 (b)		veg w/ bacon/ham	0 (a)
raisin	20 (b)		veg w/ beef	0 (a)
rye	32 (a)		veg w/ turkey/chicken	0 (a)
wheat	31 (b)		infant formula	
white	26 (a)		milk-based, rts	0 (a)
whole wheat	34 (a)		milk-based, rts, high iron	0 (a)
bread crumbs, dry, grated	38 (b)		fruits and fruit juices	
crackers			applesauce	0 (a)
cheese	9 (b)		apple jce	0 (a)
melba toast	35 (b)		banana & pineapple	0 (a)
rye wafers	24 (b)		orange jce	0 (a)
saltines	11 (a)		peaches	0 (a)
snack type	7 (b)		pears	0 (a)
snack type w/ peanut butter filling	5 (b)		prunes/plums	0 (a)
wheat	6 (b)		meats & poultry	
whole wheat	15 (b)		beef	3 (a)
english muffin	20 (b)		chicken/turkey	14 (a)
english muffin toasted	27 (b)		turkey	15 (a)
french toast, frzn	17 (b)		vegetables, str/jr	
muffin, corn	15 (b)		carrots	0 (a)
muffin, plain/blueberry	11 (a)		creamed corn	0 (a)
pancake, from mix	10 (a)		creamed spinach	0 (a)
pasta			green beans	0 (a)
macaroni, boiled	21 (b)		mixed veg	0 (a)
noodles, chow mein	43 (b)		peas	0 (a)
noodles, egg, ckd	23 (a)		sweet potatoes/squash	0 (a)
rice, brown, ckd	10 (b)			
rice, white				

21. MEATS (FLESH AVG 24, RANGE 14–33 mcg/100 g; INTERNAL ORGANS AVG 105, RANGE 22–190 mcg/100 g)

inst, ckd	4 (b)		beef	
parboiled, ckd	8 (b)		chuck roast, baked	24 (a)
reg, ckd	6 (a)		ground, extra lean, raw	14 (b)

ground, lean, broiled, med	29 (b)
ground, reg, baked	19 (a)
loin/sirloin steak, pan fried	25 (a)
rib, whole, sep lean, raw	17 (b)
round, full cut, sep lean, raw	21 (b)
round steak, stewed	28 (b)
T-bone/top loin/tenderloin/porterhouse, sep lean, raw	18 (b)
top sirloin, sep lean, broiled	33 (b)
internal organs	
kidney, beef, raw	149 (b)
kidney, lamb, raw	127 (b)
kidney, pork, raw	190 (b)
liver, beef, pan fried	58 (a)
liver, lamb, raw	82 (b)
lamb chop, pan cooked w/ fat	
pork	
backribs, sep lean & fat, roasted	39 (b)
bacon, ckd	25 (a)
blade, sep lean, roasted	42 (b)
canadian bacon	25 (b)
chop, pan fried	38 (a)
ground, ckd	35 (b)
ham, cnd	39 (b)
ham, sep lean, roasted	26 (a)
loin chops/roast, sep lean, broiled	47 (b)
loin roast, baked	37 (b)
ribs/roast, sep lean, roasted	43 (b)
sausage, ckd	19 (a)
shoulder, sep lean, broiled	39 (b)
sirloin, sep lean, broiled	52 (b)
sirloin, sep lean, roasted	43 (b)
tenderloin, sep lean, roasted	48 (b)
whole loin, sep lean roasted	35 (b)
veal cutlet, breaded, pan fried	14 (a)

22. MEAT, LUNCHEON (AVG 22, RANGE 10–58 mcg/100 g)

beef, sliced	28 (b)
bologna, beef/pork	11 (a)
chicken roll	13 (b)
frankfurter, beef/pork, boiled	10 (a)
frankfurter, chicken	18 (b)
ham, chopped	17 (b)
ham, sliced	16 (b)
kielbasa	18 (b)
liverwurst	58 (b)
pork, cnd	28 (b)
salami	15 (a)
turkey breast	31 (b)

23. MILK, MILK BEVERAGES, MILK MIXES, & YOGURT (AVG 0, RANGE 0–2 mcg/100 g as consumed)

milk, cow	
buttermilk	0 (a)
chocolate milk, lowfat	0 (a)
cocoa, from mix	0 (b)
evaporated, whole, cnd	0 (a)
lowfat, 2% fat	0 (a)
nonfat	0 (a)
nonfat, dry	27 (b)
whole, 3.3% fat	0 (a)
milk, human, mature	2 (b)
milk mix, choc flavor	0 (a)
yogurt, lowfat	0 (a)
yogurt, lowfat, fruit flavored	2 (b)
yogurt, lowfat, strawberry	0 (a)

24. NUTS & SEEDS (AVG 19, RANGE 2–78 mcg/100 g)

almonds	5 (b)
cashews, roasted	11 (b)
coconut, dried, sweetened	16 (b)
filberts (hazelnuts)	4 (b)
peanut butter	3 (a)
peanuts, roasted	4 (a)
pecans	2 (a)
soybeans, roasted	19 (b)
sunflower seed kernels, dried	60 (b)
sunflower seed kernels, roasted	78 (b)
walnuts, black	17 (b)
walnuts, english	5 (b)

25. POULTRY (AVG 30, RANGE 24–41 mcg/100 g w/o liver)

chicken	
breast, roasted	26 (a)
drumsticks/breasts, breaded & fried	24 (b)
thigh, roasted	29 (b)
chicken liver, broiled	71 (b)
turkey w/o skin	
dark meat, roasted	41 (b)
light meat, roasted	31 (a)

26. SALAD DRESSING (AVG 1, RANGE 0–2 mcg/100 g)

blue cheese	1 (b)
italian	0 (a)
mayonnaise	2 (b)
thousand island	2 (b)

27. SAUCES, CONDIMENTS, & GRAVIES (AVG 1, RANGE 0–3 mcg/100 g w/o mustard)

barbecue sce	1 (b)
brown gravy, from mix	0 (a)
catsup	0 (a)
chicken gravy	1 (b)
horseradish	3 (b)
mustard	36 (b)
soy sce	1 (b)
sweet & sour sce	0 (b)
white sce, homemade	0 (a)

28. SOUPS, CANNED (AVG 3, RANGE 0–10 mcg/100 g)

bean w/ pork/bacon, cond	6 (b)
beef bouillon, prep w/ water	0 (a)
beef noodle, cond	6 (b)
chicken broth, prep w/ water	0 (b)
chicken noodle, cond	10 (b)
chicken noodle, prep w/ water	1 (a)
clam chowder, new england, cond	8 (b)
mushroom, cream of, cond	1 (b)

tomato, cond	0 (b)	mixed veg, cnd/frzn/ckd	0 (a)
tomato, prep w/ milk	0 (a)	mung bean sprouts, cnd	1 (b)
vegetarian veg, prep w/ water	2 (b)	mushrooms, ckd/raw	12 (b)
veg beef, cond	? (b)	mushrooms, cnd	1 (a)
veg beef, prep w/ water	0 (a)	mustard greens, cnd/frzn	1 (b)
		navy beans, boiled	3 (a)

32. SUGARS, SYRUPS, & OTHER SWEETENERS (AVG 0, RANGE 0–1 mcg/100 g w/o molasses)

		onion, cnd/frzn/ckd	0 (b)
honey	0 (a)	onion, raw	0 (a)
jelly, grape	0 (a)	onion rings, frzn, heated	2 (a)
molasses	18 (b)	peas, green, cnd/frzn	0 (a)
sugar, brown	1 (b)	peas, split, raw	2 (b)
sugar, white, granulated	0 (a)	pepper, sweet, green, raw	0 (a)
syrup, pancake	1 (a)	pinto beans, boiled	6 (a)
		potato, baked/cnd/mashed	0 (a)

33. VEGETABLES, VEGETABLE PRODUCTS, & VEGETABLE SALADS (AVG 1, RANGE 0–14 mcg/100 g)

		potato, boiled	0 (a)
		potato, french fries	0 (a)
		potato, scalloped, homemade	0 (a)
asparagus, ckd/cnd/frzn	1 (a)	radishes, raw	0 (a)
beans w/ pork, cnd	2 (a)	red beans, boiled	0 (a)
beet, cnd	0 (a)	sauerkraut, cnd	0 (a)
broccoli, ckd/frzn	0 (a)	snap beans, ckd/cnd/frzn	0 (a)
broccoli, raw	3 (b)	spinach, ckd	0 (a)
cabbage, ckd/raw	0 (a)	spinach, raw	1 (b)
carrots, ckd/raw	0 (a)	soybean tofu, raw	9 (b)
cauliflower, frzn/raw	1 (a)	summer squash, boiled	0 (a)
celery, raw	0 (a)	sweet potato, candied, homemade	0 (a)
coleslaw w/ dressing, homemade	0 (a)	sweet potato, ckd/cnd	0 (a)
collards, cnd/frzn	0 (a)	tomato, cnd	0 (a)
corn, ckd/cnd/frzn	0 (a)	tomato, raw	0 (a)
corn, cream style, cnd	0 (a)	tomato sauce	0 (a)
cowpeas, boiled	1 (a)	turnip greens, frzn	1 (b)
cowpeas, cnd	2 (b)	turnip, raw	1 (b)
cowpeas, frzn, ckd	3 (b)	winter squash, boiled	0 (a)
cucumber, raw	0 (a)		
eggplant, ckd	0 (b)		

34. MISCELLANEOUS (AVG 0, RANGE 0–1 mcg/100 g w/o cocoa powder)

garlic, raw	14 (b)	cocoa powder	14 (b)
kidney beans, boiled/cnd	1 (b)	olives, ripe, cnd	1 (b)
lettuce, raw	0 (a)	pickle, dill	0 (a)
lima beans, large, boiled	1 (a)	yeast, baker's	0 (b)
lima beans, small, frzn	0 (a)		

Adapted from:
a) Pennington JAT, SA Schoen, GD Salmon, B Young, RD Johnson, RW Marts. Composition of core foods of the US food supply, 1982–1991. III. Copper, manganese, selenium, and iodine. *J Food Comp Anal* 8:171–217, 1995.

b) Gebhardt SE, JM Holden. Provisional table on the selenium content of foods. USDA Human Nutrition Information Service, HNIS/PT-109, December 1992.

Sugars[1] *(mg/100 g)*

1. BEVERAGES

brandy, cherry	32.6	fruit punch, from frzn conc	10.2
carbonated, all flavors	10.5	fruit punch, from powder	11.6
carbonated, diet, all flavors	0.9	juice drink, cherry, cnd	10.7
coffee, mocha-flavored, from inst	2.6	lemonade, from frzn conc	9.2
distilled spirits, rum/vodka	0.0	lemonade, from powder	5.5
fruit punch, cnd	11.3	liqueur, coffee	39.2

liqueur, orange	28.3
orange drink, cnd	7.2
orange drink, from frzn conc	10.0
orange drink, from powder	10.8
tea, brewed, herb	0.0
Thirst Quencher, bottled	5.9
vermouth, dry	5.5
vermouth, sweet	15.9
wine, rose	2.5
wine, sherry, med	3.6
wine, white	0.6

2. CANDY & GUM

chewing gum	68.6
chewing gum, sugarless	0.0
choc covered nougat	54.6
choc covered peanut butter nougat, caramel, & peanuts	45.1
choc, dark, sweet	48.8
choc, semi-sweet	54.0
hard candy	66.7
jelly beans	59.0
milk choc, plain	54.6
milk choc w/ almonds	48.8
milk choc w/ crisped rice	46.4
sugar-coated choc & peanut discs	47.3
sugar-coated choc discs	57.8
toffee	55.4

3. CEREALS, COOKED

farina, quick/inst	0.1
oatmeal, reg/quick	0.4
whole wheat, reg	0.4

4. CEREALS, READY-TO-EAT

bran flakes	12.1
bran flakes w/ raisins	26.6
corn flakes	6.8
crispy rice	8.8
granola w/ raisins	27.4
oat rings	2.8
puffed rice	0.1
puffed wheat	1.4
shredded wheat	0.4
wheat & malted barley nuggets	9.1
wheat flakes	7.8

5. CHEESE & CHEESE PRODUCTS

american cheese food	9.8
cheddar	1.8
cottage, creamed, 4% fat	0.6
cottage, lowfat, 0.5% fat	3.2
cream	1.7
ricotta, whole/nonfat	1.4
swiss	0.7

6. CHIPS & POPCORN

popcorn, caramel	39.3
popcorn, oil-popped	1.3

7. CREAM

whipping, unwhipped	2.8

8. DESSERTS

cake, sponge, jam filled	47.7
cookies, animal crackers	22.7
cookies, choc wafers	40.5
doughnut, cake	16.9
fruitcake	43.1
gelatin dessert, from mix	
orange	12.8
raspberry	8.7
granola bar	19.8
ice milk, soft serve w/cone	18.2
pie, snack, fruit, baked	19.8
toppings	
choc syrup	66.8
confectioner's coating	
carob	37.7
white choc	62.4
icing, choc, cnd	55.7
icing, other flavors, cnd	71.1

11. FAST FOODS

cheeseburger, reg	5.1
eggs, scrambled	0.9
english muffin w/ egg, cheese, & canadian bacon	2.0
fish sandwich	3.3
hamburger, reg	4.6
shake, all flavors	18.0
sundae, caramel	25.0
sundae, hot fudge	25.4
sundae, strawberry	27.2

14. FRUIT & VEGETABLE JUICES

apple juice, cnd	10.9
grapefruit jce, cnd	7.5
grape jce, from frzn conc	10.5
lemon jce, fresh	2.4
orange jce, fresh	10.2
orange jce, from frzn conc	10.6
pineapple jce, cnd	12.5
prune jce, bottled	13.4
tomato jce, cnd	2.9
veg jce, cnd	3.3

15. FRUITS

apple, raw	13.3
applesauce, cnd, sweetened	16.5
apricots, dried	38.9
apricots, raw	8.5
avocado, raw	0.9
banana, raw	15.6
blueberries, raw	7.3
cantaloupe, raw	8.7
cherries, sour, raw	8.1
cherries, sweet, raw	14.6
currants	8.0
dates, dried	64.2
figs, dried	66.5
fruit cocktail, jce pack, cnd	15.3
grapefruit, raw	6.2
grapes, american, raw	16.4
kiwifruit, raw	10.5

lemon, raw	2.5	cashews, dry/ oil roasted	5.1
lime, raw	0.4	chestnuts, european (italian)	11.0
nectarine, raw	8.9	coconut, dried, sweetened	34.4
peach, dried	44.6	coconut, raw	3.5
peach, jce pack, cnd	17.4	macadamia nuts, oil roasted	6.2
peach, raw	8.7	mixed nuts, oil roasted	4.0
pear, heavy syrup pack, cnd	15.2	peanut butter	7.8
pear, jce pack, cnd	9.7	peanuts, dried	4.3
pear, raw	10.5	peanuts, dry/oil roasted	4.6
pear, water pack, cnd	6.1	pecans, dried	4.3
pineapple, jce pack, cnd	14.2	pistachios, dried	6.6
pineapple, raw	11.9	pumpkin seed kernels, dried	1.0
plums, raw	7.5	sesame seeds, dried/roasted	1.2
prunes	44.0	sunflower seed kernels, dried	3.3
raisins	65.0	walnuts, english	2.1
strawberries, raw	5.8		
tangelos, raw	7.4	**32. SUGARS, SYRUPS, & OTHER SWEETENERS**	
watermelon, raw	9.0	honey	81.9

16. GRAIN FRACTIONS

wheat bran	2.2	molasses, reg	54.5
wheat flour, white	1.7	sugar, brown	89.8
wheat flour, whole wheat	2.0	sugar, white, granulated	96.8
wheat germ, crude/toasted	12.2	sugar, white, powdered	93.0
		syrup, corn, dark	37.0

17. GRAIN PRODUCTS

biscuit, from mix	4.4	syrup, corn, high fructose	74.3
bread		syrup, corn, light	63.3
white	3.8	syrup, maple	59.9
white, toasted	4.0	syrup, pancake	54.5
whole wheat	4.0		
whole wheat, toasted	4.4	**34. VEGETABLES & VEGETABLE PRODUCTS**	
cracker, rye	3.2	artichoke, boiled	1.1
english muffin, buttered	3.8	asparagus, boiled	1.6
rice, brown, ckd	0.3	beans, baked w/ pork, cnd	8.3
roll, hamburger	7.4	beans, baked w/ tomato sce, cnd	5.7
tortilla, corn	0.5	beans, common, ckd	2.2
		beet, raw	6.5

21. MEATS

pork, ham, smoked	1.0	broadbeans, ckd	1.8
pork sausage, ckd	2.6	broadbeans, immature, boiled	0.5
		broccoli, raw	1.6

22. MEATS, LUNCHEON

beef/pork spiced luncheon loaf	3.3	cabbage, chinese, raw	1.4
bologna, beef	2.0	cabbage, green, raw	3.6
frankfurter, beef/pork	2.0	cabbage, red, boiled	2.8
pastrami, beef	0.8	cabbage, red, raw	5.4
salami, beef	0.2	cabbage, savoy, raw	2.9
		carrot, boiled	4.3

23. MILK, MILK BEVERAGES, & YOGURT

buttermilk	4.8	carrot, cnd	3.3
choc malted flavor mix w/ milk	6.8	carrot, raw	6.6
milk, nonfat	4.4	cauliflower, raw	2.4
milk, nonfat, dry	50.4	celery, raw	1.0
milk, whole, 3.4% fat	5.0	chickpeas, ckd	4.8
milk, whole, dry	35.9	corn, boiled	2.6
yogurt, lowfat, plain	5.1	corn, cnd	2.8
yogurt, lowfat, strawberry	15.3	corn, frzn, boiled	1.8
		cucumber, raw	2.3
		eggplant, raw	3.4

24. NUTS, NUT PRODUCTS, & SEEDS

		endive, escarole, raw	1.1
almonds, dried/roasted	5.9	green beans (snap beans), boiled	2.3
brazilnuts, oil roasted	2.6	green beans (snap beans), cnd	1.6
		jerusalem artichoke, raw, fresh	2.5
		jerusalem artichoke, raw, stored	9.6
		kale, raw	2.2

lentils, ckd	1.8	potato, hash browns	0.2
lettuce, iceburg, raw	2.4	radishes, raw	2.6
lettuce, romaine, raw	2.0	rutabaga, raw	5.6
lima beans, ckd	2.9	soybeans, ckd	3.0
mung bean sprouts, raw	2.1	soybean tofu, raw	0.4
okra, raw	2.4	spinach, raw	0.4
onion, mature, raw	6.2	squash, summer, raw	2.1
onion, spring, raw	3.2	squash, winter, raw	3.8
parsley, raw	1.1	sweet potato, raw	5.7
peas, green, boiled	5.6	tomato, cnd	2.5
peas, green, cnd	3.5	tomato paste, cnd	12.9
peas, split, ckd	2.9	tomato, raw	2.8
pepper, sweet, green, raw	2.5	turnip, raw	3.8
potato, baked w/o skin	1.7	yam, raw	0.5
potato, french fried	0.5		

1. Total sugars includes the sum of the monosaccharides (galactose, glucose, and fructose); disaccharides (lactose, sucrose, and maltose); trioses; and tetroses. Information on total sugars is also found in the main table of this book. This supplementary table provides the 249 sugars values available from the source listed below. One hundred and seventy-five of these values have been matched to foods in the main table and are provided there in typical serving size portions.

SOURCE: Matthews RH, PR Pehrsson. Provisional Table on the Sugar Content of Selected Foods. USDA Human Nutrition Information Service. HNIS/PT-105, October 1986. (Matthews RD, PR Pehrsson. Sugar Content of Selected Foods: Individual and Total Sugars. Home Economic Research Report No 48. USDA. Washington DC. October 1986.)

Theobromine (mg)

2. CANDY & GUM

After Eight Mints—*2 mints (8 g)*	11.4
Baby Ruth—*2.1 oz bar (60 g)*	26.4
Butterfinger—*2.16 oz bar (61 g)*	20.7
choc chips, semi-sweet—*1 cup (6 oz pkg) (168 g)*	816.5
choc coated	
peanuts—*10 pieces (40 g)*	43.6
peanuts, Goobers—*1.38 oz pkg (39 g)*	42.5
raisins *10 pieces (10 g)*	12.7
raisins, Raisinets—*1.58 oz pkg (45 g)*	57.1
choc, semi-sweet—*1 oz (28 g)*	137.8
choc, sweet, dark—*1.45 oz bar (41 g)*	174.7
Special Dark, Hershey—*1.5 oz bar (41 g)*	194.0
Chunky—*1.4 oz bar (40 g)*	62.8
Crunch, Nestle—*1.4 oz bar (40 g)*	62.4
Golden Almond, Hershey—*3.2 oz bar (91 g)*	209.3
III, Hershey—*3.2 oz bar (91 g)*	162.0
Solitaires w/ almonds, Hershey—*3 oz pkg (85 g)*	124.1
Hundred Grand—*1.5 oz bar (43 g)*	31.8
Kit Kat Wafer, Hershey—*1.5 oz bar (42 g)*	42.0
Krackel choc bar, Hershey—*1.5 oz bar (41 g)*	61.5
milk choc—*1.55 oz bar (44 g)*	74.2
w/ almonds—*1.55 oz bar (44 g)*	69.5
w/ rice cereal—*1.45 oz bar (41 g)*	63.5
milk choc chips—*1 cup chips (168 g)*	283.2
Mr. Goodbar, Hershey—*1.75 oz bar (49 g)*	59.8
Peanut Butter Cups, Reese's—*2 pieces (1. 8 oz) (50 g)*	55.0
Rolo caramels w/ milk choc, Hershey—*9 pieces (1.9 oz) (53 g)*	33.9
Turtles, Demet's—*.6 oz piece (17 g)*	8.2
Twix, caramel—*2 oz pkg (2 pieces) (57 g)*	51.0

8. DESSERTS
8.6 Frozen Desserts

ice cream, choc—*½ cup (66 g)*	40.9

8.9 Granola, Cereal, and Snack Bars

peanut butter, soft w/ choc coating—*1.3 oz bar (37 g)*	15.5

8.12 Puddings, Custards, & Pie Fillings

choc, rte—*5 oz can (142 g)*	88.0

8.13 Sauces, Syrups, & Toppings for Desserts

choc fudge topping—*1 T (21 g)*	33.2

34. MISCELLANEOUS

baking choc, unsweetened—*1 oz square (28 g)*	346.4
cocoa, unsweetened, dry powder—*1 T (5 g)*	102.9
processed w/ alkali—*1 T (5 g)*	131.7

Vitamin D (IU)

4. CEREALS, READY-TO-EAT

All-Bran, Kellogg's—½ cup (1.09 oz) (31 g)	40
All-Bran w/ extra fiber, Kellogg's—½ cup (.9 oz) (26 g)	40
almond crunch w/ raisins, Healthy Choice—1 cup (2.05 oz) (58 g)	80
Alpha-Bits, Post—1 cup (1.1 oz) (32 g)	40
Apple Jacks, Kellogg's—1 cup (1.16 oz) (33 g)	40
Apple Raisin Crisp, Kellogg's—1 cup (1.87 oz) (53 g)	40
Banana Nut Crunch, Post—1 cup (2.08 oz) (59 g)	40
Basic 4, General Mills—1 cup (1.94 oz) (55 g)	40
Blueberry Morning, Post—1¼ cups (2 oz) (57 g)	40
Bran Buds, Kellogg's—⅓ cup (1.06 oz) (30 g)	40
bran flakes (40% bran), Post—⅔ cup (1 oz) (28 g)	40
Bran'ola, Post—½ cup (1.87 oz) (53 g)	40
Bran'ola Raisin, Post—½ cup (1.9 oz) (55 g)	40
Cheerios, General Mills—1 cup (1.06 oz) (30 g)	40
Cinnamon Mini-Buns, Kellogg's—¾ cup (1.06 oz) (30 g)	40
Cocoa Krispies, Kellogg's—¾ cup (1.09 oz) (31 g)	40
Cocoa Pebbles, Post—¾ cup (1.02 oz) (29 g)	40
Complete Bran Flakes, Kellogg's—¾ cup (1.02 oz) (29 g)	40
corn flakes	
Kellogg's—1 cup (1 oz) (28 g)	40
Post Toasties—1 cup (1 oz) (28 g)	40
Corn Pops, Kellogg's—1 cup (1.09 oz) (31 g)	40
Cracklin' Oat Bran, Kellogg's—¾ cup (1.7 oz) (49 g)	40
Crispix, Kellogg's—1 cup (1.02 oz) (29 g)	40
Crispy Wheaties 'n Raisins, General Mills—1 cup (1.9 oz) (55 g)	40
Double Dip Crunch, Kellogg's—¾ cup (1.02 oz) (29 g)	40
Froot Loops, Kellogg's—1 cup (1.1 oz) (32 g)	40
Frosted Bran, Kellogg's—¾ cup (1.09 oz) (31 g)	40
Frosted Flakes, Kellogg's—¾ cup (1.09 oz) (31 g)	40
Frosted Flakes, Quaker—¾ cup (1.09 oz) (31 g)	40
Frosted Krispies, Kellogg's—¾ cup (.9 oz) (26 g)	40
Fruit & Fibre w/ dates, raisins & walnuts, Post—1 cup (2.1 oz) (60 g)	60
Fruit & Fibre w/ peaches, raisins & almonds, Post—1 cup (2.1 oz) (60 g)	60
Fruit Wheats, Blueberry, Nabisco—¾ cup (1.8 oz) (51 g)	40
Strawberry, Nabisco—¾ cup (1.8 oz) (51 g)	40
Fruity Marshmallow Krispies, Kellogg's—¾ cup (1 oz) (28 g)	40
Fruity Pebbles, Post—¾ cup (.95 oz) (27 g)	40
Golden Crisp, Post—¾ cup (.95 oz) (27 g)	40
Golden Multi-Grain Flakes, Healthy Choice—¾ cup (1.09 oz) (31 g)	80
granola	
Hearty, Post—⅔ cup (2.15 oz) (61 g)	40
low-fat, Kellogg's—½ cup (1.7 oz) (49 g)	40
w/ raisins, low-fat, Kellogg's—⅔ cup (2.1 oz) (60 g)	40
Grape-Nut Flakes, Post—¾ cup (1.02 oz) (29 g)	40
Grape-Nuts, Post—½ cup (2 oz) (58 g)	40
Great Grains Crunchy Pecan, Post—⅔ cup (1.87 oz) (53 g)	40
Great Grains Raisins, Dates & Pecans, Post—⅔ cup (1.9 oz) (54 g)	60
Honey Bunches of Oats, Post—¾ cup (1.06 oz) (30 g)	40
Honey Bunches of Oats w/ almonds, Post—¾ cup (1.09 oz) (31 g)	40
Honey Crunch Corn Flakes, Kellogg's—¾ cup (1.06 oz) (30 g)	40
Honeycomb, Post—1⅓ cups (1.02 oz) (29 g)	40
Just Right w/ fiber nuggets, Kellogg's—1 cup (1.98 oz) (56 g)	40
Just Right w/ fruit & nuts, Kellogg's—1 cup (2.1 oz) (60 g)	40
King Vitaman, Quaker—1.5 cups (1.1 oz) (31 g)	42
Kix, General Mills—1⅓ cups (1.06 oz) (30 g)	40
Marshmallow Alpha-Bits, Post—1 cup (1.02 oz) (29 g)	40
muselix, apple & almond crunch, Kellogg's—¾ cup (1.87 oz) (53 g)	100
muselix, raisin & almond crunch w/ dates, Kellogg's—⅔ cup (1.9 oz) (55 g)	8
oat bran, Common Sense—¾ cup (1.06 oz) (30 g)	40
Product 19, Kellogg's—1 cup (1.06 oz) (30 g)	40
raisin bran	
Kellogg's—1 cup (2.15 oz) (61 g)	40
Post—1 cup (2.08 oz) (59 g)	60
Rice Krispies	
apple cinn, Kellogg's—¾ cup (1.02 oz) (29 g)	40
Kellogg's—1¼ cup (1.16 oz) (33 g)	40
Treats, Kellogg's—¾ cup (1.06 oz) (30 g)	40
Smacks, Kellogg's—¾ cup (.95 oz) (27 g)	40
Special K, Kellogg's—1 cup (1.09 oz) (31 g)	40
Temptations, french van almond, Kellogg's—¾ cup (.9 oz) (26 g)	40
Temptations, honey roasted pecan, Kellogg's—⅔ cup (1.02 oz) (29 g)	40
Toasted Brown Sugar Squares, Healthy Choice—1 cup (1.9 oz) (54 g)	80
Total Corn Flakes, General Mills—1.3 cups (1.06 oz) (30 g)	40
Total, General Mills—¾ cup (1.06 oz) (30 g)	40
Total Raisin Bran, General Mills—1 cup (1.9 oz) (55 g)	40
Triples, General Mills—1 cup (1.06 oz) (30 g)	40
Wheaties, General Mills—1 cup (1.06 oz) (30 g)	40

8. DESSERTS
8.9 Granola, Cereal, and Snack Bars

Breakfast Bar	
choc chip, chewy, Carnation—1.27 oz bar (36 g)	100
choc chunk granola, Carnation—1.27 oz bar (36 g)	100
honey & oats granola, Carnation—1.3 oz bar (36 g)	100
peanut butter w/ choc chips, Carnation—1.27 oz bar (36 g)	100

9. EGGS, EGG DISHES, & EGG SUBSTITUTES

egg substitutes	
Better 'n Egg, frzn, Morningstar Farms—¼ cup (57 g)	22
Scramblers, Morningstar—¼ cup (57 g)	22

11. FAST FOODS
11.8 Taco Bell

mexican pizza—1 serving (216 g)	10

17. GRAIN PRODUCTS
17.10 Pancakes

buttermilk	
mix complete, Aunt Jemima—⅓ cup (43 g)	1
mix complete, red cal, Aunt Jemima—⅓ cup (43 g)	2

23. MILK, MILK BEVERAGES, MILK MIXES & YOGURT
23.1 Milk, Cow[1]
evaporated

cnd, Carnation—*2 T (32 g)*	24
lowfat, cnd, Carnation—*2 T (32 g)*	24
nonfat, cnd, Carnation—*2 T (32 g)*	24
nonfat, dry, inst, Carnation—*⅓ cup (23 g)*	100

23.2 Milk, Cow, Beverages
instant breakfast

liquid pack, Resource—*8 fl oz (279 g)*[2]	100
rtd, cnd, Carnation—*10 fl oz can (315 g)*[3]	100

1. Milk (lowfat, nonfat, and whole) that has been fortified with vitamin D contains 100 IU vitamin D per 8 fluid ounces (400 IU per quart).

2. Includes chocolate, strawberry, and vanilla.
3. Values are averages for cafe mocha, chocolate, French vanilla, and strawberry creme.

Vitamin E (IU)

3. CEREALS, COOKED
corn grits, inst

white, enr, Quaker—*1 oz pkt dry (28 g)*	.0
white w/ butter flavor, enr, Quaker—*1 oz pkt dry (28 g)*	.2
white w/ cheddar cheese flavor, enr, Quaker—*1 oz pkt dry (28 g)*	.0
white w/ imit bacon bits, enr, Quaker—*1 oz pkt dry (28 g)*	.0
white w/ imit ham bits, enr, Quaker—*1 oz pkt dry (28 g)*	.1
corn grits, quick, yellow, enr, Quaker—*¼ cup dry (1.3 oz) (37 g)*	.1
farina, quick, enr, Quaker—*¼ cup (1.6 oz) dry (44 g)*	.1
multigrain, Quaker—*½ cup dry (40 g)*	.4
oat bran cereal, Quaker/Mother's—*1¼ cup (2 oz) dry (57 g)*	3.1

oatmeal, inst

apples & cinn, Quaker—*1.2 oz pkt dry (35 g)*	.2
choc chip cookie, Quaker Kid's Choice—*1.5 oz pkt dry (42 g)*	.3
cinn & spice, Quaker—*1.6 oz pkt dry (46 g)*	.3
cookies 'n cream, Quaker—*1.5 oz pkt dry (42 g)*	.2
fruit & cream banana, Quaker—*1.2 oz pkt dry (35 g)*	.2
fruit & cream blueberry, Quaker—*1.2 oz pkt dry (35 g)*	.2
fruity marshmallow, Quaker—*1.4 oz pkt dry (40 g)*	.2
low sodium, Quaker—*1 oz pkt dry (28 g)*	.2
maple & brown sugar, Quaker—*1.5 oz pkt dry (43 g)*	.3
oatmeal raisin cookie, Quaker Kid's Choice—*1.5 oz pkt dry (42 g)*	.2
peaches & cream, Quaker—*1.25 oz pkt dry (35 g)*	.2
radical raspberry, Quaker Kid's Choice—*1.4 oz pkt dry (40 g)*	.2
raisins & spice, Quaker—*1.5 oz pkt dry (43 g)*	.2
raisins, dates, & walnuts, Quaker—*1.3 oz pkt dry (37 g)*	.2
s'mores, Quaker Kid's Choice—*1.5 oz pkt dry (42 g)*	.2
strawberries & cream, Quaker—*1.25 oz pkt dry (35 g)*	.2
twisted strawberry & banana, Quaker—*1.4 oz pkt dry (40 g)*	.2

oatmeal, microwave

apple spice, Quaker Quick 'n Hearty—*1.6 oz pkt dry (45 g)*	.3
brown sugar cinn, Quaker Quick 'n Hearty—*1.5 oz pkt dry (42 g)*	.3
cinn double raisin, Quaker Quick 'n Hearty—*1.66 oz pkt dry (47 g)*	.3
honey bran, Quaker Quick 'n Hearty—*1.4 oz pkt dry (41 g)*	.3
Quaker Quick 'n Hearty—*1 oz pkt dry (29 g)*	.3
oatmeal, old fashioned, Quaker—*½ cup dry (40 g)*	.4
Wheat Hearts, General Mills—*¼ cup dry (36 g)*	1.2
Whole Wheat Natural, Quaker—*½ cup (1.4 oz) dry (40 g)*	.6

4. CEREALS, READY-TO-EAT

almond crunch w/ raisins, Healthy Choice—*1 cup (2.05 oz) (58 g)*	3.0
Apple Zaps, Quaker—*1 cup (1.06 oz) (30 g)*	.3
Body Buddies, Natural Fruit, General Mills—*1 cup (1.06 oz) (30 g)*	4.5

Cap'n Crunch

crunchberries/wildberry colors, Quaker—*¾ cup (1 oz) (26 g)*	.3
peanut butter, Quaker—*¾ cup (1 oz) (27 g)*	.2
Quaker—*¾ cup (1 oz) (27 g)*	.2
Cocoa Blasts, Quaker—*1 cup (1.2 oz) (33 g)*	.3
Complete Bran Flakes, Kellogg's—*¾ cup (1.02 oz) (29 g)*	7.5
Corn Quakes, Quaker—*¾ cup (1.06 oz) (30 g)*	.3
Crunchy Bran, Quaker—*¾ cup (.95 oz) (27 g)*	.2
Frosted Flakes, Quaker—*¾ cup (1.09 oz) (31 g)*	.0
Fruitany Ohs, Quaker—*1 cup (1.1 oz) (31 g)*	.3
Golden Multi-Grain Flakes, Healthy Choice—*¾ cup (1.09 oz) (31 g)*	3.0

granola

oats & honey, Quaker 100% Natural—*½ cup (1.7 oz) (48 g)*	.8
oats, honey, & raisins, Quaker 100% Natural—*½ cup (1.8 oz) (51 g)*	.7
w/ almonds, Sun Country—*½ cup (2 oz) (57 g)*	1.8

w/ raisins & dates, Sun Country—½ cup (2.1 oz) (60 g)   1.4

w/ raisins, low-fat, Kellogg's—⅔ cup (2.1 oz) (60 g)   7.5

w/ raisins, low-fat, Quaker 100% Natural—⅔ cup (1.9 oz) (55 g)   .5

Honey Graham Oh!s, Quaker—¾ cup (1 oz) (27 g)   .2

Just Right w/ fiber nuggets, Kellogg's—1 cup (1.98 oz) (56 g)   3.0

Just Right w/ fruit & nuts, Kellogg's—1 cup (2.1 oz) (60 g)   3.0

King Vitaman, Quaker—1.5 cups (1.1 oz) (31 g)   3.1

Life, oat cinn, Quaker—¾ cup (1.1 oz) (32 g)   .2

Life, Quaker—¾ cup (1.1 oz) (32 g)   .2

muselix, apple & almond crunch, Kellogg's—¾ cup (1.87 oz) (53 g)   7.5

muselix, raisin & almond crunch w/ dates, Kellogg's—⅔ cup (1.9 oz) (55 g)   7.5

Nutri-Grain, almond raisin, Kellogg's—1¼ cup (1.7 oz) (49 g)   7.5

Nutri-Grain, wheat, Kellogg's—¾ cup (1.06 oz) (30 g)   7.5

Oatmeal Squares, Quaker—1 cup (2 oz) (56 g)   3.4

Product 19, Kellogg's—1 cup (1.06 oz) (30 g)   30.0

puffed rice, Quaker—1 cup (.5 oz) (14 g)   .0

Quisp/Sweet Crunch, Quaker—1 cup (1 oz) (27 g)   .2

Sweet Puffs, Quaker—1 cup (1.2 oz) (34 g)   .5

Toasted Brown Sugar Squares, Healthy Choice—1 cup (1.9 oz) (54 g)   3.0

Total Corn Flakes, General Mills—1.3 cups (1.06 oz) (30 g)   30.0

Total, General Mills—¾ cup (1.06 oz) (30 g)   30.0

Total Raisin Bran, General Mills—1 cup (1.9 oz) (55 g)   30.0

6. CHIPS, PRETZELS, POPCORN, & OTHER SNACK FOODS

corn cakes

   blueberry crunch, Quaker—1 cake (13 g)   .0

   butter flavor, Quaker—1 cake (9 g)   .0

   caramel, Quaker—1 cake (13 g)   .0

   monterey jack, Quaker—1 cake (10 g)   .0

   strawberry crunch, Quaker—1 cake (13 g)   .0

   white cheddar, Quaker—1 cake (10 g)   .0

rice cakes

   apple cinn, mini, Quaker—5 mini cakes (14 g)   .1

   banana crunch, mini, Quaker—5 mini cakes (14 g)   .1

   banana nut, Quaker—1 cake (13 g)   .1

   caramel corn, mini, Quaker—5 mini cakes (14 g)   .1

   choc crunch, mini, Quaker—5 mini cakes (14 g)   .1

   choc crunch, Quaker—1 cake (13 g)   .1

   cinn crunch, mini, Quaker—5 mini cakes (14 g)   .2

   cinn, Quaker—1 cake (13 g)   .1

   honey nut, mini, Quaker—5 mini cakes (14 g)   .1

   monterey jack, mini, Quaker—6 mini cakes (14 g)   .1

   Quaker—1 cake (9 g)   .1

   unsalted, Quaker—1 cake (9 g)   .0

   white cheddar, mini, Quaker—6 mini cakes (14 g)   .1

8. DESSERTS
8.2 Cakes

coffee cake, easy mix, dry, Aunt Jemima—⅓ cup (1.4 oz) (39 g)   .2

8.9 Granola, Cereal, and Snack Bars

apple berry, Quaker Chewy—1 oz bar (28 g)   .1

Breakfast Bar

   choc chip, chewy, Carnation—1.27 oz bar (36 g)   7.5

choc chunk granola, Carnation—1.27 oz bar (36 g)   7.5

honey & oats granola, Carnation—1.3 oz bar (36 g)   7.5

peanut butter w/ choc chips, Carnation—1.27 oz bar (36 g)   7.5

choc chip, Quaker Chewy—1 oz bar (28 g)   .1

choc chip, Quaker Dipps—1.2 oz bar (35 g)   .3

choc chunk, low-fat, Quaker Chewy—1 oz bar (28 g)   .1

choc mint, low-fat, Quaker Chewy—1 oz bar (28 g)   .1

cookies & cream, low-fat, Quaker Chewy—1 oz bar (28 g)   .1

oatmeal cookie, low-fat, Quaker Chewy—1 oz bar (28 g)   .1

peanut butter, & choc chip, Quaker Chewy—1 oz bar (28 g)   .2

S'mores, low-fat, Quaker Chewy—1 oz bar (28 g)   .1

9. EGGS, EGG DISHES, & EGG SUBSTITUTES

egg substitutes, Better 'n Egg, frzn, Morningstar Farms—¼ cup (57 g)   1.3

10. ENTREES & MEALS
10.1 Box Mix Entrees

angel hair pasta

   w/ herb sce, dry mix, Pasta Roni—2 oz (56 g)   .1

   w/ lemon & butter, dry mix, Pasta Roni—2.5 oz (70 g)   .2

   w/ parmesan cheese, dry mix, Pasta Roni—2 oz (56 g)   .1

corkscrew pasta w/ 4 cheese sce, dry mix, Pasta Roni—2.5 oz (70 g)   .1

corkscrew pasta w/ creamy garlic sce, dry mix, Pasta Roni—2 oz (56 g)   .1

fettuccini w/ alfredo sce, dry mix, Pasta Roni—2.5 oz (70 g)   .1

lasagna w/ tomato & garden veg, dry mix, Pasta Roni—1.5 oz (42 g)   .1

linguine w/ chicken & broccoli sce, dry mix, Pasta Roni—2.5 oz (70 g)   4.1

linguine w/ creamy chicken parmesan sce, dry mix, Pasta Roni—2.5 oz (70 g)   4.0

macaroni & cheese, dry mix, Golden Grain—2 oz (56 g)   .1

pasta, broccoli au gratin, dry mix, Pasta Roni—2 oz (56 g)   .1

pasta, chicken, dry mix, Pasta Roni—2 oz (56 g)   3.3

pasta, oriental stir fry, dry mix, Pasta Roni—2 oz (56 g)   .1

pasta, parmesano, dry mix, Pasta Roni—2.5 oz (70 g)   4.1

pasta, romanoff, dry mix, Pasta Roni—2.5 oz (70 g)   .1

pasta, stroganoff, dry mix, Pasta Roni—2.5 oz (70 g)   .1

pasta w/ broccoli & mushrooms, dry mix, Pasta Roni—2.5 oz (70 g)   4.0

pasta w/ broccoli, dry mix, Pasta Roni—2 oz (56 g)   .1

penne pasta, w/ herb & butter sce, dry mix, Pasta Roni—2 oz (56 g)   .1

rigatoni w/ tomato basil sce, dry mix, Pasta Roni—1.5 oz (42 g)   .1

rigatoni w/ white cheddar & broccoli sce, dry mix, Pasta Roni—2 oz (56 g)   .1

shells w/ white cheddar, dry mix, Pasta Roni—2.5 oz (70 g)   .1

vermicelli w/ garlic & olive oil, dry mix, Pasta Roni—2.5 oz (70 g)   .2

16. GRAIN FRACTIONS

barley, pearled, med/quick, Scotch Brand—¼ cup (48 g)   .2

corn flour

   masa harina, enr, Quaker—¼ cup (31 g)   .1

   yellow, unenr, Quaker—¼ cup (31 g)   .1

cornmeal mix

   white, bolted, Aunt Jemima—3 T (25 g)   .0

white, buttermilk, self-rising, Aunt Jemima—*3 T (25 g)*	.3
cornmeal, white	
bolted, enr, self-rising, Aunt Jemima—*3 T (27 g)*	.1
degermed, enr, self-rising, Aunt Jemima—*3 T (27 g)*	.1
cornmeal, yellow, degermed, enr, Quaker—*3 T (27 g)*	.1
oat bran, dry, Quaker—*½ cup (40 g)*	.2
wheat bran	
toasted, Kretschmer—*¼ cup (.56 oz) (16 g)*	.8
unprocessed, Quaker—*⅓ cup (17 g)*	.1
wheat germ	
Honey Crunch, Kretschmer—*1⅔ T (14 g)*	4.6
toasted, Kretschmer—*2 T (13 g)*	4.9

17. GRAIN PRODUCTS
17.3 Breads, Quick

cornbread easy mix, dry, Aunt Jemima—*⅓ cup (37 g)*	.5

17.9 Muffins

corn, muffin mix, Flako—*⅓ cup (41 g)*	.6

17.10 Pancakes

buckwheat mix, Aunt Jemima—*¼ cup (34 g)*	.1
buttermilk	
mix complete, Aunt Jemima—*⅓ cup (43 g)*	.3
mix complete, red cal, Aunt Jemima—*⅓ cup (43 g)*	.2
w/ white & yellow corn flour, Aunt Jemima—*¼ cup (34 g)*	.2
plain, mix, Aunt Jemima—*⅓ cup (47 g)*	.1
whole wheat mix, Aunt Jemima—*¼ cup (38 g)*	5.6

17.11 Pasta

capellini, durum, Fideo—*⅔ cup dry (57 g)*	.1
elbow macaroni, 100% semolina, Golden Grain—*½ cup (2 oz) dry (56 g)*	.1
fettuccini	
1% egg white, Golden Grain—*1½ cups dry (56 g)*	.1
spinach, Golden Grain—*1⅓ cups dry (56 g)*	.1
noodles, egg, Golden Grain—*1¼ cups (2 oz) dry (56 g)*	.1
pasta, 1.5% egg white, Golden Grain—*1¾ cups dry (56 g)*	.1
Rainbow Radiatore, Golden Grain—*¾ cup dry (53 g)*	.1

17.12 Pastry Crust

pie crust, plain, mix, Flako—*¼ cup (25 g)*	.1

17.13 Rice & Rice Dishes

rice mix (not prepared)	
beef & mushroom, Rice-a-Roni—*2.5 oz (70 g)*	.1
beef w/ broccoli, Rice-a-Roni—*2 oz (56 g)*	.2
broccoli au gratin, Rice-a-Roni—*2.5 oz (70 g)*	1.7
broccoli rice, Rice-a-Roni—*2 oz (56 g)*	1.1
fried rice, Rice-a-Roni—*2.5 oz (70 g)*	.1
rice pilaf, Rice-a-Roni—*2.5 oz (70 g)*	1.5
rice risotto, Rice-a-Roni—*2.5 oz (70 g)*	.1
rice stroganoff, Rice-a-Roni—*2.5 oz (70 g)*	.1
rice w/ beef flavor, Rice-a-Roni—*2.5 oz (70 g)*	.1
rice w/ chicken & mushroom, Rice-a-Roni—*2.5 oz (70 g)*	.1
rice w/ chicken flavor, Rice-a-Roni—*2.5 oz (70 g)*	.1
rice w/ herbs & butter, Rice-a-Roni—*2.5 oz (70 g)*	.9
spanish rice, Rice-a-Roni—*2 oz (56 g)*	.1
white cheddar w/ herbs, Rice-a-Roni—*2.5 oz (70 g)*	1.9
yellow rice, Rice-a-Roni—*2.5 oz (70 g)*	.1

17.15 Stuffing

chicken flavor, w/ rice stuffing mix, Rice-a-Roni—*1 oz (28 g)*	.0
cornbread w/ rice stuffing mix, Rice-a-Roni—*1 oz (28 g)*	.1

19. INFANT, JUNIOR, & TODDLER FOODS
19.2 Cereals

barley, dry, Gerber—*.5 oz (15 g)*	.8
mixed, dry, Gerber—*.5 oz (15 g)*	.8
mixed w/ bananas, dry, Gerber—*.5 oz (15 g)*	.8
oatmeal, dry, Gerber—*.5 oz (15 g)*	.8
oatmeal w/ apples & cinn, inst, Gerber Granduates—*1 oz (28 g)*	1.5
oatmeal w/ bananas, dry, Gerber—*.5 oz (15 g)*	.8
rice, dry, Gerber—*.5 oz (15 g)*	.8
rice w/ apples, Gerber 2nd Foods—*.5 oz (15 g)*	.8
rice w/ bananas, dry, Gerber—*.5 oz (15 g)*	.8
rice w/ mixed fruit, dry, Gerber—*.5 oz (15 g)*	.8

23. MILK, MILK BEVERAGES, MILK MIXES & YOGURT
23.2 Milk, Cow, Beverages

instant breakfast	
liquid pack, Resource—*8 fl oz (279 g)*[1]	7.5
rtd, cnd, Carnation—*10 fl oz can (315 g)*[2]	7.5

23.3 Milk Mixes

choc milk powder	
Gerber Graduates—*.7 oz (20 g)*	2.0
Hershey—*3 T (24 g)*	.0
Instant Breakfast	
cafe mocha, Carnation—*1.3 oz pkt (37 g)*	7.5
choc malt, Carnation—*1.25 oz pkt (36 g)*	7.5
creamy milk choc, Carnation—*1.30 oz pkt (37 g)*	7.5
french van, Carnation—*1.26 oz pkt (36 g)*	7.5
strawberry, Carnation—*1.26 oz pkt (36 g)*	7.5
Instant Breakfast, no sugar added	
choc, Carnation—*.72 oz pkt (21 g)*	7.5
choc malt, Carnation—*.7 oz pkt (20 g)*	7.5
strawberry, Carnation—*.7 oz pkt (20 g)*	7.5
van, Carnation—*.7 oz pkt (20 g)*	7.5
van milk mixer, Gerber Graduates—*.7 oz (20 g)*	2.0

24. NUTS, NUT PRODUCTS, & SEEDS

peanut butter	
creamy/crunchy, Jif—*2 T (32 g)*	3.0
creamy/crunchy, red fat, Jif—*2 T (36 g)*	.9
creamy/crunchy, Simply Jif—*2 T (31 g)*	3.0
sunflower seeds/kernels, dried—*1 oz (28 g)*	41.0

1. Includes chocolate, strawberry, and vanilla.
2. Values are averages for cafe mocha, chocolate, French vanilla, and strawberry creme.

Vitamin E as Alpha-Tocopherol (mg)

1. BEVERAGES
1.4 Cereal Grain Beverages

powder—*1 t (2.3 g)*	.02

2. CANDY & GUM

Baby Ruth—*2.1 oz bar (60 g)*	1.13
Bar None—*1.5 oz bar (43 g)*	.65
Butterfinger—*2.16 oz bar (61 g)*	.97
caramel, choc flavored roll—*2.25 oz bar (64 g)*	.11
caramels—*2.5 oz (6 pieces) (71 g)*	.33
carob—*3 oz bar (87 g)*	1.96
choc coated	
fondant—*1 large patty (1.23 oz) (35 g)*	.12
peanuts—*10 pieces (40 g)*	1.02
raisins—*10 pieces (10 g)*	.10
choc, sweet, dark—*1.45 oz bar (41 g)*	.49
Special Dark, Hershey—*1.5 oz bar (41 g)*	.41
confectioner's coating	
butterscotch—*1 oz (28 g)*	.64
peanut butter—*1 oz (28 g)*	.85
white—*3 oz bar (85 g)*	1.91
Crunch, Nestle—*1.4 oz bar (40 g)*	.44
Fifth Avenue, Hershey—*2 oz bar (57 g)*	1.41
fudge	
choc—*.6 oz piece (17 g)*	.02
choc w/ nuts—*.67 oz piece (19 g)*	.08
van—*.56 oz piece (16 g)*	.03
van w/ nuts—*.53 oz piece (15 g)*	.07
Golden Almond, Solitaires w/ almonds, Hershey—*3 oz pkg (85 g)*	1.93
Hundred Grand—*1.5 oz bar (43 g)*	.32
Kit Kat Wafer, Hershey—*1.5 oz bar (42 g)*	.33
M&M's—*1.69 oz pkg (69 pieces) (48 g)*	.41
M&M's Peanut—*1.74 oz pkg (25 pieces) (49 g)*	1.05
Mars Almond—*1.76 oz bar (50 g)*	.30
milk choc—*1.55 oz bar (44 g)*	.55
w/ almonds—*1.55 oz bar (44 g)*	.83
w/ rice cereal—*1.45 oz bar (41 g)*	.51
milk choc chips—*1 cup chips (168 g)*	2.08
Milky Way—*2.15 oz bar (61 g)*	.40
Milky Way Snack Bar—*.6 oz bar (18 g)*	.12
Mounds—*1.9 oz bar (53 g)*	1.00
Mr. Goodbar, Hershey—*1.75 oz bar (49 g)*	.61
Oh Henry—*2 oz bar (57 g)*	.87
peanut bar—*1.6 oz bar (45 g)*	.44
peanut brittle—*1 oz (28 g)*	.46
Peanut Butter Cups, Reese's—*2 pieces (1. 8 oz) (50 g)*	.67
Reese's Pieces, Hershey—*1.6 oz pkg (46 g)*	.60
Rolo caramels w/ milk choc, Hershey—*9 pieces (1.9 oz) (53 g)*	.47
sesame crunch—*20 pieces (35 g)*	.35
Skittles Fruit Chews, M&M Mars—*2.3 oz (59 pieces) (65 g)*	.18
Snickers—*2.16 oz bar (61 g)*	.93
Starburst Fruit Chews—*2.07 oz pk (6 pieces) (59 g)*	.79
Three Musketeers—*2.13 oz bar (60 g)*	.28
Twix, caramel—*2 oz pkg (2 pieces) (57 g)*	.69
Twix, peanut butter—*1.77 oz pkg (2 pieces) (50 g)*	.56
Whatchamacallit, Hershey—*1.7 oz bar (48 g)*	.34

3. CEREALS, COOKED

barley, pearled, ckd—*1 cup (157 g)*	.08
buckwheat groats, roasted, ckd—*1 cup (198 g)*	.47
bulgur, ckd—*1 cup (182 g)*	.05
corn grits, inst, white, enr—*1 pkt prep (137 g)*	.36
corn grits, reg/quick, enr, ckd—*1 cup (242 g)*	.12
corn grits, reg/quick, unenr, ckd—*1 cup (242 g)*	.12
couscous, ckd—*1 cup (179 g)*	.02
Cream of Rice, ckd—*¾ cup (183 g)*	.04
Cream of Wheat	
inst, ckd—*¾ cup (181 g)*	.02
inst, mix & eat—*1 pkt prep (142 g)*	.02
quick, ckd—*¾ cup (179 g)*	.02
reg, ckd—*¾ cup (188 g)*	.02
farina	
ckd, enr—*¾ cup (175 g)*	.02
ckd, unenr—*¾ cup (175 g)*	.02
Maltex, ckd—*¾ cup (187 g)*	.69
Maypo, ckd—*¾ cup (180 g)*	1.26
millet, ckd—*1 cup (240 g)*	.43
oatmeal, inst—*1 pkt prep (177 g)*	.21
apple & cinn—*1 pkt prep (149 g)*	.12
cinn & spice—*1 pkt prep (161 g)*	.35
maple & brown sugar—*1 pkt prep (155 g)*	.16
raisins & spice—*1 pkt prep (158 g)*	.16
oatmeal, quick/reg/inst, ckd—*1 cup (234 g)*	.23
Ralston, ckd—*¾ cup (190 g)*	.19
Wheatena, ckd—*¾ cup (182 g)*	.67

4. CEREALS, READY-TO-EAT

bran 100%—*½ cup (1 oz) (28 g)*	.65
crisp rice, low Na—*1 cup (1 oz) (28 g)*	.04
crispy rice—*1 cup (1 oz) (28 g)*	.03
CW Post—*¼ cup (1 oz) (28 g)*	.20
CW Post w/ raisins—*¼ cup (1 oz) (28 g)*	.20
Frosted Rice Krinkles—*⅞ cup (1 oz) (28 g)*	.04
granola	
homemade—*¼ cup (1 oz) (28 g)*	3.61
Nature Valley—*⅓ cup (1 oz) (28 g)*	1.97
Heartland Natural—*¼ cup (1 oz) (28 g)*	.20
w/ coconut—*¼ cup (1 oz) (28 g)*	.20
w/ raisins—*¼ cup (1 oz) (28 g)*	.20
Honey Bran—*⅞ cup (1 oz) (28 g)*	.65
raisin bran, Ralston Purina—*¾ cup (1.3 oz) (38 g)*	.88
Rice Krispies, frosted, Kellogg's—*1 cup (1 oz) (28 g)*	.02
shredded wheat—*1 oz (28 g)*	.15
—*1 biscuit (.8 oz) (24 g)*	.13
Sugar Corn Pops, Kellogg's—*1 cup (1 oz) (28 g)*	.03
Sugar Frosted Flakes, Ralston Purina—*¾ cup (1 oz) (28 g)*	.07
Tasteeos, Ralston Purina—*1 ¼ cups (1 oz) (28 g)*	.20
Team Flakes, Nabisco—*1 ¼ cups (2 oz) (57 g)*	.13

5. CHEESE & CHEESE PRODUCTS
5.1 Cheese

american processed—*1 oz (28 g)*	.13
blue—*1 oz (28 g)*	.18
brick—*1 oz (28 g)*	.14
brie—*1 oz (28 g)*	.19

camembert—*1 oz (28 g)*	.19
cheddar—*1 oz (28 g)*	.10
—*3.5 oz (100 g)*	.36
—*1 cup, not packed (113 g)*	.41
low-fat—*1 oz (28 g)*	.02
low sodium—*1 oz (28 g)*	.10
colby—*1 oz (28 g)*	.10
cottage cheese	
1% fat—*1 cup (226 g)*	.25
2% fat—*1 cup (226 g)*	.13
creamed—*1 rd T (28 g)*	.03
creamed—*4 oz (113 g)*	.14
creamed—*1 cup, not packed (210 g)*	.26
creamed w/ fruit—*1 cup (226 g)*	.21
dry curd—*1 cup, not packed (145 g)*	.16
cream cheese—*1 oz (2 T) (28 g)*	.27
edam—*1 oz (28 g)*	.21
feta—*1 oz (28 g)*	.01
fontina—*1 oz (28 g)*	.10
goat, hard—*1 oz (28 g)*	.22
goat, semi-soft—*1 oz (28 g)*	.18
goat, soft—*1 oz (28 g)*	.13
gouda—*1 oz (28 g)*	.10
gruyere—*1 oz (28 g)*	.10
limburger—*1 oz (28 g)*	.18
monterey—*1 oz (28 g)*	.10
mozzarella	
low moisture—*1 oz (28 g)*	.19
part skim—*1 oz (28 g)*	.12
part skim, low moisture—*1 oz (28 g)*	.13
whole milk—*1 oz (28 g)*	.10
muenster—*1 oz (28 g)*	.13
parmesan, grated—*1 T (5 g)*	.04
parmesan, hard—*1 oz (28 g)*	.23
pimento, processed—*1 oz (28 g)*	.13
port du salut—*1 oz (28 g)*	.14
provolone—*1 oz (28 g)*	.10
queso anejo, mexican—*1 oz (28 g)*	.03
queso asadero, mexican—*1 oz (28 g)*	.03
queso chihuahua, mexican—*1 oz (28 g)*	.06
ricotta, part skim—*½ cup (124 g)*	.27
ricotta, whole milk—*½ cup (124 g)*	.43
romano—*1 oz (28 g)*	.21
swiss—*1 oz (28 g)*	.14
swiss, processed—*1 oz (28 g)*	.19
tilsit, whole milk—*1 oz (28 g)*	.20

5.2 Cheese Products

cheese food, american—*1 oz (28 g)*	.20
cheese product, mozzarella cheese substitute—*1 oz (28 g)*	.56
cheese spread, american—*1 T (16 g)*	.11
—*1 oz (28 g)*	.20

6. CHIPS, PRETZELS, POPCORN, & OTHER SNACK FOODS

banana chips—*1 oz (28 g)*	1.53
beef jerky, chopped & formed—*1 large piece (20 g)*	.10
cheese puffs/twists—*1 oz (28 g)*	1.45
corn-based snack, onion-flavor—*1 oz (28 g)*	.46
corn cakes—*2 cakes (18 g)*	.02
corn chips—*1 oz (28 g)*	.39
oriental mix, rice-based—*1 oz (28 g)*	2.39
popcorn cakes—*2 cakes (20 g)*	.02
popcorn, caramel—*1 cup (1.24 oz) (35 g)*	.42
w/ peanuts—*1 oz (28 g)*	.43
popcorn, cheese—*2.6 cups (1 oz) (28 g)*	.03
popcorn, plain	
air-popped—*3.5 cups (1 oz) (28 g)*	.03
oil-popped—*2.6 cups (1 oz) (28 g)*	.03
pork skins—*1 oz (28 g)*	.17
potato chips, barbecue—*1 oz (28 g)*	1.42
potato chips, light—*1 oz (28 g)*	.82
potato chips, light, from dried potatoes—*1 oz (28 g)*	1.42
potato chips, plain—*1 oz (28 g)*	1.38
from dried potatoes—*1 oz (28 g)*	1.38
potato sticks—*1 oz (28 g)*	1.38
pretzels—*1 oz (28 g)*	.06
rice cakes, brown—*2 cakes (18 g)*	.13
sesame sticks, wheat-based—*1 oz (28 g)*	1.11
taro chips—*12 chips (1 oz) (28 g)*	1.39
tortilla chips—*1 oz (28 g)*	.39

7. CREAMS & CREAM SUBSTITUTES

creamer, liquid/frzn w/ hydg veg oils—*½ fl oz (15 g)*[1]	.24
creamer, powdered—*1 t (2.0 g)*[2]	.01
half & half (milk & cream)—*1 T (15 g)*	.02
light (coffee/table) cream—*1 T (15 g)*	.02
medium (25% fat) cream—*1 T (15 g)*	.09
sour cream	
cultured—*1 T (12 g)*	.07
half & half, cultured—*1 T (15 g)*	.05
imitation—*1 oz (28 g)*	.04
whipped topping	
from mix, prep w/ whole milk—*1 T (4 g)*	.01
frzn—*1 T (4 g)*	.01
pressurized—*1 T (4 g)*	.01
whipping cream	
heavy, fluid—*1 T (15 g)*	.09
light, fluid—*1 T (15 g)*	.09
pressurized—*1 T (3 g)*	.02

8. DESSERTS

8.1 Brownies & Bar Cookies

brownie—*1 large brownie (2¾" x ⅞") (56 g)*	1.20

8.2 Cakes

angel food, from mix—*1/12 cake (50 g)*	.00
boston cream pie, frzn—*⅙ of 19.5 oz cake (92 g)*	.98
carrot cake, w/ cream cheese icing, homemade—*1/12 of 9" cake (111 g)*	4.69
cheesecake—*⅙ of 17 oz cake (80 g)*	.84
cherry fudge w/ choc icing—*⅛ of 20 oz cake (71 g)*	1.10
choc cake	
from mix—*1/12 of 9" cake (65 g)*	1.14
homemade—*1/12 of 9" cake (95 g)*	1.51
choc pudding type, from mix—*1/12 of 9" cake (77 g)*	1.37
coffee cake	
cheese (cream/neufchatel)—*⅙ of 16 oz cake (76 g)*	1.48
cinn w/ crumb topping—*⅑ of 20 oz cake (63 g)*	2.23
cinn w/ crumb topping, from mix—*⅛ of cake (56 g)*	.93
fruit, from mix, Aunt Jemima—*⅛ of 14 oz cake (50 g)*	.43

fruitcake—*1 piece (1.5 oz) (43 g)*	1.34
german choc w/ coconut-nut icing, from mix—*¹⁄₁₂ of 9" cake (111 g)*	1.18
gingerbread, from mix—*¹⁄₉ of 9" sq cake (67 g)*	.92
marble cake, from mix—*¹⁄₁₂ of 9" cake (73 g)*	1.38
pineapple upside-down, homemade—*¹⁄₉ of 8" cake (115 g)*	2.09
pound	
fat-free—*1 oz (28 g)*	.01
made w/ veg shortening—*¹⁄₁₀ of 10.6 oz cake (30 g)*	.77
sponge—*¹⁄₁₂ of 16 oz cake (38 g)*	.17
white	
from mix—*¹⁄₁₂ of 9" cake (62 g)*	.80
homemade—*¹⁄₁₂ of 9" cake (74 g)*	1.35
pudding type, from mix—*¹⁄₁₂ of 9" cake (69 g)*	1.18
w/ coconut icing, homemade—*¹⁄₁₂ of 9" cake (112 g)*	.15
yellow	
from mix—*¹⁄₁₂ of 9" cake (63 g)*	.98
homemade—*¹⁄₁₂ of 8" cake (68 g)*	1.40
pudding type, from mix—*¹⁄₁₂ of 9" cake (69 g)*	1.29
w/ choc icing—*¹⁄₈ of 18 oz cake (64 g)*	1.73

8.3 Cakes, Snack

choc, creme filled w/ icing—*1 snack cake (50 g)*	1.00
sponge snack cake, creme filled—*1 snack cake (43 g)*	.83

8.4 Cookies

animal crackers—*11 pieces (1 oz) (28 g)*	.52
butter cookies—*1 cookie (2" dia) (5 g)*	.02
choc chip	
(18-28% fat)—*1 cookie (2¼" dia) (10 g)*	.27
homemade w/ marg—*1 cookie (2¼" dia) (16 g)*	.47
choc coated graham crackers—*2 crackers (1 oz) (28 g)*	.47
choc sandwich	
w/ creme filling—*1 cookie (10 g)*	.30
w/ creme filling, choc coated—*1 cookie (17 g)*	.60
w/ extra creme filling—*1 cookie (13 g)*	.50
choc wafers—*5 wafers (1 oz) (28 g)*[3]	.54
fig bar—*1 bar (16 g)*	.11
fortune—*1 cookie (8 g)*	.03
gingersnaps—*4 cookies (1 oz) (28 g)*	.42
graham crackers, plain/honey—*4 crackers (1 oz) (28 g)*[4]	.54
ice cream cone	
cake/wafer—*1 cone (4 g)*	.06
sugar—*1 cone (10 g)*	.08
ladyfingers—*1 ladyfinger (11 g)*	.10
macaroon, homemade—*1 cookie (2" x ⅜") (24 g)*	.07
marshmallow, choc coated—*1 sm cookie (1¾" x ¾") (13 g)*	.25
molasses—*1 med cookie (3" x ⅜") (15 g)*	.31
oatmeal—*1 cookie (18 g)*	.51
oatmeal raisin, fat-free—*2 cookies (1 oz) (28 g)*	.04
peanut butter—*1 cookie (15 g)*	.53
sandwich—*1 cookie (14 g)*	.43
raisin, soft type—*1 cookie (15 g)*	.23
shortbread—*1 cookie (1⅝" sq) (8 g)*	.24
sugar—*1 cookie (15 g)*	.39
from refrig dough—*1 cookie (12 g)*	.38
homemade w/ marg—*1 cookie (3" dia) (14 g)*	.53
sugar wafers, w/ creme filling—*8 wafers (1 oz) (28 g)*	1.01
vanilla sandwich w/ creme filling—*1 cookie (1¾" dia) (10 g)*	.28
vanilla wafers, (12-17% fat)—*7 wafers (1 oz) (28 g)*	.38

8.5 Doughnuts

cake—*1 doughnut (47 g)*	1.62
choc coated/frosted—*1 doughnut (43 g)*	1.89
choc, sugared/glazed—*1 doughnut (42 g)*	.99
wheat, sugared/glazed—*1 doughnut (45 g)*	1.19
cruller, glazed—*1 cruller (3" dia) (41 g)*	1.04
yeast	
glazed—*1 doughnut (60 g)*	1.75
w/ creme filling—*1 doughnut (85 g)*	1.94
w/ jelly filling—*1 doughnut (85 g)*	1.83

8.6 Frozen Desserts

frozen yogurt, van, soft serve—*½ cup (72 g)*	.04
ice cream	
choc—*½ cup (66 g)*	.22
french van, soft serve—*½ cup (86 g)*	.32
sherbet, orange—*½ cup (96 g)*	.05

8.7 Fruit Cobblers & Turnovers

strudel, apple—*1 strudel (71 g)*	1.26

8.9 Granola, Cereal, and Snack Bars

peanut, hard—*.83 oz bar (24 g)*	.27

8.10 Pastries

cream puff, w/ custard filling, homemade—*1 cream puff (130 g)*	2.87
croissant—*1 med croissant (57 g)*	.25
cheese—*1 med croissant (57 g)*	.57
danish pastry	
cheese (cream/neufchatel)—*1 pastry (4¼" dia) (71 g)*	1.83
cinn—*1 pastry (4¼" dia) (65 g)*	2.01
fruit—*1 pastry (4¼" dia) (71 g)*[5]	1.25
nut—*1 pastry (4¼" dia) (65 g)*[6]	1.85
eclair, w/ custard filling & choc glaze, homemade—*1 eclair (100 g)*	2.10
sweet roll/buns, cinn raisin—*1 roll (2¾" sq) (60 g)*	1.71
toaster pastry, fruit—*1 pastry (52 g)*[7]	.97

8.11 Pies

apple, frzn—*⅛ of 9" pie (125 g)*	2.06
banana cream, homemade—*⅛ of 9" pie (148 g)*	2.18
blueberry, frzn—*⅛ of 9" pie (125 g)*	1.85
cherry, frzn—*⅛ of 9" pie (125 g)*	1.76
choc cream, frzn—*⅙ of 8" pie (113 g)*	2.70
coconut cream, frzn—*⅙ of 7" pie (64 g)*	1.03
custard, egg—*⅙ of 8" pie (105 g)*	1.25
fruit, fried—*1 snack pie (5" x 3¾") (128 g)*[8]	4.19
lemon meringue, frzn—*⅙ of 8" pie (113 g)*	1.61
mince, homemade—*⅛ of 9" pie (165 g)*	3.09
peach, frzn—*⅙ of 8" pie (117 g)*	2.01
pecan—*⅙ of 8" pie (113 g)*	2.86
pumpkin, frzn—*⅙ of 8" pie (109 g)*	1.75
van cream, homemade—*⅛ of 9" pie (126 g)*	1.70

8.12 Puddings, Custards, & Pie Fillings

choc	
from inst mix w/ whole milk—*½ cup (142 g)*	.09
from reg mix w/ whole milk—*½ cup (142 g)*	.09
rte—*5 oz can (142 g)*	.18
coconut cream, from reg mix w/ lowfat milk—*½ cup (140 g)*	.10

tapioca, rte—*5 oz can (142 g)*	.13
van	
from inst mix w/ whole milk—*½ cup (142 g)*	.09
from reg mix w/ whole milk—*½ cup (140 g)*	.08
rte—*½ cup (113 g)*	.14

8.13 Sauces, Syrups, & Toppings for Desserts

choc syrup—*2 T (1 fl oz) (38 g)*	.01
icing/frosting, rts	
coconut nut—*1/12 tub (38 g)*	.43
van creamy—*1/12 tub (38 g)*	.77
strawberry topping—*2 T (42 g)*	.06
walnut syrup topping—*2 T (41 g)*	.36

9. EGGS, EGG DISHES, & EGG SUBSTITUTES

egg, chicken	
boiled, hard/soft—*1 large (50 g)*	.53
fried—*1 large (46 g)*	.75
omelet, plain—*1 large egg (61 g)*	.79
poached—*1 large (50 g)*	.53
scrambled w/ milk—*1 large egg (61 g)*	.80
whole, fresh/frzn—*1 large (50 g)*	.53
yolk, fresh—*yolk of 1 large egg (17 g)*	.54
egg, other poultry	
duck, whole—*1 egg (70 g)*	.52
goose, whole—*1 egg (144 g)*	1.07
quail, whole—*1 egg (9 g)*	.07
egg substitutes	
frzn—*¼ cup (60 g)*[9]	1.27
liquid—*1.5 fl oz (47 g)*[10]	.23
powdered—*0.35 oz (10 g)*[11]	.16

10. ENTREES & MEALS
10.2 Canned & Shelf Stable Entrees

chili w/ beans—*1 cup (255 g)*	1.87

11. FAST FOODS
11.1 Generic

biscuit	
w/ egg, & bacon—*1 biscuit (150 g)*	2.11
w/ egg & ham—*1 biscuit (192 g)*	2.20
w/ egg & sausage—*1 biscuit (180 g)*	2.77
w/ ham—*1 biscuit (113 g)*	2.24
w/ sausage—*1 biscuit (124 g)*	3.08
cheeseburger	
large w/ lettuce & tomato—*1 sandwich (219 g)*	1.18
reg w/ double meat—*1 sandwich (155 g)*	1.19
reg w/ double meat, double-decker bun, lettuce, & tomato—*1 sandwich (228 g)*	1.98
chicken, breaded & fried, boneless pieces—*6 pieces (102 g)*	1.99
cookies, animal crackers—*1 box (67 g)*	.31
cookies, choc chip—*1 box (55 g)*	.37
egg, scrambled—*2 eggs (94 g)*	1.58
english muffin	
w/ butter—*1 muffin (63 g)*	.13
w/ cheese & sausage—*1 sandwich (115 g)*	.49
w/ egg, cheese, & canadian bacon—*1 sandwich (146 g)*	.60
fish sandwich w/ tartar sce—*1 sandwich (158 g)*	.87
fish sandwich w/ tartar sce & cheese—*1 sandwich (183 g)*	1.83
french fries, fried in veg oil—*20-25 fries (76 g)*	.14

french fries, fried in veg oil—*30-40 fries (115 g)*	.22
french toast sticks—*5 sticks (141 g)*	3.96
ham & cheese sandwich—*1 sandwich (146 g)*	.29
ham, egg, & cheese sandwich—*1 sandwich (143 g)*	.59
hamburger, reg—*1 sandwich (90 g)*	.36
hash brown potatoes—*½ cup (72 g)*	.12
ice milk, vanilla, soft serve w/ cone—*1 cone (103 g)*	.38
onion rings—*8-9 rings (83 g)*	.33
pancakes w/ butter & syrup—*3 pancakes (232 g)*	1.39
pie, fruit (apple/cherry/lemon), fried—*1 pie (85 g)*	.37
shake	
choc—*10 fl oz (283 g)*	.19
van—*10 fl oz (283 g)*	.17
sundae	
caramel—*1 sundae (155 g)*	.90
hot fudge—*1 sundae (158 g)*	.66
strawberry—*1 sundae (153 g)*	.78

11.8 Taco Bell

burrito	
bean—*1 burrito (199 g)*	.02
light chicken—*1 burrito (177 g)*	.08
seven layers—*1 burrito (284 g)*	.85
Burrito Supreme—*1 burrito (255 g)*	2.70
big beef—*1 burrito (291 g)*	3.95
fajita	
chicken—*1 fajita (220 g)*	.05
steak—*1 fajita (220 g)*	.05
Supreme, chicken—*1 fajita (255 g)*	.10
Supreme, steak—*1 fajita (255 g)*	.10
Supreme, veg—*1 fajita (255 g)*	.10
veg—*1 fajita (220 g)*	.05
mexican pizza—*1 serving (216 g)*	1.96
nachos, Supreme, big beef—*1 serving (195 g)*	1.96
pintos 'n cheese w/ red sauce—*1 serving (128 g)*	.80
sauce, guacamole—*1 serving (21 g)*	.74
soft taco—*1 taco (99 g)*	1.96
Supreme—*1 taco (135 g)*	2.01
taco—*1 taco (78 g)*	1.97
Double Decker—*1 taco (156 g)*	1.97
Supreme—*1 taco (113 g)*	2.01
Supreme, Double Decker—*1 taco (191 g)*	2.01
taco salad w/ salsa—*1 salad (464 g)*	4.48
taco salad w/ salsa & shell—*1 salad (535 g)*	4.48
tostada w/ red sce—*1 tostada (177 g)*	.11

12. FATS, OILS, & SHORTENINGS
12.1 Animal Fats

beef separable fat, ckd—*1 oz (28 g)*	.13
beef suet, raw—*1 oz (28 g)*	.43
chicken fat, raw—*1 T (13 g)*	.35
duck fat, raw—*1 T (13 g)*	.35
lamb fat, ckd—*1 oz (28 g)*	.01
lard (pork fat), raw—*1 T (13 g)*	.16
mutton tallow, raw—*1 T (13 g)*	.37
pork separable fat, ckd—*1 oz (28 g)*	.23
salt pork, raw—*1 oz (28 g)*	.14
turkey fat, raw—*1 T (13 g)*	.37

12.3 Shortenings

hydg coconut & palm kernel (for confectionery)—*1 T (13 g)*	.30

hydg soybean & cottonseed—*1 T (13 g)*	1.08
hydg soybean & cottonseed (for bread)—*1 T (13 g)*	1.06
hydg soybean & palm (household)—*1 T (13 g)*	1.08
lard & veg oil—*1 T (13 g)*	.16

12.4 Vegetable Oils & Sprays

almond oil—*1 T (14 g)*	5.50
apricot kernel oil—*1 T (14 g)*	1.21
canola oil—*1 T (14 g)*	2.93
coconut oil—*1 T (14 g)*	.04
corn oil—*1 T (14 g)*	2.96
cottonseed oil—*1 T (14 g)*	5.36
oat oil—*1 T (14 g)*	2.02
olive oil—*1 T (14 g)*	1.74
palm kernel oil—*1 T (14 g)*	.53
palm oil—*1 T (14 g)*	3.05
peanut oil—*1 T (14 g)*	1.81
safflower oil, commercial, 70% & over linoleic acid—*1 T (14 g)*	6.03
sesame oil—*1 T (14 g)*	.57
soybean (hydg) & cottonseed oil—*1 T (14 g)*	3.95
soybean lecithin—*1 T (14 g)*[12]	.72
soybean oil—*1 T (14 g)*	2.55
soybean oil, hydg—*1 T (14 g)*	2.55
sunflower oil, 60% & over linoleic acid—*1 T (14 g)*	7.08
sunflower oil, hydrg—*1 T (14 g)*	7.14
walnut oil—*1 T (14 g)*	.45
wheat germ oil—*1 T (14 g)*	26.94

13. FISH, SHELLFISH, & CRUSTACEA

abalone, raw—*3 oz (85 g)*	3.40
anchovy, cnd in olive oil—*5 anchovies (20 g)*	1.00
bass, striped, raw—*3 oz (85 g)*	.43
bluefish, raw—*3 oz (85 g)*	.43
carp, raw—*3 oz (85 g)*	.54
catfish, channel	
farmed, raw—*3 oz (85 g)*	1.02
wild, raw—*3 oz (85 g)*	.51
caviar, black & red, granular—*1 T (16 g)*	1.12
cisco, raw—*3 oz (85 g)*	.06
cisco, smoked—*3 oz (85 g)*	.17
clam liquid, cnd—*1 cup (240 g)*	2.40
clams	
cnd, drained—*3 oz (85 g)*	.85
raw—*3 oz (4 large or 9 small) (85 g)*	.85
cod, atlantic	
ckd by dry heat—*3 oz (85 g)*	.26
cnd—*3 oz (85 g)*	.17
dried & salted—*3 oz (85 g)*	.51
raw—*3 oz (85 g)*	.20
cod, pacific, raw—*3 oz (85 g)*	.20
crab, alaska king, imitation, made from surimi—*3 oz (85 g)*	.09
crab, blue	
ckd by moist heat—*3 oz (85 g)*	.85
cnd—*3 oz (85 g)*	.85
raw—*3 oz (85 g)*	.85
crayfish	
wild, ckd by moist heat—*3 oz (85 g)*	1.28
wild, raw—*3 oz (85 g)*	2.42

croaker, atlantic, raw—*3 oz (85 g)*	.85
dolphinfish, raw—*3 oz (85 g)*	.26
fish pieces, frzn, reheated—*1 piece (4" x 2' x ½") (57 g)*[13]	.78
fish sticks, frzn—*1 stick (4" x 2" x ½") (28 g)*[13]	.39
flatfish (flounder/sole)	
ckd by dry heat—*3 oz (85 g)*	1.61
raw—*3 oz (85 g)*	1.61
grouper, raw—*3 oz (85 g)*	.43
haddock	
raw—*3 oz (85 g)*	.33
smoked—*3 oz (85 g)*	.34
halibut, atlantic & pacific, ckd by dry heat—*3 oz (85 g)*	.93
halibut, atlantic & pacific, raw—*3 oz (85 g)*	.72
halibut, greenland, raw—*3 oz (85 g)*	.72
herring, atlantic	
ckd by dry heat—*3 oz (85 g)*	1.14
kippered—*1 piece (4⅜" x 1¾" x ¼") (40 g)*	.40
pickled—*1 piece (1¾" x ⅞" x ½") (15 g)*	.15
raw—*3 oz (85 g)*	.91
lingcod, raw—*3 oz (85 g)*	.20
lobster, northern, ckd by moist heat—*3 oz (85 g)*	.85
lobster, northern, raw—*3 oz (85 g)*	1.25
mackerel, atlantic, raw—*3 oz (85 g)*	1.29
mackerel, jack, cnd—*1 cup (190 g)*	2.66
mackerel, pacific, and jack, ckd by dry heat—*3 oz (85 g)*	1.09
mackerel, pacific, and jack, raw—*3 oz (85 g)*	.85
mackerel, spanish, raw—*3 oz (85 g)*	.59
mullet, striped, raw—*3 oz (85 g)*	.85
mussels, blue, raw—*3 oz (85 g)*	.63
ocean perch, atlantic, raw—*3 oz (85 g)*	1.06
octopus, ckd by moist heat—*3 oz (85 g)*	1.02
octopus, raw—*3 oz (85 g)*	1.02
oysters, eastern	
cnd—*3 oz (85 g)*	.72
wild, raw—*6 med (84 g)*	.71
oysters, pacific, raw—*3 oz (85 g)*	.72
perch, raw—*3 oz (85 g)*	.17
pike, northern, raw—*3 oz (85 g)*	.17
pike, walleye, raw—*3 oz (85 g)*	.17
pollock, atlantic, raw—*3 oz (85 g)*	.20
pollock, walleye, ckd by dry heat—*3 oz (85 g)*	.17
pollock, walleye, raw—*3 oz (85 g)*	.17
pompano, florida, raw—*3 oz (85 g)*	.15
rockfish, pacific, ckd by dry heat—*3 oz (85 g)*	1.06
rockfish, pacific, raw—*3 oz (85 g)*	1.06
roe, mixed species, raw—*1 oz (28 g)*	1.98
sablefish, raw—*3 oz (85 g)*	.43
salmon, chinook, smoked—*3 oz (85 g)*	1.15
salmon, chum, cnd w/ bone—*3 oz (85 g)*	1.36
salmon, coho	
wild, ckd by dry heat—*3 oz (85 g)*	.69
wild, raw—*3 oz (85 g)*	.55
salmon, pink	
cnd w/ bone—*3 oz (85 g)*	1.15
raw—*3 oz (85 g)*	.85
salmon, sockeye	
cnd w/ bone—*3 oz (85 g)*	1.36
raw—*3 oz (85 g)*	.85
sardines, cnd, atlantic w/ soybean oil—*2 sardines (24 g)*	.07

sardines, cnd, pacific w/ tomato sce—*1 sardine (38 g)*	1.41
scallops, mixed species, raw—*3 oz (6 large) (85 g)*	.85
scup, raw—*3 oz (85 g)*	.43
sea bass, raw—*3 oz (85 g)*	.43
seatrout, raw—*3 oz (85 g)*	.17
shad, american, raw—*3 oz (85 g)*	.85
shark, raw—*3 oz (85 g)*	.85
shrimp	
ckd by moist heat—*3 oz (15½ large) (85 g)*	.43
cnd—*3 oz (85 g)*	.79
raw—*3 oz (12 large) (85 g)*	.70
smelt, rainbow, raw—*3 oz (85 g)*	.43
snapper, raw—*3 oz (85 g)*	.43
spiny lobster, raw—*3 oz (85 g)*	1.25
spot, raw—*3 oz (85 g)*	1.32
squid, raw—*3 oz (85 g)*	1.02
sturgeon	
ckd by dry heat—*3 oz (85 g)*	.64
raw—*3 oz (85 g)*	.43
smoked—*3 oz (85 g)*	.43
swordfish, raw—*3 oz (85 g)*	.43
tilefish, raw—*3 oz (85 g)*	.30
trout, mixed species, raw—*3 oz (85 g)*	.17
trout, rainbow	
farmed, raw—*3 oz (85 g)*	.03
wild, raw—*3 oz (85 g)*	.17
tuna, bluefin, raw—*3 oz (85 g)*	.85
tuna, cnd in oil, light, drained—*3 oz (85 g)*	1.02
tuna, cnd in water, light, drained—*3 oz (85 g)*	.45
tuna, cnd in water, white, drained—*3 oz (85 g)*	1.35
tuna, yellowfin, raw—*3 oz (85 g)*	.43
whelk (sea snail), raw—*3 oz (85 g)*	.11
whitefish	
raw—*3 oz (85 g)*	.17
smoked—*3 oz (85 g)*	.17
whiting, ckd by dry heat—*3 oz (85 g)*	.26
whiting, raw—*3 oz (85 g)*	.26

14. FRUIT & VEGETABLE JUICES

acerola jce, fresh—*8 fl oz (242 g)*	.10
apple jce, cnd/bottled—*8 fl oz (248 g)*	.02
apple jce, from frzn conc—*8 fl oz (239 g)*	.02
apricot nectar, cnd—*8 fl oz (251 g)*	.20
carrot jce, cnd—*6 fl oz (184 g)*	.02
grape jce, from frzn conc, sweetened—*8 fl oz (250 g)*	.13
grapefruit jce	
cnd—*8 fl oz (247 g)*	.12
cnd, sweetened—*8 fl oz (250 g)*	.13
fresh—*8 fl oz (247 g)*	.12
from frzn conc—*8 fl oz (247 g)*	.12
lemon jce	
cnd/bottled—*1 T (15 g)*	.01
fresh—*1 T (15 g)*	.01
fresh—*8 fl oz (244 g)*	.22
frzn, single-strength—*1 T (15 g)*	.01
lime jce	
cnd/bottled—*1 T (15 g)*	.01
fresh—*1 T (15 g)*	.01
fresh—*8 fl oz (246 g)*	.22

orange grapefruit jce, cnd—*8 fl oz (247 g)*	.17
orange jce	
cnd—*8 fl oz (249 g)*	.22
fresh—*8 fl oz (248 g)*	.22
from frzn conc—*8 fl oz (249 g)*	.47
papaya nectar, cnd—*8 fl oz (250 g)*	.05
passion fruit jce, purple, fresh—*8 fl oz (247 g)*	.12
passion fruit jce, yellow, fresh—*8 fl oz (247 g)*	.12
peach nectar, cnd—*8 fl oz (249 g)*	.02
pear nectar, cnd—*8 fl oz (250 g)*	.25
pineapple jce, cnd—*8 fl oz (250 g)*	.05
pineapple jce, from frzn conc—*8 fl oz (250 g)*	.03
prune jce, cnd—*8 fl oz (256 g)*	.03
tangerine jce	
cnd, sweetened—*8 fl oz (249 g)*	.22
fresh—*8 fl oz (247 g)*	.22
tomato jce—*6 fl oz (182 g)*	1.66
veg jce cocktail, cnd—*6 fl oz (182 g)*	.58

15. FRUITS

acerola, raw—*1 cup (98 g)*	.13
apple	
boiled, w/o skin—*1 cup (171 g)*	.02
cnd, sliced, sweetened—*½ cup (102 g)*	.01
dried, sulfured—*10 rings (64 g)*	.35
micro ckd w/o skin—*1 cup (170 g)*	.02
raw, w/o skin—*1 med (128 g)*	.10
raw, w/ skin—*1 med (138 g)*	.44
applesauce, cnd	
sweetened—*½ cup (128 g)*	.01
unsweetened—*½ cup (122 g)*	.01
apricots	
cnd, heavy syrup—*4 halves (90 g)*	.80
cnd, jce pack—*3 halves (84 g)*	.75
cnd, light syrup—*3 halves (85 g)*	.76
cnd, water pack—*4 halves (90 g)*	.80
dried, sulfured—*10 halves (35 g)*	.52
frzn, sweetened—*½ cup (121 g)*	1.08
raw—*3 med (106 g)*	.94
avocado, raw, calif—*1 med (173 g)*	2.32
banana, raw—*1 med (114 g)*	.31
blackberries	
cnd, heavy syrup—*½ cup (128 g)*	.91
frzn, unsweetened—*1 cup (151 g)*	1.07
raw—*½ cup (72 g)*	.51
blueberries	
cnd, heavy syrup—*½ cup (128 g)*	1.28
frzn, sweetened—*1 cup (230 g)*	1.63
raw—*1 cup (145 g)*	1.45
boysenberries, cnd, heavy syrup—*½ cup (128 g)*	.91
boysenberries, frzn, unsweetened—*1 cup (132 g)*	.59
breadfruit, raw—*¼ small (96 g)*	1.08
cantaloupe, raw—*1 cup pieces (160 g)*	.24
carambola, raw—*1 med (127 g)*	.47
casaba melon, raw—*1 cup pieces (170 g)*	.26
cherries, sour	
cnd, heavy syrup—*½ cup (128 g)*	.17
cnd, water pack—*½ cup (122 g)*	.16
raw—*10 cherries (68 g)*	.09

cherries, sweet
   cnd, heavy syrup—½ cup (129 g) .08
   cnd, jce pack—½ cup (125 g) .13
   cnd, water pack—½ cup (124 g) .16
   frzn, sweetened—1 cup (259 g) .34
   raw—10 cherries (68 g) .09
cranberries, raw—1 cup whole (95 g) .10
cranberry sce, jelled, cnd—½ cup (138 g) .14
currants
   european black, raw—½ cup (56 g) .06
   red & white, raw—½ cup (56 g) .06
   zante, dried—½ cup (72 g)[14] .07
dates, dried—10 dates (83 g) .08
elderberries, raw—1 cup (145 g) 1.45
figs
   cnd, heavy syrup—3 figs (85 g) .76
   raw—1 med (50 g) .45
fruit cocktail
   cnd, heavy syrup—½ cup (128 g)[15] .37
   cnd, jce pack—½ cup (124 g) .25
   cnd, water pack—½ cup (122 g) .35
fruit salad
   cnd, heavy syrup—½ cup (128 g)[16] .59
   cnd, tropical, heavy syrup—½ cup (128 g)[17] .64
fruit snack, fruit roll—1 large roll (.74 oz) (21 g) .06
gooseberries, cnd, light syrup—½ cup (126 g) .47
gooseberries, raw—1 cup (150 g) .55
grapefruit
   cnd, jce pack—½ cup (124 g) .31
   cnd, light syrup—½ cup (127 g) .32
   raw, pink & red—½ med (123 g) .31
   raw, white—½ med (118 g) .29
grapes
   american (slip skin), raw—1 cup (92 g) .31
   european (adherent skin), raw—1 cup (160 g) 1.12
   thompson seedless, cnd, heavy syrup—½ cup (128 g) .90
guava, raw—1 med (90 g) 1.01
honeydew melon, raw—1 cup cube (170 g) .26
jackfruit, raw—3.5 oz (99 g) .15
kiwifruit, raw—1 med (76 g) .85
kumquats, raw—1 med (19 g) .05
lemon peel—1 T (6 g) .01
lemon, raw—1 med (58 g) .14
lime, raw—1 med (67 g) .16
loganberries, frzn—1 cup (147 g) 3.25
loquats, raw—6 med (100 g) .89
lychees, dried—3.5 oz (99 g) .69
lychees, raw—10 med (100 g) .70
mammy apple, raw—⅛ med (100 g) .59
mandarin oranges, cnd, jce pack—½ cup (124 g) .62
mandarin oranges, cnd, light syrup—½ cup (126 g) .43
mango, raw—1 med (207 g) 2.32
melon balls (cantaloupe & honeydew), frzn—1 cup (173 g) .26
mulberries, raw—1 cup (140 g) .63
nectarine, raw—1 med (136 g) 1.21
orange peel—1 T (6 g) .01
papaya, raw—1 med (304 g) 3.40
passion fruit (grandilla), purple, raw—1 med (18 g) .20
peach

   cnd, heavy syrup—1 cup (256 g) 2.28
   cnd, heavy syrup, spiced—1 med (88 g) .78
   cnd, jce pack—1 cup (248 g) 3.72
   cnd, light syrup—1 cup (251 g) 2.23
   cnd, water pack—1 cup (244 g) 2.17
   frzn, sweetened—1 cup (250 g) 2.23
   raw—1 med (87 g) .61
pear
   cnd, heavy pack—1 cup (255 g) 1.27
   cnd, jce pack—1 cup (248 g) 1.24
   cnd, light syrup—1 cup (251 g) 1.25
   cnd, water pack—1 cup (244 g) 1.22
   raw—1 med (166 g) .83
pear, asian, raw—1 pear (2½" high, 2½" dia) (122 g) .61
persimmon, japanese, raw—1 med (168 g) .99
pineapple
   cnd, heavy syrup—1 cup pieces (255 g) .26
   cnd, jce pack—1 cup pieces (250 g) .25
   raw—1 cup pieces (155 g) .16
plantain, ckd—1 cup slices (154 g) .22
plums
   cnd, heavy syrup—3 plums (133 g) .93
   cnd, jce pack—3 plums (95 g) .66
   raw—1 med (66 g) .40
pomegranate, raw—1 med (154 g) .85
pricklypear, raw—1 med (103 g) .01
prunes, dried—10 prunes (84 g) 1.22
quince, raw—1 med (92 g) .51
raisins
   golden seedless—⅔ cup (100 g) .70
   seeded—⅔ cup (100 g) .70
   seedless—⅔ cup (100 g) .70
raspberries
   cnd, heavy syrup—½ cup (128 g) .58
   frzn, sweetened—⅖ cup (100 g) .45
   raw—1 cup (123 g) .55
sapodilla, raw—1 med (170 g) .42
soursop, raw—1 cup (225 g) .90
strawberries
   frzn, sweetened—1 cup (255 g) .69
   frzn, unsweetened—1 cup (149 g) .40
   raw—1 cup (149 g) .21
sugar apple, raw—1 med (155 g) .91
tamarind, raw—1 cup (120 g) .84
tangerine, raw—1 med (84 g) .20
watermelon, raw—1 cup (160 g) .24

16. GRAIN FRACTIONS

amaranth—1 cup (195 g) 2.01
buckwheat flour, whole groat—1 cup (120 g) 1.24
carob (St. Johnsbread) flour—1 cup (103 g) .65
corn bran—⅓ cup (25 g) .58
corn flour, masa harina, enr—1 cup (114 g) .28
corn flour, whole grain—1 cup (117 g) .29
cornmeal, white, degermed, enr—1 cup (138 g) .46
cornmeal, whole grain—1 cup (122 g) .82
cracker meal—1 cup (115 g) .06
oat bran, raw—⅓ cup (31 g) .53
oats, reg/quick/inst, dry—⅓ cup (.95 oz) (27 g) .19
potato flour—½ cup (90 g) .23

rice bran—*1 oz (28 g)*	1.72
rice flour, brown—*1 cup (158 g)*	1.14
rice flour, white—*1 cup (163 g)*	.21
rye flour	
dark—*1 cup (128 g)*	3.30
light/—*1 cup (102 g)*	.57
medium—*1 cup (102 g)*	1.36
semolina, enr—*½ cup (84 g)*	.05
soy flour	
defatted—*1 cup (85 g)*	.17
full fat—*1 cup (85 g)*	1.66
low fat—*1 cup (88 g)*	.17
triticale flour, whole grain—*1 cup (130 g)*	2.48
wheat bran—*½ cup (30 g)*	.70
wheat flour, white	
all purpose, enr—*1 cup (125 g)*	.07
bread, enr—*1 cup (137 g)*	.07
cake, enr—*1 cup (109 g)*	.07
self-rising, enr—*1 cup (125 g)*	.07
wheat flour, whole wheat—*1 cup (120 g)*	1.48
wheat germ, toasted—*¼ cup (29 g)*	5.26

17. GRAIN PRODUCTS
17.1 Bagels

cinn raisin—*1 bagel (3½")* (71 g)	.12
oat bran—*1 bagel (3½")* (71 g)	.17
plain/onion/poppy seed/sesame seed—*1 bagel (3½")* *(71 g)*	.02

17.2 Biscuits

plain/buttermilk	
—*1 biscuit (2½" x 1") (35 g)*	1.01
from refrig dough (12 -28% fat)—*1 biscuit (2½" x 1") (27 g)*	.49
from refrig dough (2 -12% fat)—*1 biscuit (2¼" x 1") (21 g)*	.21
homemade—*1 biscuit (2½" x 1½") (60 g)*	1.45

17.3 Breads, Quick

banana, homemade w/ marg—*1 slice (4⅜" x 2½" x ½") (60 g)*	1.07
boston brown, cnd—*1 slice (3½" x 2") (45 g)*	.13
hush puppy, homemade—*1 hush puppy (2¼" x 1¼") (22 g)*	.23

17.4 Breads, Yeast & Unleavened

bread crumbs, dry, grated—*1 cup (108 g)*	.95
cracked wheat—*1 slice (25 g)*	.14
egg—*1 slice (5" x 3" x ½") (40 g)*	.31
french/vienna/sourdough—*1 med slice (4¾" x 4" x ½") (25 g)*	.06
indian (navajo) fry—*5" dia (90 g)*	1.67
irish soda, homemade—*1 slice (60 g)*	.63
italian—*1 slice (4½" x 3¼" x ¾") (30 g)*	.08
mixed grain/whole grain/7-grain—*1 slice (26 g)*	.16
oat bran—*1 slice (30 g)*	.12
oatmeal—*1 slice (27 g)*	.09
pita	
white—*1 pita (6½" dia) (60 g)*	.02
whole wheat—*1 pita (6½" dia) (64 g)*	.60
protein/gluten—*1 slice (19 g)*	.01
pumpernickel—*1 slice (5" x 4" x ⅜") (32 g)*	.16

raisin—*1 slice (26 g)*	.20
rice bran—*1 slice (27 g)*	.19
rye, american—*1 slice (5" x 4" x ½") (32 g)*	.18
wheat bran—*1 slice (36 g)*	.24
wheat germ—*1 slice (28 g)*	.24
wheat/wheat berry—*1 slice (25 g)*	.14
white—*1 slice (25 g)*	.07
whole wheat—*1 slice (28 g)*	.29
homemade—*1 slice (46 g)*	.65

17.5 Breadsticks

plain—*2 breadsticks (20 g)*	.29

17.6 Crackers & Croutons

cheese—*14 1" sq crackers (14 g)*	.14
cheese w/ peanut butter filling—*1 sandwich (7 g)*	.31
croutons, seasoned—*1 cup (40 g)*	.63
matzo—*1 matzo (1 oz) (28 g)*	.11
whole wheat—*1 matzo (1 oz) (28 g)*	.38
melba toast—*1 toast (5 g)*	.01
rye/pumpernickel)—*1 toast (19 g)*	.26
milk—*1 cracker (12 g)*	.28
round—*1 cracker (3 g)*	.13
rye, crispbread—*1 cracker (10 g)*	.14
rye wafers—*1 triple cracker (25 g)*	.50
saltines—*1 saltine (3 g)*	.05
fat-free, low-sodium—*3 crackers (15 g)*	.01
wheat—*7 crackers (14 g)*	.56
whole wheat—*1 sq cracker (4 g)*	.16

17.7 English Muffins

mixed grain/granola—*1 muffin (66 g)*	.76
plain—*1 muffin (57 g)*	.07
raisin cinn/apple cinn—*1 muffin (57 g)*	.10
wheat—*1 muffin (57 g)*	.18
whole wheat—*1 muffin (66 g)*	.46

17.8 French Toast

frzn—*1 slice (59 g)*	.25

17.9 Muffins

blueberry—*1 muffin (2½" x 2¼") (57 g)*	.60
corn—*1 muffin (2½" x 2¼") (57 g)*	.70
oat bran—*1 muffin (2½" x 2¼") (57 g)*	1.24
toaster muffin	
blueberry—*1 muffin (31 g)*	.24
wheat bran raisin—*1 muffin (34 g)*	.42

17.10 Pancakes

plain, frzn—*4" pancake (36 g)*	.27

17.11 Pasta

corn, ckd—*1 cup (140 g)*	.46
macaroni	
enr, ckd—*1 cup (140 g)*	.04
veg, ckd—*1 cup (134 g)*	.05
whole wheat, ckd—*1 cup (140 g)*	.14
noodles, chow mein—*1 cup (45 g)*	.07
noodles, egg	
& spinach, ckd—*1 cup (160 g)*	.08
enr, ckd—*1 cup (160 g)*	.08
spaghetti	
enr, ckd—*1 cup (140 g)*	.08

protein-fortified, ckd—*1 cup (140 g)*	.08
whole wheat, ckd—*1 cup (140 g)*	.07

17.12 Pastry Crust
cream puff shell, homemade—*1 shell (66 g)*	2.55
phyllo dough—*1 sheet (16½" x 12") (19 g)*	.19
pie crust, graham, homemade—*⅛ of 9" crust (30 g)*	1.23
pie crust, plain, frzn—*⅛ of 9" crust (16 g)*	.82
puff pastry, frzn—*1 pastry (40 g)*	.95
wonton wrappers—*1 wrapper (7" sq) (8 g)*	.01

17.13 Rice & Rice Dishes
brown rice, long grain, ckd—*1 cup (195 g)*	1.40
white rice	
glutinous, ckd—*1 cup (241 g)*	.07
long grain, enr, ckd—*1 cup (158 g)*	.08
long grain, inst, ckd—*1 cup (165 g)*	.08
long grain, parboiled, ckd—*1 cup (175 g)*	.09
wild rice, ckd—*1 cup (164 g)*	.38

17.14 Rolls
dinner—*1 roll (28 g)*	.22
egg—*1 roll (2½") (35 g)*	.25
homemade w/ lowfat milk—*1 roll (2½") (35 g)*	.39
french—*1 roll (38 g)*	.14
hamburger/hot dog—*1 roll (43 g)*	.20
hamburger/hotdog, mixed-grain—*1 roll (43 g)*	.31
hard/kaiser—*1 roll (3½" dia) (57 g)*	.10
oat bran—*1 roll (33 g)*	.15
popover, homemade w/ lowfat milk—*1 popover (2¾" x 4") (40 g)*	.43
rye—*1 roll (28 g)*	.16
wheat—*1 roll (28 g)*	.30
whole wheat—*1 roll (28 g)*	.35

17.15 Stuffing
bread, from mix—*½ cup (100 g)*	1.40
cornbread, from mix—*½ cup (100 g)*	1.39

17.16 Tortillas
corn—*1 med (6-7" dia) (25 g)*	.04
taco shell—*1 med (5" dia) (13 g)*	.39
flour—*7-8" dia (35 g)*	.44

17.17 Waffles
plain, frzn—*1 waffle (4" sq) (33 g)*	.27

19. INFANT, JUNIOR, & TODDLER FOODS
19.1 Baked Products
baby cookie—*.2 oz cookie (7 g)*	.03
baby pretzel—*.2 oz pretzel (6 g)*	.01
teething biscuit—*.4 oz biscuit (11 g)*	.05
zwieback toast—*.2 oz piece (7 g)*	.03

19.2 Cereals
barley, dry—*1 T (2.4 g)*	.01
cereal & egg yolks, jr—*1 jar (213 g)*	.58
cereal & egg yolks, str—*1 jar (128 g)*	.35
cereal, egg yolks, & bacon, str—*1 jar (128 g)*	.35
high protein, dry—*1 T (2.4 g)*	.01
high protein w/ apple & orange, dry—*1 T (2.4 g)*	.01
mixed, dry—*1 T (2.4 g)*	.01

mixed w/ applesce & bananas	
jr—*1 jar (170 g)*	.46
str—*1 jar (113 g)*	.44
mixed w/ bananas, dry—*1 T (2.4 g)*	.01
oatmeal, dry—*1 T (2.4 g)*	.01
oatmeal w/ applesce & bananas	
jr—*1 jar (170 g)*	.46
str—*1 jar (113 g)*	.43
oatmeal w/ bananas, dry—*1 T (2.4 g)*	.01
rice, dry—*1 T (2.4 g)*	.01
rice w/ applesce & bananas, str—*1 jar (113 g)*	.36
rice w/ bananas, dry—*1 T (2.4 g)*	.01
rice w/ mixed fruit, jr—*1 jar (170 g)*	.12

19.3 Desserts
cherry van pudding	
jr—*1 jar (170 g)*	.39
str—*1 jar (113 g)*	.26
dutch apple	
jr—*1 jar (170 g)*	.39
str—*1 jar (113 g)*	.68
fruit dessert	
jr—*1 jar (170 g)*	.39
str—*1 jar (113 g)*	.26
orange pudding, str—*1 jar (113 g)*	.26
peach cobbler	
jr—*1 jar (170 g)*	.39
str—*1 jar (113 g)*	.26
pineapple pudding, jr—*1 jar (170 g)*	.39
pineapple pudding, str—*1 jar (113 g)*	.26
van custard pudding	
jr—*1 jar (170 g)*	.39
str—*1 jar (113 g)*	.26

19.4 Dinners
beef & egg noodles	
jr—*1 jar (213 g)*	.85
str—*1 jar (128 g)*	.31
beef stew, toddler—*1 jar (177 g)*	.42
chicken & noodles	
jr—*1 jar (213 g)*	.51
str—*1 jar (128 g)*	.31
chicken soup, str—*1 jar (128 g)*	.31
chicken stew, toddler—*1 jar (170 g)*	.41
macaroni & cheese	
jr—*1 jar (213 g)*	.51
str—*1 jar (128 g)*	.31
macaroni, tomato, & beef	
jr—*1 jar (213 g)*	.51
str—*1 jar (128 g)*	.31
spaghetti, tomato, & beef, jr—*1 jar (213 g)*	.51
turkey & rice	
jr—*1 jar (213 g)*	.51
str—*1 jar (128 g)*	.31
veg & bacon	
jr—*1 jar (213 g)*	.51
str—*1 jar (128 g)*	.31
veg & beef	
jr—*1 jar (213 g)*	.51
str—*1 jar (128 g)*	.31

veg & chicken
  jr—1 jar (213 g) .51
  str—1 jar (128 g) .31
veg & ham
  jr—1 jar (213 g) .51
  str—1 jar (128 g) .31
veg & lamb
  jr—1 jar (213 g) .51
  str—1 jar (128 g) .31
veg & turkey
  jr—1 jar (213 g) .51
  str—1 jar (128 g) .31

19.5 Fruit Juices
apple, str—1 jar (130 g) .78
apple cherry, str—1 jar (130 g) .01
apple grape, str—1 jar (130 g) .78
apple peach, str—1 jar (130 g) .01
apple plum, str—1 jar (130 g) .01
apple prune, str—1 jar (130 g) .47
mixed fruit, str—1 jar (130 g) .26
orange—1 jar (130 g) .78
orange apple-banana—1 jar (130 g) .78
orange apricot—1 jar (130 g) .78
orange pineapple—1 jar (130 g) .78

19.6 Fruits
apple blueberry
  jr—1 jar (170 g) 1.02
  str—1 jar (113 g) .68
apple raspberry, jr—1 jar (170 g) 1.02
apple raspberry, str—1 jar (113 g) .68
applesauce
  jr—1 jar (213 g) 1.28
  str—1 jar (128 g) .77
applesauce & apricots
  jr—1 jar (170 g) 1.02
  str—1 jar (113 g) .68
applesauce & cherries
  jr—1 jar (170 g) 1.02
  str—1 jar (113 g) .68
applesauce & pineapple, jr—1 jar (213 g) 1.28
applesauce & pineapple, str—1 jar (128 g) .77
apricots w/ tapioca, jr—1 jar (170 g) 1.02
apricots w/ tapioca, str—1 jar (113 g) .68
bananas w/ pineapple & tapioca, jr—1 jar (170 g) 1.02
bananas w/ pineapple & tapioca, str—1 jar (113 g) .68
bananas w/ tapioca, jr—1 jar (170 g) 1.02
bananas w/ tapioca, str—1 jar (113 g) .68
mango w/ tapioca, str—1 jar (113 g) .68
peaches
  jr—1 jar (170 g) 1.02
  str—1 jar (113 g) .68
pears
  jr—1 jar (213 g) 1.28
  str—1 jar (128 g) .77
pears & pineapple
  jr—1 jar (213 g) 1.28
  str—1 jar (128 g) .77

plums w/ tapioca, jr—1 jar (170 g) 1.02
plums w/ tapioca, str—1 jar (135 g) .81
prunes w/ tapioca, jr—1 jar (170 g) 1.02
prunes w/ tapioca, str—1 jar (113 g) .68

19.7 Meats
beef
  jr—1 jar (99 g) .40
  str—1 jar (99 g) .40
chicken
  jr—1 jar (99 g) .40
  str—1 jar (99 g) .40
chicken sticks, jr—1 jar (71 g) .28
ham
  jr—1 jar (99 g) .40
  str—1 jar (99 g) .40
lamb
  jr—1 jar (99 g) .40
  str—1 jar (99 g) .40
meat sticks, jr—1 jar (71 g) .28
pork, str—1 jar (99 g) .40
turkey
  jr—1 jar (99 g) .40
  str—1 jar (99 g) .40
turkey sticks, jr—1 jar (71 g) .28
veal
  jr—1 jar (99 g) .40
  str—1 jar (99 g) .40

19.8 Vegetables
beets, str—1 jar (128 g) .67
carrots
  jr—1 jar (213 g) 1.11
  str—1 jar (128 g) .67
corn, creamed
  jr—1 jar (213 g) 1.11
  str—1 jar (128 g) .67
garden veg, str—1 jar (128 g) .67
green beans
  creamed, jr—1 jar (213 g) 1.11
  jr—1 jar (206 g) 1.07
  str—1 jar (128 g) .67
mixed veg
  jr—1 jar (213 g) 1.11
  str—1 jar (128 g) .67
peas
  creamed, str—1 jar (128 g) .67
  str—1 jar (128 g) .67
spinach, creamed, str—1 jar (128 g) .67
squash
  jr—1 jar (213 g) 1.11
  str—1 jar (128 g) .67
sweet potatoes
  jr—1 jar (170 g) .88
  str—1 jar (113 g) .59

20. MEAT ANALOGUE PRODUCTS
bacon, simulated meat product—1 strip (8 g) .55
sausage, simulated meat product—1 link (25 g) .53
sausage, simulated meat product—1 patty (38 g) .80

21. MEATS
21.1 Beef

breakfast strips, ckd—*3 slices (34 g)*	.07
brisket, whole	
sep lean & fat, braised, 0" fat trim—*3.5 oz (100 g)*	.19
sep lean & fat, braised, ¼" fat trim—*3.5 oz (100 g)*	.24
sep lean, braised, 0" fat trim—*3.5 oz (100 g)*	.14
sep lean, braised, ¼" fat trim—*3.5 oz (100 g)*	.14
chuck arm pot roast, sep lean	
braised, choice, ¼" fat trim—*3.5 oz (100 g)*	.14
braised, select, ¼" fat trim—*3.5 oz (100 g)*	.14
chuck arm pot roast, sep lean & fat	
braised, choice, ¼" fat trim—*3.5 oz (100 g)*	.23
braised, select, ¼" fat trim—*3.5 oz (100 g)*	.21
chuck blade roast, sep lean	
braised, choice, ¼" fat trim—*3.5 oz (100 g)*	.14
braised, select, ¼" fat trim—*3.5 oz (100 g)*	.14
chuck blade roast, sep lean & fat	
braised, choice, ¼" fat trim—*3.5 oz (100 g)*	.23
braised, select, ¼" fat trim—*3.5 oz (100 g)*	.23
corned beef, cured brisket, ckd—*3.5 oz (100 g)*	.16
flank, choice, sep lean, braised, 0" fat trim—*3.5 oz (100 g)*	.14
ground, extra lean	
broiled, med—*3.5 oz (100 g)*	.18
broiled, well done—*3.5 oz (100 g)*	.18
pan fried, med—*3.5 oz (100 g)*	.18
ground, lean	
broiled, med—*3.5 oz (100 g)*	.20
broiled, well done—*3.5 oz (100 g)*	.20
ground, regular	
broiled, med—*3.5 oz (100 g)*	.23
broiled, well done—*3.5 oz (100 g)*	.23
pan fried, med—*3.5 oz (100 g)*	.23
rib, shortribs, sep lean & fat, braised—*3.5 oz (100 g)*	.29
rib, shortribs, sep lean, braised—*3.5 oz (100 g)*	.14
rib, small end (ribs 10-12), sep lean, select, roasted, ¼" fat trim—*3.5 oz (100 g)*	.14
rib, whole (ribs 6-12), sep lean, choice, roasted, ¼" fat trim—*3.5 oz (100 g)*	.14
round, bottom, sep lean & fat, choice, braised, ¼" fat trim—*3.5 oz (100 g)*	.18
round, full cut	
sep lean & fat, choice, broiled, ¼" fat trim—*3.5 oz (100 g)*	.19
sep lean, choice, broiled, ¼" fat trim—*3.5 oz (100 g)*	.14
round, tip, sep lean	
roasted, choice, ¼" fat trim—*3.5 oz (100 g)*	.14
roasted, select, ¼" fat trim—*3.5 oz (100 g)*	.14
round, tip, sep lean & fat	
roasted, choice, ¼" fat trim—*3.5 oz (100 g)*	.18
roasted, select, ¼" fat trim—*3.5 oz (100 g)*	.17
round, top, sep lean, choice, pan fried, ¼" fat trim—*3.5 oz (100 g)*	.14
round, top, sep lean & fat, choice, pan fried, ¼" fat trim—*3.5 oz (100 g)*	.18
short loin porterhouse steak, ¼" fat trim, broiled, sep lean & fat—*3.5 oz (100 g)*	.22
short loin porterhouse steak, ¼" fat trim, broiled, sep lean—*3.5 oz (100 g)*	.14
short loin T-bone steak, ¼" fat trim, broiled, sep lean & fat—*3.5 oz (100 g)*	.21
short loin T-bone steak, ¼" fat trim, broiled, sep lean—*3.5 oz (100 g)*	.14
tenderloin, sep lean, prime, roasted, ¼" fat trim—*3.5 oz (100 g)*	.14
top sirloin, sep lean	
choice, broiled, ¼" fat trim—*3.5 oz (100 g)*	.14
choice, pan fried, ¼" fat trim—*3.5 oz (100 g)*	.14
select, broiled, ¼" fat trim—*3.5 oz (100 g)*	.14
top sirloin, sep lean & fat	
choice, broiled, ¼" fat trim—*3.5 oz (100 g)*	.21
choice, pan fried, ¼" fat trim—*3.5 oz (100 g)*	.21
select, broiled, ¼" fat trim—*3.5 oz (100 g)*	.21

21.2 Game Meats

bear, simmered—*3.5 oz (100 g)*	.26
beaver, roasted—*3.5 oz (100 g)*	.79
bison, roasted—*3.5 oz (100 g)*	.14
boar, wild, roasted—*3.5 oz (100 g)*	.26
caribou, roasted—*3.5 oz (100 g)*	.03
eel, ckd by dry heat—*3 oz (85 g)*	4.33
eel, raw—*3 oz (85 g)*	3.40
goat, roasted—*3.5 oz (100 g)*	.05
moose, roasted—*3.5 oz (100 g)*	.20
opossum, roasted—*3.5 oz (100 g)*	.79
rabbit, domesticated, stewed—*3.5 oz (100 g)*	.79
rabbit, wild, stewed—*3.5 oz (100 g)*	.79
raccoon, roasted—*3.5 oz (100 g)*	.79
squirrel, roasted—*3.5 oz (100 g)*	.75

21.3 Lamb

domestic, foreshank, choice, braised, sep lean & fat—*3.5 oz (100 g)*	.18
domestic, foreshank, choice, braised, sep lean—*3.5 oz (100 g)*	.20
domestic, ground, broiled—*3.5 oz (100 g)*	.25
domestic, leg	
shank half, choice, roasted, sep lean—*3.5 oz (100 g)*	.18
shank half, choice, roasted, sep lean & fat—*3.5 oz (100 g)*	.16
sirloin half, choice, roasted, sep lean—*3.5 oz (100 g)*	.17
sirloin half, choice, roasted, sep lean & fat—*3.5 oz (100 g)*	.13
whole (shank & sirloin), choice, roasted, sep lean—*3.5 oz (100 g)*	.18
whole (shank & sirloin), choice, roasted, sep lean & fat—*3.5 oz (100 g)*	.15
domestic, leg & shoulder, cubed for stew or kabob, sep lean, braised—*3.5 oz (100 g)*	.20
domestic, leg & shoulder, cubed for stew or kabob, sep lean, broiled—*3.5 oz (100 g)*	.20
domestic, loin	
sep lean & fat, choice, broiled—*3.5 oz (100 g)*	.13
sep lean & fat, choice, roasted—*3.5 oz (100 g)*	.11
sep lean, choice, broiled—*3.5 oz (100 g)*	.16
sep lean, choice, roasted—*3.5 oz (100 g)*	.16
domestic, rib	
sep lean & fat, choice, broiled—*3.5 oz (100 g)*	.12
sep lean & fat, choice, roasted—*3.5 oz (100 g)*	.10
sep lean, choice, broiled—*3.5 oz (100 g)*	.18
sep lean, choice, roasted—*3.5 oz (100 g)*	.15
domestic, shoulder, arm	
sep lean & fat, choice, braised—*3.5 oz (100 g)*	.15

sep lean & fat, choice, broiled—*3.5 oz (100 g)*	.13
sep lean & fat, choice, roasted—*3.5 oz (100 g)*	.14
sep lean, choice, braised—*3.5 oz (100 g)*	.18
sep lean, choice, broiled—*3.5 oz (100 g)*	.20
sep lean, choice, roasted—*3.5 oz (100 g)*	.17
domestic, shoulder, blade	
sep lean & fat, choice, braised—*3.5 oz (100 g)*	.16
sep lean & fat, choice, broiled—*3.5 oz (100 g)*	.15
sep lean & fat, choice, roasted—*3.5 oz (100 g)*	.14
sep lean, choice, braised—*3.5 oz (100 g)*	.20
sep lean, choice, broiled—*3.5 oz (100 g)*	.17
sep lean, choice, roasted—*3.5 oz (100 g)*	.17
domestic, shoulder, whole (arm & blade)	
sep lean & fat, choice, braised—*3.5 oz (100 g)*	.16
sep lean & fat, choice, broiled—*3.5 oz (100 g)*	.16
sep lean & fat, choice, roasted—*3.5 oz (100 g)*	.14
sep lean, choice, braised—*3.5 oz (100 g)*	.20
sep lean, choice, broiled—*3.5 oz (100 g)*	.20
sep lean, choice, roasted—*3.5 oz (100 g)*	.18
New Zealand, imported	
composite of trimmed retail cuts, sep lean & fat, ckd—*3.5 oz (100 g)*	.14
composite of trimmed retail cuts, sep lean, ckd—*3.5 oz (100 g)*	.19
foreshank, sep lean & fat, braised—*3.5 oz (100 g)*	.18
foreshank, sep lean, braised—*3.5 oz (100 g)*	.20
leg, whole (shank & sirloin), sep lean & fat, roasted—*3.5 oz (100 g)*	.15
leg, whole (shank & sirloin), sep lean, roasted—*3.5 oz (100 g)*	.18
loin, sep lean & fat, broiled—*3.5 oz (100 g)*	.13
loin, sep lean, broiled—*3.5 oz (100 g)*	.16
rib, sep lean & fat, roasted—*3.5 oz (100 g)*	.10
rib, sep lean, roasted—*3.5 oz (100 g)*	.15

21.4 Pork

arm picnic	
cured, sep lean & fat, roasted—*3.5 oz (100 g)*	.26
cured, sep lean, roasted—*3.5 oz (100 g)*	.26
lean, braised—*3.5 oz (100 g)*	.26
sep lean & fat, braised—*3.5 oz (100 g)*	.26
bacon, canadian style, grilled—*2 slices (47 g)*	.12
bacon, canadian style, unheated—*2 slices (57 g)*	.15
bacon, cured	
broiled/pan fried—*3 med slices (19 g)*	.10
broiled/pan fried—*4.48 oz (yield from 1 lb raw) (127 g)*	.69
raw—*3 med slices (68 g)*	.33
blade roll, cured, sep lean & fat, roasted—*3.5 oz (100 g)*	.26
boston blade (steaks/roasts)	
lean & fat, braised—*3.5 oz (100 g)*	.26
lean & fat, broiled—*3.5 oz (100 g)*	.26
lean & fat, roasted—*3.5 oz (100 g)*	.26
lean, braised—*3.5 oz (100 g)*	.26
lean, broiled—*3.5 oz (100 g)*	.26
lean, roasted—*3.5 oz (100 g)*	.26
breakfast strips, ckd—*3 slices (34 g)*	.10
center loin (loin chops/roasts), sep lean	
braised—*3.5 oz (100 g)*	.26
pan fried—*3.5 oz (100 g)*	.26
center loin (loin chops/roasts), sep lean & fat, pan fried—*3.5 oz (100 g)*	.26

center rib (rib chops/roasts), sep lean	
braised—*3.5 oz (100 g)*	.26
pan fried—*3.5 oz (100 g)*	.26
center rib (rib chops/roasts), sep lean & fat, pan fried—*3.5 oz (100 g)*	.26
ham, cured (fully cooked as purchased)	
lean (4-5% fat), cnd—*3.5 oz (100 g)*	.26
lean (4-5% fat), roasted—*3.5 oz (100 g)*	.26
patties, grilled—*1 patty (60 g)*	.16
reg (11-13% fat), cnd—*3.5 oz (100 g)*	.26
reg (11-13% fat), roasted—*3.5 oz (100 g)*	.26
whole, sep lean & fat, roasted—*3.5 oz (100 g)*	.26
whole, sep lean, roasted—*3.5 oz (100 g)*	.26
whole, sep lean, unheated—*3.5 oz (100 g)*	.26
leg, sep lean & fat, roasted—*3.5 oz (100 g)*	.26
leg, sep lean, roasted—*3.5 oz (100 g)*	.26
loin blade (chops & roasts), sep lean	
braised—*3.5 oz (100 g)*	.26
pan fried—*3.5 oz (100 g)*	.26
loin blade (chops & roasts), sep lean & fat	
braised—*3.5 oz (100 g)*	.26
pan fried—*3.5 oz (100 g)*	.26
loin, sep lean	
braised—*3.5 oz (100 g)*	.26
broiled—*3.5 oz (100 g)*	.26
roasted—*3.5 oz (100 g)*	.26
loin, sep lean & fat	
braised—*3.5 oz (100 g)*	.26
broiled—*3.5 oz (100 g)*	.26
roasted—*3.5 oz (100 g)*	.26
rump, sep lean & fat, roasted—*3.5 oz (100 g)*	.26
sausage	
fresh, ckd—*1 link (13 g)*	.02
fresh, ckd—*1 patty (27 g)*	.04
fresh, w/ beef, ckd—*1 link (13 g)*	.03
shank, sep lean, roasted—*3.5 oz (100 g)*	.26
shoulder, sep lean & fat, roasted—*3.5 oz (100 g)*	.26
shoulder, sep lean, roasted—*3.5 oz (100 g)*	.26
sirloin (chops & roasts), sep lean	
broiled—*3.5 oz (100 g)*	.26
roasted—*3.5 oz (100 g)*	.26
sirloin (chops & roasts), sep lean & fat	
braised—*3.5 oz (100 g)*	.26
broiled—*3.5 oz (100 g)*	.26
roasted—*3.5 oz (100 g)*	.26
tenderloin, sep lean & fat, roasted—*3.5 oz (100 g)*	.26
tenderloin, sep lean, roasted—*3.5 oz (100 g)*	.26
top loin (chops & roasts), sep lean	
broiled—*3.5 oz (100 g)*	.26
pan fried—*3.5 oz (100 g)*	.26
top loin (chops & roasts), sep lean & fat, pan fried—*3.5 oz (100 g)*	.26

21.5 Veal

ground, broiled—*3.5 oz (100 g)*	.15
leg & shoulder, cubed for stew, sep lean, braised—*3.5 oz (100 g)*	.45

leg (top round), sep lean	
braised—*3.5 oz (100 g)*	.50
pan fried, breaded—*3.5 oz (100 g)*	.53
pan fried, not breaded—*3.5 oz (100 g)*	.42
roasted—*3.5 oz (100 g)*	.55
leg (top round), sep lean & fat,	
braised—*3.5 oz (100 g)*	.49
pan fried, breaded—*3.5 oz (100 g)*	.53
pan fried, not breaded—*3.5 oz (100 g)*	.42
roasted—*3.5 oz (100 g)*	.49
loin	
sep lean & fat, braised—*3.5 oz (100 g)*	.40
sep lean & fat, roasted—*3.5 oz (100 g)*	.44
sep lean, braised—*3.5 oz (100 g)*	.42
sep lean, roasted—*3.5 oz (100 g)*	.49
rib	
sep lean & fat, braised—*3.5 oz (100 g)*	.34
sep lean & fat, roasted—*3.5 oz (100 g)*	.35
sep lean, braised—*3.5 oz (100 g)*	.35
sep lean, roasted—*3.5 oz (100 g)*	.36
shoulder, arm	
sep lean & fat, braised—*3.5 oz (100 g)*	.46
sep lean & fat, roasted—*3.5 oz (100 g)*	.46
sep lean, braised—*3.5 oz (100 g)*	.47
sep lean, roasted—*3.5 oz (100 g)*	.50
shoulder, blade	
sep lean & fat, braised—*3.5 oz (100 g)*	.44
sep lean & fat, roasted—*3.5 oz (100 g)*	.47
sep lean, braised—*3.5 oz (100 g)*	.45
sep lean, roasted—*3.5 oz (100 g)*	.50
shoulder, whole (arm & blade)	
sep lean & fat, braised—*3.5 oz (100 g)*	.42
sep lean & fat, roasted—*3.5 oz (100 g)*	.46
sep lean, braised—*3.5 oz (100 g)*	.45
sep lean, roasted—*3.5 oz (100 g)*	.50
sirloin	
sep lean & fat, braised—*3.5 oz (100 g)*	.41
sep lean & fat, roasted—*3.5 oz (100 g)*	.42
sep lean, braised—*3.5 oz (100 g)*	.44
sep lean, roasted—*3.5 oz (100 g)*	.46

21.6 Variety Cuts & Internal Organs

belly, pork, raw—*1 oz (28 g)*	.13
brain	
beef, simmered—*3.5 oz (100 g)*	2.30
lamb, braised—*3.5 oz (100 g)*	1.53
chitterlings, pork, simmered—*3.5 oz (100 g)*	.26
ears, pork, simmered—*1 ear (111 g)*	.29
feet, pork, cured, pickled—*3.5 oz (100 g)*	.26
feet, pork, simmered—*3.5 oz (100 g)*	.26
heart, beef, simmered—*3.5 oz (100 g)*	.72
jowl, pork, raw—*3.5 oz (100 g)*	.29
kidneys, beef, simmered—*3.5 oz (100 g)*	.18
liver	
beef, pan fried—*3.5 oz (100 g)*	.64
lamb, braised—*3.5 oz (100 g)*	.70
lamb, pan fried—*3.5 oz (100 g)*	.70
pork, braised—*3.5 oz (100 g)*	.47
veal, braised—*3.5 oz (100 g)*	.34
veal, pan fried—*3.5 oz (100 g)*	.50

lungs, pork, braised—*3.5 oz (100 g)*	.26
stomach, pork, raw—*3.5 oz (100 g)*	.29
tail, pork, simmered—*3.5 oz (100 g)*	.26
thymus, veal, braised—*3.5 oz (100 g)*	.77
tongue, beef, simmered—*3.5 oz (100 g)*	.35
tripe, beef, raw—*3.5 oz (100 g)*	.08

22. MEATS, LUNCHEON

beef, loaved lunch meat—*1 oz slice (28 g)*	.06
beef, thin sliced lunch meat—*5 slices (21 g)*	.04
blood sausage (blood pudding)—*1 slice (25 g)*	.06
bockwurst (pork, veal, milk), raw—*1 link (65 g)*	.09
bologna, beef—*1 slice (23 g)*	.04
bologna, beef & pork—*1 slice (23 g)*	.05
bologna, pork—*1 slice (23 g)*	.06
bologna, turkey—*1 slice (28 g)*	.15
bratwurst, pork, ckd—*1 link (85 g)*	.21
braunschweiger (pork liver sausage)—*1 slice (18 g)*	.06
chicken roll, light meat—*2 slices (57 g)*	.15
chorizo (pork & beef)—*1 link (60 g)*	.13
corned beef, loaf, jellied—*1 oz slice (28 g)*	.05
frankfurter	
beef—*1 frank (8 per 1 lb pkg) (57 g)*	.11
beef—*1 frank (10 per 1 lb pkg) (45 g)*	.09
beef & pork—*1 frank (57 g)*	.14
chicken—*1 frank (45 g)*	.10
turkey—*1 frank (45 g)*	.28
ham & cheese loaf/roll—*1 oz slice (28 g)*	.08
ham, cured	
chopped, cnd—*1 slice (21 g)*	.05
sliced, lean (5% fat)—*1 oz slice (28 g)*	.08
sliced, reg (11% fat)—*1 oz slice (28 g)*	.08
ham salad spread—*1 oz (28 g)*	.49
headcheese (pork)—*1 oz slice (28 g)*	.07
honey loaf (pork & beef)—*1 slice (28 g)*	.06
honey roll sausage (beef)—*1 slice (23 g)*	.03
italian sausage, pork, ckd—*1 link (67 g)*	.17
kielbasa/kolbassy (pork & beef w/ nfdm)—*1 slice (26 g)*	.06
knockwurst/knackwurst (pork & beef)—*1 slice (68 g)*	.39
lebanon bologna (beef)—*1 slice (23 g)*	.04
liver pate, chicken, cnd—*1 oz (28 g)*	.28
mortadella (beef & pork)—*1 slice (15 g)*	.03
New England Brand Sausage (pork & beef)—*1 slice (23 g)*	.05
old fashioned loaf (pork & beef), Dutch Brand—*1 oz slice (28 g)*	.06
olive loaf (pork)—*1 oz slice (28 g)*	.07
peppered loaf (pork & beef)—*1 slice (28 g)*	.06
pepperoni (pork & beef)—*1 slice (6 g)*	.01
pickle & pimento loaf (pork)—*1 oz slice (28 g)*	.07
pork & beef lunch meat—*1 slice (28 g)*	.06
pork lunch meat, cnd—*1 slice (21 g)*	.05
poultry (chicken/turkey) salad spread—*1 oz (28 g)*	.62
salami, beef—*1 slice (23 g)*	.04
salami, beef & pork—*1 slice (23 g)*	.05
salami, beerwurst, beef—*1 slice (23 g)*	.04
salami, dry/hard, pork—*1 slice (10 g)*	.03
salami, dry/hard, pork & beef—*1 slice (10 g)*	.03
salami, turkey, ckd—*2 slices (57 g)*	.32
smoked link sausage, pork—*1 link (68 g)*	.17

smoked link sausage, pork & beef—*1 link (68 g)*	.15
w/ american cheese—*1 link (43 g)*	.14
w/ flour & nfdm—*1 link (68 g)*	.15
thuringer (cervelat/summer sausage), beef & pork—*1 slice (23 g)*	.05
turkey breast—*1 slice (21 g)*	.02
turkey ham (cured thigh meat)—*2 slices (57 g)*	.36
turkey pastrami—*2 slices (57 g)*	.12
turkey roll, light & dark meat—*2 slices (57 g)*	.19
turkey roll, light meat—*2 slices (57 g)*	.08
vienna sausage, beef & pork, cnd—*1 sausage (16 g)*	.04

23. MILK, MILK BEVERAGES, MILK MIXES & YOGURT
23.1 Milk, Cow

buttermilk, cultured—*8 fl oz (245 g)*	.15
buttermilk, dry—*1 T (7 g)*	.03
condensed, sweetened, cnd—*1 fl oz (38 g)*	.08
evaporated	
nonfat, cnd—*1 fl oz (32 g)*	.00
whole, cnd—*1 fl oz (32 g)*	.06
whole, cnd—*4 fl oz (126 g)*	.23
lowfat	
1% fat—*8 fl oz (244 g)*	.10
1% fat w/ nfdm—*8 fl oz (245 g)*	.10
2% fat—*8 fl oz (244 g)*	.17
2% fat w/ nfdm—*8 fl oz (245 g)*	.17
nonfat—*8 fl oz (245 g)*	.10
dry—*¼ cup (30 g)*	.01
dry, Ca reduced—*1 oz (28 g)*	.00
dry, inst—*1⅓ cups (3.2 oz pkt) (91 g)*[18]	.02
w/ nfdm—*8 fl oz (245 g)*	.10
whole	
3.3% fat—*8 fl oz (244 g)*	.24
3.7% fat—*8 fl oz (244 g)*	.24
dry—*¼ cup (32 g)*	.35
low sodium—*8 fl oz (244 g)*	.24

23.2 Milk, Cow, Beverages

choc milk	
1% fat milk—*8 fl oz (250 g)*	.07
2% fat milk—*8 fl oz (250 g)*	.13
whole milk—*8 fl oz (250 g)*	.23
cocoa (hot choc), prep w/ 2% milk—*8 fl oz (250 g)*	.26
eggnog, nonalcoholic—*8 fl oz (254 g)*	.58

23.3 Milk Mixes

choc milk powder—*2-3 hp t (22 g)*	.09
malted—*.75 oz (3 hp t) (21 g)*	.08
malted w/ added nutrients, powder—*.75 oz (4-5 hp t) (21 g)*	.08
cocoa mix, powder—*1 oz pkt (3-4 hp t) (28 g)*	.04
aspartame sweetened—*.53 oz pkt (15 g)*	.06
eggnog mix, powder, nonalcoholic—*2 hp T (28 g)*	.02
malted milk powder—*.75 oz (3 hp t) (21 g)*	.08
w/ added nutrients—*¾ oz (4-5 hp t) (21 g)*	.08

23.4 Milk, Other

goat milk—*8 fl oz (244 g)*	.22
human milk—*1 fl oz (31 g)*	.28
soy milk—*8 fl oz (240 g)*	.02

23.5 Yogurt

lowfat	
coffee/van flavor w/ nfdm—*8 fl oz (227 g)*	.08
fruit flavor w/ nfdm—*8 fl oz (227 g)*	.07
plain w/ nfdm—*8 fl oz (227 g)*	.10
nonfat, plain w/ nfdm—*8 fl oz (227 g)*	.01
whole, plain—*8 fl oz (227 g)*	.20

24. NUTS, NUT PRODUCTS, & SEEDS

almond butter—*1 T (16 g)*	3.25
almond paste—*1 oz (28 g)*	5.74
almonds	
dried—*1 oz (24 nuts) (28 g)*	6.72
dry roasted—*1 oz (28 g)*	1.57
oil roasted, unblanched—*1 oz (22 nuts) (28 g)*	1.55
toasted, unblanched—*1 oz (28 g)*	4.54
brazilnuts, dried—*1 oz (8 med nuts) (28 g)*	2.15
butternuts, dried—*1 oz (28 g)*	.99
cashew butter—*1 oz (28 g)*	.44
cashews	
dry roasted—*1 oz (28 g)*	.16
oil roasted—*1 oz (18 med nuts) (28 g)*	.44
chestnuts, european	
dried—*1 oz (28 g)*	.34
roasted—*1 oz (3½ nuts) (28 g)*	.34
coconut	
dried—*1 oz (28 g)*	.38
dried, sweetened, flaked, cnd—*4 oz (114 g)*	.83
dried, sweetened, flaked, packaged—*1 cup (74 g)*	.54
dried, sweetened, shredded—*1 cup (93 g)*	1.26
raw—*1 piece (2" x 2" x ½") (45 g)*	.33
coconut cream, raw—*1 cup (240 g)*[19]	1.75
coconut cream, sweetened, cnd—*1 cup (296 g)*	2.16
coconut milk, raw—*1 cup (240 g)*[20]	1.75
cornuts—*1 oz (28 g)*	.29
cottonseed flour, partially defatted—*1 T (5 g)*	.01
cottonseed kernels, roasted—*1 T (10 g)*	.03
filberts (hazelnuts)	
dried—*1 oz (28 g)*	6.78
dry roasted—*1 oz (28 g)*	6.78
oil roasted—*1 oz (28 g)*	6.78
ginkgo nuts, cnd—*1 oz (14 med nuts) (28 g)*	.99
hickorynuts, dried—*1 oz (28 g)*	1.48
macadamia nuts	
dried—*1 oz (28 g)*	.12
oil roasted—*1 oz (10-12 nuts) (28 g)*	.12
mixed nuts	
dry roasted—*1 oz (28 g)*[21]	1.70
oil roasted—*1 oz (28 g)*[22]	1.70
w/o peanuts, oil roasted—*1 oz (28 g)*	1.70
peanut butter, creamy/smooth—*2 T (32 g)*	3.20
peanut flour, defatted—*1 oz (28 g)*	.01
peanuts	
boiled—*½ cup (32 g)*	1.01
dry roasted—*1 oz (28 g)*	2.10
oil roasted—*1 oz (28 g)*	2.10
unroasted—*1 oz (28 g)*	2.59
pecans	
dried—*1 oz (31 large nuts) (28 g)*	.88

dry roasted—*1 oz (28 g)*	.88
pine nuts, pignolia, dried—*1 oz (28 g)*	.99
pistachios	
dried—*1 oz (47 nuts) (28 g)*	1.48
dry roasted—*1 oz (28 g)*	1.48
pumpkin & squash seeds, dried—*1 oz (142 seeds) (28 g)*	.28
pumpkin & squash seeds, roasted—*1 oz (28 g)*	.28
sesame butter (tahini), from roasted & toasted kernels—*1 T (15 g)*	.34
sesame seeds	
kernels, dried—*1 T (8 g)*	.18
kernels, toasted—*1 oz (28 g)*	.64
whole, dried—*1 T (9 g)*	.20
soybean nuts, roasted—*½ cup (86 g)*	1.68
sunflower seed flour, partially defatted—*1 T (5 g)*	.08
sunflower seeds/kernels	
dry roasted—*1 oz (28 g)*	14.25
oil roasted—*1 oz (28 g)*	14.25
walnuts	
black, dried—*1 oz (28 g)*	.74
english/persian, dried—*1 oz (14 halves) (28 g)*	.74

25. POULTRY
25.1 Chicken, Broiler/Fryer

dark meat w/o skin	
roasted—*3.5 oz (100 g)*	.27
stewed—*3.5 oz (100 g)*	.27
light & dark meat w/o skin	
flour coated & fried—*3.5 oz (100 g)*	.46
roasted—*3.5 oz (100 g)*	.27
stewed—*3.5 oz (100 g)*	.27
light & dark meat w/ skin	
batter dipped & fried—*3.5 oz (100 g)*	1.24
flour coated & fried—*3.5 oz (100 g)*	.63
roasted—*3.5 oz (100 g)*	.27
stewed—*3.5 oz (100 g)*	.27
light meat w/o skin	
roasted—*3.5 oz (100 g)*	.27
stewed—*3.5 oz (100 g)*	.27
light meat w/ skin	
flour coated & fried—*3.5 oz (100 g)*	.57
stewed—*3.5 oz (100 g)*	.27

25.2 Chicken, Broiler/Fryer Parts

breast w/o skin	
flour coated & fried—*½ breast (86 g)*	.36
roasted—*½ breast (86 g)*	.23
stewed—*½ breast (95 g)*	.25
breast w/ skin	
roasted—*½ breast (98 g)*	.26
stewed—*½ breast (110 g)*	.29
drumstick w/o skin, roasted—*1 drumstick (44 g)*	.12
drumstick w/ skin	
roasted—*1 drumstick (52 g)*	.14
stewed—*1 drumstick (57 g)*	.15
leg w/o skin, stewed—*1 leg (101 g)*	.27
leg w/ skin	
roasted—*1 leg (114 g)*	.30
stewed—*1 leg (125 g)*	.33
neck w/o skin, simmered—*1 neck (18 g)*	.05

neck w/ skin, simmered—*1 neck (38 g)*	.10
thigh w/o skin, roasted—*1 thigh (52 g)*	.14
thigh w/ skin	
roasted—*1 thigh (62 g)*	.16
stewed—*1 thigh (68 g)*	.18
wing w/ skin	
roasted—*1 wing (34 g)*	.09
stewed—*1 wing (40 g)*	.11

25.3 Chicken, Capon, Roaster, & Stewer

roaster	
light & dark meat w/ skin, roasted—*3.5 oz (100 g)*	.27
light meat w/o skin, roasted—*3.5 oz (100 g)*	.27
stewer, light & dark meat w/ skin, stewed—*3.5 oz (100 g)*	.27

25.4 Chicken, Unspecified

chunks, w/ broth, cnd—*5 oz can (142 g)*	.30

25.5 Duck, Goose, & Other Poultry

cornish game hen, w/o skin, roasted—*½ bird (110 g)*	.29
cornish game hen, w/ skin, roasted—*½ bird (114 g)*	.30
duck w/o skin, roasted—*3.5 oz (100 g)*	.70
duck w/ skin, roasted—*3.5 oz (100 g)*	.70
goose w/ skin, roasted—*3.5 oz (100 g)*	1.74
pheasant w/ skin, raw—*3.5 oz (100 g)*	.30

25.6 Internal Organs

giblets	
chicken, simmered—*3.5 oz (100 g)*	1.30
turkey, simmered—*3.5 oz (100 g)*	1.46
gizzard	
chicken, simmered—*3.5 oz (100 g)*	1.19
turkey, simmered—*3.5 oz (100 g)*	.16
heart, turkey, simmered—*3.5 oz (100 g)*	.16
liver	
chicken, simmered—*3.5 oz (100 g)*	1.44
turkey, simmered—*3.5 oz (100 g)*	2.90

25.7 Turkey

dark meat w/o skin, roasted—*3.5 oz (100 g)*	.64
dark meat w/ skin, roasted—*3.5 oz (100 g)*	.61
ground, ckd—*3 oz patty (82 g)*	.28
light & dark meat	
seasoned, frzn, roasted—*3.5 oz (100 g)*	.38
w/o skin, roasted—*3.5 oz (100 g)*	.33
w/ skin, roasted—*3.5 oz (100 g)*	.34
light meat w/o skin, roasted—*3.5 oz (100 g)*	.09
light meat w/ skin, roasted—*3.5 oz (100 g)*	.13
patty, breaded & fried—*1 patty (94 g)*	2.25

26. SALAD DRESSINGS
26.1 Low & Reduced Calorie

french—*1 T (16 g)*	.19
italian—*1 T (15 g)*	.22
russian—*1 T (16 g)*	.12
thousand island—*1 T (15 g)*	.18

26.2 Regular

blue (bleu) cheese—*1 T (15 g)*	1.40
ckd, homemade—*1 T (16 g)*	.30
french—*1 T (16 g)*	1.35

italian—*1 T (15 g)*	1.55
mayonnaise type—*1 T (15 g)*	.60
russian—*1 T (15 g)*	1.53
thousand island—*1 T (16 g)*	.18
vinegar & oil, homemade—*1 T (16 g)*	1.41

27. SAUCES, CONDIMENTS, & GRAVIES
27.1 Gravies

beef, cnd—*½ can (117 g)*	.07
brown, mix—*amt to make 1 cup (22 g)*	.08
chicken, cnd—*½ can (119 g)*	.19
mushroom, mix—*amt to make 1 cup (21 g)*	.03
pork, mix—*amt to make 1 cup (21 g)*	.10
turkey, cnd—*½ can (149 g)*	.09

27.2 Sauces & Condiments

barbeque sce—*1 T (16 g)*	.18
catsup (ketchup)—*1 T (15 g)*	.22
hollandaise sce, mix w/ butterfat—*1 pkt (34 g)*	.31
spaghetti sce—*1 cup (249 g)*	3.12
tomato sce—*½ cup (122 g)*	1.71
w/ onions, green peppers, & celery—*½ cup (122 g)*	1.81
white sce	
med, homemade—*½ cup (125 g)*[23]	1.70
thick, homemade—*½ cup (125 g)*	2.35
thin, homemade—*½ cup (125 g)*	.89

28. SOUPS
28.1 Canned, Condensed

celery, crm of—*1 can (305 g)*	.46
cheese—*1 can (257 g)*	.41
chicken, crm of—*1 can (305 g)*	.40
mushroom, crm of—*1 can (305 g)*	3.17
tomato—*1 can (305 g)*	6.16

28.2 Canned, Condensed, Prepared With Milk

asparagus, crm of—*1 cup (248 g)*	.84
celery, crm of—*1 cup (248 g)*	.97
cheese—*1 cup (251 g)*	.25
chicken, crm of—*1 cup (248 g)*	.24
clam chowder, new england—*1 cup (248 g)*	.15
mushroom, crm of—*1 cup (248 g)*	1.34
onion, crm of—*1 cup (248 g)*	.07
pea, green—*1 cup (254 g)*	.18
potato, crm of—*1 cup (248 g)*[24]	.10
shrimp, crm of—*1 cup (248 g)*	.87
tomato—*1 cup (248 g)*	2.60

28.3 Canned, Condensed, Prepared With Water

asparagus, crm of—*1 cup (244 g)*	.66
bean w/ bacon—*1 cup (253 g)*	.08
beef noodle—*1 cup (244 g)*	.00
black bean—*1 cup (247 g)*	.07
celery, crm of—*1 cup (244 g)*	.90
chicken & dumplings—*1 cup (241 g)*	.14
chicken broth—*1 cup (244 g)*	.04
chicken, crm of—*1 cup (244 g)*	.20
chicken gumbo—*1 cup (244 g)*	.04
chicken noodle—*1 cup (241 g)*[25]	.07
chicken rice—*1 cup (241 g)*	.05
chicken veg—*1 cup (241 g)*	.08

chili beef—*1 cup (250 g)*	.18
clam chowder, manhattan style—*1 cup (244 g)*	.73
clam chowder, new england style—*1 cup (244 g)*	.08
minestrone—*1 cup (241 g)*	.07
mushroom, crm of—*1 cup (244 g)*	1.24
onion—*1 cup (241 g)*	.29
pea, green—*1 cup (250 g)*	.10
pepperpot—*1 cup (241 g)*	.09
potato, crm of—*1 cup (244 g)*[24]	.02
scotch broth—*1 cup (241 g)*	.07
shrimp, crm of—*1 cup (244 g)*	.83
tomato—*1 cup (244 g)*	2.49
tomato beef w/ noodle—*1 cup (244 g)*	.78
tomato rice—*1 cup (247 g)*	.79
turkey noodle—*1 cup (244 g)*	.06
turkey veg—*1 cup (241 g)*	.14
veg beef—*1 cup (244 g)*[26]	.32
veg vegetarian—*1 cup (241 g)*	.80
veg w/ beef broth—*1 cup (241 g)*	.31

28.4 Canned, Ready-To-Serve

beef, chunky—*1 cup (240 g)*	.17
chicken, chunky—*1 cup (251 g)*	.18
chicken noodle, chunky—*1 cup (240 g)*	.79
chicken rice, chunky—*1 cup (240 g)*	.09
clam chowder, manhattan style, chunky—*1 cup (240 g)*	.10
gazpacho—*1 cup (244 g)*	.46
minestrone, chunky—*1 cup (240 g)*	.72
split pea w/ ham, chunky—*1 cup (240 g)*	.14
veg, chunky—*1 cup (240 g)*	.60

28.5 Dehydrated

beef broth cube—*1 cube (6 g)*	.01
onion—*amt for 6 fl oz (7 g)*	.08
oxtail—*amt for 8 fl oz (17 g)*	.07
pea, green/split—*amt for 6 fl oz (28 g)*	.10
tomato—*amt for 8 fl oz (23 g)*	.69
tomato veg—*amt for 8 fl oz (39 g)*	1.20

28.6 Dehydrated, Reconstituted

bean w/ bacon—*1 cup (265 g)*	.26
beef broth/ bouillon—*1 cup (245 g)*	.02
beef noodle—*1 cup (251 g)*[27]	.03
chicken broth/bouillon—*1 cup (244 g)*[28]	.02
chicken, crm of—*1 cup (261 g)*	.15
chicken noodle—*1 cup (252 g)*[29]	.03
chicken rice—*1 cup (253 g)*	.04
leek—*1 cup (254 g)*	.15
mushroom—*1 cup (253 g)*	.63
onion—*1 cup (246 g)*[30]	.10
oxtail—*1 cup (253 g)*	.08
pea, green/split—*1 cup (271 g)*[31]	.14
tomato—*1 cup (265 g)*[32]	.85
tomato veg—*1 cup (253 g)*[33]	.81
veg, crm of—*1 cup (260 g)*	1.24

30. SPICES, HERBS, & FLAVORINGS

allspice, ground—*1 t (2.0 g)*	.02
anise seed—*1 t (2.0 g)*	.02
basil, ground—*1 t (1.0 g)*	.02
bay leaf, crumbled—*1 t (1.0 g)*	.02

caraway seed—*1 t (2.0 g)*	.05
celery seed—*1 t (2.0 g)*	.02
chervil, dried—*1 t (1.0 g)*	.02
chili powder—*1 t (3 g)*[34]	.03
chives	
freeze-dried—*¼ cup (0.8 g)*	.02
raw—*1 T chopped (3 g)*	.01
cinnamon, ground—*1 t (2.0 g)*	.00
cloves, ground—*1 t (2.0 g)*	.03
coriander (cilantro)	
leaf, dried—*1 t (1.0 g)*	.01
leaf, fresh—*¼ cup (4 g)*	.10
cumin seed—*1 t (2.0 g)*	.02
curry powder—*1 t (2.0 g)*	.01
dill seed—*1 t (2.0 g)*	.02
garlic powder—*1 t (3 g)*	.00
ginger, fresh—*¼ cup slices (24 g)*	.06
ginger, ground—*1 t (2.0 g)*	.01
mace, ground—*1 t (2.0 g)*	.05
marjoram, dried—*1 t (1.0 g)*	.02
mustard seed, yellow—*1 t (3 g)*	.07
nutmeg, ground—*1 t (2.0 g)*	.05
onion powder—*1 t (2.0 g)*	.00
oregano, ground—*1 t (2.0 g)*	.03
paprika—*1 t (2.0 g)*	.01
parsley, dried—*1 t (1.0 g)*	.02
parsley, fresh—*½ cup chopped (30 g)*	.54
pepper	
black—*1 t (2.0 g)*	.02
red/cayenne—*1 t (2.0 g)*	.10
white—*1 t (2.0 g)*	.05
poppy seed—*1 t (3 g)*	.08
poultry seasoning—*1 t (2.0 g)*[35]	.03
pumpkin pie spice—*1 t (2.0 g)*[36]	.02
saffron—*1 t (1.0 g)*	.02
sage, ground—*1 t (1.0 g)*	.02
tarragon, ground—*1 t (2.0 g)*	.03
thyme, ground—*1 t (1.0 g)*	.02
turmeric, ground—*1 t (2.0 g)*	.00

31. SPREADS

butter—*1 t (5 g)*	.08
—*1 T (15 g)*	.24
sweet (unsalted)—*1 t (5 g)*	.08
sweet (unsalted)—*1 T (15 g)*	.24
whipped—*1 t (4 g)*	.06
whipped—*1 T (11 g)*	.17
mayonnaise	
imitation, soybean—*1 T (15 g)*	.96
soybean—*1 T (14 g)*	1.65
sandwich spread—*1 T (15 g)*	1.05

32. SUGARS, SYRUPS, & OTHER SWEETENERS

apple butter—*1 T (18 g)*	.00

33. VEGETABLES, VEGETABLE PRODUCTS, & VEGETABLE SALADS

alfalfa sprouts, raw—*1 cup (33 g)*	
artichoke, boiled—*1 med (300 g)*	.57
artichoke, frzn, boiled—*2.8 oz (80 g)*	.15
arugula, raw—*½ cup (10 g)*	.04
asparagus	
boiled—*½ cup (6 spears) (90 g)*	.34
cnd—*½ cup (121 g)*	.52
frzn, boiled—*4 spears (60 g)*	.75
balsam pear, leafy tips, boiled—*1 cup (58 g)*	.29
balsam pear, pods, boiled—*½ cup pieces (62 g)*	.43
bamboo shoots	
cnd—*1 cup (131 g)*	.50
raw—*½ cup (76 g)*	.76
beans, vegetarian, cnd—*1 cup (254 g)*	1.35
beans w/ pork	
in sweet sce, cnd—*1 cup (253 g)*	1.37
in tomato sce, cnd—*1 cup (253 g)*	1.37
beet greens, boiled—*½ cup (72 g)*	.22
beets	
boiled—*½ cup slices (85 g)*	.26
cnd—*½ cup slices (85 g)*	.26
black turtle beans, boiled—*1 cup (185 g)*	.57
broadbeans, boiled—*1 cup (170 g)*	.15
broccoli	
boiled—*½ cup (78 g)*	1.32
chopped, frzn, boiled—*½ cup (92 g)*	1.52
raw—*½ cup chopped (44 g)*	.73
spears, frzn, boiled—*½ cup (92 g)*	.95
brussels sprouts	
boiled—*½ cup (78 g)*	.66
frzn, boiled—*½ cup (78 g)*	.45
burdock root, boiled—*1 cup (125 g)*	.24
cabbage, chinese	
pak-choi, boiled—*½ cup shredded (85 g)*	.10
pak-choi, raw—*½ cup shredded (35 g)*	.04
pe-tsai, raw—*½ cup shredded (38 g)*	.05
cabbage, green, boiled—*½ cup shredded (75 g)*	.08
cabbage, green, raw—*½ cup shredded (35 g)*	.04
cabbage, red, boiled—*½ cup shredded (75 g)*	.09
cabbage, red, raw—*½ cup shredded (35 g)*	.04
cabbage, savoy, raw—*½ cup shredded (35 g)*	.04
carrots	
boiled—*½ cup slices (78 g)*	.33
cnd—*½ cup slices (73 g)*	.31
frzn, boiled—*½ cup slices (73 g)*	.31
raw—*1 med (72 g)*	.33
cassava, raw—*3.5 oz (100 g)*	.19
cauliflower	
boiled—*½ cup pieces (62 g)*	.02
frzn, boiled—*½ cup pieces (90 g)*	.04
raw—*½ cup pieces (50 g)*	.02
cauliflower, green, raw—*½ cup pieces (50 g)*	.02
celeriac, raw—*3.5 oz (100 g)*	.36
celery, boiled—*½ cup diced (75 g)*	.27
celery, raw—*1 stalk (7.5" long) (40 g)*	.14
chard, swiss, boiled—*½ cup chopped (88 g)*	1.66
chickpeas (garbanzo beans)	
boiled—*1 cup (164 g)*	.57
hummus—*1 cup (246 g)*[37]	2.46
chicory greens, raw—*½ cup chopped (90 g)*	2.03
chrysanthemum, garland, boiled—*1 cup pieces (100 g)*	2.50
collards, boiled—*1 cup chopped (128 g)*	1.13
collards, frzn, boiled—*½ cup chopped (85 g)*	.42

corn, yellow

    boiled—½ cup (82 g)   .07

    cnd—½ cup (82 g)   .12

    cnd, vacuum pack—½ cup (105 g)   .09

    creamstyle, cnd—½ cup (82 g)   .07

    frzn, boiled—½ cup (82 g)   .07

cowpeas (blackeye peas)

    boiled, frzn—½ cup (85 g)   .33

    boiled, immature—1 cup (165 g)   .36

cucumber, raw—½ cup sl (⅙ cucumber) (52 g)   .04

dandelion greens, boiled—½ cup (52 g)   1.30

dandelion greens, raw—½ cup chopped (28 g)   .70

eggplant

    boiled—½ cup (48 g)   .01

    raw—½ cup (41 g)   .01

endive, raw—½ cup chopped (25 g)   .11

garden cress, boiled—½ cup (68 g)   .48

garden cress, raw—½ cup (25 g)   .17

garlic, raw—3 cloves (9 g)   .00

green beans (snap beans)[38]

    boiled—½ cup (62 g)[38]   .09

    cnd—½ cup (68 g)   .10

    frzn, boiled—½ cup (68 g)   .10

hominy, cnd, white—1 cup (160 g)   .08

horseradish tree, leafy tips, boiled—1 cup chopped (42 g)   .04

horseradish tree, pods, boiled—1 cup slices (118 g)   .11

jerusalem artichoke, raw—½ cup slices (75 g)   .14

jute, potherb, boiled—½ cup (43 g)   .30

kale, boiled—½ cup chopped (65 g)   .55

kale, frzn, boiled—½ cup chopped (65 g)   .12

kidney beans, red

    boiled—1 cup (177 g)   .14

    calif, boiled—1 cup (177 g)   .09

kohlrabi, boiled—½ cup slices (82 g)   1.37

lambsquarters, boiled—½ cup chopped (90 g)   1.21

leeks, raw—¼ cup chopped (26 g)   .24

lentils, boiled—1 cup (198 g)   .22

lettuce

    butterhead, raw—2 leaves (15 g)[39]   .07

    cos/romaine, raw—½ cup shredded (28 g)   .12

    iceberg, raw—1 leaf (20 g)[40]   .06

    looseleaf, raw—½ cup shredded (28 g)   .12

lima beans

    baby, frzn, boiled, immature—½ cup (90 g)   .58

    boiled—1 cup (188 g)   .34

    fordhook, frzn, boiled—½ cup (85 g)   .25

lotus root, boiled—10 slices (89 g)   .01

mixed veg

    cnd—½ cup (82 g)[41]   .49

    frzn—½ cup (91 g)[42]   .33

mung bean sprouts

    ckd—½ cup (62 g)   .01

    cnd—½ cup (62 g)   .01

    raw—½ cup (52 g)   .01

mung beans, boiled—1 cup (202 g)   1.03

mungo beans, boiled—1 cup (202 g)   .30

mushrooms

    boiled—½ cup pieces (78 g)   .09

    cnd—½ cup pieces (78 g)   .09

    raw—½ cup pieces (35 g)[43]   .04

    shitake, ckd—4 mushrooms (72 g)   .09

    shitake, dried—4 mushrooms (15 g)   .02

mustard greens, boiled—½ cup chopped (70 g)   1.41

mustard greens, frzn, boiled—½ cup chopped (75 g)   1.30

navy beans, cnd—1 cup (262 g)   1.00

nopales, ckd—1 cup (149 g)   .00

nopales, raw—1 cup (86 g)   .00

okra

    boiled—½ cup slices (80 g)   .55

    raw—½ cup slices (50 g)   .34

onions

    boiled—½ cup chopped (105 g)   .14

    boiled, frzn—3.5 oz (100 g)   .19

    cnd—½ cup chopped (112 g)   .08

    dehydrated flakes—¼ cup (14 g)   .19

    raw—½ cup chopped (80 g)   .10

onions, spring, raw—½ cup chopped (50 g)   .07

parsnips, boiled—½ cup slices (78 g)   .78

peas & carrots, frzn—½ cup (80 g)   .26

peas & onions, frzn, boiled—½ cup (90 g)   .14

peas, green

    cnd—½ cup (85 g)   .32

    frzn, boiled—½ cup (80 g)   .14

peas, split, boiled—1 cup (196 g)   .76

peppers, hot chili

    cnd—½ cup chopped (68 g)   .47

    raw—1 pepper (45 g)   .31

    red, sun-dried—10 peppers (5 g)   .16

peppers, jalapeno, cnd—½ cup chopped (68 g)   .47

peppers, sweet

    boiled—½ cup chopped (68 g)   .47

    freeze-dried—¼ cup (1.6 g)   .06

    raw—½ cup chopped (50 g)   .34

pimientos, cnd—1 T (12 g)   .08

pink beans, boiled—1 cup (169 g)   .66

pinto beans

    boiled—1 cup (171 g)   1.61

    cnd—1 cup (240 g)   2.26

poi—½ cup (120 g)   .22

pokeberry shoots, boiled—½ cup (82 g)   .70

potato, baked

    w/o skin—1 potato (156 g)   .06

    w/ skin—1 potato (202 g)   .10

potato, boiled w/o skin—1 potato (135 g)   .07

potato, cnd w/o skin—½ cup (90 g)   .05

potato puffs, frzn, prep—½ cup (62 g)   .03

potato, raw w/o skin—1 potato (112 g)   .07

potatoes, fried, fries, frzn, heated—10 pieces (50 g)   .10

potatoes, hash brown

    frzn, prep—½ cup (78 g)[44]   .15

    homemade—½ cup (78 g)[44]   .15

potatoes, mashed

    from flakes—½ cup (105 g)[45]   .73

    homemade—½ cup (105 g)[46]   .32

potatoes, scalloped, from mix—⅙ of 5.5 oz pkg (137 g)[47]   .21

pumpkin

    boiled—½ cup mashed (122 g)   1.29

    cnd—½ cup (122 g)   1.29

pumpkin flowers, boiled—½ cup (67 g)   .03

pumpkin leaves, boiled—1 cup (71 g)   .68

radicchio, raw—½ cup shredded (20 g)	.45	cnd, syrup pack—½ cup (98 g)	.27
radish, oriental, raw—½ cup slices (44 g)[48]	.00	taro, ckd—½ cup slices (66 g)	.29
radish, raw—10 radishes (45 g)	.00	tomatillos, raw—1 med (34 g)	.13
rhubarb, frzn, ckd, sweetened—½ cup (120 g)	.24	tomato, green, raw—1 tomato (123 g)	.47
rhubarb, frzn, raw—1 cup (137 g)	.27	tomato paste, cnd—½ cup (131 g)	5.63
rutabaga, boiled—½ cup cubes (85 g)	.13	tomato puree, cnd—1 cup (250 g)	6.30
salsify, boiled—½ cup slices (68 g)	.13	tomato, red, boiled—½ cup (120 g)	.46
sauerkraut, cnd—½ cup (118 g)	.12	tomato, red, raw—1 tomato (123 g)	.47
seaweed		tomato, red, stewed, cnd—½ cup (128 g)	.49
agar, dried—3.5 oz (100 g)	5.00	tomato, red, sun-dried—1 cup (54 g)	.01
agar, raw—3.5 oz (100 g)	.87	tomato, red, whole, peeled, cnd—½ cup (120 g)	.38
irishmoss, raw—3.5 oz (100 g)	.87	tree fern, ckd—½ cup chopped (71 g)	.53
kelp (kombu/tangle), raw—3.5 oz (100 g)	.87	turnip, boiled—½ cup cup (78 g)	.02
laver (nori), raw—3.5 oz (100 g)	1.00	turnip, frzn, boiled—3.5 oz (100 g)	.03
spirulina, dried—3.5 oz (100 g)	5.00	turnip greens	
wakame, raw—3.5 oz (100 g)	1.00	boiled—½ cup chopped (72 g)	1.24
shellie beans, cnd—½ cup (122 g)	.04	frzn, boiled—½ cup (82 g)	2.39
soybean product, miso—½ cup (138 g)	.01	raw—½ cup chopped (28 g)	.81
soybean product, natto—½ cup (88 g)	.01	turnip greens & turnips, frzn, boiled—3.5 oz (100 g)	.23
soybean product, tofu		water chestnuts, chinese	
fried—1 piece (13 g)	.00	cnd—½ cup slices (70 g)	.35
raw—½ cup (124 g)	.01	raw—½ cup slices (62 g)	.74
soybeans, green, boiled—½ cup (90 g)	.01	watercress, raw—½ cup chopped (17 g)	.17
soybeans, mature		waxgourd, boiled—½ cup cubes (87 g)[49]	.34
boiled—1 cup (172 g)	3.35	white beans, boiled—1 cup (179 g)	.39
sprouted, steamed—½ cup (47 g)	.00	yam, boiled/baked—½ cup cubes (68 g)	.11
spinach			
boiled—½ cup (90 g)	.86	**34. MISCELLANEOUS**	
cnd—½ cup (107 g)	1.39	baking choc, unsweetened—1 oz square (28 g)	.34
frzn, boiled—½ cup (95 g)	.91	baking powder, low sodium—1 t (5 g)	.00
raw—½ cup chopped (28 g)	.53	cocoa, unsweetened, dry powder—1 T (5 g)	.02
squash, summer, all varieties, boiled—½ cup slices (90 g)	.11	processed w/ alkali—1 T (5 g)	.02
squash, summer, all varieties, raw—½ cup slices (65 g)	.08	olives, pickled, ripe, manzanillo/mission	
squash, summer, crookneck		—1 small (3.2 g)	.10
boiled—½ cup slices (90 g)	.11	—1 med (4.1 g)	.12
cnd—½ cup slices (108 g)	.13	—1 large (4.4 g)	.13
frzn, boiled—½ cup slices (96 g)	.27	—1 extra large (6.0 g)	.18
squash, summer, scallop, boiled—½ cup slices (90 g)	.11	olives, pickled, ripe, sevillano/ascolano	
squash, summer, zucchini		—1 jumbo (8 g)	.25
boiled—½ cup slices (90 g)	.11	—1 colossal (11 g)	.34
frzn, boiled—½ cup slices (112 g)	.34	—1 super colossal (15 g)	.46
raw—½ cup slices (65 g)	.08	pickle relish, sweet—1 T (15 g)	.01
squash, winter,		pickles, dill—1 slice (6 g)	.01
all varieties, baked—½ cup cubes (102 g)	.12	—1 large (3¾" long x 1¼" dia) (65 g)	.10
all varieties, raw—½ cup cubes (58 g)	.07	pickles, sour—1 med (3¾" long, 1½" dia) (35 g)	.06
hubbard, boiled, mashed—½ cup (118 g)	.14	pickles, sweet—1 large (3" long, ¾" dia) (35 g)	.06
spaghetti, boiled/baked—½ cup (78 g)	.09	tomato powder—3.5 oz (100 g)	.51
succotash, frzn, boiled—½ cup (85 g)	.31	whey	
swamp cabbage, boiled—½ cup chopped (49 g)	.01	acid, dry—1 T (3 g)	.00
sweet potato		acid, fluid—1 cup (246 g)	.00
baked, frzn—½ cup cubes (88 g)	.24	sweet, dry—1 T (8 g)	.00
baked w/ skin—1 sweet potato (114 g)	.32	sweet, fluid—1 cup (246 g)	.02
boiled w/o skin—½ cup mashed (164 g)	.46	yeast	
cnd—1 cup pieces (200 g)	.50	bakers, active dry—1 pkg (¼ oz) (7 g)	.01
cnd, mashed—1 cup (255 g)	.69	bakers, compressed—1 cake (.6 oz) (17 g)	.01

1. Contains hydrogenated vegetable oil and soy protein; vegetable oils are usually soybean, cottonseed, safflower, or blends thereof.

2. Contains lauric acid oils and sodium caseinate; lauric oils include modified coconut oil, hydrogenated coconut oil, and/or palm kernel oil.

3. 28 wafers (168 g) = 1½ cups wafer crumbs.
4. Nine crackers (126 g) are equivalent to 1½ cups of cracker crumbs.
5. Includes apple, cinnamon, raisin, lemon, raspberry, and strawberry.
6. Includes almond, raisin nut, and cinnamon nut.
7. Includes apple, blueberry, cherry, and strawberry.
8. Includes apple, blueberry, cherry, lemon, peach, and strawberry.
9. Contains egg whites, corn oil, and nonfat dry milk.
10. Contains egg white, hydrogenated soybean oil, and soy protein.
11. Contains egg white solids, whole egg solids, sweet whey solids, nonfat dry milk, and soy protein.
12. 70% soybean phosphatide in 30% oil.
13. Prepared from walleye pollock, bread crumbs, egg, milk, and salt.
14. Dried black corinth grapes; not related to european black, red, or white currants.
15. Peaches, pears, grapes, pineapples, and cherries.
16. Peaches, pears, apricots, pineapples, and cherries.
17. Pineapples, papayas, pineapple juice, bananas, guava puree, cherries, and passion fruit juice.
18. Reconstitutes to 1 quart of fluid nonfat milk.
19. Liquid expressed from grated coconut.
20. Liquid expressed from grated coconut and coconut water.
21. Cashew, almonds, peanuts, filberts, and pecans.
22. Cashews, peanuts, brazilnuts, filberts, almonds, and pecans.
23. Contains lowfat milk, margarine, flour, and salt.
24. Includes vichyssoise.
25. Includes chicken alphabet, chicken noodle-o's, chicken with stars, and curly noodle with chicken.
26. Includes beef, beef vegetable, and barley and vegetable beef.
27. Includes beef and macaroni and beef flavored noodle.
28. Includes chicken consomme.
29. Includes chicken broth with noodles.
30. Includes french onion.
31. Includes pea with ham.
32. Includes cream of tomato.
33. Includes Italian vegetable and spring vegetable.
34. Contains red pepper, cumin, oregano, salt, and garlic powder.
35. Contains white pepper, sage, thyme, marjoram, savory, ginger, allspice, and nutmeg.
36. Contains cinnamon, ginger, nutmeg, allspice, and cloves.
37. Made with chickpeas, lemon juice, tahini, olive oil, and garlic.
38. Includes Italian, green, and yellow varieties.
39. Includes Boston and Bibb types.
40. Includes crisphead types.
41. Carrots, green peas, snap beans, and lima beans.
42. Corn, lima beans, snap beans, green peas, and carrots.
43. Agaricus bisporus.
44. Pan fried in vegetable oil.
45. Whole milk and butter added.
46. Whole milk and margarine added.
47. Water, whole milk, and butter added.
48. Includes daikon (Japanese) and Chinese radishes.
49. Chinese preserving melon.

Vitamin K (mcg)[1]

BEVERAGES	
coffee, dry—*1 rd t (1.8 g)*	0.7
tea, green, dry—*1 oz (28 g)*	199

EGGS, CHICKEN	
whole, fresh/frzn—*1 large (50 g)*	25
yolk, fresh—*yolk of 1 large egg (17 g)*	25

FATS & OILS	
Vegetable Oils	
coconut oil—*1 T (14 g)*	1
corn oil—*1 T (14 g)*	8
cottonseed oil—*1 T (14 g)*	0
olive oil—*1 T (14 g)*	0
palm oil—*1 T (14 g)*	1
peanut oil—*1 T (14 g)*	0
safflower oil, linolcic—*1 T (14 g)*	0
safflower oil, oleic—*1 T (14 g)*	0.4
soybean oil—*1 T (14 g)*	76

FRUITS	
apple, raw w/skin—*1 med (138 g)*	4
orange, raw—*1 med (131 g)*	7
strawberries, raw—*1 cup (149 g)*	21

GRAIN FRACTIONS	
oats, dry—*1 oz (28 g)*	18
wheat bran—*1 oz (28 g)*	23
wheat flour, whole wheat—*1 cup (120 g)*	36
wheat germ—*1 oz (28 g)*	10

INFANT FORMULAS[1]	
concentrate, reconstituted—*1 fl oz (30 g)*	4
powder, reconstituted—*1 fl oz (30 g)*	5
ready-to-feed—*1 fl oz (30 g)*	4

MEATS	
Beef	
ground, regular, raw—*3.5 oz (100 g)*	4

Variety Cuts	
heart, beef, raw—*3.5 oz (100 g)*	0
kidneys, beef, raw—*3.5 oz (100 g)*	0
liver, raw	
beef—*3.5 oz (100 g)*	104
chicken—*3.5 oz (100 g)*	80
lamb—*3.5 oz (100 g)*	0
pigeon—*3.5 oz (100 g)*	0
pork—*3.5 oz (100 oz)*	88
rabbit—*3.5 oz (100 g)*	35
turkey—*3.5 oz (100 g)*	0
veal—*3.5 oz (100 g)*	27

MILK, COW	
skim—*8 fl oz (245 g)*	10
skim, dry—*¼ cup (30 g)*	3
whole, 3.7% fat—*8 fl oz (244 g)*	10

MILK, OTHER	
human—*1 fl oz (30 g)*	0.6

SWEETENERS

honey—*1 T (21 g)*	5

VEGETABLES

asparagus spears	16
frzn, boiled—*4 spears (60 g)*	16
raw—*4 spears (58 g)*	23
beet, raw—*½ cup (68 g)*	3
broccoli	
raw—*½ cup chopped (44 g)*	58
frzn—*½ cup (92 g)*	63
cabbage, green, raw—*½ cup shredded (35 g)*	52
carrot, raw—*1 med (72 g)*	9
cauliflower, raw—*½ cup pieces (50 g)*	96
chickpeas (garbanzo beans)	
mature seeds, dry—*1 oz (28 g)*	74
sprouted seeds, raw—*1 oz (28 g)*	13
corn, yellow, raw—*1 oz (28 g)*	2
cucumber, raw—*½ cup slices (⅙ cucumber) (52 g)*	3
green beans (snap beans)	
frzn, boiled—*½ cup (68 g)*	22
raw—*1 oz (28 g)*	8
lentils	
mature seeds, dry—*1 oz (28 g)*	62
sprouted seeds, raw—*1 oz (28 g)*	11
lettuce, iceberg, raw—*1 leaf (20 g)*	22

mung beans	
mature seeds, dry—*1 oz (28 g)*	48
sprouted seeds, raw—*½ cup (52 g)*	17
mushrooms, raw—*½ cup pieces (35 g)*	3
nettle leaves, raw—*1 oz (28 g)*	104
peas	
mature, seeds, dry—*1 oz (28 g)*	23
sprouted seeds, raw—*1 oz (28 g)*	7
potato	
raw—*1 potato (112 g)*	18
baked—*1 potato (156 g)*	6
seaweed	
dulse, dried—*3.5 oz (100 g)*	1700
rockweed, dried—*3.5 oz (100 g)*	1700
seagrass—*3.5 oz (100 g)*	246
sea lettuce—*3.5 oz (100 g)*	68
soybeans, mature, raw—*1 oz (28 g)*	53
spinach	
raw—*½ cup chopped (28 g)*	74
frzn—*½ cup (95 g)*	131
tomato	
green, raw—*1 tomato (123 g)*	58
red, raw—*1 tomato (123 g)*	28
turnip greens, raw—*½ cup chopped (28 g)*	182
watercress, raw—*½ cup chopped (17 g)*	10

1. Vitamin K values are listed in Section 18 of the main table for specific infant formulas and in Section 29 for special dietary foods.

SOURCE: Weihrauch JL. Provisional table on the vitamin K content of foods. USDA. Washington DC. June 1986.

For additional information see:
Booth SL, JAT Pennington, JA Sadowski. Dihypero-phylloquinone. Primary food sources and estimated dietary intakes in the American diet. *Lipids* 11:715–720, 1996.

Booth SL, JAP Pennington, JA Sadowski. Food sources and dietary intakes of phylloquinone in the American diet: Data from the FDA Total Diet Study. *J Am Diet Assoc* 96:149–154, 1996.

Booth SL, JA Sadowski, JAT Pennington. The phylloquinone (vitamin K) contents of foods in the USFDA Total Diet Study. *J Am Food Chem* 43:1574–1579, 1995.

Sources Consulted for the Seventeenth Edition (reference code):

1. Adams CF. *Nutritive Value of American Foods in Common Units.* Agriculture Handbook No 456. USDA. November 1975 (456).

2. Booth SL, JAT Pennington, JA Sadowski. Dihydro-phylloquinone: Primary food sources and estimated dietary intakes in the American diet. *Lipids* 11:715–720, 1996.

3. Booth SL, JAT Pennington, JA Sadowski. Food sources and dietary intakes of phylloquinone in the American diet: Data from the FDA Total Diet Study. *J Am Diet Assoc* 96:149–154, 1996.

4. Booth SL, JA Sadowski, JAT Pennington. The phylloquinone (vitamin K) content of foods in the USFDA Total Diet Study. *J Agr Food Chem* 43:1574–1579, 1995.

5. *Code of Federal Regulations, Food and Drugs,* Title 21, Part 101.9, Nutrition labeling of food. The Office of the Federal Register, National Archives and Records Administration. Washington DC. US Government Printing Office. 1996.

6. Gebhardt SE, JM Holden. Provisional table on the selenium content of foods. USDA Human Nutrition Information Service, HNIS/PT-109, December 1992.

7. Grand AN, LN Bell. Caffeine content of fountain and private-label store brand carbonated beverages. *J Am Diet Assoc* 97:179–182, 1997.

8. King I, MT Childs, C Dorsett, JG Ostrander, ER Monsen. Shellfish: proximate composition, minerals, fatty acids, and sterols. *J Am Diet Assoc* 90:677, 1990 (L).

9. Matthews RH, PR Pehrsson. Provisional table on the sugar content of selected foods. USDA Human Nutrition Information Service. HNIS/PT-105, October 1986. [Matthews RD, PR Pehrsson. Sugar Content of Selected Foods: Individual and Total Sugars. Home Economics Research Report No. 48. USDA. Washington DC. October 1986.]

10. Nettleton JA, WH Allen Jr, LV Klatt, WMN Ratnayake, RG Ackman. Nutrients and chemical residues in one-to-two-pound Mississippi farm-raised channel catfish (Ictalurus punctatus). *J Food Sci* 55:954 1990 (L).

11. Pennington JAT, SA Schoen, GD Salmon, B Young, RD Johnson, RW Marts. Composition of core foods of the US food supply, 1982–1991. III. Copper, manganese, selenium, and iodine. *J Food Comp Anal* 8:171–217, 1995.

12. Perry CA, J Dwyer, JA Gelfand, RR Couris, WW McCloskey. Health effects of salicylates in foods and drugs. *Nutr Rev* 54:225–240, 1996.

13. Randolph S, M Snyder. *The Seafood List.* US Government Printing Office. Washington DC. 1993.

14. Ranhotra GS, JA Gelroth. Stability of enrichment vitamins in bread and cookies. *Cereal Chem* 63:401–403, 1986 (L).

15. Ranhotra GS, JA Gelroth, K Astroth. Total and soluble fiber in selected bakery and other cereal products. *Cereal Chem* 67:499–501, 1990 (L).

16. *Recommended Dietary Allowances,* 10th edition. National Academy Press, Washington DC. 1989.

17. Swain AR, SP Dutton, AS Truswell. Salicylates in foods. *J Am Diet Assoc* 85:950–960, 1985.

18. USDA. Nutrient Data Base for Standard Reference, Release 11 (SR11). http://www.nal.usda.gov/fnic/foodcomp. Nutrient Data Laboratory, USDA, Riverdale, MD. 1996 (801 through 821).

19. USDA, US DHHS. *Nutrition and Your Health: Dietary Guidelines for Americans,* fourth edition. Home and Garden Bulletin No. 232. 1995.

20. Weihrauch JL. Provisional table on the vitamin K content of foods. USDA. Washington DC. June 1986.

21. 92 food companies and trade associations (I).

Latin Names for Plants and Animals Used as Foods or Food Ingredients

FOOD NAME	LATIN NAME	FOOD NAME	LATIN NAME
abalone, mixed species	*Haliotis* spp.	burbot	*Lota lota*
acerola	*Malpighia punicifolia*	burdock	*Arctium lappa*
acorn	*Quercus* spp.	butterbur (fuki)	*Petasites japonicus*
adzuki beans	*Vigna angularis*	butterfish	*Peprilus triacanthus*
alewife	*Alosa pseudoharengus*	butternut	*Juglans cinerea*
alfalfa	*Medicago sativa*	cabbage (green, red, savoy)	*Brassica oleracea* (Capitata group)
allspice	*Pimenta dioica*		
almond	*Prunus dulcis*	cabbage, chinese	*Brassica rapa* (Chinensis group)
amaranth	*Amaranthus* spp.	cacao	*Theobroma cacao*
anchovy, european	*Engraulis encrasicholus*	cantaloupe	*Cucumis melo*
anise seed	*Pimpinella anisum*	carambola	*Averrhoa carambola*
apple	*Malus sylvestris*	caraway seed	*Carum carvi*
apricot	*Prunus armeniaca*	cardamom	*Elettaria cardamomum*
arrowhead	*Sagittaria latifolia*	cardoon	*Cynara cardunculus*
artichoke (globe, french)	*Cynara scolymus*	caribou	*Rangifer caribou*
asparagus	*Asparagus officinalis*	carissa	*Carissa macrocarpa*
avocado (california, florida)	*Persea americana*	carob	*Ceratonia siliqua*
babassu	*Orbignya barbosiana*	carp	*Cyprinus carpio*
banana	*Musa X paradisiaca*	carrot	*Daucus carota*
balsam pear	*Momordica charantia*	casaba melon	*Cucumis melo*
bamboo	*Phyllostachys* spp.	cashews	*Anacardium occidentale*
barley	*Hordeum vulgare*	cassava	*Manihot esculenta*
barracuda	*Sphyraena* spp.	catfish, channel	*Ictalurus punctatus*
basil	*Ocimum basilicum*	cauliflower	*Brassica oleracea* (Botrytis group)
bass, freshwater, mixed species	Percichthyidae and Centrarchidae	celeriac	*Apium graveolens*
		celery	*Apium graveolens*
bass, striped	*Morone saxatilis*	celtuce	*Lactuca sativa*
bay leaf	*Laurus nobilis*	chayote	*Sechium edule*
beans (black, cranberry, navy, pink, pinto, snap, white, yellow)	*Phaseolus vulgaris*	cherimoya	*Annona cherimola*
		chervil	*Anthriscus cerefolium*
		cherries, sour	*Prunus cerasus*
bear	*Ursus* spp.	cherries, sweet	*Prunus avium*
beaver	*Castor canadensis*	chestnuts, chinese	*Castanea mollissima*
beechnut	*Fagus* spp.	chestnuts, european	*Castanea sativa*
beet	*Beta vulgaris*	chestnuts, japanese	*Castanea crenata*
bison	*Bison americanus*	chia seeds	*Salvia* spp.
black beans	*Phaseolus vulgaris*	chicken	*Gallus domesticus*
blackberries	*Rubus* spp.	chickpeas	*Cicer arientinum*
blueberries	*Vaccinium* spp.	chicory	*Cichorium intybus*
bluefish	*Pomatomus saltatrix*	chicory, witloof	*Cichorium intybus*
boar, wild	*Sus scofa*	chives	*Allium scheonoprasum*
bonito	*Sarda* spp.	chrysanthemum	*Chrysanthemum coronarium*
borage	*Borago officinalis*	cinnamon	*Cinnamonum verum* (*C. zeylanicum*) and *Cinnamomum aromaticum* (*C. cassia*)
boysenberries	*Rubus ursinus* var. (loganobaccus)		
brazilnuts	*Bertholletia excelsa*	cisco	*Coregonus artedil*
breadfruit	*Artocapus altilis*	clam, mixed species	*Lamellibranchia* spp.
breadnuttree	*Brosimum alicastrum*	cloves	*Syzgium aromaticum*
broadbeans	*Vicia faba*	coconut	*Cocos nucifera*
broccoli	*Brassica oleracea* (Botrytis group)	cod, Atlantic	*Gadus mortha*
brussels sprouts	*Brassica oleracea* (Gemmifera group)	cod, Pacific	*Gadus macrocephalus*
		collards	*Brassica oleracea* (Acephala group)
buckwheat	*Fagopyrum esculentum*		
buffalo, water	*Babalus bubalis*	coriander	*Coriandrum sativum*
bullhead	*Ameiurus* spp.	corn (field, sweet)	*Zea mays mays*

FOOD NAME	LATIN NAME	FOOD NAME	LATIN NAME
cornsalad	*Valeriznella locusta*	grouper, mixed species	*Epinephelus* spp.
cottonseed	*Gossypium* spp.	guava	*Psidium guajava*
cow	*Bos taurus*	guava, strawberry	*Psidium cattlejanum*
cowpeas, catjang	*Vigna unguiculata cylindrica*	guinea (bird)	*Numida meleagris*
cowpeas	*Vigna unguiculata unguiculata*	haddock	*Melanogrammus aeglefinus*
crabapples	*Malus* spp.	halibut, atlantic and pacific	*Hippoglossus hippoglossus* and
crab, alaska king	*Paralithodes camtschatica*		*Hippoglossus stenolepis*
crab, blue	*Callinectes sapidus*	halibut, greenland	*Reinhardtius hippoglossoides*
crab, dungeness	*Cancer magister*	hazelnut (filbert)	*Corylus avellana*
crab, queen	*Chionoectes opilio*	herring, atlantic	*Clupea harengus harengus*
cranberry beans	*Phaseolus vulgaris*	herring, pacific	*Clupea harengus pallasi*
cranberries	*Vaccinium macrocarpon*	hickorynut	*Carya* spp.
crayfish, mixed species	*Astacus* spp., *Orconectes* spp.,	honeydew melon	*Cucumis melo*
	Procambarus spp.	horse	*Equus caballus*
croaker, atlantic	*Micropogonias undulatus*	horseradish	*Moringa oleifera*
cucumber	*Cucumis sativus*	hyacinth beans	*Dolichos purpureus, Dolichos*
cumin seed	*Cuminum cyminum*		*lablab*
currants (european black, red,		jackfruit	*Artocarpus heterophyllus*
and white)	*Ribes nigrum*	java plum	*Syzygium cumini*
currants, zante	*Vitis vinifera*	jerusalem artichoke	*Helianthus tuberosus*
cusk	*Brosme brosme*	jew's ear (pepeao)	*Auricularia polytricha*
custard apple	*Annona reticulata*	jujube	*Ziziphus jujuba*
cuttlefish, mixed species	*Sepiidae*	jute, potherb	*Corchorus olitorius*
dandelion	*Taraxacum officinale*	kale	*Brassica oleracea* (Acephala
dates	*Phoenix dactylifera*		group)
deer	*Odocoileus* spp.	kale, scotch	*Brassica napus* (Pabularia group)
dill weed	*Anethum graveolens*	kidney beans	*Phaseolus vulgaris*
dock	*Rumex* spp.	kingfish	*Menticirrhus* spp.
dolphinfish	*Coryphaena hippurus*	kiwifruit	*Actinidia chinensis*
drum, freshwater	*Aplodinotus grunniens*	kohlrabi	*Brassica oleracea* (Gongylodes
duck, domesticated	*Anas platyrhynchos*		group)
duck, wild	*Anas boschas*	kumquat	*Fortunella* spp.
eel, mixed species	*Anguilla* spp.	lamb	*Ovis aries*
eggplant	*Solanum malongena*	lambsquarters	*Chenopodium album*
elderberries	*Sambucus* spp.	leek	*Allium ampeloprasum*
elk	*Cervus alces*	lemon	*Citrus limon*
endive	*Cichorium endivia*	lentils	*Lens culinaris*
eppaw	*Perideridia oregana*	lettuce (butterhead, cos/	
fennel	*Foeniculum vulgare*	romaine, iceberg, looseleaf)	*Latuca sativa*
fenugreek	*Trigonella foenum-graecum*	lima beans (large, baby)	*Phaseolus lunatus*
fig	*Ficus carica*	lime	*Citrus aurantiifolia*
flatfish	Bothidae and Pleuronectidae	ling	*Molva molva*
frog	*Rana* spp.	lingcod	*Ophiodon elongatus*
garden cress	*Lepidium sativum*	linseed	*Linum usitatissimum*
garlic	*Allium sativum*	lobster, northern	*Homarus americanus*
ginger	*Zingiber officinale*	loganberries	*Rubus ursinus* var. (loganbaccus)
ginkgo	*Ginkgo biloba*	longan	*Dimocarpus longan*
goat	*Capra* spp.	loquat	*Eriobotrya japonica*
goose	*Anser anser*	lotus	*Nelumbo nucifera*
gooseberries	*Ribes* spp.	lupins	*Lupinus albus*
gourd, dishcloth (towel-gourd)	*Luffa aegyptiaca*	lychee	*Litchi chinensis*
gourd, white-flowered		macadamia nut	*Macadamia integrifolia* or
(calabash gourd)	*Lagenaria siceraria*		*Macadmaia tetraphylla*
grapefruit (pink, red, and		mace	*Myristica fragrans*
white)	*Citrus paradisi*	mackerel, atlantic	*Scomber scombrus*
grapes, american	*Vitis* spp.	mackerel, jack	*Trachurus symmetricus*
grapes, european	*Vitis vinifera*	mackerel, king	*Scombermorus cavalla*
great northern beans	*Phaseolus vulgaris*	mackerel, pacific & jack	*Scomber* spp. *Trachurus* spp.
groundcherries	*Physalis* spp.	mackerel, spanish	*Scombermorus maculatus*

FOOD NAME	LATIN NAME	FOOD NAME	LATIN NAME
mammy apple	*Mammea americana*	perch, mixed species	*Morone americana* and *Perca flavenscens*
mango	*Mangifera indica*	persimmon, japanese	*Diospyros kaki*
marjoram	*Majorana hortensis*	persimmon, native	*Diospyros virginiana*
menhaden	*brevoortia* spp.	pheasant	*Phasianus colchicus*
milkfish	*Chanos chanos*	pig	*Sus scrofa*
millet	*Panicum miliaceum*	pigeonpeas	*Cajanus cajan*
monkfish	*Lophius piscatorius*	pike, northern	*Esox lucius*
moose	*Alces americana*	pike/pickerel	*Esox niger*
mothbeans	*Vigna aconitifolia*	pike, walleye	*Stizostedion vitreum vitreum*
mountain yam, hawaii	*Dioscorea pentaphylla*		
mulberries	*Morus nigra*	pilinuts, canarytree	*Canarium ovatum*
mullet, striped	*Mugil cephalus*	pineapple	*Ananas comosus*
mung beans	*Vigna radiata*	pine nut, pignolia	*Pinus pinea*
mungo beans	*Vigna mungo*	pine nut, pinyon	*Pinus edulis*
mushrooms	*Agaricus bisporus*	pink beans	*Phaseolus vulgaris*
muskrat	*Ondatra zibethica*	pinto beans	*Phaseolus vulgaris*
mussel, blue	*Mytilus edulis*	pistachio nut	*Pistacia vera*
mustard greens	*Brassica juncea*	pitanga	*Eugenia uniflora*
mustardseed	*Sinapis alba*	plantain	*Musa X paradisiaca*
mustard spinach (tendergreen)	*Brassica rapa* (Perviridis group)	plum	*Prunus* spp.
navy beans	*Phaseolus vulgaris*	pokeberry	*Phytolacca americana*
nectarine	*Prunus persica* var. (nectarina)	pollock, atlantic	*Pollachius virens*
new zealand spinach	*Tetragonia tetragonioides*	pollock, walleye	*Theragra chalcogramma*
nopales	*Nopalea cochenillifera*	potato	*Solanum tuberosum*
nutmeg	*Myristica fragrans*	pomegranate	*Punica granatum*
oat	*Avena sativa*	pompano, florida	*Trachinotus carolinus*
ocean perch, atlantic	*Sebastes marinus*	poppyseed	*Papaver somniferum*
octopus	*Octopus vulgaris*	pout, ocean	*Macrozoarces americanus*
oheloberries	*Vaccinium reticulatum*	pricklypear	*Opuntia* spp.
okra	*Abelmoschus esculentus*	prune	*Prunus domestica*
olive	*Olea europaea*	pummelo	*Citrus grandis*
onion	*Allium cepa*	pumpkin	*Cucurbita* spp.
onion, spring	*Allium cepa* or *Allium fistulosum*	purslane	*Portulaca oleracea*
onion, welsh	*Allium fistulosum*	quail	*Bonsas umbellus, Colinus virginianus*
opossum	*Didelphis virginiana*		
orange (navel, valencia)	*Citrus sinensis*	quinoa	*Chenopodium quinia*
orange roughy	*Hopolostethus atlanticus*	quince	*Cydonia oblonga*
oregano	*Origanum vulgare*	rabbit, domesticated	*Oryetolagus euniculus*
oyster, eastern	*Crassostrea virginica*	rabbit, wild	*Sylvilagus floridanus*
oyster, pacific	*Crassostrea gigas*	raccoon	*Procyon lotor*
palm	*Elaeis guineensis*	radish	*Raphanus sativus*
papaya	*Carica papaya*	radish, oriental (daikon, chinese)	*Raphanus sativus* (Longipinratus group)
paprika	*Capsicum annuum*		
parsley	*Petroselinum crispum*	radish, white icicle	*Raphanus sativus*
parsnip	*Pastinaca sativa*	raisins	*Vitis vinifera*
passion fruit, purple	*Passiflora edulis*	rapeseed	*Brassica* spp.
passion fruit, yellow	*Passiflora laurifolia*	raspberries	*Rubus* spp.
peach	*Prunus persica*	rice	*Oryza sativa*
peanuts (spanish, valencia, virginia)	*Arachis hypogaea*	rhubarb	*Rheum rhabarbaum*
		reindeer	*Rangifer* spp.
pear	*Pyrus communis*	rockfish, pacific, mixed species	*Sebastes* spp.
peas (green, split)	*Pisum sativum*		
pecan	*Carya illinoensis*	rose apple	*Syzgium jambos*
pepeao	*Auricularia polytricha*	roselle	*Hibiscus sabdariffa*
pepper, black and white	*Piper nigrum*	rosemary	*Rosmarinus officinalis*
pepper, red/cayenne	*Capsicum frutescens* and *Capsicum annuum*	rutabaga	*Brassica napus* (Napobrassica group)
peppers, hot chili (green, red)	*Capsicum frutescens*	rye	*Secale cereale*
peppers, sweet (green, red)	*Capsicum annuum*	sablefish	*Anoplopoma fimbria*

FOOD NAME	LATIN NAME	FOOD NAME	LATIN NAME
safflower	*Carthamus tinctorius*	squirrel	*Sciurus vulgaris*
saffron	*Crocus sativus*	strawberries	*Fragaria X ananassa*
sage	*Salvia officinalis*	sturgeon, mixed species	*Acipenser* spp.
salmon, atlantic	*Salmo salar*	sucker, white	*Catostomus commersoni*
salmon, chinook	*Oncorhynchus tshawytscha*	sugar apple	*Annona squamosa*
salmon, chum	*Oncorhynchus keta*	sunfish, pumpkinseed	*Lepomis gibbosus*
salmon, coho	*Oncorhynchus kisutch*	sunflower	*Helianthus annuus*
salmon, pink	*Oncorhynchus gorbuscha*	swamp cabbage	*Ipomoea aquatic*
salmon, sockeye	*Oncorhynchus nerka*	sweetpotato	*Ipomoea batatas*
salsify	*Tragopogon porrifolius*	swiss chard	*Beta vulgaris* (Cicla group)
sapodilla	*Manikara zapota*	swordfish	*Xiphias gladius*
sapote	*Pouteria sapota*	tamarind	*Tamarindus indica*
sardine, atlantic	*Clupea harengus harengus*	tangerine	*Citrus reticulata*
sardine, pacific	*Sardinops* spp.	taro	*Colocasia esculenta*
savory	*Satureja hortensis*	tarragon	*Artemisia dracunculus*
scallop, mixed species	*Pectinidae*	tautog	*Tautoga onitis*
scup	*Stenotomus chrysops*	tea	*Camellia sinensis*
sea bass, mixed species	*Centropristes striata* and *Lateolabrax japonicus*	thyme	*Thymus vulgaris*
		tilefish	*Lopholatilus chamaeleonticeps*
seatrout, mixed species	*Cynoscion* spp.	tomato	*Lycopersicon esculentum*
seaweed, agar	*Eucheuma* spp.	tomcod	*Microgadus* spp.
seaweed, irishmoss	*Chandrus crispus*	triticale	*X Triticosecale rimpaui*
seaweed, kelp (kombu, tangle)	*Laminaria* spp.	trout, dolly varden	*Salvelinus malma*
seaweed, laver (nori)	*Porphyra laciniata*	trout, mixed species	*Salmonidae*
seaweed, spirulina	*Spirulina* spp.	trout, rainbow	*Salmo gairdneri*
seaweed, wakame	*Undaria* spp.	tuna, bluefin	*Thunnus thynnus*
sesame	*Sesamum indicum*	tuna, skipjack	*Euthynnus pelamis*
sesbania	*Sesbania* spp.	tuna, yellowfin	*Thunnus albacares*
shad, american	*Alosa sapidissima*	turbot, European	*Scophthalmus maximus*
shallot	*Allium ascalonicum*	turkey	*Meleagris gallopavo*
shark, mixed species	*Squaliformes*	tumeric	*Curcuma domestics*
sheanut	*Butyrospermum paradoxum*	turnip	*Brassica rapa* (Rapifera group)
sheep	*Ovis aries*	turtle	*Chelonia mydas*
sheepshead	*Archosargus probatocephalus*	vinespinach	*Basella alba*
shrimp, mixed species	Penaeidae and Pandalidae	walnut (english, persian)	*Juglans regia*
sisymbrium seeds	*Sisymbrium* spp.	waterchestnuts, chinese	*Eleocharis dulcis*
skate	*Raja* spp.	watercress	*Nasturtium officiale*
smelt, rainbow	*Osmerus mordax*	watermelon	*Citrullus lanatus*
snap beans (italian, green, yellow)	*Phaseolus vulgaris*	waxgourd (Chinese preserving melon)	*Benincasa hispida*
snapper, mixed species	*Lutjanidae*	whale	*Balaena glacialis, balaenoptera borealis, balaenoptera physalus, balaenoptera musculus, Physeter catadon*
sorghum	*Sorghum* spp.		
Soursop	*Annona muricata*		
soybeans	*Glycine max*	wheat, durum	*Triticum durum*
spinach	*Spinacia oleracea*	wheat (hard red spring, hard red winter, soft white)	*Triticum aestivum*
spiny lobster, mixed species	*Jasus* spp. and *Panulirus* spp.	whelk	*Buccinidae*
spot	*Leiostomus xanthuras*	whitefish, mixed species	*Coregonus* spp.
squash, summer (crookneck, straightneck, scallop, zucchini)	*Cucurbita* spp.	white perch	*Morone americana*
		whiting, mixed species	*Gadidae*
squash, winter	*Cucurbita* spp.	wild rice	*Zizania* spp.
squash, winter, acorn	*Cucurbita maxima*	winged beans	*Psophocarpus tetragonolobus*
squash, winter, butternut	*Cucurbita moschata*	wolffish, atlantic	*Anarhichas lupus*
squash, winter, hubbard	*Cucurbita maxima*	yam	*Diosorea* spp.
squash, winter, spaghetti	*Cucurbita* spp.	yambean	*Pachyrhizus* spp.
squid, mixed species	Loligoidae and Ommastrephidae	yardlong bean	*Vigna unguiculata sesquipedalis*
		yellowtail	*Seriola* spp.

Food Name Synonyms and Cross References[1]

SYNONYM	FOOD NAME USED IN THE 17TH EDITION (PREFERRED TERM IN INDEX)	SYNONYM	FOOD NAME USED IN THE 17TH EDITION (PREFERRED TERM IN INDEX)
albacore	tuna, white	cervelat	thuringer (cervelat/summer sausage)
ahi	tuna, yellowfin	cheesefurter	smoked link sausage with cheese
aku	tuna, skipjack	cheese smokie	smoked link sausage with cheese
apple, mammy	mammy apple	chicken frank	frankfurter, chicken
artichoke, Jerusalem	jerusalem artichoke	chicken frankfurter	frankfurter, chicken
Asian pears	pears, asian	chicken hot dog	frankfurter, chicken
asparagus beans	yardlong beans	chicken spread	meat spread, chicken
aubergine	eggplant	Chinese cabbage	cabbage, chinese
awa	milkfish	Chinese gooseberries	kiwifruit
baked beans	beans, baked	Chinese parsley	coriander
Barbados cherry	acerola	Chinese pears	pears, asian
basella	vinespinach	Chinese preserving melon	waxgourd
bean of malacca	cashews	chinook salmon	salmon, chinook
beans, black	black beans	chocolate, dark	chocolate, sweet, dark
beans, black turtle soup	black turtle soup beans	chocolate, milk	milk chocolate
beans, cranberry	cranberry beans	chub	cisco, smoked [fish]
beans, French	french beans	Colorado pinyon pines	pine nuts/pinyon nuts
beans, goa	winged beans	confectioner's sugar	powdered sugar
beans, great northern	great northern beans	cotto salami	salami
beans, hyacinth	hyacinth beans	creamnuts	brazilnuts
beans, kidney	kidney beans	creme caramel	pudding, flan/creme caramel
beans, lima	lima beans	crowder peas	cowpeas
beans, mung	mung beans	custard	pudding, custard
beans, navy	navy beans	dark chocolate	chocolate, sweet, dark
beans, pink	pink beans	daikon	radishes, oriental
beans, pinto	pinto beans	dasheen	taro
beans, Roman	cranberry beans	dishcloth gourd	gourd, dishcloth
beans, shellie	shellie beans	custard	pudding, custard
beans, white, small	white beans, small	dogfish	shark, mixed species
beans, winged	winged beans	Dutch brand loaf	old fashioned loaf [luncheon meat]
beans, yardlong	yardlong beans		
beans, yellow	yellow beans	egg custard	pudding, egg custard
beer salami	salami, beerwurst	endive, Belgian	chicory, witloof
beerwurst	salami, beerwurst	European chestnuts	chestnuts, european
bengal gram	chickpeas	falafel	broadbeans, falafel
benniseeds	sesame seeds	farina	Cream of Wheat
bittergourd	balsam pear pods	fava beans	broadbeans
bittermelon	balsam pear pods	flan	pudding, flan/creme caramel
black-eyed peas	cowpeas	flounder	flatfish
blood pudding	blood sausage	fondant, chocolate coated	chocolate coated fondant
bologna, Lebanon	lebanon bologna	frosting	icing
breakfast sausage	beef sausage; pork sausage	fuyu	soybean product, tofu, salted and fermented
brinjal	eggplant		
brown and serve sausage	beef sausage; pork sausage	garbanzo beans	chickpeas
bullock's heart	custard apple	garland, chrysanthemum	chrysanthemum, garland
bushnuts	macadamia nuts	gingelly	sesame seeds
butterbeans	lima beans	goa beans	winged beans
cabbage salad	coleslaw	golden gram	chickpeas
cabbage, swamp	swamp cabbage	goobers/goober peas	peanuts
cacao butter	cocoa oil	goosefish	monkfish
cannellini beans	kidney beans	granadilla	passion fruit
cape gooseberries	groundcherries	green gram	mung beans
carambola	starfruit		
catfish, ocean	wolffish		

SYNONYM	FOOD NAME USED IN THE 17TH EDITION (PREFERRED TERM IN INDEX)	SYNONYM	FOOD NAME USED IN THE 17TH EDITION (PREFERRED TERM IN INDEX)
Greenland halibut	halibut, greenland	paranuts	brazilnuts
groundnuts	peanuts	pastrami, turkey	turkey pastrami
gumbo	okra	pate	liver pate
hake	whiting (fish)	pear pods, balsam	balsam pear pods
ham and cheese roll	ham and cheese loaf/roll	pectin	fruit pectin
ham and cheese spread	meat spread, ham and cheese	penoche	fudge, brown sugar with nuts
ham salad spread	meat spread, ham salad	pepeao	jew's ear
hazelnuts	filberts	pe-tsai	cabbage, chinese
heart nuts	cashew nuts	pickerel	pike (fish)
herring, Atlantic, canned	sardine, atlantic, canned	pigeon	squab
herring, lake	cisco	pignolis	pine nuts/pignolia
highball	bourbon and water	pignolias	pine nuts/pignolia
hot chocolate	cocoa	pignons	pine nuts/pignolia
hot dog	frankfurter	pinocchios	pine nuts/pinyon
hummus	chickpeas, hummus	pinyons	pine nuts/pinyon
ice pop	ice, water	pistache nuts	pistachio nuts
Italian chestnuts	chestnuts, european	pistachia nuts	pistachio nuts
Italian stone pines	pine nuts/pignolia	poha	groundcherries
jack	mackerel, pacific and jack, mixed species	pollock, Alaskan	pollock, walleye
jambolan	java plum	popsicle	ice, water
Japanese pears	pears, asian	porgy	scup (fish)
Kool Pop	ice, water	pork liver sausage	braunschweiger
kolbassy	kielbasa/kolbassy	poultry salad sandwich spread	meat spread, poultry salad
koyadefu	soybean product, tofu, dried	Queensland nuts	macadamia nuts
knackwurst	knockwurst/knackwurst	Raisinets	chocolate coated raisins, Raisinets
lard	pork fat	rajah	skate (fish)
litchis	lychees	ramons	breadnuttree seeds
liver sausage, braunschweiger	braunschweiger	redfish	ocean perch, atlantic
liverwurst	liver sausage	red gram	pigeon peas
long walnuts	butternuts	Reese's Peanut Butter Cups	Peanut Butter Cups, Reese's
lox	salmon, chinook, smoked	Roman beans	cranberry beans
mahimahi	dolphinfish	roughy, orange	orange roughy
mahongany apples	cashews	salmon, keta	salmon, chum
mamey	mammy apple	salmon, red	salmon, sockeye
mammee apple	mammy apple	sausage, blood	blood sausage
manioc	cassava	sausage, liver	liver sausage
marmalade plum	sapotes	scrod	cod, atlantic
matai	waterchestnuts, chinese	semi-sweet chocolate	chocolate, semi-sweet
miso	soybean product, miso	shoyu	soy sauce made with soy and wheat
mousse	pudding, chocolate mousse	sim-sim	sesame seeds
muffins, english	english muffins	skipjack tuna	tuna, skipjack
muskmelon	cantaloupe	snail, sea	whelk, unspecified
natal plum	carissa	snap beans	green beans/wax beans
natto	soybean product, natto	snow peas	peas, edible-podded
Nestle Crunch	Crunch, Nestle	sole	flatfish
nutmeg butter	nutmeg oil	sorbet	ice, water
nut pines	pine nuts/pinyon	sorrel	dock
ocean catfish	wolffish	southern peas	cowpeas
okara	tofu, okara	soybean curd	soybean product, tofu
oranges, Mandarin	mandarin oranges	Special Dark chocolate	chocolate, sweet, Special Dark
Oriental radishes	radishes, oriental	spinach, mustard	mustard spinach
oysterplant	salsify	sprouts	specific mature seeds, sprouted (eg, alfalfa seeds, sprouted)
Pacific mackerel	mackerel, pacific & jack, mixed species		
pak-choi	cabbage, chinese	squash seeds	pumpkin and squash seeds

SYNONYM	FOOD NAME USED IN THE 17TH EDITION (PREFERRED TERM IN INDEX)	SYNONYM	FOOD NAME USED IN THE 17TH EDITION (PREFERRED TERM IN INDEX)
St. John's bread	carob	tofu	soybean product, tofu
stone pines	pine nuts/pignolia	towelgourd	gourd, dishcloth
string beans	green beans	turbot, domestic species	halibut, greenland
sugar snap peas	snow peas	turtle soup black beans	black turtle soup beans
summer sausage	thuringer (cervelat/summer sausage)	vegetable oyster	salsify
		vegetables, mixed	mixed vegetables
sunchoke	jerusalem artichoke	walleye	pollock, walleye
surinam cherry	pitanga	water convulvolus	swamp cabbage
swedes	turnips	wiener	frankfurter
sweet chestnuts	chestnuts, european	West Indian cherry	acerola
sweetsop	sugar apple	witloof chicory	chicory, witloof
Swiss chard	chard, swiss	yambean	jicama
tamari	soy sauce made with soy	yellowfin tuna	tuna, yellowfin
tangerines, canned	mandarin oranges	yokan	adzuki beans with sugar
tempeh	soybean product, tempeh	York Peppermint Patty	Peppermint Patty, York
tendergreen	mustard spinach		

1. To assist users in locating foods in the database. The list provides a food name synonym or a food name with a different arrangement of terms in the left-hand column and the "preferred" food name (ie, the name used in the 17th edition). The preferred food name is listed in the index with the page numbers of its location.

Bibliography for Food Composition Data
(January 1992-February 1997)

Agbor-Egbe T, S Treche. Evaluation of the chemical composition of **Cameroonian yam germplasm.** *J Food Comp Anal* 8:274–284, 1995.

Akinwunmi I, LD Thompson, CB Ramsey. Marbling, fat trim and doneness effects on sensory attributes, cooking loss and composition of cooked **beef steaks.** *J Food Sci* 58:242–244, 1993.

Akoh CC, Nwosu CV. **Fatty acid** composition of **melon seed oil lipids and phospholipids.** *J Am Oil Chem Soc* 69:314–316, 1992.

Almazan AM. Antinutritional factors in **sweet potato greens.** *J Food Comp Anal* 8:363–368, 1995.

Almazan AM, F Begum. **Nutrients and antinutrients** in **peanut greens.** *J Food Comp Anal* 9:375–383, 1997.

Anderson RA, NA Bryden, KY Patterson, C Veillon, MB Andon, PB Moser-Veillon. **Breast milk chromium** and its association with chromium intake, chromium excretion, and serum chromium. *Am J Clin Nutr* 57:519–523, 1993.

Appel BR, JK Kahlon, J Ferguson, AJ Quattrone, SA Book. Potential **lead** exposures from lead crystal decanters. *Am J Pub Health* 82:1671–1673, 1992.

Arbuckle LD, MJ MacKinnon, SM Innis. **Formula 18:2 (n-6) and 18:3 (n-3)** content and ratio influence long-chain polyunsaturated fatty acids in the developing piglet liver and central nervous system. *J Nutr* 124:289–298, 1994 (**fatty acid** composition of **soy milk and formulas**).

Badiani A, P Anfossi, L Fioretini, PP Gatta, M Manfredini, N Nanni, S Stipa, B Tolomelli. Nutritional composition of cultured **sturgeon** (Acipenser spp). *J Food Comp Anal* 9:171–190, 1996.

Barclay MNI, A MacPherson, J Dixon. **Selenium** content of selected **baby food cereals and juices.** *J Food Comp Anal* 8:307–318, 1995.

Barshick, S-A, SM Smith, MV Buchanan, MR Guerin. Determination of **benzene** content in food using a novel blender purge and trap GC/MS method. *J Food Comp Anal* 8:244–257, 1995.

Behrens WA, R Madere. **Ascorbic acid, isoascorbic acid, dehydroascorbic acid, and dehydroisoascorbic acid** in selected food products. *J Food Comp Anal* 7:158–170, 1995.

Belinshy DL, HV Kuhnlein, F Yeboah, AF Penn, HM Chan. Composition of **fish** consumed by the James Bay Cree. *J Food Comp Anal* 9:148–162, 1996.

Blank ML, EA Cress, ZL Smith, F Snyder. **Meats and fish** consumed in the American diet contain substantial amounts of **ether-linked phospholipids.** *J Nutr* 122:1656–1662, 1992.

Booth S, R Bressani, T Johns. Nutrient content of selected indigenous **leafy vegetables** consumed by the Kekchi people of Alta Verapaz, **Guatemala.** *J Food Comp Anal* 5:25–34, 1992.

Booth SL, JAT Pennington, JA Sadowski. **Dihydro-phylloquinone:** Primary food sources and estimated dietary intakes in the American diet. *Lipids* 11:715–720, 1996.

Booth SL, JAT Pennington, JA Sadowski. Food sources and dietary intakes of **phylloquinone** in the American diet: Data from the FDA Total Diet Study. *J Am Diet Assoc* 96:149–154, 1996.

Booth SL, JA Sadowski, JAT Pennington. The **phylloquinone (vitamin K)** content of foods in the USFDA Total Diet Study. *J Agr Food Chem* 43:1574–1579, 1995.

Brandolini V, E Menziani, D Mazzotta, P Cabras, B Tosi, G Lodi. Use of AMD-HPTLC for **carbohydrate** monitoring in **beers.** *J Food Comp Anal* 8:336–343, 1995.

Brule D, G Sarwar, L Savoie. Changes in serum and urinary uric acid levels in normal human subjects fed **purine-rich foods** containing different amounts of **adenine and hypoxanthine.** *J Am Col Nutr* 11:353–358, 1992.

Candela M, I Astiasaran, J Bello. Effect of frying on the **fatty acid** profile of some **meat dishes.** *J Food Comp Anal* 9:277–282, 1996.

Caragay AB. **Cancer-preventive** foods and **ingredients.** *Food Tech* 46:65–68, 1992.

Chang JHP, DK Lunt, SB Smith. **Fatty acid** composition and fatty acid elongase and stearoyl-CoA desaturase activities in tissues of **steers** fed high oleate sunflower seed. *J Nutr* 122:2074–2080, 1992.

Chang M-CJ, JW Bailey, JL Collins. Dietary **tannins** from **cowpeas** and **tea** transiently alter apparent calcium absorption but not absorption and utilization of protein in rats. *J Nutr* 124:283–288, 1994.

Chan W, J Brown, DH Buss. **Miscellaneous Foods.** Supplement to McCance & Widdowson's The Composition of Foods. The Royal Society of Chemistry Information Services. Cambridge, England. 1994.

Chauhan GS, Eskin NAM, Tkachuk R. Nutrients and antinutrients in **quinoa seed.** *Cereal Chem* 69:85–88, 1992.

Chen H-Y, G Hwang. Estimation of the dietary **riboflavin** required to maximize tissue riboflavin concentration in **juvenile shrimp** (Penaeus monodon). *J Nutr* 122:2474–2478, 1992.

Chin SF, W Liu, JM Storkson, YL Ha, MW Pariza. Dietary sources of **conjugated dienoic isomers of linoleic acid,** a newly recognized class of anticarcinogens. *J Food Comp Anal* 5:185–197, 1992.

Chug-Ajuja JK, JM Holden, MR Forman, AR Mangels, GR Beecher, E Lanza. The development and application of a **carotenoid** database for **fruits, vegetables,** and selected **multicomponent foods.** *J Am Diet Assoc* 93:318–323, 1993.

Chulei R, L Xiaofang, M Hongsheng, M Xiulan, L Guizheng, D Gianhong, CA DeFrancesco, WE Conner. **Milk** composition in **women** from five different regions of **China:** The great diversity of milk **fatty acids.** *J Nutr* 125:2993–2998, 1995.

Cobos A, LDL Hoz, MI Camero, JA Ordonez. **Fatty acid** composition of meat from **rabbits** fed diets with high levels of fat. *J Food Comp Anal* 7:291–300, 1994.

Coburn SP, JD Mahuren, TA Pauly, KL Ericson, DW Townsend. **Alkaline phosphatase** activity and **pyridoxal phosphate** concentrations in the **milk of various species.** *J Nutr* 122:2348–2353, 1992.

Coppa GV, O Gabrielli, P Pierani, C Catassi, A Carlucci, PL Giorgi. Changes in **carbohydrate** composition in **human milk** over 4 months of lactation. *Pediatrics* 91:637–641, 1993.

Cormier A, G Vautour, J Allard. **Canada**-wide survey of the nutritional composition of six **retail pork cuts.** *J Food Comp Anal* 9:255–268, 1996.

Cross KC, SJ Weese, J Johnson, SS Gropper. Soluble **galactose** content of selected **baby food cereals and juices.** *J Food Comp Anal* 8:319–325, 1995.

Dagnelie PC, WA van Staveren, AH Roos, LGMT Tuinstra, J Burema. Nutrients and contaminants in **human milk** from mothers on macrobiotic and omnivorous diets. *Eur J Clin Nutr* 46:355–366, 1992.

Dewailly E, P Ayotte, C Laliberte, J-P Weber, S Gingras, AJ Nantel. **Polycholorinated biphenyl** (PCB) and **dicholorodiphenyl dichloroethylene** (DDE) concentrations in the **breast milk** of women in **Quebec.** *Am J Pub Health* 86:1241–1246, 1996.

Dignan CA, BA Burlingame, JM Arthur, RJ Quigley, GC Milligan. **The Pacific Islands Food** Composition Tables. Swiftprint. Parmerston North, New Zealand. 1994.

Dreher ML, CV Maher, P Kearney. The traditional and emerging role of **nuts** in healthful diets. *Nutr Rev* 54:241–245, 1996.

Dusdieker LB, PH Stumbo, BC Kross, CI Dungy. Does increased nitrate ingestion elevate **nitrate levels in human milk?** *Arch Ped Adol Med* 150:311–314, 1996.

Elkins ER, A Matthys, R Lyon, CJ Huang. Characterization of commercially produced **apple juice concentrate.** *J Food Comp Anal* 9:43–56, 1996.

Faustman C, MC Yin, DB Nadeau. Color stability, lipid stability, and **nutrient composition** of red and white veal. *J Food Sci* 57:302–304, 311, 1992.

Foulke JE. **Urethane** in **alcoholic beverages** under investigation. *FDA Consumer* 27:19–23, 1992.

Fretzdorff B, J-M Brummer. Reduction of **phytic acid** during breadmaking of **whole-meal bread.** *Cereal Chem* 69:266–270, 1992.

Gardner DR, RA Sanders, DE Henry, DH Tallmadge, HW Wharton. Characterization of used **frying oils.** Part 1: Isolation and identification of compound classes. *J Am Oil Chem Soc* 69:499–508, 1992.

Gelardi RC, MF Holick, TC Chen. **Vitamin D** content of **infant formula.** (letter). *New Eng J Med* 327:894–895, 1992.

Goihl DM, KB Harris, JW Savell, HR Cross. Location of **fat migration** during cooking of **beef loin steaks** with external fat still attached. *J Food Comp Anal* 5:246–251, 1992.

Graham HN. **Green tea** composition, consumption, and polyphenol chemistry. Physiological and pharmacological effects of **Camellia sinensis** (tea): 1st Intl Symposium. *Prev Med* 21:334–350, 1992.

Grand AN, LN Bell. **Caffeine** content of **fountain and private-label store brand carbonated beverages.** *J Am Diet Assoc* 97:179–182, 1997.

Grooper SS, KC Gross, SJ Olds. **Galactose** content of selected **fruit and vegetable baby foods:** Implications for infants on galactose-restricted diets. *J Am Diet Assoc* 93:328–330, 1993.

Gross KC, SJ Weese, J Johnson, SS Gropper. Soluble **galactose** content of selected **baby food cereals and juices.** *J Food Comp Anal* 8:319–323, 1995.

Guardiola F, R Codony, M Rafecas, J Boatella, A Lopez. **Fatty acid** composition and nutritional value of **fresh eggs**, from large- and small-scale farms. *J Food Comp Anal* 7:171–188, 1995.

Hagg M, J Kumpulainen. **Thiamine and riboflavin** contents in Finnish **pig, heifer, and cow livers and in pork loin.** *J Food Comp Anal* 7:301–307, 1994.

Hagg M, S Ylikoski, J Kumpulainen. **Vitamin C and alpha- and beta-carotene** contents in **vegetables** consumed in **Finland** during 1988–1989 and 1992–1993. *J Food Comp Anal* 7:252–259, 1994.

Hagg M, S Ylikoski, J Kumpulainen. **Vitamin C** content in **fruits and berries** consumed in **Finland.** *J Food Comp Anal* 8:12–20, 1995.

Haight KG, BH Gump. **Red and white grape juice** concentrate component ranges. *J Food Comp Anal* 8:71–77, 1995.

Hardisson A, AG Padron, I Frias, JI Reguera. The evaluation of the content of **nitrates and nitrites** in food products for infants. *J Food Comp Anal* 9:13–17, 1996.

Hamaker BR, C Valles, R Gilman, RM Hardmeier, D Clark, HH Garcia, AE Gonzales, I Kohlstad, M Castro, R Valdivia, T Rodriquez, M Lescano. **Amino acid and fatty acid** profiles of the **Inca peanut** (Plukenetia volubilis). *Cereal Chem* 69:423–428, 1992.

Harris KB, TJ Harberson, JW Savell, HR Cross, SB Smith. Influences of quality grade, external fat level, and degree of doneness on **beef steak fatty acids.** *J Food Comp Anal* 5:84–89, 1992.

Heinonen M, A-M Lampi, L Hyvonen, D Homer. The **fatty acid** and **cholesterol** content of the average **Finnish diet.** *J Food Comp Anal* 5:198–208, 1992.

Henry DE, DH Tallmadge, RA Sanders, DR Gardner. Characterization of used **frying oils.** Part 2: Comparison of **olestra** and **triglyceride.** *J Am Oil Chem Soc* 69:509–519, 1992.

Hernandez-Perez, J Frias, R Rabanal, C Vidal-Valverde. **Proximate composition** of "mocan" (Visnea mocanera L.f.): A fruit consumed by **Canary** natives. *J Food Comp Anal* 7:203–207, 1995.

Holick MF, Q Shao, WW Liu, TC Chen. The **vitamin D** content of **fortified milk and infant formula.** *New Eng J Med* 326:1178–1181, 1992.

Holland B, J Brown, DH Buss. **Fish and Fish Products.** The third supplement to McCance & Widdowson's The Composition of Foods (5th ed). Royal Society of Chemistry Information Services. Cambridge, England. 1993.

Holland B, AA Welch, DH Buss. **Vegetable Dishes.** The second supplement to McCance & Widdowson's The Composition of Foods (5th ed). Royal Society of Chemistry Information Services. Cambridge, England. 1992.

Holland B, ID Unwin, DH Buss. **Fruit and Nuts.** The first supplement to McCance & Widdowson's The Composition of Foods (5th ed). Royal Society of Chemistry Information Services. Cambridge, England. 1992.

Holmes-McNary MQ, W-L Cheng, M-H Mar, S Fussell, SH Zeisel. **Choline** and choline esters in **human** and rat **milk** and in **infant formulas.** *Am J Clin Nutr* 64:572–576, 1996.

Hong J-H, K Yasumoto. Near-infrared spectroscopic analysis of **heme and nonheme iron** in raw **meats.** *J Food Comp Anal* 9:127–134, 1996.

Hsieh HM, Y Pomeranz, BG Swanson. Composition, cooking time, and maturation of **azuki (Vigna angularis) and common beans.** *Cereal Chem* 69:244–248, 1992.

Jackson MB, CJ Lammi-Keefe, RG Jensen, SC Couch, AM Ferris. Total **lipid and fatty acid** composition of **milk from women** with and without insulin-dependent diabetes mellitus. *Am J Clin Nutr* 60:353–361, 1994.

Jensen RG (ed). *Handbook of* **Milk** *Composition.* Academic Press. Orlando, FL, 1996.

Kamel BS, Y Kakuda. Characterization of the **seed oil and meal** from **apricot, cherry, nectarine, peach, and plum.** *J Am Oil Chem Soc* 69:492–494, 1992.

Karakoltsidis PA, A Zotos, SM Constantinides. Composition of the commercially important **Mediterranean finfish, crustaceans, and molluscs.** *J Food Comp Anal* 8:258–273, 1995.

Keizer SE, RS Gibson, DL O'Commor. Postpartum **folic acid** supplementation of adolescents: impact on maternal folate and zinc status and **milk composition.** *Am J Clin Nutr* 62:377–384, 1995.

Klein GL. **Aluminum** in **parenteral solutions** revisited—Again. *Am J Clin Nutr* 61:449–456, 1995.

Kneale CR, RL Hood. The **biotin** content of **Australian bread and crumpets.** *Aust J Nutr Diet* 49:85–86, 1992.

Koziol MJ. Chemical composition and nutritional evaluation of **quinoa (Chenopodium quinoa Willd.).** *J Food Comp Anal* 5:35–68, 1992.

Kuhnlein HV, D Appavoo, N Morrison, R Soueida, P Pierrot. Use and nutrient composition of **traditional Sahtu (Hareskin) Dene/Metis foods.** *J Food Comp Anal* 7:144–157, 1995.

Kuhnlein HV, R Soueida. Use and nutrient composition of traditional **Baffin Inuit foods.** *J Food Comp Anal* 5:112–126, 1992.

Kuhnlein HV, F Yeboah, M Sedgemore, S Sedgemore, HM Chan. Nutritional qualities of **Ooligan grease:** A traditional food fat of **British Columbia** First Nations. *J Food Comp Anal* 9:18–31, 1996.

L'Abbe MR, KD Trick, A Koshy. The **selenium** content of **Canadian infant formulas and breast milk.** *J Food Comp Anal* 9:119–126, 1996.

Lake R, B Thomson, G Devane, P Scholes. **Trans fatty acid** content of selected **New Zealand foods.** *J Food Comp Anal* 9:365–374, 1997.

Lee TA, R Kempthorne, JK Hardy. Compositional changes in **brewed coffee** as a function of brewing time. *J Food Sci* 57:1417–1419, 1992.

Li BW. Comparison of three methods and two cooking times in the determination of **total dietary fiber** content of **dried legumes.** *J Food Comp Anal* 8:27–31, 1995.

Livsmedels Tabell, Energi-och Naringsamnen (**Swedish Food** Composition Tables, Energy and Nutrients). Livsmedelsverket. Uppsala, Sweden. 1996.

Love JA, KJ Prusa. Nutrient composition and sensory attributes of **cooked ground beef:** Effects of fat content, cooking method, and water rinsing. *J Am Diet Assoc* 92:1367–1371, 1992.

Maia EL, DB Rodriguez-Amaya, MRB Franco. **Fatty acids** of the total, neutral, and phospholipids of the **Brazilian freshwater fish Prochilodus scrofa.** *J Food Comp Anal* 7:240–251, 1994.

Mangels AR, JM Holden, GR Beecher, MR Forman, E Lanza. **Carotenoid** content of **fruits and vegetables:** An evaluation of analytic data. *J Am Diet Assoc* 93:284–296, 1993.

Marlett JA. The content and composition of **dietary fiber** in 117 frequently consumed foods. *J Am Diet Assoc* 92:175–186, 1992.

Marlett JA, Vollendorf NW. **Dietary fiber** content and composition of different forms of **fruits.** *Food Chem* 51:39–44, 1994.

Marlett JA, Vollendorf NW. **Dietary Fiber** content and composition of **vegetables** determined by two methods of analysis. *J Agr Food Chem* 41:1608–1612, 1993.

Marlett JA, Vollendorf NW. **Dietary fiber** content of **cereal and grain products** determined by enzymatic-chemical and enzymatic-gravimetric methods. *J Food Comp Anal* 7:23–36, 1994.

Marsden J, R Pesselman. **Nitrosamines** in food-contact netting: Regulatory and analytical changes. *Food Tech* 47:131–134, 1993.

Massey LK, HR-S Smith, RAL Sutton. Effect of dietary **oxalate** and **calcium** on urinary oxalate and risk of formation of calcium oxalate kidney stones. *J Am Diet Assoc* 93:901–906, 1993.

Mattila P, V Piironen, E Uusi-Rauva, P Koivistoinen. **Cholescalciferol and 25-hydroxycholecalciferol** contents in **fish and fish products.** *J Food Comp Anal* 8:232–243, 1995.

Medrano A, TA Masoud, MC Martinez. **Mineral** and **proximate** composition of **borage.** *J Food Comp Anal* 5:313–318, 1992.

Miller-Ihli NJ. Atomic absorption and atomic emission spectrometry for the determination of the **trace element** content of selected **fruits** consumed in the United States. *J Food Comp Anal* 9:301–311, 1997.

Miller-Ihli, NJ. Graphite furnace atomic absorption spectrometry for the determination of the **chromium** content of selected **US foods.** *J Food Comp Anal* 9:290–300, 1997.

Mitchell GE, RL McLauchlan, AR Isaacs, DJ Williams, SM Nottingham. Effect of low dose irradiation on composition of **tropical fruits and vegetables.** *J Food Comp Anal* 5:291–311, 1992.

Mizutani T, A Kimizuka, K Ruddle, N Ishige. Chemical components of **fermented fish products.** *J Food Comp Anal* 5:152–159, 1992.

Mock DM, NI Mock, SE Langbehn. **Biotin** in **human milk:** Methods, location, and chemical form. *J Nutr* 122:535–545, 1992.

Moreno-Rojas R, MA Amaro-Lopez, G Zurera-Cosano. **Mineral elements** distribution in fresh **asparagus.** *J Food Comp Anal* 5:168–171, 1992.

Morris ER, AD Hill. **Inositol phosphate, calcium, magnesium, and zinc** contents of selected **breakfast cereals.** *J Food Comp Anal* 8:3–11, 1995.

Morris ER, AD Hill. **Inositol phosphate** content of selected **dry beans, peas, and lentils,** raw and cooked. *J Food Comp Anal* 9:2–12, 1996.

Mukhtar H, ZY Wang, SK Katiyar, R Agarwal. **Tea components:** Antimutagenic and anticarcinogenic effects. Physiological and pharmacological effects of **Camellia sinensis** (tea): 1st Intl Symposium. *Prev Med* 21:351–360, 1992.

Musaiger AO. **Traditional Foods** *in the* **Arabian Gulf Countries.** FAO/RNEA, Cairo, Egypt and Arabian Gulf University, Bahrain. Arabian Printing & Publishing House, Bahrain. 1993.

Naghii MR, PML Wall, S Samman. The **boron** content of **selected foods** and the estimation of its daily intake among free-living subjects. *J Am Col Nutr* 15:614–619, 1996.

Nettleton JA, Exler J. **Nutrients in wild and farmed fish and shellfish.** *J Food Sci* 57:257–260, 1992.

Noakes M, PJ Nestel, PM Clifton. Modifying the **fatty acid** profile of **dairy products** through feedlot technology lowers plasma cholesterol of humans consuming the products. *Am J Clin Nutr* 63:42–46, 1996.

Papadopoulos LS, SC Nowak, RK Miller, HR Cross, JW Savell, DJ Brauchi, LW Scott. Development and preparation of **lean meat products.** *J Am Diet Assoc* 92:1358–1364, 1992.

Pennington JAT, SA Schoen. Estimates of dietary **aluminum** exposure. *Food Additives Contam* 12:119–128, 1995.

Pennington JAT, SA Schoen, GD Salmon, B Young, RD Johnson, RW Marts. Composition of core foods of the U.S. food supply, 1982–91. II. **Calcium, magnesium, iron, and zinc.** *J Food Comp Anal* 8:129–170, 1995.

Pennington JAT, SA Schoen, GD Salmon, B Young, RD Johnson, RW Marts. Composition of core foods of the U.S. food supply, 1982–91. III. **Copper, manganese, selenium, and iodine.** *J Food Comp Anal* 8:171–217, 1995.

Pennington JAT, SA Schoen, GD Salmon, B Young, RD Johnson, RW Marts. Composition of core foods of the U.S. food supply, 1982–91. I. **Sodium, phosphorus, and potassium.** *J Food Comp Anal* 8:91–128, 1995.

Pennington JAT, VL Wilkening. Nutrition labeling of **raw fruit, vegetables, and fish.** *J Am Diet Assoc* 92:1250–1257, 1992.

Perlmutter CA, MB Gregoire. Comparison of nutrient content of two types of **frozen meals** for a nutrition program for the elderly. *J Am Diet Assoc* 93:587–588, 1993.

Perry CA, J Dwyer, JA Gelfand, RR Couris, WW McCloskey. Health effects of **salicylates** in **foods and drugs.** *Nutr Rev* 54:225–240, 1996.

Pietschnig B, F Haschke, H Vanura, M Shearer, V Veitl, S Kellner, E Schuster. **Vitamin K in breast milk:** No influence of maternal dietary intake. *Eur J Clin Nutr* 47:209–215, 1993.

Plaami S, J Kumpulainen. **Inositol phosphate** content of some **cereal-based foods.** *J Food Comp Anal* 8:324–335, 1995.

Plaami S, J Kumpulainen. **Soluble and insoluble dietary fiber** contents of various **breads, pastas, and rye flours** on the **Finnish** market, 1990–1991. *J Food Comp Anal* 7:134–143, 1995.

Plessi M, A Monzani. **Aluminium** determination in **bottled mineral waters** by electrothermal atomic absorption spectrometry. *J Food Comp Anal* 8:21–26, 1995.

Pollack PF, Koldovsky O, Nishioka K. **Polyamines** in **human** and rat **milk** and in **infant formulas.** *Am J Clin Nutr* 56:371–375, 1992.

Polo MV, MJ Lagarda, R Farre. The effect of freezing on **mineral element** content of **vegetables.** *J Food Comp Anal* 5:77–83, 1992.

Prentice A, LMA Jarjou, TJ Cole, DM Sirling, B Dibba, S Fairweather-Tait. Calcium requirements of lactating **Gambian** mothers: effects of a calcium supplement on **breast-milk calcium** concentration, maternal bone mineral content, and urinary calcium excretion. *Am J Clin Nutr* 62:58–67, 1995.

Pringuez E, I Saude, C Hulen. Improvement of standard method IDF 95A:1984 for determination of the **nitrate and nitrite** contents of **dried milk.** *J Food Comp Anal* 8:344–350, 1995.

Prosky L, JW DeVries. *Controlling* **Dietary Fiber** in Food Products. Van Nostrand Reinhold. NY. 1992.

Proulx WR, CM Weaver, MA Bock. Trypsin inhibitor activity and **tannin** content do not affect calcium bioavailability of three commonly consumed **legumes.** *J Food Sci* 58:382–384, 1993.

Pylypiw HM, MJI Mattina, V Agarwal, L Hankin. **Pesticides** and **alcohol** in **imported and domestic wine** sold in Connecticut. *J Food Protection* 55:220–221, 1992.

Ranhotra GS, JA Gelroth, BK Glaser, KJ Lorenz. Nutrient composition of **spelt wheat.** *J Food Comp Anal* 9:81–84, 1996.

Raper NR, FJ Cronin, J Exler. **Omega-3 fatty acid** content of the US food supply *J Am Col Nutr* 11:304–308, 1992.

Ravai M. **Caneberries,** An important food in a healthy diet. *Nutr Today* 31:143–147, 1996.

Riha WE, WL Wendorff, S Rank. **Benzo(a)pyrene** content of **smoked and smoke-flavored cheese products** sold in Wisconsin. *J Food Prot* 55:636–638, 1992.

Rodrigo M, MJ Lazaro, A Alvarruiz, V Giner. Composition of **capers** (**Capparis spinosa**): Influence of cultivar, size and harvest date. *J Food Sci* 57:1152–1154, 1992.

Rodriguez-Amaya, DB. Assessment of the **provitamin A** contents of foods—The **Brazilian** experience. *J Food Comp Anal* 9:196–230, 1996.

Ros G, P Abellan, F Rincon, MJ Periago. **Electrolyte composition** of **meat-based infant beikosts.** *J Food Comp Anal* 7:282–290, 1994.

Ruel MT, KG Dewey, C Martinez, R Flores, KH Brown. Validation of single daytime samples of **human milk** to estimate the 24-h concentration of **lipids** in urban **Guatemalan** mothers. *Am J Clin Nutr* 65:439–444, 1997.

Sales J, D Marais, M Kruger. Fat content, **caloric value, cholesterol** content, and **fatty acid** composition of raw and cooked **ostrich meat.** *J Food Comp Anal* 9:85–89, 1996.

Sanchez-Castille CP, PJS Dewey, ML Solano, S Finney, WPT James. Preliminary data: The **dietary fiber content** (nonstarch polysaccharides) of **Mexican fruits and vegetables.** *J Food Comp Anal* 8:284–294, 1995.

Sankaran K, A Papageorgiou, A Ninan, R Sankaran. A randomized, controlled evaluation of two commercially available **human breast milk fortifiers** in healthy preterm neonates. *J Am Diet Assoc* 96:1145–1149, 1996.

Sheppard AJ, JL Weihrauch, JAT Pennington. Analysis and distribution of **vitamin E in vegetable oils and foods.** In: *Vitamin E in Health and Disease.* L Packer, J Fuchs (eds). Marcel Dekker, Inc. NY, 1992, p 9–31.

Siddhuraju P, K Vijayakumari, K Janardhanan. Nutritional and antinutritional properties of the underexploited **legumes Cassia laevigata Willd. and Tamarindus Indica L.** *J Food Comp Anal* 8:351–362, 1995.

Silka M, A Terrab, PB Swan, PVJ Hegarty. Composition of selected **Moroccan cereals and legumes:** Comparison with the FAO table for use in Africa. *J Food Comp Anal* 8:62–70, 1995.

Silva ML, FX Malcata, G De Revel. Volatile contents of **grape marcs** in **Portugal.** *J Food Comp Anal* 9:72–80, 1996.

Simopoulos AP (ed). **Plants** in *Human Nutrition.* Karger Publishers, Inc., Farmington, CT 1995.

Simopoulos AP, HA Norman, JE Gillaspy, JA Duke. Common **purslane:** A source of **omega-3 fatty acids and antioxidants.** *J Am Col Nutr* 11:374–382, 1992.

Sinclair A, GA Dunstan, JM Naughton, AJ Sanigorski, K O'Dea. The **lipid content and fatty acid** composition of **commercial marine and freshwater fish and molluscs** from temperate **Australian** waters. *Aust J Nutr Diet* 49:77–84, 1992.

Stich HF. Teas and **tea components** as inhibitors of carcinogen formation in model systems and man. Physiological and pharmacological effects of **Camellia sinensis** (tea): 1st Intl Symposium. *Prev Med* 21:377–384, 1992.

Sundberg B, H Falk. Composition and properties of **bread and porridge** prepared from different types of barley four. *Am J Clin Nutr* 59 (suppl):780S, 1994.

Swize SS, KB Harris, JW Savell, HR Cross. **Cholesterol** content of lean and fat from **beef, pork, and lamb cuts.** *J Food Comp Anal* 5:160–167, 1992.

Szabo AS, DW Golightly. Determination of **boron** in **liquid nutritional foods** by ICP-AES. *J Food Comp Anal* 8:220–231, 1995.

Torelm I, R Danielsson, S Danfors, A Bruce. Variations in **major nutrients and minerals** due to standardized preparation for **dishes and raw ingredients.** 1. Losses and gains in preparation. *J Food Comp Anal* 9:312–330, 1997.

Troutt ES, MC Hunt, DE Johnson, JR Claus, DH Krofp, S Stroda. Chemical, physical, and sensory characterization of **ground beef** containing 5 to 30 percent fat. *J Food Sci* 57:25–29, 1992.

Ukoha AI, PC Onyenekwe, AU Ezealor, JA Elegbede. **Proximate and elemental** composition of the **double-spurred francolin** (Francolinus bicalcaratus). *J Food Comp Anal* 5:323–327, 1992.

Urgert R, N Essed, G Weg, TG Kosmeijer-Schuil, MB Katan. Separate effects of the **coffee diterpenes cafestol and kahweol** on serum lipids and liver aminotransferases. *Am J Clin Nutr* 65:519–524, 1997.

van Beusekom CM, TA Zeegers, IA Martini, HJR Velvis, GHA Visser, JJ van Doormaal, FAJ Muskiet. **Milk** of patients with tightly controlled insulin-dependent diabetes mellitus has normal **macronutrient** and **fatty acid** composition. *Am J Clin Nutr* 57:938–943, 1993.

Van Elswyk ME, AR Sams, PS Hargis. Composition, functionality, and sensory evaluation of **eggs** from hens fed dietary menhaden oil. *J Food Sci* 57:342–344, 349, 1992.

Vidal-Valverde C, J Frias, S Valverde. Changes in the **carbohydrate** composition of **legumes** after soaking and cooking. *J Am Diet Assoc* 93:547–550, 1993.

Voi AL, M Impembo, G Fascanaro, D Castaldo. Chemical characterization of **apricot puree.** *J Food Comp Anal* 8:78–85, 1995.

Vollendorf NW, JA Marlett. Comparison of two methods of **fiber** analysis of 58 foods. *J Food Comp Anal* 6:203–214, 1993.

Vollendorf NW, JA Marlett. **Dietary fiber** content and composition in **home-prepared and commercially baked products:** Analysis and prediction. *Cereal Chem* 77:99–105, 1994.

Watkins BA, RG Elkin. Dietary modulation of **oleic and stearic acids** in **egg yolks.** *J Food Comp Anal* 5:209–215, 1992.

Wolff RL. **Trans-polyunsaturated fatty acids** in French edible **rapeseed and soybean oils.** *J Am Oil Chem Soc* 69:106–110, 1992.

Wolf WR, JM Holden, A Schubert, DG Lurie, J Woolson-Doherty. **Selenium** content of selected foods important for improved assessment of dietary intake. *J Food Comp Anal* 5:2–9, 1992.

Wooten K, RA Shulze, RW Lancey, M Lietzow, MC Linder. **Ceruloplasmin** is found in **milk** and amniotic fluid and may have a nutritional role. *Nutr Biochem* 7:632–639, 1996.

Yazzie D, DJ VanderJagt, A Pastuszyn, A Okolo, RH Glew. The **amino acid and mineral** content of **baobab (Adansonia digitata L.) leaves.** *J Food Comp Anal* 7:189–193, 1995.

Yoshida H, M Tatsumi, G Kajimoto. Influence of fatty acids on the **tocopherol** stability in **vegetable oils** during microwave heating. *J Am Oil Chem Soc* 69:119–125, 1992.

Zhou JR, EJ Fordyce, V Raboy, DB Dickinson, M-S Wong, RA Burns, JW Erdman. Reduction of **phytic acid** in **soybean products** improves **zinc** bioavailability in rats. *J Nutr* 122:2466–2473, 1992.

Index